CARCINOGENS IN INDUSTRY AND THE ENVIRONMENT

POLLUTION ENGINEERING AND TECHNOLOGY

A Series of Reference Books and Textbooks

EDITOR

PAUL N. CHEREMISINOFF

Associate Professor
of Environmental Engineering
New Jersey Institute of Technology
Newark, New Jersey

1. Energy from Solid Wastes, *Paul N. Cheremisinoff and Angelo C. Morresi*
2. Air Pollution Control and Design Handbook (in two parts), *edited by Paul N Cheremisinoff and Richard A. Young*
3. Wastewater Renovation and Reuse, *edited by Frank M. D'Itri*
4. Water and Wastewater Treatment: Calculations for Chemical and Physical Processes, *Michael J. Humenick, Jr.*
5. Biofouling Control Procedures, *edited by Loren D. Jensen*
6. Managing the Heavy Metals on the Land, *G. W. Leeper*
7. Combustion and Incineration Processes: Applications in Environmental Engineering, *Walter R. Niessen*
8. Electrostatic Precipitation, *Sabert Oglesby, Jr. and Grady B. Nichols*
9. Benzene: Basic and Hazardous Properties, *Paul N. Cheremisinoff and Angelo C. Morresi*
10. Air Pollution Control Engineering: Basic Calculations for Particulate Collection, *William Licht*
11. Solid Waste Conversion to Energy: Current European and U.S. Practice, *Harvey Alter and J. J. Dunn, Jr.*
12. Biological Wastewater Treatment: Theory and Applications, *C. P. Leslie Grady, Jr. and Henry C. Lim*
13. Chemicals in the Environment: Distribution · Transport · Fate · Analysis, *W. Brock Neely*
14. Sludge Treatment, *edited by W. Wesley Eckenfelder, Jr. and Chakra J. Santhanam*
15. Wastewater Treatment and Disposal: Engineering and Ecology in Pollution, *S. J. Arceivala*
16. Carcinogens in Industry and the Environment, *edited by James M. Sontag*

Additional Volumes in Preparation

CARCINOGENS IN INDUSTRY AND THE ENVIRONMENT

Edited by

James M. Sontag

National Cancer Institute
National Institutes of Health
Bethesda, Maryland

MARCEL DEKKER, INC. *New York and Basel*

Library of Congress Cataloging in Publication Data

Main entry under title:

1. Carcinogens. 2. Environmentally induced diseases.

(Pollution Engineering and Technology; 16)
Includes index.
1. Carcinogens. 2. Environmentally induced diseases.
3. Industrial hygiene. I. Sontag, James M. [date].
II. Series.
RC268.6.C37 363.1'79 81-5484
ISBN 0-8247-1021-5 AACR2

MARCEL DEKKER, INC.
270 Madison Avenue, New York, New York 10016

Current printing (last digit):
10 9 8 7 6 5 4 3 2 1

PRINTED IN THE UNITED STATES OF AMERICA

Foreword

Awareness that the environment plays a role in cancer development dates back to the early documented evidence of cancer of the scrotum among chimney sweeps, cancer of the face among sailors exposed to strong sunlight, urinary bladder cancer among workers exposed to certain intermediates in the synthetic dye industry, and so on. Yet little attention has been paid, until recently, to the possibility of extrapolating this evidence in a broader sense for the purpose of eradicating the disease by preventive measures. Even with the establishment of experimental carcinogenesis in animals—a relatively recent development—research had been devoted largely to mechanisms of action of carcinogens rather than to immediate practical application. The time, it seemed, was not yet ripe for substantial implementation of the available knowledge, except in a few specific areas, notably in relation to industrial occupations.

What was lacking was knowledge of the extent to which human cancer *in general* is attributable to environmental factors. And here epidemiological studies began to supply the relevant information, by bringing to light striking differences in tumor incidence among various populations, related to their habits and, more particularly, according to their geographical location. It thus became apparent that the environment plays a far more important role in human cancer development than had previously been supposed.

In consequence of this newly accumulated information, there has been a dramatic change in outlook in recent years, resulting in much greater emphasis on practical exploitation of the knowledge and on efforts to devise rapid methods of identifying carcinogens in our environment. This book reflects this new orientation in thinking, planning, and application.

If epidemiological studies revealed the *scope* of environmental carcinogenesis in human beings, the experimental studies in other animals provided most of the information about the *complexity* of carcinogenic action.

We now know that some carcinogens can operate on virtually any tissue in the body in most species of animals, that others have a more limited range of action with respect to organ or species response, and that still others are virtually single-organ carcinogens and effective in very few species. With some carcinogens repeated administrations of large doses for long periods are needed for tumor induction; with others a single exposure to a very small dose is sufficient. (This variation is partly explained by differences in metabolic activation among carcinogens, on the one hand, and detoxication differences among compounds on the other, with the relative proportion of the two competing processes determing the effective dose for carcinogenic action; and this proportion may vary according to species, strain, or individual.) Again, some carcinogens act fairly quickly, others very slowly. And finally, cocarcinogenic factors, and more specifically, promoting or "precipitating" action following a subeffective dose of carcinogen, or after the action of a pure initiator, can be decisive in determining whether a tumor will develop. These are but a few of the important variables that must be taken into account in assessing carcinogenic risks for humans.

The important role of cocarcinogenesis in human cancer development is only now beginning to be recognized. The implications are far reaching, and since existing methods of assay are only capable of detecting "complete" carcinogens, and in the case of the short-term Ames' test can only recognize the initiating phase of carcinogenesis, new testing procedures will have to be devised to cope with the important problem of "cofactors."

We turn next to the implementation of the knowledge about environmental carcinogenesis, in terms of potential and realizable cancer prevention in humans.

A policy of cancer prevention is most easily formulated for carcinogenic hazards in industry. The workers at risk can be more easily traced than people in the general population, and so can the various products to which they are exposed. Thus, carefully conducted statistical surveys of cancer incidences among the employees and systematic carcinogenicity testing of the suspected products enable one eventually to establish the causal association and to assess the degree of risk. The implementation of preventive measures is then the primary responsibility of the industry concerned, though often calling for governmental legislation for proper enforcement.

The situation is more complicated for carcinogens of occupational origin outside industrial establishments. The people at risk are more widely dispersed among the general population, and the suspected (or unsuspected) carcinogens to which they are exposed are less easily traced. Elaborate statistical surveys are, therefore, called for here, and possibly more extensive carcinogenicity testing, to establish a true association and to assess the degree of risk involved. Implementation of preventive measures is, in such cases, largely the responsibility of public health authorities, at both the regional and national levels.

By far the most difficult problem (and numerically perhaps the most important) is concerned with environmental carcinogens that are not industrial or occupational (or, as in the case of pollutants, indirect products of industrial or occupational processes). The difficulties here involve not only procedure—discovering who are the people at risk, identifying the incriminating substances, and recognizing cocarcinogenic, promoting, and other "associated" factors—but also the means of implementing preventive measures, because cancer prevention, in such cases, is to a large extent in everyone's hands and public education on the subject is therefore critical.

This problem further poses a number of conflicting problems which have not yet been properly resolved, and to which serious attention must be paid.

Public education on the subject of potential carcinogenic risks—in relation to certain habits, such as cigarette smoking, and to pollution, food additives, contaminants, and other elements in our environment, whether naturally occurring or caused by people—is likely to be counterproductive if one fails to discriminate between serious hazards and those of marginal risks. People are already heard to say that if almost everything is potentially dangerous, why bother to take any precautions? (This also applies, incidentally, to the more technical debates about, and preoccupation with, "safe" (minimal) doses of carcinogenic exposure, often overlooking the fact that the real dangers lie at the other extreme. Note, in this connection, the sobering comment by A. C. Kolbye, Jr. [1976, Oncology 33:90] that a precipitous rush to "zero tolerance" for all animal carcinogens may impair our efforts to prevent the worst "causes" of cancer induction in humans.) On the other hand, to withhold or limit information to the public about potential carcinogenic hazards would be inexcusable.

A properly balanced program of public education about carcinogenic risks has not yet been devised (e.g., the poor results so far obtained from intensive efforts in public education to wean the public from cigarette smoking!). Related to the problem of public education is the need to provide authoritative responses to recurrent scares in the lay press about causes of cancer, some of which may be justified, others grossly exaggerated, and still others completely without foundation. The public should be kept properly informed and be spared unnecessary anguish and, at the same time, encouraged to exercise reasonable vigilance when it is appropriate.

Isaac Berenblum
The Weizmann Institute of Science
Rehovot, Israel

Preface

An increasing number of carcinogens are being identified in our environment. Frequently, it is difficult to understand the human significance of these carcinogens because their relationship to humans may be obscure. A major objective of this book is to clarify this relationship by sorting out carcinogens according to where they are found and how they are used. In addition, the book attempts to address some of the critical social and scientific issues associated with environmental carcinogens.

The book's early chapters deal with the cost and social implications of cancer, as well as with the identification and evaluation of carcinogens. Subsequent chapters address specific categories of carcinogens found in industry and the environment. The chapter on the research chemical N-2-fluorenylacetamide (Chapter 14) is included to show the tremendous effort and variety of scientific disciplines required to understand how carcinogens produce their effects. The last chapter is on ionizing radiation, a physical carcinogen of concern to all sectors and at all levels of society.

This compilation by authorities in the field presents a detailed, up-to-date account of carcinogens in the environment. It is hoped that the information provided will be useful to researchers and other workers in areas of public health and will serve as a basis for actions directed toward cancer prevention in humans.

James M. Sontag

Contents

Contributors

JOSEPH C. ARCOS* Professor, Department of Medicine, Tulane University School of Medicine; Biochemistry Section, Seamen's Memorial Research Laboratory, U.S. Public Health Service Hospital, New Orleans, Louisiana

NICHOLAS A. ASHFORD Assistant Director, Center for Policy Alternatives, and Associate Professor, Department of Technology and Policy, Massachusetts Institute of Technology, Cambridge, Massachusetts

GEORGE W. CASARETT Professor, Department of Radiation Biology and Biophysics, University of Rochester School of Medicine, Rochester, New York

DAVID BARRINGER CLAYSON Deputy Director, Eppley Institute for Research in Cancer and Allied Diseases, University of Nebraska Medical Center, Omaha, Nebraska

DAVID J. CLEGG Head, Bureau of Chemical Safety, Food Directorate, Pesticide Section, Toxicological Evaluation Division, Health and Welfare Canada, Ottawa, Ontario, Canada

D. EARLE COFFIN Director, Bureau of Nutritional Sciences, Food Directorate, Health Protection Branch, Health and Welfare Canada, Ottawa, Ontario, Canada

PAUL B. FISHER Associate Professor, Department of Biology, Bronx Community College of the City University of New York, New York; Department of Microbiology Cancer Center, Institute of Cancer Research, Columbia University College of Physicians and Surgeons, New York, New York

DAVID W. GAYLOR Director, Division of Biometry, National Center for Toxicological Research, Jefferson, Arkansas

BERNARD M. GOLDSCHMIDT Associate Professor, Institute of Environmental Medicine, New York University Medical Center, New York, New York

---

Present affiliations:
*Senior Environmental Health Scientist, Chemical Hazard Identification Branch (TS-792), Assessment Division, Office of Toxic Substances, Environmental Protection Agency, Washington, D.C.

HAROLD C. GRICE* Director, Bureau of Chemical Safety, Health Protection Branch, Health and Welfare Canada, Ottawa, Ontario, Canada

THOMAS A. HODGSON Economist, Office of Health Research, Statistics, and Technology, National Center for Health Statistics, Department of Health and Human Services, Hyattsville, Maryland

DAVID G. HOEL Chief, Biometry Branch, National Institute of Environmental Health Sciences, Research Triangle Park, North Carolina

NEIL B. JURINSKI† Industrial Hygiene Consultant, Tracor Jitco, Inc., Rockville, Maryland

DONALD V. LASSITER‡ Environmental Health Scientist, Environmental Health Associates, Inc., Berkeley, California

MEI-TEIN LO Toxicologist, Toxicological Evaluation Division, Food Directorate, Health Protection Branch, Health and Welfare Canada, Ottawa, Ontario, Canada

PRABHAKAR D. LOTLIKAR Associate Professor, Department of Biochemistry, Fels Research Institute, Temple University Medical School, Philadelphia, Pennsylvania

FRANCIS N. MARZULLI** Senior Scientist, Toxicology Division, Bureau of Foods, Food and Drug Association, Washington, D.C.

EDWARD J. MIDDLETON Head, Food Additives, Bureau of Health, Food Directorate, Toxicological Evaluation Division, Health Protection Branch, Health and Welfare Canada, Ottawa, Ontario, Canada

DOROTHY P. RICE Director, National Center for Health Statistics, U.S. Department of Health and Human Services, Hyattsville, Maryland

ADRIANNE E. ROGERS Senior Research Scientist, Department of Nutrition and Food Science, Massachusetts Institute of Technology, Cambridge, Massachusetts

EMIL SANDI Head, Food Contaminants Section, Toxicological Evaluation Division, Food Directorate, Health and Welfare Canada, Ottawa, Ontario, Canada

PETER M. SCOTT Research Scientist, Health Protection Branch, Health and Welfare Canada, Ottawa, Ontario, Canada

NRISINHA P. SEN Research Scientist, Bureau of Chemical Safety, Food Directorate, Health Protection Branch, Health and Welfare Canada, Ottawa, Ontario, Canada

BARRY L. SMITH Adviser, Legislative Policy, Food Directorate, Health Protection Branch, Health and Welfare Canada, Ottawa, Ontario, Canada

JAMES M. SONTAG Assistant Director, Interagency Affairs, Office of the Director, National Cancer Institute, National Institutes of Health, Bethesda, Maryland

---

Present affiliations:
*Toxicology Consultant, F.D.C. Consultants, Inc., Nepean, Ontario, Canada
†President, NuChemCo, Inc., Burke, Virginia
‡Consultant, Environmental/Occupational Health, San Jose, California
**Senior Toxicologist, National Academy of Sciences, Washington, D.C.

I. BERNARD WEINSTEIN Professor, Department of Medicine and Environmental Science, Division of Environmental Sciences and Cancer Center, Institute of Cancer Research, Columbia University College of Physicians and Surgeons, New York, New York

ELIZABETH K. WEISBURGER Chief, Laboratory of Carcinogen Metabolism, Division of Cancer Cause and Prevention, National Cancer Institute, National Institutes of Health, Bethesda, Maryland

JAMES R. WITHEY Research Scientist, Health Protection Branch, Health and Welfare Canada, Ottawa, Ontario, Canada

YIN-TAK WOO* Instructor, Department of Medicine, Tulane University Medical Center; Biochemistry Section, Seamen's Memorial Research Laboratory, U.S. Public Health Service Hospital, New Orleans, Louisiana

---

Present affiliation:
*Senior Toxicologist, Health Hazard Assessment Group, JRB Associates, Inc., McLean, Virginia

1

Introduction

JAMES M. SONTAG / National Cancer Institute, Bethesda, Maryland

It is now commonplace to hear or read that up to 90% of all human cancers are attributable to environmental factors (Boyland, 1969; Higginson, 1972; Doll, 1977). The basis for the claim is founded on worldwide epidemiologic studies showing different incidences for the same types of cancer. After considering genetic and other factors that might account for the differences, it has become clear that variations in cancer incidence are inextricably linked to the environments in which the populations live. The identification of the major environmental factors linked to human cancer is important for prevention and intervention efforts.

In speaking of environmental factors, it is important to understand the frame of reference. Frequently, environmental factors have been thought of simply as synthetic industrial chemicals. Besides man-made chemicals (e.g., industrial intermediates, agricultural chemicals, drugs, food additives, and other societally important chemicals), environmental factors include sunlight, alcoholic beverages, tobacco products, medical treatments, dietary components, and any other component of the human environment. It is thus important to have a holistic perspective in understanding the significance of the statement that up to 90% of all cancers have an environmental association.

It is likely that many, if not most, of the major environmental factors contributing to the overall cancer burden are not complete carcinogens in themselves (see Chapter 8). In other words, they must act together and/or in combination with other environmental factors before they produce their carcinogenic effect. Such factors may naturally occur together, as in the diet, or may result from discrete but coincidental exposures, as with smoking and drinking alcoholic beverages. Individual genetic susceptibility also plays an important but as yet ill-defined role. Because of the complexity of these relationships, good model systems and methods still have not been developed which would lead to the identification and understanding of interactions of these environmental factors. Thus, efforts have been mainly focused on the identification of individual environmental substances that may pose carcinogenic hazards. Although these efforts may identify only a small fraction of environmental contributors to human cancer, the knowledge learned through them is adding to the science base which, together with other efforts in carcinogenesis research, ultimately should provide the clues and answers leading to cancer prevention.

I. IDENTIFICATION OF CARCINOGENS

Epidemiologic studies provide the most convincing evidence that a substance is a human carcinogen. Such studies, however, have severe limitations which restrict their usefulness. It is not until after the "body count" has been made that an effect can be identified by epidemiology. As a result, people may be exposed to a carcinogenic agent for decades before it is identified and control actions are instigated. Ideally, the potential hazard of a substance should be known before the occurrence of human exposure.

Epidemiologic studies are limited by the long latency periods (10-40 years) between first exposure to a substance and the appearance of cancer. By the time an effect is observed, it may be impossible to track down the etiologic agents in the cancer patient's past. Epidemiologic studies also may be confounded by the inability to find adequate control populations against which to compare exposed groups. Even when using an acceptable cohort, an increased cancer incidence may easily be missed when the increase is of a relatively common type of cancer, for example, lung, colon, or breast (in females). For these and other reasons, animal studies are the most desirable and feasible means of identifying potential human carcinogens.

Laboratory animals have been used since the early part of the century to identify chemical carcinogens. In 1918 Yamagiwa and Itchikawa induced skin tumors in rabbits after continued application of coal tar. Since that time, of the few thousand chemicals that have been adequately tested, several hundred entities have been reported to be carcinogenic (Maugh, 1978a). Small rodents have been the most widely used animal models to detect and identify carcinogens.

The validity of laboratory animals is confirmed by the fact that all human carcinogens identified epidemiologically, with the exception of only a few compounds, also induce cancer in animal models (Tomatis et al, 1978). In a number of instances, a substance was identified first as an animal carcinogen and only later found to be a human carcinogen as well. For the many carcinogens thus far identified only in animals, the possible untoward human effects are unknown. However, given the almost perfect correlation between known human carcinogens and their carcinogenicity in animal models, unless proven otherwise, it is prudent to treat all animal carcinogens as if they were confirmed human carcinogens.

II. EXPERIMENTAL CONSIDERATIONS

The choice of animal models, study size, conditions of test, and other experimental factors are often dictated by practical considerations. Details of experimental designs, study conduct, pathology protocols, and other aspects of carcinogenesis bioassay can be found in a number of publications (Berenblum, 1969; Sontag et al., 1976; Weisburger, 1976; Page, 1977; Sontag, 1977; Food Safety Council, 1978). The conceptual basis for certain bioassay practices is now given.

A. Animal Model

Rats, mice, and hamsters are the most commonly used and accepted animal models for carcinogenesis bioassay. Over the years they have proven to be reliable and sensitive models for detecting carcinogens representing a variety of chemical classes. In instances of human carcinogens, one or more of the species usually respond with the same tumor type as found in people. The historical data accumulated on each species, and strains within species, are important in defining the peculiar characteristics of each animal model, as well as in providing a baseline of spontaneous tumor incidence. The latter may be particularly important in evaluating rare tumors occurring in nonstatistically significant incidences among treated animals. Other considerations for using small rodents include their size, ease of handling, reproductivity, hardiness, longevity, sensitivity, and relatively cheap cost.

B. Dose Levels

Chemicals are frequently tested at dose levels several orders of magnitude higher than concentrations to which humans are exposed. Although attempts have been made to discredit this practice, there are sound and valid reasons to support it. First, it should be noted that most chemicals tested at the "maximum tolerated dose" have not been proven to be carcinogenic. Thus, the intrinsic carcinogenicity of chemicals is not linked to dosage, although the expression of carcinogenicity in animals is related. Second, a great deal more confidence can be placed in the safety of a substance if it is shown not to be carcinogenic when tested at high concentrations.

The major reason for testing at high dosages relates to the sensitivity of the test system. The probability of detecting a carcinogenic response is linked to the "potency" of a chemical; the less potent the chemical, the smaller the probability of detecting an effect in an animal group of constant size. The probability diminishes as the test population becomes smaller. In a typical bioassay, a group of 200-400 test animals serves as a surrogate for as many as 220 million Americans. If the animals are exposed to the low levels at which most human exposures occur, the probability of detecting the response in such a small test population becomes remote, even for relatively potent carcinogens. To increase the sensitivity of the test system, hence the probability of detection, "maximum tolerated doses" are administered. Results from studies, in which high dose levels are used to compensate for the relative insensitivity of test systems, are valid qualitative indicators of potential human risk.

C. Duration of Study

Typical bioassay studies are conducted over the majority of the test animals' life span. In the case of rats and mice, the chronic study period lasts for a minimum of 24 months and for hamsters, at least 18 months. Treatment of the animals continues over the entire study period. This practice maximizes the intake of the substance, thus adding to the sensitivity of the study. Also, greater confidence can be given to the validity of "negative" results, if no effect is found after the study is completed.

D. Route of Exposure

Questions have arisen regarding the inappropriateness of testing chemicals by routes other than those by which humans are exposed. The necessity to use alternative routes may result for a number of reasons. First, animals may not eat a substance normally ingested by humans because of its disagreeable odor or taste; it therefore must be force fed through a stomach tube. The instability of other substances requires that they be administered immediately after preparation, thereby influencing the route of exposure used. The cost of administering a substance by a particular route also is a factor in selecting which is to be employed. (Inhalation studies may cost almost twice as much as feeding studies.) A critical factor in selecting an experimental route of exposure is evidence that it would not produce a different general effect from the one expected by the route comparable to the one by which humans are exposed. In this regard, data on qualitative and quantitative absorption patterns by the different routes are important in determining comparability.

Humans are often exposed to a substance by more than a single route. A colorant, for example, may be ingested in foods by the general public, inhaled by workers manufacturing or processing the substance, and contacted on the skin by others using it in vocational pursuits. In the final analysis, it may make no difference whether the route of exposure is inhalation, ingestion, or skin if systemic absorption occurs by all three routes.

E. Statistical Analysis

The basis for determining if a substance is carcinogenic often relies solely on the statistical analysis of results. Such an analysis must allow for a number of factors that may bias the conclusions one way or another. The importance of proper statistical analysis is so critical that Chapter 5 is devoted solely to this topic.

III. MAGNITUDE OF THE PROBLEM

The cost of cancer to society is enormous. Costs have implications not only to cancer victims, but also to federal, state, and local governments, industrial and worker communities, and the general public. These implications are discussed in Chapters 2-4.

The number of chemicals in common use has been estimated to be more than 60,000 (Maugh, 1978b). A 1978 inventory by the U.S. Environmental Protection Agency identified more than 44,000 chemicals with "significant" commercial production (U.S. Environmental Protection Agency, 1979). Using today's testing standards it is clearly impossible to study the carcinogenicity of all existing chemicals and those to be developed; the resource requirements would be overwhelming. Thus, there is a need to apply reliable, rapid, and inexpensive screening techniques to identify substances having the greatest likelihood of being carcinogenic; these then can be tested by traditional methods. The importance of screening techniques and progress in their development is described in Chapter 6.

REFERENCES

Berenblum, I. (1969). Carcinogenicity Testing, Vol. 2, UICC Technical Report Series. International Union Against Cancer, Geneva, Switzerland.

Boyland, E. (1969). The correlation of experimental carcinogenesis and cancer in man. In Progress in Experimental Tumor Research, Vol. 11, F. Homburger (Ed.). Karger, New York, pp. 222-234.

Doll, R. (1977). Introduction. In Origins of Human Cancer, Book A, H. H. Hiatt, J. D. Watson, and J. A. Winsten (Eds.). Cold Spring Harbor Laboratory, Cold Spring Harbor, N.Y., pp. 1327-1338.

Food Safety Council, the Scientific Committee (1978). Proposed system for food safety assessment. Food Cosmet. Toxicol. 16:1-136.

Higginson, J. (1972). The role of geographical pathology in environmental carcinogenesis. In Proceedings of the 1971 Symposium on Fundamental Cancer Research, Environment and Cancer, R. L. Clark (Ed.). Williams and Wilkins, Baltimore, pp. 69-92.

Maugh, T. H., II (1978a). Chemical carcinogens: the scientific basis for regulation. Science 201:1200-1205.

Maugh, T. H., II (1978b). Chemicals: How many are there? Science 199:162.

Page, N. P. (1977). Current concepts of a bioassay program in environmental carcinogenesis. In Environmental Cancer, H. F. Kraybill and M. A. Mehlman (Eds.). Adv. Mod. Toxicol. pp. 87-172.

Sontag, J. M. (1977). Aspects in carcinogen bioassay. In Origins of Human Cancer, Book C, H. H. Hiatt, J. D. Watson, and J. A. Winsten (Eds.). Cold Spring Harbor Laboratory, Cold Spring Harbor, N.Y., pp. 1327-1338.

Sontag, J. M., Page, N. P., and Saffiotti, U. (1976). Guidelines for Carcinogen Bioassay in Small Rodents. DHEW Publication No. (NIH)76-801, U.S. Government Printing Office, Washington, D.C.

Tomatis, L., Agthe, C., Bartsch, H., Huff, J., Montesano, R., Saracci, R., Walker, E., and Wilbourn, J. (1978). Evaluation of the carcinogenicity of chemicals: A review of the monograph program of the International Agency for Research in Cancer (1971 to 1977). Cancer Res. 38:877-885.

U.S. Environmental Protection Agency (1979). Availability of TSCA initial inventory, Fed. Reg. 44(95):28559.

Weisburger, J. H. (1976). Bioassay and tests for chemical carcinogens. In Chemical Carcinogens, ACS Monograph 173, C. E. Searle (Ed.). American Chemical Society, Washington, D.C.

Yamagiwa, K., and Itchikawa, K. (1918). Experimental study of the pathogenesis of carcinoma. J. Cancer Res. 3:1.

2

Social and Economic Implications of Cancer in the United States

DOROTHY P. RICE and THOMAS A. HODGSON / National Center for Health Statistics, Hyattsville, Maryland

I. INTRODUCTION

Death rates reported to the World Health Organization by member countries reveal that for most countries in North America, Europe, and Oceania, cancer is the second leading cause of death [1]. Among 27 selected countries, the proportion of all deaths in 1971 that were classified as malignant neoplasms ranged from 13 to 24% with a median of 19%. For the leading cause of death, heart diseases, the proportion ranged from 20 to 40%, with a median of 31% [2]. Standardized death rates for cancer in 1972 at ages 45 years and over ranged

---

Presented to the Expert Committee on Cancer Statistics of the World Health Organization and International Agency for Research on Cancer at Madrid, Spain, June 20-26, 1978.

from 411 to 843 per 100,000 among males and from 313 to 601 per 100,000 among females, with a general level of cancer mortality in these countries of 600 for males and 450 for females [1].

Cancer usually strikes those who are middle-aged and older. But even in the less developed countries of Africa, South and Middle America, and Asia, where the proportion of the population surviving to late adult life is lower and economic development has not progressed as far, cancer may be the fifth or sixth leading cause of death [1]. In 1971 the median proportion of all deaths that were due to malignant neoplasms in 11 selected countries of these continents was 11%, compared to the median for heart diseases of 13.5% [3].

It is estimated that in the United States over one million persons will have been diagnosed as having cancer in 1979 (including 300,000 new cases of nonmelanoma skin cancer), and 400,000 persons will die of the disease [4]. The social and economic implications of cancer for fictims and the society at large are pain, suffering, disability, and death; millions of years of life are lost; vast amounts of human and economic resources are devoted to detection, diagnosis, and treatment; and billions of dollars of economic output are foregone annually because of lost human resources. Goals in the fight against cancer, and other diseases as well, are prevention before the disease strikes, cure with minimum untoward effects when it occurs, and maximum quality of life if cure is not possible. Faced with limited resources and a multiplicity of diseases and other social problems demanding attention, it is essential to know and understand the magnitude of the economic and social costs of cancer and their relationship to the total burden on society.

A. Social Costs and Quality of Life

While it has long been recognized that there are certain "noneconomic" effects of illness and disease, pain and suffering foremost among them, in recent years there has been increased interest in this aspect of disease cost. Social costs refer to psychosocial deteriorations that are brought about by disease [5]. Persons exposed to social costs include cancer victims; children, spouses, and siblings of victims; friends and co-workers of victims; and care givers. They number several million persons in the United States [5]. Recent research has studied the influence of mortality on the family and its life cycle [6,7]. Mortality has direct consequences for the family, affecting, for example, duration of marriage and age at widowhood. In the long run, large reductions in mortality can influence behavioral patterns. To a large extent, however, studies in the area of economic costs are refinements of an accepted methodology, but measures and methodology for social costs remain to be developed.

Cancer, especially advanced cancer, may bring about personal catastrophes that are not reflected in the direct and indirect economic costs of cancer that have been estimated to this date. A cancer victim may suffer loss of a body part or speech, disfigurement, disability, impending death, pain, and grief. The victim and those around him or her may be forced into economic dependence and social isolation, unwanted job changes, loss of opportunities for promotion and education, relocation of living quarters, and other undesired changes in life plans. The environment created by cancer induces anxiety, reduced self-esteem and feeling of well-being, resentment, and emotional problems that often require psychotherapy. Mental illness may develop, leading to family conflict, antisocial behavior, and suicide. The cancer victim and others may experience marked personality changes and reduced sexual function. Disrupted development and delinquency may occur among children. Cancer frequently reduces the quality of life beyond the restorative capability of current rehabilitation efforts. The combination of financial strain and psychosocial problems is especially devastating.

The social costs just listed have been documented in numerous studies and appear to be widespread. Cancer Care, Inc. and the National Cancer Foundation, Inc. found that most families with a member suffering from advanced cancer needed help to maintain family stability. Two-thirds of the families studied reported emotional or adjustment problems on the part of family members, and one-third underwent changes in life plans such as changing employment [8]. Fortunately, quality of life for cancer patients is recognized as an important issue and considerable attention is being given to it [9-12].

Although quantifying social costs has been rather intractable, some progress has been made. Translating qualitative social costs into money costs by using market values or shadow prices* of imputed costs, it has been estimated that social costs vary quite a bit by form of cancer and may greatly exceed direct and indirect economic costs if the social cost of death is included. Excluding the cost of extinction produces a money value for social costs that resembles direct economic costs of cancer.† Although these estimates need refinement, they point out the importance of social costs and the misallocation of resources that may occur when only economic costs are considered.

Increased effort is needed to refine the methodology and develop the necessary data. Frequently, there is little observable difference in the effectiveness of alternative treatments for cancer (simple versus radical mastectomy, for example), at least in terms of survival and recurrence rates. In these circumstances it would be especially helpful to quantify and compare the quality of life under alternative treatments. Quality of life information could also be integrated with survival probabilities to determine the treatment giving the maximum utility when comparing alternatives involving a trade-off between increased probability of survival, or the length of survival, and reduced quality of life [13].

Indicators must be developed and data collected to estimate quality of life and social costs. The state of the art is still in a rather primitive stage but has begun to attract attention [14-19]. The impact of sickness on a person in terms of his or her own sense of well-being, including evaluations of the well-being of family and associates in addition to the individual having the illness, must be measured. For cancer, indicators must reflect the reduced self-esteem, emotional problems, pain, and suffering caused by loss of body part, disability, social isolation, economic dependence, impending death, and the otherwise reduced quality of life that often accompanies cancer.

Although direct measures of social costs and quality of life are not available, and considerable methodological research and data collection are necessary if social costs are to be adequately quantified, the situation is not completely hopeless. A number of scales have been developed to assess the rehabilitation of patients by measuring functional status. The Performance Status Scale assesses mobility and ability to carry out usual roles. More comprehensive measures of functional status are the Pulses Functional Profile and the Barthel Index [20]. Pain and suffering can be measured by duration and severity of pain as indicated by the potency of drugs needed for relief. Suicide and mental illness or psychiatric care can indicate grief, worry, and emotional stress. These can be shadow-priced by the cost of drugs used to relieve pain and the cost of psychotherapy used to relieve emotional problems. Dollar values have also been estimated, albeit crudely, for other social costs [13], including disrupted child development and limitations on sex life. With quantification of quality of life in money terms, quality of life, quantity of life, and direct and indirect economic costs will all be expressed in terms of a common denominator and can be compared and combined to obtain the total cost of cancer.

Initial efforts at measuring perceptions of the quality of life are encouraging [15,21-25]. Also of interest is the Sickness Impact Profile, developed at the University of Washington

---

*Shadow prices are accounting prices attached to goods and services for which there are no market prices. These shadow prices are the costs incurred in obtaining the items in question.

†The minimum annual social costs of cancer are estimated to be about $2.5 billion, excluding extinction costs, and about $138 billion if costs of extinction are included. The dollar magnitudes of these costs have undoubtedly increased since this research was published in 1975. Abt's estimates include the social costs incurred by victims, spouses, children, parents, siblings, friends, co-workers, and care givers resulting from extinction, mental illness, family conflict, antisocial behavior, sexual loss, grief, limited consciousness, segregation, isolation, and discrimination associated with cancer.

and the Group Health Cooperative of Puget Sound, which attempts to measure behavioral expressions of sickness [19]. Construction of quality of life indicators requires surveys of affected individuals, and the task is not easy. Questions of quality of life are difficult to answer and involve painful and emotional topics. The surveys have to be very carefully constructed. National household interview surveys already in existence, such as those conducted by the National Center for Health Statistics (Health Interview Survey) and the Health Care Financing Administration (Current Medicare Survey), cancer registries, and patient self-help groups like Lost Chord Clubs (laryngectomy patients), Reach to Recovery (mastectomy patients), and Ostomy Clubs, all represent possible vehicles for collecting information on quality of life and social costs.

The Commission on Cancer of the American College of Surgeons has recognized the need for data on quality of survival. It required as of January 1973 that each hospital cancer registry evaluate performance status of patients in order to gain approval by the American College of Surgeons [11]. As a result, the Department of Clinical Statistics at Memorial Hospital for Cancer and Allied Diseases in New York requires information on quality of survival from all cancer patients. Each year the respondents provide information on employment, functional capabilities, and whether, after treatment, they have realized their potential for employability and resumed normal functions in the family and community. Such surveys, already producing valuable information, might be expanded to obtain additional data on the patient and to begin ascertaining the impact of cancer on others besides the patient exposed to cancer [11].

Nevertheless, estimation of social costs is a hope for the future. The remainder of this chapter focuses on economic costs—discussing recent estimates of economic costs including some methodological aspects, and providing new information on certain costs by cancer site.

B. Economic Costs

Cancer like other diseases produces economic as well as social costs. Direct economic costs are those connected with prevention, diagnosis, and treatment. These costs include expenditures for hospital and nursing home care, physicians' and nurses' services, drugs, medical research, training of medical personnel, construction of facilities, and other expenditures such as those for public health education. Indirect costs are the losses in output as time is lost from work because of mortality, morbidity, and disability. Economic costs represent foregone alternatives, the direct costs being the value of resources which could be allocated to other uses in the absence of disease, and the indirect costs being the value of idle resources and lost output [26].

Section II discusses economic costs of neoplasms in 1975 and their relationship to total costs for all illnesses, and summarizes the assumptions and principles of economics used to calculate indirect costs. Section III presents costs of short-term hospital care, physicians' services, and mortality by cancer site. Section IV provides a summary and conclusion, and the appendix explains methodology.

II. ECONOMIC COSTS IN 1975

The most recent national estimates of costs of disease in the United States are for fiscal year 1975 [27]. These calculations follow closely, with some modifications, the methodology pioneered by Rice [28] more than a decade ago and recently updated by Cooper and Rice [29]. In 1975 the total estimated cost of illness ranged from $239 to $323 billion, depending on the discount rate employed, with neoplasms (benign and malignant) accounting for $19 to $28 billion, or 8-9% of total costs. Thus, neoplasms make up one of the most costly disease categories, surpassed only by diseases of the circulatory system (18-19% of total costs), and by accidents, poisonings, and violence (12-18% of total costs). Costs of neoplasms are

TABLE 1 Estimated Direct Expenditures and Percent Distribution for All Diseases and Neoplasms, and Expenditures for Neoplasms, as a Percent of All Diseases, According to Type of Expenditures, Fiscal Year 1975

	Expenditures				
	All diseases[a]		Neoplasms		Neoplasms as a % of all diseases
	Amount in millions	% distribution	Amount in millions	% distribution	
Total	$99,373.2[b]	100.0	$5,278.9	100.0	5.3
Hospital care	46,414.9	46.7	4,134.2	78.3	8.9
Physicians' services	22,099.9	22.2	671.2	12.7	3.0
Other professional services	1,453.5	1.5	50.1	1.0	3.4
Drugs and drug sundries	10,604.9	10.7	202.7	3.8	1.9
Nursing home care	9,000.0	9.1	220.7	4.2	2.5
Dentists' services	7,500.0	7.5	—	—	—
Eyeglasses and appliances	2,300.0	2.3	—	—	—

[a]Based on Social Security Administration's preliminary estimates for fiscal year 1975.

[b]Excludes unallocated expenditures for prepayment and administration, government public health activities, other health services, research, and construction.

Source: From Ref. 27.

similar in magnitude to those for mental disorders and diseases of the respiratory and digestive systems.

A. Direct Costs

Direct costs of neoplasms totaled $5.3 billion in fiscal 1975, representing 5.3% of the total direct expenditures for medical care (Table 1). Hospital care expenditures of $4.1 billion accounted for 78% of the total direct costs of neoplasms, and an estimated $671 million, almost 13% of the total, was spent on physicians' services. The remaining 9% of direct expenditures were incurred for other professional services, drugs and drug sundries, and nursing home care. Thus, by far the largest share of expenses connected with the prevention, diagnosis, and treatment of neoplasms is that incurred for hospital care (Fig. 1). This is quite different from the distribution of direct costs for all diseases taken together. While the amount spent on hospital care for all diseases is the largest component of direct costs, it accounts for only 47% of the total expenditures, and significantly larger proportions were spent on other types of care for all diseases than for neoplasms. As shown in the appendix, however, the figure for physicians' services for neoplasms ($671 million) is a serious underestimate of expenditures.

B. Indirect Costs

Illness and death due to cancer prevent people from leading their accustomed productive lives in terms of working and keeping house. They may lose time from their activities, be forced out of the labor force, or become institutionalized. Persons dying of cancer in a given year would otherwise be expected to live into the future with an estimated life expectancy. The value of current and future output lost because of cessation or reduction of productive activity due to morbidity and mortality is an indirect cost of cancer. The calculation of the loss of output resulting from mortality and morbidity involves the application of several assumptions and principles of economics, which we now summarize.

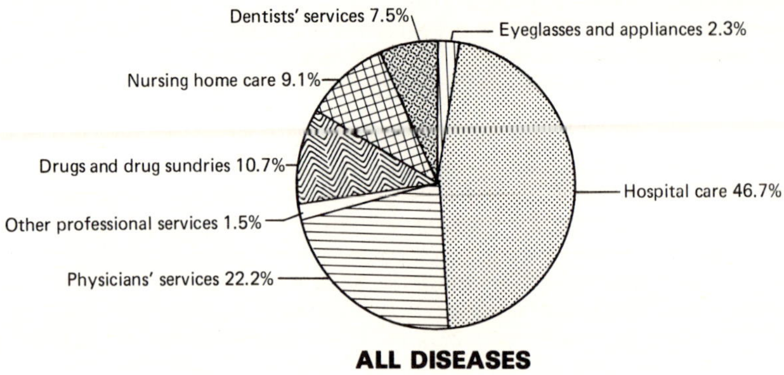

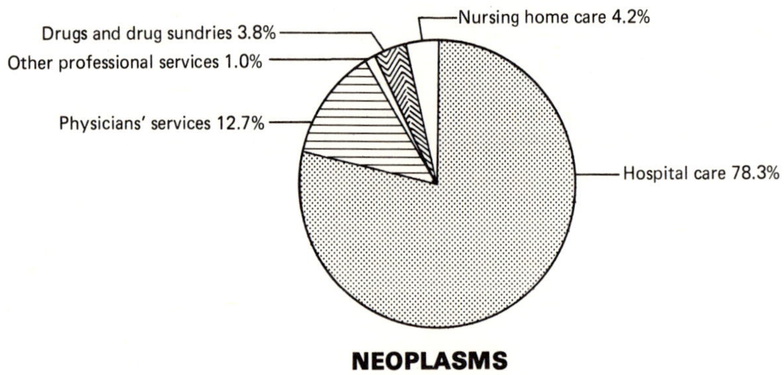

FIGURE 1 Direct expenditures: distribution by type of expenditure, fiscal year 1975.

1. Earnings

The appropriate measure of output loss for individuals is earnings, and the proper measure of expected earnings is the arithmetic average or mean. In this report output losses are based upon annual mean earnings by age and sex provided by the Bureau of Labor Statistics [27], adjusted for wage supplements such as employer contributions for social insurance, private pensions, and welfare funds.

Cross-sectional profiles of mean earnings by age for each sex are used to estimate lifetime earnings. In applying these cross-sectional data, it is assumed that the future pattern of earnings for an average individual within a sex group will follow the pattern reported by the Bureau of Labor Statistics during the base year 1975. This model recognizes that the average individual may expect his or her own earnings to increase with age and experience, in accordance with the cross-sectional data for 1975.

The use of these average earnings based on cross-sectional surveys would understate the present value of expected lifetime earnings if future economic growth patterns were not taken into account. However, an average annual rate of gain in productivity is projected and applied as a partial offset to the discount rate.

2. The Discount Rate

The calculation of the present value of expected lifetime earnings raises questions about the importance of discounting and choosing the appropriate discount rate. From the economist's viewpoint, the arithmetic sum of lifetime earnings overstates the present value of an individual. Determining the present value of the future earnings stream is the correct way to measure the economic value over a period of time; discounting converts a stream of earnings into its present value.

Economists agree that comparison of streams of earnings over varying time spans should employ the process of discounting, but there is no agreement on the discount rate to be used [30-31]. The higher the discount rate, the lower the present value of a given money stream. With a high rate of discount, earnings far into the future yield a relatively small present value. Conversely, lowering the discount rate increases the present value of these future earnings.

Two basic concepts behind the rationale for choosing a discount rate are the opportunity cost concept and subjective time preference. Opportunity cost refers to the notion that resources should be valued according to what they could earn in alternative uses, assuming that the alternative uses are productive and resources so used today will generate a larger or more highly valued output in the future. The rate of return on corporate earnings and the government borrowing rate have been suggested as two measures of the discount rate. Time preference refers to the usual preference for a dollar now compared to a dollar in the future, a preference that cannot be measured directly.

The discount rate should be the result of a balance between opportunity cost and time preference. How to arrive at this balance is not specified, however, and the usual practice is to present a number of alternative rates. The 6% and 10% rates in this report provide a range that encompasses the rates generally in use today for costs of disease. It is usually, if not always, assumed that a single discount rate applies to all subgroups of a population. There is evidence, however, that discount rates vary significantly with age, income, sex,

TABLE 2 Present Value of Lifetime Earnings Discounted at 6% and 10%, According to Sex and Age, Fiscal Year 1975

Age (years)	Present value of lifetime earnings: 6% discount, Male	6% discount, Female	10% discount, Male	10% discount, Female
Under 1	$129,435	$ 96,303	$ 37,659	$ 29,802
1-4	129,794	97,284	38,036	30,223
5-9	157,381	118,002	55,705	44,285
10-14	191,965	143,745	82,066	65,164
15-19	230,812	171,067	117,367	91,810
20-24	263,308	188,384	152,964	113,891
25-29	274,496	185,581	173,868	119,888
30-34	263,864	170,571	176,882	114,057
35-39	241,464	152,391	170,362	105,802
40-44	210,785	132,100	156,719	95,489
45-49	171,975	110,049	134,756	83,230
50-54	127,682	85,799	105,213	67,962
55-59	83,144	60,224	72,093	49,846
60-64	42,318	35,957	38,439	30,676
65-69	15,698	18,995	14,048	16,238
70-74	7,239	10,672	6,579	9,351
75-79	3,268	5,541	3,018	4,981
80-84	1,499	2,771	1,410	2,565
85 and over	610	1,183	610	1,103

Source: Present values at 6% are unpublished data obtained from the Public Services Laboratory, Georgetown University, Washington, D.C. Present values at 10% are from Ref. 27.

and race [32]. Mortality also varies according to these factors, and the effect on costs of assuming a uniform discount rate is not known. A uniform rate is a simplification required by limitations of data.

The discount rate can be adjusted for expected changes in productivity. An increase in productivity of 20% a year, for example, can be incorporated into the discounting calculations to obtain a net effective discount rate. Thus, a 6% discount rate adjusted for a rise in productivity of 2.0% per year will yield an effective discount rate of approximately 4% (1.06/1.02 = 1.078). The present value of lifetime earnings by age and sex for discount rates of 6 and 10%, adjusted for an annual increase in productivity of 2.0% per year, are given in Table 2 and Fig. 2.

3. Employment

The estimate of lifetime earnings takes into account varying work-experience rates. The assumption is that an individual will be working and productive during his or her lifetime in accordance with the current pattern of work experience for his or her sex and age group. For this calculation, work-experience rates for 1975 published by the Bureau of Labor Statistics were used [27]. Unfortunately, 1975 was a year of high unemployment. With less than full employment, the estimated cost of illness is lower than it would be under full employment because losses due to illness cannot be isolated from losses due to unemployment. To overcome this downward bias in the estimate of illness costs, work-experience rates during a year of full employment should be used.

4. Household Work

Marketplace earnings underestimate the loss resulting from illness of women, and the value of household work must be added to earnings. Based on a time-motion study of housewives [33], the relevant market wages for various services performed were multiplied by the time required for doing that service to obtain an estimate of the cost of replacing the housewife's duties with person-hours from the labor force. This takes into account the housewife's age, number of children, and age of youngest child. The value of household work was imputed for all women ever married until age 65, and beyond age 65 for women with spouses present and female heads of household. It was also imputed for married men with spouses present. Imputed household values plus marketplace earnings give total earnings, which were used to compute the present value of lifetime earnings [27].

5. Consumption

In the past it has been questioned whether the cost of morbidity and mortality due to illness is an individual's output or the individual's output minus his consumption [34-36]. Our concern is with the cost of illness to society. The individual, and not just the output he or she contributes in excess of consumption, is valued by society, so it is now generally agreed among economists that consumption should not be deducted [37].

6. Life Expectancy

Lifetime earnings data were calculated using modified generation life tables. These tables assume life expectancy changes between the years 1975 and 2050, with each cohort having a different mortality experience [27].

7. Value of Human Life

One, if not the chief, issue with respect to indirect costs is how to value life. The method in this report is referred to as the "human capital" approach because it views an employed person as producing a stream of output over the years that is valued at the individual's earnings. The main criticism of this methodology is that it excludes intangibles, only counting earnings, and undervalues some groups relative to others because earnings may not reflect

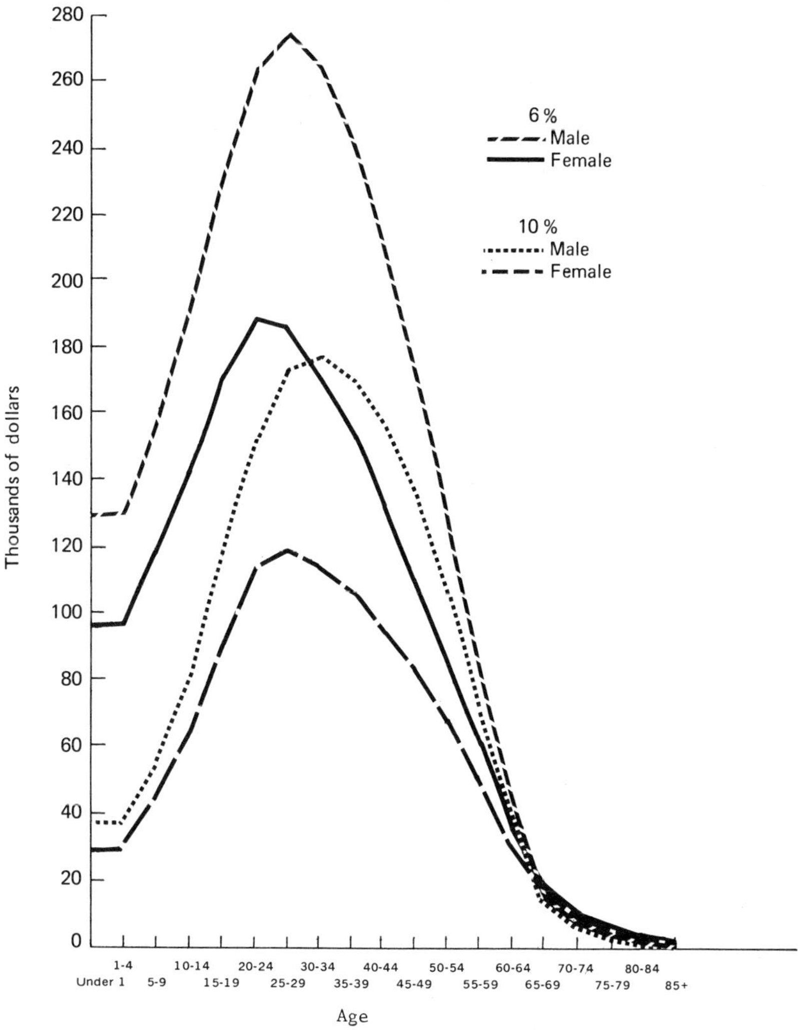

FIGURE 2 Present value of lifetime earnings, discounted at 6% and 10% by age according to sex, fiscal year 1975. (Source: Present values at 6% are unpublished data obtained from the Public Services Laboratory, Georgetown University, Washington, D.C. Present values at 10% are from Ref. 27.

TABLE 3 Number and Percent Distribution of Deaths, Estimated Total Person-Years Lost, and Discounted Earnings at 6 and 10%, for All Diseases and Neoplasms, According to Age and Sex, Fiscal Year 1975[a]

	Age							
Characteristic	All ages	Under 45 years	45-64 years	65 years and over	All ages	Under 45 years	45-64 years	65 years and over
	Number in thousands				Percent distribution			
Deaths								
All diseases								
Both sexes	1,936	232	463	1,241	100	12	24	64
Male	1,071	151	297	624	100	14	28	58
Female	865	81	166	617	100	9	19	71
Neoplasms								
Both sexes	366	23	131	211	100	6	36	58
Male	199	11	71	117	100	6	36	59
Female	166	12	60	94	100	7	36	57
Years Lost								
All diseases								
Both sexes	35,005	15,479	9,248	10,378	100	44	26	29
Male	17,344	8,217	3,770	5,357	100	47	22	31
Female	17,661	7,262	5,478	4,921	100	41	31	28
Neoplasms								
Both sexes	5,545	1,013	2,552	1,981	100	18	46	36
Male	2,770	549	1,244	966	100	20	45	35
Female	2,775	464	1,308	1,004	100	17	47	36
	Amount in millions				Percent distribution			
Lost Earnings Discounted at 6%								
All diseases								
Both sexes	$87,926	$43,268	$37,062	$ 7,596	100	49	42	9
Male	62,328	32,093	26,499	3,736	100	51	43	6
Female	25,598	11,176	10,563	3,860	100	44	41	15
Neoplasms								
Both sexes	15,974	4,342	9,972	1,661	100	27	62	10
Male	9,454	2,537	6,082	835	100	27	64	9
Female	6,520	1,805	3,890	825	100	28	60	13
Lost Earnings Discounted at 10%								
All diseases								
Both sexes	65,527	24,984	30,763	6,781	100	40	49	11
Male	44,210	18,590	22,249	3,371	100	42	50	8
Female	18,318	6,394	8,514	3,410	100	35	46	19
Neoplasms								
Both sexes	12,549	2,816	8,257	1,476	100	22	66	12
Male	7,508	1,624	5,129	755	100	22	68	10
Female	5,041	1,192	3,128	721	100	24	62	14

[a]Deaths are those for calendar year 1974.

Note: Numbers and percents may not add to totals due to rounding.

Source: Deaths, years lost, and lost earnings discounted at 10% are from Ref. 27.

one's ability to produce. Thus, men are more highly valued than women, whites more than blacks, and the middle-aged more than the young and elderly, with some of the differences the result of racial and sexual discrimination.

An alternative approach favored by some is that of "willingness to pay." This method values human life according to the amount people are willing to spend to obtain reductions in the probability of death. Objections to this approach are that the value of individual lives depends on the income distribution, with the rich able to pay more than the poor, and that it is exceedingly difficult for persons to place a value on small reductions in the probability of death. One of the few attempts to apply "willingness to pay" was in a study of heart and circulatory disease [38]. The human capital approach is still most often used. It provides valuable information based upon reliable statistics, so long as one realizes its limitations.

8. Findings

Number of deaths, person-years lost, and lost earnings in 1975 for all diseases and neoplasms by age and sex are shown in Table 3. Twenty percent more males than females died of neoplasms compared to 24% more for all diseases. But owing to the longer life expectancy among women, total person-years lost were about the same for each sex. Men, however, accounted for a much larger share of lost earnings due to lower labor force participation rates among women, lower earnings for women who do work, and still lower values imputed for women keeping house. For all diseases, mortality costs for males were significantly higher than for females, comprising 71% and 29%, respectively (Fig. 3). For neoplasms the difference was less, mortality costs for males comprising 59% of the total. This difference in mortality costs by sex is mostly due to a difference in age at death for females dying

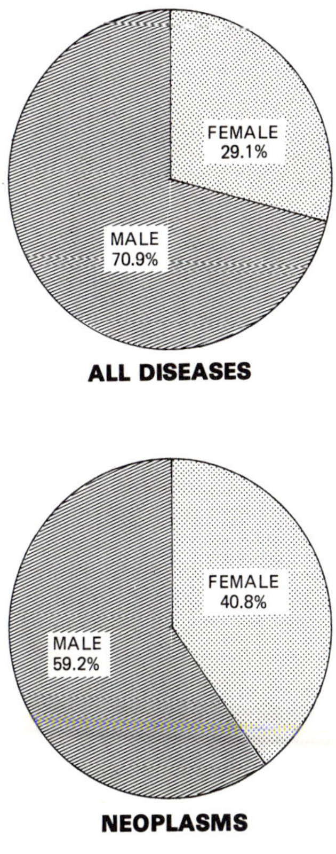

FIGURE 3 Indirect costs of mortality: distribution by sex at 6% discount rate, fiscal year 1975.

TABLE 4 Estimated Indirect Costs and Percent Distributions of All Diseases and Neoplasms by Discount Rate, According to Type of Cost and Demographic Characteristic, Fiscal Year 1975

Disease category, type of cost, and demographic characteristic	Indirect costs: 10% discount: Amount in millions	10% discount: Percent distribution by type of cost	10% discount: Percent distribution by demographic characteristic	6% discount: Amount in millions	6% discount: Percent distribution by of cost	6% discount: Percent distribution by demographic characteristic
All diseases						
Total	$120,375	100.0	—	$145,774	100.0	—
Morbidity	57,846	48.1	100.0	57,846	39.7	100.0
Currently employed	21,303	17.7	36.8	21,303	14.6	36.8
Females keeping house	4,384	3.6	7.6	4,384	3.0	7.6
Unable to work	24,410	20.3	42.2	24,410	16.7	42.2
Institutionalized	7,750	6.4	13.4	7,750	5.3	13.4
Mortality	62,529	51.9	100.0	87,925	60.3	100.0
Male	44,210	36.7	70.7	62,328	42.8	70.9
Female	18,318	15.2	29.3	25,598	17.6	29.1
Neoplasms						
Total	$ 13,654	100.0	—	$ 17,079	100.0	—
Morbidity	1,105	8.1	100.0	1,105	6.5	100.0
Currently employed	422	3.1	38.2	422	2.5	38.2
Females keeping house	194	1.4	17.6	194	1.1	17.6
Unable to work	440	3.2	39.8	440	2.6	39.8
Institutionalized	49	0.4	4.4	49	0.3	4.4
Mortality	12,549	91.9	100.0	15,974	93.5	100.0
Male	7,508	55.0	59.8	9,454	55.4	59.2
Female	5,041	36.9	40.2	6,520	38.2	40.8

Note: Numbers and percents may not add to totals due to rounding.

Source: From Ref. 27.

of neoplasms and females dying of all diseases. Forty-three percent of women whose deaths were caused by neoplasms were under 65 years of age, the most productive years, while the corresponding figure for all diseases is only 28%.

Estimates of the total indirect costs of neoplasms and all diseases are given in Table 4. A much larger proportion of indirect costs was due to mortality for neoplasms than for all diseases: 94% versus 60%, at a 6% discount rate (Fig. 4). Morbidity accounted for only a small proportion of the indirect costs of neoplasms (6%). This disparity between neoplasms and all diseases in the distribution of indirect costs results directly from a similar disparity in person-years lost due to morbidity and mortality. For neoplasms only 2% of all person-years lost resulted from morbidity, while 14% of person-years lost were due to morbidity for all diseases. That neoplasms cause a relatively greater burden from mortality compared to morbidity than do all diseases together is further evidenced by the following statistics. Neoplasms account for 16% of person-years lost due to mortality from all diseases but only 2% of person-years lost due to morbidity. Also, data from the National Center for Health Statistics show that while malignant neoplasms account for 18% of all deaths, only 1% of all persons with limitations of activity report malignant neoplasms as the cause.

Morbidity costs for the currently employed and those unable to work each accounted for almost 40% of morbidity losses for neoplasms as well as for all diseases, with the remaining one-fifth split between females keeping house and the institutionalized population. A final point to note is that while a change in the discount rate produces a change in the amount of mortality costs and the relative contribution of mortality and morbidity to total costs, it produces almost no change in the proportion of mortality costs attributed to men and women.

The dollar amounts and percentage distribution of total economic costs in fiscal year 1975 are given in Table 5 by type of cost for all diseases and neoplasms. The total cost of neoplasms was $19 billion or $22 billion in fiscal year 1975 depending on whether mortality costs are discounted at 6% or 10%. The indirect cost of mortality was by far the largest component of economic costs of neoplasms, accounting for 71% of the total at a 6% discount rate. Morbidity contributed a very small share, only 5%, and direct costs made up 24% of the total (Fig. 5). In contrast, for all diseases, mortality contributed only 36%, morbidity accounted for 24%, and direct costs were 40% of the total, at a 6% discount rate.

Table 5 shows the significant impact of the discount rate on costs. The lower the discount rate, the higher the present value of future earnings lost due to mortality. Although only the indirect cost of mortality is affected by changes in the discount rate, the resulting change in mortality cost is large and produces significant shifts in the proportional distribution of costs.

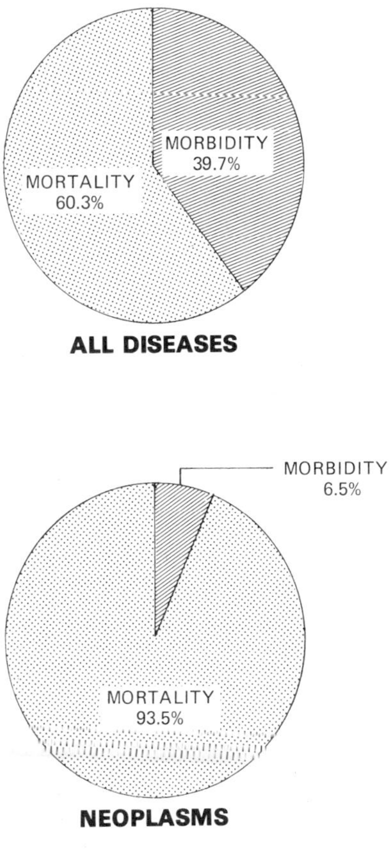

FIGURE 4 Indirect costs: distribution by type of cost at 6% discount rate, fiscal year 1975.

TABLE 5 Estimated Costs and Percent Distribution for All Diseases and Neoplasms, and Neoplasms as a Percent of All Diseases, According to Type of Cost and Discount Rate, Fiscal Year 1975

Disease category and discount rate	Type of cost				
	All costs	Direct cost[a]	Indirect cost		
			Total	Morbidity	Mortality
	Amount in millions				
All diseases					
10% discount	$219,749	$99,374	$120,375	$57,846	$62,529
6% discount	245,145	99,374	145,771	57,846	87,925
Neoplasms					
10% discount	18,933	5,279	13,654	1,105	12,549
6% discount	22,358	5,279	17,079	1,105	15,974
	% distribution				
All diseases					
10% discount	100.0	45.2	54.8	26.3	28.5
6% discount	100.0	40.5	59.5	23.6	35.9
Neoplasms					
10% discount	100.0	27.9	72.1	5.8	66.3
6% discount	100.0	23.6	76.4	4.9	71.5
	% of costs of all diseases				
Neoplasms					
10% discount	8.6	5.3	11.3	1.9	20.1
6% discount	9.1	5.3	11.7	1.9	18.2

[a]Excludes unallocated expenditures for prepayment and administration, government public health activities, other health services, research, and construction.

Source: From Ref. 27.

Neoplasms were responsible for about 9% of the total costs of all diseases in fiscal year 1975. Direct costs of neoplasms were 5% of all direct costs, and morbidity due to neoplasms contributed 2% of all costs associated with morbidity. Neoplasms represented a much larger share of costs associated with mortality, however; between 18 and 20%.

III. ECONOMIC COSTS OF CANCER BY SITE

Cancer is not a single disease, but a group of diseases. These have in common the uncontrolled growth of abnormal cells, but there are great differences among various forms of cancer. Causes, appearance, and behavior are dissimilar [39]. Survival rates show considerable variation according to organ of origin. Cancers of the pancreas are highly fatal, with 5-year survival rates of only 1%. The 5-year survival rate for breast cancer, on the other hand, is around 65% [40]. Trends in age-adjusted death rates also vary for different sites. In the United States age-adjusted death rates for malignant neoplasms of the respiratory system have increased dramatically, rising from 21.6 deaths per 100,000 white males and 4.6 per 100,000 white females in 1950 to 54.6 deaths per 100,000 white males and 13.8 per 100,000 white females in 1975. During this same period age-adjusted death rates for

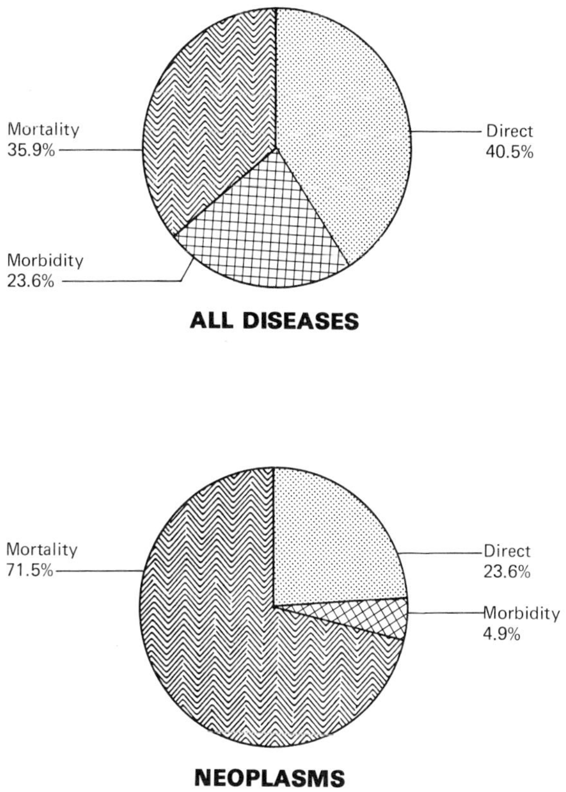

FIGURE 5 Economic costs: distribution by type of cost at 6% discount rate, fiscal year 1975.

cancers of the digestive organs and peritoneum decreased from 54.0 to 40.2 deaths per 100,000 white males and from 41.1 to 26.4 deaths per 100,000 white females [41]. Expenditures for resources in the form of hospital care and physician's services for prevention, diagnosis, and treatment of cancer, and the number of person-years and value of output lost due to premature mortality also vary significantly among cancer sites.

For these reasons, it is important to distringuish among cancer sites, and in this section we present estimates by cancer site of expenditures in 1975 for short-stay hospital care and physicians' services, and indirect costs of mortality. Together, these three categories account for 90% of total economic costs of meoplasms. The two largest of the remaining categories of costs, those arising from morbidity and nursing home care, account for 5-7% of total costs, but cannot be estimated by cancer site.

A. Short-Term Hospital Care

Table 6 presents the distribution of days of care for patients discharged from short-stay hospitals in 1975 according to cancer site, age, and sex. Patients with neoplasms spent more than 25.5 million days in short-stay hospitals in 1975. About 56% of these days (14.3 million) were used by persons under age 65, and 58% (14.9 million) were used by females. Eighty-three percent of days for benign neoplasms were used by those under age 65 and 78%

TABLE 6 Days of Care for Patients with Neoplasms Discharged from Short-Stay Hospitals, According to Sex, Age, and Site, Calendar Year 1975

Site	Total	Sex: Male	Sex: Female	Age: Under 65 years	Age: 65 years and over
	Days of care in short-stay hospitals in thousands				
All neoplasms	25,505.1	10,610.7	14,894.4	14,301.2	11,203.9
Malignant neoplasms	20,611.6	9,520.9	11,090.7	10,212.8	10,398.8
Buccal cavity and pharynx	394.5	265.9	a	233.6	a
Stomach	570.0	339.4	230.6	253.8	361.1
Intestine and rectum	2,629.1	1,310.0	1,319.1	1,001.3	1,627.8
Other digestive organs	958.8	445.3	513.5	327.3	631.5
Trachea, lung, and bronchus	2,366.5	1,690.5	675.9	1,252.9	1,113.6
Other respiratory organs	291.7	237.6	a	a	a
Skin	503.9	265.2	238.8	291.2	212.7
Breast	2,464.7	a	2,429.1	1,536.7	928.0
Cervix uteri	743.1	—	743.1	654.7	a
Other parts of uterus	482.3	—	482.3	279.4	202.9
Other female genital organs	605.9	—	605.9	345.8	260.1
Male genital organs	1,190.1	1,190.1	—	266.3	923.8
Urinary organs	1,113.6	787.3	326.3	406.7	706.9
Other and unspecified sites	4,109.0	1,934.1	2,174.8	2,008.7	2,100.2
Leukemia	683.6	371.2	312.4	378.9	304.7
Other lymphatic and hematopoietic tissues	1,504.7	648.6	856.1	857.5	647.2
Benign neoplasms and neoplasms of unspecified nature	4,893.5	1,089.8	3,803.7	4,088.4	805.1

[a]Figure does not meet standards of reliability or precision (more than 30% relative standard error).

Note: Numbers may not add to totals due to rounding.

Source: Hospital Discharge Survey, National Center for Health Statistics.

by females. For malignant neoplasms, the older age group accounted for slightly more days than those under age 65, while utilization by females exceeded that by males by about 7.5 percentage points.

More days of care were used by persons over age 65 for malignant neoplasms of the stomach, intestine and rectum, other digestive organs, male genital organs, and urinary organs. Younger persons accounted for more days of care for malignant neoplasms of the buccal cavity and pharynx, skin, breast, female genital organs, leukemia and other lymphatic and hematopoietic tissues, and benign neoplasms. Days of care for patients with cancers of the trachea, lung, and bronchus, and of other and unspecified sites were almost evenly distributed by age. For patients under age 65, 71% of hospital days were for malignant neoplasms, while for those age 65 and over the figure was 93%. About one-third of days used by the younger patients were for malignant neoplasms of the intestine and rectum, respiratory organs, breast, and lymphatic and hematopoietic tissues, while these sites plus male genital organs accounted for almost 50% of the days reported for patients age 65 and over.

Excluding neoplasms of the breast and genital systems, males accounted for more of the days resulting from cancer of the buccal cavity and pharynx, stomach, respiratory system, urinary organs, and leukemia. Females used more days of care for other digestive organs, other lymphatic and hematopoietic tissues, and benign neoplasms, while there was little difference in utilization between the sexes for cancers of the intestine and rectum, skin, and other and unspecified sites.

Expenditures for short-stay hospital care are shown in Table 7. (See the appendix for an explanation of the methodology that resulted in a significantly higher estimate than that made by Georgetown University for short-term hospital care.) The total spent for all neoplasms in 1975 was estimated at $4.1 billion, with 78%, or $3.2 billion, spent for malignant neoplasms. Average daily charges for hospital care vary according to the site of the neoplasm and are somewhat higher for patients under age 65. Nevertheless, the primary determinant of the distribution of expenditures among sites and between the two age groups and sexes is the number of days of care. Expenditures follow closely the distribution of days of care, and the comments about hospital days also apply to expenditures.

TABLE 7 Estimated Hospital Expenditures for Patients with Neoplasms Discharged from Short-Stay Hospitals, According to Sex, Age, and Site, Calendar Year 1975

		Sex		Age	
	Total	Male	Female	Under 65 years	65 years and over
	Expenditures for short-stay hospitals in millions				
All neoplasms	$4,131.6	$1,761.2	$2,370.4	$2,477.1	$1,654.5
Malignant neoplasms	3,215.7	1,542.1	1,673.6	1,699.6	1,516.1
Buccal cavity and pharynx	67.0	46.5	a	41.2	a
Stomach	93.2	56.9	36.4	43.3	49.9
Intestine and rectum	425.3	221.8	203.5	170.3	255.0
Other digestive organs	151.0	73.3	77.7	55.1	95.9
Trachea, lung, and bronchus	379.5	273.6	105.9	211.3	168.3
Other respiratory organs	47.4	39.1	a	a	a
Skin	84.4	45.6	38.8	53.5	30.9
Breast	344.3	a	339.0	219.2	125.0
Cervix uteri	124.4	—	124.4	112.2	a
Other parts of uterus	78.0	—	78.0	48.3	29.7
Other female genital organs	95.5	—	95.5	59.6	35.9
Male genital organs	169.4	169.4	—	42.2	127.2
Urinary organs	177.7	128.1	49.7	70.4	107.3
Other and unspecified sites	593.1	292.1	301.1	313.0	280.1
Leukemia	130.7	75.6	55.1	80.9	49.8
Other lymphatic and hematopoietic tissues	254.9	114.9	140.0	159.4	95.5
Benign neoplasms and neoplasms of unspecified nature	915.8	219.1	696.8	777.4	138.4

[a]Figure does not meet standards of reliability or precision (more than 30% relative standard error).

Note: Amounts may not add to totals due to rounding.

Sources: Days of care, from the Hospital Discharge Survey of the National Center for Health Statistics; Health Care Financing Administration for average per diem charges to Medicare patients; Third National Cancer Survey of the National Cancer Institute for ratio of average daily hospital payments for patients under age 65 to payments for patients 65 and over.

TABLE 8 Estimated Expenditures for Physicians' Services Due to Neoplasms and Percent Distributions, According to Site and Type of Visit, Calendar Year 1975

Site	Type of visit											
			Inpatient hospital				Inpatient hospital				Inpatient hospital	
	Total	Office and other[a]	Medical	Surgical	Total	Office and other[a]	Medical	Surgical	Total	Office and other[a]	Medical	Surgical
	Expenditures in millions				% distribution by site				% distribution by type of visit			
All neoplasms	$1,245.6	$299.2	$274.1	$672.3	100.0	100.0	100.0	100.0	100.0	24.0	22.0	54.0
Digestive organs	114.1	14.0	36.2	63.9	9.2	4.7	13.2	9.5	100.0	12.3	31.7	56.0
Respiratory organs	78.0	10.0	25.5	42.4	6.3	3.4	9.3	6.3	100.0	12.9	32.7	54.4
Skin	46.1	19.4	2.5	24.2	3.7	6.5	0.9	3.6	100.0	42.1	5.4	52.5
Breast	84.3	15.4	17.8	51.1	6.8	5.1	6.5	7.6	100.0	18.3	21.1	60.6
Female genital organs	73.9	8.0	8.8	57.1	5.9	2.7	3.2	8.5	100.0	10.8	11.9	77.3
Male genital organs	51.2	10.2	14.8	26.2	4.1	3.4	5.4	3.9	100.0	19.9	28.9	51.2
Leukemia	23.9	8.6	9.9	5.4	1.9	2.9	3.6	0.8	100.0	36.0	41.4	22.6
All other malignant neoplasms	259.1	50.0	97.5	111.6	20.8	16.7	35.6	16.6	100.0	19.3	37.6	43.1
Benign neoplasms and neoplasms of unspecified sites	514.9	163.4	61.1	290.4	41.3	54.6	22.3	43.2	100.0	31.7	11.9	56.4

[a]Other includes home, telephones, nursing home, and other.

Note: Numbers and percents may not add to totals due to rounding.

Source: Health Care Financing Administration for total expenditures for physicians' services; National Disease Therapeutic Index for physicians' visits by site; James R. Cantwell, editor, Profiles of Medical Practice, American Medical Association, Chicago, 1976 for average fees; and Hospital Discharge Survey, National Center for Health Statistics for number of short-stay hospital discharges with surgery by site.

B. Physicians' Services

Costs of physicians' care in 1975 for neoplasms are estimated at more than $1.2 billion as shown in Table 8. (See the appendix for an explanation of the methodology that resulted in significantly higher estimates than those made by Georgetown University.) Over half of this total, $672 million or 54%, was for surgery in the hospital. The remainder was almost equally divided between medical care in the hospital ($274 million) and office and other visits ($299 million). This pattern of expenditures did not prevail among all cancer sites, however. Although surgery accounted for over half the expenditures for most sites, surgery produced only 23% of the total for leukemia. At the other extreme, 77% of the total for cancers of female genital organs was surgery connected. Relatively small amounts were spent for medical care in the hospital for some sites, such as cancers of the skin (5% of the total for this site), female genital organs (12%), and benign neoplasms (12%), while 41% of the total spent for leukemia and almost one-third of expenditures for digestive and respiratory organs were for medical care in the hospital. With respect to amounts spent for office and other types of visits, cancers of the female genital, digestive, and respiratory organs required relatively small expenditures (11-13% of their totals), while for benign neoplasms, leukemia, and skin cancers, 32, 36, and 42% of expenditures, respectively, were for office and other visits.

Benign neoplasms accounted for 55% of the amount spent for office and other visits for all neoplasms, 22% of the cost of medical care in the hospital, and 43% of the total for surgery. Except for the residual category of "all other malignant neoplasms" and medical care in the hospital for cancer of the digestive system, no other site accounted for as much as 10% of expenditures when viewed according to place of visit. Furthermore, there is no discernible pattern of expenditures by site according to place of visit.

C. Mortality

Tables 9 and 10 present data on deaths from neoplasms in 1975 by age, sex, cancer site, and color. There were almost 371,000 deaths, 54% being deaths of males and 46% deaths of females (Table 9). The majority of persons who died, 59%, were age 65 or older at time of death, while 35% were 45-64 years of age, and 6% were under age 45 (Table 9).

Deaths due to cancers of the breast, digestive, respiratory, and genital organs encompass about 70% of all deaths from neoplasms among both men and women. For males the leading causes of death were cancers of the respiratory organs (33.2%), digestive organs (26.1%), and genital organs (10.1%). Among females the rank order is digestive organs (27.8%), breast (19.1%), genital organs (13.4%), and respiratory organs (11.6%). Except for breast cancer and several sites, such as intestine and rectum, for which the numbers of male and female deaths were almost equal, there were more deaths reported for males than females for each site. Male deaths were especially predominant for neoplasms of the buccal cavity and pharynx, stomach, respiratory organs, and urinary organs, accounting for 60% or more of all deaths reported for each of these sites. Except for cancers of the respiratory system and the small number of men who died of breast cancer, women tended to be older than men at age of death for most cancer sites.

Cancer of the sites listed here as the leading causes of death for males and for females were also the leading causes of death for ages 45-64 and 65 and over. For persons under age 45, leukemia, other lymphatic and hematopoietic tissues, and other and unspecified sites made a significant contribution to mortality of both sexes. In the 65 and over age group, higher than average proportions of deaths were due to neoplasms of the digestive organs, urinary organs, and male genital organs. Deaths from skin cancers, leukemia, cancers of other lymphatic and hematopoietic tissues, other and unspecified sites, and benign neoplasms, on the other hand, occurred with relatively high proportions at ages under 65 years.

About 89% of persons dying because of neoplasms in 1975 were white (Table 10). The distribution of deaths by color varied according to cancer site, with the ratio of white to total

TABLE 9 Deaths from Neoplasma, According to Sex, Age, and Site, Calendar Year 1975

Site	Both sexes				Male				Female			
	All ages[a]	Under 45 years	45–64 years	65 years and over	All ages[a]	Under 45 years	45–64 years	65 years and over	All ages[a]	Under 45 years	45–64 years	65 years and over
	Deaths in thousands											
All neoplasms	370.6	22.8	130.0	217.8	201.9	11.1	70.2	120.6	168.8	11.7	59.8	97.3
Malignant neoplasms	365.7	22.0	128.4	215.3	199.4	10.7	69.4	119.4	156.2	11.3	59.0	95.9
Buccal cavity and pharynx	8.1	0.3	3.8	4.0	5.7	0.2	2.7	2.8	2.4	0.1	1.1	1.3
Stomach	15.0	0.5	4.3	10.3	9.0	0.3	2.8	5.9	6.0	0.2	1.5	4.4
Intestine and rectum	50.1	1.4	13.7	35.0	24.2	0.7	7.1	16.4	25.9	0.7	6.6	18.6
Other digestive organs	34.6	0.9	11.6	22.0	19.6	0.6	7.4	11.7	15.0	0.3	4.3	10.3
Trachea, lung, and bronchus	82.0	2.7	36.5	42.9	63.4	1.7	27.4	34.3	18.6	0.9	9.1	8.6
Other respiratory organs	4.6	0.2	2.0	2.4	3.7	0.2	1.6	1.9	1.0	0.1	0.4	0.5
Bone, connective, and other soft tissue	3.2	0.8	1.0	1.4	1.7	0.5	0.5	0.7	1.5	0.4	0.5	0.7
Skin	5.3	0.9	1.9	2.5	3.1	0.5	1.2	1.3	2.2	0.4	0.7	1.1
Breast	32.4	2.7	14.5	15.2	0.3	0.0	0.1	0.2	32.2	2.7	14.4	15.0
Cervix uteri	5.6	0.9	2.5	2.2	—	—	—	—	5.6	0.9	2.5	2.2
Other parts of uterus	5.6	0.2	1.8	3.7	—	—	—	—	5.6	0.2	1.8	3.7
Other female genital organs	11.4	0.7	5.0	5.8	—	—	—	—	11.4	0.7	5.0	5.8
Male genital organs	20.4	0.6	2.6	17.3	20.4	0.6	2.6	17.3	—	—	—	—
Urinary organs	16.5	0.5	4.6	11.4	11.0	0.3	3.2	7.5	5.5	0.2	1.3	4.0
Other and unspecified sites	36.1	3.5	12.7	19.9	18.3	1.9	7.0	9.4	17.8	1.6	5.7	10.4
Leukemia	14.8	3.0	3.5	8.2	8.4	1.7	2.1	4.6	6.4	1.3	1.4	3.6
Other lymphatic and hematopoietic tissues	20.0	2.3	6.5	11.2	10.8	1.4	3.8	5.6	9.2	0.8	2.7	5.6
Benign neoplasms and neoplasms of unspecified nature	4.9	0.8	1.6	2.5	2.4	0.4	0.9	1.2	2.5	0.4	0.3	1.3

[a]Totals include persons of unknown ages.

Note: Numbers may not add to totals due to rounding.

Source: Division of Vital Statistics, National Center for Health Statistics.

TABLE 10 Deaths from Neoplasms and Percent Distributions, According to Site and Color, Calendar Year 1975

Site	Color								
	Total	White	All other	Total	White	All other	Total	White	All other
	Deaths in thousands			% distribution by site			% distribution by color		
All neoplasms	370.6	329.9	40.8	100.0	100.0	100.0	100.0	89.0	11.0
Malignant neoplasms	365.7	325.5	40.2	98.7	98.7	98.5	100.0	89.0	11.0
Buccal cavity and pharynx	8.1	7.1	1.1	2.2	2.1	2.6	100.0	86.6	13.4
Stomach	15.0	12.6	2.4	4.0	3.8	5.8	100.0	84.0	16.0
Intestine and rectum	50.1	45.7	4.4	13.5	13.8	10.7	100.0	91.2	8.8
Other digestive organs	34.6	29.8	4.8	9.3	9.0	11.8	100.0	86.1	13.9
Trachea, lung, and bronchus	82.0	73.3	8.8	22.1	22.2	21.5	100.0	89.3	10.7
Other respiratory organs	4.6	4.0	0.6	1.3	1.2	1.5	100.0	87.0	13.0
Bone, connective, and other soft tissue	3.2	2.8	0.4	0.9	0.9	0.9	100.0	87.5	12.5
Skin	5.3	5.1	0.2	1.4	1.5	0.4	100.0	96.2	3.8
Breast	32.4	29.6	2.9	8.8	9.0	7.0	100.0	91.1	8.9
Cervix uteri	5.6	4.3	1.3	1.5	1.3	3.1	100.0	76.8	23.2
Other parts of uterus	5.6	4.9	0.8	1.5	1.5	1.8	100.0	86.0	14.0
Other female genital organs	11.4	10.6	0.9	3.1	3.2	2.1	100.0	92.2	7.8
Male genital organs	20.4	17.2	3.2	5.5	5.2	7.8	100.0	84.3	15.7
Urinary organs	16.5	15.2	1.3	4.5	4.6	3.2	100.0	92.1	7.9
Other and unspecified sites	36.1	31.9	4.2	9.7	9.7	10.4	100.0	88.4	11.6
Leukemia	14.8	13.5	1.2	4.0	4.1	3.0	100.0	91.8	8.2
Other lymphatic and hematopoietic tissues	20.0	18.1	1.9	5.4	5.5	4.6	100.0	90.5	9.5
Benign neoplasms and neoplasms of unspecified nature	4.9	4.3	0.6	1.3	1.3	1.5	100.0	87.8	12.2

Note: Numbers and percents may not add to totals due to rounding.

Source: Division of Vital Statistics, National Center for Health Statistics.

mortality highest for skin cancer (96% white) and lowest for cancer of the cervix uteri (77% white).

The number of person-years lost because of premature mortality is given in Table 11 by age at death, sex, and site. The distributions of person-years lost by cancer site are similar to those for deaths for each age and sex. But there are noticeable differences in the age and sex distributions of person-years lost and the number of deaths, since more person-years are lost when a death occurs at a younger age and women have longer life expectancy than men. Almost 60% of deaths from neoplasms occurred at ages 65 and over, but these deaths produced only 36% of person-years lost. The 35% of deaths occurring at ages 45-64 resulted in 47% of person-years lost, while deaths under age 45, 6% of the total, caused 17% of lost person-years.

Just as the age distribution of deaths varies according to cancer site, so does the age distribution of person-years lost. Age distributions by site are similar for males and females, but there is not a single pattern among the sites. For example, over half the person-years lost because of leukemia resulted from deaths of persons under age 45; while the majority of person-years lost due to cancers of the buccal cavity and pharynx, respiratory organs, breast, and certain female genital organs were in the 45-64 age group; and 67% of years lost because of neoplasms of male genital organs occurred among persons age 65 and over at time of death.

Although more males than females died of cancer (54.5%), they contributed a little less than half of all person-years lost (48.1%), owing mostly to the higher life expectancy among women. Still, except for breast cancer and malignant neoplasms of the intestine and rectum, person-years lost by males exceeded or were only slightly less than years lost by females. Years lost by males exceeded those lost by females by the largest amounts for cancers of the buccal cavity and pharynx, respiratory, and urinary organs.

Another way of looking at the relationship among deaths, person-years lost, and age is to consider person-years lost per death (Table 12). This ranged in 1975 from a low of 10.1 years per death associated with male genital organs to a high of 24.3 years per death for bone, connective, and other soft tissue, with an average of 16.1 years for all sites combined. The number of person-years per death also equaled or exceeded 20 years for the breast, cervix uteri, leukemia, and benign neoplasms. Years lost per female death exceeded years lost per male death for every site, the average difference being 4.1 years. Excluding breast cancers, the sex difference in years lost per death was largest for the trachea, lung, and bronchus (5.3 years) and smallest for benign neoplasms (1.2 years).

For all neoplasms, there were 43.5 years lost per death at ages under 45, 21.5 years lost per death at ages 45-64, and 9.9 years at age 65 and over (Table 12). Although years lost per death must decrease as age at death increases, there is considerable variation among sites within each age group, especially under age 65. The expected years lost to a person dying of leukemia at less than 45 years of age was almost 53 years in 1975, while the average person under age 45 who died of cancer of the trachea, lung, or bronchus lost an estimated 34.8 years. For deaths between ages 45-64, the average years lost ranged from a low of 17.3 for male genital organs to 30.5 for benign neoplasms. These figures vary somewhat when males and females are considered separately.

Multiplying number of deaths by present discounted values of lifetime earnings (both specified by age and sex) gives present discounted values of earnings lost due to premature mortality. These total $15.9 billion at a 6% discount rate and average almost $43,000 for each death due to neoplasms. Lost earnings are shown by age, sex, and site in Table 13 at a 6% discount rate. The age distributions of lost earnings vary according to cancer site, depending on the age distribution of deaths for each site, but are similar for males and females.

Although almost 60% of all deaths from neoplasms in 1975 occurred at age 65 and over, this age group accounted for only 36% of person-years lost and 11% of lost earnings (Fig. 6), reflecting the lower life expectancy and earnings of the elderly. Those 45-64 years of age contributed 35% of deaths from neoplasms, 47% of person-years lost, and 62% of lost earnings.

TABLE 11 Person-Years Lost Due to Neoplasms, According to Sex, Age, and Site, Calendar Year 1975

Site	Both sexes				Male				Female			
	All ages	Under 45 years	45-64 years	65 years and over	All ages	Under 45 years	45-64 years	65 years and over	All ages	Under 45 years	45-64 years	65 years and over
	Person-years lost in thousands											
All neoplasms	5,954.4	992.9	2,796.6	2,164.9	2,864.9	458.5	1,324.8	1,081.6	3,089.5	534.4	1,471.8	1,083.3
Malignant neoplasms	5,839.5	952.7	2,746.8	2,139.8	2,809.6	438.3	1,300.0	1,071.2	3,029.9	514.4	1,446.8	1,068.6
Buccal cavity and pharynx	130.4	12.1	77.8	40.5	85.3	7.5	51.6	26.2	45.1	4.6	26.2	14.3
Stomach	201.3	16.8	87.8	96.7	112.4	8.9	52.3	51.2	88.9	7.9	35.5	45.5
Intestine and rectum	682.7	53.6	289.1	340.1	299.6	26.0	131.5	142.2	383.1	27.6	157.6	197.9
Other digestive organs	493.4	35.9	235.9	221.4	266.3	21.3	137.4	107.5	227.1	14.6	98.5	113.9
Trachea, lung, and bronchus	1,261.4	92.3	736.4	432.6	898.5	57.1	513.3	328.0	362.9	35.2	223.1	104.6
Other respiratory organs	72.0	8.2	40.4	23.3	53.3	5.8	29.6	17.8	18.7	2.4	10.8	5.5
Bone, connective, and other soft tissue	78.0	42.8	21.2	14.1	38.3	22.1	10.1	6.2	39.7	20.7	11.1	7.9
Skin	101.9	36.7	41.8	23.5	56.0	20.3	24.3	11.5	45.9	16.4	17.5	12.0
Breast	648.8	109.3	365.5	174.1	3.7	0.5	1.8	1.4	645.1	108.8	363.7	172.7
Cervix uteri	124.7	35.8	63.4	25.5	—	—	—	—	124.7	35.8	63.4	25.5
Other parts of uterus	90.6	6.8	41.9	41.9	—	—	—	—	90.6	6.8	41.9	41.9
Other female genital organs	220.3	28.9	123.4	68.0	—	—	—	—	220.3	28.9	123.4	68.0
Male genital organs	207.1	23.7	44.1	139.3	207.1	23.7	44.1	139.3	—	—	—	—
Urinary organs	220.6	21.5	92.4	106.7	136.2	11.3	60.2	64.7	84.4	10.2	32.2	42.0
Other and unspecified sites	641.0	166.1	273.2	201.7	304.9	85.6	133.1	86.3	336.1	80.5	140.1	115.4
Leukemia	312.7	161.1	74.9	76.7	164.6	86.7	39.2	38.7	148.1	74.4	35.7	38.0
Other lymphatic and hematopoietic tissues	352.6	101.1	137.6	113.8	183.3	61.5	71.5	50.3	169.3	39.6	66.1	63.5
Benign neoplasms and neoplasms of unspecified nature	114.9	40.2	49.7	25.0	53.3	20.2	24.8	10.3	59.6	20.0	24.9	14.7

Note: Numbers may not add to totals due to rounding.

Source Number of deaths and current life tables for 1975 from the Division of Vital Statistics, National Center for Health Statistics.

TABLE 12 Person-Years Lost per Death Due to Neoplasms, According to Sex, Age, and Site, Calendar Year 1975

Site	Both sexes				Male				Female			
	All ages	Under 45 years	45-64 years	65 years and over	All ages	Under 45 years	45-64 years	65 years and over	All ages	Under 45 years	45-64 years	65 years and over
	Person-years lost per death											
All neoplasms	16.1	43.5	21.5	9.9	14.2	41.3	18.9	9.0	18.3	45.6	24.6	11.1
Malignant neoplasms	16.0	43.3	21.4	9.9	14.1	41.1	18.7	9.0	18.2	45.4	24.5	11.1
Buccal cavity and pharynx	16.0	38.5	20.6	10.0	15.0	35.9	19.1	9.4	18.4	43.8	24.4	11.3
Stomach	13.4	37.2	20.5	9.4	12.6	34.1	18.6	8.7	14.8	41.4	24.1	10.4
Intestine and rectum	13.6	38.3	21.1	9.7	12.4	35.8	18.6	8.7	14.8	40.9	23.9	10.6
Other digestive organs	14.3	38.4	20.3	10.1	13.6	35.9	18.7	9.2	15.2	42.7	23.0	11.0
Trachea, lung and bronchus	15.4	34.8	20.2	10.1	14.2	32.7	18.7	9.6	19.5	39.0	24.6	12.1
Other respiratory organs	15.5	38.9	19.9	9.7	14.6	36.7	18.7	9.3	19.1	45.3	24.4	11.3
Bone, connective, and other soft tissue	24.3	51.4	21.9	10.0	23.0	47.5	19.6	9.1	25.7	56.3	24.4	11.0
Skin	19.3	40.6	21.9	9.5	18.2	37.9	20.0	8.7	20.9	44.7	25.3	10.5
Breast	20.0	40.2	25.1	11.5	13.4	35.7	18.2	8.5	20.1	40.3	25.2	11.5
Cervix uteri	22.5	41.3	25.6	11.5	—	—	—	—	22.5	41.3	25.6	11.5
Other parts of uterus	16.2	42.0	23.7	11.4	—	—	—	—	16.2	42.0	23.7	11.4
Other female genital organs	19.3	42.6	24.9	11.7	—	—	—	—	19.3	42.6	24.9	11.7
Male genital organs	10.1	42.6	17.3	8.0	10.1	42.6	17.3	8.0	—	—	—	—
Urinary organs	13.3	43.3	20.1	9.3	12.4	38.7	18.5	8.7	15.3	50.0	24.0	10.6
Other and unspecified sites	17.8	47.4	21.5	10.1	16.6	44.5	19.1	9.1	18.9	50.9	24.4	11.1
Leukemia	21.2	52.9	21.3	9.4	19.6	49.7	19.0	8.5	23.2	57.0	24.7	10.5
Other lymphatic and hematopoietic tissues	17.7	44.7	21.2	10.2	17.0	42.7	19.0	9.0	18.4	48.2	24.2	11.3
Benign neoplasms and neoplasms of unspecified nature	23.2	49.5	30.5	10.0	22.6	47.8	29.1	8.8	23.8	51.4	32.0	11.0

Source: Number of deaths and current life tables for 1975 from the Division of Vital Statistics, National Center for Health Statistics.

TABLE 13 Present Discounted Value of Lost Earnings Due to Neoplasms at 6% Discount Rate, According to Sex, Age, and Site, Calendar Year 1975

	Both sexes				Male				Female			
	All ages	Under 45 years	45-64 years	65 years and over	All ages	Under 45 years	45-64 years	65 years and over	All ages	Under 45 years	45-64 years	65 years and over
	Lost earnings in millions											
All neoplasms	$15,868.7	$4,252.0	$9,914.5	$1,702.2	$9,406.8	$2,511.9	$6,035.7	$859.2	$6,461.9	$1,740.1	$3,878.8	$843.0
Malignant neoplasms	15,529.8	4,103.0	9,743.9	1,682.9	9,203.8	2,420.7	5,931.9	851.1	6,326.0	1,682.3	3,812.0	831.8
Buccal cavity and pharynx	408.4	63.0	311.0	34.4	312.9	47.2	242.7	22.9	95.5	15.8	68.3	11.5
Stomach	486.8	88.7	327.5	70.6	334.7	60.1	236.1	38.5	152.1	28.6	91.4	32.1
Intestine and rectum	1,510.3	269.4	990.1	250.8	868.1	170.2	590.8	107.1	642.2	99.2	399.3	143.7
Other organs	1,228.7	185.0	869.6	174.2	845.5	134.5	623.9	87.2	383.2	50.5	245.7	87.0
Trachea, lung, and bronchus	3,826.1	516.9	2,929.5	379.6	3,020.3	389.5	2,341.9	288.9	805.8	127.4	587.6	90.7
Other respiratory organs	226.3	43.9	162.9	19.5	135.9	36.1	134.7	15.1	40.4	7.8	28.2	4.4
Bone, connective, and other soft tissue	254.5	165.2	78.2	11.1	162.1	107.7	49.4	5.0	92.4	57.5	28.8	6.1
Skin	376.5	189.3	169.8	17.4	261.2	130.8	121.7	8.7	115.3	58.5	48.1	8.7
Breast	1,536.6	398.4	996.7	141.5	12.6	3.2	8.3	1.1	1,524.0	395.2	988.4	140.4
Cervix uteri	327.0	130.2	176.0	20.8	—	—	—	—	327.0	130.2	176.0	20.8
Other parts of uterus	163.0	24.4	105.0	33.6	—	—	—	—	163.0	24.4	105.0	33.6
Other female genital organs	488.9	101.2	331.0	56.6	—	—	—	—	488.9	101.2	331.0	56.6
Male genital organs	402.3	140.2	172.9	89.2	402.3	140.2	172.9	89.2	—	—	—	—
Urinary organs	521.9	91.9	351.5	78.5	380.5	62.9	269.4	48.2	141.4	29.0	82.1	30.3
Other and unspecified sites	1,807.2	657.4	989.8	160.0	1,118.7	424.2	623.4	71.1	688.5	233.2	366.4	88.9
Leukemia	897.6	565.6	277.6	54.6	583.4	373.1	182.7	27.7	314.2	192.5	94.9	26.9
Other lymphatic and hematopoietic tissues	1,067.6	472.3	504.8	90.5	715.5	341.0	334.0	40.5	352.1	131.3	170.8	50.0
Benign neoplasms and neoplasms of unspecified nature	338.9	148.9	170.6	19.3	203.0	91.1	103.8	8.1	135.9	57.8	66.8	11.2

Note: Numbers may not add to totals due to rounding.

Source: Number of deaths from the Division of Vital Statistics, National Center for Health Statistics and present values of lifetime earnings from the Public Services Laboratory, Georgetown University, Washington, D.C.

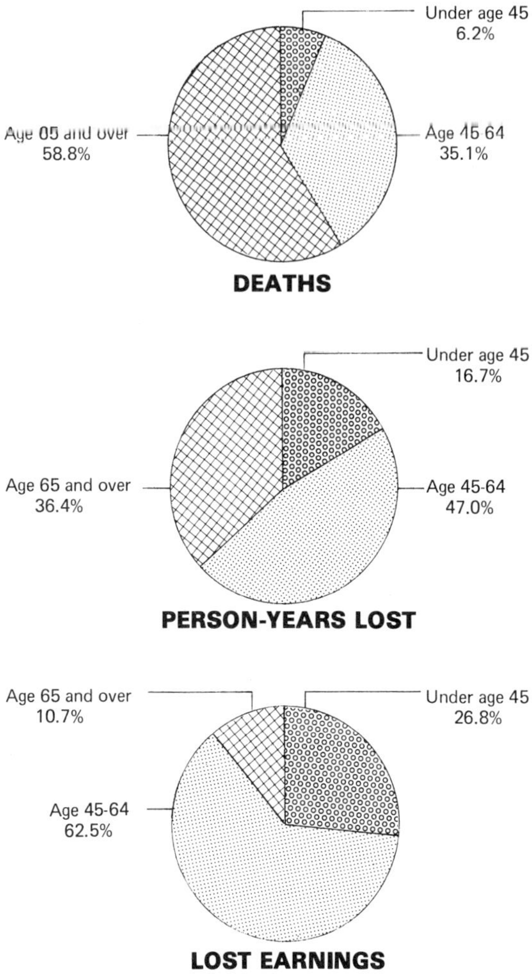

FIGURE 6 Mortality losses: distribution by age of number of deaths, person-years lost, and lost earnings at 6% for all neoplasms, 1975.

This is an age at which an individual who dies might otherwise have had a significant number of productive years remaining and earnings are relatively high, thus explaining the high proportions of lost years and earnings for this group. Persons under age 45 at time of death were responsible for 6% of deaths, 17% of years lost, and 27% of lost earnings. Individuals under age 45 have many productive years at high earnings remaining, so that years lost and the mortality costs are quite high relative to the number of deaths.

For all enoplasms, lost earnings are distributed approximately 60% among males and 40% among females. The male-female distribution of lost earnings varies according to site, but except for those sites specific to women, intestine and rectum, and benign neoplasms, over 60% of lost earnings result from deaths of males.

It must be remembered, however, that an inherent limitation of this approach to valuing life is the difference in economic reward accruing to groups distinguished by characteristics such as sex and race. The amount of earnings lost to women is less than that lost to men, even though women account for over half of all person-years lost. As seen in Fig. 7, 46% of deaths from neoplasms occurred among women, producing 52% of person-years lost but only 41% of lost earnings. This occurs because earnings of men exceed those of women at each age and also because of the longer life expectancy of women. The longer length of life for women serves to decrease, ceteris paribus, the value, in terms of earnings, of a year lost to women compared to men since those additional years of life experienced by the average woman produce only small amounts of earnings.

The distributions of deaths, person-years lost, and lost earnings among selected cancer sites are shown in Fig. 8. For the most part, the proportions attributed to a given cancer site are similar. Neoplasms of the respiratory organs and neoplasms of other and unspecified sites each accounted for approximately one-fourth of all deaths, person-years lost, and lost earnings. Cancers of the digestive organs were responsible for 26.8% of deaths, 23.2% of person-years lost, and 20.3% of lost earnings. For cancers of the breast and female genital organs, the respective percentages are 14.9, 18.7, and 15.9; and for lymphatic and hematopoietic tissues the figures are 9.4% of deaths, 11.2% of person-years lost, and 12.4% of lost earnings.

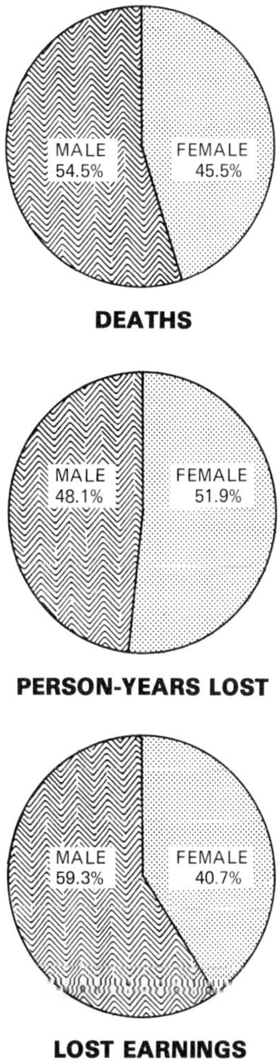

FIGURE 7 Mortality losses: distribution by sex of number of deaths, person-years lost, and lost earnings at 6% for all neoplasms, 1975.

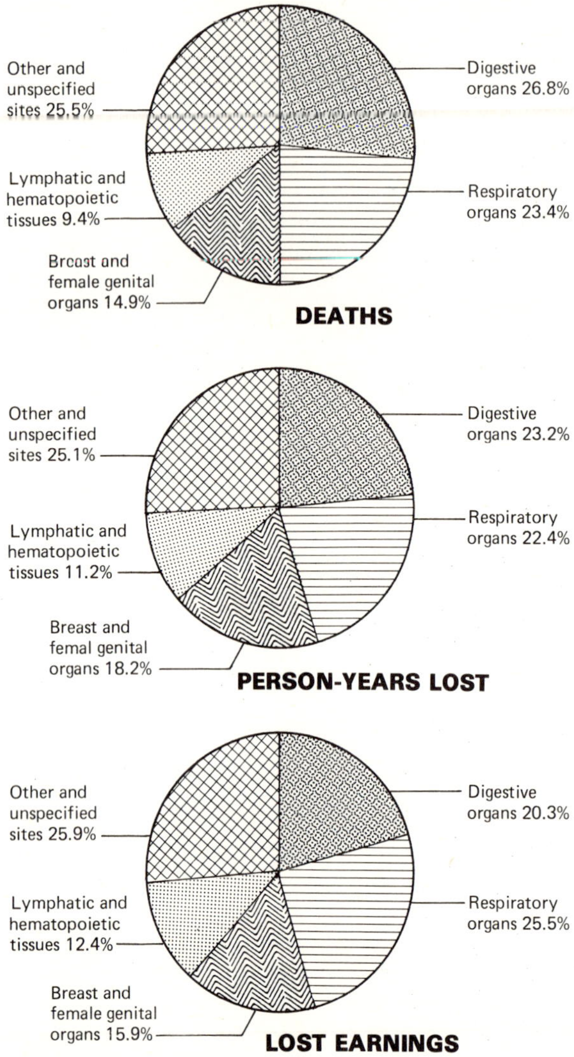

FIGURE 8 Mortality losses: distribution by cancer site of number of deaths, person-years lost, and lost earnings at 6% for all neoplasms, 1975.

D. Economic Costs

Table 14 summarizes estimated expenditures in 1975 for short-stay hospital care, expenditures for physicians' services, and indirect costs of mortality by cancer site. Expenditures for direct costs reflect the amount and cost per unit of medical care; indirect mortality costs reflect the number, age, and sex distribution of deaths, labor force participation, and earnings. It is estimated that in 1975 more than $4.1 billion was spent on hospital care for neoplasms and over $1.2 billion for physicians' services. Indirect costs of mortality were $12.4 billion at a 10% discount rate or $15.9 billion at 6%.

TABLE 14 Estimated Expenditures Due to Neoplasms and Percent Distributions for Short-Stay Hospital Care and Physicians' Services, and Indirect Costs of Mortality at 6 and 10% Discount Rates, According to Site, Calendar Year 1975

	Expenditures		Indirect costs of mortality	
	Short-stay hospital care	Physicians' services	6% discount	10% discount
	Amount in millions			
All neoplasms	$4,131.6	$1,245.6	$15,868.7	$12,448.0
Digestive organs	669.5	114.1	3,225.8	2,641.6
Respiratory organs	426.9	78.0	4,052.4	3,344.2
Skin	84.4	46.1	376.5	282.7
Breast	344.3	84.3	1,536.6	1,199.7
Female genital organs	297.9	73.9	978.9	763.2
Male genital organs	169.4	51.2	402.3	319.4
Leukemia	130.7	23.9	897.6	595.0
All other malignant neoplasms	1,092.7	259.1	4,059.6	3,089.0
Benign and unspecified neoplasms	915.8	514.9	338.9	213.2
	% distribution			
All neoplasms	100.0	100.0	100.0	100.0
Digestive organs	16.2	9.2	20.3	21.2
Respiratory organs	10.3	6.3	25.5	26.9
Skin	2.0	3.7	2.4	2.3
Breast	8.3	6.8	9.7	9.6
Female genital organs	7.2	5.9	6.2	6.1
Male genital organs	4.1	4.1	2.5	2.6
Leukemia	3.2	1.9	5.7	4.8
All other malignant neoplasms	26.4	20.8	25.6	24.8
Benign and unspecified neoplasms	22.2	41.3	2.1	1.7

Note: Numbers and percents may not add to totals due to rounding.

Source: Table 7 for expenditures for short-stay hospital care; Table 8 for expenditures for physicians' services; Table 13 for indirect costs of mortality at 6%; same sources as in Table 13 for indirect costs of mortality at 10%.

Aside from the residual category, cancers of the digestive and respiratory organs resulted in the highest economic costs. Cancers of the digestive system accounted for 16% of expenditures for hospital care, 9% of those for physicians' services, and 20% of mortality costs for neoplasms. Cancers of the respiratory system resulted in fewer expenditures for hospital care (10% of the total) and physicians' services (6%), but were responsible for one-fourth of mortality costs. These figures reflect the relatively high use of medical care and large number of deaths due to cancers of these sites. Although overall there were 15% more deaths from cancers of the digestive organs, deaths from cancers of the respiratory system occurred more frequently among men than women and at younger ages. Consequently, the average indirect cost per cancer death was higher for the respiratory system than for the digestive system, both because more productive years were lost and because earnings are higher for men than women. This is clearly shown in the detailed tables already discussed.

Cancers of the breast and female genital organs and benign neoplasms resulted in lower expenditures, but these amounted to about one-third to one-half the costs of cancers of digestive and respiratory organs. The remaining cancer sites, namely cancers of the skin, male genital organs, and leukemia, accounted for relatively small amounts of cost compared to other sites. Benign neoplasms are unique in that direct costs exceeded mortality costs because of the very low mortality for this site. Benign neoplasms accounted for 22% of all short-stay hospital costs and 41% of costs of physicians' care, but only 2% of mortality costs. Although indirect costs vary by considerable amounts for different discount rates, decreasing as the discount rate increases, the percentage distributions of mortality costs among sites are similar.

IV. SUMMARY AND CONCLUSION

We have discussed the direct and indirect economic costs resulting from the prevalence of neoplasms in 1975 in the United States. These costs include expenditures for hospital care, physicians' services, and other health care used in prevention, diagnosis, and treatment, and also include the value of output lost due to morbidity and premature mortality.

Neoplasms accounted for 9% of the total costs estimated for all illnesses. Over $4.1 billion was spent for an estimated 25.5 million days of nonfederal short-stay hospital care. In addition, care was received by cancer patients in other types of hospitals such as Veterans Administration hospitals. Expenditures in these hospitals amounted to almost 15% of the sum for nonfederal short-stay hospitals and bring the total cost of hospital care for neoplasms to about $4.7 billion. An additional $1.2 billion was spent for physicians' services, with $672 million or 54% of this total for surgery in the hospital and the remainder almost equally divided between medical care in the hospital ($274 million) and office and other visits ($299 million). Almost 371,000 persons died from neoplasms in 1975. This premature mortality resulted in an average of 16.1 person years and almost $43,000 lost per death. Total mortality costs amounted to $15.9 billion at a 6% discount rate based upon the human capital approach to valuing lives.

Over the years, the cost of neoplasms has increased relative to that of most other diseases. Neoplasms accounted for 1% of the total costs of all diseases in 1900 [42], 4% in 1930 [43], and 9% in 1975 [27]. Direct costs of neoplasms as a percent of all direct costs almost doubled between 1900 and 1975, increasing from 2.3 to 4.5%. More than three-fourths of the total cost of neoplasms are indirect costs, and these have increased by the largest amount, from 0.9% of all indirect costs in 1900 to 4.3% in 1930, and to 11.2% in 1975. This increase in the cost of neoplasms relative to all other diseases results from the increasing importance of neoplasms as a cause of death. In 1900 neoplasms were the tenth leading cause of death and accounted for less than 3% of all deaths [42]. In 1930, deaths from neoplasms were 9% of all deaths and the sixth leading cause of death [43]. By 1975, only the number of deaths from diseases of the circulatory system exceeded the number due to neoplasms, and neoplasms accounted for 19% of all deaths [27].

Future levels of the costs of neoplasms depend on a number of factors, including incidence, mortality, and survival rates; utilization and cost of medical care; economic variables such as employment and earnings; and the size and age distribution of the population. The net impact on the future level of costs is uncertain, since some factors are working to increase and others to decrease costs, and projection of trends in the future requires considerable conjecture.

Incidence, prevalence, and mortality are three common measures of disease. Although there is no nationwide reporting of cancer incidence in the United States, surveys conducted by the National Cancer Institute in 1937, 1947, and 1969 show a rising trend in age-adjusted rates for men and a falling trend for women [44]. The changes over time differ among sites, however. For some sites, such as the stomach and uterus, cancer has decreased significantly. Equally dramatic changes, but in the opposite direction, are observed for cancers of the lung. Time trends in mortality rates for the United States released by the National

Center for Health Statistics, although much lower, parallel the trends in incidence rates by cancer site [41].

Other things equal, the absolute level of direct and indirect economic costs will rise with increases in incidence and mortality as more medical care is used and output lost increases. Without any increase in incidence or mortality, the increasing size and aging of the population will tend to increase both the absolute cost of cancer, and the cost of cancer relative to the cost of diseases that occur mainly at younger ages, since cancer is mostly a disease of middle and old age. Under alternative assumptions about future fertility, mortality, and net immigration, the Bureau of the Census projects future population. Of three projections, the middle one estimates that the United States' population will increase from 217 million persons in 1977 to 260 million persons in the year 2000 [45]. While total population will increase by 20%, the population age 45 and over will increase by 35%, from 67.2 million to 91.0 million people. During this period, the population will grow older as median age rises from 29.4 to 35.5 years and the proportion age 45 and over increases from 31% in 1977 to 35% in 2000.

For all cancer patients combined, there has been a small improvement in relative survival rates in the past 20 years, with the increase in survival depending on cancer site [46]. Among the 10 leading cancer sites, the greatest improvements in 5-year relative survival rates were for cancers of the bladder and prostate. Cancers of the breast and rectum also show some improvement, especially among black patients. Improvements in survival rates may have a mixed effect upon costs. Indirect costs of mortality will decrease, but this may be offset to some extent if increases in use of medical care and indirect losses due to morbidity accompany increases in survival time.

Given the amount of illness that exists, the use and cost of medical care for prevention, diagnosis, and treatment will affect the magnitude of direct costs. Medical care prices have been rising rapidly in the United States since the Economic Stabilization Program ended in April 1974. During the period 1974-1976, physicians' fees rose 25% and hospital service charges for a semiprivate room increased 33%, as measured by annual averages of the Consumer Price Index [47]. There are many components to medical care utilization. Hospital care, for example, includes room and board, and miscellaneous services such as laboratory tests, medications, intensive care, and surgical facilities. Variation in use of these hospital services will be reflected in the cost of a hospital stay. For example, the average length of stay for malignant neoplasms in nonfederal short-stay hospitals has decreased slowly but steadily in recent years, declining 1.4 days from 14.1 days in 1971 to 12.7 days in 1976 [48].

Cancer therapy has changed significantly over the years, and it is likely that change will continue to take place. Studying a small number of selected illnesses during two time periods, Scitovsky and McCall found changes in treatment could be cost raising or cost saving [49].* In the years between 1951 and 1964, there was a consistent decrease in average length of hospital stay, and this was the main cost-saving change observed. Between 1951 and 1964, however, savings due to reduced length of hospital stay were outweighed by increases in costs due to increases in the number of diagnostic tests and therapeutic procedures per case, greater use of specialists, and substitution of inpatient for outpatient care. During the period 1964-1971, average length of stay continued to decline, while the average number of diagnostic tests increased. Whereas in the earlier period the net effect of changes in treatment was cost raising for the illnesses studied, in the latter period, the net effect was cost raising for some conditions and cost saving for others. The reasons for cost savings vary, although shorter lengths of stay occurred for all illnesses studied. In addition there was a shift to lower priced tests for cancer of the breast and a decline in the number of physician visits, X rays, and laboratory tests for treating a case of duodenal ulcer. This study shows the cost of treating an illness may increase or decrease as the method of treatment changes.

---

*"Changes in treatment" refers to all changes in inputs of medical services, including new techniques or drugs, increases or decreases in the use of specialists, laboratory tests, days of hospital stay, and substitution, for example, of outpatient for inpatient care.

Indirect economic costs are directly related to levels of employment and earnings. Since 1970 the proportion employed of the civilian population between ages 18 and 65 has consistently been near 70%, varying only from a low of 69.1% to a high of 71.2% [47]. Earnings of wage and salary workers, on the other hand, have been increasing steadily for at least a decade, paralleling the general inflation that has taken place in the United States economy. Between 1967 and 1976, median weekly earnings of wage and salary workers increased at an average annual rate of 6.8% [50].

Future economic costs depend on the extent of cancer illness, cancer therapies and the attendant use of medical care, medical care prices, and economic variables such as employment and earnings. Our brief description of recent trends indicates the changes that can occur, often quite rapidly. Measures that increase (greater exposure to environmental carcinogens, for example) or decrease (reduced smoking) the incidence of cancer will have a like effect on the direct and indirect costs that accompany morbidity and mortality, whereas new forms of therapy may be cost raising or cost saving. It is likely that at some point in time scientific breakthroughs in prevention and treatment will reduce the threat of cancer. In some cases already existing knowledge, if implemented, would result in significant reductions in mortality. For example, mortality from lung cancer is many times higher in cigarette smokers than lifelong nonsmokers. Ex-smokers also benefit, as mortality from lung cancer in this group decreases steadily with length of time since having stopped smoking [51].

It would be speculative, however, to anticipate future trends and the net effect of changes in several factors. A recent effort to project cancer mortality in year 2000 by a Delphi technic [52] illustrates the uncertainty involved in projecting future trends. A panel of experts was asked to predict death rates from cancer by the year 2000. The seven responses ranged from a 20% increase in current death rates to a 90% reduction in cancer mortality. The expert predicting a 90% reduction expected new developments in detection and therapy, a decrease in the proportion of the population that smokes, and an increase in the use of low-tar cigarettes. The expert predicting an increase in mortality believed increases in occupational exposure to chemicals, air and water pollution, food additives, and nuclear radiation, will result in higher mortality rates. The median response predicts a 6.5% decrease in total cancer deaths from the number that will occur if 1974 death rates apply in the year 2000, and the average of the middle five responses predicts a 16% decrease in cancer deaths. These projections of future cancer mortality from a panel including clinicians, administrators of cancer clinics, researchers, and epidemiologist-biostatisticans are quite varied.

Economic costs are potential benefits of reduced cancer morbidity and mortality. Direct costs represent resources that could be allocated to other uses, and indirect costs are the value of idle resources and lost output. Knowledge of the costs of specific diseases is an aid to more rational decision-making with respect to allocating scarce resources among competing ends.

Economic costs are, however, an incomplete measure of the burden of disease. The quality of life is very important, and it is hoped that rapid progress can be made in measuring social costs of illness and disease. Further work is also needed on economic costs. We have no knowledge of the future costs of morbidity; estimates are lacking for the costs associated with incidence of disease; and alternative approaches to valuing life, such as willingness to pay, need refinement. Nevertheless, the methodology employed, pending improvements and refinements, is a means for estimating a large part of the burden of disease and provides consistent estimates across the spectrum of disease categories.

APPENDIX: METHODOLOGY

A. Direct Costs

The methodology and data employed in estimating economic costs of disease have been explained in detail by Rice [28], Cooper and Rice [29], and Paringer and Berk [27]. National health expenditures, by type of expenditure, have been published annually by the Social Security

Administration and will be released by the Health Care Financing Administration in the future. Total expenditures for hospital care, physicians' services, and the other direct costs of illness are distributed by diagnosis according to utilization and costs, using consistent data sources for each diagnosis. Expenditures in community hospitals, for example, are allocated to a diagnosis in proportion to the number of days of care attributable to the diagnosis weighted by the expense per patient day. Similar procedures are applied to the other categories of direct costs to distribute the total among diagnoses. In each case, utilization, weighted by unit cost when possible, determines the share of total expenses assigned to each diagnosis.

The cancer sites discussed in this report and their ICDA-8 codes (Eighth Revision International Classification of Diseases, Adapted for Use in the United States) are:

Site	ICDA Code
Buccal cavity and pharynx	140-149
Digestive organs and peritoneum:	
Stomach	151
Intestine and rectum	152-154
Other	150, 155-159
Respiratory system	
Trachea, lung, and bronchus	162
Other	160-161, 163
Bone, connective, and other soft tissue	170-171
Breast	174
Genital organs, female:	
Cervix uteri	180
Other parts of uterus	181-182
Other	183-184
Genital organs, male	185-187
Urinary organs	188-189
Skin	172-173
Other and unspecified sites	190-199
Lymphatic and hematopoietic tissues:	
Leukemia	204-207
Other	200-203, 208-209
Benign neoplasms and neoplasms of unspecified nature	210-228, 230-239

1. Hospital Care by Cancer Site

Expenditures in short-stay hospitals are estimated by multiplying the number of days of care, as estimated by the Hospital Discharge Survey of the National Center for Health Statistics, by the average cost per day. For the population age 65 and over, average per diem charges to a large sample of Medicare patients are used as the average cost per day.* For those under age 65, an estimate of average costs is obtained by adjusting average Medicare charges by the ratio of average daily payment for patients under age 65 at time of diagnosis to average daily payment for patients age 65 and over observed in the Third National Cancer Survey of the National Cancer Institute [53]. This procedure is repeated for each cancer site.

Expenditures in nonfederal short-stay hospitals for all neoplasms obtained by this method are about 13% higher than the share of hospital expenditures in Table 1 attributed to short-stay hospitals. Of the $4.1 billion for hospital care in Table 1, only $3.6 billion was spent in short-stay hospitals; the remainder being the cost of care in other types of hospitals such as those of the Veterans Administration. Most of this difference between expenditures in short-stay hospitals in Tables 1 and 7 can be explained, however. Since the computation of the estimates in Table 1, the Health Care Financing Administration has revised upward by

*Unpublished data are provided by the Health Care Financing Administration.

4% its estimate of national health expenditures for hospital care in fiscal year 1975, the figure used to obtain expenditures in Table 1. Furthermore, estimates in this section are for calendar year 1975 rather than fiscal 1975. Hospital care expenditures increased 15% between fiscal 1975 and fiscal 1976[54]. If this increase were uniform over time, expenditures in calendar 1975 would be 7-8% greater than in fiscal 1975. Thus, all but 1-2% of the difference in the two estimates can be explained. The two estimating procedures yield quite consistent results.

2. Physicians' Services by Cancer Site

In previous studies the magnitude of expenditures for physicians' services by diagnosis were determined by distributing the Social Security Administration's estimate of national expenditures [54] according to the proportion of physician visits reported for each diagnosis by the National Disease and Therapeutic Index.* This report assumes that every visit has the same cost; office and hospital visits are given equal weight, for example. Furthermore, national expenditures for physicians' services include payments for surgery, which are also allocated to diagnoses according to the relative number of physicians' visits. This method understates expenditures on physicians' services related to neoplasms because the estimate does not reflect that neoplasms account for a higher proportion of all hospital visits than of total visits, and hospital visits are somewhat more expensive than office visits. Also, the proportion of short-term hospital discharges with surgery having a diagnosis classified under neoplasms is significantly higher than the proportion of physician visits reported for neoplasms. Equal weighting of the cost of hospital versus office visits and of the relative shares among diagnoses of surgical and nonsurgical expenditures results in an underestimate of expenditures for physicians' services related to neoplasms.

For this paper, we have estimated expenditures for physicians' services by the following method. Total expenditures for physicians' services in calendar year 1975 (obtained by personal communication with Robert H. Gibson) were separated into those resulting from surgery in the hospital and other expenditures. The proportions used were those observed for the year 1970 in a survey of utilization and expenditures conducted by the Center for Health Administration Studies at the University of Chicago and the National Opinion Research Center [55]. This survey found that 24% of expenditures were for surgery in the hospital.

Next, nonsurgery expenditures for all diseases were split into those for inpatient medical care and those for office and other types of visits, taking into account both the number of visits and differences in average fees for each type.† Total expenditures for each place of visit were then distributed among sites according to the proportion of visits reported for each site. Finally, expenditures for in-hospital surgery were allocated by site according to the proportion of all short-stay hospital discharges with surgery reported for each site by the Hospital Discharge Survey of the National Center for Health Statistics. This assumes equal charges for in-hospital surgery for every site and probably introduces some bias into the allocation of expenditures for surgery among sites.

By this method, the cost of physicians' services for neoplasms was estimated at $1.25 billion (Table 14), a cost 85% and $574 million higher than the figure in Table 1. Ten percent of the increase ($60 million) is due to using calendar 1975 rather than fiscal 1975 expenditures, 3% ($18 million) results from introducing the place and relative cost of visits, and 87% ($497 million) occurs because expenditures for surgery were distributed according to the number of hospital discharges with surgery as opposed to the number of physicians' visits.

It is likely that even this revised estimate understates expenditures on physician's services for neoplasms because the amount of surgery performed has increased since 1970

*The National Disease and Therapeutic Index is a product of Medical Business Services, a division of IMS America, Ltd., Ambler, Pennsylvania.

†Average fees used are those found in J. R. Cantwell (Ed.), Profile of Medical Practice, 1975-1976 edition, American Medical Association, Chicago, 1976.

more than the number of physician visits. Between 1971 and 1975, there was a 5.7% increase in physician visits and a 22% increase in the number of short-stay hospital discharges with surgery.* Consequently, expenditures for surgery probably account for more than one-quarter of all expenditures on physicians' services in 1975, so the share of expenditures allocated to neoplasms, which is surgery intensive compared to all other diseases, is underestimated. Neoplasms lose 8 cents for every dollar of expenditures in 1975 that has incorrectly been attributed to nonsurgical visits, because the revised estimating procedure awards 11% of surgical and 3% of nonsurgical expenditures to neoplasms. It is unfortunate that an up-to-date figure for the distribution of physicians' expenditures between surgery and nonsurgery visits is not available.

3. Further Considerations

Another aspect of the methodology for estimating direct costs should be pointed out. The existence of multiple diseases causes some difficulty in distributing expenditures by diagnosis. Hospital days, for example, are allocated according to the primary diagnosis, but other accompanying conditions influence the length of stay in the hospital and the cost. The bias introduced by assigning the total cost of a hospital episode to the illness indicated by the first-listed diagnosis when a portion of the cost is due to the presence of other conditions has not yet been investigated.

The aforementioned methodology does not account for all economic costs incurred because of cancer. Excluded are transportation costs of persons receiving care and visiting patients; costs of extra household help for the patient and family; expenditures for retraining or reeducation, special diets, and special housing facilities; free or reduced fee care provided as charity by hospitals and other institutions, physicians, family, and friends; subsudies provided to cancer patients in the form of fixed hospital rates, with less ill patients sharing costs of those more ill who use more nursing time and ancillary services; free care provided by institutions and medical personnel as part of their teaching or research function; and losses in the form of reduced capital gains due to forced sale of assets. Inclusion of these costs would provide more complete estimates of cancer costs, but at the present time we do not know their magnitude. A recent study estimated some of the nonhealth sector costs that can be identified. Although not a complete evaluation, it was found that nonhealth sector costs add at least 12% to the total cost of all illnesses [56]. Unfortunately, costs were not estimated by disease category and it is not known what proportion of nonhealth sector costs are due to neoplasms.

Finally, we point out here some extensions of the usual treatment of direct economic costs which could provide additional insight into disease costs. These are: (1) costs distributed by stage or extent of disease at initial diagnosis (e.g., localized or not), by method of treatment (surgery, radiotherapy, chemotherapy, etc.), or by provider characteristics such as physician's experience treating cancer, hospital services available, and whether the institution specializes in cancer care; (2) costs distributed over diagnosis, treatment, and rehabilitation; (3) costs arising from complications of the disease and side effects of treatment; (4) costs per person with cancer, including lifetime costs of the disease. Estimates of the omissions and extensions cited here have not yet appeared in the literature, and at least some of the required data have not been readily available. However, a study investigating some of these aspects of direct costs is now underway in the United States [57].

B. Indirect Costs

Indirect economic costs result from morbidity and mortality. Estimates of morbidity losses are made separately for those currently employed, housekeepers, persons unable to work

---

*Data are from the Health Interview Survey and Hospital Discharge Survey of the National Center for Health Statistics.

because of ill health, and the institutionalized population. Days lost from work among the currently employed are converted to years lost by age and sex and multiplied by age- and sex-specific estimates of average annual earnings to obtain lost earnings for this group. Days of bed-disability suffered by women usually keeping house are also converted to years and multiplied by age-specific values of housewives' services to obtain morbidity costs for this group. The number of persons unable to work by age and sex is multiplied by employment rates and average annual earnings and by housekeeping rates and housekeeping values to determine indirect morbidity costs among members of this group. A similar procedure is applied to the institutionalized population to estimate morbidity costs by institution. These separate components of morbidity costs are aggregated to obtain a total cost figure.

1. Mortality Costs by Cancer Site

To obtain indirect costs of mortality by cancer site, the numbers of deaths for each site in 1975 by age and sex are multiplied by the present value of lifetime earnings, also by age and sex. Person-years lost due to premature mortality are the product of number of deaths and life expectancy at the midyear of the age group. This method takes into account the life expectancy, labor force participation and housekeeping rates, earnings and imputed values of housekeeping services, and discount rate for each age and sex group. Estimates for 1975 in this paper include in the present value of future earnings imputed housekeeping values for women and men in the labor force who have household responsibilities.

For these calculations, present values of lifetime earnings were those developed by Selma Mushkin at the Public Services Laboratory, Georgetown University, and mortality data were provided by the Division of Vital Statistics, National Center for Health Statistics. Two different life tables are employed in this report. All lifetime earnings data and estimated person-years lost in Table 3 are based upon modified generation life tables developed at the Public Services Laboratory at Georgetown University. Person-years lost by cancer site in Table 11 are based upon a current life table for 1975 provided by the Division of Vital Statistics, NCHS. A full explanation of the methodology and data used to compute indirect cost can be found in Cooper and Rice [29] and Paringer and Berk [27].

2. Measures of Indirect Costs

This methodology provides an estimate of the economic burden, discounted to 1975, resulting from the prevalence of disease in 1975. Included are costs of resources used during the year for prevention, diagnosis, and treatment; output lost during the year because of morbidity; and output lost due to deaths in 1975. Because a death in 1975 means lost output in future years, the present discounted value of the future losses is also counted.

It is important to note that, unlike the estimates for mortality, those for morbidity do not include the present discounted value of future losses resulting from disease in 1975 that may cause decreased productivity and lost earnings in future years. Other effects of disease besides death may decrease future output—for example, the lost output of a professional singer after a laryngectomy. This decreased output should be included in our cost estimates. Unfortunately, we do not have the data for this component, and the extent of the underestimate because of its omission is not known. It must be emphasized that the omission is the present cost of future losses resulting from morbidity in 1975, and not the present cost of future morbidity that may arise from disease that has its onset in 1975. The latter is not relevant to the cost measures in this report, but is important in another context discussed later.

In addition to the costs associated with the prevalence of disease in 1975, we might be interested in the cost of disease from onset until cure or death. This requires knowing the incidence of disease in 1975 and the likely course of the disease, including treatments required, morbidity, and mortality. For any new case in 1975, both direct and indirect costs may occur in 1975 and subsequent years. Because of illness beginning in 1975, a person may require treatment for a number of years, lose time from work during this period, and eventually die of the disease. The total cost is the sum of the present discounted values of all direct costs and earnings lost because of morbidity and death. This value is the best measure of the savings, or benefits, of preventing a new case of the disease.

A third cost that may be of interest is the economic burden of disease that is actually born in 1975. This consists of direct costs in 1975, indirect costs of morbidity and mortality incurred in 1975, and the value of output lost in 1975 because of morbidity and mortality in previous years, but excludes present discounted values of future losses of earnings due to morbidity and mortality in 1975.

Each of these three measures of costs of disease provides different information, and which one is most appropriate depends on the question being asked. Usually, the cost of disease prevalence is estimated. The cost of disease incidence is more difficult to estimate, requiring projections of treatment and disability over the course of the disease, time between onset and death, whether death is related to the disease being studied, and the impact of disability and death on earnings. The third cost measure is rarely estimated, but was calculated for cardiovascular diseases and cancer in 1962 [58].

REFERENCES

1. Bernard Benjamin. Trends and differentials in lung cancer mortality. World Health Stat. Rep. 30 (2): 1977.
2. The ten leading causes of death for selected countries in North America, Europe, and Oceania, 1969, 1970, and 1971. World Health Stat. Rep. 27 (9): 1974.
3. The ten leading causes of death for selected countries in Africa, South and Central America and Asia, 1969-1971. World Health Stat. Rep. (3-4): 1974.
4. 1979 cancer facts and figures. American Cancer Society, New York, 1978.
5. C. C. Abt. The social costs of cancer. Soc. Indic. Res. 2: 175-190 (1975).
6. Mortality and the life cycle of the family. Some implications of recent research. World Health Stat. Rep. 29 (4): 220-234 (1976)
7. G. Feichtinger and H. Hansluwka. The Impact of Mortality on the Life Cycle of the Family. IUSSP Conference, Mexico City, 1977.
8. <u>The Impact, Costs and Consequences of Catastrophic Illness on Patients and Families</u>. Cancer Care and The National Cancer Foundation, New York, March 1973.
9. B. McPeek, J. P. Gilbert, and F. Mosteller. The end result: quality of life. In <u>Costs, Risks, and Benefits of Surgery</u>, J. P. Bunker, B. A. Barnes, F. Mosteller (Eds.), University Press, New York, 1977.
10. E. F. Cooper. Community services in support of the cancer patient. In <u>Cancer Epidemiology and Prevention</u>, D. Schottenfeld (Ed.). Thomas, Springfield, Ill., 1975.
11. D. Schottenfeld and G. F. Robbins. Quality of survival among patients who have had radical mastectomy. Cancer 26 (3): 650-655 (September 1970).
12. J. E. Healey, Jr. <u>Ecology of the Cancer Patient</u>, Interdisciplinary Communication Associates, Washington, D.C., 1970.
13. C. C. Abt. The issue of social costs in cost-benefit analysis of surgery. In <u>Costs, Risks, and Benefits of Surgery</u>, J. P. Bunker, G. A. Barnes, and F. Mosteller (Eds.). Oxford University Press, New York, 1977.
14. F. M. Andrews and S. B. Withey. Developing measures of perceived life quality: results from several national surveys. Soc. Indic. Res. 1: 1-26 (1974).
15. F. M. Andrews. Social indicators of perceived life quality. Soc. Indic. Res. 1: 279-299 (1974).
16. M. Bunge. What is a quality of life indicator. Soc. Indic. Res. 2: 65-79 (1975).
17. R. B. D'Agostino. Social indicators: a statistician's view. Soc. Indic. Res. 1: 459-484 (1975).
18. H. S. Eisenberg and I. S. Goldenberg. Measurement of quality of survival of breast cancer patients. <u>Clinical Evaluation in Breast Cancer</u>, Academic Press, New York, 1966, 93-100.
19. J. Elinson. Toward sociomedical health indicators. Soc. Indic. Res. 1: 59-71 (1974).

20. C. V. Granger and D. S. Greer. Functional status measurement and medical rehabilitation outcomes. Arch. Phys. Med. Rehabil. 57:103-109 (March 1976).
21. C. Liu. Quality of life indicators: a preliminary investigation. Soc. Indic. Res. 1: 187-208 (1974).
22. S. McCall. Quality of life. Soc. Indic. Res. 2:229-248 (1975).
23. W. L. Rodgers and P. E. Converse. Measures of the perceived overall quality of life. Soc. Indic. Res. 2:127-152 (1975).
24. M. E. Switzer. After cancer—the quality of survival. Reprinted by DHEW Vocational Rehabilitation Administration from Rehabil. Rec. 7 (1): January-February 1966.
25. R. E. Ziller. Self-other orientations and quality of life. Soc. Indic. Res. 1:301-327 (1974).
26. T. A. Hodgson, Jr. The economic costs of cancer. Chapter 1 in Cancer Epidemiology and Prevention, D. Schottenfeld (Ed.). Charles C. Thomas, Springfield, Ill., 1975.
27. L. Paringer and A. Berk. Costs of illness and disease fiscal year 1975. Report Number Two, Public Services Laboratory, Georgetown University, Washington, D.C., January 4, 1977.
28. D. P. Rice. Estimating the cost of illness. Public Health Service Publication No. 947-6, Washington, D.C., May 1966.
29. B. S. Cooper and D. P. Rice. The economic cost of illness revisited. Soc. Secur. Bull. 39(2):21-36 (February 1976).
30. H. E. Klarman. The Economics of Health, Columbia University Press, New York, 1975.
31. P. D. Henderson. Investment criteria for public enterprises. In Public Enterprise, R. Turvey (Ed.). Penguin, New York, 1968.
32. H. Gilman. Determinants of personal discount rates and their implications for social and economic policies. Presented before the National Economists Club, Washington, D.C., 1977.
33. K. E. Walker and W. H. Gauger. The dollar value of household work. Information Bulletin No. 60, New York College of Human Ecology, Ithaca, N.Y., 1973.
34. B. A. Weisbrod. Economics of Public Health, University of Pennsylvania Press, Philadelphia, 1961.
35. L. I. Dublin and A. J. Lotka. The Money Value of Man, Ronald Press, Philadelphia, 1946.
36. R. Fein. Economics of Mental Illness, Basic Books, New York, 1958.
37. E. J. Mishan. Evaluation of life and limb. J. Pol. Econ. 79 (4):1971.
38. J. P. Acton. Measuring the social impact of heart and circulatory disease programs: preliminary framework and estimates. Rand Corporation, Santa Monica, April 1975.
39. M. B. Shimkin. Science and cancer. DHEW Publication No. (NIH)75-568, 2nd Revision, Washington, D.C., 1973, p. 4.
40. 1977 cancer facts and figures. American Cancer Society, New York, 1976.
41. D. P. Rice. Statement Before the Intergovernmental Relations and Human Resources Subcommittee Committee on Government Operations, United States House of Representatives, June 14, 1977.
42. A. Berk and L. Paringer. Costs of illness and disease, 1900. Report Number B5, Public Services Laboratory, Georgetown University, Washington, D.C., August 1977.
43. A. Berk and L. Paringer. Costs of illness and disease fiscal year 1930. Report Number Four, Public Services Laboratory, Georgetown University, Washington, D.C., January 24, 1977.
44. D. L. Levin, S. S. Devesa, J. D. Godwin, D. T. Silverman, Cancer Rates and Risks, 2nd edition, DHEW Publication No. (NIH)76-691, U.S. Government Printing Office, Washington, D.C., 1974.
45. Projections of the population of the United States: 1977 to 2050. Current Population Reports, Series P-25, No. 704, U.S. Bureau of the Census, U.S. Government Printing Office, Washington, D.C., 1977.

46. Cancer patient survival report number 5. DHEW Publication No. (NIH)77-992, U.S. Department of Health, Education, and Welfare, Washington, D.C., 1976.
47. Soc. Secur. Bull. 40 (12): December 1977.
48. Vital and health statistics, Series 13. U.S. Department of Health, Education and Welfare, Washington, D.C., June 1978.
49. A. A. Scitovsky and N. McCall. Changes in the costs of treatment of selected illnesses 1951-1964-1971. DHEW Publication NO+ (HRA)77-3161, U.S. Government Printing Office, Washington, D.C., 1977.
50. Weekly and hourly earnings data from the current population survey. Special Labor Force Report 195, Bureau of Labor Statistics, U.S. Department of Labor, Washington, D.C., 1977.
51. R. Doll and R. Peto. Mortality in relation to smoking: 20 years' observations on male British doctors. Br. Med. J. 2(6051):1525-1536 (December 1976).
52. D. P. Wagner. Projected mortality in the year 2000 due to cancer. Report Number B6, Public Services Laboratory, Georgetown University, Washington, D.C., 1977.
53. J. Scotto and L. Chiazze. Third national cancer survey: hospitalizations and payments to hospitals, part A: summary. DHEW Publication No. (NIH)76-1094, U.S. Government Printing Office, Washington, D.C., March 1976.
54. R. M. Gibson and M. S. Mueller. National health expenditures, fiscal year 1976. Soc. Secur. Bull. 40(4): April 1977.
55. R. Andersen, J. Lion, O. W. Anderson. Two Decades of Health Services: Social Survey Trends in Use and Expenditure. Ballinger, Cambridge, Mass., 1976.
56. S. J. Mushkin and J. S. Landefeld. Non-health sector costs of illness. Report Number A7, Public Services Laboratory, Georgetown University, Washington, D.C., January 25, 1978.
57. J. Cromwell, R. Friedman, P. Gertman, I. B. Mitchell, R. Taber, G. F. Vanderschmidt. The Measurement of the Cost of Cancer Care. Abt Associates and Boston University Cancer Research Center, Cambridge and Boston, Mass., 1976.
58. D. P. Rice. Economic costs of cardiovascular diseases and cancer, 1962. Public Health Service Publication No. 947-5, Washington, D.C., May 1965.

3

Legal Implications of Working with Carcinogens

NICHOLAS A. ASHFORD / Massachusetts Institute of Technology, Cambridge, Massachusetts

I. INTRODUCTION

Health, safety, and environmental legislation of the 1970s has focused increasing attention on chemical carcinogens. Carcinogens in general use are regulated under a variety of acts, including the Occupational Safety and Health Act (OSHAct, 1972), the Consumer Product Safety Act (CPSAct, 1972), and the Toxic Substances Control Act (TSCAct, 1976). In addition, special-use products such as pesticides, pharmaceuticals, and food additives are regulated under legislation especially enacted to deal with those substances. Each of these acts is administered by regulatory agencies which establish the legal norm for qualification of human carcinogens and evaluate evidence to define a human carcinogenic risk requiring regulation. Different legislation sometimes contains different norms or bestows a differing degree of discretion to the relevant regulatory agency to establish the norm. Thus, what constitutes a carcinogen for food additives under the Delaney Amendment to the Food, Drug, and Cosmetic Act may not be regulated as a carcinogen under the Consumer Product Safety Act. While there is an organizational unification of the animal-testing activities in the government under the recently formed National Toxicology Program, there is no uniform policy for defining what constitutes a carcinogen for legal or regulatory purposes (Science, 1979). Through the Interagency Regulatory Liaison Group (IRLG), consisting of the Occupational Safety and Health Administration (OSHA), the Environmental Protection Agency (EPA), the Consumer Product Safety Commission (CPSC), the Food and Drug Administration (FDA), and the Food Safety and Quality Services of the Department of Agriculture (FSQS), a more uniform carcinogen policy is being attempted. However, the differences among the legislative mandates embodied in the various acts will require important distinctions to remain. Whatever legal norm is developed, the legal standard of proof to determine human carcinogenicity is likely to differ from scientific standards of proof of causality. The legal determination of human carcinogenicity often depends on information that is "on the frontiers of scientific knowledge" (Society of the Plastics Industry v. OSHA, 1975) and is a legislative policy decision.

This chapter focuses on the responsibilities placed upon government, employers, and employees by existing common law, recent legislation, and resulting regulations of occupational and environmental carcinogens. The chapter also addresses important rights of scientists, employees, consumers, and the general public, which can be individually or collectively exercised to ensure adequate protection from exposure to carcinogenic substances. The discussion of rights is important not only for the protection of those who are or may be exposed to carcinogens, but also because the issue of rights is necessary for an undertaking of the dimensions of legal liability.

II. ACTIVITIES AND RESPONSIBILITIES OF THE FEDERAL GOVERNMENT

In this section we emphasize the activities and responsibilities of the federal government under the OSHAct, the TSCAct, and the CPSAct. The interested reader is referred elsewhere for discussion of the important regulatory systems controlling carcinogens, such as food additives, pesticides, and pharmaceuticals (Ashford et al., 1979). The disposal of hazardous wastes, including carcinogens, is regulated under the Resource Conservation and Recovery Act (RCRAct, 1976). Regulations defining what is meant by carcinogenic substances have not yet been promulgated under this act, although they are long overdue.

The governmental activities discussed in this section include (1) the recognition of carcinogenic risks for workers, consumers, and society, and (2) the setting of standards for reducing exposure to suspect carcinogens. Legislation imposes requirements on manufacturers and employers to provide information concerning carcinogenic risks to government. The obligations of the various federal agencies to disclose this information and information from nonindustry sources are more fully discussed in Sec. III.

A. Recognizing Carcinogenic Risks

1. Research

A number of government agencies have recently conducted or supported research relevant to the epidemiology of occupational and environmental cancer including the National Institute for Occupational Safety and Health (NIOSH), the National Cancer Institute (NCI), and the National Institute for Environmental Health Science (NIEHS). The major responsibility in the occupational cancer area lies with NIOSH, which has conducted a number of epidemiological studies on industrial populations exposed to known carcinogens (National Cancer Institute, 1978). In 1978 NIOSH and the Cancer Control and Prevention Program of NCI administered a $3 million budget for joint research in occupational cancer epidemiology (Testimony and Budget Justification, 1977). NIOSH is currently conducting epidemiological studies on a number of industrial populations thought to be exposed to occupational carcinogens, including workers in the organic dye, leather products, rock wool, and oil shale industries (National Institute for Occupational Safety and Health, 1978). In addition, NIOSH also has authority to conduct hazard investigations of individual firms at the request of employees, unions, or employers. The Environmental Protection Agency (EPA) is also conducting some epidemiological investigations of industrial populations exposed to carcinogens (U.S. Department of Housing and Urban Development, 1979). In the environmental cancer area, both NIEHS and NCI undertake epidemiological investigation of the general population (Mason et al., 1975).

Until recently essentially all of the federally conducted animal carcinogenicity bioassays were conducted as part of the National Cancer Institute's bioassay program. Problems that arose relating to coordination of the bioassay program with the needs of various federal regulatory agencies, and with the management of the program itself, led to the formation last year of the National Toxicology Program (NTP). The NTP will take over all responsibility for conducting animal bioassays, and will coordinate research efforts in the area of animal bioassays performed in NCI, NIEHS, FDA, and NIOSH (Rall, 1979, private communication). It will be headed by the director of NIEHS. The $40 million allocated for the program this year will come from the budgets of the four agencies involved. The executive committee of the NTP will include members from all of the federal regulatory agencies to ensure that bioassay priorities can be set in response to regulatory needs.

Much research is now being conducted by federal regulatory agencies making use of in vitro mutagenesis assays as an indication of carcinogenic activity. Among the government agencies supporting research about in vitro tests or their application are NCI, in the Cancer Cause and Prevention Program; EPA, in the Toxic Substances Program; NIEHS; and the National Science Foundation, in the Applied Science and Research Applications Program. The Division of Biomedical and Behavioral Sciences in NIOSH has recently awarded a number of contracts which will involve the use of in vitro tests as part of studies assessing carcinogenicity of a number of different families or compounds.

A number of efforts are now under way to develop methods by which the carcinogenic activity of a given chemical compound can be predicted from its chemical structure, either because of its relationship to other compounds of known activity, or in light of chemical theories of carcinogenicity. However, no regulatory agency is yet ready to base any regulatory action solely on considerations of chemical structure. The FDA did, however, recently sponsor a symposium dealing with the question of structure-activity relationships among carcinogens and mutagens (Food and Drug Administration, 1977).

2. Identifying Carcinogenic Risks in the Field

The identification of carcinogenic hazards in the workplace, consumer products, or the general environment may be initiated by findings in animal or in vitro tests, or may occur independently, as the result of a chance observation of a suggestive pattern of excess cancer incidence among workers, consumers, or in a geographically defined population. However, governmental programs do exist which aggressively seek to identify both the extent of chemical exposure to workers, consumers, and the society and populations at risk.

The federal government is currently engaged in a broad spectrum of activities aimed at improving the ability of employers, employees, and consumers to determine the nature of the chemical products they sell, work with, or buy. A number of legal authorities exist, or are being developed, to deal with the problem of chemical exposure produced by products designated as trade secrets; these include labeling standards and disclosure requirements. They are discussed in Sec. III.

To aid in the better characterization of workplace chemical exposures, NIOSH has conducted the National Occupational Hazard Survey, during which lists of commonly occurring chemical exposures associated with a very wide range of commercial processes and activities were compiled (National Institute for Occupational Safety and Health, 1974). NIOSH is planning a second survey in the near future. NIOSH is also now completing a trade name product data base which would make available to employers, workers, and consumers the ingredients of various trade name products encountered during the survey that were not considered proprietary data (National Institute for Occupational Safety and Health, 1978). NIOSH criteria documents, recommending standards for OSHA to adopt related to specific processes or industries, can also provide useful information resources relating to chemical exposures.

OSHA is also involved in activities to identify chemicals in the workplace through its New Directions Program (Occupational Safety and Health Reporter, 1978). This is a program of grants to unions, trade associations, and research and educational institutions for the purpose of improving institutional capability in occupational safety and health, so that workers and employers can be better informed about occupational health issues, including the nature of chemical exposures in the workplace. Grants totaling \$3.4 million were disbursed in 1978. The program funding was to have been expanded to \$6.4 million in 1979, including \$700,000 contributed by NCI specifically for the development of programs dealing with occupational cancer (Harris, 1979, private communication), but the Office of Management and Budget did not allocate any program funds for that year. NIOSH also provides training to workers responsible for occupational safety and health.

In the field of analytical methods development, NIOSH is conducting ongoing research programs related to occupational chemical exposures. Presently research related to personal gas and aerosol dosimeters is being performed. Also being investigated is the development of analytical methods applicable to the detection and quantification of a number of organic and inorganic carcinogens (National Institute for Occupational Safety and Health, 1978). In addition, the EPA is conducting research relating to the development of analytical techniques applicable to carcinogens present in the general environment.

Presently there does not seem to be a lack of published information relating to the known carcinogenic properties of chemical compounds. There are numerous reviews and compilations of data available in the open literature, for example, the IARC Monographs (International Agency for Research on Cancer, 1972), the Survey of Compounds that Have Been Tested for Carcinogenic Activity (U.S. Department of Health, Education, and Welfare, 1975), and the NIOSH Toxic Substances List (U.S. Department of Health, Education, and Welfare, 1976), to name only a few, relating to the carcinogenicity of chemical compounds, and several computer data services (TOXLINE, for example) carrying up-to-date information about the carcinogenic properties of chemical substances. In addition, the 1978 amendments to the Communities Mental Health Centers Act require the Secretary of Health, Education, and Welfare to compile an annual report containing a list of all known or suspect carcinogens to which significant numbers of people are exposed (Community Mental Health Centers Act, 1978).

In cases in which new chemical substances are produced, and only the management of the firm involved has any information relating to the carcinogenic properties of that substance, testing and disclosure requirements under the TSCAct may be used to assure that the government, exposed workers, consumers, and the general public have access to the relevant information.

Government programs aimed at facilitating the process whereby suggestive evidence of cancer hazards is followed up by epidemiological investigations have taken a number of approaches. First, in cases in which the suggestive evidence of an industry-wide cancer hazard is present, or in which the small size of firms in an industry has created difficulties in generating sufficient resources to conduct epidemiological investigations, NIOSH itself has taken on the responsibility for conducting the follow-up process. NIOSH is currently conducting morbidity and mortality studies on working populations in a number of industries (including leather workers, brake lining manufacturers, and others) and cross-industry studies of workers exposed to substances thought to present occupational cancer risks (including urethane, styrene, and toluene) (National Institute for Occupational Safety and Health, 1978).

A major barrier to the conduct of retrospective studies of cancer incidence in working population arises from the necessity to locate workers many years after exposure, often long after they have retired or died. Locating workers and/or determining the causes of death under these conditions commonly accounts for a substantial proportion of the time and expense involved in conducting studies of occupational cancer incidence.

These difficulties often make it impossible for individual firms to conduct epidemiological investigations, and the problem is often exacerbated by failure to preserve employment and exposure records for a sufficient length of time. Thus, the federal government has often had to assume the burden for conducting research of this nature, as already discussed. The government is currently involved in a number of activities that could facilitate this research.

First, both the OSHA regulations relating to specific carcinogens and the proposed record keeping requirement contain provisions requiring that exposure, medical, and employment records of exposed workers be preserved by employers for a long enough period of time so that they could be readily available for use in epidemiological investigations. In addition, the Department of Labor has conducted a feasibility study of a system whereby Social Security Administration data could be quickly and easily accessed and used to relate patterns in occupational disease incidence to employment at particular establishments during particular time periods (Morsch, 1978). Finally, the Health Services Research, Health Statistics, and Health Care Technology Act of 1978 passed in November 1978 provides funds to the secretary of Health, Education, and Welfare for the purposes of studying the development of a coordinated federal system for tracing persons exposed to high-risk substances or occupations. The development of such a system could greatly facilitate the ease with which suggestive evidence of occupational cancer could be followed up, could help provide a much better measure of the magnitude of the occupational cancer problem in general, and could also probably be used to investigate much more easily the problem of multiple exposures to occupational carcinogens.

The discovery of occupational cancer traceable to the manufacture of a particular product may reveal a similar risk for consumer purchasers of that product. Unfortunately, it is usually difficult to obtain exposure data or identify the consumer population at risk. Thus, governmental activities are generally limited to publicizing the danger and recalling the products, when possible.

B. Standard-Setting

There are three kinds of standards that limit worker, consumer, and societal exposures to carcinogens:

- Workplace-exposure standards
- Product-safety standards
- Standards limiting environmental contamination

Workplace-exposure standards place limits on daily worker exposure levels. Selected precautionary work practices can be required in workplaces where carcinogen exposure is possible. Such requirements are generally monitored by air sampling in workplaces and enforced by industrial hygiene inspections (primarily the responsibility of OSHA).

Product-safety standards place limits on the composition of products used in industry. Such requirements become a duty of the manufacturers of those products, enforced by pre-market clearance procedures and seizure of noncomplying products in interstate commerce (primarily the responsibility of EPA and CPSC; additionally, however, under OSHA's generic carcinogen policy, OSHA may essentially effectuate product-safety regulations by promulgating "no permissible exposure" limits for cancer-causing substances which are known to have technically satisfactory substitutes in particular uses).

Promulgation of either product-safety or workplace standards is usually preceded by informational efforts. For example, NCI issues press releases on recent bioassay results and cancer control monographs. NIOSH issues bulletins, "Special Hazard Reviews," and criteria documents.

Standards limiting environmental contamination include concentration and effluent restrictions on air pollutants under the Clean Air Act (1970); water quality standards and emission limitations on water pollutants under the Clean Water Act (1972) and Safe Drinking Water Act (1974); and limits on hazardous waste disposal under the RCRAct. EPA and local environmental authorities exercise authority over this legislation.

OSHA regulations limiting the concentration of carcinogenic substances in workplace air (and specifying certain other work practices) are the control method of choice for hazards in industrial locations which can be efficiently policed by OSHA industrial hygiene inspectors. Because of the limited number of OSHA hygienists, however, OSHA's capability for intensive inspection is limited to industries in which large numbers of workers are exposed in a relatively small number of moderate- to large-sized establishments (e.g., steel mills for coke oven emissions, polyvinyl chloride polymerization plants for vinyl chloride, oil refineries for benzene). At least for the foreseeable future, OSHA will not have the resources to provide effective inspection coverage of such dispersed industries as dry cleaning and auto repair garages.

Moreover, most of the hazards that occur in industries dominated by very small establishments could be regulated more efficiently in another way. For example, in the case of dry cleaners, where some solvents are now suspected to be carcinogenic, it is likely to be easier to eliminate the problem by appropriate limitations on the composition of dry-cleaning solvents and/or the design of dry-cleaning equipment. Such requirements could be mandated by EPA under the TSCAct for the manufacturers of dry-cleaning solvents and equipment. The resulting change in technology could be fairly easily monitored by a limited program of testing such products. Similarly, for any of the numerous chemical products used in auto repair which eventually are shown to have carcinogenic ingredients, it will probably be far more efficient for CPSC or EPA to impose product-composition requirements on manufacturers than to control usage in garages. (CPSC can exercise jurisdiction only if the products in industrial use are also consumer products.) The product-safety approach is thus useful in places where OSHA is likely to be ineffective. On the other hand, for dangerous chemicals which are not products but by-products or intermediates in selected industrial manufacturing operations, the OSHA exposure-limit approach is clearly essential.

1. Workplace-Exposure Standards

Although the OSHAct imposes a "general duty" on employers to provide safe workplaces, the most direct and effective method for controlling carcinogens to date has been through the promulgation of specific standards controlling exposures. The OSHAct provides three mechanisms for establishing health standards.

As an interim measure to get initial enforcement activity started, Sec. 6(a) of the Act allowed OSHA to adopt existing consensus standards which had been previously developed by voluntary standard-setting groups. These include the Threshold Limit Values (TLVs) of the American Conference of Governmental Industrial Hygienists (American Conference of Governmental Industrial Hygienists, 1978). Nearly all current OSHA regulations were adopted in this way. New standards must go through a more elaborate process specified in Sec. 6(b) of the act, or an emergency process outlined in Sec. 6(c).

Section 6(b)(5) of the OSHAct requires OSHA, in promulgating a standard for a toxic substance, to set the standard which

> most adequately assures, to the extent feasible, on the basis of the best available evidence, that no employee will suffer material impairment of health or functional capacity even if such employee has regular exposure to the hazard dealt with by such standard for the period of his working life [emphasis added].

Under Sec. 6(c) of the OSHAct, if the secretary finds that employees are exposed to grave danger from a newly determined hazard, an emergency temporary standard may be issued. Such a standard is not subject to the hearing requirements of the Administrative Procedure Act and is effective immediately upon publication in the Federal Register. However, the emergency standard promulgated must be necessary to protect employees from such danger. An emergency temporary standard may remain in effect for 6 months; thereafter, the secretary must adopt a permanent standard or the protection of the temporary standard will cease.

In 1971 OSHA adopted approximately 400 TLVs as Sec. 6(a) health standards. At the time OSHA refused to incorporate the ACGIH standards for carcinogens (Ashford, 1976), although OSHA's 6(a) standards may inadvertently include some substances that are now suspect carcinogens. Thus, standards for carcinogens must be regulated through either the 6(b) permanent standard or 6(c) emergency temporary standard routes.

There have been only seven completed rule-makings for carcinogens under Sec. 6(b), of which five have occurred by the emergency 6(c) route. The list of controlled substances is found in Table 1.

Several factors are important in evaluating whether OSHA standards effectively reduce worker exposure to carcinogens. Probably the most serious problem at present is the limited number of standards set relative to the number of known carcinogens to which workers are exposed. Promulgating a permanent health standard under Sec. 6(b) is a time-consuming

TABLE 1 OSHA Rule-Making Proceedings for Carcinogenic Materials

	Year promulgated
Asbestos[a]	1972
"14 Carcinogens"	1974
4-nitrobiphenyl; alpha-napthylamine; 4,4'-methylene bis (2-chloroaniline); methyl chloromethyl ether; 3,3'-dichlorobenzidine; bis-chloromethyl ether; beta-naphthylamine; benzidine; 4-aminodiphenyl; ethyleneimine; beta-propiolactone; 2-acetylaminofluorene; 4-dimethylaminoazobenzene; N-nitrosidimethylamine	
Vinyl chloride	1975
Coke oven emissions	1976
Benzene	1977[b]
Acrylonitrile	1978
Arsenic	1978[b]

[a]The cancer-causing properties of asbestos were not used as a basis for rule-making for the asbestos standard of 1972. More recently, greatly strengthened regulation of asbestos has been suggested by NIOSH and OSHA leaders, in recognition of the cancer hazard. Thus the standard-setting process for asbestos cannot be considered complete as of now.

[b]Judicial review still pending.

and resource-draining procedure. OSHA must demonstrate the technological feasibility of meeting the desired exposure limits established (this process also involves some consideration of economic factors) and must prove that the substance regulated is harmful (i.e., carcinogenic). According to a recent court decision reviewing the benzene standard (*American Petroleum Institute* v. *OSHA*, 1978), OSHA may also have to quantify the benefits of its standards, a difficult, highly uncertain, and time-consuming procedure. Economic impact analyses are also required by executive order and are carefully scrutinized by the Council on Wage and Price Stability, adding to the length of the standard-setting process. Extensive hearings are conducted in which almost any "evidence" is permitted to be included. Thus, the same scientific issues (e.g., the validity of animal tests to predict human carcinogens) come up again and again, contributing to a lengthy and resource-consuming process. Every carcinogen standard that has been promulgated except one has been litigated in court, thus further extending the process.

It is difficult to believe that the drafters of the OSHAct anticipated that the progress in setting standards would be as slow as it has been. It is possible that the magnitude of the technical problems involved in regulating exposures to workplace chemicals was not appreciated since the major thrust of the act, and of occupational safety and health efforts at that time, was directed toward the abatement of hazards related to industrial accidents. Also, at the time of the passage of the OSHAct only a few substances present in the workplace were "known" to produce a significant cancer hazard. (The 1968 ACGIH list of toxic substances appendix of carcinogenic substances contained only 10 substances.)

Given the present state of knowledge, the present rate of output of standards for the control of occupational carcinogens is clearly inadequate to deal with the hundreds of compounds with carcinogenic properties known to be present in the working environment. The slow output of OSHA standards has in fact been one of the important rate-limiting steps in the control of occupational carcinogens.

Apart from the limited number of standards set, another factor that is important in evaluating the effectiveness of standards in reducing worker exposure is the level of protection afforded by those standards promulgated. There is no known safe level of exposure to carcinogens. However, OSHA is required by the OSHAct to set standards that are "feasible." Thus, zero exposure levels have not been established, both because at some point exposure reduction would not be feasible, and because in some cases no monitoring devices are available to detect (and enforce) very low levels of exposure that might be achieved.

In setting standards for workplace carcinogen exposure, OSHA is supposed to be guided, at least in part, by technical advice and information furnished by the National Institute of Occupational Safety and Health (Occupational Safety and Health Act, 1972). The functions of NIOSH as envisioned in the OSHAct are, generally, to conduct research dealing with occupational safety and health and to develop recommended safety and health standards relating to physical and chemical hazards in the workplace (National Institute for Occupational Safety and Health, 1978).

NIOSH has conducted a number of epidemiological studies related to specific hazards, completed the National Occupational Hazard Survey, and performed other research related to occupational safety and health. In addition, NIOSH has developed recommended standards and supporting information (criteria documents) for more than 100 specific occupational hazards, some of which are carcinogens.

On October 4, 1977, OSHA issued a proposed generic standard for regulating toxic substances with suspected carcinogenic activity (Federal Register, October 1977). The purposes of the regulation were to increase the speed and efficiency with which OSHA could deal with occupational carcinogens. The proposed regulation would specifically: (1) establish scientifically based criteria for the identification and classification of potential workplace cancer hazards, (2) establish procedures and timetables for OSHA, and (3) establish model standards for use in future rule-makings.

On January 22, 1980, more than two years after the issuance of the proposed standard, OSHA issued a final standard for regulating toxic substances with suspected carcinogenic activity. The general carcinogen standard establishes procedures by which OSHA would classify substances present in U.S. workplaces into one of two categories, based on the strength of evidence supporting carcinogenicity. Substances for which evidence is strong (data from human studies, positive results from one animal species plus other supporting data such as positive results in short-term tests) would be classified as Class I suspect carcinogens. The permanent standard for a Class I suspect carcinogen would require that exposure to the substance in question be reduced to the maximum extent feasible. Moreover, no exposures would be allowed for Class I substances in uses for which less hazardous substitutes are available. Substances for which evidence of carcinogenicity is less conclusive (such as unsupported results in a single animal species) would be classified as Class II suspect carcinogens. OSHA would issue permanent standards for Class II carcinogens mandating exposure limits "as appropriated and consistent with statutory requirements."

The proposed generic standard also contains model standards for Class I and II of suspect carcinogens. The model standard contains descriptions of work and hygiene practices, maximum exposure limits, provisions for personal protective equipment, as well as exposure-monitoring and medical recordkeeping requirements. The standards embody OSHA's policy that engineering controls are inherently more effective and reliable than personal protective equipment for the reduction of exposure.

Unlike the proposed standards, the final standard does not require that OSHA immediately begin regulatory proceedings upon classification of a substance as a Class I suspect carcinogen. Instead, the standard requires OSHA to publish two priority lists containing about 10 substances each, selected from the previously determined list of candidates for regulation as Class I and Class II carcinogens, every six months. These priority lists are intended as a non-binding indication of those substances that OSHA intends to regulate in the near future. The criteria for placing chemicals on a priority list include the number of workers exposed, the level of exposure, the levels of exposure reported to cause cancer in man or animals, whether the molecular structure of the compound is similar to that of other known carcinogens, and the degree to which regulation could be expected to reduce occupational and environmental exposure. OSHA is not required by law to regulate all chemicals on the priority list, nor are they limited to regulating only substances on the priority lists.

The major goal of the generic standard is to expedite the lengthy standard promulgation process for carcinogens on a substance-by-substance basis. Resolving certain scientific issues (thus foreclosing their being raised in future regulatory proceedings as a general issue) and standardizing the form of carcinogen regulation should contribute to a more efficient and effective rule-making process.

Among the important scientific issues "resolved" by the OSHA generic standard are:

1. Positive results in human epidemiological studies alone, or positive results in at least one animal bioassay meeting certain minimum standards of quality and in the presence of supporting evidence, will suffice to establish the "inference" that a substance is a carcinogen.
2. Negative results in animal bioassays or human epidemiological studies will not be considered in deciding whether a chemical is a carcinogen if positive results have been obtained in either an animal bioassay or epidemiological study, unless the negative studies meet stringent quality standards.
3. In animal bioassays, any tumor produced (including benign tumors), or an increase in the incidence of tumors which occur spontaneously, or the occurrence of tumors at the site of application of a substance by inhalation or oral routes, will establish the inference that the substance is a carcinogen.
4. Tumors induced in animals at high dosage levels (including the maximum tolerated dose) will be considered evidence of carcinogenicity of that substance, unless strong

evidence can be supplied that the metabolism of the substance in question is such that at low dose, no carcinogenic metabolites are produced.

The positions taken by OSHA regarding the resolution of these issues seem to represent a reasonable consensus of the state-of-the-art in carcinogenicity testing. The resolution of these issues once and for all in court could, if it occurs, greatly reduce the time and resources required of OSHA in addressing these topics during regulatory proceedings. It is not yet clear to what extent the remaining allowable areas for discussion will result in lengthy and protracted regulatory proceedings. Besides the remaining scientific issues related to the determination of carcinogenicity, OSHA will still be required to determine what level of control is feasible, and this is likely to remain a lengthy and difficult process, subject to delay by court challenge.

During the process of developing the proposed generic standards, OSHA and NIOSH developed lists of chemical substances likely to be classified as Class I suspect carcinogens. Each agency arrived at a list of about 250 substances. It is thus clear that some method is necessary for expediting the process by which standards are set if a reasonable effort is to be made to protect workers against exposures to a large proportion of all the known hazards. Even with the streamlined procedure, it is not likely that this can be accomplished for many years. On the other hand, large numbers of workers are exposed to only a few of these substances, and the publication of OSHA's priority lists will serve as warning to employers and employees alike that certain substances are thought to present serious hazards and are likely to be regulated in the near future. Such warnings can be expected to result in voluntary efforts to reduce exposure, and this voluntary effort will probably be an important part of the total "benefits," in terms of reduced exposure, which will result from the generic carcinogen standard.

Aside from standards set by OSHA to limit worker exposure to carcinogens, it is possible that EPA could also take action that would limit such exposures. Section 9(a) of the TSCAct requires that the administrator of EPA notify other federal agencies if he or she becomes aware of chemical hazards that could be best dealt with under legislation administered by another agency. Thus, the data gathered by EPA under the wide information-gathering power of the TSCAct could be used to inform OSHA of important occupational chemical hazards. Once notified of the existence of the hazard, OSHA would be required either to take regulatory action to control the hazard or to publish reasons in the Federal Register explaining why it feels such action is not necessary. Once OSHA begins regulatory proceedings or determines that they are not necessary, EPA may not take any regulatory action with regard to the same hazard (Toxic Substances Control Act, Sec. 6(a)(2), 1976).

It is not clear to what extent EPA could step in to regulate occupational hazards if there were a disagreement as to whether a hazard were present. If OSHA were unable to act expeditiously to abate a hazard, regulation under the TSCAct could be an effective way to supplement OSHA's limited standard-setting capability. EPA's effectiveness might be limited, however, by its available resources to enforce regulations under the TSCAct.

In cases in which chemical substances present hazards to the general public as well as to workers, the potential for action by EPA under the TSCAct is greater. Section 9(d) requires that the administrator consult and coordinate with other regulatory bodies so as not to impose unnecessary burdens on regulated firms. In the case of a hazardous substance that is both an occupational hazard and a hazard to the general environment, it could well be that the regulatory strategy that would best assure that workers and the public were protected and be least burdensome to employers would be a strategy in which all aspects of the chemical hazard were regulated by EPA under the TSCAct. With the concurrence of OSHA, EPA could set both maximum permissible workplace exposures and external emission standards and enforce them jointly. Such an approach would help regulators to estimate the total cost of environmental regulations to firms and coordinate efforts designed to regulate hazards produced by the same chemical in different settings, thus fulfilling two of the major aims of the TSCAct. It should be remembered, however, that allowing the extensive regulation of occupational hazards under the TSCAct could involve a substantial shift in the criteria used to design and evaluate occupational health standards. The OSHAct requires that standards for exposure to toxic substances be set in such a fashion so as to protect workers to the maximum extent that is feasible. In contrast, the TSCAct requires that specific consideration be given to the costs and benefits of the regulation in setting standards. Thus, an occupational standard set under the TSCAct might well allow more exposure than one promulgated under the OSHAct. Whether or not this is desirable would depend on the extent to which similar occupational standards set by EPA and OSHA would actually differ in their degree of protection, and to what extent this difference is felt to be justifiable on economic grounds.

In addition to regulatory activities, the data gathering and dissemination provisions of Sec. 10 of the TSCAct could be of great significance for OSHA standard-setting activities. Section 10 of the TSCAct requires that EPA set up an interagency committee for the purpose of information dissemination, and that it assemble a data system for the purpose of making data obtained under the TSCAct available to other regulatory agencies.

2. Product-Safety Standards

Through the TSCAct, EPA appears to have the broadest authority of the three agencies to develop product-safety standards to protect both consumers and workers. Under Sec. 6 of the TSCAct, EPA may ban a substance or limit: (1) the amount of the substance that may be manufactured, (2) its concentration, and/or (3) its use. EPA is authorized to set these product-safety standards if the agency finds that there is a "reasonable basis to conclude" that the use of the substance presents or will present an unreasonable risk of injury to health or the environment. The standard must be set to protect adequately against the risk, using the least burdensome requirements. In promulgating standards, EPA must consider the health effects of the substance, the magnitude of exposure, the benefits of the substance, the availability of substitutes, and, to a certain extent, the economic consequences of the standard. Standards dealing with occupational carcinogens that could not be effectively regulated by OSHA could clearly be developed under this section. EPA has not yet exercised this authority.

The Consumer Product Safety Act (1972) authorizes the CPSC to regulate consumer products. The agency is authorized to promulgate standards regulating the composition, packaging, and labeling of consumer products. Requirements must be "reasonably necessary to prevent or reduce an unreasonable risk of injury" (Sec. 7(a)(1)) associated with the product. The CPSC may ban products which present an unreasonable risk if no feasible standard would adequately protect the public from the substance (Sec. 8).

While the CPSC has no direct authority to regulate workplace hazards, the agency could directly influence workplace carcinogen exposures in two ways: (1) a product sold as a consumer product is also used in workplaces, and the manufacturer may change the composition of the product to reduce consumer exposures to carcinogens in response to CPSC regulation; and (2) banning carcinogenic consumer products eliminates hazardous exposures of workers engaged in the manufacture of the product. Similarly, CPSC standards that reduce the amount of a carcinogenic substance in a product could also lead to reduced exposures of workers engaged in the manufacture of the product.

In June 1978 the CPSC issued a policy for classifying and regulating carcinogens (Federal Register, June 1978). According to the policy, known carcinogens will not be permitted to be intentionally added to consumer products if the carcinogens can be absorbed, inhaled, or ingested. When reasonable substitutes exist, the carcinogens must be gradually phased out. If there are no reasonable substitutes available and elimination of the product would lead to unacceptable economic and social costs, the carcinogens must be reduced to the lowest attainable level until substitutes are identified.

The first substance that the CPSC has attempted to regulate under this policy is perchloroethylene, a dry-cleaning agent that poses an occupational hazard to persons in the dry-cleaning business. However, in November 1978 the CPSC was enjoined from implementing the policy because it failed to follow the Administrative Procedure Act's requirements for notice and hearing prior to the adoption of its cancer policy (Dow Chemical v. CPSC, 1978). Although the CPSC initially appealed this decision, it subsequently withdrew both the appeal and its entire carcinogen policy (Federal Register, 1979). It took this step to avoid protracted litigation and because it felt that the existing legal authority provided an adequate basis on which to regulate carcinogens. However, the commission did indicate its strong support for the Interagency Regulatory Liaison Group (ILRG) carcinogen policy, in which it will participate.

If a CPSC cancer policy is eventually implemented, workers as well as consumers may benefit. For example, the CPSC may regulate typewriter correction fluid which now contains trichloroethylene. Rather than market two separate products, one for consumers and another for workplace use, the manufacturer may choose to manufacture only the safer product needed to comply with CPSC requirements. Thus, office workers would also receive increased protection.

OSHA's generic cancer standard would prohibit worker exposures to Class I carcinogens if less hazardous substitutes were available. A no-permissible-exposure level could be achieved through use of a contained system or as a result of a ban. A ban would result in the protection of both workers and consumers. The OSHAct does not explicitly give OSHA authority to ban a substance and the issue has never been directly tested in the courts. However, the third circuit in the no-hands-in-die case, commented in nonbinding language that very hazardous industrial activities with little social utility might properly be prohibited if there was no technologically feasible method of eliminating them (AFL-CIO v. Brennan, 1975). The equivalent of a ban could be accomplished by setting a standard at a "no detectable level," while technically not banning the substance.

3. Standards Limiting Environmental Contamination

Very few substances are currently regulated as carcinogens through the Clean Air and Clean Water Acts. The acts include air pollution control of vinyl chloride and asbestos, and water pollution control of aldrin, dieldrin, and benzidine. Under court order, EPA will also regulate water pollution by acrylonitrile, arsenic compounds, asbestos, benzene, carbon tetrachloride, chlorinated benzenes and ethanes, chloroform, chromium, nickel and selium compounds, vinyl chloride, and trichloroethylene.

The contamination of the drinking water supply occurs through direct disposal of carcinogens, indirect contamination through the leaching of materials contained in hazardous waste disposal sites, and subsequent chlorination of organic chemicals by municipal water treatment plants. This drinking water contamination problem is thought to be the most serious threat to the general public arising from chemical carcinogens. The federal efforts to date have been entirely inadequate. Regulations defining what constitutes a "carcinogen" for regulation of hazardous waste disposal under the RCRAct have not been issued. Activities for control of environmental contamination will be expected to increase slowly. Therefore, efforts to control the nature of industrial products under the OSHAct, the TSCAct, and the CPSCAct are most crucial to prevent subsequent contamination of the environment by carcinogenic products, and resulting danger to the general public.

III. RESPONSIBILITIES OF EMPLOYERS AND MANUFACTURERS

A. Statutory Requirements for Reducing Exposure to Carcinogens

1. Complying with Standards and the Duty to Limit Exposure

We discussed in Sec. II the activities of several regulatory agencies in setting permissible exposure standards for carcinogens and in banning carcinogen-containing products in industrial and commercial uses. Employers and manufacturers are responsible for complying with those standards. In addition, a general duty to provide a safe workplace is imposed on employers.

If an OSHA inspection reveals high levels of exposure to a carcinogen not regulated by a specific standard, the agency may attempt to issue a citation under the general duty clause of the OSHAct to control exposures. Section 5(a)(1) states:

> Each employer shall furnish to each of his employees employment and a place of employment which are free from recognized hazards that are causing or are likely to cause death or serious physical harm to his employees [emphasis added].

The burden of proving a violation of the general duty clause is on OSHA. If a criteria document or other reputable scientific studies showing that the substance is carcinogenic exist, OSHA should not have much difficulty proving that the substance is likely to cause death or serious physical harm. However, proving that the hazard was "recognized" is more difficult. A hazard is considered "recognized" if (1) it is common knowledge in the employer's industry, or (2) the employer had actual knowledge of the hazardous condition. Whether a hazard is recognized by industry can be determined by the common knowledge of safety experts who are familiar with the industry (National Realty and Construction Co. v. OSHRC, 1973), ANSI standards, or state or local safety laws (Rothstein, 1978). If an employer has actual knowledge of a hazard and means of abating it, he or she may be successfully cited and required to take abatement measures that go beyond those generally recognized as necessary by the industry (Southern Railway Co., 1975). Hazards that are only detectable through instrumentation, as well as those detectable through the senses, may be recognized (American Smelting and Refining Co. v. OSHRC, 1974).

Citations issued under the general duty clause will be more effective for controlling carcinogens which are recognized by the industry. The general duty clause is less useful in situations in which the carcinogenic problem is not widely known. However, this latter problem might be circumvented in the following way. An OSHA industrial hygienist detects a suspected carcinogenic hazard in the workplace during inspection and informs the employer of the hazard and abatement methods. A follow-up inspection is made after a reasonable period of time for implementing controls has expired. Since the employer now has actual knowledge of the hazard, a citation for failure to reduce the hazard should, theoretically, be successful (Rothstein, 1978).

It is possible that the mere classification of a chemical as a carcinogen by OSHA, NIOSH, or NCI, or by the secretary of HEW under the annual list of carcinogens he or she is required to compile (Community Mental Health Centers Act, 1978) would render it a "recognized hazard." Thus, even if the OSHA generic carcinogen standard is not enacted, classification by an appropriate agency could allow considerable enforcement activity by OSHA using the general duty clause, rather than substance-specific standards.

The general duty obligation is particularly relevant to carcinogen exposure in the laboratory. OSHA had at one time proposed specific laboratory standards for handling chemical carcinogens when it proposed its final exposure regulations on 14 carcinogens (Long, 1975). The Third Circuit Court of Appeals, however, remanded them to OSHA because OSHA had failed to give notice of its intent to promulgate them. The court also vacated the standard on MOCA (4,4'-methylene bis-2-chloroaniline) on procedural grounds. The standards will eventually be issued. In the meantime, laboratories must continue to provide protection for these substances because of the general duty obligation and the fact that these substances are considered to be "recognized hazards" (Occupational Safety and Health Reporter, 1976).

2. Reducing Exposure to Carcinogens by Developing New Technology

Recognizing that the reduction of toxic hazards might require changes in manufacturing processes and practices, both the OSHAct and the TSCAct give the agencies charged with their enforcement the power to require changes in process and production technologies to differing extents. The OSHAct is the older of the two statutes, and the degree to which it can require that new technologies be developed and implemented has been the subject of numerous court cases. In all the cases addressing this issue, the courts have consistently characterized it as a "technology-forcing" piece of legislation (<u>AFL-CIO</u> v. <u>Brennan</u>, 1975). The interpretation of this phrase, however, is far from complete. At a minimum, it is clear that OSHA is not limited to mandating the institution of technology which is "fully developed" (<u>Society of the Plastics Industry</u> v. <u>OSHA</u>, 1975). This means that OSHA can go further than simply requiring the diffusion of an already fully commercialized technology to firms that were not using it. Rather, standards may in effect require "improvements in <u>existing</u> technology" (emphasis added) (<u>Society of the Plastics Industry</u> v. <u>OSHA</u>, 1975). Thus, requirements for changes of a more than incremental nature and changes in fairly early stages of development are apparently feasible within the meaning of the act.

Furthermore, the courts have realized that in determining the feasibility of change, OSHA can look to the stage of development of new technologies and is permitted to make reasoned judgments (i.e., predictions), about the future of technology. Thus, the secretary should look to both "existing capabilities and imminent advances in the art" (<u>AFL-CIO</u> v. <u>Brennan</u>, 1975). Similarly, a finding that a technical advance is feasible can be made on the basis of evidence that a technology is in the "experimental" stage (<u>American Iron and Steel Institute</u> et al. v. <u>OSHA</u>, 1978).

Although OSHA derives substantial leeway from these cases as to the <u>amount</u> of new technology it can mandate, there is a constraint on its authority to determine <u>how</u> the development may take place. Specifically, in the coke oven case, the court invalidated OSHA's requirement that R&D be undertaken when compliance was not achieved after implementation of the required controls. The rationale for the court's action appears to be that the requirement was too speculative and open ended. The case does not, however, stand for the proposition that OSHA cannot de facto require R&D because of the stringency of a promulgated standard. On the contrary, if the need for R&D arises in order to comply (which, of course, is not always the case, especially when already-developed technology can be purchased), it <u>may</u> of course be performed. It is not the <u>need</u> for R&D to which the court was objecting in the coke oven decision but rather, simply, the unavoidable "affirmative duty" to perform it.

While OSHA's authority to insist, via its standard-setting, upon significant technological change is clear, the cases do not offer much guidance as to the frame of reference for determining "newness." In the intraindustry context, it is clear that mandatory diffusion of the latest techniques is appropriate. This interpretation, offered in the <u>AFL-CIO</u> v. <u>Brennan</u> case, relies upon the act's legislative history, which expresses the intent of Congress to bring lagging firms up to the standards of the more progressive members (U.S. Code Cong. & Admin. News, 1970). The legislative history specifically recognizes that without regulation, firms that provide safe and healthful workplaces suffer a competitive disadvantage until the recalcitrant employers change their practices, and that therefore a purpose of regulation is to diffuse the best practices throughout the industry. Going further, the vinyl chloride and coke oven cases both recognize the necessity and feasibility of requiring technology that surpasses that currently in use in even the leading firms. Because the degree of newness involved in any such change is likely to be different for different industries or different firms within the same industry, the cases permit standards to be drafted to take such factors into account.

In sum, it is possible to say that the courts have consistently permitted OSHA to require different degrees of "new" technology. However, the extent of this authority is not clear, because no specific outer bound has been put on the degree of newness permissible, except by virtue of the necessity for "feasible" standards.

While there is at present little case law that defines the degree to which EPA action under the TSCAct can be used to force the development of new technologies, it is clear that many of the regulatory actions allowed under the TSCAct have great potential for influencing manufacturers to search for substitutes for dangerous products and process technologies.

Under Sec. 6(A) of the TSCAct, the Administrator of EPA, upon finding that there is a reasonable basis to conclude that an activity presents an unreasonable risk of injury to health or the environment, may:

1. Prohibit the manufacture, use, or disposal of the substance in question, either totally, or for a given application
2. Limit the amount of the substance produced or used
3. Require that dangerous substances be labeled, and that records be kept to assure that dangerous exposures do not arise
4. Require that manufacturers of dangerous substances notify users of the product of the danger and repurchase the products from users, if requested

Clearly, any of these regulated measures could influence manufacturers to search for new technologies if the requirements imposed were onerous enough to render the existing technology too expensive to be used profitably. In addition, the administrator may require that the manufacturer adopt or revise quality control measures if necessary to limit harmful effects of the substances in question. Thus, EPA can essentially order a specific process change. It thus appears that Sec. 6 of the TSCAct does give the administrator wide power to require the development of new technology, and the rigorous use of this power could greatly decrease the extent to which workers, consumers, and society are exposed to carcinogens.

B. Statutory Requirements for the Generation and Disclosure of Information

1. Data on the Carcinogenic Potential of Chemical Substances

A number of federal statutes attempt to deal with the problem of assuring that all the available data concerning carcinogenicity are made available to regulating agencies and other parties involved in making decisions regarding the abatement of occupational and environmental cancer hazards. Perhaps the most comprehensive statute in this area is the TSCAct. Regulations promulgated under the act should expand the available knowledge about the carcinogenic potential of substances in future regulatory proceedings. Carcinogenicity data, including in vitro test results, can be required as part of the premarket notification procedure for new substances. Decisions are now being made as to the policy concerning the amount of data required with each premarket notification. Limited regulatory and testing resources probably indicate that, in the vast majority of cases for new substances, at most, in vitro data will be required. However, any data voluntarily generated must be divulged to EPA, whether specifically requested or not.

For existing chemicals EPA can similarly require testing, but it may have to resort to the use of court orders to get the desirable tests performed. For chemicals already in use in which there may be indications of carcinogenic potential, when tests are required, the majority are likely to be animal tests or epidemiological investigations.

The act gives wide discretion to the EPA administrator in disclosing confidential data, allowing disclosures to any government employee or government contractor in connection with activities necessary to fulfill the act, or to any person if the administrator determines that disclosure is necessary to protect health or the environment from unreasonable risk, or generally in the course of any proceeding under the act (Toxic Substances Control Act, Sec. 14a). Thus, theoretically at least, the administrator of EPA could disclose carcinogenicity test data directly to workers, unions, or consumers, although in practice EPA might defer any action to OSHA or CPSC, since, as will be further discussed, there is some conflict between the public disclosure provisions of the TSCAct and the OSHAct or the CPSAct.

In addition, Sec. 8e of the TSCAct requires manufacturers to provide the administrator with "information which reasonably supports the conclusion that [a] substance or mixture presents a substantial risk to health or the environment" which would almost certainly include results of animal or in vitro tests or epidemiological studies indicating that a given substance might present a cancer risk. The language of this provision has been criticized as being much too vague to provide industry with workable guidelines as to what information should be supplied (Zener, 1977), and it is probable that clarifying regulations would be helpful.

A third important provision is Sec. 26(a)(2), which requires other federal agencies to release their data to EPA to assist it in the implementation of the TSCAct. Although one could argue that these data are then subject to the public disclosure provisions of the act, many of the other regulatory statutes under which the data were collected forbid such disclosure. This creates a legal conflict for EPA. The Toxic Substances Strategy Committee has recommended that new legislation be enacted to resolve the conflict.

Although the TSCAct's disclosure provisions are certainly broad on their face, certain difficulties have arisen in implementing them. These are exemplified by the Polaroid case, which suggests that due care must be taken to balance the need for trade secret protection against the public need to know. Although this case did not concern test data, if trade secrets were involved, the same considerations would likely apply.

Unlike the TSCAct, which provides EPA with direct authority to obtain carcinogenicity data, OSHA has only indirect capability in this area. Although OSHA has no authority to require testing by employers, it does require that employers post notice to workers exposed to regulated carcinogens and to some "suspect carcinogens." This is at least an indirect way to inform workers about the results of carcinogenicity tests. Unfortunately, it only applies to the relatively few toxic substances which are the subject of specific regulations, since the general duty clause of the OSHAct only requires that employers furnish a workplace free from recognized hazards, and places no affirmative duty on employers to generate data on the carcinogenicity of unregulated chemicals. It also does not appear that NIOSH has specifically been granted the power to require the submission of carcinogenicity test results on particular substances by employers. Sections 20 and 22 of the OSHAct, which deal with the duties and powers of NIOSH, specifically mention its authority to obtain exposure and medical records from employers, but do not mention toxicity data. In any event, it does not appear that NIOSH has ever attempted to obtain carcinogenity test results (at least, not animal test results) from private firms, and its right to do so has not been established in court. In practice, this is not likely to impede the dissemination of carcinogenicity test results produced by industry, since the inventory and premanufacturing notification requirement under the TSCAct, combined with the requirements for interagency coordination on data sharing, allows the EPA great latitude to assure that government agencies and concerned parties have access to carcinogenicity data. It is possible that occasionally the disclosure of carcinogenicity test results by a firm would require the disclosure of information which could be classified as a trade secret, however. In such cases, the freedom with which such information could be disseminated by government agencies might be greatly curtailed.

2. Health and Exposure Records Relating to Occupational Carcinogens

Two statutes, the TSCAct and the OSHAct, define the extent to which OSHA, NIOSH, and EPA have authority to require the compilation of health and exposure records relating to occupational carcinogens, and define the conditions under which these records must be made available to the various agencies. The most detailed health and exposure data that currently must be kept are specified in OSHA standards for specific toxic hazards (currently 20 carcinogenic compounds and a carcinogenic mixture are regulated through this process). Some standards require employers to provide medical exams and to monitor individuals' exposures to contaminants. The earliest OSHA carcinogen standard, dealing with 14 highly carcinogenic industrial chemicals (29 C.F.R. 1910.1003-1016), contains no monitoring requirements <u>per se</u> and does not prescribe any analytical techniques for monitoring. The standard does require, however, that all firms using the substance must notify OSHA; that "regulated areas" be set aside where these compounds are used; that access to these areas be limited to as few employees as possible; that a continuous record of those allowed in regulated areas be kept and preserved for 20 years; and that in case the firm goes out of business, the roster of presumably exposed employees must be forwarded to the director of NIOSH. The standard for exposure to coke oven emissions requires that exposure records be kept for 40 years.

Some of the later standards, such as the regulation governing acrylonitrile (29 C.F.R. 1910.1045), require exposure monitoring and record-keeping related to carcinogen exposure. The standards for vinyl chloride (29 C.F.R. 1910.1017), inorganic arsenic (29 C.F.R. 1910.1018), and benzene* (29 C.F.R. 1010.1028) require monitoring at specific intervals, usually monthly, if exposures are above an "action level" (usually one-half the maximum exposure level allowed by the standard), and less often, usually quarterly, otherwise. They also establish regulated areas and, with the exception of arsenic and benzene, require the maintenance of rosters of employees allowed in the regulated areas. In the benzene standard, an estimate of the number of potentially exposed workers is required. Most of the standards require that employees be informed of monitoring results, and several specify accuracy requirements for monitoring techniques. In addition, the OSHAct requires worker notification of exposures for any standards for which monitoring and record-keeping are required.

<u>None</u> of the regulations governing toxic substances, adopted earlier under the OSHAct through Sec. 6(a) (the 387 TLVs), <u>requires</u> monitoring that could be of any use in determining which employees were subject to a given level of exposure to a given agent. Some of these classical toxic materials may well turn out to be carcinogens, for example, cadmium. The regulations only require that exposures everywhere in the workplace be limited below a certain level. It is likely that in most cases monitoring is performed, if at all, only in those areas known to have the highest exposures. Which workers are exposed in these areas and the general exposures that occur in other parts of the establishment is not likely to be known. OSHA has initiated the Standards Completion Project, which adds monitoring and recording requirements to the 387 TLVs.

OSHA's access to medical records rule requires that employers in general industry, construction, and maritime operations furnish to employees, employee representatives, and OSHA a wide range of existing employer-kept records. These records, which are to be retained for a minimum of 30 years, include medical records covering pre-employment and episodic physical examinations, laboratory test results, and employee medical complaints, as well as exposure records covering past or present exposure to toxic agents. If firms consider these access and record-keeping requirements to be sufficiently onerous, they might well decide to not keep some health and exposure records that they otherwise would have. This might not be a serious problem in the case of carcinogens if the generic carcinogen policy is upheld, since it would require that health and exposure records related to all Class I carcinogens be kept.

*The OSHA regulation for benzene was vacated by the Fifth Circuit Court of Appeals for failure to adequately quantify the benefits of the maximum allowable exposure level; the case was upheld by the Supreme Court.

NIOSH also has specific authority to require employers to make, keep, and make available to NIOSH records of employee exposure to substances which it believes have a potential for causing harm to workers (Occupational Safety and Health Act, Section 20(a)(5), 1972). For the most part, NIOSH has exercised this authority in the context of conducting epidemiological research related to the establishment of associations between particular exposures and disease incidence.

Section 20a of the OSHAct allows NIOSH to acquire health and exposure records for the purpose of conducting research related to occupational disease. In cases in which the data are of aggregate or summary nature and individuals are not identified by name, NIOSH's right to acquire it is relatively clear and has been affirmed in court (General Motors Corp. v. Finklea, 1978). In cases in which data are involved which include specific identification of individuals by name or by some other method, the situation is slightly more complicated. In such cases issues relating to the worker's constitutional right to privacy must be considered. A recent court case (E. I. Dupont de Nemours and Co. v. Finklea, 1977) has upheld NIOSH's right to obtain individual health records if such information were necessary for NIOSH to conduct its statutory mission, even if the workers involved refused to give their permission. NIOSH was required, however, to take extreme care to assure that such data were accessible only to the persons directly involved in conducting the investigations, and to assure that adequate precautions were taken to see that no data relating to specific individuals were released outside of NIOSH.

Section 8 of the TSCAct also imposes specific duties on manufacturers with regard to exposure records. Under Sec. 8a employers may be required to furnish records relating to the number of workers exposed, and the degree and duration of exposure. In the case of manufacturers who intend to produce a given substance, estimates of these data must be furnished. Manufacturers may also be required to furnish all available data relating to adverse effects of exposure (Sec. 8c, and must communicate to EPA any information which suggests that a given substance presents a substantial risk of injury to health or the environment (Sec. 8e).

All of the provisions of Sec. 8 of the TSCAct that apply to the obligations of manufacturers to furnish exposure data to EPA also apply to health data in roughly the same fashion. Employers may be required to furnish health records to the EPA either for existing chemicals or for new chemical uses (Sec. 8a). Also, data on "significant adverse health effects," which EPA could require of any manufacturer, also could presumably include employee health records (Sec. 8c), as could data relating to the possibility of a substance presenting a substantial risk to health or the environment (Sec. 8e).

Thus, the two major statutes relevant to occupational safety and health provide extensive authority for the various agencies involved to obtain health and exposure data relating to individual workers. It is, unfortunately, not clear to what extent the various agencies can share data for the purpose of informing workers of hazards or coordinating efforts to detect and abate health hazards. The reason for this is that the two laws differ in the degree to which they allow the dissemination of such data, and the circumstances under which such data can be made public. The TSCAct, for instance, allows the administrator to disclose any data obtained under the act to federal employees for the purpose of performing his or her duty, or to disclose data in the course of regulatory proceedings, or to disclose data when it is determined that disclosure is necessary to protect against an unreasonable risk of injury to health or the environment (Sec. 14). The conditions under which OSHA and NIOSH may disclose data, on the other hand, are much more narrowly defined, and thus the requirement in Sec. 26(a)(2) of the TSCAct requiring that other agencies furnish data to the EPA for purposes of implementing and enforcing the act could well produce serious conflicts, which would probably have to be resolved by the passage of additional legislation (Subcommittee on Trade Secrets and Confidentiality, 1978). At present the EPA and other regulatory agencies are in the process of deciding how best to reconcile differences in policy relating to the use of health and exposure records, and to coordinate efforts to assure that such data are used effectively to reduce health hazards produced by toxic exposures in the workplace.

3. Data Related to Products or Processes

The degree to which data concerning the chemical nature of products or the processes by which products are made are available to regulatory agencies will strongly affect the ability of the agencies to formulate effective policies for the reduction of worker and consumer exposure to toxic substances, including carcinogens. Knowledge of the chemical constituents of a product can help indicate whether either the workers making the product or the users of the product (who may be workers using the product as part of their jobs) are being exposed to chemical hazards. In addition, knowledge about the particular process used to make a product can be very useful in estimating the degree of hazard experienced by workers and in suggesting strategies for abating the hazard.

Recent research by NIOSH has found that about 70% of the chemical exposures that occur in the workplace arise out of worker exposures to tradename products, the ingredients of which are not known to the employers of the exposed workers (Finklea, 1977). It was also found that at least 300,000 workers were being exposed to products containing OSHA-regulated carcinogens. It is not known how many workers are being exposed to ingredients of products that are known to be carcinogens, but which are not the subject of OSHA regulation, although the number is almost certainly much greater.

Details of manufacturing processes are also of great importance in detecting and abating carcinogenic hazards. For agencies attempting to formulate regulations to abate hazards, the availability of such data greatly simplifies the task of estimating the compliance costs and economic impact of standards. In addition, the general availability of process data enables firms and agencies to identify the lowest cost abatement strategies, or to find suitable safe alternative technologies. The availability of knowledge of this type to workers or their unions is also important if they are to meaningfully take part in the processes by which hazards are detected and abated.

Specific information related to the chemical composition of products or the nature of manufacturing processes is often not easily available outside of the industry that makes the products or uses the process, and occasionally it is not even available outside of a particular firm. The reason for this is that much of this kind of information is proprietary data, claimed by its owner to be trade secrets, which are protected not only by state laws, but also by virtually every federal regulatory statute (including the TSCAct and the OSHAct), to one degree or another.

The existence of trade secret protection impedes the identification of hazardous chemical exposures even as it rewards the holder of the secret. This is not so much a problem to the government directly in its regulatory function, because the right of the government to have access to these secrets when the public welfare demands it is well established. However, trade secrets do create significant problems for workers, consumers, and employers seeking to identify tradename chemical substances, and for the government in its attempts to disseminate such information to the public and to share information among agencies.

The issue of trade secrets is dealt with directly by both the OSHAct and the TSCAct. The OSHAct (Sec. 15) clearly allows OSHA access to trade secrets, but provides for the preservation of their confidentiality and does not allow their release except to other officers and employees of the federal government concerned with implementing the act. In addition, the right of NIOSH to obtain trade secret data relating to product ingredient lists has been upheld in court subject to similar constraints (U.S. v. McGee Industries, 1977). In contrast, the TSCAct's public disclosure provisions (Section 14a) are quite liberal, allowing disclosure of confidential information to other environmental regulatory agencies, government contractors, and to the public if necessary to protect against unreasonable risks.

Thus, a difficult problem has arisen in the context of agency sharing of trade secret data. An interagency task force on this issue has concluded that the various environmental and other statutes bearing on the problem are so in conflict that the issue cannot be resolved without new legislation specifically addressing the issue of trade secrets (Subcommittee on Trade Secrets and Confidentiality, 1978).

Whether or not the agency may disclose trade secret data under specific circumstances, the existence of a trade secret imposes some obligation on the government to attempt to prevent the secret from falling into the hands of a competitor. Thus, "protective orders" are routinely issued by agencies when releasing trade secrets. The issue of what constitutes an appropriate protective order can be challenged before regulatory action, and has been in several circumstances (Reynolds Metals Co., 1978, and Polaroid Corp. v. Costle, 1978), thereby delaying government or public access to the data.

The trade secret problem, in sum, is not so much a barrier to government identification of hazardous chemicals as to the knowledge of those hazards on the part of workers, consumers, and employers. Because of trade secret protection, these individuals often cannot obtain chemical identification directly from chemical manufacturers or processors. Moreover, because of the government's obligation to protect trade secrets, it often cannot serve as an alternative source of information. This problem may diminish considerably as the TSCAct's broad disclosure provisions are implemented; however, the implementation of those provisions will require considerable delicacy in balancing the public's need to know with the trade secret holder's legitimate right to protect his commercial interests.

A number of government efforts in the area of dissemination of product and process information are currently under way. NIOSH is continuing its efforts to discover the chemical composition of products to which workers are exposed, by requesting such data from manufacturers and challenging trade secret classifications in court when it thinks such action is necessary (Finklea, 1977) and is currently developing a computer data base of tradename product composition to enable much more rapid determination of whether or not a given product contains carcinogenic ingredients (National Institute for Occupational Safety and Health, 1978).

OSHA has drafted, but not formally proposed, a labeling standard that would require that all chemicals present in the workplace be identified and that all products or substances presenting a toxic hazard to workers be labeled to that effect (Federal Register, January 1977). In addition, Sec. 6(a)(3) of the TSCAct authorizes EPA to require manufacturers to label substances with "clear and adequate warnings" when necessary to protect adequately against an unreasonable risk of injury to health. Section 14(a)(3) authorizes EPA to release trade secret information when necessary to protect against unreasonable health risks. Clearly, requiring manufacturers to identify carcinogens and to specify the percentage of the product containing the carcinogen would be very useful in protecting workers from exposure and in selecting safer substitutes. It is not clear from the language of the TSCAct whether EPA can promulgate a generic standard which would require all manufacturers of products containing carcinogens to provide this information on a label or whether labeling standards must be considered on a case-by-case basis. The EPA is currently investigating this issue. In addition, Section 6(a)(7) of the TSCAct requires manufacturers of products to give notice to distributors, purchasers, and the public of any unreasonable risk of injury presented by the product due to toxic ingredients if the administrator determines that such a hazard exists. The CPSC also has the power to require the labeling of products, and could conceivably have some impact in this area.

The TSCAct may also be useful in allowing federal agencies to obtain process data that would be useful in helping to identify and abate carcinogenic hazards. In principal, any data submitted to EPA under any of the reporting requirements of the act can be disclosed to OSHA for regulatory purposes. In practice, however, the previously mentioned problems relating to trade secret protection may interfere with EPA's ability to share information with other agencies. EPA could, of course, use such information for its own regulatory purposes, which could also help reduce workers exposure to carcinogens.

C. Common Law Duties

The duties that the common law imposes upon employers or manufacturers are grounded in the same legal principles that pertain to the daily affairs of ordinary individuals. Simply stated, the law of torts demands that people conduct their affairs using "reasonable care under the circumstances." When this duty to act with care has been breached, the law considers the person to be "at fault" or "negligent," and individuals who have been harmed as a result can recover money damages from the negligent party as compensation for their injuries. The determination of what constitutes negligence is a factual question, usually decided by a jury.

Because of the special relationship between employees and employers, a discrete set of common law rules, based on the aforementioned general concepts, has arisen with respect to workplace injury and disease. Similarly, there are detailed rules governing a manufacturer's duty to sell safe products to the public. Although there are still only a few cases in which the law in either area has actually dealt with carcinogens, as the social consciousness about cancer increases, more cases will undoubtedly arise. These will be based on the existing principles but will move the law in new directions, imposing new duties in new circumstances. Although this movement makes tort law somewhat unpredictable, it also results in an extraordinary flexibility, allowing the legal system to adapt to changed conditions. Moreover, because the ultimate standards of legal responsibility are determined by juries, the system allows for the prevailing social attitudes of common people to define the measure of legally acceptable risk.

Employers have a general, common law duty to furnish their employees with a safe and healthful workplace. They have other, more specific responsibilities, such as the duty to warn of hazards that they know or should know are present in the workplace. Employers are also liable for the torts of their agents and thus may be held legally accountable for the failure of their employees or contractors to act with reasonable care. For example, the failure of a company physician to warn an employee of a precancerous condition could lead to liability on the part of the employer for the damage that results to the employee.

Although the common law places strict duties on the employer with respect to the safety and health of employees, employees often are unable to sue their employers for violating these duties, because of the workers' compensation system. Workers' compensation statutes in all states modify the common law by providing the principal worker "remedy" for workplace injury or disease in the form of monetary compensation, according to schedules established by workers' compensation agencies. In exchange for this compensation, which is awarded without regard to the negligence of employer or employee, employees are barred, in general, from suing their employers.

Workers' compensation systems, however, have provided notoriously inadequate compensation for occupational disease—particularly workplace cancer. Moreover, these systems were only intended to be a worker's exclusive remedy for certain kinds of actions. Thus, there are still a variety of circumstances under which employers may be held liable to employees. Most states allow tort suits irrespective of worker's compensation, in instances of "gross negligence," such as knowingly exposing workers to a carcinogen. Another instance in which employers may still be sued is if they act in more than one capacity vis à vis the employee—for example, when the employer is also the manufacturer of a hazardous product and the employee also a consumer of that product. Similarly, liability may arise out of obligations the employer assumes that are not within the ordinary course of employment—for example, the provision of medical services. This source of liability is likely to increase in proportion to the increase in employer-provided medical services.

Manufacturers and sellers of consumer products have a general legal duty to consumers to provide products that are "reasonably safe" and not "defective." There is also a general duty to warn consumers of unsafe aspects of products so that they can protect themselves from harm. The law in this area, which is known as "products liability," has developed a set of specialized concepts called "strict liability." Under this doctrine, manufacturers can be held liable irrespective of their own negligence or nonnegligence in production and irrespective of the consumer's behavior—if their product is defective or unreasonably dangerous. Defects in design, as well as manufacturing defects, may give rise to liability. Furthermore, a defect may remain "latent" for many years and still give rise to liability when its discovery causes injury.

One of the important determinants of legal liability is the "state of the art" and manufacturer knowledge about product hazards. (This issue is also important for employers.) Liability will almost certainly arise when the manufacturer has actual knowledge of a defect and takes no steps to minimize its harmful consequences. However, manufacturers (or employers) can also be held liable for defects that they "should have known" about even when there is no actual knowledge. In general, manufacturers are presumed in law to have the level of knowledge of an "expert" in the field and they have a duty to seek out the latest information about hazards inherent in their products. Thus, advances in the state of the art lead to corresponding increases in the duty of care. On the other hand, compliance with "custom" in the industry is often used as a defense in negligence actions. However, this defense will not succeed when the defendant's knowledge exceeds custom, or when the industry custom is itself unreasonable.

Regulatory actions can raise the standard of care applicable in tort. For example, when violation of a regulatory standard results in an injury, negligence is usually automatically assumed (Arthur v. Flota Mercante, 1973). Moreover, failure on the part of a manufacturer to eliminate the use of a substance shown by government tests to be a carcinogen is likely to be persuasive evidence of negligence, even if no regulatory standard has been established. This kind of interaction between regulation and tort law is likely to be important now, as OSHA, CPSC, and EPA implement carcinogen policies.

IV. RESPONSIBILITIES OF EMPLOYEES

The legal responsibility of individual employees for the control of carcinogens arises both from statutory duties placed on them and their employers, and from the common law. The statutory responsibilities imposed by legislation and regulation technically apply to employers or corporations, but must, of course, actually be fulfilled by real individuals. Although, in general, legal responsibility for compliance rests with the business, not its employees, under certain circumstances, private individuals acting on behalf of the firm may run the risk of legal liability.

Most regulatory statutes, including both the OSHAct and the TSCAct, contain criminal penalties for "knowing" or "willful" violations. These apply to any "person," including employees. For example, under the TSCAct, the knowing or willful failure to file a report or maintain records as required by the act can result in fines of up to $25,000 per day and up to one year imprisonment. Although these penalties apply only to knowing failure to comply, the U.S. Supreme Court has found that knowing failure to supervise compliance efforts properly can give rise to criminal penalties under the Food, Drug, and Cosmetic Act (U.S. v. Park, 1975).

Employees have a general duty to their employers to carry out their assigned functions with the exercise of due care. This is an implied term of their employment contract, which can give rise to legal liability running from the employee to the employer. For example, if a supervisory employee negligently fails to limit workplace exposures to a hazardous substance and this results in an OSHA citation and fine, the employer may be able to recover these damages from the employee. Similarly, an employer could recover for tort judgments against him or her that resulted from an employee's negligence.

Employees also have a general common law duty to exercise reasonable care toward their coemployees and toward the public in general. The condition of employment does not alter this responsibility. In the case of coemployees, for example, there may be a duty to warn of exposures to carcinogens or a duty on the part of a supervisory employee to comply with all relevant regulations for the protection of fellow workers. If the supervisory employee has special skills or knowledge (for example, if he or she were a toxicologist or biochemist), the duty may be more extensive than otherwise. For example, a chemist might be expected to recognize the danger of using benzene and be expected to do what is within his or her control to limit exposure of fellow employees. The fact that officers of the corporation may have ordered the supervisor not to comply with a standard or take protective action would not be a defense to a negligence action against him or her by an injured worker. The workers' compensation system, however, may provide a shield if it does not allow suits between fellow employees. This is the case in about two-thirds of the states.

The responsibilities of employees to consumers or the public rests on the same duty of reasonable care. For example, if it could be proved that an employee's negligence was responsible for a product defect, any injured consumer could sue that employee personally. Such suits are rare. This is because of the difficulty of proof they present and because the consumer also has a right of action against the employer, from whom recovery is likely to be easier. Suits against employees are not unheard of, however, particularly in the special circumstance under which the employee is responsible for performing acts on which the public safety depends (AmJur, Section 151), for example, checking for product defects.

V. RIGHTS OF EMPLOYEES, CONSUMERS, AND THE GENERAL PUBLIC

A. Rights Against Regulatory Agencies to Bring the Enforcement Machinery into Play

Regulatory legislation defines new legal duties that are imposed on employers and manufacturers. The legislation also provides for affected individuals, such as workers, consumers, or the general public, to actively participate in the setting and enforcement of standards, often through the taking of legal action to require the regulatory agencies to exercise their authority.

Employees can play an important role in facilitating the abatement of carcinogenic exposures. OSHA's limited enforcement personnel and difficulties in standard promulgation make employee involvement essential if protection from occupational carcinogens is to be achieved. The OSHAct provides employees with a number of rights. Important among these is the employee right to request an OSHA inspection. Any employee or employee representative who believes that a violation of a safety or health standard, or of the general duty obligation, has occurred which threatens physical harm or which is imminently dangerous, may request an inspection by OSHA in writing. A signed letter must be sent to OSHA detailing specific information about the alleged violation. OSHA gives a copy to the employer prior to the inspection, and the employee need not notify the employer of this request to OSHA. Moreover, the employee's name must be withheld by the secretary if the employee so requests. A special investigation must be made if the secretary determines that there are reasonable grounds to believe that a violation or danger exists. However, if the secretary finds that there are no reasonable grounds to believe that a violation exists, notification of this finding must be given to the complainant.

Other important rights of employees include limited participation in the monitoring of hazards and the right to have a representative accompany an OSHA inspector on his or her inspection. An employee may also sue the Department of Labor in certain circumstances. For example, suits have frequently been brought by labor groups to force OSHA to promulgate standards for carcinogens. In situations involving imminent danger which would reasonably be expected to cause death or serious physical harm, workers may also sue the secretary of labor for failing to obtain an injunction against the employer to eliminate the hazard (Occupational Safety and Health Act, Sec. 13, 1972). Exposure to high levels of carcinogens would certainly be deemed to be an "imminent danger." The difficulty with utilizing this section is that harmful exposures may continue until the two-step abatement process occurs. (See the discussion later in this section on the employee's right, under the OSHAct and labor law, to walk off the job when exposed to dangerous levels of carcinogens.)

Protection of employee rights under the OSHAct is provided in Sec. 11c, which prohibits discrimination against an employee for exercising his or her rights under the act. Thus, if an employer fires an employee for filing a complaint with OSHA because he or she believes that workplace exposure to carcinogens is hazardous, the employee can request OSHA to bring an action against the employer for reinstatement and back pay.

Consumers and the general public also have general rights under the CPSAct and the TSCAct to go to court to require CPSC and EPA to take appropriate protective action against carcinogenic and other risks. The TSCAct offers two mechanisms. Section 21 authorizes individuals to petition EPA to set standards, require testing, reporting, and so on. If EPA denies or fails to respond to the petition, the petitioners could bring a suit against the agency. The court can award the costs of the suit and attorneys' fees when appropriate. Workers or consumers concerned about occupational or consumer product exposures to carcinogens could find this authority useful in several ways. For example, they could petition EPA to ban a substance or set product-safety standards for carcinogens that would be most effectively regulated by such standards. (Note, however, that Sec. 21 authorizes the court to permit EPA to defer action on a petition if the court determines (1) that the risks alleged by the petitioners are less than those against which EPA is authorized to take action, and (2) that EPA has insufficient resources to act on the petitioners' request.) For substances believed to be suspect carcinogens, workers and consumers might petition EPA to require manufacturers to test the substances.

B. Rights to Privately Enforce Health, Safety, and Environmental Legislation

Employees are, of course, closely tied to the employer or manufacturer who uses or produces carcinogenic substances. It is understandable that the legal avenues they might pursue in seeking enforcement of the OSHAct are carefully defined, so as not to conflict with the extensive labor law governing management-labor relations. This may be one of the reasons that the OSHAct does not allow private individuals to enforce it or claim damages for its violation. Other statutes, however, do allow private enforcement to supplement the efforts of the government. The TSCAct (Sec. 20) allows any citizen to sue <u>any person</u> to require him or her to comply with the act (and its implementing regulations) or to restrain violations of it. The CPSAct (Sec. 23) goes even farther, allowing injured persons to collect monetary damages for violations of government product-safety rules in addition to allowing for private enforcement. These provisions can greatly increase the effectiveness of whatever carcinogen policies are adopted under these acts.

Under Sec. 20 of the TSCAct, petitioners may bring civil actions against <u>persons</u> violating the act and against EPA for failing to perform any nondiscretionary duty. Thus, if EPA had promulgated product-safety standards for certain carcinogens, <u>workers</u> could sue manufacturers and/or their employers, when appropriate, under the TSCAct for violating these standards, even if they could not do so under the OSHAct.

C. Rights to Sue for Damages Under Common Law

The establishment of a common law legal duty on the part of one person to exercise care toward another gives rise both to a corresponding right to enforce exercise of the duty and to a right to recover damages for its violation. The employer's duty to provide a safe workplace and the manufacturer's duty to make safe products were discussed in Sec. III.C. The ability of the tort system to translate theoretical rights into realities is particularly limited in the area of exposure to carcinogens. As a general principle, the plaintiff in a tort action must prove that there is a close causal connection (proximate cause) between the defendant's breach of legal duty and the harm complained of. Such proof is often impossible for cancer, because the disease typically has multiple causes and long latency periods. As a result, only a few workers (mostly in cases of asbestos exposure) have been able to meet the burden of proof necessary to gain recovery for occupational cancer, and almost no consumers have been able to do so. However, the common law does change, and these suits are becoming more commonplace. Increased suits, especially against supervisory personnel or product managers, may serve an important deterrent role in altering the practices of employees responsible for carcinogenic substances.

D. Rights to Injunctive Relief

Bringing an action to recover damages for harm caused by tortious conduct is only one way a consumer or worker can assert his or her legal rights. In addition, injunctive actions may be brought. In an injunctive action, the remedy requested is for the court to prevent harm before it occurs. For example, in one 1976 case in New Jersey, a company was ordered to prevent exposure to cigarette smoke in order to safeguard one employee's right to a safe and healthy workplace (Shimp v. New Jersey Bell Telephone Company, 1976). Injunctive actions face a variety of technical legal difficulties and have been quite uncommon in the tort area. Nevertheless, they may be used increasingly in the future as a means of enforcing various rights—for example, the right of a worker to have access to exposure data and medical records (Blumrosen et al., 1976). The reader may wish to refer to Sec. III.B, in which we discussed how disclosure requirements imposed on employers, manufacturers, and the government give rise to workers' and consumers' "right to know."

E. The Right to Refuse Hazardous Work

One of the most important protections employees have is the right to refuse work assignments when the assignment will expose them to harmful carcinogenic exposures (Ashford and Katz, 1977). As already discussed, workers may sue the Department of Labor to force it to obtain an injunction restraining employers from exposing them to "imminent hazards." However, if workers rely exclusively on this remedy, they will continue to obtain harmful exposures during the time it takes the courts and OSHA to act. (Furthermore, it is not clear how high exposures to carcinogens would need to be in order to meet the Sec. 13a test of an imminent hazard.) Clearly, the best recourse would be a right to refuse immediately the hazardous work assignment. However, without legal protection, the employee who refuses to work under these circumstances may be fired. This section discusses three legal mechanisms under labor law and the OSHAct that provide employees with the right to refuse hazardous work under certain limited circumstances.

1. Section 7 of the Labor Management Relations Act

Section 7 of the Labor Management Relations Act guarantees employees the right to engage in "concerted activities" for the purpose of collective bargaining or other mutual aid or protection. Concerted activities are protected by Sec. 8(a)(1) of the act, which forbids employers to interfere with employees' exercise of the Sec. 7 rights. Discharge of an employee or other discriminatory action taken by the employer would constitute an unfair labor practice. The National Labor Relations Board is empowered to prevent employers from engaging in such unfair practices and can force reinstatement of discharged employees with back pay.

Both nonunion and union employees whose collective bargaining agreements specifically exclude health and safety issues can be protected under Sec. 7 from employer reprisals for concerted activity of a work stoppage over unsafe conditions. (Walkoffs by a minority of union employees in derogation of the union and in conflict with the union's exclusive representation would not be protected by Sec. 7 (NLRB v. Sunbeam Lighting Co., 1963). Scrutiny need not be given to the nature or extent of the hazard over which a Sec. 7 health or safety walkout is concerned. The subjective belief that a condition is unsafe is all that is needed. Known carcinogens clearly meet this test; more importantly, because certainty of carcinogenicity is not required, workers could be protected from suspected carcinogens or substances for which data on carcinogenicity are not yet completely developed. Hence, workers fearful of carcinogenic exposure would receive protection from discrimination under Sec. 7 if they refused to work with potentially carcinogenic substances.

Individuals who walk off the job can still be protected under the doctrine of "concerted" activity if the individual is acting for the mutual benefit of other employees (NLRB v. Interbow Contractors, Inc., 1967, NLRB v. C & I Air Conditioning, Inc., 1973, Shelly and Anderson Furniture Co., Inc. v. NLRB, 1974). Interest of fellow workers in the work stoppage would be evidence of a concerted purpose.

2. Section 502 of the Labor Management Relations Act

In addition to the "concerted activities" protected under Secs. 7 and 8, Sec. 502 of the Labor Management Relations Act explicitly protects workers who refuse work because of abnormally dangerous working conditions:

> nor shall the quitting of labor by an employee or employees in good faith because of abnormally dangerous working conditions for work at the place of employment be deemed a strike under this Act.

This section is useful for activities not covered under Sec. 7, specifically actions by organized workers subject to collective bargaining agreements which (1) have not explicitly excluded health and safety issues from arbitration, and/or (2) contain a no-strike clause. However, the situations in which workers could refuse to work for fear of exposure to harmful levels of carcinogens is more limited under Sec. 502. In contrast to Sec. 7, the exposures must be "abnormally dangerous." Thus, if exposures to harmful levels of carcinogens not regulated by standards are normal for the job, a work stoppage would not be protected (Anaconda Aluminum, 1972). Furthermore, the test of "abnormal danger" is an objective test determined by the National Labor Relations Board (Redwing Carriers, 1961). Thus, employees risk penalties if their judgment regarding the extent of the hazard and the increase in the risk differs from that of the board.

3. Section 11c of the OSHAct

OSHA has interpreted the OSHAct to include a limited right to refuse hazardous work to union and nonunion workers alike. OSHA regulations state:

> occasions might arise when an employee is confronted with a choice between not performing assigned tasks or subjecting himself to serious injury or death arising from a hazardous condition at the workplace. If the employee, with no reasonable alternative, refuses in good faith to expose himself to the dangerous condition, he would be protected against subsequent discrimination. The condition causing the employee's apprehension of death or injury must be of such a nature that a reasonable person, under the circumstances then confronting the employee, would conclude that there is a real danger of death or serious injury and that there is insufficient time, due to the urgency of the situation, to eliminate the danger through resort to regular statutory enforcement channels. In addition, in such circumstances, the employee, where possible, must also have sought from his employer, and been unable to obtain, a correction of the dangerous condition [29 C.F.R. 1977.12(b)(2)].

If an employer discriminated against an employee who came within the scope of protection of these regulations, OSHA could seek relief in court under Sec. 11c to have the employee reinstated with back pay.

The Sec. 11c protection would appear to be most useful to unionized workers whose activities would not be protected under Sec. 7 of the Labor Management Relations Act. The Sec. 11c standard is, in some respects, less stringent than that available under Sec. 502. Section 11c could offer protection to workers engaged in inherently dangerous activities (continuous or frequent exposure to dangerous levels of carcinogens) who would not be protected by the "abnormally dangerous" standard under Sec. 502. In addition, the "reasonable men" standard for determining danger under Sec. 11c is conceivably less stringent than the objective standard set forth in Section 502, although the case has not yet been litigated.

However, in certain situations, Sec. 502 may offer greater protection to the unionized worker than Sec. 11c. For example, if the workplace carcinogens are governed by an OSHA standard and environmental monitoring equipment has been installed, a worker who one day notices the monitor revealing exposures greatly in excess of the standard would have objective proof that abnormally dangerous conditions exist. Under Sec. 502, the worker could immediately walk off the job and be protected. However, under Sec. 11c, he or she would have had to (1) try to contact the employer to obtain abatement, and (2) determine that there was insufficient time to eliminate the danger through the normal administrative process.

The validity of the Sec. 11c regulations was upheld by the Supreme Court in a unanimous opinion in Whirlpool Corporation v. Marshall (1980). (See Ashford and Katz, 1977 for a fuller discussion.)

F. Using Collective Bargaining to Reduce Workplace Exposures to Carcinogens

Collective bargaining may provide unionized employees with more protection from health and safety dangers than underbudgeted OSHA efforts in some instances. The OSHAct has been important in providing a basis for union demands that basic safety and health standards be included in collective bargaining contracts. Prior to the OSHAct, collective bargaining did not adequately focus on or protect employee safety and health. Safety and health issues had low priority on the bargaining agenda and were often bartered for more pressing objectives. Recent developments indicate that this unfortunate state of affairs may now be changing for the better, due in large measure to the stimulus provided by the OSHAct.

The number of union contracts including health and safety clauses has increased substantially in recent years. In a recent summary, occupational safety and health provisions appeared in 82% of the sample contracts, compared to 65% in the 1970 study (Kelley, unpublished). Among the provisions included are sophisticated procedures for the resolution of safety and health disputes; specification of standards for particular problems; periodic company or consultant inspections for health hazards; requirements that the company inform workers of the generic names and toxicity, if known, of chemicals in the plant; environmental monitoring rights for the union; support for research into occupational health hazards; provisions for worker safety training; union involvement in work practices; engineering controls to minimize health hazards; and provisions for payment of wages for time lost due to injury or presence of a health hazard. Any of these provisions would be useful for controlling occupational carcinogens. Workers could use the collective bargaining process to obtain protection from carcinogens not yet regulated by OSHA or other agencies. In addition, by incorporating existing OSHA standards into the collective bargaining agreement, the worker obtains a new mechanism for enforcement. The employer's failure to comply with the standard would, thus, constitute a breach of contract. Thus, in addition to OSHA enforcement actions, the union could file a grievance for violation of the contract. If the employer continues to refuse to abate the hazard, the union (or individual workers) can resort to the National Labor Relations Board for relief. In the case of extremely hazardous conditions, the union may wish to take advantage of Sec. 301 of the National Labor Relations Act and seek an injunction from the U.S. District Court for immediate abatement as required by adherence to the contract.

The discussion in Sec. V.E.3 highlighted some of the difficulties in obtaining protection for workers who refuse to perform hazardous work through provisions of the OSHAct and labor law. One remedy for these problems would be to insert a specific provision in the collective bargaining agreement to protect workers who refuse to perform hazardous work. If employees are discriminated against for walking off the job when subject to dangerous exposures to carcinogens, the unions can bring an action for reinstatement and back pay on behalf of workers under Sec. 301 of the Labor Management Relations Act.

VI. ETHICAL CONSIDERATIONS

The discussion in this chapter has focused on the legal duties and rights of government, manufacturers, employers, employees, consumers, and the general public. It is clear that the regulatory machinery is responding to the problems of chemical carcinogens very slowly. Many substances that undoubtedly will be regulated are not yet regulated. Thus, while technically no legal responsibility may exist for the various parties to act, a case can be made for an ethical responsibility. It is hoped that the reader is persuaded of the serious nature of human exposure to carcinogens and of the existence of a moral obligation to reduce that exposure whenever possible, independent of the existence of a legal responsibility or liability.

REFERENCES

AFL-CIO v. Brennan, 530 F.2d 109 (3rd Cir., 1975).

American Conference of Governmental Industrial Hygienists (1978). Threshold Limit Values of Airborne Contaminants and Physical Agents With Intended Changes Adopted by ACGIH for 1978, Cincinnati, Ohio.

American Iron and Steel Institute et al. v. OSHA, 577 F.2d 825 (3rd Cir., 1978).

American Jurisprudence, Master and Servant, Sec. 451.

American Petroleum Institute v. OSHA, 6 OSHC 1959 (5th Cir., 1978).

American Smelting and Refining Co. v. OSHRC, 501 F.2d 504, 511 (8th Cir., 1974).

Anaconda Aluminum, 197 NLRB 336 (1972).

Aqua Slide 'n' Dive Corp. v. CPSC, 569 F.2d 831 (1978).

Arthur v. Flota Mercante Gran Centro Americana, S.A., 487 F.2d 561 (5th Cir., 1973).

Ashford, N. A. (1976). Crisis in the Workplace: Occupational Disease and Injury. MIT Press, Cambridge, Mass., p. 154.

Ashford, N. A., and Katz, Jr. (1977). Unsafe working conditions: employee rights under the labor management relations act and the occupational safety and health act. Notre Dame Lawyer (52)802.

Ashford, N. A., Zolt, E. M., Hattis, D., Katz, J., Heaton, G. R., and Priest, W. C. (1979). Evaluating chemical regulations: trade-off analysis and impact assessment for environmental decision-making. Final report to the Council on Environmental Quality and the U.S. Environmental Protection Agency, Contract No. EQ4ACA35, Center for Policy Alternatives, Cambridge, Mass.

Blumrosen, P., Ackerman, D., Kligerman, J., VanSchaick, P., and Sheehy, K. (1976). Injunctions against occupational hazards: the right to work under safe conditions. Calif. L. Rev. 64:702.

Clean Air Act, 42 U.S.C. 7401 et seq. (1970).

Clean Water Act (Federal Water Pollution Control Act), 33 U.S.C. 1251 et seq. (1972).

29 Code of Federal Regulations 1910.1003-1016.

29 Code of Federal Regulations 1910.1017.

29 Code of Federal Regulations 1910.1018.

29 Code of Federal Regulations 1910.1028.

29 Code of Federal Regulations 1910.1045.

29 Code of Federal Regulations 1977.12(b)(2).

Community Mental Health Centers Act, amendments, PL 95-622, Sec. 62(b)(4) (1978).

Consumer Product Safety Act, PL 92-573 (October 27, 1972), amended in PL 94-284, May 11, 1978.

Dow Chemical v. CPSC, 459 F. Supp. 378 (W.D. La., 1978).

E. I. Dupont de Nemours and Co. v. Finklea, 422 F. Supp. 821 (D.C. W. Va., 1977).

42 Federal Register 5372, January 28, 1977.

42 Federal Register 54148, October 4, 1977.

43 Federal Register 25658, June 13, 1978.

43 Federal Register 31371, July 21, 1978.

44 Federal Register 23821, April 23, 1979.

Finklea, J. F. (1977). Monitoring of industrial workers exposed to carcinogens. Hearings before the Subcommittee on Labor of the Committee on Human Resources of the U.S. Senate, May 9.

Food and Drug Administration (1977). Structural correlates of carcinogenicity and mutagenecity. Summer Symposium, Office of Science, Washington, D.C.

General Motors Corp. v. Finklea 6 OSHC 1976 (S.D. Ohio, 1978).

Harris, L. (1979). Private communication. Occupational Safety and Health Administration, Washington, D.C.

Health Services Research, Health Statistics, and Health Care Technology Act, PL 95-623 (1978).

International Agency for Research on Cancer (1971). Monographs on the evaluation of carcinogenic risk of chemicals to man. From IARC Working Group on the Evaluation of the Carcinogenic Risk of Chemicals to Man, 13-17 December, Geneva, Switzerland. (Vol. 1, Lyon, France, 1971.)

Kelley, T. (year). Recent contractural developments in safety and health. Unpublished paper.

Labor Management Relations Act, PL80-101 (1947), as amended by PL 86-257 (1959) and PL 93-360 (1974).

Long, J. R. (1975). Tighter safety rules ahead for academic labs. Chem. Eng. News July 14, p. 21.

Mason, T. J., McKay, F., Hoover, R., Blot, W. J., and Fraumeni, J. F. (1975). Atlas of cancer mortality for U.S. counties: 1950-1969. DHEW Publication No. (NIH)75-780, U.S. Government Printing Office, Washington, D.C.

Morsch, W. (1978). Use of social security data for analysis of occupational disease. Report to assistant secretary of labor for policy evaluation and research, July 7, Washington, D.C.

National Cancer Institute (1978). Estimates of the fraction of cancer in the United States related to occupational factors. National Institute of Environmental Health Sciences, National Institute for Occupational Safety and Health, September 15, Washington, D.C.

National Institute for Occupational Safety and Health (1974). National occupational hazard survey. DHEW Publication No. (NIOSH)74-127, U.S. Government Printing Office, Washington, D.C.

National Institute for Occupational Safety and Health (1978). Program of the national institute for occupational safety and health—program plans by program area for FY1979. DHEW Publication No. (NIOSH)79-103, October, U.S. Government Printing Office, Washington, D.C.

National Labor Relations Board v. C & I Air Conditioning, Inc., 486 F.2d 977 (9th Cir., 1973).

National Labor Relations Board v. Interbow Contractors, Inc., 388 F.2d 495 (2nd Cir., 1967).

National Labor Relations Board v. Sunbeam Lighting Co., 318 F.2d 661 (7th Cir., 1963).

National Realty and Construction Co. v. OSHRC, 489 F.2d 1257, 1265-66 (D.C. Cir., 1973).

Occupational Safety and Health Act, PL 91-596 (1972).

Occupational Safety and Health Reporter (1976). 6 (9):268.

Occupational Safety and Health Reporter (1978). Current report. October 12:536, 662-664.

Polaroid Corporation v. Costle, 11 ERC 2134 (D.C. Mass., 1978).

Redwing Carriers, 130 NLRB 1208 (1961).

Resource Conservation and Recovery Act, 42 U.S.C. 6901 et seq. (1976).

Reynolds Metals Co. (OSHRC), 6 OSHC 1667 (1978).

Rothstein, M. A. (1978). Occupational Safety and Health Law. West, St. Paul, Minn.

Safe Drinking Water Act, PL 93-523 (1974), as amended by PL 95-190 (1977).

Science (1979). How to assess cancer risks. 204:811.

Shelly and Anderson Furniture Co., Inc. v. NLRB, 497 F.2d 1202 (1974).

Shimp v. New Jersey Bell Telephone Co., 145 N.J. Super. 516, 368 A.2d 408 (1976).

Society of the Plastics Industry v. OSHA, 509 F.2d 1301 (2d Cir., 1975).

Southern Railway Co., 20 OSHRC 691, 30 OSHC 1657 (1975).

Subcommittee on Trade Secrets and Confidentiality of the Toxic Substances Strategy Committee (1978). Initial report, June 14, Washington, D.C.

Testimony and Budget Justification (1977). Hearings before the House Appropriations Subcommittee, U.S. Departments of Labor and Health, Education, and Welfare, Washington, D.C.

Toxic Substances Control Act, 15 U.S.C. 2601 et seq. (1976).

U.S. Code Cong. & Admin. News 5180, S. Rep. No. 91-1282, 91st Cong., 2d Sess. (1970).

U.S. Department of Health, Education, and Welfare (1976). NIOSH toxic substances list. DHEW Publication No. (NIOSH)76-207, June, U.S. Government Printing Office, Washington, D.C.

U.S. Department of Health, Education, and Welfare (1975). Survey of compounds which have been tested for carcinogenic activity. DHEW/PHS Public Health Service Report No. 149, U.S. Government Printing Office, Washington, D.C.

U.S. Department of Housing and Urban Development (1979). Independent Agencies Appropriation for 1979, hearings before a subcommittee on appropriations, U.S. House of Representatives, Budget Request and Justification, Washington, D.C.

U.S. v. McGee Industries, 439 F. Supp. 296 (D.C. Pa., 1977).

U.S. v. Park, 421 U.S. 658 (1975).

Whirlpool Corporation v. Marshall, 100 S.Ct. 883 (1980).

Zener, R. B. (1977). The toxic substances control act: federal regulation of commercial chemicals. The Business Lawyer 30:1185.

4

Safety and Control Implications of Industrial Carcinogens

NEIL B. JURINSKI* / Tracor Jitco, Inc., Rockville, Maryland
DONALD V. LASSITER† / Environmental Health Associates, Berkeley, California

I. INTRODUCTION

Health risk associated with the manufacture or use of carcinogenic substances has become one of the most controversial issues in private and public life today. This issue reaches into every sector of our environment, including home products, workplace chemicals, food and drugs ingested, water supplies, and the air we breathe. Existence of carcinogenic substances

---

Present affiliation:
*NuChemCo, Inc., Burke, Virginia
†Consultant, Environmental/Occupational Health, San Jose, California

in the workplace, whether in a manufacturing process, in a disposal process, or perhaps, only in a laboratory facility designed to perform experimental animal testing to determine carcinogenicity of chemical substances, ensures the possibility of human exposure to such substances. Hence, it is absolutely essential that methods and techniques to minimize such possibilities of exposure be developed.

As research into cancer cause and prevention continues, our knowledge increases regarding the frequency and distribution of cancer occurrence. There is an increasing body of evidence that distribution by occupation or geography of certain types of cancer may provide clues to specific etiologic agents [1]. This concept is further reinforced when the cancer statistics by county [2] are analyzed or examined graphically by mapping techniques [3].

The variety of causative agents suspected of initiating cancer are multitudinous and include foods, chemicals, viruses, and physical agents such as radioactivity and ultraviolet radiation. Development of safe work practices and environmentally acceptable discharge procedures presents a constant challenge.

Control processes and procedures developed to meet this challenge must begin with organized approaches to evaluation of the carcinogencity of specific substances and the opportunities that exist throughout the environment for possible exposures. Such an evaluation process should be applied to both the occupational and the environmental sphere of operations. There is no prevailing reason to distinguish between the acute toxic property of a substance and its carcinogenic properties in conducting such a hazard evaluation. An example of the type of systematic approach to be employed is presented in Fig. 1, which illustrates an occupational hazard evaluation system flowchart. By performing the operations illustrated, one may survey the status of compliance with safe practices in an occupational situation. This procedure allows documentation of carcinogenic hazards, along with toxic and physical hazards, and enables early recognition of those work sites and work operations that should be given a high level of scrutiny. It is essential in development of a sound control program that particular attention be given to the total control problem to avoid unnecessary concentration on relatively minor problem areas.

Control of chemical substances considered to be carcinogenic has been largely voluntary until passage of the Occupational Safety and Health Act of 1970 (OSHAct) and subsequent regulations promulgated under the authority of this act. Hence, in the years prior to passage of the act, although the federal Food and Drug Administration (FDA) had been active in establishing standards regulating additives to food, drugs, and cosmetics with regard to possible carcinogenic activity, and although the Environmental Protection Agency (EPA) possessed authority under several of its statutory provisions to regulate chemicals in the environment, it was only in 1972 that stringent exposure controls were established for certain chemical substances manufactured or used in the workplace. Prior to that time only the State of Pennsylvania had established stringent guidelines with respect to chemical substances believed to be carcinogenic. However, widespread attention to the presence of carcinogenic substances in the general workplace environment became of considerable importance only with promulgation, in 1972, of emergency temporary standards regulating occupational exposure to 14 chemical substances by the Occupational Safety and Health Administration (OSHA):

1. 2-Acetylaminofluorene
2. 4-Aminodiphenyl
3. Benzidine
4. 3,3'-Dichlorobenzidine
5. 4-Dimethylaminoazobenzene
6. Alpha-naphthylamine
7. Beta-naphthylamine
8. 4-Nitrobiphenyl
9. N-Nitrosodimethylamine
10. Beta-propiolactone
11. Bis(chloromethyl) ether
12. Chloromethyl methyl ether
13. 4,4'-Methylene-bis(2-chloroaniline)
14. Ethyleneimine

Many questions of both scientific and political natures were raised during the rule-making procedures for regulatory control of the 14 chemical substances. A similar situation surrounded promulgation of an emergency temporary standard for vinyl chloride several years later. A central feature of these questions or concepts was a report to the Surgeon General of the U.S. Public Health Service in 1970 (prepared by the Ad Hoc Committee on the Evaluation of Low Levels of Environmental Chemical Carcinogens). Conclusions contained in the report addressed such considerations as tumor latency, dose response, and extrapolation of findings produced in experimental animals to humans. Although the scientific controversy concerning initiation of carcinogenesis had been in progress for some time, it was primarily the impetus of the Occupational Safety and Health Act, with its mandate to protect workers from all health hazards, that set in motion the train of events that today has embroiled health agencies, labor, industry, and the federal courts in long, and often protracted, legal battles. At stake is the answer to the question of how one decides that a given chemical substance represents a carcinogenic hazard for exposed humans.

A variety of schemes have been developed by various authors in attempts to classify relative carcinogenicity of chemical substances that may be present in the workplace. Examples of such classification schemes include those developed by Eckardt [4], Hueper and Conway [5], the ACGIH [6], Dinmann [7], Cole and Goldman [8], Rose [9], and recently by Lassiter [10]. Most of these schemes attempt to weigh carcinogenic hazard or risk in terms of perceived carcinogenicity. This quantity-perceived carcinogenicity can be an important consideration in development of control measures for chemical substances based on degree of such carcinogenicity. Simple stated, this concept dictates establishment of at least minimal control of any chemical substance considered to possess biologic activity in the oncogenic sense, and would require extremely stringent exposure control for substances possessing considerable such activity. The objective of a system of exposure controls based on a classification scheme of perceived carcinogenicity is to ensure that proper consideration, in terms of necessary exposure controls, is given to any substance demonstrating oncogenic properties and not to limit such considerations only to highly carcinogenic substances.

In the United States the practical situation concerned with industrial control of occupational exposures to carcinogenic substances is mediated both by regulatory standards promulgated by OSHA and by voluntarily established controls developed by the affected industry itself. Hence, in the case of substances or processes regulated by mandatory standards, industry has little leeway except to abide by such standards. In the case of chemical substances which industry, itself, may consider to possess oncogenic activity, but which are not presently regulated by legal standards, industry has the option of providing controls consistent with degree of perceived carcinogenic hazard or of waiting for mandatory standards to take effect. Although the latter situation was once commonplace, industry would be hard pressed today to explain why appropriate action was not taken to protect exposed employees on recognition that certain chemical substances, previously considered safe were now, for whatever reason, considered to possess carcinogenic activity.

In previous years the initial indication that a particular chemical substance posed carcinogenic risk for humans was usually based on results of an epidemiologic investigation of an exposed worker population. This fact can be appreciated when one reviews the various lists of "known" or "recognized" human carcinogens developed by organizations such as the National Cancer Institute (NCI) and the International Agency for Research on Cancer (IARC). Of the many chemicals that have been associated with human cancers, only a very small number are so intimately related that there is general agreement concerning their human carcinogenicity. Many other chemicals are associated with human cancers on the basis of positive results obtained from experimental animal investigations and, perhaps, less definitive observations of increased cancer risk in exposed worker populations. In this context, then, the role of experimental animal investigations, including the bioassay of suspected carcinogenic substances, is one of creating an early awareness of the possibility of carcinogenic hazard to humans. Similarly, mutagenicity testing procedures likewise may provide an even earlier indication of possible carcinogenic risk.

In instances in which either animal experimentation or epidemiologic investigations provide substantive evidence that workers exposed to specific chemical substances or particular processes may be at excess risk of cancer because of such exposure, the responsibility

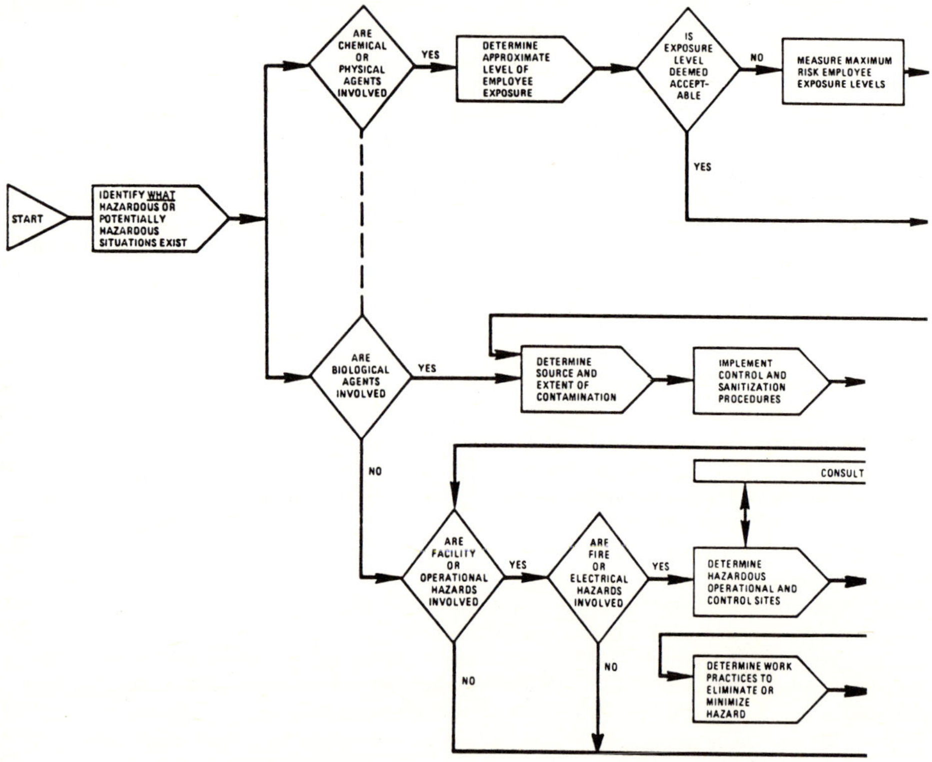

FIGURE 1 Occupational hazard evaluation system. EL, exposure level; AL, action level; PEL, permissible exposure level; SOP, standard operating procedure.

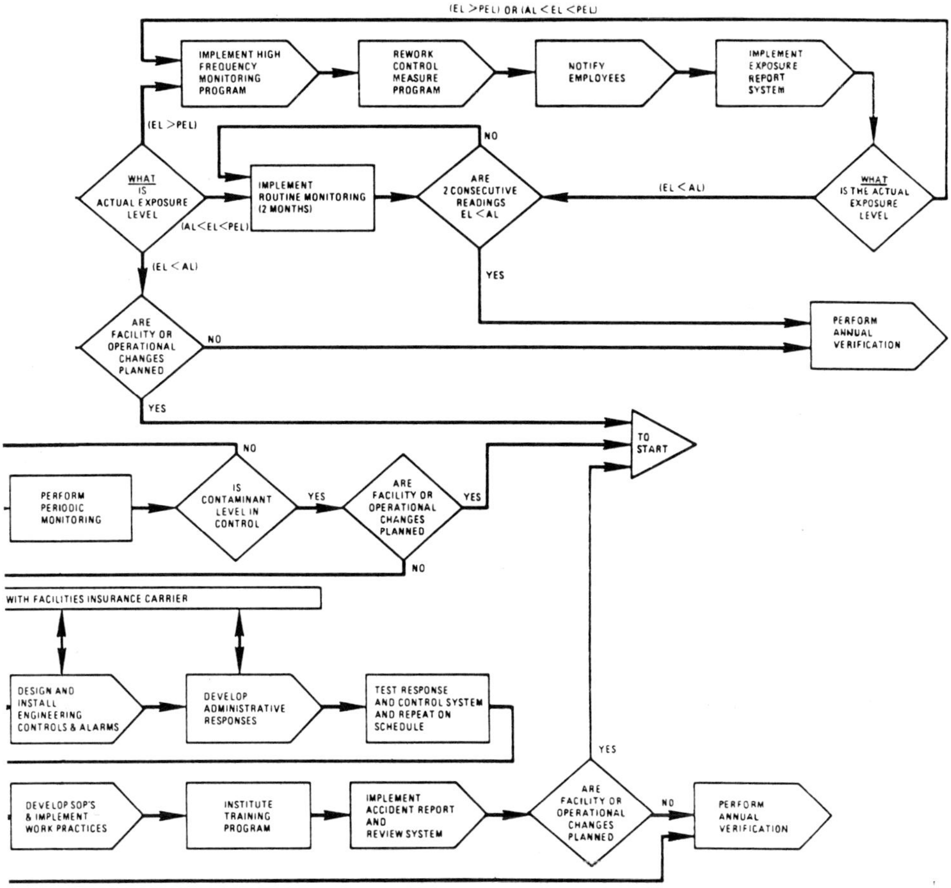

FIGURE 1 (continued)

of employers and regulatory agencies to control exposures is clear. In the case of the OSHAct of 1970, control measures required by OSHA under the act have as their primary objective control of worker exposure to a defined chemical substance or group of substances. Hence, regulatory control of occupational exposures to such substances as asbestos, various aromatic amines, arsenic, vinyl chloride, bis(chloromethyl)ether, and benzene, in the United States and elsewhere, represent examples of control of specific chemical substances based, primarily, on epidemiologic evidence.

Problems associated with hazard evaluations involving long latency periods, or with pure versus mixed chemical exposure histories of workers, often have effectively served to mask individual agents of etiology such that regulatory and research agencies, alike, frequently will be required to utilize a "black box" approach in development of exposure control methodologies. Under such circumstances the workplace can be evaluated in much the same manner as the "black box" approach to problem-solving utilized by the physical scientist and engineer, in which definitive resolution of inputs resulting in an observed output may not be possible prior to complete understanding of the various mechanisms that are at work inside the "black box." In this example, outputs of the "black box," which affect workers in their occupational environment, may include observation of normally, rare tumors or of increases in observed to expected ratios of more common tumors in an exposed worker population.

The classic examples of scrotal cancer among chimney sweeps and of urinary bladder tumors in dyestuffs workers exposed to a variety of aromatic amines, as well as the more recent examples of excess lung cancer among coke oven workers [11] and chloromethylation workers [12] amply illustrate the necessity of exposure controls even when a state of contemporary ignorance may exist concerning agents of definitive etiology. In such situations controls must be process or activity oriented on a scale sufficiently broad to include all suspected agents of etiology. Thus, in the example of worker exposure to coke oven emissions, it was not necessary for OSHA to undertake the task of defining etiology in order to require control of hazardous exposures, although for research agencies such tasks may be of high-priority concern. Naturally, this conceptual approach to regulatory control of exposure to occupational carcinogens on an industry or process basis does not begin to detail the complexities and problems associated with such attendant matters as (1) the scientific and legal basis of proposed regulations, (2) methodologies for engineering controls, (3) sampling and analytical technology, (4) componments of medical surveillance programs, or (5) even the growing field of what has been labeled "political oncology."

At a time when concepts of dose-response relationships, of animal-to-human extrapolations, and of "safe" levels of exposure determinations represent the principal concerns for establishing "thresholds" of tumorgenic response in man, one threshold that is commonly overlooked is the threshold for regulatory activity.

This approach embodies the principle of risk minimization, and it allows a regulatory agency a wide policy range in developing standards by assuring that practically any standard promulgated will, to some degree, accomplish the objective by minimizing risk of cancer for all workers covered by the standard, assuming, of course, the existence of an operative dose-response relationship. An additional advantage of this regulatory concept is that the scientific evidence necessary to support rule-making on the basis of industry or process control may be the results of a single epidemiologic investigation—if such an investigation is scientifically and statistically valid.

Although full application of this regulatory concept would possibly result in promulgation of a large number of regulations designed to minimize recognized cancer risks, and although most of such regulations would provide, perhaps, for only a minimum of exposure controls, medical surveillance, and employee exposure monitoring, this situation would be far more preferable to one of uncontrolled exposures. The concept is also consistent with application of present knowledge concerning the scope and nature of occupationally related cancer and with the spirit and intent of the OSHAct of 1970. In any event, it is paramount that during the regulatory process those chemicals or processes being considered for regulatory control are clearly specified in order that specific regulatory control measures can be tailored to the circumstances of exposure and are not simply generically mandated based on broad concepts of carcinogenicity for ease of promulgation.

II. OCCUPATIONAL PROCEDURES AND WORK PRACTICES

A. Hazard Recognition Program

The key aspect of any program dealing with hazard recognition lies in the organization of the hazard search. Observing a potential hazard is not the same as recognizing it as such. Many times the eye of an experienced observer will identify a hazard which occupants in the area do not consider to be unsafe. Alternatively, a person who has performed a task repeatedly may be aware of hidden hazards that the visiting observer will not detect. Thus, it becomes imperative in developing a hazard recognition program to include both types of observers.

1. Inventory of Hazards

A formalized detailed hazard inventory should be planned for any workplace that is handling carcinogenic materials. This program should be structured such that persons having no special expertise in control technology can participate. The basic data required include listing for each operation potential carcinogenic exposures and the number of persons considered to be at risk. Once such an inventory of potential exposures has been developed for a facility, it can be distributed to employees in various work areas for them to correlate with whatever operations they perform. Such exposure data, once obtained, then can provide the basis for considering what engineering controls, protective devices, work practices, and types of medical surveillance are needed for persons in the various areas. Such data can also identify the magnitude of problem areas requiring resolutions on a priority basis.

Figure 2 presents an example of a chemical hazards coding form which has been used for an inventory of operations in laboratories performing cancer research programs [13]. Each of the entries (except for numerical answers) was obtained from a collection of precoded possibilities. In actual practice the workers in the separate laboratory areas performed an initial compilation of operations with associated exposures, and also completed the other information indicated. After this initial survey was compiled, the data were used as the basis for a verification survey by a professionally trained individual. This procedure permitted addressing the most pressing problems first and effected a more efficient utilization of this person's time.

2. Estimation of Exposures

The extent of exposure to hazardous chemical substances and physical/biologic agents can vary markedly among individuals. Routes of exposure to chemical substances include inhalation of contaminated air, absorption through skin, and ingestion via food, drink, cosmetics, or smoking materials. Personal work habits of individuals can alter by factors of 10-100 the actual exposure to a workplace contaminant. Simple variations in laboratory procedures, such as the position of the head or the lack of skill in pouring, exemplify aberrations in personal work practices which should be observed. A qualitative estimate of an individual's exposure, thus, can be very imprecise, and one must rely on actual samples of air from the workers' breathing zone to have a valid measure of the true exposure.

Sampling and analysis of contaminant levels to obtain data on worker exposures fall into the domain of industrial hygiene. A comprehensive discussion of this area is beyond the scope of this chapter, and the reader is referred to any of the numerous works on this topic. Recent work by Leidel et al. [14] has attempted to increase the statistical reliability of results associated with the selected sampling strategy. Of primary concern is the necessity of maintaining complete records of accuracy of the entire sampling and analysis procedure.

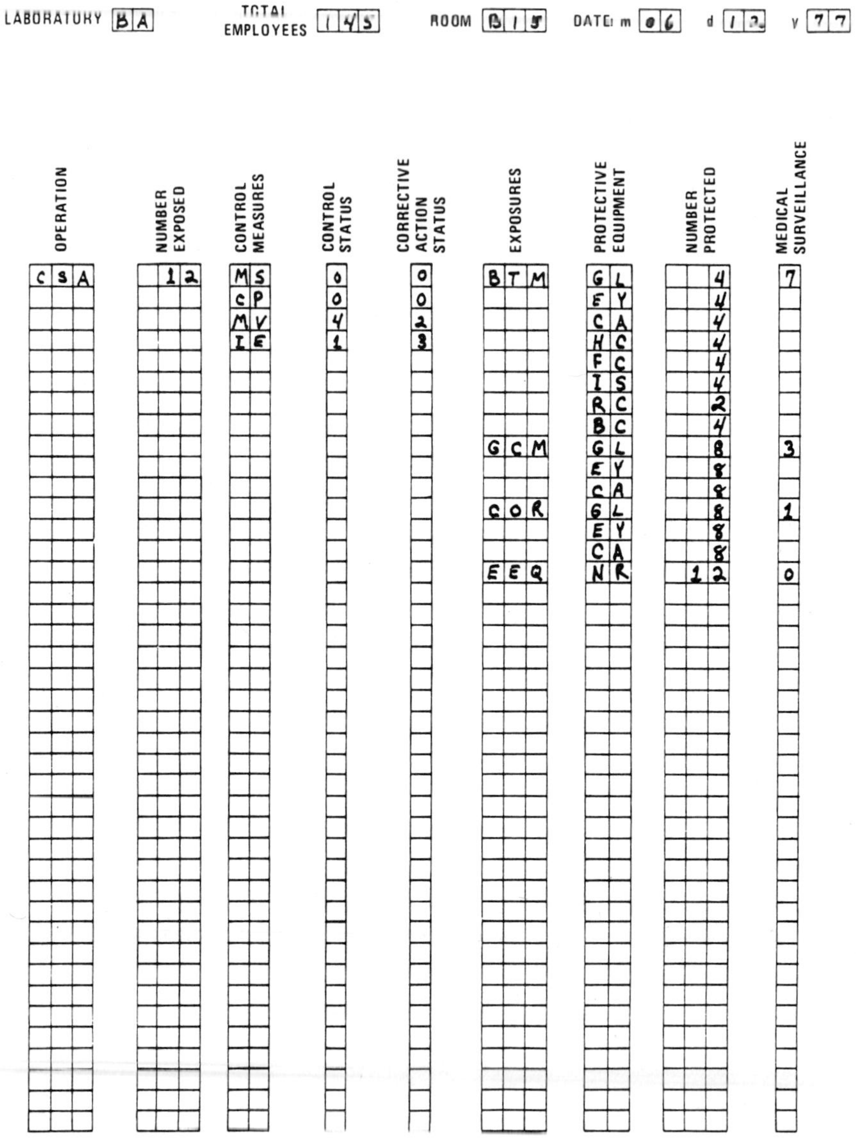

LABORATORY BA TOTAL EMPLOYEES 145 ROOM B15 DATE m 06 d 12 y 77

OPERATION	NUMBER EXPOSED	CONTROL MEASURES	CONTROL STATUS	CORRECTIVE ACTION STATUS	EXPOSURES	PROTECTIVE EQUIPMENT	NUMBER PROTECTED	MEDICAL SURVEILLANCE
CSA	12	MS	0	0	BTM	GL	4	7
		CP	0	0		EY	4	
		MV	4	2		CA	4	
		IE	1	3		HC	4	
						FC	4	
						IS	4	
						RC	2	
						BC	4	
					GCM	GL	8	3
						EY	8	
						CA	8	
					COR	GL	8	1
						EY	8	
						CA	8	
					EEQ	NR	12	0

FIGURE 2 Worker hazard inventory program.

B. Hazard Control Program

Once a hazard has been recognized, it becomes essential to determine the extent to which it is controlled, that is, the extent of exposure risk associated with the hazard. The process of separating a carcinogen from potentially exposed persons forms the basis for control technology and may be accomplished by administrative procedures, engineering techniques, protective equipment, or a combination of these techniques.

1. Relative Severity Ranking

A number of factors should be considered in establishing priorities for resolution of the identified hazards. Data on many of these factors can be accumulated during performance of a hazard inventory. Both the number of persons potentially exposed to a chemical substance as well as the number of the potentially exposed persons who have and use protective equipment should be ascertained. The difference in these two numbers is the number of persons potentially exposed, yet unprotected.

It is also necessary to estimate the probability that a potential exposure event could actually occur. Development of such an estimate involves consideration of many risk factors, including equipment malfunction, human error, natural events such as wind damage, floods, and so on. In addition, attempt should be made to rank the importance of the occurrence of these probabilities.

A final factor requiring consideration is an estimate of the severity of consequences of various exposures. Here the aspect of reversibility of effects or the treatability of symptoms is evaluated. The current status of knowledge concerning cancer cause and treatment makes it difficult to rank severity; however, the concept can be perceived by analogy with other toxic effects that may be lethal or nonlethal, and which may exhibit a no-effect exposure threshold.

Once the three factors, (1) number of unprotected people, (2) probability of event, and (3) severity of consequences, have been determined for all the types of operations and exposures in a facility,* it becomes possible to compare the hazards associated with each on a common basis. This procedure often requires a subjective evaluation based on scientific knowledge, assessment of risk, and many imponderables.

2. Control Technology Effectiveness

The previously described exercise allows one to establish a ranked order of hazards. Ameliorative control strategies must then address the question of comparing the effectiveness of various engineering techniques, work practices, and training methods conceived to reduce the hazard. Answers should be obtained for the following questions: (1) How long would it take to implement the control measure? (2) What would be the change in the number of persons exposed? (3) What would be the cost of implementing the control? (4) What would be the reduction in probability of occurrence and duration of exposure? (5) What would be the reduction in concentration during exposure? The answers to these questions can assist in establishing the magnitude of an increase in personnel protection which could be accomplished within a given time period by expenditure of a certain level of financial resources. By comparing different combinations of control measures it should become evident how to maximize the effectiveness of the Hazard Control Program through allocation of available resources.

C. Medical Surveillance Program

The difficulties that surround the establishment of effective medical surveillance are primarily attributable to the dearth of adequate diagnostic procedures with predictive capability.

---

*For purposes of this discussion, exposure refers to any exposure, irrespective of concentration, that is, a zero-exposure concept. If actual concentrations are considered, another factor is introduced.

Many forms of cancer are known to have extremely long latency periods prior to appearance of identifiable clinical symptoms. Until such time as medically acceptable predictive tests can be developed, there will exist an unknown element of risk for anyone exposed.

It is definitely essential to establish an individual's physical status prior to exposure to obtain a baseline reference point for various physiologic indicators of medical significance. Medical findings in future physical examinations can then be related to a common basis for comparison.

The type of medical testing employed should be patterned to detect abnormality in a target organ such as urinary bladder exfoliate cytology, sputum cytology, respiratory function analysis, liver function analysis, and so on, as appropriate.

D. Administrative Control Program

The use of recognized or suspected carcinogens within an industrial environment requires a high degree of administrative control in addition to engineering and personal control systems. The basis for the administrative control program should be establishment of a system to account for the total quantity of material, its distribution throughout the use cycle, and those persons with access and/or exposure to the material.

1. Material Balance Records

A material inventory system should be developed for each recognized or suspected carcinogen manufactured or used (as opposed to a process intermediate, which is consumed as it is produced). This inventory should be similar in nature to systems commonly in use which provide accountability for precious metals, radioactive isotopes, ethyl alcohol, narcotics, and so on. The inventory should identify all users, the quantity and intent each of use, and physical locations where the substance is in use. This inventory will provide a check on the medical surveillance program to ensure that persons actually using the carcinogen, or in a location where the material is being used, are included in a medical testing program appropriate to their activity and possible exposure. For those operations in which an existing inventory control system for products is in effect, this system should not be difficult to implement and can probably be incorporated within existing programs.

The final item of the inventory control system involved identification of process losses and discharge points. These two items will provide an assessment of workplace exposure and environmental discharge exposure. Monthly maintenance of these inventory records can serve to establish the degree of control over release of the carcinogenic material and to assist in documenting compliance with discharge regulations, providing that the rate and method of discharge are known.

2. Material Flowcharts

Another aspect of the administrative control program concerns the use of material flowcharts. For an industrial process it is frequently possible to quantify the amount of a particular material present at each step of the process for a specified flow rate or production rate. For each carcinogenic material used in a process, a process chart should be developed which presents the expected quantity of material present at each point and the upper and lower bounds (if known). The purpose of the chart would be to allow for rapid assessment of hazard potential in the event of an accident or emergency such as fire, explosion, or major leakage. It is essential that adequate protection for emergency crews, which can only be accomplished properly through advance planning, be afforded.

The material flowcharts can serve as sources of supplementary information for the material inventory. For carcinogenic materials that are merely process intermediates, such flowcharts may be the only quantifiable source of data for identifying the degree of risk present in an operation.

E. Controlled Access Area

The word "safe" is a relative term that requires a value judgment pertaining to the acceptability of a certain level of risk. One obviously simple way of reducing risk is to reduce the number of persons exposed to a carcinogenic hazard through control of access to any area in which the hazard is found. Administrative control measures are most frequently employed, although there is growing use of automated, computer-based, limited-access systems utilizing a machine readable identification card. Consideration should be given to each facility to determine how an effective control program can best be implemented.

1. Personal Protective Equipment

Personal protective equipment should be designed to prevent exposure and to prevent spread of contamination from one work site to another. Routes of exposure may include inhalation, ingestion, or skin adsorption, or any combination of these routes. Contaminant spread is usually caused when contaminated footwear, gloves, or hands transfer a carcinogenic material from one site to another. Protective equipment use practices must be developed to address protection of both people and uncontaminated areas. Unfortunately, only limited information is available with respect to the extent of protection afforded by such items as protective gloves [15,16] or hand lotions [17].

Clothing items utilized for worker protection should cover all exposed skin areas which have a probability of contact with carcinogenic materials. Items such as coveralls, gloves, caps or bonnets, and shoe coverings should be routinely considered for use. Removal techniques for used clothing should be developed to prevent skin contact when exiting an area. Skin should only come into contact with the "clean" side of a garment. Collection stations for contaminated items must be available for items awaiting disposal or cleaning. For certain particularly dirty operations, it may be necessary to resort to full-body protective suits with an air supply system.

Facial protection required will vary considerably, depending on the physical state of the material in question. For very volatile materials it may be necessary to employ a full-face covering in the form of an air-supplied hood or a full-face respirator with an organic vapor cartridge. Eye protection should always be employed as a minimum.

A program for respiratory protection should be given strict attention. The subject is too broad to be given comprehensive coverage here, and the reader is referred to specific works in this field (see especially Pritchard [18]). One aspect of a respiratory protection program that is frequently overlooked is the associated involvement with the medical surveillance program. It is not a satisfactory practice to require a worker to utilize a respiratory protective device for normal duty unless the individual has been examined by a physician and is found fit to work utilizing such an apparatus. Certain workers may have respiratory impairments that would prevent them from being able to work under these conditions, and a properly designed medical program would protect such workers.

Persons required to work in designated areas that require respiratory protection should be trained in proper fitting, use, cleaning, and maintenance of their equipment. Consideration should be given to setting up a centralized maintenance program for all respiratory protective devices. Each individual should be instructed in performance of qualitative leak tests, as well as in the need for frequent visual inspection of all parts. In addition, the various types of respirator cartridges must be described, and instruction should be given concerning the frequency of changing absorbing/filtering units.

2. Isolation Areas

Carcinogenic substances and operations that require special containment measures because of special properties such as high volatility or extreme carcinogenic potency should be identified. The isolation area may be as small as a glove box or as large as an entire building. In such areas rigorous measures must be taken to maintain the integrity of the barrier separating the worker from the carcinogenic material, and either the worker or the carcinogen may be inside the protective container.

For large-scale operations involving entire buildings process control rooms must be constructed to achieve isolation, normally through ventilation controls, with the contaminated area kept under a relative negative pressure. Access to contaminated areas should be only via an airlock with a mechanism to ensure that one door is closed before the next one can be opened. When airline supplied units are in use it is essential that an observer be stationed outside the area who can implement a rescue and recovery action if needed. Sufficient protective equipment must be on hand to provide for such emergency situations. For large facilities it may be practical to utilize a closed circuit television system to monitor multiple operations. If the operational area requires transfer of airline connections within a contaminated area, provision should be made to prevent worker exposure through contaminated hose couplings.

3. Sanitation Facilities

Because carcinogenic materials may enter the environment in a variety of physical states, it is necessary to review the entire sanitation program. Liquid and solid wastes require special consideration because normal municipal systems are not designed to treat safely highly hazardous materials, hence, special consideration must be given to pretreatment of liquid wastes or special disposal techniques for solid wastes. Workplaces that use launderable protective clothing should determine that the contaminated clothing is not processed by an unknowing and unskilled party. A commercial laundry may be acceptable if it can establish proper handling procedures.

Restrooms in a controlled access area are another potentially troublesome area concerning contamination. Procedures should be established and room should be provided for removal of any contaminated outerwear to keep toilet facilities free from contamination. Drinking water supplied to these areas should be from foot-operated fountains, which should be operated several seconds prior to use to flush away possible contaminants. Water supply lines to fountains or to restrooms in such areas should come from a main outside the controlled area and should have check valves to prevent possible backflush of contaminants into the water supply system. Check valves should be present also on any process water supply line for the controlled areas.

Work practices, including cleaning of rooms and halls in a controlled facility, must be performed in a manner to avoid contaminant spread. For example, wet mopping techniques should be used to prevent spread of airborne contaminant particles. Use of a central vacuum system, in which the power unit is located in a place where the filtered exhaust air cannot cause contaminant spread, should be considered.

4. Engineering and Maintenance

The best method for achieving a safe facility is to provide essential features and engineering systems in the design phase. Many facilities have structural features in their design which are not conducive to strict control. Some general concepts that should be considered are (1) that contaminated areas should be contiguous to one another to facilitate sharing of utilities, (2) that areas with pressure differentials should be arranged to keep airflows in a linear direction; (3) that exhaust air crossovers with damper controls should be considered to provide backup ventilation in case of equipment malfunction; and (4) that emergency standby generators with automatic cut-ins be on hand to maintain system integrity in the event of blackouts.

Obviously, the types of systems described are quite costly to install and maintain. However, it must be emphasized that, in general, engineering controls are somewhat less prone to human error than either administrative or protective equipment controls.

A good preventive maintenance program can do much to maintain a system operational. A documented schedule for lubrication of bearings, belt replacement, pump maintenance, and visual inspection of mechanical systems should be established and documented. Through proper design, maintenance areas can be kept external to the controlled access areas, thereby reducing the requirement for maintenance personnel to use protective equipment only to those times when entry into a contaminated system is required; for example, when a pump replacement is needed. Attention should be given to providing all maintenance personnel with instruction and training concerning the nature of carcinogenic hazards existing in the controlled area, control measures in force, and proper use of protective equipment. Because maintenance personnel frequently service highly contaminated areas, they should also be included in a medical surveillance program.

5. Monitoring

The effectiveness of control systems in maintaining a workplace free from recognized carcinogenic hazards requires documentation. The foregoing statement is simple, but considerable planning is required to establish a valid, ongoing monitoring system. Types of monitoring systems may range in complexity from a continuous, on-line system with automatic alarm set points, to manual grab sampling and subsequent analysis of the process stream. Whatever the system, documentation of the accuracy and reproducibility of the measurements is necessary. Accuracy is determined by comparison with a defined standard, and reproducibility is determined by the capability of replicate measurements to be repeated. When a monitoring method is employed which requires sample collection, it is necessary to evaluate the total recovery efficiency of the sampling and analytical techniques and apply this factor to the measured results.

Records of all monitoring programs must be retained to permit subsequent documentation of worker exposure in controlled areas monitored. The system of records must, therefore, permit establishment of a link among actual exposure concentrations, sample calibration, and quality assurance of samples that were analyzed during the time period in question. The standard procedures for sampling and analysis should always be included in the documentation.

F. Education

1. Although regulatory standards promulgated by the Occupational Safety and Health Administration (OSHA) require training of employees regarding hazards in the workplace, few details are available concerning performance of this responsibility. Most employers believe that an on-the-job training (OJT) program is most effective and efficient. However, difficulties with such practices normally center on the absence of adequate documentation of the performance and thoroughness of such training. Many times in an OJT session, the instructor (often a fellow employee) merely passes on poor work practices to the new employee, thereby perpetuating such procedures.

Any facility manufacturing or using carcinogenic substances should develop and implement a formalized program of instruction designed to cover all situations and operations in which the employee may become exposed to such substances. Persons required to attend these sessions should include both new employees, as well as those already familiar with operations, to accomplish a continuing education program. In bringing together a mixture of new and old employees in the training sessions, resulting discussions will reveal potentially poor work practices and, perhaps, provide the foundation for their amelioration.

2. An important aspect of any employee education program is preparation of effective responses to emergency conditions. In developing anticipatory emergency programs, it is very important and extremely valuable to utilize the experience and knowledge of the more senior employees in providing a thorough listing of possible emergencies. Once developed, the safety and production staffs should develop response tactics to adequately cover each contingency. Containment methods are crucial factors in control of carcinogenic substances, and the volume of reaction vessels and storage tanks should be listed and used for determining spill containments or diked areas. Past experiences in Italy, associated with dioxin release,

or in the United States, associated with grain elevator explosions, indicate the nature of problems to be addressed with respect to requirements for pressure relief values and associated recovery systems.

3. Written Standard Operating Procedures (SOPs) are an invaluable means of obtaining an organized control program for the workplace. These procedures can comprise the basis and documentation for a formalized program for training of new employees. SOPs can also be utilized effectively for identifying those operations with inherent carcinogenic hazards, thereby calling the attention of the operator to critical process steps. Whenever SOPs are employed the procedures should be dated and reviewed annually to ensure that actual work practices are consistent with those prescribed in the SOP.

G. Record-keeping

The monitoring and control activities already discussed, including hazard recognition, hazard control, medical surveillance, material control, area control, and employee training can result in generation of large amounts of data which, when considered in total, can provide extensive documentation of the health and safety program of the facility and attendant responsibilities. These records, obviously, are of great value for both operational and legal purposes and, for that reason, require that a prudent records control program be implemented including a backup records system. Normally, original copies of records are reserved for legal purposes and duplicate copies serve operational purposes. In circumstances under which frequent retrieval of old data is normal, an automated information storage and retrieval system should be considered for daily operations. Many commercially available systems are capable of providing this type of information control and can be tailored to individual needs at relatively moderate costs.

III. ENVIRONMENTAL POLLUTION AND EFFLUENT PROBLEMS

Control of the release of carcinogenic substances into the general environment is receiving much attention and increasing concern. Numerous regulatory agencies, acting under increasingly strict legislative dates, are likewise becoming more stringent in promulgation of regulations and their enforcement. The magnitude of problems created by past spills, such as with mercury, PCBs, dioxin, and kepone, is so great that resultant unfavorable public opinion makes the prudent consideration of control actions increasingly more cost effective.

A. Airborne Emissions

Technology for control of pollutant emissions from manufacturing processes has rapidly progressed during the past decade, and the environmental controls industry has fluorished, spurred on by new environmental laws and regulations. However, in some instances control devices have not performed according to specifications, thereby generating a certain degree of disenchantment. In the realm of airborne emissions, contaminants can be characterized as either gaseous or condensed (solid particulates and liquids) phase. Condensates have, historically, been the most easily controlled because they have more mass, and hence, are subject to physical separation techniques such as filtration and impaction. Accordingly, gaseous phase contaminants are viewed as more difficult to remove from a process stream because of the requirement for gas-liquid or gas-solid adsorption units or for incineration of the exhaust gas stream.

Many new installations have incorporated carbon absorption filter units, or some similar solid absorbent phase, to remove gaseous contaminants. Such units require periodic replacement of the absorbent as its absorbing capacity is approached. Several major operating difficulties that exist with units of this nature include determination of absorbing capacity, monitoring of contaminants breakthrough, and disposal of spent contaminated units.

Defining useful capacity of an absorbent bed is difficult and empirical in nature. In practice, one normally would monitor for some predefined level of contaminant breakthrough sufficient to initiate a change. Variations in air velocity, temperature, humidity, channeling, and presence of cocontaminants are factors that can affect predictions of the necessity to change absorbents. For insuring a "zero-discharge" contaminant level it is necessary to utilize two units in tandem to provide backup for the initial unit when it becomes saturated or when it is being replaced or regenerated.

Disposal of a spent bed of solid absorbent from an air filtering unit presents a solid waste problem. Thus, contaminants that were once airborne are now "stored" on a bed of charcoal or resin and, if not properly handled, could desorb back into the environment.

B. Water Contamination

Legislation and regulations in the field of water pollution control have tended to separate waste waters from drinking waters. The density of living patterns associated with modern civilization has rendered this distinction somewhat blurred because of the high degree of water reuse prior to discharge into the oceans.

Although many carcinogenic materials are appreciably soluble in water, they are not readily removed by normal purification processes such as filtration and coagulation. Most municipal water systems are designed to remove bacteria, some inorganic ions, and particulates, but are not designed to remove soluble organic compounds. However, s small number of facilities have installed carbon beds and/or ozonation units to process organics and viruses. It is, of course, in these latter two classes that substances are formed which are most frequently associated with cancer. As the nature and causes of cancer are more fully understood, additional emphasis will, undoubtedly, be placed on development of more sophisticated process technologies. The EPA has taken the position that carbon adsorption systems may be required for use in municipal water supply systems to meet compliance standards for allowable levels of organic chemicals under the Safe Drinking Water Standards.

Treatment of liquid wastes prior to discharge or reuse once again raises the problem associated with disposal of spent solid waste collection units. These units are even more hazardous than the original liquid stream because the process of concentration of organic carcinogens (for which they were designed) converts them into potentially dangerous items.

A survey should be performed in any facility engaged in the manufacture or use of carcinogenic substances to determine actual and potential process losses. The survey should be structured to consider carcinogenic substances on a mass balance basis to determine quantities used and/or produced and routes of entry and exit of all known process steps, including flow volumes for each step. Analysis of these data could perhaps identify in particular a large-volume, noncontaminated stream, which could be isolated from the several processes, thereby reducing the total stream load while increasing contaminant concentration at the treatment unit, whether it be an adsorption bed, a reaction vessel, or an incinerator. Such segregation of processes would help to reduce treatment costs in two ways: (1) a smaller size treatment unit could be used, and (2) it would normally be easier to achieve a higher degree of removal of contaminants from a waste stream (i.e., it is easier to go from one part per thousand to one part per million, than it is to go from one part per million to one part per billion, even though the reduction factor is the same in both cases). To obtain a goal of "zero discharge" such segregation tactics may be absolutely essential.

C. Waste Material Control

1. Process loss control programs to minimize and contain spills and leaks are developed with the recognition that accidents, although abnormal occurrences, actually do occur. The prudent course of action is to plan for the event by anticipating the consequences, as much as possible, and then to take appropriate anticipatory actions to reduce and minimize the possibility of the occurrence of such unfortunate events. It is not difficult to understand

that a loss control program is more straightforward for a manufacturing process than for a facility such as a research laboratory. In a manufacturing facility in which one can easily observe unit processes and contents it is easy to envision the possibility of a tank rupture or failure of a pump seal, gasket, or valve, and hence, to plan for such events. Action plans organized with such considerations in mind have led, commonly, to use of dikes or of other containment devices including lined emergency holding ponds. It is, of course, much more difficult to implement such contaminant programs in facilities in which the nature of the work is constantly changing, such as in a pilot plant or a research laboratory. In these instances identification of problems can only be performed, properly, by persons possessing much experience in the general laboratory environment who also have some knowledge of the nature of the specific operations and processes at the facility.

2. Much of the research work now being performed in the field of cancer research utilizes experimental animal-testing facilities in order to investigate in a scientifically systematic manner the thousands of chemicals that may cause—or cure—cancer. Such exposure experimentation necessitates development of safe procedures for the study of these substances over extended periods of time [19]. In most situations there are no known biological indicators or symptoms that can provide a measure of the adequacy of the control procedures. Instead, in the dearth of such diagnostic tools, one is forced to exercise prudent judgment as to how to perform the test protocols in such a manner as to prevent release.

Obviously, performance of animal exposure investigations involving carcinogenic substances generates contaminated wastes. It is necessary that all waste streams are considered, including gaseous, solid, and liquid. A complicating factor in disposal of solid wastes is the occasional presence of animal tissue, which can be difficult to incinerate. High-temperature incineration appears to be the most effective method for a final disposition of most waste carcinogenic materials, because very few satisfactory landfill operations exist which could, otherwise, accommodate such wastes. For purposes of disposal of carcinogenic waste materials an adequate sanitary landfill operation must have no significant degree of leaching or migration of disposed substances through the soil, and it must be routinely monitored for leachate flow. Only a rudimentary knowledge exists to define leachate contaminant attenuation obtainable with different landfill liners. Open dumps or improperly supervised landfills are not satisfactory means for disposal of carcinogenic wastes. To minimize the volume of hazardous waste handling problems, it is essential to develop separation procedures to collect all noncontaminated wastes separately.

D. Materials of Commerce

1. Routine transportation of chemical substances, some of which are carcinogenic, occurs daily on a worldwide basis and is not, necessarily, cause for alarm. Chemical transport by common carrier is a vital part of our economy, and methods for performing this activity in a responsible manner are well established, although the potential for accidental spills or releases is everpresent. Considerable effort has surrounded the installation of control and recovery equipment at transfer stations where materials are pumped and conveyed from one container to another. However, because many of these control/recovery systems are of an "add on" variety, rather than integral components of original systems, many shortcomings exist. Although technological advancements in the materials handling field have greatly reduced the potential for spills in many cases, methodologies for complete containment often defy facile resolution. One major difficulty with such systems concerns development of "fail-safe" techniques to insure that their proper operations cannot be an optional feature or ignored by the transfer operator. Much additional work and innovation research will certainly be required prior to justification of claims of achieving complete containment of carcinogenic substances in major industrial processes.

2. With the exception of certain classes of products such as foods, drugs, cosmetics, and pesticides, consumer products have only very recently become subject to federal regulatory control. Now, however, substances or physical agents that are potentially carcinogenic

and have previously been uncontrolled, are being closely scrutinized. The problem of hazard recognition is extremely difficult in the consumer product area because of the absence of adequate information concerning chemical composition. For example, one can imagine the immense difficulty in defining the many process chemicals, present in only trace amounts, that might still be present following manufacture of a decorative plastic bracelet. Complete knowledge of such contaminants would require complete understanding of the nature of production process involving dyes, resins, and polymerization catalysts, as well as processing aids such as mold release agents, and so on. Further complicating this situation is the fact that most of these materials are, themselves, a multicomponent formulation. Obviously, even providing a comprehensive list of all of these materials to a consumer will not result in significant increases in development of safety practices proportionate to the work required to implement them.

Likewise, regulations that are intended to advance technology, such as those associated with development of fire-retardant sleepwear, often can generate new problems in related areas due to secondary, or even tertiary effects. As regulations force new products, or product modifications, onto the market to displace existing ones, situations are created in which associated control technologies have not had sufficient time to fully evolve, or in which possible health hazards are not fully realized, thus causing to surface many problems of this nature. Hence, as more materials are suspected of being possible carcinogens many existing products will require reformulation to remove questionable components. Thus, a great need is created with respect to promptly and adequately informing manufacturers, users, and the general public concerning carcinogenic risks associated with exposure to previously unsuspected chemical substances. It is unfortunate that transmission of information of this nature seldom is performed with recognition of the effects on the target audience. Because of this situation, the general public, and often manufacturers as well, are faced with the problem of accepting risks which they do not have the education or ability to adequately assess.

E. Monitoring Pollutants

With the exception of gross spill situations, practically all monitoring of pollutants is performed using instrumentation capable of detecting trace quantities. Even detection of oil spills on the open sea often requires use of trace analysis because of the great dilutory effect of the ocean. A major difficulty in obtaining trace measurements concerns the confidence that a measurement is "true." Every measuring device is characterized by a level of uncertainty, or noise, that prevents obtaining a definite "zero" reading. This noise signal is statistically related and varies both with time and between identical measuring units. Normally, a defined statistical threshold is required to distinguish between a "true" reading and a random noise signal. A commonly used threshold involves evaluation of the instrument noise level, measuring only those signals that are three or more times in excess of the noise level. This noise threshold value then becomes the limit of detectability characteristic of the monitoring unit.

Further measurement complications arise in the environmental areas because of background concentrations of particular natural substances. Specific information concerning natural background levels of most chemical substances and their physical properties is practically nonexistent. Natural background levels can vary with regard to geographical location, time of day, and season of year, in addition to many human events [20]. However, it is not possible to determine whether a single high concentration of a trace contaminant is of concern or whether the concentration falls within the normal statistical and/or seasonal fluctuations of background readings, unless statistical/seasonal variations are known. An example of the importance of knowing environmental background levels concerned the high mercury levels found in fish that were, thus, suspected of being contaminated by a human pollution source. However, analysis of a 200 year old fish specimen from a museum yielded mercury levels in the same concentration range. This finding obviously obscured the cause-and-effect interpretation that was assumed. Similarly, changing concentrations of chlorinated hydrocarbons in tap water demonstrate seasonal as well as short-term variations (G. Esposito, USAEHA, personal communication).

The preceding discussion of monitoring and detection problems associated with instrumentation and background "noise" is particularly appropriate for carcinogenic substances. In addition to such considerations are problems associated with interfering substances, that is, other materials present in the analyzed sample that can produce either a positive or a negative interference with the measured signal. When monitoring for the total amount of a chemical substance present, the task usually is not overcomplicated because a number of detection devices are available. However, problems may be encountered in attempting to distinguish among different states of the same element or among compounds of similar chemical classes. For example, the analysis of hexavalent chromium in the presence of trivalent chromium, or the analysis of low levels of benzene in the presence of toluene, can cause difficult analytical problems.

A valid monitoring program for any carcinogen must include a measure of the quality of the analyses. Calibration standards, calibration analyses, and intermittent, unknown blind samples must be introduced to verify the reliability of the program. Requirement of a quality assurance program dictates that the analyst have a reference sample of the material to be analyzed in order to calibrate the monitor. Provision must be made to ensure safe and proper procedures for such calibration.

Finally, only rudimentary knowledge is available concerning transport and degradation processes for carcinogenic materials throughout the environment. In brief, when a particular contaminant concentration is detected at one point, we are still unable to predict, accurately, what concentrations are to be encountered at other points in the ecosystem of man and what interrelationships may be expected with other components present.

F. Record-keeping

The tasks and responsibilities associated with record-keeping with respect to manufacture and/or use of carcinogenic substances are multiplying. Practically all activities concerned with carcinogens are subject to some kind of control program, whether mandated by law or by prudence. Each employer who operates a facility in which carcinogens are produced, used or consumed, transported, or disposed of in any process or operation has legal obligations to his employees and to the surrounding environment. The employer must be able to document the state of compliance and responsible, competent actions.

Protection of such records is of vital concern. A system must be devised that can insure retention of the information for extended periods of time (e.g., 40 years for medical records in the OSHA Coke Oven Emission Standard), and yet be available for ready access to review by legal, medical, or regulatory personnel. Microfilm or machine-based data systems appear to present the best answers to the hardware needs for a records control system. Absence of an adequate system can commit much of a company's personnel resources in the event of an environmental crisis concerning its activities. The area of records control is one of increasing federal regulation and will most likely continue in that direction for several years.

Of paramount importance in establishing any record-keeping system in the medical, occupational, or environmental area is the necessity of first performing an internal audit of personnel procedures, operations, and chemical substances. Only after such an audit has been performed can the essential elements that should be incorporated into the records control system be identified. Retaining too much information can be just as useless and confusing as retaining too little. Hence, one must initially establish what information <u>must</u> be collected and retained and for <u>what</u> purposes before designing a records control system to permit storage and retrieval of information.

REFERENCES

1. T. J. Mason. Statistics point to high cancer localities. Occup. Health and Saf. 46 (3): 44-48 (1977).
2. T. J. Mason and F. W. McKay. U.S. cancer mortality by county: 1950-1969. DHEW Publication No. (NIH)74-615, U.S. Government Printing Office, Washington, D.C.
3. T. J. Mason, F. W. McKay, R. Hoover, W. J. Blot, and J. F. Fraumeni. Atlas of cancer mortality for U.S. counties, 1950-1969. DHEW Publication No. (NIH)75-780, U.S. Government Printing Office, Washington, D.C., 0000.
4. R. E. Eckardt. Industrial Carcinogens. Grune and Stratton, New York, 1959.
5. W. C. Hueper and W. D. Conway. Chemical Carcinogenesis and Cancers. Thomas, Springfield, Ill., 1964.
6. Threshold Limit Values for 1978. American Conference of Governmental Industrial Hygienists, 1978.
7. B. D. Dinman. The Nature of Occupational Cancer. Thomas, Springfield, Ill., 1974.
8. P. Cole and M. B. Goldman. Occupation. In Persons at High Risk of Cancer—An Approach to Cancer Etiology and Control, J. F. Fraumeni, Jr. (Ed.). Academic Press, New York, 1975, pp. 167-183.
9. V. E. Rose. Standards for the control of carcinogens in the workplace. J. Occup. Med. 18:81-89 (1976).
10. D. L. Lassiter. Occupational carcinogenesis. In Advances in Modern Toxicology Environmental Cancer, Vol. 3, H. F. Kraybill and M. A. Mehlman (Eds.). Hemisphere, Washington, D.C., 1977, pp. 63-86.
11. C. K. Redmond, A. Ciocco, J. W. Lloyd, and H. W. Rush. Long-term mortality study of steelworkers. VI. Mortality from malignant neoplasms among coke oven workers. J. Occup. Med. 14:621-629 (1972).
12. W. G. Figueroa, R. Raszkowski, and W. Weiss. Lung cancer in chloromethyl methyl ether workers. N. Engl. J. Occup. Med. 288:1096-1097 (1973).
13. D. R. Voss, K. W. Vorpahl, D. L. Royse, and N. B. Jurinski. Worker Hazard Inventory Program. American Industrial Hygiene Conference, Los Angeles, May 1978.
14. N. A. Leidel, K. A. Busch, and J. R. Lynch. Occupational exposure sampling strategy manual. DHEW (NIOSH) Publication No. 77-173, U.S. Government Printing Office, Washington, D.C., January 1977.
15. R. W. Weeks and B. J. Dean. Permeation of methanolic aromatic amine solutions through commercially available glove materials. Am. Ind. Hyg. Assoc. J. 38:712-725 (1977).
16. E. B. Sansone and Y. B. Tewari. The permeability of laboratory gloves to selected solvents. Am. Ind. Hyg. Assoc. J. 39:169-174 (1978).
17. N. P. Langford. Fluorochemical resin complexes for use in solvent repellent hand creams. Am. Ind. Hyg. Assoc. J. 39:33-40 (1978).
18. J. A. Pritchard. A guide to industrial respiratory protection. DHEW (NIOSH) Publication No. 76-189, U.S. Government Printing Office, Washington, D.C., June 1976.
19. N. B. Jurinski. Health and Safety Plan, Occupational and Environmental Hygiene. NCI Carcinogenesis Bioassay Program, November 1977.
20. J. R. Schubel. The physical and chemical characteristics of the Chesapeake Bay. J. Wash. Acad. Sci., 62:56-87 (1972).

5

Statistical Analysis of Carcinogenesis Data from Chronic Animal Studies

DAVID W. GAYLOR / National Center for Toxicological Research, Jefferson, Arkansas
DAVID G. HOEL / National Institute of Environmental Health Sciences, Research Triangle Park, North Carolina

I. INTRODUCTION

Lifetime animal experiments are difficult to analyze because competing causes of death that may not be related to a tumor type under study alter the pattern of the time of occurrences of the tumor. Nevertheless, a common format for presenting tumor data is simply to report the proportion of animals possessing particular tumor types over the duration of the study. This proportion may contain a mixture of three types of tumor observations: (1) the tumor causes the death of an animal and is subsequently observed upon necropsy, (2) an animal dies because of some cause other than a particular tumor type, and the tumor is observed upon necropsy, or (3) the tumor is observed to be present upon necropsy of an animal at the time of a scheduled sacrifice, this sacrifice generally being at the termination of an experiment.

Simply combining tumors observed under these three distinct situations makes interpretation difficult and in fact misleading if the mortality pattern is altered by the toxicity of the chemical under study.

Use of serial sacrifices, or perhaps a terminal sacrifice, provides an opportunity to compare the prevalence of tumors in various groups of animals unperturbed by mortality. However, sacrifice data do not provide an opportunity to study the effect of a chemical on survival, nor can causes of death be studied. Utilizing all the animals from a survival study, including sacrificed animals, the net probability of death due to a tumor type under certain biological assumptions can be estimated as though that were the only cause of death acting on a group of animals. By comparison of these net probabilities for control and chemically treated groups of animals, statistical tests for differences in tumor rates can be performed.

For tumors that do not cause death, methods of analyses based on life table techniques are not appropriate. These tumors are observed conditionally as a result of other events occurring first: (1) death of an animal due to another cause, or (2) a scheduled sacrifice. To estimate the incidence of nonlethal tumors, it is necessary to assume that the cause of death is unrelated to the presence of the tumor.

The analysis of a survival study is limited by the quantity and quality of data. Such studies must include the age of each animal at the beginning of the experiment, its age at time of removal from the experiment, reason for removal (dead, moribund, scheduled sacrifice, or missing), tumors observed by both gross and microscopic examination, and if possible the cause of death. Admittedly, determination of the exact cause of death may be subjective, but it is necessary only to attempt to identify probable causes of death for those diseases under study. All other causes of death need not be identified and can be lumped together in one category.

The techniques discussed in this chapter address only the question of whether administration of a chemical to a group of animals results in an increase in tumors. No attempt is made to discuss the relevance of animal results to the human population. Nor is any attempt made here to discuss the potential risks at low levels of exposure which may be more akin to human exposure levels than the high doses generally used in animal experiments.

II. SACRIFICED ANIMALS: COMPARISON OF TREATED AND CONTROL GROUPS

A. Single Terminal Sacrifice

First, consider a typical experiment in which there is only a single terminal sacrifice. Here the proportion of animals with tumors in treated and control groups can be compared for survivors at the time of sacrifice. Obviously, one major shortcoming of a comparison only at the time of sacrifice is that it ignores all the time-to-tumor information available from animals dying during the course of the experiment. The advantage is that the statistical comparison of terminal animals is easy to perform and the interpretation is simply a comparison between treated and control animals for the prevalence of the tumor type among survivors. Of course, the outcome is highly dependent on the time of the terminal sacrifice. If the time is too short, tumors may not have had sufficient time to develop. If the time is too long, survival may be low, resulting in small sample sizes, or the background rate in the controls may become high, making it difficult to ascertain if an increase in tumors occurred in the treated group. Techniques for using the total data from all animals—dead, moribund, or sacrificed—are discussed in later sections.

Let r_c represent the number of animals possessing the tumor type in n_c control animals surviving to the time of termination of a study. Similarly, let r_t be the number of tumor-bearing animals in n_t treated animals. The data may be displayed in a 2×2 (two-by-two) array, where $n = n_c + n_t$.

	Tumor absent	Tumor present	Total
Control	$n_c - r_c$	r_c	n_c
Treated	$n_t - r_t$	r_t	n_t
Total	$n - r_c - r_t$	$r_c + r_t$	n

Fisher's exact test, conditional on the total number of tumor-bearing animals observed in the two groups, gives, for the one-sided significance probability level,

$$P = \sum_{i=0}^{r_c} \frac{n_c!\,n_t!\,(r_c + r_t)!\,(n - r_c - r_t)!}{n!\,(n_c - r_c + i)!\,(r_c - i)!\,(n_t - r_t - i)!\,(r_t + i)!} \tag{1}$$

For example, suppose 6 out of 30 treated animals and 1 out of 28 control animals exhibited a certain tumor type. The 2×2 array would appear as

	Tumor absent	Tumor present	Total
Control	27	1	28
Treated	24	6	30
Total	51	7	58

The significance level probability given by Fisher's exact conditional test is

$$P = \frac{28!\,30!\,7!\,51!}{58!\,27!\,1!\,24!\,6!} + \frac{28!\,30!\,7!\,51!}{58!\,28!\,0!\,23!\,7!} = 0.062 \tag{2}$$

Statistically, this is saying that, given the observance of 7 tumor-bearing animals, the probability of observing 6 or more tumor-bearing animals among the 30 treated animals due to chance alone is 0.062.

Cochran (1954) recommends using Fisher's exact test if $n < 20$ or when $20 < n < 40$, if the smallest expected value in the 2×2 table is less than 5. Otherwise, the following approximate chi-square test, which is somewhat easier to calculate, may be used:

$$\chi^2 = \frac{[\,|(n_c - r_c)r_t - (n_t - r_t)r_c| - n/2]^2 \times n}{n_c \times n_t \times (r_c + r_t) \times (n - r_c - r_t)} \tag{3}$$

Then the approximate probability that the proportion of tumor-bearing animals in the treated group exceeds the controls due to chance alone is given by the probability that the standard normal deviate exceeds $\sqrt{\chi^2}$. For the above example:

$$\chi^2 = \frac{(|27 \times 6 - 24 \times 1| - 29)^2 \times 58}{28 \times 30 \times 7 \times 51} = 2.30 \tag{4}$$

The probability that a value as large as 2.3 could arise by chance is given approximately by the probability that the standard normal deviate exceeds $\sqrt{2.30} = 1.52$, which is 0.064, which in this case is nearly the same as the Fisher's exact conditional probability of 0.062.

As stated earlier, this analysis ignores the results in nonsacrificed animals and only considers the prevalence of tumors at a single point in time. Fisher's exact test or the approximate chi-square test are often inappropriately applied to the total number of animals accruing tumors over the duration of an experiment. This is not correct because it requires that each animal has an equally likely chance of developing a tumor. Obviously, this requirement is not satisfied when animals die at different points in time. If the mortality pattern, apart from the tumor type under investigation, is essentially the same for the two groups, then the test can be used. Techniques for analyzing tumor data accruing over time are discussed in Secs. III and IV.

B. Combining Data from Several Sacrifices

When observations are taken at two or more points in time or from two or more experiments, a 2×2 array can be constructed for each set of sacrifice data. A procedure is given by Cochran (1954) for combining data from two or more independent 2×2 arrays. The test gives appropriate weight to tables with large sample sizes and is sensitive if differences between treated and controls are constant on a logit scale. A difference on a logit scale considers

$$\ell n \frac{p_{ti}}{1 - p_{ti}} - \ell n \frac{p_{ci}}{1 - p_{ci}} \tag{5}$$

where p_{ti} and p_{ci} are the proportions of tumor-bearing animals for the treated and control animals, respectively, in the ith array. This approach alleviates the difficulties that arise in detecting small differences as p approaches either 0 or 1. Mantel and Haenszel (1959) modified the Cochran test to provide a better approximation for small sample sizes and to provide a correction for continuity. Let r_{ci} be the number of control animals with the tumor of interest for the ith array, r_{ti} number of treated animals with tumors, n_{ci} total number of control animals, and $n_i = n_{ci} + n_{ti}$ the total number of animals. The expected number of treated animals with tumors for the ith array is then $E(r_{ti}) = n_{ti}(r_{ci} + r_{ti})/n_i$ under the null hypothesis that the proportion of animals with tumors is the same for both treated and control groups. Cochran's test (1954) is based on the standard normal deviate

$$Z = \frac{\Sigma_i r_{ti} - \Sigma_i E(r_{ti})}{[\Sigma_i n_{ci} n_{ti}(r_{ci} + r_{ti})(n_i - r_{ci} - r_{ti})/n_i^3]^{\frac{1}{2}}} \tag{6}$$

The modification given by Mantel and Haenszel (1959) is

$$Z = \frac{|\Sigma_i r_{ti} - \Sigma_i E(r_{ti})| - 0.5}{[\Sigma_i n_{ci} n_{ti}(r_{ci} + r_{ti})(n_i - r_{ci} - r_{ti})/n_i^2(n_i - 1)]^{\frac{1}{2}}} \tag{7}$$

C. Linear Trend

In the case in which several doses are employed, it is of interest to determine if there is a tendency for the proportion of animals with tumor type(s) to increase with dose for surviving animals examined at a given point in time. Armitage (1955) gives a test for a linear trend of proportion versus dose. Cox (1958) proposed the use of the logistic model as a basis for developing a regression test. Let P_i be the probability an animal receiving a dose d_i has a tumor, where $i = 0, 1, \ldots, r$,

$$P_i = \frac{e^{\alpha+\beta d_i}}{1 + e^{\alpha+\beta d_i}} \tag{8}$$

where α and β are unknown parameters. We wish to test the homogeneity of the P_i, that is, $H_0: \beta = 0$, against the alternative hypothesis of a positive linear trend ($\beta > 0$) in the logit scale, $\ln[P_i/(1 - P_i)]$.

An asymptotic test for positive trend is based on the normal deviate

$$Z = \frac{\Sigma x_i d_i - \dfrac{(x.\Sigma n_i d_i)}{n.} - \dfrac{\Delta}{2}}{\left[\dfrac{x.(n. - x.)}{n.(n. - 1)} \Sigma n_i (d_i - \bar{d})^2\right]^{\frac{1}{2}}}$$

where

x_i = number of tumor bearing animals in group i at the time of sacrifice
n_i = number of animals in group i at the time of sacrifice
$x. = \Sigma x_i$
$n. = \Sigma n_i$
$\bar{d} = \Sigma n_i d_i / n.$
$\Delta/2$ = continuity correction

If doses are equally spaced on an arithmetic scale, then Δ is the difference between adjacent doses. When the doses are not equally spaced, the minimum and maximum differences between adjacent doses can be used for Δ in order to obtain a range on the test statistic Z, as suggested by Thomas et al. (1977).

In order to check on the logistic assumption, a chi-square statistic with (r - 1) degrees to test for departure from linearity is given by

$$\chi_{r-1}^2 = \frac{n.(n. - 1)}{x.(n. - x.)}\left[\sum \frac{x_i^2}{n_i} - \frac{x.^2}{n.}\right] - Z^2 \tag{10}$$

Recall that the animals dying during the course of the experiment again have not been utilized. Trend tests utilizing all animals making adjustments for time to tumor death are given in Sec. III.C.

III. TIME-TO-TUMOR OBSERVATION (LETHAL TUMORS)

A. Estimation

In Sec. II only observations from animals sacrificed at specific points in time were used. The data from animals dying between sacrifice periods were not used, which could result in a considerable loss of information. In this section the data from all animals receiving pathological examinations are used regardless of the reason for removal from the experiment: dead, moribund, or sacrificed. An important distinction between this section and Sec. IV is that we are now considering lethal tumors. In the lethal case, statistical analyses based on life table techniques should be employed. It is necessary to determine if the tumor types under consideration are the probable cause of death for each animal in which those tumor types are observed. All other causes of death can be combined and the exact cause need not be established. However, it is assumed that the competing causes, tumor versus nontumor death, are independent. Obviously, the cause of death for sacrificed animals is the sacrifice and not the tumor types, even if they are present upon necropsy.

We present a nonparametric procedure due to Kaplan and Meier (1958) for estimating the net probabilities of a lethal tumor as a function of time for censored data. The net probability is the probability of death due to a specific tumor type as if that cause of death were the only risk acting. That is, the analysis adjusts for competing causes of death. In order to perform these analyses, it is necessary to assume that the lethal tumor behaves independently of other principal diseases causing death. Let

Q(t) = prob (an animal will die before time t if R is the only risk operating)

For an experiment of size n, suppose the ages of death are $t_1 \leq t_2 \leq \ldots \leq t_n$. The estimator of Q(t) given by Kaplan and Meier (1958) is the step function:

$$\hat{Q}(t) = 1 - \Pi_r\left(\frac{n - r}{n - r + 1}\right) \tag{11}$$

where r assumes values for which $t_r \leq t$, and t_r is an age associated with an animal dying from the cause of death R.

A simple example serves to demonstrate the ease of obtaining the Kaplan-Meier time-to-tumor curves in the presence of competing causes of death. The simple example also demonstrates how misleading gross unadjusted tumor rates ignoring time to tumor can be.

TABLE 1 Experimental Data and Adjusted Type A Tumor Rates

	Controls			Treated		
Rank (r)	Age at death (days)	Cause of death	$\hat{Q}(t)$	Age at death (days)	Cause of death	$\hat{Q}(t)$
1	180	O	O	210	O	O
2	256	O	O	264	O	O
3	378	O	O	299	O	O
4	454	O	O	320	O	O
5	488	O	O	385	O	O
6	505	B	O	389	A	0.143
7	520	B	O	407	A	0.286
8	579	A	0.200[a]	444	O	0.286
9	601	B	0.200	492	A	0.464
10	687	A	0.467[b]	588	A	0.643
11	730[c]	T/A	0.467	650	B	0.643
12	730[c]	T/B	0.467	730[c]	T/O	0.643

[a] $1 - 4/5 = 0.200$.

[b] $1 - 4/5 \times 2/3 = 0.467$.

[c] Terminal sacrifice.

A sample of only 12 animals is used so that the reader may follow the calculations readily. Equal sample sizes were used but are not necessary. The time to death (time on experiment) and cause of death for each animal are given in Table 1, where A and B refer to the type of tumor causing death, O refers to other causes of death, and T/A, T/B, and T/O refer to terminal sacrifice animals with type A, type B, or no tumors present, respectively; the adjusted tumor rates $\hat{Q}(t)$ will be discussed later.

Gross tumor rates totaled over the experiment ignoring time to tumor frequently are presented as a means of summarizing data, as shown in Table 2. Often, as in this example, the gross tumor rates inadequately summarize the data.

A cursory examination of these results would lead one to erroneously conclude that this experiment demonstrated no increase in tumor type A due to the treatment and possibly a decrease in tumor type B. Further examination of the data indicates that type A tumors are occurring earlier in the treated group, indicating the need for a more detailed analysis incorporating the time to tumors.

Assuming independence of tumor type A, type B, and other causes of death, the adjusted Kaplan-Meier type A rates are calculated in Table 1 for control and treated animals. Note that for the terminal sacrifice animals the adjusted tumor rate does not increase even if a tumor is present because the cause of death is the scheduled sacrifice and not the tumor. Note that $\hat{Q}(t)$ increases only when an animal dies because of the tumor in question. For example, there are no tumor type A deaths in the control animals up to 579 days. At 579

TABLE 2 Prevalence of Tumors

Tumor type	Controls	Treated
A	3/12 = 25.0%	4/12 = 33.3%
B	4/12 = 33.3%	1/12 = 8.3%

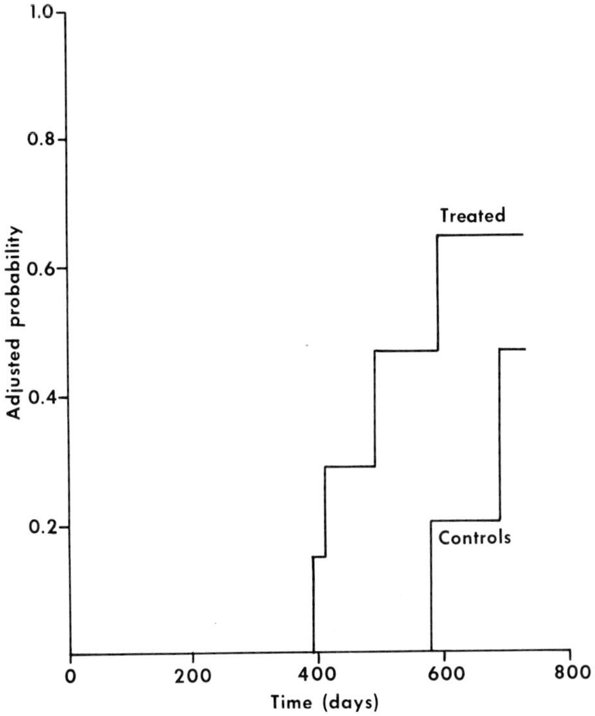

FIGURE 1 Cumulative probability of tumor type A adjusted for competing causes of death.

TABLE 3 Unadjusted and Adjusted, $\hat{Q}(t)$, Tumor Rates

Tumor type A					
Controls			Treated		
Days	Unadjusted	Adjusted	Days	Unadjusted	Adjusted
579	0.083	0.200	389	0.083	0.143
687	0.167	0.467	407	0.167	0.286
			492	0.250	0.464
			588	0.333	0.643

Tumor type B					
Controls			Treated		
Days	Unadjusted	Adjusted	Days	Unadjusted	Adjusted
505	0.083	0.143	650	0.083	0.500
520	0.167	0.286			
601	0.250	0.464			

TABLE 4 Unadjusted and Adjusted Rates for Tumor Types A or B

Controls			Treated		
Days	Unadjusted	Adjusted	Days	Unadjusted	Adjusted
505	0.083	0.143	389	0.083	0.143
520	0.167	0.286	407	0.167	0.286
579	0.250	0.429	492	0.250	0.464
601	0.333	0.571	588	0.333	0.643
687	0.417	0.714	650	0.417	0.821

days, among the five animals reaching this age, four animals have not died due to tumor type A and one died giving $\hat{Q}(t) = 0.200$ (Table 1). At 687 days, the joint probability of control survivors not dying due to tumor type A is $4/5 \times 2/3$ giving $\hat{Q}(t) = 0.467$.

Note the considerable differences between the crude unadjusted rates, which are the proportion of the total number of animals in a group with a tumor type by a specific time, and adjusted cumulative mortality rates. Recall that comparing the final unadjusted proportion of treated animals with tumor type A (4/12 = 33%) with the controls (3/12 = 25%) did not indicate any statistically significant increase. An examination of the adjusted cumulative mortality rates, Fig. 1, shows that tumor type A is occurring earlier in the treated group resulting in higher tumor rates at any given time.

Recall that the final unadjusted proportion of animals with tumor type B exhibited a decrease in the treated animals. However, the adjusted tumor rate of the treated animals is 0.500 compared with 0.464 for the control animals at 730 days (Table 3).

If tumor types A and B are not considered to be independent of each other, but independent of other causes of death, then the two tumor types can be combined. The unadjusted and adjusted tumor rates for types A and B combined are given in Table 4.

B. Treated Versus Control

1. Generalized Kruskal-Wallis Test

Breslow (1970) gives a generalization of the Kruskal-Wallis test, which extends Gehan's (1965) generalization of Wilcoxon's test, for testing the equality of continuous distribution functions when observations are subject to arbitrary right censorship. The asymptotic nonparametric test for randomly censored data given by Breslow (1970), which corrects for independent competing causes of death, applies only to lethal tumors.

A simple algorithm for calculating the Breslow test statistic for a comparison of two groups is given by Tarone and Ware (1977). Let R_k denote the total number of animals at risk at time t_k and A_k denote the proportion of R_k that belongs to the treated group. Let S_{1k} and S_{2k} denote the number of tumors observed in the treated and control groups respectively at time t_k. Let $S_k = S_{1k} + S_{2k}$, $E_k = S_k A_k$, $W_k = R_k(S_{1k} - E_k)$ and $V_k^2 = R_k^2 S_k A_k(1 - A_k)(R_k - S_k)/(R_k - 1)$. Define $W = \Sigma W_k$ and $V^2 = \Sigma V_k^2$. Under the null hypothesis of no difference between the treated and control animals with respect to the risk R, W is approximately normally distributed with zero mean and standard deviation V. The null hypothesis is rejected if

$$\frac{|W|}{V} \geq Z \tag{12}$$

where Z is the standard normal deviate corresponding to the desired level of significance.

2. Cox Test

In order to obtain estimates of time-to-tumor curves and perform statistical tests comparing these curves as well as testing for dose trend for lethal tumors, it is convenient to construct

TABLE 5 Illustrative Data for a Carcinogenesis Experiment

Group (i)	Dose (d_i)	Day of removal with tumor (*) or death due to tumor (**)
0	0	180, 196, 219, 244, 245, 279, 296,* 301, 340,** 360, 360*
1	d_1	197, 219, 228, 240, 287, 287,* 299, 304, 333, 360*
2	d_2	154, 177, 179, 191, 210, 222,* 231,** 240,* 255**
3	d_3	143, 188, 191, 196,* 196,** 217, 231,** 239,* 242**

life tables. This was not done in the previous example employing the generalized Kruskal-Wallis test for comparing a treated and control group because of the convenient algorithm available for that test. For the remainder of the techniques discussed in this section it is useful to consider a life table framework. Consider the data in Table 5 in which the day of removal from the experiment is recorded for each animal. An (*) indicates the tumor of interest was present but did not kill the animal and (**) indicates that the tumor of interest was the probable cause of death.

The general life table format for an animal carcinogenesis experiment is shown in Table 6. A line is added each time an animal dies due to the tumor type under consideration. That is, each tumor death establishes a new time interval. This is unlike the life tables for large human populations in which time generally is divided into intervals a priori. The number of deaths in the ith group at the kth time of tumor death due to the tumor type(s) in all groups is denoted by x_{ik} (typically $x_{ik} = 0$ or 1, depending on the absence or presence of a death due to the tumor). The number of animals surviving to the kth tumor death time in the ith group is n_{ik}. Summation over i is denoted by a dot giving $x_{\cdot k}$ as the number of deaths due to the tumor type(s) and $n_{\cdot k}$ as the number of animals in the experiment surviving at the kth time a tumor death occurred. The illustrative data given in Table 5 are displayed in the standard life table format in Table 7.

A test for comparing two or more censored distributions was developed by Cox (1972). For the special case of comparing a treated and control distribution of a lethal tumor type adjusted for censoring from other causes of death, the test is based on x_{ik}, the number of tumor deaths in the ith group (i = 0 for controls and i = 1 for treated) at the kth point in time at which tumors of the type(s) of interest kill animals in either group. A moribund animal removed from an experiment because it is not expected to live will be treated as an animal dying on the day of removal. Removing moribund animals is practiced to reduce autolysis. However, premature removal of animals will bias survival and time-to-tumor curves. The number of animals at risk, survivors, in the ith group is n_{ik} at the kth time of occurrence of death to an animal in either group due to the tumor type(s) of interest. The test proposed

TABLE 6 General Life Table Format

Tumor death k^{th} time	Group 0	1 . . . i . . . r	Totals $x_{\cdot k}/n_{\cdot k}$
1	x_{01}	x_{11} . . . x_{i1} . . . x_{r1}	$x_{\cdot 1}/n_{\cdot 1}$
⋮			
k	x_{0k}	x_{1k} . . . x_{ik} . . . x_{rk}	$x_{\cdot k}/n_{\cdot k}$
⋮			
s	x_{0s}	x_{1s} . . . x_{is} . . . x_{rs}	$x_{\cdot s}/n_{\cdot s}$

TABLE 7 Number of Tumor Deaths, x_{ik}, over Survivors at k^{th} Time of Tumor Death

Tumor k	Death time	0	1	2	3	Total $x_{\cdot k}/n_{\cdot k}$
1	196	0/10	0.10	0/5	1/6	1/31
2	231	0/8	0/7	1/3	1/3	2/21
3	242	0/8	0/6	0/1	1/1	1/16
4	255	0/6	0/6	1/1	0/0	1/13
5	340	1/3	0/1	0/0	0/0	1/4

by Cox (1972) is conditional on $x_{\cdot k} = \Sigma x_{ik}$, n_{0k}, and n_{1k}. The expected number of these tumor deaths under the null hypothesis in the treated group at the kth time of a death is

$$E(X_{1k}) = \frac{n_{1k}\, x_{\cdot k}}{n_{\cdot k}} \tag{13}$$

where $n_{\cdot k} = \Sigma n_{ik}$. For large samples an approximate chi-square test statistic with one degree of freedom is given by

$$\chi_1^2 = \frac{[\Sigma_k x_{1k} - \Sigma_k E(x_{1k})]^2}{\Sigma_k \dfrac{n_{1k}(n_{\cdot k} - n_{1k}) x_{\cdot k}(n_{\cdot k} - x_{\cdot k})}{n_{\cdot k}^2 (n_{\cdot k} - 1)}} \tag{14}$$

for $n_{\cdot k} > 1$. This is also the log rank statistic given by Peto and Peto (1972). The above test has been shown to have certain optimal properties for testing survival curves having hazard functions (the probability of a tumor at time t among the survivors at time t) which are multiples of each other. The former test based on the W statistic by Breslow (1970) gives more weight to early tumor deaths and is shown to be more powerful for testing against certain alternatives where ratios of the hazard functions are not constant; see Lee et al. 1975) and Tarone and Ware (1977).

3. Peto Test

Peto (1974) proposed dividing the data into a number of short-time intervals, generally no longer than one week. The number of animals dying due to a particular tumor type in the jth interval (x_{ij}) divided by the number of animals (n_{ij}) alive at the beginning of the jth interval are calculated for each group. The expected values E_{ij} are computed for the ith group for the jth time interval under the null hypothesis that the proportions of animals dying in each group are equal within each time interval. An approximate chi-square test for equivalency of deaths due to the tumor among groups, with r degrees of freedom, is

$$\chi^2 = \sum_i \frac{(\Sigma_j O_{ij} - \Sigma_j E_{ij})^2}{\Sigma_j E_{ij}} \tag{15}$$

where O_{ij} is the observed number of animals dying due to the tumor type in the ith group ($i = 0, 1, 2, \ldots, r$) during the jth interval. Peto and Pike (1973) discuss the conservatism of the approximate test.

C. Test for Trend

When there are more than two dose levels d_i ($i = 0, 1, \ldots, r$), Thomas et al. (1977) and Tarone and Ware (1977) give a one degree of freedom chi-square linear trend test based on the W statistic of Breslow (1970)

$$\chi_i^2 = \frac{\left(\Sigma_{i=0}^{r} d_i W_i\right)^2}{\Sigma_{i=0}^{r} \Sigma_{j=0}^{r} V(W_{ij}) d_i d_j} \tag{16}$$

where

$$W_i = \sum_k (n_{\cdot k}\, x_{ik} - x_{\cdot k}\, n_{ik}) \tag{17}$$

and

$$V(W_{ij}) = \sum_k \frac{n_{ik}(n_{\cdot k}\,\delta_{ij} - n_{jk}) x_{\cdot k}(n_{\cdot k} - x_{\cdot k})}{n_{\cdot k} - 1} \tag{18}$$

where $\delta_{ij} = 1$ for $i = j$ and $\delta_{ij} = 0$ for $i \neq j$ and $n_{\cdot k} > 1$. Thomas et al. (1977) also give a test for departure from trend.

Using the regression model proposed by Cox (1972), where the hazard function for the ith dose group is $\lambda_i(t) = \lambda_0(t) \exp \beta d_i$, a test for linear trend in $\ell n\, \lambda_i(t)$, i.e., $H_0 : \beta = 0$ for censored data adjusted for competing causes of death, is given by Tarone (1975) and is identical to the analogous contingency table test of Mantel (1963). The asymptotic one degree of freedom chi-square test given by Tarone (1975) is

$$\chi_i^2 = \frac{\left(\Sigma_{i=0}^{r} (O_i - E_i) d_i\right)^2}{\Sigma_{i=0}^{r} \Sigma_{j=0}^{r} V_{ij} d_i d_j} \tag{19}$$

where $O_i = \Sigma_k x_{ik}$ is the total number of animals in the ith dose group killed by the tumor type(s) under investigation, and $E_i = \Sigma_k n_{ik}\, x_{\cdot k}/n_{\cdot k}$ is the total expected number in the ith dose group totaled over all the times at which tumor deaths of the type(s) occurred in the course of the experiment in any dose group, and

$$V_{ij} = \sum_k \frac{n_{ik}(n_{\cdot k}\,\delta_{ij} - n_{jk}) x_{\cdot k}(n_{\cdot k} - x_{\cdot k})}{n_{\cdot k}^2 (n_{\cdot k} - 1)} \tag{20}$$

where $\delta_{ij} = 1$ for $i = j$, and $\delta_{ij} = 0$ for $i \neq j$, and $n_{\cdot k} > 1$.

Failure to detect a trend does not necessarily indicate that a chemical under test is not carcinogenic. The number of animals per dose may not be large enough to detect a trend, particularly in view of the complicating effects introduced by competing causes of death. Chemical carcinogens frequently exhibit rather steep dose response curves. To observe this effect requires a very judicious choice of doses. If the doses chosen are too low, sufficient tumors will not be observed to indicate the presence of a trend. Likewise, if the doses chosen are too high, an apparent plateau may be reached or competing causes of death may obliterate any trend.

Patel and Hoel (1973) have developed a test for monotone dose response. Their test is also based on the W statistic of Breslow (1970). Let

$$T = \sum_{i=0}^{r-1} \sum_{j=i+1}^{r} W_{ij} \tag{21}$$

$$\nu = \min\{n_{io}\} \tag{22}$$

then the test statistic is

$$\frac{\nu^{1/2}\, T}{\hat{\sigma}} \tag{23}$$

and is assumed to be approximately normally distributed in small samples. The estimated variance $\hat{\sigma}$ is complicated to calculate and the reader is referred to Patel and Hoel (1973) for the specific method. The test does have the advantage of not having been adversely affected if the doses exhibit a plateauing of the response.

IV. TIME-TO-TUMOR OBSERVATION (NONLETHAL TUMORS)

A. Estimation

Sufficient attention is not often paid to the reason of the discovery of tumors. Lethal tumors that kill an animal and are verified to be the probable cause of death lend themselves to the life table type analyses discussed in Sec. III. However, a nonlethal or incidental tumor that is discovered upon necropsy as a result of sacrifice or death of the animal due to some other cause requires statistical analyses not based upon life table techniques devised for lethal tumors. Competing causes of death are not a factor if it can be assumed that the occurrence of a nonlethal tumor is independent of death. Thus, the prevalence of a nonlethal tumor may be estimated from animals dying during the course of the study as well as from scheduled sacrifices.

A simple method can be used for estimating the prevalence of animals bearing certain tumor types during various time intervals. If r_j out of n_j animals necropsied bear the tumor types in the jth time interval, the estimate of its prevalence is given by

$$\hat{P}_j = \frac{r_j}{n_j} \tag{24}$$

A dilemma arises with this estimator for animal studies. The time intervals must be short enough so that the probability of a tumor arising over the time interval remains relatively constant, but the time interval must be long enough to include enough animals to obtain somewhat stable estimates. The proportions of tumors between a control and treated group can be compared for the jth time interval by Fisher's exact test or the approximate chi-square test as described in Sec. II.A. The data may be combined into a single test over all corresponding time intervals by the Mantel-Haenszel procedure (1959) described in Sec. II.B.

With the typically small numbers of animals used in carcinogenesis tests, dividing data into time intervals often is not very satisfactory. Hoel and Walburg (1972) present a noninterval estimator for nonlethal tumors. Let P(t) represent the proportion of animals possessing a nonlethal tumor at time t. Assuming that the tumors do not disappear, then P(t) is a nondecreasing function of time. Recall that it has been assumed that the time of death is independent of the presence of the nonlethal tumor. To obtain an estimate of P(t), all of the necropsied animals are ordered by age at death, regardless of the cause of death (including scheduled sacrifices). Starting with the earliest death with the nonlethal tumor, let $a_1 \geq 1$ be the number of successive deaths with the tumor. Next let $b_1 \geq 1$ be the number of successive deaths without the tumor followed by $a_2 \geq 1$ with the tumor, and so on, to the end of the experiment. Estimates of P(t) are obtained from $P_i = a_i/(a_i + b_i)$, combining adjacent a_i and b_i, if necessary, such that $P_1 \leq P_2 \leq P_3 \leq \cdots \leq P_n$; an algorithm for this solution is given by Hoel and Walburg (1972).

B. Treated Versus Control

Peto (1974) also presented an interval technique for comparing treatment groups for nonlethal or incidentally observed tumors. For comparison of a control and treated group, let r_{ij} be the number of incidental nonlethal tumors of the tumor type(s) under consideration observed in the ith group (i = 0 controls and i = 1 treated) for the jth time period (j = 1, 2, . . . , s) in n_{ij} necropsied animals. The basic data for nonlethal tumors can be summarized as in Table 8. Under the null hypothesis of no difference between treated and control animals, the expected number of incidental nonlethal tumors in the ith group for the jth time period is

TABLE 8 Tabulation of Nonlethal Tumor-Bearing Animals, r_{ij}, over Number of Animals Examined, n_{ij}

Group	Period 1 . . . Period j . . . Period s			Totals
Control	r_{01}/n_{01}	. . . r_{0j}/n_{0j}	. . . r_{0s}/n_{0s}	$r_{0\cdot}/n_{0\cdot}$
Treated	r_{11}/n_{11}	. . . r_{1j}/n_{1j}	. . . r_{1s}/n_{1s}	$r_{1\cdot}/n_{1\cdot}$
Totals	$r_{\cdot 1}/n_{\cdot 1}$	. . . $r_{\cdot j}/n_{\cdot j}$	. . . $r_{\cdot s}/n_{\cdot s}$	$r_{\cdot\cdot}/n_{\cdot\cdot}$

$$E(r_{ij}) = \frac{n_{ij}\, r_{\cdot j}}{n_{\cdot j}} \tag{25}$$

Over all time periods the observed number of incidental nonlethal tumors is $r_{i\cdot}$ with an expected value of

$$E(r_{i\cdot}) = \frac{\Sigma_{j=1}^{s} n_{ij}\, r_{\cdot j}}{n_{\cdot j}} \tag{26}$$

An approximate one degree of freedom chi-square test is given by

$$\chi_1^2 = \frac{[r_{0\cdot} - E(r_{0\cdot})]^2}{E(r_{0\cdot})} + \frac{[r_{1\cdot} - E(r_{1\cdot})]^2}{E(r_{1\cdot})} \tag{27}$$

The conservatism of this test is discussed in Peto and Pike (1973).

To illustrate the procedure suggested by Peto (1974) for nonlethal incidental tumors, consider the illustrative data presented in Table 9.

The expected values for the number of nonlethal tumors in each group for each time period are given in Table 10.

The approximate one degree of freedom chi-square test for a difference between the treated and control animals is

$$\chi_1^2 = \frac{(3 - 6.467)^2}{6.467} + \frac{(9 - 5.533)^2}{5.533} = 4.03 \tag{28}$$

TABLE 9 Illustrative Data of the Occurrence of Incidental Nonlethal Tumors Among Dying Animals

Group	Period 1	Period 2	Period 3	Period 4	Period 5	Totals
Control	0/3	0/4	1/6	0/6	2/5	3/24
Treated	0/2	1/2	2/4	2/6	4/5	9/19
Total	0/5	1/6	3/10	2/12	6/10	12/43

TABLE 10 Expected Numbers of Incidental Nonlethal Tumors Among Dying Animals

Group	Period 1	Period 2	Period 3	Period 4	Period 5	Totals
Control	0.000	0.667	1.800	1.000	3.000	6.467
Treated	0.000	0.333	1.200	1.000	3.000	5.533

which is significant at the $P < 0.05$ level. In such an experiment, one is probably more interested in the alternative hypothesis that the treatment with a chemical causes an increase in tumors. Thus, $\sqrt{\chi_1^2} = 2.01$ is a normal deviate with a one-sided significance level of $P < 0.03$. Note the ability of this test in this example to detect a difference with relatively few animals.

V. DISCUSSION

The techniques discussed in this chapter have focused on procedures to determine if a chemical results in an increase in tumors in experimental animals. No attempt has been made to estimate dose response curves or to extrapolate from the generally high experimental doses used to lower doses that might be experienced by humans. Also, a good deal of recent statistical literature is devoted to fitting various mathematical models to experimental data in order to describe time-to-tumor functions. We have avoided that problem and emphasized ascertaining if a carcinogenic effect has been demonstrated in a test population of animals. Tests for trends in dose have been introduced to strengthen those conclusions when warranted.

Unfortunately, Fisher's exact test or the corresponding chi-square approximation have been inappropriately used on many occasions to compare the proportion of tumors in two groups. This test does not take into account tumor rates varying over time or pertubations caused by death of the animals. We have presented techniques that adjust the data for changing mortality patterns and have emphasized the important distinction between lethal tumors that kill an animal (in which case life table analyses may be employed) and nonlethal tumors which are only discovered at necropsy after an animal dies of other causes (in which case alternative techniques must be employed). Tumors that can be observed upon palpation, such as large mammary tumors, may be treated statistically as lethal tumors if these observations result in the removal of an animal from an experiment.

Serial sacrifice experiments are sometimes employed to study the progression of a tumorigenic process with time, particularly so that animals can be examined at early ages before many deaths occur. If the tumor is nonlethal and independent of other lethal diseases the data from sacrificed and dying animals can be combined with an interval technique. For lethal tumors serial sacrifices are treated simply as competing causes of death and the presence of tumors in these animals is ignored. Perhaps this information would not be ignored if the pathologists could predict that the animal would eventually die because of the presence of the tumor, if a competing cause had not resulted in death. The potential use of such information requires further statistical research.

Any analysis of lethal and nonlethal tumors is open to controversy, particularly because of the difficulty of determining the cause of death of an animal (Gart, 1975).

It should be mentioned that the competing risk methodology that has been used throughout this chapter is dependent on the assumption of disease independence. J. Neyman and other investigators at the University of California at Berkeley have been exploring models that do not require this assumption of independence. Specifically, they have been considering models that assume that an animal is in a given disease state at any point in time, and Markov transitions between disease states are assumed. This approach is so far fairly complicated and not yet ready for routine data analysis. It does, however, hold promise for future methodologies.

Important problems regarding the design of carcinogenesis experiments remain: number of animals per dose, number of doses, spacing of doses, duration of study, sampling of tissues and organs, and so on. The solutions to these problems depend on the purpose of a study. Screening experiments emphasize the use of high doses, extrapolation experiments may employ lower doses, and research experiments designed to study dose response relationships and correlations with other factors require different protocols. No attempt was made here to investigate these important and relatively unexplored areas.

Finally, a word of caution is needed in interpreting results from small experiments. Only relatively potent carcinogens can be expected to be detected. On the other hand, because of the large number of tissues examined and the use of more than one dose level, strain, or sex, numerous statistical comparisons may be employed in one study resulting in several opportunities to obtain false positive results. Fears et al. (1977) discuss these problems in the context of the current National Cancer Institute Bioassay Screening Program.

REFERENCES

Armitage, P. (1955). Tests for linear trends in proportions and frequencies. Biometrics 11:375-386.

Breslow, N. (1970). A generalized Kruskal-Wallis test for comparing k samples subject to unequal patterns of censorship. Biometrika 57:579-594.

Cochran, W. G. (1954). Some methods for strengthening the common χ^2 tests. Biometrics 10:417-451.

Cox, D. R. (1958). The regression analysis of binary sequences. J. R. Stat. Soc. (Series B) 20:215-242.

Cox, D. R. (1972). Regression models and life tables. J. R. Stat. Soc. (Series B) 34: 187-220.

Fears, T. R., Tarone, R. E., and Chu, K. C. (1977). False-positive and false-negative rates for carcinogenicity screens. Cancer Res. 37:1941-1945.

Gart, J. J. (1975). Letter to the editor. Br. J. Cancer 31:696-697.

Gehan, E. (1965). A generalized Wilcoxon test for comparing arbitrarily single censored samples. Biometrika 52:203-223.

Hoel, D. G., and Walburg, H. E. (1972). Statistical analysis of survival experiments. J. Natl. Cancer Inst. 49:361-372.

Kaplan, E. L., and Meier, P. (1958). Nonparametric estimation from incomplete observations. J. Am. Stat. Assoc. 53:457-481.

Lee, E. T., Desu, M. M., and Gehan, E. (1975). A Monte Carlo study of the power of some two sample tests. Biometrika 62:425-432.

Mantel, N. (1963). Chi-square tests with one degree of freedom: extensions of the Mantel-Haenszel procedure. J. Am. Stat. Assoc. 58:690-700.

Mantel, N., and Haenszel, W. (1959). Statistical aspects of the analysis of data from retrospective studies of diseases. J. Natl. Cancer Inst. 22:719-748.

Patel, K. M., and Hoel, D. G. (1973). A generalized Jonckheere k-sample test against ordered alternatives when observations are subject to arbitrary right censorship. Commun. Stat. 2:373-380.

Peto, R. (1974). Guidelines on the analysis of tumor rates and death rates in experimental animals. Br. J. Cancer 29:101-105.

Peto, R., and Peto, J. (1972). Asymptotically efficient rank invariant test procedures. J. R. Stat. Soc. (Series A) 135:185-206.

Peto, R., and Pike, M. C. (1973). Conservatism of the approximation $\Sigma(O - E)^2/E$ in the logrank test for survival data or tumor incidence data. Biometrics 29:579-584.

Tarone, R. E. (1975). Tests for trend in life table analysis. Biometrika 62:679-682.

Tarone, R. E., and Ware, J. (1977). On distribution-free tests for equality of survival distributions. Biometrika 64:156-160.

Thomas, D. G., Breslow, N., and Gart, J. J. (1977). Trend and homogeneity analyses of proportions and life table data. Comput. Biomed. Res. 10:373-381.

6

In Vitro Screening Tests for Potential Carcinogens

PAUL B. FISHER and I. BERNARD WEINSTEIN / Columbia University College of Physicians and Surgeons, New York, New York

---

Research support was supplied by Contract No. NO-1-CP-2-3234 and Grant No. CA-21111-02 from the National Cancer Institute and Research Grant RD-50 from the American Cancer Society.

I. OVERVIEW OF IN VITRO SCREENING TESTS FOR CARCINOGENS

A. Introduction—General Aspects

Epidemiological evidence suggests that 70-90% of all human cancers result from exposure to environmental agents (Haenszel and Kurihara, 1968; Haenszel, 1961). Table 1 presents a list of the approximately 30 compounds that are now known to cause human cancer. (For a detailed discussion see Tomatis, 1977; Tomatis et al., 1978.) These do not, however, account for the majority of human cancers, and thus many of the major human carcinogens have not yet been identified. With the increasing exposure of humans to newly synthesized agents introduced into our foods, drugs, consumer products, and general environment, there is also an urgent need to develop reliable assay systems for detecting whether any of these agents are potential carcinogens and for estimating their possible risks to humans (Cornfield, 1977). The rationale behind carcinogen screening programs, therefore, is to have an efficient and reliable system of identifying compounds that have carcinogenic potential. Positive compounds must then be assessed in terms of their possible risks to humans and the feasibility of preventing human exposure, or at least reducing the quantity or the degree of human exposure. If these goals are achieved, then it is likely that the current high incidence of human cancer will be substantially reduced and the possible introduction of new and potent carcinogens into the human environment will be avoided.

The ability of a compound to induce cancer in experimental animals is generally viewed as an indication of potential hazard to humans. As a result of the long latent period between application of the carcinogen and tumor formation in vivo, tests have been modified to increase the incidence of tumor formation and reduce the latency time. This modification has been accomplished by utilizing sensitive strains of animals and applying maximally tolerated doses of the test compound. The results obtained using small groups of animals (usually a few hundred or fewer) must often then be interpreted in terms of the potential hazards of possible exposure of millions of humans to much lower levels of this material and over longer periods of time. Quantitative extrapolations of this type are fraught with considerable uncertainties because (1) one seldom has dose response data over a wide range of doses (since this requires large numbers of animals), and (2) marked variations exist between species in terms of carcinogen susceptibility (Weinhouse, 1977; Clayson, 1977). Other problems in interpreting animal carcinogenicity data include: (1) the uncertainty of extrapolating from results obtained with high dosage (done to increase the sensitivity of the assay) to what would happen at low dosage; (2) the validity of comparing test results obtained in one or a few animal species to humans and the problem of comparing genetically inbred animal populations to human populations that have extensive genetic diversity; (3) the shorter life span of test animals in comparison with humans; and (4) the difficulty in comparing results obtained using defined exposures of animal populations to the human situation in which individuals are exposed to a spectrum of physiological and environmental factors that may modify host response. Other limitations of assays for carcinogens in the intact animal include: the large expense required to test the multitude of newly synthesized compounds as well as those already present in our environment and the need for specialized personnel to initiate and maintain large-scale animal studies (Clayson, 1977). For all of these reasons the development of well-validated, short-term, in vitro screening tests has become a necessary complement to animal studies in the evaluation of an immense number of environmental agents for possible carcinogenicity.

In developing short-term in vitro screening tests for chemical carcinogens one must be cognizant of certain fundamental aspects of the carcinogenic process. These aspects include the following:

1. Human and animal carcinogens are extremely diverse in terms of their sources and chemical structures (Table 1). The screening tests must be capable, therefore, of detecting a broad spectrum of chemical structures.
2. Many carcinogens are initially inactive and require metabolic activation.

TABLE 1 Chemicals Recognized as Carcinogens in Humans

Chemical	Site of cancer
Chemical mixtures	
Soots, tars, oils	Skin, lungs
Cigarette smoke	Lungs
Industrial chemicals	
2-Naphthylamine	Urinary bladder
Benzidine	Urinary bladder
4-Aminobiphenyl	Urinary bladder
Chloromethyl methyl ether	Lungs
Nickel compounds	Lungs, nasal sinuses
Chromium compounds	Lungs
Asbestos	Lungs, mesothelia
Arsenic compounds	Skin, lungs
Vinyl chloride	Liver
Drugs	
N,N-bis(2-chloroethyl)-2-naphthylamine	Urinary bladder
Bis(2-chloroethyl)sulfide (mustard gas)	Lungs
Diethylstibestrol	Vagina
Phenacetin	Renal pelvis
Birth control pills	Benign hepatomas
Naturally occurring compounds	
Betal nuts	Buccal mucosa
Aflatoxins	Liver
Potent carcinogens in animals to which humans are exposed	
Sterigmatocystin	Liver
Cycasin	Liver
Safrole	Liver
Pyrrolizidine alkaloids	Liver
Nitroso compounds	Esophagus, liver, kidney, stomach

Source: Modified from Heidelberger, 1973; see also Tomatis, 1977; Tomatis et al., 1978; Althouse et al., 1979; and Montesano et al., 1980.

3. Cancer induction usually occurs in multiple steps. The individual steps may be elicited by different types of agents and occur via different mechanisms.

Carcinogens such as benzo(a)pyrene (BP) and 2-fluorenylacetamide (2-FAA) are not capable of inducing neoplasia unless they are first enzymatically converted into reactive electrophilic species (Gelboin, 1969; Miller, 1970; Miller and Miller, 1969, 1971; Grover et al., 1971). The parent compound is called, therefore, a "procarcinogen." Once metabolically converted to a "proximate" carcinogen, and then to a highly reactive or "ultimate" carcinogen, it can react with nucleophilic residues in cellular macromolecules (proteins and nucleic acids) to form covalent adducts (Miller and Miller, 1969, 1971; Brookes and Lawley, 1971; Weinstein, 1978; Miller, 1978). Different species of animals vary in their enzymatic capacity to activate or detoxify potential carcinogens, and this is an important variable in terms of host susceptibility. This variable is clearly shown in the case of the potent human urinary bladder carcinogen 4-aminobiphenyl (4-ABP) which induced bladder tumors in dogs, but not in monkeys or hamsters. With other animal species 4-ABP induces hepatomas (mouse) or mammary tumors (rat), reflecting possible differences in tissue-specific metabolic activation systems (Clayson, 1977).

The concept that cancer induction results from more than one step is most clearly demonstrated in mouse skin carcinogenesis (for review see Berenblum, 1969, 1975; Slaga et al., 1978), although this principle certainly extends to other species and tissues (Neish et al., 1967; Warwick, 1967; Berenblum, 1969; Foulds, 1969; Cairns, 1975a; Peraino et al., 1970; Slaga et al., 1978). In mouse skin carcinogenesis two descrete stages have been defined, one termed "initiation" and the other "promotion." It appears that initiating agents produce a stable alteration in the cellular genome but that these potentially neoplastic cells do not give rise to tumors unless a second agent, the promoter, is applied repeatedly to the same tissue. At high doses certain initiating agents can also act as "complete carcinogens." On the other hand, even when applied to tissues at high dosage and in the absence of prior exposure of the tissue to an initiating agent, tumor promoters do not produce a significant increase in tumor incidence. Other properties of tumor promoters are described in detail in a separate section of this chapter. In designing an effective in vitro screening program in terms of cancer prevention, tests must be used that will detect not only complete carcinogens, but also compounds that exhibit initiating or promoting activity, or act as cofactors through other mechanisms. An example of the latter is the interaction between a chemical and a viral agent in the induction of cell transformation. In vitro systems that assay for this type of combination are described later in this chapter.

Freeman (1978) has previously discussed some of the advantages and disadvantages of in vitro carcinogen assays when compared to animal assays. Advantages of in vitro assays include: shorter time required to conduct assays; reduced expense in performing tests; reduced space requirements for conducting experiments and maintaining test systems; ability to utilize human cells as potential assay systems or as sources of metabolizing enzymes; the relative ease of doing dose response curves, which in animal bioassays would usually be prohibitive in terms of numbers of animals; and the smaller quantities, often microgram amounts, of the test agents required for assays. Disadvantages in utilizing short-term in vitro screening assays include:

- The need for specialized expertise and facilities in microbial and tissue culture methods
- Problems in cell line stability after repeated subcultures
- Background levels of spontaneous mutations and transformation, especially if proper precautions are not followed in cell line maintenance
- Absence of chemical carcinogen activation mechanisms in many cell types carried in vitro
- The need for in vitro activation systems that can metabolize a wide variety of chemical compounds in a manner analogous to that occurring in vivo, which may not always be the case with an arbitrary liver microsomal "S-9" preparation
- The problem of distinguishing induced mutations or transformation from toxicity and cell selection
- Variability among species, individuals within a species, etc. which may extend to cell cultures obtained from these organisms
- And the developmental nature of the tests, most of which require further validation using larger numbers and different classes of known carcinogens and noncarcinogens

Some of these types of problems are not, of course, unique to in vitro test systems. Animal assays are fraught with the problems of spontaneous tumor incidence; variations among species, tissues, and individuals in terms of metabolism and other susceptibility factors; the definition of endpoints (interpretation of pathology, benign versus malignant tumors, etc.); accurate quantitation; and the problem of extrapolation of the results to the human. It is likely, therefore, that in many cases more precise evaluation of the potential human hazards of an agent can be obtained by a combination of animal and in vitro assays (Berky and Sherrod, 1978).

B. Types of In Vitro and Short-Term Assay Systems

Recognizing the limitations of animal studies and the fact that it is simply not feasible to depend only on animal tests to assess environmental and industrial chemicals for carcinogenicity has led to the recent development of a large number of in vitro tests for potential carcinogens (Table 2). Other short-term tests done in vivo rather than in vitro have exploited carcinogen induced changes in sperm structure (Wyrobek and Bruce, 1975; Moutschen and Colizzi, 1975) and mutations in drosophila (Mollet and Wurgler, 1974; Mollet and Weilenmann, 1976; Vogel, 1977) as endpoints. Although they are not discussed in this chapter, the following systems in the intact animal have also demonstrated promise as useful short-term screening tests for carcinogens:

- In vivo tests utilizing mice, such as the induction of pulmonary adenomas in strain A mice (Stoner et al., 1973; Shimkin and Stoner, 1975)
- The induction of hyperplastic liver nodules in rats (Tatematsu et al., 1977)
- Initiation-promotion studies on mouse skin (Slaga et al., 1978)
- The dominant lethal assay (Epstein et al., 1972)
- Specific locus test (Searle, 1975; Russell, 1977)
- Somatic mutation test (Fahrig, 1977)
- Dominant mutations resulting in skeletal malformations (Selby and Selby, 1977)
- Micronucleus test (Schmid, 1975)
- Heritable translocation test (Generoso, 1973)
- Sister chromatid exchange (Lambert et al., 1978)

Previous authors have evaluated the relative merits of some of these tests. Stoltz et al. (1974) reviewed short-term carcinogenicity assays that utilized the following endpoints: accelerated tumor formation in the animal, teratogenesis, induction of chromosome aberrations, mutagenesis, DNA repair synthesis, in vitro cell transformation, interactions with nucleic acids, or cytological alterations. Based on the overall relevance to carcinogenesis and practical applicability they suggested that three of the tests, mutagenesis, DNA repair synthesis, and in vitro cell transformation, offer promise as useful screening tests. A critical parameter is the ability of the short-term tests to distinguish between known carcinogens and noncarcinogens. Purchase et al. (1976) evaluated six short-term tests using 120 test compounds, 58 of which were known carcinogens. The tests included

- Bacterial mutagenesis utilizing the *Salmonella typhimurium*/microsome assay (Ames test)
- A mammalian cell transformation assay based on growth in soft agar
- Ribosomal loss from rat liver rough endoplasmic reticulum (Rabin's test)
- The implant test based on analysis of the fibrous capsule and surrounding tissue following surgical implantation of millipore filter discs containing the test compound
- The sebaceous gland test, which monitors a decrease in the ratio of sebaceous glands to hair follicles on treated mouse skin
- The tetrazolium reduction test based on increased reduction of tetrazolium to formazan by treated mouse skin

The two most accurate predictors of carcinogenic or noncarcinogenic potential were the Ames and the mammalian cell transformation tests. Both of these assays were 91% accurate in identifying carcinogens and 93% (Ames) or 97% (cell transformation) accurate in their lack of response to noncarcinogens. The usefulness of these two test systems was further indicated by their ability to distinguish between pairs of structurally similar carcinogens and noncarcinogens. With the exception of β- and α-naphthylamine, which were both negative in cell transformation analysis but positive (β-naphthylamine) and negative (α-naphthylamine) in the Ames assay, both systems discriminated between eight structurally matched pairs of carcinogens and noncarcinogens. Both the Ames and cell transformation assays accurately predicted the carcinogenic activity or lack of activity of 106 of the 120 compounds (88%). Two compounds gave false negatives in both assays, diethylstilbestrol and vinyl chloride (the latter

TABLE 2 Short-Term In Vitro Test Systems for Mutagens and Carcinogens[a]

System	Basis of test (parameter monitored)	References
I. Microbial		
A. Bacterial mutagenesis		
1. Salmonella typhimurium (with microsome activation)	Histidine auxotrophs	Ames et al., 1975; McCann et al., 1975a, McCann and Ames, 1976a
2. Salmonella typhimurium	8-azaguanine resistance	Shopek et al., 1978
3. Escherichia coli (K-12)	Inductest (prophage induction) Mutatest (forward mutation in prophage immunity region)	Moreau et al., 1976; Moreau and Devoret, 1977
4. Escherichia coli (K-12/343/13)	Arginine auxotrophs	Mohn et al., 1974
5. Escherichia coli (WP-2)	Tryptophan auxotrophs	Green and Muriel, 1976
6. Escherichia coli (REC$^-$)	Repair deficient strain (growth inhibition)	Ichinotsubo et al., 1977
7. Bacillus subtilis	Histidine auxotroph reversion	Tanooka, 1977
8. Bacillus subtilis	Sporulation gene mutation	MacGregor and Sacks, 1976
B. Yeast and molds		
1. Saccharomyces cerevisiae	Mutation, gene conversion, and mitotic recombination	Zimmermann, 1975
2. Neurospora crassa (ad-3)	Adenine auxotrophs	Ong and deSerres, 1972
3. Aspergillus sps.	Mutation and recombination	Kafer et al., 1976
II. Mammalian cell cultures		
A. Alterations in growth properties and transformation		
1. Early-passage Syrian hamster embryo	Morphological transformation	Pienta et al., 1977; Dunkel et al., 1977
2. Guinea pig embryo	Growth in agar	Evans and DiPaolo, 1975, 1976; Evans et al., 1977
3. Rat embryo	Morphological transformation, tumorigenesis	Namba et al., 1969; Rhim and Huebner, 1973, Freeman et al., 1975
4. Rat or mouse embryo infected with murine leukemia virus	Morphological transformation	Freeman et al., 1973; Rhim et al., 1974
5. Rat embryo infected with adenovirus	Epithelial-transformed colonies	DiPaolo and Casto, 1976; Fisher et al., 1978

6. Syrian hamster embryo infected with adenovirus	Epithelioid transformed foci	Casto et al., 1976, 1978
7. Mouse embryo C3H 10T1/2	Morphological transformation	Reznikoff et al., 1973a, 1973b
8. Balb 3T3 mouse embryo	Morphological transformation	DiPaolo et al., 1972b; Kakunaga, 1973
9. BHK 21 (Syrian hamster newborn kidneys)	Growth in agar	Bouck and diMayorca, 1976; Styles, 1977
10. Human diploid fibroblasts	Morphological transformation	Kakunaga, 1977, 1978
11. Mouse prostate (adult)	Morphological transformation	Chen and Heidelberger, 1969c
12. Rat liver (epithelial cells)	Growth in agar, cytologic changes, tumorigenesis	Katsuta and Takaoka, 1968, 1972; Namba et al., 1969; Williams et al., 1973; Montesano et al., 1973; Yamaguchi and Weinstein, 1975
13. Mouse epidermal cultures	Growth in agar, tumorigenesis	Colburn et al., 1978a
B. Specific gene mutations		
1. Chinese hamster ovary (CHO)	HGPRT locus mutation	O'Neill et al., 1977a
2. Chinese hamster lung (V79)	HGPRT locus mutation	Krahn and Heidelberger, 1977; Chu and Malling, 1968
3. Human lymphoblast	HGPRT locus mutation	Thilly et al., 1976
4. Human fibroblast	APRT locus mutation	DeMars, 1974
5. Mouse lymphoma (L-5178Y)	Mutation from TK^+ to TK^-	Clive and Spector, 1975
6. Mouse lymphoma (L-5178Y)	Alanine auxotrophs	Nakamura et al., 1977
7. Rat liver epithelial cells	8-azaguanine resistance	San and Williams, 1977
C. Chromosome analysis		
1. Chinese hamster ovary (CHO) and lung (V79)	Sister chromatid exchange	Perry and Evans, 1975; Popescu et al., 1977; Carrano et al., 1978
2. Normal and Xeroderma pigmentosum human fibroblasts	Sister chromatid exchange	Wolff et al., 1977
3. Human peripheral blood lymphocytes	Chromosome aberrations	Evans and O'Riordan, 1975
D. DNA damage and repair		
1. Chinese hamster lung (V79)	DNA damage—alkaline elution assay	Swenberg et al., 1976
2. HeLa cell (human carcinoma)	DNA synthesis inhibition	Painter, 1977; Painter and Howard, 1978
3. Syrian hamster embryo	DNA-mutagen binding	Ivanovic et al., 1978a; 1978b
4. Rat hepatocytes (primary)	Unscheduled DNA synthesis	Williams, 1977
5. Mouse testicular	Unscheduled DNA synthesis	Beikirch, 1977
6. Human skin fibroblasts	Sucrose sedimentation profiles	Stich et al., 1976
7. Human skin fibroblasts	Unscheduled DNA synthesis (autoradiography)	San and Stich, 1975; Stich et al. 1977

TABLE 2 (continued)

System	Basis of test (parameter monitored)	References
8. Human skin fibroblasts	In vitro cell-free DNA repair synthesis	Ciarrocchi and Linn, 1978
9. Normal and Xeroderma pigmentosum human fibroblasts	DNA repair and cytotoxicity	Maher et al., 1977
E. Biochemical assays		
1. Canine kidney cells	Prostaglandin synthesis	Levine, 1977
2. Rat liber	Degranulation of rough endoplasmic reticulum (Rabin's test)	Purchase et al., 1976
3. Viral and chemical transformed 3T3	Fluorescence analysis of cell surface and DNA	Hawkes and Bartholomew, 1977
F. Assays for promoters[c]		
1. Chicken embryo fibroblasts and HeLa cells	Plasminogen activator production	Wigler and Weinstein, 1976, Wigler et al., 1978; Weinstein et al., 1977
2. Mouse skin	Ornithine decarboxylase induction	Boutwell, 1977
3. Mouse epidermal cell cultures	Ornithine decarboxylase induction	Yuspa et al., 1976
4. Rat embryo fibroblasts	Fluorescence polarization	Fisher et al., 1979a; Weinstein et al., 1978b
5. Murine erythroleukemia cells	Inhibition of differentiation	Rovera et al., 1977; Yamasaki et al., 1977
6. Chicken embryo myoblast and chondroblast cultures	Inhibition of differentiation	Cohen et al., 1977; Pacifici and Holtzer, 1977
7. B-16 melanoma cells	Inhibition of differentiation	Mufson et al., 1979
8. Neuroblastoma cells	Inhibition of differentiation	Ishii et al., 1978
9. 3T3 fibroblast conversion to adipose like cells	Inhibition of differentiation	Diamond et al., 1977

[a]Modified from a list kindly provided by J. McCann, M. Hollstein, and W. Nichols. See also Hollstein et al., 1979, and Montesano et al., 1980.

[b]For further details see Table 4.

[c]See Table 8 and text.

was, however, positive when tested as a vapor in the Ames assay (Purchase et al., 1976; Bartsch et al., 1976). The remaining 12 compounds, which gave false responses in both assays, includes six established carcinogens and six putative noncarcinogens. If one combined the results obtained using both test systems, all of the known carcinogens (except diethylstilbestrol and vinyl chloride) were detected and six false positives were generated. For a comprehensive review of the relative merits of a number of in vitro assays and the application of these tests to the evaluation of the potential carcinogenicity of saccharine the reader is also referred to an office of Technology Assessment Report, Cancer Testing Technology and Saccharin (1977).

Because of the breadth of the subject and the fact that it is undergoing rapid changes and developments, it would be impossible in this chapter to review all of the short-term in vitro tests in detail. We will, therefore, concentrate on only a selected few of the in vitro tests that we feel currently warrant emphasis. These tests include certain mutagenesis (both bacterial and mammalian somatic cell), DNA damage and repair, and cell transformation assays. The latter systems are discussed in greatest detail because we believe they provide the closest model to the process of carcinogenesis in the intact animal. For other recent reviews of short-term tests the reader is referred to the following references: Ames and McCann, 1976; Hollstein et al., 1979; Montesano et al., 1980; Nagao and Sugimura, 1978.

II. MUTAGENESIS ASSAYS

A. Introduction—General Aspects

Although the critical event in carcinogenesis is not presently known, evidence implicating mutational changes has been presented (Fahmy and Fahmy, 1970; Knudson, 1971, Weinstein, 1976; Cairns, 1975b). In addition, even if it is eventually established that certain tumors are induced by nonmutational mechanisms, the ability of agents to function as mutagens provides a sensitive assay for their ability to form covalent adducts with cellular macromolecules, a property frequently associated with known carcinogens (Miller, 1978). The ability of carcinogens to induce mutational change in microbial, insect, and mammalian systems has, therefore, been exploited as an endpoint in short-term bioassays. A wide spectrum of carcinogens has been shown to be mutagenic, including

- Direct-acting alkylating agents, such as nitrogen mustards, nitrosamines, epoxides, etc. (Malling and de Serres, 1969; Drake, 1970; Barthelmess, 1970; Fishbein et al., 1970; Miller and Miller, 1971; Ames, 1971; Ames et al., 1972a; McCann et al., 1975a; McCann and Ames, 1976a, 1976b)
- Metabolically activated polycyclic hydrocarbons (Maher et al., 1971; Huberman et al., 1971a; Miller and Miller, 1971; Ames et al., 1972b; McCann et al., 1975a; Levin et al., 1976; Wood et al., 1976)
- Aminoazo dyes (Maher et al., 1968; Miller and Miller, 1971; McCann et al., 1975a)
- Aromatic amines (Maher et al., 1968, 1970; Mukai and Troll, 1969; Miller and Miller, 1971; Ames et al., 1972a; McCann et al., 1975a)
- Carbamates (Fahmy and Fahmy, 1970; Miller and Miller, 1971; McCann et al., 1975a)
- Nitrosamines (Malling and de Serres, 1969; Miller and Miller, 1971; McCann et al., 1975a; Bartsch et al., 1980)
- Aflatoxins (Maher and Summers, 1970; McCann et al., 1975a)

Although a direct link between mutagenesis and carcinogenesis in humans is not presently available, short-term genetic assays based on mutation offer tremendous potential as prescreens for these agents in our environment (Bartsch et al., 1980).

The ability of carcinogens to induce DNA damage (Lieberman et al., 1971; Lieberman and Poirier, 1973; Cleaver, 1973; San and Stich, 1975; Stich et al., 1977) and chromosomal alterations (Kato et al., 1969; Stich and San, 1970; Perry and Evans, 1975; Ishidate and Odashima, 1977) has also been used as a predictor of carcinogenic potential. The DNA repair assay is based on the assumption that: (1) carcinogens interact with DNA; (2) damage induced by carcinogens is repaired in normal cells, and (3) DNA repair can be monitored by an unscheduled incorporation of DNA precursors (Cleaver, 1970; Regan et al., 1971; Stoltz et al., 1974; San and Stich, 1975; Stich et al., 1977). This type of repair synthesis has been monitored using alkaline sucrose gradients (Laishes and Stich, 1973a, 1973b) and autoradiography (Stich and San, 1970). With the advent of improved techniques to distinguish among chromosomes and to map their banding patterns (Sumner et al., 1971; Caspersson et al., 1971) and sensitive assays for sister chromatid exchange (Perry and Evans, 1975), the analysis of chromosomal damage following carcinogen treatment can now be evaluated more accurately. DNA repair and chromosomal analysis are quick and simple techniques that may be useful as part of a regimen of in vitro carcinogen prescreening tests.

B. Microbial Systems

At the present time, the most extensively studied and utilized short-term mutagenic assay system employs histidine requiring bacterial mutants of *S. typhimurium* in combination with a mammalian microsomal activation system (Ames, 1971, 1972; Ames et al., 1972a, 1972b, 1975; Ames and McCann, 1976; McCann et al., 1975a, 1975b; McCann and Ames, 1976a, 1976b, 1977; McCann, 1978). The success of this assay can largely be attributed to the ability of a variety of known carcinogenic agents to induce, via mutagenic action, reversion of the histidine requiring mutants to a normal prototroph. The basic *Salmonella* tester strains are sensitive to DNA base-pair substitution (TA1535) and to frameshift mutations (TA1537 and TA1538). A significant increase in the sensitivity of the tester strains has been accomplished by incorporating two additional mutations in these systems: loss of the lipopolysaccharide permeability barrier (rfa) and loss of the excision repair system (uvrB). An additional improvement in the ability of the *Salmonella* system to detect environmental carcinogens has been the development of strains TA100 and TA98 by the introduction of a resistance transfer factor (R plasmid) to the standard tester strains TA1535 and TA1538, respectively (McCann et al., 1975b). The newer tester strains exhibit an enhanced mutagenic response when exposed, in the presence of rat or human microsomal enzymes (S-9 mix), to such potent carcinogens as aflatoxin B1 (AFB1), BP and 7,12-dimethylbenz(a)anthracene (DMBA). TA100 has also proven useful in demonstrating the activity of nitrofuran and other carcinogens, which were not easily detected by the standard tester strains (Ames and McCann, 1976).

The ability of the *Salmonella*/microsome test to distinguish between carcinogens and noncarcinogens from a diverse group of chemical compounds has been demonstrated by McCann et al. (1975a). Approximately 300 chemicals were tested using the standard tester strains (Ames et al., 1973), the improved strains (Ames et al., 1975), and the R factor tester strains (McCann et al., 1975b). Both carcinogens and putative noncarcinogens were tested with and without a mammalian liver microsomal activating system. The classes of compounds tested by McCann et al. (1975a) included aromatic amines, alkyl halides, polycyclic aromatics, esters, epoxides, carbamates, nitro aromatics and heterocycles, miscellaneous aliphatics and aromatics, nitrosamines, fungal toxins, antibiotics, mixtures (cigarette smoke condensate), miscellaneous heterocycles, miscellaneous nitrogen compounds, azo dyes, and diazo compounds. A high correlation (90%) between carcinogenicity and mutagenicity was obtained. Thus, 156 out of 174 known carcinogens scored positive as mutagens and 96 out of 108 noncarcinogens did not induce mutations. More recently 855 chemicals were assayed in a modified Ames test for bacterial mutagens and 182 were found to be mutagenic (McMahon et al., 1979).

The *Salmonella*/microsome test (Ames assay) has generated both false-negative and false-positive results when applied to diverse groups of carcinogens and noncarcinogens (McCann et al., 1975a; Ames and McCann, 1976; McCann and Ames, 1977). The known carcinogens auramine, carbon tetrachloride, dieldrin, thiourea, urethan, thioacetamine, acetamide, ethionine, safrole, 1'-hydroxysafrole, diethylstilbestrol, cycasin, sodium phenobarbital, amitrole, 1,2-dimethylhydrazine, natulan (procarbasine), as well as metal carcinogens such as lead acetate and titanocene dichloride, have thus far not been mutagenic in this assay. Apparently false-positive compounds, that is, compounds found to be mutagenic in this assay but apparently negative as carcinogens in animal studies, include 4-acetylaminofluorene, 2-aminobiphenyl, ICR-191, folpet, 3-hydroxybenzo(a)pyrene, dibenz(a,h)anthracene-5, 6-oxide, styrene oxide, glycidol, 5-nitro-2-furamidoxime, 1-[(5-nitrofurfurylidene)-amino]-hydantoin, 5-nitro-2-furoic acid, sodium azide, sodium nitrite, and N-hydroxy-4-aminoazobenzene. It has been suggested by McCann and Ames (1976a) that both false negatives and positives may be explainable by either inadequate in vivo animal carcinogenicity testing or the inability of the in vitro metabolic activating system to convert the test substance into active electrophilic species (ultimate carcinogens).

False negatives can also be generated in the Ames assay, as well as in other short-term in vitro tests and in vivo animal studies, as a result of toxicity of the test compound. Excessive toxicity can preclude the use of high enough levels of the test agent to induce mutation in Salmonella or cause cancer in a particular animal assay. A greater proportion of false negatives are probably produced as a result of technical problems involved in using in vitro metabolic activation systems. If the carcinogen is not metabolically activated by the particular S-9 system used, a false negative will result. At present very little biochemical information is available on the effects of species, tissues, inducers, assay conditions, cofactors, and so on, on the quantitative and qualitative aspects of activation and detoxification of chemically diverse chemicals in these systems. Potential problems in attempting to extrapolate in vitro mutagenicity data to in vivo carcinogenicity when using the Ames assay and different S-9 fractions and different activation systems have been presented and discussed by Ashby and Styles (1978a, 1978b). They point out that the choice of species or organ from which the S-9 fraction is prepared, the inducing agent, the amount of S-9, the concentration of cofactors, and other variables of the assay system can influence the results obtained with different compounds. They caution that these variables may make attempts at quantitative evaluation of mutagenic and carcinogenic potency particularly difficult.

It would, of course, be extremely desirable to be able to use the Ames assay, and other short-term tests, not only to obtain yes or no answers but to obtain data on the relative potency of positive compounds that relate to carcinogenic potency. In animal assays carcinogens can vary a millionfold in terms of potency. Society may often be faced with the necessity of choosing the compound that appears to be a very weak carcinogen, over a related potent one, for uses in which a substitute with zero mutagenic or carcinogenic activity is not feasible or possible. Meselson and Russell (1977) have found a good but not perfect correlation for 14 compounds in terms of mutagenic potency in the Ames assay and in animal carcinogenesis assays. Ames and co-workers are attempting to extend this correlation (Ames and Hooper, 1978). The data cited in the correlation of Meselson and Russell, however, are very limited and do not include several striking exceptions. Bartsch et al. (1979) found that the mutagenic activities in the Ames assay of a series of hydrocarbons (BA, 7MeBA, BP, 3-MCA, DMBA) did not correlate with their activities as initiating agents in mouse skin or their extents of DNA binding on mouse skin. On the other hand, microsome-mediated mutagenicities of the corresponding "Bay-region" dihydrodiols did correlate with the latter parameters in mouse skin. These results suggest that the Ames assay may not give precise information on relative potencies because of variations between the in vitro system and intact tissue in terms of metabolic activation. Obviously much more work remains to be done in this important area.

Even with continued improvements of the Ames assay, development of new tester strains and advances in in vitro metabolic activation systems, certain classes of compounds may still generate false negatives. Hormones, tumor promoters, various cofactors, physical agents, indirectly acting materials, and certain specific carcinogens will probably fall into this category. The first examples leading to false negatives, namely, hormones, tumor promoters, and various cofactors, are not generally mutagenic and appear to enhance carcinogenesis via other modes of action. Similarly, there may be classes of compounds that are carcinogenic because they exert damage to eukaryotic chromosomes (perhaps by impairing the mitotic apparatus), act during germ cell formation (meiotic segregation), interfere with normal embryological development, or damage other functions not present in prokaryotes.

These agents will also lead to false negatives in the Ames assay. Studies designed, therefore, to detect these classes of compounds and to develop assay systems to monitor their presence in the environment are extremely important for a comprehensive carcinogen screening program. The use of simple eukaryotic systems such as yeast and molds may be useful for detecting some but not all of such compounds.

False positives in the Ames assay may result from bacterial activation of a chemical, unphysiologic conditions of metabolic activation, the absence of repair mechanisms in bacterial systems normally present in mammalian systems, inadequate animal carcinogenicity data, and mutagenic impurities in the test compounds (McCann and Ames, 1977). The presence of enzyme-activating systems in bacteria, which may be absent or unexpressed in mammals, can lead to incorrect results using the Ames assay. Although there are only a few examples, this may be the case with various compounds containing a nitro group and 2-acetylaminofluorene (AAF)-like carcinogens (McCann and Ames, 1976a). Tester strains utilized in the Ames assay carry mutations that impair their capacity for excision repair and/or appear to increase their capacity for error-prone repair (Ames et al., 1975). These mutational modifications increase the mutagenic sensitivity of the Salmonella/microsome system, but may generate false positives, especially with compounds that would otherwise be very weak mutagens. Improperly conducted animal tests or limited data may lead to the conclusion that a compound is noncarcinogenic, whereas additional testing might prove otherwise. This is a major problem, especially when dealing with weak carcinogens not detected because of the lack of sensitivity of the animal tests or when dealing with compounds which have a limited host range. Under these circumstances, the Ames assay, instead of registering a false positive, would actually provide evidence that a compound previously thought to be noncarcinogenic actually has carcinogenic potential.

The presence of impurities in the test compound is another important consideration when using the Ames test. Even a small quantity of a potent carcinogen contaminating an excess of the noncarcinogenic compound might be detected because of the increased sensitivity of the tester strains. The ability of the Ames test to detect small quantities of a potent carcinogenic impurity in a complex mixture, however, may be an extremely useful indicator of the carcinogenic potential of cosmetic products, food additives, impure chemicals and drugs, and other complex materials to which humans are exposed.

A major problem in attempting to directly extrapolate from in vitro mutagenicity data to animal and human carcinogenicity risks has been the absence of a direct correlation between mutagenic and carcinogenic potency. In the whole animal a spectrum of modifying factors is present, including species and individual differences in absorption, distribution, metabolic activation, metabolic deactivation, and excretion of potential carcinogens (Stoltz et al., 1974; Ashby and Styles, 1978a, 1978b). These factors may influence the amount of active electrophiles that reach the target tissue and cellular macromolecules in the whole animal (Miller and Miller, 1967). The known species and tissue specificity of certain chemical carcinogens, as well as marked differences in potencies of the same agent in different species, also makes a direct extrapolation between in vitro and in vivo data difficult, especially if only one type of activation system is used in vitro (Montesano, 1978). As mentioned, Meselson and Russell (1977) have demonstrated a correlation between the carcinogenic and mutagenic potency of certain compounds. Their study, however, included only about 14 compounds, and other compounds did not show this correlation. Further studies of this aspect are required before reliable extrapolations on new compounds can be made with confidence.

Despite these reservations, there is no doubt that the Ames assay represents an extremely useful method for detecting mutagens and potential carcinogens in our environment. Because the test system is simple and economical to use it permits large-scale prescreening of new industrial compounds. Recent studies indicate that it may also be useful for detecting mutagens in human feces (Bruce et al., 1977) and urine (Durston and Ames, 1974; Yamasaki and Ames, 1977) as a result of the ingestion of carcinogens or endogenous metabolism. The assay is also proving to be highly useful in research studies concerned with mechanisms involved in metabolic activation of procarcinogens into ultimate carcinogens (see, for example, Wood et al., 1976).

Although the Ames assay has been the most extensively validated system, other bacterial and fungal mutagenesis assays have also proven to be extremely useful (Table 2). Poirier (1976) has reported a comparison of in vitro mutagenic testing of 95 compounds, including procarcinogens, ultimate carcinogens, and structurally similar noncarcinogens, in five histidine requiring mutants of _S. typhimurium_—TA1530, TA1535, TA1536, TA1537, and TA1538 (Ames, 1971)—to results obtained with the polymerase A-deficient mutants of _Escherichia coli_ (pol A$^-$) and the _Saccharomyces cerevisiae_ (D-3) system (Slater et al., 1971). TA1530, TA1535, TA1538, and D-3 were also tested using an in vivo "host-mediated activation system" (Legator and Malling, 1971). The latter assay involved the administration of the test compounds to animals containing the indicator organisms in their peritoneal cavity. Host-mediated activation was not found useful as a short-term assay because of the greater difficulty in using the assay, when compared with the in vitro assays, and the fact that this test detected less than one-half of the known carcinogens. The classes of compounds summarized by Poirier (1976) included aromatic hydrocarbons, aromatic amines, nitrosamines, alkylating agents, and miscellaneous compounds (including metals, acylating agents, heterocyclic and benzylic compounds, hydrazine, urethan, and ethionine). No single microbial system was adequate for screening all the known compounds. For example, the carcinogen thioacetamide was not mutagenic in the _Salmonella_ strains tested or the _Saccharomyces_ system, but was active in the _E. coli_ pol A$^-$ system. The _Sacchoramyces_ D-3 and _E. coli_ pol A$^-$ systems accurately detected approximately 50% of the carcinogens and 25 % of the noncarcinogens. Combining the results obtained using the _Salmonella_ and _E. coli_ pol A$^-$ systems, more than 95% of the ultimate carcinogens and 80% of the procarcinogens belonging to the aromatic hydrocarbons, aromatic amines, nitrosamines, and alkylating agents were detected. Several compounds, however, generated false positive or negative results when using the Ames _Salmonella_ assay. Mutagenic compounds that are currently classified as noncarcinogens included 4-acetylaminofluorene, 1-anthramine, 1,2-epoxybutane, glycidol, BUdR, and hydroxylamine. Known carcinogens which were not mutagenic included metals, bis(p-dimethylamine)diphenylmethane, ethionine, thiourea, and urethan. The majority of false negatives resulted with chemicals whose mode of carcinogenic action was not known. These results clearly emphasize the importance of continued research on the problem of metabolic activation and the usefulness of particular types of assays for the detection of specific chemical classes of compounds (Ashby and Purchase, 1977).

C. Mammalian Mutagenesis Systems

The ability of mutagens and carcinogens to induce specific mutations (Chu, 1971; Sato et al., 1972, Clive, 1974; Fischer et al., 1974; Huberman, 1976; Krahn and Heidelberger, 1977; O'Neill and Hsie, 1977; O'Neill et al., 1977b) in mammalian cell cultures represents another useful short-term screening system for potential carcinogens (Table 2). A problem in utilizing mammalian cells to monitor point mutations is the complexity of the eukaryotic genome and the small number of well-characterized genetic mutants currently available. The three mammalian cell cultures that have been tested against a large number of carcinogens and noncarcinogens are the mouse lymphoma cell line L-5178Y (Clive, 1974; Fischer et al., 1974) and the Chinese hamster cell lines CHO and V-79 (Huberman, 1976, Krahn and Heidelberger, 1977; O'Neill et al., 1977a, 1977b). In one study the L-5178Y cell line was examined for mutability to drug resistance to cytosine arabinoside, methotrexate, and thymidine (Poirier, 1976). With a list of 95 carcinogens and noncarcinogens there was a high proportion of false positives. On the other hand, Clive has found a good correlation between tumorigenic potency and mutagenic potency at the thymidine kinase locus (1979). Several laboratories are currently further evaluating this system. It is of interest that diethylstilboestrol was reported positive in this system, although it is negative in the Ames assay (Clive et al., 1979).

In the Chinese hamster cell lines, V79 and CHO, a variety of mutagenic and carcinogenic agents induce specific gene mutations (Huberman et al., 1971a; Huberman and Sachs, 1973; Huberman and Sachs, 1974; O'Neill and Hsie, 1977). Metabolic activation is necessary for many of these compounds to exert their mutagenic effect (Huberman et al., 1971b; Huberman and Sachs, 1973; Huberman, 1975; Krahn and Heidelberger, 1977; O'Neill et al., 1977b). One approach is to use Syrian hamster embryo cells as metabolizer cells and Chinese hamster lung (V79) cells as the target cells in which mutations are scored. Although V79 cells are susceptible to mutagens they are deficient in metabolic activation. Utilizing this system, polycyclic aromatic hydrocarbons with varying degrees of carcinogenicity were tested by Huberman (1976) for their ability to induce mutations in V79 affecting the surface membrane (ouabain resistance), purine metabolism (8-azaguanine resistance), and protein synthesis (reversion to temperature resistance by temperature sensitive leucyl-transfer RNA synthetase mutants). A good correlation between known carcinogenicity and mutation induction at all three genetic loci was found with DMBA, BP, MC, and 7-methylbenz(a)anthracene (7-MBA). The noncarcinogenic polycyclics, pyrene (PY), phenanthrene (PH), and chrysene (CH) were not mutagenic toward V79 cells. An increase in the mutagenicity of the polycyclic hydrocarbons was observed after exposure of the cells to aminophylline, a cyclic nucleotide phosphodiesterase inhibitor known to induce enzymes metabolizing BP and related compounds (Yamasaki et al., 1975). Cell-mediated mutagenesis of mammalian cells with or without addition of inducers may, therefore, represent a useful short-term assay for detecting polycyclic hydrocarbon carcinogens. It remains to be determined, however, if this system will be useful for monitoring other classes of carcinogens in our environment. Recently reported innovations in this type of system include the use of primary rat liver cell cultures (Langenbach et al., 1978) or human bronchial explants (Hsu et al., 1978) as sources of metabolizer cells. Thus the system has the potential of dealing with the problem of species and tissue specificity of carcinogen activation.

Mutagenesis of V79 cells to 6-thioguanine resistance, which correlates with a loss or alteration in hypoxanthine-guanine phosphoribosyl transferase (HGPRT) activity, has been demonstrated after treatment of the cultures with AFB1, AFB2, BP, MC, and DMBA (Krahn and Heidelberger, 1977). The mutagenic activity of the latter compounds was dependent on metabolic activation, which was supplied by incorporating a rat liver S-9 microsomal fraction and cofactors into the assay. A good correlation between carcinogenicity and mutagenicity was found, with the exception of the compounds dibenz(a,h)anthracene (DB(a,h)A) and dibenz(a,c)anthracene (DB(a,c)A). These two isomers of dibenzanthracene (DBA) exhibited a reverse order of activity when compared to previous animal carcinogenicity studies. DB(a,c)A was more cytotoxic and mutagenic than its structural analogue DB(a,h)A. Although additional problems may be encountered in using the S-9 fraction (see also discussion of this aspect under Sec. II.B) the V79 + S9 technique warrants further study with a larger number of carcinogens and noncarcinogens to determine its validity as a carcinogen prescreen.

The Chinese hamster ovary cell line (CHO) represents one of the best genetically characterized mammalian cell culture systems (Puck et al., 1958; Kao and Puck, 1967, 1969; Siminovitch, 1976). CHO cells exhibit a rapid population doubling time (12-13 hr), can be grown in monolayer on plastic or glass substratums as well as in suspension culture, have a high cloning efficiency, and have a stable karyotype of 20 or 21 chromosomes. They have also been utilized to isolate a large number of recessive mutants (Kao and Puck, 1967, 1969; Hsie et al., 1975a, 1975b; Siminovitch, 1976; O'Neill et al., 1977a, 1977b; O'Neill and Hsie, 1977). Optimal 6-thioguanine selection conditions for mutation induction at the HGPRT locus have been determined, resulting in greater than 98% recovery of mutant clones with altered enzyme activity (O'Neill et al., 1977a). This CHO/HGPRT system has been used to demonstrate the mutagenicity of a spectrum of physical agents, such as ultraviolet light and X rays; organic chemicals, such as N-methyl-N'-nitrosoguanidine (MNNG), ethyl methanesulfonate (EMS), ICR 191; and metallic compounds (O'Neill et al., 1977a, 1977b, 1978). By incorporating a rat liver microsomal enzyme preparation or using host-mediated activation by BALB/c athymic mice, the procarcinogen dimethylnitrosamine (DMN) has also been shown to be mutagenic toward CHO cells (O'Neill et al., 1977b). This well-defined mammalian locus-specific mutation system is presently being tested using a broad spectrum of carcinogens and noncarcinogens (A. W. Hsie, 1979, personal communication), and offers considerable promise as an in vitro mammalian mutagenesis assay.

Compared to bacterial genetics the subject of mammalian somatic cell genetics is still in its infancy. One should not overlook, however, the potential advantages of mammalian systems for mutagenicity assays and as complements to the bacterial systems for the following reasons:

1. Because of major differences in chromosome structure and replication, and other factors, the process of mutagenesis in the more complex eukaryotic cell may be quite different than in procaryotic organisms.
2. Most bacterial systems employ reverse mutations, whereas forward mutation may be more applicable to mammalian carcinogenesis.
3. The uptake of test compounds by mammalian cells may differ from that of bacteria.
4. Intact mammalian cells may metabolize carcinogens by mechanisms different from those utilizing the S-9 type enzyme preparations.
5. Mammalian cell culture systems can undergo DNA repair after carcinogen-induced damage (Setlow et al., 1977); this process may be different from that in bacteria and the currently used bacterial tester strains are actually repair deficient to enhance their sensitivity to mutagenic agents. There is evidence that DNA repair is an important determinant of cancer induction in humans (for review see Setlow et al., 1977).
6. By developing mammalian cell culture systems which can score for both mutagenesis and cell transformation (Barrett and Ts'o, 1978; Barrett et al., 1978; Huberman, 1975; Huberman et al., 1976), mammalian cells may provide more insight into the carcinogenic process than bacteria.

For all of these reasons, as well as other yet to be discovered aspects of genetic toxicology, a comprehensive carcinogen-screening program should include mammalian cell mutagenesis assays. These assays may also be more suitable for quantitative assessments of the risk to humans of carcinogenic and mutagenic agents in our environment than bacterial mutagenesis assays, and this aspect warrants further study.

III. DNA DAMAGE AND REPAIR AND A DNA MONITOR ASSAY

A. Introduction

As discussed in earlier sections of this chapter, it appears that most carcinogens form electrophiles that covalently bind to DNA, and to other cellular macromolecules, and that this aspect is a critical event in the carcinogenic process (for review see Weinstein, 1978, and Miller, 1978). In a sense, the bacterial and mutagenesis assays already described represent bioassays for these biochemical events. With advances in our understanding of the biochemistry of carcinogen-induced damage to DNA, and of the DNA repair mechanisms that respond to this damage, methods have become available to examine more directly these aspects of carcinogen action. Since some of these methods are relatively simple and extremely sensitive they provide a new generation of short-term assays for potential mutagens and carcinogens.

B. DNA Repair Assays

The ability of carcinogens to induce DNA repair synthesis, as measured by an unscheduled (i.e., nonreplicative) incorporation of ^{3}H-thymidine into DNA, and DNA single-strand breaks, as monitored by alkaline sucrose gradient ultracentrifugation techniques, in cultured human and Syrian hamster fibroblasts has been tested as a potential in vitro carcinogen bioassay system (Stich et al., 1971, 1973, 1976, 1977; Stich and San, 1973). Stich et al. (1976) tested 96 compounds, consisting of 31 direct-acting carcinogens, 38 precarcinogens, 24 noncarcinogens, and three mutagens (classified as noncarcinogens) for their ability to induce unscheduled

DNA synthesis in fibroblastic cells. A good but not absolute correlation between known carcinogenic potential and induction of DNA repair synthesis was observed. None of the noncarcinogens and none of the noncarcinogenic mutagens (acriflavine neutral, daunomycin, or ethidium bromide) induced DNA repair synthesis. Actually, more recent studies indicate that daunomycin is carcinogenic (Adamson and Sieber, 1977). A spectrum of procarcinogens, however, even with a metabolic activation system containing the S-9 or 105,000 g supernatant fractions from the liver or other organs of mammals, birds, or fish, including BA, dibenzanthracene (DBA), BP, MC, AAF, 4-acetylamino-trans-stilbene, 4-acetylaminophenanthrene, 4-aminobenzene, safrole, AFG1, luteoskyrin, rugulosin, nitrofurantoin, nitrofurazone, and N-[4-(5-nitro-2-furyl)-2-thiazolyl] formamide, failed to induce unscheduled DNA repair synthesis. In addition, the carcinogens, methylazoxymethylacetate, methylazoxymethanol, n-butyl nitrosourea, trimethylurea, 3-hydroxy-xanthine, 3-hydroxy-guanine, and guanine-3-N-oxide, were also negative in this assay. It is not clear whether the inability of the various procarcinogens to induce DNA repair synthesis was due to inadequate metabolic activation of these compounds to proximate carcinogens or the possibility that in this system not all agents that damage DNA produce detectable induction of an excision type of DNA repair (Stich et al., 1976). This system, therefore, requires further modification and validation before it can be considered for use as a short-term assay.

Primary hepatocyte cell cultures have been found to retain a large number of liver specific functions (Bissel et al., 1973; Lin and Snodgrass, 1975; Michalopoulos and Pitot, 1975). In addition, since there is negligible cell replication in these cultures unscheduled ^{3}H-thymidine incorporation can be measured against an essentially zero background. These properties have been exploited by Williams (1977) to test the effect of five different classes of procarcinogens, including mycotoxins (AFB1, AFB2, AFG1), polycyclic hydrocarbons (DMBA), nitrosamines (DMN), aromatic amines (2FAA), and azo dyes (aminoazobenzene (AB), 2-methyl-dimethylaminoazobenzene, 4'-methyl-dimethyl-aminoazobenzene, 3'-methyl-dimethylaminoazobenzene, and a direct-acting carcinogen, MNNG, on unscheduled DNA synthesis in primary rat liver cell cultures. A good correlation between known carcinogenic activity and induction of DNA repair synthesis, as measured by ^{3}H-thymidine incorporation, was found, with the exception of the weak carcinogen BA, which was negative in this assay. This system should prove useful not only as a short-term screening assay, but also as a means of investigating in vitro liver-specific aspects of metabolic activation and deactivation of carcinogens.

An alkaline elution technique has been employed to monitor DNA damage in Chinese hamster V79 cells exposed in cell culture to various noncarcinogens, ultimate, proximate, and procarcinogens, in the presence or absence of a liver microsomal activating system (Swenberg et al., 1976). Forty-three compounds were tested in this assay, including alkylating agents—MNNG, methylnitrosourea (MNU), EMS, β-propiolactone, propyleneamine, diethylnitrosamine (DENA), and DMN; polycyclic aromatic hydrocarbons-BP, benzo(e)pyrene (B(e)P), DMBA, MC, PH, and anthracene; amines—benzidine, 4-ABP, AAF, n-hydroxyacetylaminofluorene (N-OH-AFF), N-acetoxy-acetylaminofluorene (N-OAc-AAF), aniline, and pararosaniline; and miscellaneous compounds—AFB1, 4-nitroquinoline-1-oxide (4NQO), safrole, 1-hydroxysafrole, 1-acetoxysafrole, captan, DDT, dinitrophenol, cyclophosphamide, ethionine, methionine, phenobarbital, aspirin, caffeine, EDTA, ethanol, acetone, dimethylsulfoxide, propylene glycol, and benzene. Although there was not a direct correlation between in vivo carcinogenic potential and the degree of alteration in the DNA elution profile, a good qualitative indication of carcinogenic potential was demonstrated. Thus, all of the ultimate carcinogens and the majority of procarcinogens, except safrole, 1'-OH safrole, DDT, dieldren, and cyclophosphamide, induced DNA damage, whereas none of the noncarcinogens induced DNA damage when measured by the alkaline elution assay. In the presence of rat liver microsomes, safrole and cyclophoshamide did have an effect on DNA elution but only at drug concentrations resulting in low cell viability. This assay system appears promising but requires further validation with a larger number of compounds.

Analysis of DNA repair and DNA fragmentation may ultimately become important components in a short-term in vitro carcinogenic screening program. The unscheduled incorporation of ^{3}H-thymidine into DNA, as detected by autoradiography, provides information about carcinogen induced damage in individual cells within the population, while sucrose gradient techniques provide information about large numbers of cells within the population. Both techniques have problems, including: (1) the lack of a direct correlation between carcinogenic potency and the degree of induced DNA repair; (2) nonspecific toxicity of test compounds which can also lead to an increase in DNA repair and fragmentation; (3) artifacts in the sedimentation or alkaline elution profiles of cellular DNA as a result of improper handling of cells, inadequate cell lysis, or nuclease activity, (4) failure of the system to adequately activate procarcinogens into ultimate carcinogens, thus resulting in false negatives; and (5) the types of DNA repair manifest in certain rodent cell cultures may not be the same as those in human cells. A distinct advantage of DNA repair and fragmentation as a potential short-term screening assay is the ability of this system to directly monitor DNA-carcinogen interactions in animal and human cells both in cell culture and in the intact host. Sarma et al. (1975) have demonstrated that several carcinogens administered to rats cause damage to liver DNA as measured by alkaline sucrose gradients. By utilizing genetically abnormal cells from patients with an increased predisposition to cancer—for example, Xeroderma pigmentosum, Fanconi's anemia, and so on, and differentiated cell types from various organs known to be sensitive to in vivo cancer development—the sensitivity and utility of DNA repair and fragmentation systems as prescreens for carcinogens, and also for assays of variations in host cell responses to DNA damage, may be greatly enhanced.

Recent observations have indicated that various chemical mutagens and carcinogens induce an increase in sister chromatid exchange (SCE) in eukaryotic chromosomes (Latt, 1974; Perry and Evans, 1975; Natarajan et al., 1976; Ueda et al., 1976; Wolff et al., 1977; Wolff, 1977). Perry and Evans (1975) examined SCE in CHO cells treated with adriamycin (AM), mitomycin C (MMC), MNNG, quinacrine mustard, 4NQO, nitrogen mustard (NM), diepoxy-butane, Hoechst 33258, bleomycin (BLM), MMS, β-propiolactone, EMS, cyclophosphamide (CP), and maleic hydrazide (MH). With the exception of AM and BM, low concentrations (10^{-7}-10^{-3} M, depending on the compound) of the test agents resulted in approximately a 10-fold increase in SCEs, without inducing chromosomal aberrations. MH, which is not mutagenic in mammalian cells, and CP, which requires metabolic activation, did not induce an increase in SCEs in CHO cells. A rat liver microsomal activation system has been used to demonstrate that DENA, DMN, and CP can induce an increase in SCEs in CHO cells (Natarajan et al., 1976; Stetka and Wolff, 1976). Further research using a much wider spectrum of compounds is needed before SCE can be considered for use as routine short-term in vitro carcinogen screening system.

C. A DNA Monitor Assay and Effects on DNA Synthesis

A biochemical approach to the detection of potential carcinogens is to determine by chemical methods whether exposure of cells or tissues to the compound in question results in the formation of a covalent adduct of that compound or its derivatives with the DNA of the target cells. We refer to this approach as the "DNA monitor assay." It is based on the assumption that compounds that form such adducts are likely to be mutagenic and carcinogenic. A positive result, therefore, would provide a warning that the compound requires further evaluation as a potential carcinogen. The assumptions underlying this approach relate to the electrophile theory of carcinogenesis (Miller, 1978) and are similar to those underlying the Ames and other mutagenesis assays, except that the endpoint is covalent binding to DNA, rather than mutagenesis.

This approach has the following advantages:

1. It can be applied to cells and tissues in which mutagenesis assays may not be possible, for example tissues in the intact animal or primary explants and cell cultures from animal or human sources.
2. It can provide quantitative information on the extent to which an agent modifies cellular DNA over a period of time, and under physiologic conditions of activation

pathways, competing pathways, inactivation pathways, and DNA repair mechanisms characteristic of cells or tissue in which the assay is done.

3. In cases in which the structure of the DNA adduct can be determined one might obtain information on the nature of the DNA damage, as well as clues to the mechanism of metabolic activation of the compound.
4. Utilizing blood leukocytes or biopsy material it may be possible to determine whether humans exposed to a given occupation or environment have foreign residues covalently bound to their nucleic acids, thus signaling the potential dangers of such an environment.

The major technical limitation of this approach is that following exposure of tissue or cell cultures to known carcinogens the amounts of carcinogen or its metabolites covalently bound to cellular nucleic acids are extremely small, in the range of about one residue of the carcinogen moiety per 10^4-10^5 nucleic acid bases (Weinstein, 1976). On the other hand, with the advent of radioactively labeled compounds of high specific activity, highly sensitive spectral methods, and high resolution chromatographic techniques, detection at this low level can be achieved with many compounds. As a matter of fact, by a combination of in vitro techniques the complete chemical structures of several carcinogen-DNA adducts have been elucidated (Weinstein, 1978), and it is likely that this list will expand rapidly.

The specific methods for the DNA monitor assay must be tailored to the compound in question. If it can be radioactively labeled, then covalent binding to cellular DNA can easily be detected by the radioactivity of DNA extracted and purified from the exposed cells. If the compound is not radioactive, it may have absorption, fluorescence, or other spectral properties that can be exploited. It is possible, for example, to detect by fluorescence emission the presence of covalently bound derivatives of BP, and certain other polycyclic aromatic hydrocarbons, on DNA obtained from cells or tissues exposed to the parent compound (Daudel et al., 1975; Ivanovic et al., 1976; Vigny et al., 1977; Ivanovic et al., 1978a). Highly sensitive radioimmunoassays have been developed for O^6-ethylguanine (Müller and Rajewsky, 1980), AAF-guanine (Poirier et al., 1977), and BP-guanine (Poirier et al., 1980), and this approach can be expanded to detect the binding of other carcinogens to cellular DNA. High-pressure liquid chromatographic (HPLC) techniques greatly facilitate separation of the small amounts of carcinogen-modified nucleosides from the natural nucleosides present in cellular RNA and DNA (Jeffrey et al., 1976; Jeffrey et al., 1977). Utilizing HPLC one can detect by ultraviolet (UV) absorbence as little as 0.1 nmol of certain carcinogen-nucleoside adducts (A. Jeffrey and I. B. Weinstein, unpublished studies). This corresponds to the amount of BPDE-deoxyguanosine present in 1 mg of cellular DNA (equivalent to about 1 g wt weight of cells) following the exposure of cell cultures to BP (Ivanovic et al., 1978b). With improved instrumentation and fluorescence or other spectral techniques even lesser amounts of cellular DNA are required with this and other carcinogens. We must stress that in employing this approach the DNA obtained from cells must be highly purified and extensively extracted to avoid contaminants and the presence of materials not actually bound covalently to the DNA (Ivanovic et al., 1976).

Although this approach has not been studied extensively and has not been validated with a known list of carcinogens and noncarcinogens, we have included it because we believe it warrants intensive evaluation and application.

Closely related to this approach are biochemical assays in mammalian cells based on the functional effects of carcinogen damage to cellular DNA. It is well known that the exposure of cells to carcinogens frequently causes a rapid inhibition of DNA and RNA synthesis (Weinstein, 1976). Painter and Howard (1978) have examined 16 compounds and found a good correlation between carcinogenic potency and inhibition of DNA synthesis in human HeLa cell cultures. This type of relatively simple test warrants further evaluation.

Loeb and his associates have suggested that alterations in the fidelity of DNA synthesis in vitro can be used as a screening test for suspected mutagens or carcinogens (Sirover and Loeb, 1976). They have found that all 10 salts of known metal carcinogens decreased the fidelity of DNA synthesis in a subcellular system employing DNA polymerase (E.C. 2,7,7,7) from avian myeloblastosis virus (AMV) and synthetic homopolymer templates. The assay measures the extent of incorporation of noncomplementary nucleotides. In contrast, 17 non-carcinogenic metal salts did not affect fidelity. This test may be particularly useful for screening metal compounds since thus far the S. typhimurium assay has not been successfully applied to this class of compounds. Since a template modified with β-propiolactone (Sirover and Loeb, 1976) and templates containing sites of depurination (Shearman and Loeb, 1977) also gave decreased fidelity in this system, this approach might also be used for the assay of certain alkylating carcinogens that lead to either spontaneous or enzyme-mediated depurination.

IV. ASSAYS FOR TRANSFORMATION AND RELATED CHANGES IN MAMMALIAN CELL CULTURES

A. General Aspects

Mammalian cell culture systems offer great promise for investigating the mechanisms involved in chemical carcinogenesis and as short-term bioassay systems for monitoring environmental carcinogens (Heidelberger, 1973; Stoltz et al., 1974; Purchase et al., 1976). The majority of systems used to assess the carcinogenic potential of chemicals have utilized fibroblast cell cultures derived from embryo cultures or established cell lines (Table 3). Normal cells derived from embryo tissue exhibit a finite life span in culture and contact inhibition of growth upon reaching confluency (Sanford, 1974). However, when certain embryonic cells or established cell lines (i.e., 3T3, 10T1/2) are infected with DNA tumor viruses, such as SV_{40} or polyoma, or exposed to chemical carcinogens, a portion of the cell population becomes morphologically transformed with the potential to grow indefinitely in vitro (Tooze, 1973; Heidelberger, 1973). Table 4 summarizes the phenotypic properties often associated with transformed fibroblasts and epithelial cells in culture. There is considerable variation in the expression of these properties between individual transformed clones, and thus far no single in vitro property can be used to define transformation. The ultimate criterion, of course, is tumorigenicity in histocompatible or immunosuppressed hosts, and cells that have acquired this property are said to have undergone "malignant transformation." At the present time, the best correlation between an in vitro parameter and in vivo tumorigenicity, in both fibroblast and epithelial cell transformants, is loss of anchorage dependence (growth in agar or methylcellulose suspension) (Freedman and Shin, 1974; Shin et al., 1975; Weinstein et al., 1976; Montesano et al., 1977), but here too exceptions have been noted (Stiles et al., 1975; Shields, 1976).

For short-term bioassays fibroblastic cells offer certain advantages over epithelial cells. Chemical carcinogen-induced transformation of rodent fibroblast cell cultures generally requires only a single exposure to the carcinogen, exhibits a short lag period (1-6 weeks), occurs at high efficiency (generally 0.1-20%), and can easily be scored by morphological criteria. In contrast, chemical transformation of most rodent epithelial cell cultures requires continuous or repeated exposure to the carcinogen, exhibits long lag periods (8-36 weeks), occurs at a low frequency, and is not characterized by a distinctive change in morphology (for review, see Weinstein et al., 1976). Although epithelial cultures are not currently useful for short-term bioassays, their continued study is warranted by the fact that over 85% of human cancers develop from epithelial rather than fibroblastic tissues (Higginson and Muir, 1973; Cairns, 1975a, 1975b), and the tumor cell phenotype of transformed fibroblastic cells may not accurately reflect the properties of tumorigenic epithelial (i.e., carcinoma) cells.

B. Syrian Hamster Embryo Cultures

The first definitive demonstration of carcinogen-induced morphological transformation of fibroblast cells in culture is credited to Berwald and Sachs (1963). Following treatment of Syrian hamster embryo cells with the chemical carcinogens benzo(a)pyrene (BP) or 3-

TABLE 3 Cell Culture Systems Utilized to Demonstrate the Carcinogenic Potential of Chemicals

Type of system	Usual endpoint	Scoring time	References
A. Primary or secondary embryo cultures			
1. Syrian hamster	Morphological transformation	8–10 days	Berwald and Sachs, 1963; DiPaolo et al., 1969b, 1971b, 1972a; Pienta et al., 1977
2. Guinea pig	Growth in agar	4 months	Evans and DiPaolo, 1975, 1976; Evans et al., 1977
3. Rat	Morphological transformation, tumorigenesis	130 days	Namba et al., 1969
4. Rat or mouse infected with murine leukemia virus	Morphological transformation	3–8 weeks	Freeman et al., 1970, 1973; Price et al., 1971; Rhim et al., 1971, 1974
5. Rat infected with adenovirus	Morphological transformation (epithelial colonies)	25–30 days	DiPaolo and Casto, 1976
		28–42 days	Fisher et al., 1978
6. Syrian hamster infected with adenovirus	Morphological transformation (epithelial colonies)	25–30 days	Casto, 1973; Casto et al., 1973, 1976, 1978
B. Fibroblast cell cultures			
1. Human skin fibroblasts	Morphological transformation	7–14 weeks	Kakunaga, 1977, 1978
C. Fibroblast cell lines			
1. Mouse prostate (adult)	Morphological transformation	4–6 weeks	Chen and Heidelberger, 1969c; Marquardt et al., 1972; Marquardt, 1974
2. 3T3[a]	Morphological transformation	10–28 weeks	DiPaolo et al., 1972b, Kakunaga, 1973
3. $10T\frac{1}{2}$[b]	Morphological transformation	4–6 weeks	Reznikoff et al., 1973a, 1973b

4. BHK 21[c]	Growth in agar	2-4 weeks	Bouck and diMayorca, 1976; Styles, 1977
5. Continuous rat embryo cell line (Fischer rat embryo[d])	Morphological transformation, tumorigenesis	40-43 days	Rhim and Huebner, 1973; Freeman et al., 1975
D. Epithelial cell cultures			
1. Rat liver	Growth in agar, cytologic changes, tumorigenesis	8-36 weeks	Katsuta and Takaoka, 1968, 1972; Namba et al., 1969; Williams et al., 1973; Yamaguchi and Weinstein, 1975; Montesano et al., 1977
2. Mouse epidermis	Growth in agar, morphological alterations, tumorigenesis	12-16 weeks	Colburn et al., 1978b, 1978c

[a]Cell line established from Balb C mouse embryos.

[b]Cell line established from C3H mouse embryos.

[c]Established from newborn Syrian hamster kidneys.

[d]Transformation occurred in later-passage cultures treated with carcinogens.

TABLE 4 Properties of Malignantly Transformed Rodent Cells in Culture[a]

Cell properties	Fibroblasts[b]	Epithelial cells[b]
Morphological changes (refractile, rounded cells); crisscross orientation	+	-
Increased saturation density, piling up, loss of density-dependent inhibition of growth	+	±
Decreased serum requirement	+	?
Growth in agar or methocel	+	+
Tumorigenicity	+	+
Altered cell-surface glycoproteins and glycolipids	+	+
Lectin agglutination	+	+
Increased membrane transport	+	±
Decreased cAMP	+	?
Increased protease production	+	±
Decreased microfilament sheaths	+	?

[a]In most cases, particularly with epithelial cells, only a few cell types have been studied (for related references, see text). Note also that some of these properties can be dissociated from one another during transformation, reversion (Risser and Pollack, 1974), or cell hybridization (see, for example, Stanbridge and Wilkinson, 1978), and that no single in vitro property is a hallmark of tumorigenicity.

[b](+) indicates that the property usually (but not always) applies to the transformed cells; (-) indicates that it does not apply, (±) indicates that it has been shown to apply in a few cases, and (?) indicates that studies are not sufficient to tell if it does or does not apply.

Source: Modified from Weinstein et al., 1976.

methylcholanthrene (MC), they observed the formation of fusiform cells which grew in an irregular crisscross pattern. In contrast, Syrian hamster embryo cells exposed to urethan or solvent controls did not undergo morphological transformation, implicating the carcinogens as the cause of the alterations observed in treated cultures.

Berwald and Sachs (1965) extended their initial observations and obtained both fibroblastic and epithelioid transformed hamster embryo cells after treatment with the carcinogens BP, MC, 7-12 dimethylbenz(a)anthracene (DMBA), and 10-methylbenz(a)anthracene (10-MBA), but not with the noncarcinogenic compounds 8-methylbenz(a)anthracene (8-MBA), chrysene (CH), or pyrene (PY). The transformed cells formed stable clones that grew in a random pattern, were capable of continued in vitro propagation, were resistant to the toxic effect of BP when treated at a later stage of growth in culture, and produced progressively growing tumors (predominantly fibrosarcomas) when inoculated subcutaneously into adult hamsters. They further demonstrated that Syrian hamster embryo cultures were preferable to SWR mouse-embryo cells for studies on in vitro carcinogenesis. The hamster cells did not undergo appreciable spontaneous transformation, whereas spontaneous transformants capable of inducing tumors in adult SWR mice were obtained in control mouse embryo cultures after continued in vitro passage. These studies were of fundamental importance because they demonstrated the feasibility of utilizing a quantitative in vitro mammalian cell culture assay system for assessing chemical carcinogenic activity and demonstrated that in vitro transformation correlated with in vivo tumorigenicity.

The relationship between BP induced cytotoxicity and transformation of Syrian hamster embryo cells was investigated by Huberman and Sachs (1966). They presented evidence indicating that BP induced transformation followed "one-hit" kinetics and that cytotoxicity and transformation were two different events. Transformed hamster clones were isolated after a single exposure of normal cells that were either resistant or susceptible to BP-induced cytotoxicity. A spectrum of normal clones was isolated which exhibited a differential response to BP, ranging from resistance to transformation to 0.7-60.8% transformed clones. In addition, treatment of cloned populations of hamster cells resulted in four morphological types of transformed colonies, each reflecting the morphology of the parental normal cell type. These results suggest both a hereditary and physiological state of cell competence for transformation and further indicate a differential sensitivity to chemical transformation of cells within the heterogeneous hamster embryo cell population.

Morphological transformation of Syrian hamster embryo cells by the carcinogen 4-nitroquinoline-N-oxide (4NQO) was independently demonstrated by two Japanese groups in 1966 (Kamahora and Kakunaga, 1966; Sato and Kuroki, 1966). Subsequent studies demonstrated that 4NQO-induced morphologically transformed cells were capable of inducing tumors when injected either subcutaneously or in the cheek pouch of adult Syrian hamsters (Kamahora and Kakunaga, 1966; Kakunaga and Kamahora, 1968; Kuroki and Sato, 1968). A dose and time course relationship in 4NQO transformation of hamster cells was demonstrated by Kamahora and Kahunaga (1966). Treatment with 5×10^{-7} M 4NQO for 8 days resulted in transformation, whereas 10^{-6} or 10^{-7} M 4NQO for 1-8 days, 5×10^{-7} 4NQO for 1 or 3 days, 6 nitroquinoline-1-oxide (6NQO—a noncarcinogenic derivative), and untreated cultures failed to result in morphological transformation. The ability of the active metabolite of 4NQO, 4-hydroxyaminoquinoline-1-oxide (4HAQO), to induce malignant transformation of hamster embryo cells was also demonstrated (Kuroki et al., 1967). In a more detailed followup study Kuroki and Sato (1968) demonstrated morphological transformation and malignancy with 4NQO and its carcinogenic derivatives, 4 HAQO and 6-chloro 4-nitroquinoline-1-oxide (6-chloro4NQO), but not with two noncarcinogenic derivatives of 4NQO. They also demonstrated spontaneous transformation and neoplastic development of one culture of hamster embryo cells after 300 days in vitro. This rare transformation event did not affect the validity of this assay system since carcinogen induced transformation occurred approximately 20-80 days after carcinogen treatment. Kuroki and Sato (1968) also demonstrated that under certain circumstances carcinogen-induced morphological transformation preceded, by as much as 50-100 days of cultivation, the ability to induce fibrosarcomas upon inoculation into hamsters. These types of studies further supported the concept that cell culture systems could be used to investigate mechanisms of chemical carcinogenesis and were useful in discriminating between known carcinogenic and noncarcinogenic compounds.

DiPaolo and co-workers (1969a, 1969b, 1971a, 1971b, 1972a, 1973) have also studied the Syrian hamster embryo system as a model for in vitro chemical carcinogenesis. They obtained morphologically altered clones of cells from both random-bred and inbred hamster embryos by treatment with various known chemical carcinogens, but not with noncarcinogenic compounds or in acetone control cultures (DiPaolo et al., 1969a). A good correlation between carcinogenic activity in the animal and in vitro transformation efficiency was found; DMBA, MC, and BP were the most active and benzo(e)pyrene (B(e)P), benz(a)anthracene (BA), and dibenz(a,c)anthracene (DBA) were the least active in their assay system. In addition, toxicity increased with the concentration of test compound and was related to carcinogenic potency, and the absolute number of altered clones (per constant carcinogen concentration) increased with the number of cells initially exposed.

The ability of independently isolated morphologically transformed clones induced by BP, when grown up into cell lines, to produce fibrosarcomas after injection intradermally or subcutaneously into weanling hamsters was demonstrated by DiPaolo et al. (1969b). In this study PY-treated controls did not exhibit morphological transformation or tumorigenicity. DiPaolo et al. (1971a) also performed karyological studies on BP-, MC-, and DMBA-transformed hamster embryo clones. They were unable, however, to demonstrate a specific karytopic change characteristic of carcinogen transformation. Subsequent studies by this group (DiPaolo et al., 1971b) indicated that the transformation frequency with BP in hamster embryo cells was proportional to the dose of carcinogen and that transformation was absent in control cultures. The authors interpreted this as evidence that transformation was the result of induction by the carcinogen rather than selection.

DiPaolo et al. (1972a) used the Syrian hamster system for monitoring transformation by various classes of chemicals other than polycyclic hydrocarbons. Direct transformation was obtained using aflatoxin B1 (AFB1), 11-methylcyclopenta(a)-phenanthrene, N-methyl-N'-nitro-N-nitrosoguanidine (MNNG), methylazoxymethanol (MAM), and N-2-fluorenylacetamide (FAA) and its metabolites, but not with urethan, N-hydroxyurethan, or diethylnitrosamine (DENA). The importance of metabolic activation of certain compounds in transformation was also indicated. The compound FAA had only weak transforming activity, whereas the more active metabolites N-hydroxy FAA and N-acetoxy FAA were 4- and 30-fold more active, respectively, than FAA in their transforming activity. In fact, N-acetoxy FAA, which is considered an ultimate carcinogen, was even more active than AFB1. Direct evidence for activation in the intact animal has been shown for the compounds DENA and urethan (DiPaolo et al., 1972a, 1973). When these compounds were injected intraperitoneally into pregnant hamsters on day-12 and on day-14 embryo cultures, transformation was observed in isolated clones; whereas, direct exposure of hamster embryo cells to these compounds in vitro failed to induce morphological transformation. In the case of urethan, two isolated clones were developed into cell lines and these produced fibrosarcomas in hamsters. These studies further demonstrate the validity of using the Syrian hamster embryo system as an in vitro model for chemical carcinogenesis and also illustrate that these cell cultures are capable of activating several but not all types of carcinogens.

Further evidence indicating the importance of metabolic activation of polycyclic hydrocarbons with respect to cell toxicity and malignant transformation of Syrian hamster embryo cells has been presented by Grover et al. (1971) and Huberman et al. (1972). The K-region epoxides and cis-dihydrodiols obtained from BA and DBA were more active in inducing malignant transformation than were the parent hydrocarbons and K-region phenols (Grover et al., 1971), whereas three K-region derivatives of BA and DBA (cis-5,6-dihydrodiols, 5,6-oxide, and 5-hydroxy) exhibited increased toxicity in comparison with BA and DBA. The K-region phenols, 5-hydroxy BA or DBA, were the most toxic compounds tested, although they failed to transform hamster embryo cells. These findings provided additional evidence that toxicity and transformation are not directly related processes. Huberman et al. (1972) demonstrated that the 5,6-epoxides (K-region) of DBA and BA were more active in inducing malignant transformation in hamster embryo cells than the corresponding parent hydrocarbons or the K-region 5,6-cis- and trans-dihydrodiols and phenols. The K-region epoxide of BA, BA-5,6-epoxide, was more cytotoxic and produced more transformation than the non-K-region BA-8,9-epoxide. In addition, the K-region epoxides of phenanthrene and CH induced transformation, whereas the parent hydrocarbons did not, when compared to acetone controls. These types of studies provided evidence that epoxide derivatives of polycyclic aromatic hydrocarbons have biologic activity, although subsequent studies have indicated that non-K-region dihydrodiol epoxides of BP (BP 7,8-dihydrodiol-9,10-oxide, "BPDE") are the major metabolites of BP responsible for carcinogenicity (for review of this aspect see Weinstein et al., 1978a). In recent studies Mager et al. (1977) compared the frequency of transformation of secondary Syrian hamster embryo cells exposed to BP and six of its metabolites. The trans-7,8-dihydrodiol was more active than the 4,5- or 9,10-dihydrodiols, or the parent compound BP in inducing transformation. BPDE I (the isomer in which 7,8-diol and 9,10-oxide are on opposite sides of the ring system) was more active than BPDE II (the isomer in which the 7,8-diol and 9,10-oxides are on the same side of the ring system) and was also more active than the 4,5-epoxide, indicating that BPDE I is the most potent metabolite of BP with respect to cell transformation.

Variations in the response of different preparations of early-passage Syrian hamster embryo cells to transformation by MC and BP have been demonstrated by Pienta et al. (1977). In order to improve the reliability and reproducibility of the transformation assay, different batches of cryopreserved primary hamster embryo cells were screened and those giving uniform transformation after repeated trials with MC and BP were utilized to test 97 compounds for transforming ability (Pienta et al., 1977; Dunkel et al., 1977). A 90.8% positive

TABLE 5 Correlation of Reported Carcinogenic Activity of Chemicals Tested in the Hamster Embryo Cell In Vitro Carcinogenesis Bioassay

Chemical class	Reported activity	Number tested	Concurrence	False negatives	False positives
I. Direct alkylating agents	Carcinogen	9	9/9	0	—
	Noncarcinogen	1	1/1	—	0
II. Polycyclic hydrocarbons and derivatives	Carcinogen	6	6/6	0	—
	Noncarcinogen	6	6/6	—	0
III. Nitrosamines	Carcinogen	3	2/3	1	—
	Noncarcinogen	1	1/1	—	0
IV. Aromatic amines and aminoazo dyes	Carcinogen	16	13/16	3	—
	Noncarcinogen	7	7/7	—	0
V. Miscellaneous compounds	Carcinogen	20	16/20	4	—
	Noncarcinogen	6	6/6	—	0
Total		75	67/75 (89%)	8	0

Source: Reproduced by permission from Dunkel et al., 1977.

correlation between morphological transformation and the reported carcinogenic activity of all of the chemicals tested was achieved. A 100% positive correlation was found with direct-alkylating agents, polycyclic hydrocarbons and derivatives and solvents. An approximately 85% positive correlation was shown with nitrosamines and amides, aromatic amines and amino dyes, and miscellaneous compounds (Table 5). The reliability of this assay was shown by the absence of false positives using 21 noncarcinogens, and apparently no spontaneous transformation was observed (Dunkel et al., 1977). The ability of morphological transformation in culture to predict tumorigenic potential was also demonstrated by tumorigenicity assays using weanling hamsters.

With respect to the problem of detecting potential metal carcinogens, DiPaolo and Casto (1979) have reported morphologic transformation of Syrian hamster embryo cells by some inorganic salts of nickel, cadmium, chromium, beryllium, and arsenic, but not salts of iron, titanium, tungstate, zinc, aluminum, and nickel sulfide amorphous.

Transformation of these cells by tryptophan pyrolysis products has also been reported (Takayama et al., 1978), thus extending this assay to the detection of potential carcinogens in pyrolysis products of food.

C. Mouse Prostate Fibroblastic Cell Lines

Chen and Heidelberger (1969a, 1969b, 1969c) developed an in vitro quantitative malignant transformation assay for carcinogenic hydrocarbons utilizing adult C3H mouse ventral prostate cell lines. MC-treated cultures formed randomly oriented, piled-up colonies of transformed cells after approximately 100 days in culture (Chen and Heidelberger, 1969b), whereas spontaneous transformation in control cultures did not occur until 261, 344, and 570 days in culture (Chen and Heidelberger, 1969a). The transformed cells did not show density-dependent inhibition of growth, were resistant to the toxicity of MC, and as few as 1000 cells produced 100% incidence of fibrosarcomas in unconditioned mice. In contrast, control cells did not produce tumors even when 10^6 cells were injected subcutaneously into irradiated C3H mice (Chen and Heidelberger, 1969b). A good quantitative correlation between carcinogenic activity and in vivo transforming ability of various polycyclic hydrocarbons in the C3H mouse prostate cell system was also demonstrated (Chen and Heidelberger, 1969c). The potent carcinogens

4-fluoro-1-methyl-1,2-benz(a)anthracene (4-F-1-Me-BA), BP, DMBA, and MC produced maximum transformation with frequencies of 35, 28, 26, and 16 transformed colonies per 7000 cells, respectively. The moderately active initiating carcinogen, 1,2,5,6-dibenz(a)anthracene (1,2,5,6-DBA) resulted in four transformed colonies per seven dishes, and the noncarcinogenic compounds PY, 3-fluoro-10-methyl-1,2-benz(a)anthracene (3-F-10-Me-BA), and 1,2,3,4-dibenz(a)anthracene (1,2,3,4-DBA) failed to produce any transformed colonies.

The mouse prostate cell culture system has also been useful in demonstrating the importance of metabolic activation of hydrocarbons and the role of the cell cycle in the in vitro transformation process. Grover et al. (1971) obtained higher levels of transformation with the K-region epoxides of MCA and BA than with the respective parent compounds. In contrast, the non-K-region cis-dihydrodiols and trans-dihydrodiols of BA, DBA, and MCA were inactive in transforming G23 mouse ventral prostate cells (Marquardt et al., 1972). These findings provided further support of the concept that epoxides are the metabolically activated intermediate of BA, DBA, and MCA responsible for in vitro malignant transformation, although, as already mentioned, subsequent studies indicated that the major in vivo intermediate is not a simple K-region epoxide. The importance of the cell cycle in in vitro transformation of mouse prostate cells with DMBA-5,6-oxide and MNNG has been demonstrated by Marquardt (1974). (See also studies by Peterson et al., 1974.) Both agents were inactive in transformation assays when applied during the G2 and M phase of the cell cycle, but were capable of inducing malignant transformation during the S phase. It is interesting to note that unlike transformation, toxicity was found to be similar during the various stages of the cell cycle, again indicating that transforming ability and toxicity are not directly related.

D. Mouse 3T3 Fibroblast

The 3T3 line has also been used as a quantitative assay system for monitoring malignant transformation in vitro. DiPaolo et al. (1972b) obtained transformation of sublines of the BALB/3T3 mouse fibroblast cell line after a single 48-hour exposure to polycyclic hydrocarbons (DMBA, MCA, and BP), AFB1, N-acetoxy FAA, and MNNG, but not with noncarcinogens (acetone, anthracene, PH) or DENA. Transformation followed one-hit kinetics, with higher levels of carcinogen resulting in increased transformation and reduced cloning efficiency. Malignant transformation was demonstrated using 23 independently isolated clones transformed with the carcinogens DMBA, BP, or MNNG. Injection of 10^6 cells subcutaneously into nonirradiated and irradiated BALB/c mice resulted in palpable tumors after 2-3 weeks with incidences of 10-50% and 50-100%, respectively. In contrast, untreated BALB/3T3 cells and PY- and anthracene-treated cells failed to induce tumors even when 10^8 cells were injected into mice. The ability of MC and 4NQO to induce malignant transformation in A31-714 cells, a subclone of BALB/3T3 cells, has also been demonstrated by Kakunaga (1973). Carcinogen-transformed clones exhibited an altered morphology, increased saturation density, growth in soft agar, and the capacity to induce fibrosarcomas in both newborn and adult mice. The noncarcinogenic substances DMSO, 4-nitroquinoline (4NQ), 4-aminoquinoline-1-oxide (4AQO), and PH did not induce transformation in this system.

E. The 10T1/2 Cell Line

Another quantitative in vitro transformation assay system for chemical carcinogens which utilizes a mouse fibroblast cell line was developed by Heidelberger and co-workers (Reznikoff et al., 1973a, 1973b). This group isolated a cloned cell line from C3H mouse embryos, C3H 10T1/2 CL8, which exhibited a high degree of contact inhibition at confluency, and a low incidence of spontaneous transformation. Exposure to the polycyclic hydrocarbons MC, DBA, and DMBA resulted in a high frequency of malignant transformation. This system has also been utilized to demonstrate the carcinogenic potential of alkylating agents (Bertram and Heidelberger, 1974; Benedict et al., 1977), X rays (Terzaghi and Little, 1975), ultraviolet light (Mondal and Heidelberger, 1976), cigarette smoke condensates (Benedict et al., 1975), and various cancer-chemotherapeutic drugs (Jones et al., 1976; Benedict et al., 1977).

Unlike the mouse prostate system (Marquardt, 1974), MNNG transformation was highest in the 10T1/2 system when exposure was initiated during the late G1, as opposed to S1, phase of the cell cycle (Peterson et al., 1974). In contrast, 5-fluorodeoxyuridine and 1-β-D-arabinofuranosylcytosine were maximally active in inducing transformation of 10T1/2 cells during the S phase of the cell cycle (Jones et al., 1976). The reasons for these differences in cell cycle dependence between the mouse prostate and 10T1/2 when each was studied with the same carcinogen, and when 10T1/2 cells are exposed to different agents is presently unknown. The latter differences may reflect variations in the mechanism by which different carcinogens induce transformation. Precise interpretations of some of these results are also complicated by the severe toxicity in the MNNG studies (Peterson et al., 1974).

F. The BHK Cell Line

The Syrian hamster fibroblast cell line, BHK 21 clone 13, has also proven useful as a system for quantitating malignant transformation after a single exposure to carcinogens (DiMayorca et al., 1973; Bouck and DiMayorca, 1976; Ishii et al., 1977; Styles, 1977) or ultraviolet irradiation (Ishii et al., 1977). The basic assay involves exposing BHK 21 cells to the test compound for 20 min to 4 hr, followed by seeding one aliquot in liquid media for determining plating efficiency and survival and another aliquot in soft agar for determining the transformation frequency. The ability to directly plate cells in agar and score for transformation makes this a very easy to score and quantitative assay system. Studies by DiMayorca and co-workers (DiMayorca et al., 1973) have demonstrated that certain transformants resulting from treatment with the carcinogens DENA, nitrosomethylurea (NMU), or 4NQO exhibit a strict in vitro temperature dependence. At 38.5°C certain carcinogen-transformed clones grow in agar and display the transformed phenotype, whereas at 32°C they exhibit a more normal phenotype. Transformants that are heat sensitive with respect to expression of growth in agar have also been isolated (for review see Basilico, 1977). Evidence has been presented that the carcinogens induce somatic mutations and that expression of the normal phenotype can be cold sensitive, heat sensitive, or unexpressed in isolated clones and that these properties are dependent on the type and dose of carcinogen administered (Bouck and DiMayorca, 1976). Studies on the nature of the altered gene products required for maintenance of the normal and transformed phenotype make this a valuable system for elucidating the molecular mechanism(s) involved in the expression of chemically induced transformation in BHK 21 cells. Styles (1977) has used a modified BHK 21 carcinogen assay system in which the cells are exposed to the test agent in the presence of a rat liver postmitochondrial supernatant fraction and cofactors (S-9 mix) to aid metabolism and then scored for survival and growth in agar. A dose response curve for transformation was calculated and a fivefold increase in transformation frequency at the LD_{50} (concentration producing 50% lethality) for a given compound was regarded as a positive test result. Using this procedure over 120 compounds were tested, 58 of which were known carcinogens, and the assay was found to be more than 90% accurate in distinguishing between carcinogens and noncarcinogens (Purchase et al., 1976). Five false negatives, including β-naphthylamine, vinyl chloride, and diethylstilbestrol, and only two false positives were obtained with this cell transformation assay. Few details, however, of the results by Purchase et al. were given in their publication. A limitation of this system is that most clones of BHK cells already grow in agar and are tumorigenic.

G. Guinea Pig and Human Fibroblasts

Guinea pig fetal cell strains (Evans and DiPaolo, 1975; 1976; Evans et al., 1977) have been found to exhibit a much greater delay in the time course of cell transformation by chemical carcinogens than hamster, rat, or mouse cell cultures. With the guinea pig cell strains (which have the advantage of being diploid) morphological alterations, growth in 0.35% agar, and tumor formation in irradiated syngeneic newborn guinea pigs resulted only after 5-18 months following exposure to MC, BP, MNNG, DMBA, AFB1, or DENA (Evans and DiPaolo, 1975; 1976; Evans et al., 1977). In this system certain changes in growth properties, including saturation density, plating efficiency, and average population doubling time, and the chromosomal composition of transformed cells did not correlate with tumorigenic potential. However, a good correlation between growth in soft agar, which developed subsequent to or at the same time as appearance of morphological transformation, and the ability to induce tumor formation in syngeneic hosts was observed.

It would of course be highly desirable to have a human cell culture system sensitive to in vitro transformation by chemical carcinogens. Recently Kakunaga (1977, 1978) has reported morphological transformation of normal human diploid fibroblast cells. The transformation was first observed 7-14 weeks (5 to 10 passages) following exposure to a dose of 4NQO or MNNG which caused about a 70% reduction in cell survival. Morphologically altered clones had increased saturation densities and grew in soft agar, and certain clones induced tumors in nude mice. Transformation was obtained in a mass culture, rather than a clonal or focus assay, and required at least 13 cell generations with repeated subculturing. The frequency of transformation was extremely low, estimated at 1×10^{-7} per treated cell, and low concentrations of 4NQO or MC failed to induce transformation. Thus, because of the long lag and low efficiency of transformation this human cell system is not yet applicable as a short-term predictive test for carcinogenicity. Another system for in vitro transformation of human cells has been recently reported (Milo and DiPaolo, 1978) and warrant further study.

H. Epithelial Cell Systems

As discussed in the introduction, since the majority of human tumors arise from epithelial tissues, it would be highly desirable to utilize epithelial cell cultures for the detection of possible human carcinogens. Unfortunately, at the present time epithelial cell culture systems are not useful for the routine assay of potential carcinogens for three major reasons. (1) There are currently very few normal epithelial cultures that are generally available, that can be serially passaged, and that grow under simple and defined conditions. (2) Transformation of epithelial cultures to tumorigenicity following exposure to known carcinogens occurs with a long lag (many weeks to months) and with such a low efficiency that it cannot be readily reproduced or quantitated. (3) There are few objective and well validated in vitro markers of transformation of epithelial cell cultures. Epithelial cell cultures are useful, however, for studies concerned with the mechanism of chemical carcinogenesis (for review see Weinstein et al., 1976). Some examples of results obtained with epithelial cell cultures exposed to chemical carcinogens are now described.

Katsuta and Takaoka (1968, 1972) obtained malignant conversion of normal diploid strains of rat liver parenchymal cells with single or multiple exposures of 3.3×10^{-6} M 4NQO. Transformed cells did not exhibit distinctive changes in morphology but were capable of inducing carcinomas in rats after approximately 4 months following carcinogen treatment, whereas control cultures under similar conditions did not induce tumor formation. Montesano et al. (1973) demonstrated that repeated exposure of rat liver epithelial cell lines to dimethylnitrosamine (DMN) or MNNG resulted in the development of cells capable of growth in soft agar and tumor formation in rats. The development of malignant potential was not observed until a minimum of 8 (MNNG) or 15 weeks (DMN) following cessation of carcinogen treatment and did not result in distinctive morphological changes. When injected into rats, the DMN treated cells produced adenocarcinomas while the MNNG treated cells produced both fibrosarcomas and carcinomas. Malignant conversion of rat liver epithelial cell lines after prolonged exposure to AFB, DMN, MNU, N-hydroxy FAA, or DMBA has also been reported by Williams et al. (1973). The treated cells, although capable of inducing carcinomas when injected into X rayed syngeneic rats, revealed only minor and no consistent morphological alterations when examined in cell culture.

Montesano et al. (1977) examined three parameters of 22 rat liver epithelial cell cultures: cytology, growth in soft agar, and production of extracellular plasminogen activator

(PA), and correlated these with their tumorigenic potential. Cytologic diagnosis and growth in agar, but not PA, correlated with tumorigenesis. Of the cytologic parameters evaluated, the two that correlated best with tumorigenic potential were increased cytoplasmic basophilia and an increased nuclear: cytoplasmic ratio. H. S. Smith (1979, personal communication) in studies with epithelial cell lines established from human carcinomas and nonmalignant tissues, and in studies with mouse epithelial cell lines, found that loss of anchorage dependence generally correlated with malignancy, whereas the production of PA did not. A similar correlation between growth in 0.33% agar and tumorigenesis of BALB/c mouse primary epidermal cell cultures transformed by MNNG has been demonstrated by Colburn et al. (1978b; 1978c). In this system no discrete morphological alterations were observed and shorter population doubling times of transformants did not correlate with tumorigenicity, whereas anchorage independent growth did correlate with malignancy.

Mammalian cell mutants temperature sensitive (TS) in the maintenance of the transformed state have proven invaluable for studying the mechanisms of cell transformation. Yamaguchi and Weinstein (1975) have isolated such TS mutants from epithelial cells transformed by the carcinogen N-acetoxy-2-acetylaminofluorene (N-Ac-AAF). The original source of this mutant was a transformed rat liver epithelial cell line, W-8, obtained following a single exposure of normal K-16 cells to 0.5 μg/ml of N-acetoxy-AAF. The parental K-16 cells were incapable of growth in agar at either 36° C or 40° C and were not tumorigenic. In contrast, W-8 cells grew in agar at both 36° C and 40° C, piled up at confluency, and were tumorigenic. TS-223 and other TS cell mutants proved to be temperature sensitive for maintenance of transformation as demonstrated by reduced cloning efficiency in agar, reduced plating efficiency in liquid medium, reduced saturation density, and a more normal morphology at confluency when grown at 40° C rather than 36° C. This TS system represents a valuable model for investigating those biochemical alterations required for expression of the transformed phenotype in epithelial cell cultures.

A potentially interesting system for detecting polycyclic hydrocarbon carcinogens, which utilizes prostaglandin synthesis as an endpoint, has been developed by Levine (1977). Briefly, 2×10^5 MDCK cells, an epithelial cell line derived from dog kidney, are exposed to the putative carcinogen for 24 hr, grown for an additional 24 hr in media lacking the test compound and assayed by radioimmunoassay with antisera to $PGF_{2\alpha}$ and PGE_2. A positive correlation between carcinogenic activity and prostaglandin synthesis was observed with BP, DMBA, MC, 7-MBA, 5 methylchrysene, 3 methylchrysene, chrysene, AFB, and 1,2,7,8-diepoxyoctane. On the other hand, neither the aromatic amines nor the nitrosamines, at 0.5 μg/ml, affected prostaglandin synthesis. The importance of metabolic activation of polycyclic hydrocarbons by the microsomal monooxygenase system was demonstrated by the ability of 7,8-benzoflavone (an inhibitor of this type of metabolic activation) to block the prostaglandin stimulating activity of BP, DMBA, and AFB1. In contrast, the inhibitors of microsomal monooxygenases, metyrapone, and SKF 525-A, inhibited BP-induced stimulation of prostaglandin synthesis by 20%, and an inhibitor of epoxide hydrase (1,2-epoxy 3,3,3-trichloropropane) had no effect. Further studies are needed with more compounds and other cell types to determine if this simple and rapid biochemical test is useful as a reliable short-term screening test for polycyclic aromatic hydrocarbon carcinogens and possibly certain other classes of carcinogens.

I. Systems Employing Viruses Plus Chemical Carcinogens

Enhanced tumorigenesis has been shown to occur in animals exposed to both a chemical carcinogen and either RNA or DNA viruses (Table 6). This observation was extended to cells in culture using combinations of a chemical carcinogen with murine leukemia virus (Freeman et al., 1970, 1973; Price et al., 1971; Rhim et al., 1971, 1974), adenovirus (Casto, 1973; Casto et al., 1973, DiPaolo and Casto, 1976; Fisher et al., 1970) or SV_{40} virus (Diamond et al., 1974a). Carcinogen enhancement of transformation in cell culture has been shown to exhibit different temporal relationship with RNA and DNA tumor viruses. In the case of the RNA leukemia virus, transformation occurred when the carcinogen was added

TABLE 6 Synergistic Interactions Between Viruses and Chemical Carcinogens

Virus	Carcinogen	Systems	References
In animals			
Papilloma	PAH[a]	Rabbit skin	Rous and Kidd, 1938
Fibroma	PAH	Rabbit skin	Ahlstrom and Andrewes, 1938; Andrewes et al., 1937
Fowl pox	PAH	Chicken	Duran-Reynals, 1952
Vaccinia	PAH	Mouse skin	Duran-Reynals, 1962
West Nile	PAH	Mouse skin	Tanaka and Southam, 1962
Polyoma	PAH	Mouse	Berenblum, 1963; Chieco-Bianchi et al., 1963
Murine leukemia	Urethan	Mouse	Salaman et al., 1963
In cell culture			
Murine leukemia:		Rat embryo cells Mouse embryo cells	Freeman et al., 1970; Rhim et al, 1971; Price et al., 1971;
	PAH, azo dyes, aromatic amines, etc.	Rat embryo cells	Freeman et al., 1973 Rhim et al., 1974
Adenoviruses:			
Simian adenovirus 7	PAH, wide spectrum of carcinogens including metals, azo dyes, aromatic amines, etc.	Hamster embryo cells Rat embryo cells	Casto, 1973; Casto et al., 1973; DiPaolo and Casto, 1976; Casto et al., 1978
Human adenovirus 5	PAH	Rat embryo cells	Fisher et al., 1978, 1980
SV_{40}	4NQO[b]	Chinese hamster embryo cells	Diamond et al., 1974a

[a]PAH = polycyclic aromatic hydrocarbons.

[b]4NQO = 4-nitroquinoline 1-oxide.

after viral infection, whereas in the DNA virus systems synergisms occurred when the carcinogens were administered shortly before viral infection. Rhim et al. (1974) and Price et al. (1971) demonstrated that DENA and MC treatment of murine leukemia virus infected rat embryo cells resulted in morphological transformation, whereas carcinogen-treated uninfected cultures and cultures infected only with virus did not exhibit transformation. These studies were extended by Rhim et al. (1971) using DMBA and rat cells chronically infected with Rauscher leukemia virus. Only cultures previously infected with the virus underwent transformation when exposed to the carcinogen, and the transformed cells produced sarcomas when injected into newborn rats.

The possibility of utilizing morphological transformation of murine leukemia virus-infected embryo cells as a short-term screening system for carcinogens has been explored by Freeman et al. (1973) and Rhim et al. (1974). Freeman et al. (1973) tested a list of 30 compounds, including PAHs, azo dyes, aromatic amines, and miscellaneous compounds for their ability to induce morphological transformation of Fischer rat embryo cells chronically infected with Rauscher leukemia virus. In general, a good correlation between carcinogenic potential and transformation was found. This assay system, however, was highly dependent on the dose of compound tested, not readily quantitatable (with respect to the number of transformed foci per carcinogen dose) and gave variable responses with certain test compounds. Noncarcinogenic compounds, such as anthracene (one of six tests), phenanthrene (one of five tests) and fluoranthene (one of four tests), were occasionally positive; weakly active carcinogens, such as 3-aminofluorene, 4-aminobiphenyl, and acetamide (three of five tests), were sometimes negative; and certain active carcinogens, such as N-hydroxy-FAA or FAA (three tests) and propane sulfone (two of four tests), were found to be negative in this assay. Rhim et al. (1974) tested the effect of different classes of chemical carcinogens (PAH, azo dyes, aromatic amines, nitrosamines, and urethans) and noncarcinogenic analogs, on transformation of NIH Swiss mouse embryo cells infected with the AKR leukemia virus. Problems found in the Rauscher leukemia virus infected rat embryo system were also apparent in this study. The system was not readily quantitatable and produced both false-negative and false-positive results. The active carcinogens N-hydroxy-FAA, DBA, and 3-methyl-4-dimethylaminoazobenzene did not induce transformation, but the inactive compounds phenanthrene (one of two tests) and 2-biphenylamine induced transformation. Thus, at the present time neither of the above two systems appear to be reliable short-term screening assays for chemical carcinogens.

Enhanced viral transformation by the combined action of chemical carcinogens and DNA viruses has also been observed, both in the intact animal and in cell culture (Table 6). Casto et al. (1973) obtained increased frequencies of simian adenovirus 7 (SA7) transformation of primary hamster embryo cells by pretreatment of the cells with BP, MC, DMBA, or DBA 18 hr prior to viral infection. In contrast, treatment of cells 5 hr after infection actually inhibited transformation. Noncarcinogenic PAHs (PY, phenanthrene, and perylene) failed to stimulate transformation. In this system, levels of carcinogens higher than those required to induce maximal enhancement generally led to a decrease or complete inhibition of viral transformation. The carcinogens that have given transformation in this system include polycyclic aromatic hydrocarbons, azo dyes, aromatic amines, mycotoxins, metals, and so on (Casto et al., 1978) (Table 6). It should be mentioned, however, that with certain compounds marked enhancement was obtained only under conditions of appreciable toxicity and false negatives have resulted with DENA, DMN, urethan, red dye 2, trichloroethylene, chloroform, dioxane, and FAA (Casto et al., 1978).

Fisher et al. (1978) found enhanced transformation of rat embryo cells by a temperature-sensitive mutant of human adenovirus type 5 (H5ts125), which is defective in DNA replication (Ginsberg et al., 1974), when the cells were pretreated with DMBA or BP, 18 hr prior to viral infection. As with the SA7 system, under the conditions employed the carcinogen alone did not produce transformation. Enhanced viral transformation was found even at carcinogen concentrations resulting in less than a 10% decrease in survival, indicating that toxicity was not a prerequisite for the enhancement. Diamond et al. (1974a) obtained enhanced SV_{40} transformation of Chinese hamster embryo cells when the cells were treated with 4NQO 2 or 7 hr prior to viral infection or up to 8 hr post infection.

The mechanism(s) involved in chemical carcinogen-induced enhancement of DNA virus transformation are not known with certainty. A few studies have addressed this question. Casto et al. (1976) studied the relationship between time of initial exposure to the chemical, DNA repair, and enhancement of viral transformation by carcinogens and mutagens. Three interactions were observed that were dependent on the compound tested: AFB1, BP, MC, and DMBA enhanced SA7 transformation only when added to cells prior to virus infection; cytosine arabinoside, caffeine, and 6 acetoxy-benzo(a)pyrene gave maximal enhancement when added after virus infection; and β-propiolactone, methyl methanesulfonate, N-Ac-FAA, MNNG, and methylazoxymethanol acetate enhanced transformation when added before or after virus infection. A direct correlation between enhancement of SA7 virus transformation and the ability of certain chemicals to induce scissions in DNA (as measured by DNA sedimentation in alkaline sucrose gradients) and unscheduled DNA (repair) synthesis in hamster cells was observed (Casto et al., 1976). However, certain compounds, for example, benzo(e)pyrene, cytosine arabinoside, and caffeine, resulted in enhanced SA7 transformation without altering DNA sedimentation profiles or inducing unscheduled DNA synthesis. From these and other studies Casto et al. (1976) have postulated that enhanced viral transformation induced by agents causing DNA damage may be due to the availability of additional integration sites for viral DNA insertion resulting from the repair process. The mechanism of enhancement by those compounds that do not appear to induce excision DNA repair is not known.

Hirai et al. (1974) have observed that the enhanced transformation of Chinese hamster embryo cells resulting from treatment with 4NQO prior to SV_{40} infection is associated with increased nuclear penetration of SV_{40} DNA and an increase in the total amount of SV_{40} DNA integrated into cellular DNA. However, they were unable to distinguish if there was an increase in the absolute number of SV_{40} genomes integrated per cell or if more cells contained integrated genomes. Nucleic acid hybridization studies of rat embryo cells transformed by adenovirus H5ts125, with or without exposure of the cells to BP or DMBA prior to infection with virus, revealed similar patterns of integrated viral sequences in both types of transformed cells (Dorsch-Häsler et al., 1980). Hatch et al. (1978) compared the properties of hamster embryo cells transformed by SA7 virus with and without prior exposure of the cells to MCA, BP, or DMBA. In general, the ability of cells to express virus-specified antigens, grow in soft agar, and induce sarcomas in hamster was found to be similar in all of the transformants. However, some transformants obtained from cells treated with both chemical carcinogen and virus exhibited a higher incidence of tumor formation than cells exposed to virus alone. In separate experiments hamster cells were first transformed by MCA and then infected with SA7 virus, resulting in conversion from a fibroblastic to an epithelioid morphology. The latter cells were more tumorigenic than cells transformed by SA7 alone but less than those transformed by MCA alone. Transformed rat embryo clones obtained after exposing cells to the H5ts125 virus, with or without pretreatment with carcinogens, were found to be similar with respect to a spectrum of properties, including population doubling time, saturating density, growth in reduced serum, cloning efficiency in liquid media, level of LETS protein, and plasminogen activator production. The only discernible differences were the temporal acquisition of the ability to grow in agar and cell surface glycoproteins (Fisher et al., 1979b; 1979c; Goldstein and Fisher, 1980). Clones derived from cells exposed to chemical carcinogen plus virus generally exhibited these altered properties after a shorter time in culture than those derived from cells exposed to virus alone (Fisher et al., 1979b; Fisher and Weinstein, 1980).

Taken together, the above studies suggest that carcinogen-enhanced DNA virus transformation does not result from an increase in the number or types of viral DNA sequences integrated in individual cells. It seems more likely that the carcinogen may enhance the number of cells that acquire integrated sequences. In some cases exposure of cells to the carcinogen enhanced expression of transformation associated properties, including tumorigenicity, but this was not always the case.

The aforementioned types of cell culture systems should be useful for further studies on the interactions between chemical and viral agents in cancer induction and with further refinements may represent useful short-term carcinogen bioassay systems.

J. Advantages and Limitations of the Various Cell Culture Transformation Systems: Future Directions

It is apparent that each of the aforementioned mammalian cell culture systems have advantages and disadvantages as assays for potential environmental carcinogens.

The hamster embryo system, and similar systems, have the following advantages: (1) the cells are diploid; (2) they metabolize and activate many, although not all, classes of carcinogens; (3) since they are not a cell line, they are less likely to be subject to artifacts resulting from long-term cell culture; and (4) the system can be scored for morphologic transformation within 7-10 days after exposure to the carcinogen. The major limitations of this system are: (1) the scoring of morphologically transformed foci requires considerable experience, and a simpler, more objective parameter, would be desirable; and (2) there can be considerable variation in this system with different batches of embryo cultures.

The $10T\frac{1}{2}$ cell line and certain other closely related fibroblast cell lines have the following advantages: (1) being a cloned cell line the response is less variable; and (2) foci of transformation are more easily scored. The disadvantages are the following: (1) since the cells are aneuploid and represent a cell line, they may differ appreciably from completely normal cells; it has been shown, for example, that the 3T3 cell line is tumorigenic when the cells are allowed to attach to glass fibers and then implanted subcutaneously (Boone, 1975); and the BHK cells are known to be weakly tumorigenic and many BHK clones spontaneously grow in agar; and (2) these cells are less active in carcinogen metabolism than primary or secondary cultures. Although they activate polycyclic aromatic hydrocarbons, they do not appear to activate aromatic amines, nitrosamines, or aflatoxin.

The systems employing both virus infection and carcinogen exposure of cells in culture are useful for studying such interactions, but some of the results obtained thus far raise the question of whether they will yield an excessive number of false positives.

Further work is needed to improve the metabolic activation systems which convert procarcinogens to reactive electrophiles and ultimate carcinogens. With these improvements certain compounds that now produce false negatives should score positive, thus improving the overall validity of these in vitro systems. Several current approaches are in progress to facilitate the conversion of procarcinogens to ultimate carcinogens in cell culture. One is to include at the time of addition of the test compound the microsomal fraction (so-called "S-9") of liver or other tissues (either rodent or human) and cofactors, to the target cells in which transformation is scored (Dunkel et al., 1977; Benedict et al., 1978). Another is to add intact "metabolizer cells," known to have the capacity to activate the carcinogen, to the target cells. Similar approaches have been used to enhance mutagenesis in mammalian cell cultures (Huberman and Sachs, 1974; Huberman, 1976; O'Neill et al., 1977b) and show promise in transformation assays (C. Heidelberger, 1980, personal communication).

Recent studies indicate that through the use of feeder layer cultures, or conditioned medium it is possible to grow well-differentiated epidermal cell cultures (Rheinwald and Green, 1975). These approaches should facilitate the establishment of other epithelial cell culture systems for use in carcinogenesis bioassays.

It seems likely that, as with animal bioassay systems, no single cell culture system will be capable of detecting and providing information on the relative potency of diverse types of chemical carcinogens. Major variables between systems will exist in terms of uptake, metabolism, activation, and detoxification of various carcinogens; types of macromolecular damage that may occur and the efficiency and fidelity of DNA repair; chromosomal stability; the role of endogenous and exogenous viral genomes as possible cofactors in the transformation process; the reliability of specific in vitro markers of transformation as predictors of tumorigenicity; and other aspects. A major limitation of cell culture systems, and indeed of all laboratory assays for chemical carcinogens, including animal tumorigenicity assays, is their validity in terms of predicting which chemicals are likely to be important human carcinogens. In this regard it would be desirable to have more efficient and reproducible systems utilizing human cell cultures. For reasons already mentioned in this chapter, it would also be desirable to have better epithelial cell culture systems. Although these are desirable goals, we would emphasize that even when they are achieved, no single human cell culture system, fibroblastic or epithelial, will be capable of detecting all classes of carcinogens. This can be anticipated because of differences in carcinogen metabolism and DNA repair among different human tissues, differences among individuals, and the probable alterations of cellular capacities as a consequence of in vitro culture.

The above comments are not meant to indicate that mammalian cell culture systems will not be useful in the screening of carcinogens. On the contrary, it is likely that they will play a prominent role in this area. As with other assays, the proper interpretation of the results obtained, both positive and negative, and their extrapolation to the human, will depend on a thorough understanding of the limitations of each assay. In this complex area cell culture transformation assays should be part of a panel of other short-term tests, and in many cases this panel will have to include tumorigenesis assays in the whole animal.

V. THE ACTION OF TUMOR PROMOTERS IN CELL CULTURE

It is well recognized that the carcinogenic process is often multifactor in terms of its etiology and multistep in its evolution. This concept is clearly demonstrated by the "two-stage" mouse skin carcinogenesis assay in which application of a subcarcinogenic dose of an "initiating agent" followed by repeated application of a "promoting agent" (which itself is not carcinogenic) results in multiple skin neoplasms (for review see Berenblum, 1975). The most potent tumor-promoting agents in the mouse skin system are 12-0-tetradecanoyl-phorbol-13-acetate (TPA) and related plant diterpenes (for reviews see Van Duuren, 1969; Boutwell, 1974; Hecker, 1975). Table 7 contrasts the major biologic properties of initiating and promoting agents. It is apparent that they act by quite different mechanisms and, therefore, different types of short-term in vitro tests will be required for their detection (Table 1). A major difference that bears emphasis is that promoters, in contrast to initiating carcinogens, do not appear to damage DNA or to be mutagenic.

Most of the short-term in vitro tests discussed in the preceding sections of this chapter are designed to detect initiating carcinogens, via the transformation of mammalian cell cultures, mutagenesis in either bacterial or mammalian cell cultures, DNA damage and repair, chromosome damage, and sister chromatid exchange, and so on, but not promoting agents. Recent studies indicate that TPA and related phorbol esters enhance the in vitro transformation of fibroblast cultures previously exposed to carcinogenic PAHs (Lasne et al., 1974; Mondal et al., 1976), ultraviolet light (Mondal and Heidelberger, 1976), X ray (Kennedy et al., 1978), an adenovirus (Fisher et al., 1978), or Epstein-Barr virus (Yamamoto and zur Hausen, 1979). In addition, TPA has been shown to induce a spectrum of changes in cell culture which mimic those seen in cells transformed either by chemical carcinogens or viruses (Table 8). (For reviews see Weinstein et al., 1977, 1978b, 1978c, 1979).

Lasne et al. (1974) compared the occurrence of transformation in rat embryo fibroblasts exposed to 1 μg/ml BP and then serially passaged in the presence or absence of 0.01 μg/ml TPA. Very few transformants were noted in any of the cultures at passage 20. By passage 34, however, a marked increase in the number of transformants was found in both types of cultures, and the incidence of transformation was highest in those cultures exposed to BP and then grown continuously in TPA. In addition, the combined treatment resulted in transformants that acquired the ability to grow earlier and more efficiently in agar and were generally more tumorigenic than cells exposed only to BP. Interpretation of these results is complicated by the fact that a clonal assay was not used, and, because of the prolonged serial passage, selection may have played a role in the results obtained. Mondal et al. (1976) demonstrated enhanced transformation in a clonal assay when 10T1/2 cells were exposed to

TABLE 7 A Comparison of Biologic Properties of Initiating Agents and Promoting Agents

Initiating agents	Promoting agents
1. Carcinogenic by themselves—"solitary carcinogens."	1. Not carcinogenic alone.
2. Must be given before promoting agent.	2. Must be given after the initiating agent.
3. Single exposure is sufficient.	3. Require prolonged exposure.
4. Action is "irreversible" and additive.	4. Action is reversible (at early stage) and not additive.
5. No apparent threshold.	5. Probable threshold.
6. Yield electrophiles that bind covalently to cell macromolecules.	6. No evidence of covalent binding.
7. Mutagenic.	7. Not Mutagenic.

Source: For details see Weinstein et al., 1978b.

TABLE 8 A Comparison of the Effects of 12-0-Tetradecanoyl-phorbol-13-acetate (TPA) on Mouse Skin and in Cell Culture

	Mouse skin	Cell culture[b]
Cell surface effects		
↑ Phospholipid synthesis	+	+
↑ Membrane transport	+	+
Altered glycoproteins	N.D.[a]	+
Membrane fluorescence polarization	N.D.	+
Macromolecular synthesis		
↓ DNA synthesis (early)	+	+
↑ RNA, protein, DNA synthesis	+	+
Specific biochemical		
↑ Histone phosphorylation	+	N.D.
↑ Ornithine decarboxylase	+	+
↑ Plasminogen activator	N.D.	+
↑ Prostaglandin synthesis	N.D.	+
Physiologic		
↑ Saturation density	N.D.	+
Morphology	+	+
Inhibits differentiation	+	+
Hyperplasia or mitogenesis	+	+
Promotion	+	+

[a]N.D. indicates not done or not applicable.

[b]It should be stressed that not all cell cultures show these responses.

Source: For references see text and Weinstein et al., 1978b, 1978c.

low concentrations of MC, BP, or DMBA, followed after 4 days by continuous growth in media containing 0.1 μg/ml TPA, or other phorbol esters active as tumor promoters, but not with the inactive analog phorbol. A strict temporal relationship was observed between application of the initiators and exposure to promoters. TPA failed to enhance transformation when added prior to the initiators and actually inhibited transformation when added immediately after PAH treatment. The optimum enhancement was found when continuous exposure to TPA was begun about 4 days after exposure to the initiator. TPA has also been found to enhance adenovirus transformation of rat embryo cells by a mutant of human adenovirus H5ts125, with or without exposure of the cells to PAH carcinogens prior to infection with virus (Fisher et al., 1978). In this viral-promoter system enhancement was observed when TPA was added continuously to the culture medium beginning 1-7 days after virus infection, but not when added 14 or 21 days post infection. Evidence was obtained that TPA-enhanced transformation resulted from the promoter's ability to facilitate expression of the transformed state rather than an effect on virus uptake or integration (Fisher and Weinstein, 1980, Fisher, 1980; Fisher et al., 1979d).

As shown in Table 8, TPA induces a number of changes in cell culture which resemble those seen when this compound is applied to mouse skin. The spectrum of TPA-induced alterations in cell culture includes changes in morphology and growth (Diamond et al., 1974b; Weinstein et al., 1978b, 1978c), cell surface properties (Blumberg et al., 1976; Pietropaolo et al., 1977), 2-deoxyglucose transport (Driedger and Blumberg, 1977), and plasminogen activator production (Wigler and Weinstein, 1976; Weinstein et al., 1977, 1978b, 1978c). It is interesting that these changes mimic those associated with cell transformation by viral or chemical agents. The reversibility of TPA's action in cell culture makes this compound extremely useful for studying regulation of phenotypic properties normally associated with the transformed state and their role in growth control (Weinstein et al., 1978c, 1979).

Specific biochemical and physiological changes induced by TPA and related plant diterpenes may prove useful as short-term screening tests for this class of promoters. Wigler and Weinstein (1976) demonstrated that TPA induces approximately a 10-fold increase in plasminogen activator (PA) production in early passage chick embryo fibroblasts (CEF) and human tumor cells (HeLa). TPA-induced PA synthesis in CEF cells was observed with concentrations as low as 5×10^{-9} M (3 ng/ml) and as early as 3 hr after treatment. The induction was completely blocked by actinomycin D and cycloheximide, indicating the importance of RNA and protein synthesis in this process. Structure function studies (Weinstein et al., 1977, 1978b; Wigler et al., 1978) have shown an excellent correlation between PA induction and tumor-promoting activities of a wide range of plant diterpenes. However, PA induction did not result from treatment with the promoting agents anthralin, cantharidin, and tween-60; or asbestos fibers, amosite, crocidilite, and chrysotile. Thus induction of PA synthesis is a useful screening test for detecting tumor promoters structurally related to the phorbol esters, although it may not detect other classes of tumor promoters.

Another biochemical change found to occur following treatment of mouse skin or exposure of various cell types in culture to TPA is induction of the enzyme ornithine decarboxylase (ODC) (O'Brien et al., 1975; Yuspa et al., 1976; Boutwell, 1977). When a series of phorbol esters was studied there was a good correlation between tumor promotion activity on mouse skin and the ability to induce ODC synthesis in mouse skin and in cell culture (Yuspa et al., 1976; O'Brien and Diamond, 1978; Boutwell, 1977). One exception is the compound 4-O-MeTPA, which has been reported to be a weak tumor promoter on mouse skin but induces both PA (Weinstein et al., 1977, 1978b) and ODC (Yuspa et al., 1976) synthesis in cell culture. Other classes of promoters remain to be tested to determine if ODC induction can be used for their rapid detection.

We have recently demonstrated that TPA and related plant diterpenes alter the physical structure of cell membranes (Fisher et al., 1979a). These studies were based on changes in the fluorescence polarization of a lipid-specific probe, 1-6-diphenyl-1,3,5-hexatriene (DPH), in early passage rat embryo cells. Active tumor promoters induced a decrease in fluorescence polarization of DPH after 1 hr of treatment (maximal effect between 3 and 4 hr post treatment) at levels as low as 10^{-9}-10^{-10} M. This change in fluorescence was not inhibited by actinomycin D or cycloheximide, and no decrease was found after treatment with the inactive analogs phorbol and 4α-phorbol-12,13-didecanoate (4αPDD). These results suggest a specific interaction with membranes as the primary effect in the action of tumor promoters. Several other early effects on membrane structure and function have been noted (Sivak and Van Duuren, 1971; Suss et al., 1972; Blumberg et al., 1976; Weinstein et al., 1978b; Lee and Weinstein, 1978; Wenner et al., 1978) in cells treated with TPA (see also Table 8).

A second category of effects of the phorbol esters in cell culture is inhibition of terminal differentiation. This effect has been observed with a variety of cell types and with diverse programs of differentiation. Thus, TPA is a potent inhibitor of terminal differentiation of murine erythroleukemia cell cultures (Rovera et al., 1977; Yamasaki et al., 1977); chick embryo myoblast, and chondroblast cultures (Cohen et al., 1977; Pacifici and Holtzer, 1977); B 16 melanoma cells (Mufson et al., 1979); neuroblastoma cultures (Ishii et al., 1978); and the conversion of 3T3 fibroblasts to adiposelike cells (Diamond et al., 1977). These findings support the concept that an important action of tumor promoters in carcinogenesis is to block terminal differentiation in initiated stem cells, thus allowing them to divide exponentially and generate a clone that can ultimately become a tumor (Weinstein and Wigler, 1977; Yamasaki et al., 1979). In the majority of differentiating systems that have been studied, a good correlation was found between the tumor-promoting ability of compounds on mouse skin and their ability to inhibit differentiation. Differentiating cell culture systems may also prove, therefore, to be useful short-term bioassay screens for tumor promoters.

We have emphasized the importance of the interaction between multiple factors in the carcinogenic process. Rapid short-term tests are now available for the in vitro assay of the plant diterpene class of tumor promoters and for the study of interactions among viruses, carcinogens, and these tumor promoters. There is also a need to develop short-term in vitro assays for other classes of tumor promoters, for hormones, and for other cofactors important in the complex process of carcinogenesis as it occurs in experimental animals and in humans.

ACKNOWLEDGMENT

The dedication of Evelyn Emeric in typing this chapter and its many revisions is deeply appreciated.

REFERENCES

Adamson, R. H., and Sieber, S. M. (1977). Antineoplastic agents as potential carcinogens. In The Origins of Human Cancer, H. H. Hiatt, J. D. Watson, and J. A. Winston (Eds.). Cold Spring Harbor Conference on Cell Proliferation, IV, Cold Spring Harbor, N.Y., pp. 429-443.

Ahlstrom, C. G., and Andrewes, C. H. (1938). Fibroma virus infection in tarred rabbits. J. Path. Bact. 47:65-86.

Althouse, R., Tomatis, L., Huff, J., and Wilbourn, J. (1979). Chemicals and Industrial Processes Associated with Cancer in Humans. IARC Scientific Publication, Monographs 1-20, Supplement No. 1, Lyon, France.

Ames, B. N. (1971). The detection of chemical mutagens with enteric bacteria. In Chemical Mutagens, Principles and Methods for Their Detection, Vol. I, A. Hollaender (Ed.). Plenum Press, New York, pp. 267-282.

Ames, B. N. (1972). A bacterial system for detecting mutagens and carcinogens. In Mutagenic Effects of Environmental Contaminants, E. Sutton and M. Harris (Eds.). Academic Press, New York, pp. 57-66.

Ames, B. N., Gurney, E. G., Miller, J. A., and Bartsch, H. (1972a). Carcinogens as frameshift mutagens: metabolites and derivatives of 2-acetyl-aminofluorene and other aromatic amine carcinogens. Proc. Natl. Acad. Sci. USA 69:3128-3132.

Ames, B. and Hooper, K. (1978). Does carcinogenic potency correlate with mutagenic potency in the Ames assay? Nature 274:19-20.

Ames, B. N., Lee, F. D., and Durston, W. E. (1973). An improved bacterial test system for the detection and classification of mutagens and carcinogens. Proc. Natl. Acad. Sci. USA 70:782-786.

Ames, B. N., and McCann, J. (1976). Carcinogens are mutagens: a simple test system. In Screening Tests in Chemical Carcinogenesis, R. Montesano, H. Bartsch, and L. Tomatis (Eds.). IARC Scientific Publication No. 12, Lyon, France, pp. 493-501.

Ames, B. N., McCann, J., and Yamasaki, E. (1975). Methods for detecting carcinogens and mutagens with the Salmonella/mammalian microsome mutagenicity test. Mutat. Res. 31:347-364.

Ames, B. N., Sims, P., and Grover, P. L. (1972b). Epoxides of carcinogenic polycyclic hydrocarbons are frameshift mutagens. Science 176:47-49.

Andrewes, C. H., Ahlstrom, C. G., Foulds, L., and Gye, W. E. (1937). Reaction of tarred rabbits to the infectious fibroma virus. Lancet ii:893-895.

Ashby, J., and Purchase, I. F. (1977). The selection of appropriate chemical class controls for use with short-term tests for potential carcinogenicity. Ann. Occup. Hyg. 20:297-301.

Ashby, J., and Styles, J. A. (1978a). Does carcinogenic potency correlate with mutagenic potency in the Ames assay? Nature 271:452-455.

Ashby, J., and Styles, J. A. (1978b). Factors influencing mutagenic potency in vitro. Nature 274: 20-22.

Barrett, J. C., Bias, N. E., and Ts'o, P. O. (1978). A mammalian cellular system for the concomitant study of neoplastic transformation and somatic mutation. Mutat. Res. 50: 121-136.

Barrett, J. C., and Ts'o, P. O. (1978). Relationship between somatic mutation and neoplastic transformation. Proc. Natl. Acad. Sci. USA 75: 3297-3301.

Barthelmess, A. (1970). Mutagenic substances in the human environment. In Chemical Mutagenesis in Mammals and Man, F. Vogel (Ed.). Springer-Verlag, Berlin and New York, pp. 69-147.

Bartsch, H., Malaveille, C., Camus, A. M., Martel-Planche, G., Brun, A., Hautefeuille, A., Sabadie, N., Barbin, A., Kuroki, T., Drevon, C., Piccoli, C., and Montesano, R. (1980). Validation and comparative studies on 180 chemicals with S. typhimurium strains and V79 Chinese hamster cells in the presence of various metabolizing systems. Mutat. Res. 76 (1): 1-50.

Bartsch, H., Malaveille, C., and Montesano, R. (1976). The predictive value of tissue-mediated mutagenicity assay to assess the carcinogenic risk of chemicals. In Screening Tests in Chemical Carcinogenesis, R. Montesano, H. Bartsch, and L. Tomatis (Eds.). IARC Scientific Publication No. 12, Lyon, France, pp. 467-486.

Bartsch, H., Malaveille, C., Tierney, B., Grover, P. L., and Sims, P. (1979). The association of bacterial mutagenicity of hydrocarbon-derived "Bay region" dihydrodiols with the Iball indices for carcinogenicity and with the extents of DNA-binding in mouse skin of the parent hydrocarbons. Chem. Biol. Interact. 26: 185-196.

Basilico, C. (1977). Temperature sensitive mutations in animal cells. Adv. Cancer Res. 24: 223-266.

Beikirch, H. (1977). Induction of unscheduled DNA synthesis by chemical mutagens in testicular cells of the mouse in vitro. Arch. Toxicol. 37: 195-201.

Benedict, W. F., Banerjee, A., Gardner, A., and Jones, P. A. (1977). Induction of morphological transformation in mouse C3H/10T1/2 clone 8 cells and chromosomal damage in hamster A (T_1)Cl-3 cells by cancer chemo-therapeutic agents. Cancer Res. 37: 2202-2208.

Benedict, W. F., Banerjee, A., and Venkatesan, N. (1978). Cyclophosphamide-induced oncogenic transformation, chromosomal breakage and sister chromatid exchange following microsomal activation. Cancer Res. 38: 2922-2924.

Benedict, W. G., Rucker, N., Faust, J., and Kouri, R. E. (1975). Malignant transformation of mouse cells by cigarette smoke condensate. Cancer Res. 35: 857-860.

Berenblum, I. (1963). The possible role of a "transmissible factor" in leukemia induction by radiation plus urethan. In Viruses, Nucleic Acids and Cancer, 17th Annual Symposium on Fundamental Cancer Research, M. D. Anderson Tumor Institute, Univ. of Texas. Williams and Wilkins, Baltimore, Md., pp. 529-543.

Berenblum, I. (1969). A re-evaluation of the concept of cocarcinogenesis. Prog. Exp. Tumor Res. 11: 21-30.

Berenblum, I. (1975). Origin of the concept of sequential stages of skin carcinogenesis. In Cancer 1, F. F. Becker (Ed.). Plenum Press, New York, pp. 323-344.

Berky, J., and Sherrod, P. C. (1978). Short Term in Vitro Testing for Carcinogenesis, Mutagenesis and Toxicity. Collected Proceedings of the First and Second Working Conferences of Toxicity Testing In Vitro, 1975/1976. The Franklin Institute Press, Philadelphia, pp. 1-438.

Bertram, J. S., and Heidelberger, C. (1974). Cell cycle dependency of oncogenic transformation induced by N-methyl-N'-nitro-N-nitrosoguanidine in culture. Cancer Res. 34: 526-537.

Berwald, Y., and Sachs, L. (1963). In vitro cell transformation with chemical carcinogens. Nature 200: 1182-1184.

Berwald, Y., and Sachs, L. (1965). In vitro transformation of normal cells to tumor cells by carcinogenic hydrocarbons. J. Natl. Cancer Inst. 35: 641-661.

Bissel, D. M., Hammaker, L. E., and Meyer, U. A. (1973). Parenchymal cells from adult rat liver in nonproliferating monolayer culture. I. Functional studies. J. Cell Biol. 59: 722-734.

Blumberg, P. M., Driedger, P. E., and Rossow, P. W. (1976). Effect of a phorbol ester on a transformation sensitive surface protein of chick fibroblasts. Nature 264: 446-447.

Boone, C. W. (1975). Malignant hemangioendotheliomas produced by subcutaneous inoculation of Balb/3T3 cells attached to glass beads. Science 188: 68-70.

Bouck, N., and diMayorca, G. (1976). Somatic mutation as the basis for malignant transformation of BHK cells by chemical carcinogens. Nature 264: 722-727.

Boutwell, R. K. (1974). The function and mechanism of promoters of carcinogenesis. CRC Crit. Rev. Toxicol. 2:419-443.

Boutwell, R. K. (1977). The role of the induction of ornithine decarboxylase in tumor promotion. In The Origins of Human Cancer, H. H. Hiatt, J. D. Watson, and J. A. Winston (Eds.). Cold Spring Harbor Conference on Cell Proliferation, IV, Cold Spring Harbor, N.Y., pp. 773-783.

Brookes, P., and Lawley, P. D. (1971). Effects on DNA: chemical methods. In Chemical Mutagens, Principles and Methods for Their Detection, Vol. I, A. Hollaender (Ed.). Plenum Press, New York, pp. 121-144.

Bruce, W. R., Varghese, A. J., Furrer, R., and Land, P. C. (1977). A mutagen in the feces of normal humans. In The Origins of Human Cancer, H. H. Hiatt, J. D. Watson, and J. A. Winston (Eds.). Cold Spring Harbor Conference on Cell Proliferation, IV. Cold Spring Harbor, N.Y., pp. 1641-1646.

Cairns, J. (1975a). The cancer problem. Sci. Am. 233: 64-72, 77-78.

Cairns, J. (1975b). Mutation selection and the natural history of cancer. Nature 255: 197-200.

Cancer Testing Technology and Saccharin (1977). OTA Congress of the United States Office of Technology Assessment, Washington, D.C., pp. 1-149.

Carrano, A. V., Thompson, L. H., Lindl, P. A., and Minkler, J. L. (1978). Sister chromatid exchange as an indicator of mutagenesis. Nature 271: 551-553.

Caspersson, T., Lomakka, G., and Zech, L. (1971). The 24 fluorescent patterns of the human metaphase chromosomes—distinguishing characters and variability. Hereditas 67: 89-102.

Casto, B. C. (1973). Enhancement of adenovirus transformation by treatment of hamster cells with ultraviolet-irradiation, DNA base analogs, and dibenz(a,h)anthracene. Cancer Res. 33: 402-407.

Casto, B. C., Janosko, N., Meyers, J., and DiPaolo, J. A. (1978). Comparison of in vitro tests in Syrian hamster cells for detection of carcinogens. Proc. Am. Assoc. Cancer Res. 19: 331 (Abst.).

Casto, B. C., Pieczynski, W. J., and DiPaolo, J. A. (1973). Enhancement of adenovirus transformation by pretreatment of hamster cells with carcinogenic polycyclic hydrocarbons. Cancer Res. 33: 819-824.

Casto, B. C., Pieczynski, W. J., Janosko, N., and DiPaolo, J. A. (1976). Significance of treatment interval and DNA repair in the enhancement of viral transformation by chemical carcinogens and mutagens. Chem. Biol. Interact. 13: 105-125.

Chen, T. T., and Heidelberger, C. (1969a). Cultivation in vitro of cells derived from adult C3H mouse ventral prostate. J. Natl. Cancer Inst. 42: 903-914.

Chen, T. T., and Heidelberger, C. (1969b). In vitro malignant transformation of cells derived from mouse prostate in the presence of 3-methylcholantrene. J. Natl. Cancer Inst. 42: 915-925.

Chen, T. T., and Heidelberger, C. (1969c). Quantitative studies on the malignant transformation of mouse prostate cells by carcinogenic hydrocarbons in vitro. Int. J. Cancer 4: 166-178.

Chieco-Bianchi, L., Fiore-Donati, L., de Benedictus, G., and Tridente, G. (1963). Influence of urethan on susceptibility to leukemia induction by Graffi virus in adult mice. Nature 199: 292-293.

Chu, E. H., and Malling, H. V. (1968). Mammalian cell genetics. II. Chemical induction of specific locus mutations in Chinese hamster cells in vitro. Proc. Natl. Acad. Sci. USA 61: 1306-1312.

Chu, H. Y. (1971). Induction and analysis of gene mutations in mammalian cells in culture. In Chemical Mutagens: Principles and Methods for Their Detection, Vol. 2, A. Hollaender (Ed.). Plenum Press, New York, pp. 411-444.

Ciarrocchi, G., and Linn, S. (1978). A cell-free assay measuring repair DNA synthesis in human fibroblasts. Proc. Natl. Acad. Sci. USA 75: 1887-1891.

Clayson, D. B. (1977). Principles underlying testing for carcinogenicity. In The Cancer Bulletin, R. L. Clark (Ed.). Medical Arts Publishing Foundation, Houston, Tex., 29: 161-166.

Cleaver, J. E. (1970). Repair of damages in human and other eukaryotic cells. In Nucleic Acid-Protein Interactions, D. W. Ribbons, J. F. Woessner, and J. Schultz (Eds.). North-Holland, Amsterdam, pp. 7-11.

Cleaver, J. E. (1973). DNA repair with purines and pyrimidines in radiation and carcinogen damaged normal and Xeroderma pigmentosum human cells. Cancer Res. 33: 362-369.

Clive, D. (1974). Mutagenicity of thioxanthenes (hycanthone, lucanthone and four indazole derivatives) at the TK locus in cultured mammalian cells. Mutat. Res. 26: 307-318.

Clive, D., Johnson, K. O., Spector, J. F., Batson, A. G., Brown, M. M. (1979). Validation and characterization of the L5178Y/Tk^{+-} mouse lymphoma assay system. Mutat. Res. 59: 61-108.

Clive, D., and Spector, J. F. (1975). Laboratory procedure for assessing specific locus mutations at the TK locus in cultured L-5178Y mouse lymphoma cells. Mutat. Res. 31: 17-29.

Cohen, R., Pacifici, M., Rubenstein, N., Biehl, J., and Holtzer, H. (1977). Effect of a tumor promoter on myogenesis. Nature 266: 538-540.

Colburn, N. H., Bormer, F., and Warren, L. (1978a). Tumor promoting phorbol esters induce anchorage independent growth in some epidermal cell strains. Proc. Am. Assoc. Cancer Res. 19: 65 (Abst.).

Colburn, N. H., Vorder Bruegge, W. F., Bates, J. R., Gray, R. H., Rossen, J. D., Kelsey, W. H., and Shimada, T. (1978b). Correlation of anchorage-independent growth with timorigenicity of chemically transformed mouse epidermal cells. Cancer Res. 38: 624-634.

Colburn, N. H., Vorder Bruegge, W. F., Bates, J., and Yuspa, S. H. (1978c). Epidermal cell transformation in vitro. In Mechanisms of Tumor Promotion and Cocarcinogenesis, Carcinogenesis, Vol. 2, T. J. Slaga, A. Sivak, and R. K. Boutwell (Eds.). Raven Press, New York, pp. 257-275.

Cornfield, J. (1977). Carcinogenic risk assessment. Science 198: 693-699.

Daudel, P., Duquesne, M., Vigny, P., Grover, P. L., and Sims, P. (1975). Fluorescent spectral evidence that benzo(a)pyrene-DNA products in mouse skin arise from diol-epoxides. FEBS Lett. 51: 250-253.

DeMars, R. (1974). Resistance of cultured human fibroblasts and other cells to purine and pyrimidine analogues in relation to mutagenesis detection. Mutat. Res. 24: 335-364.

Diamond, L., Knorr, R., and Shimizu, Y. (1974a). Enhancement of simian virus 40-induced transformation of Chinese hamster embryo cells by 4-nitroquinoline 1-oxide. Cancer Res. 34: 2599-2604.

Diamond, L., O'Brien, S., Donaldson, C., and Shimizu, Y. (1974b). Growth stimulation of human diploid fibroblasts by the tumor promoter, 12-O-tetradecanoyl-phorbol-13-acetate. Int. J. Cancer 13: 721-730.

Diamond, L., O'Brien, T. G., and Rovera, G. (1977). Inhibition of adipose conversion of 3T3 fibroblasts by tumor promoters. Nature 269:247-249.

DiMayorca, G., Greenblatt, M., Trauthen, T., Soller, A., and Giordano, R. (1973). Malignant transformation of BHK 21 clone 13 cells in vitro by nitrosamines—a conditional state. Proc. Natl. Acad. Sci. USA 70:46-49.

DiPaolo, J. A., and Casto, B. C. (1976). In vitro transformation: Interaction of chemical carcinogens with viruses and physical agents. In Screening Tests in Chemical Carcinogenesis, R. Montesano, H. Bartsch, and L. Tomatis (Eds.). IARC Scientific Publication No. 12, Lyon, France, pp. 355-381.

DiPaolo, J. A., and Casto, B. C. (1979). Quantitative studies of in vitro morphological transformation of Syrian hamster cells by inorganic metal salts. Cancer Res. 39:1008-1013.

DiPaolo, J. A., Donovan, P., and Nelson, R. (1969a). Quantitative studies of in vitro transformation by chemical carcinogens. J. Natl. Cancer Inst. 42:867-876.

DiPaolo, J. A., Nelson, R. L., and Donovan, P. J. (1969b). Sarcoma-producing cell lines derived from clones transformed in vitro by benzo(a)pyrene. Science 165:917-918.

DiPaolo, J. A., Nelson, R. L., and Donovan, P. J. (1971a). Morphological, oncogenic, and karyological characteristics of Syrian hamster embryo cells transformed in vitro by carcinogenic polycyclic hydrocarbons. Cancer Res. 31:1118-1127.

DiPaolo, J. A., Donovan, P. J., and Nelson, R. L. (1971b). In vitro transformation of hamster cells by polycyclic hydrocarbons: factors influencing the number of cells transformed. Nature New Biol. 230:240-242.

DiPaolo, J. A., Nelson, R. L., and Donovan, P. J. (1972a). In vitro transformation of Syrian hamster embryo cells by diverse chemical carcinogens. Nature 235:278-280.

DiPaolo, J. A., Nelson, R. L., and Donovan, P. J. (1973). Host-mediated in vivo-in vitro assay for chemical carcinogenesis. Arch. Pathol. Lab. Med. 95:380-385.

DiPaolo, J. A., Takano, K., and Popescu, N. C. (1972b). Quantitation of chemically induced neoplastic transformation of Balb/3T3 cloned cell lines. Cancer Res. 32:2686-2695.

Dorsch-Häsler, K., Fisher, P. B., Weinstein, I. B., and Ginsberg, H. S. (1980). Patterns of viral DNA integration in cells transformed by wild type or DNA-binding protein mutants of type 5 adenovirus and the effect of chemical carcinogens on integration. J. Virol. 34: 305-314.

Drake, J. W. (1970). The Molecular Basis of Mutation. Holden-Day, San Francisco, pp. 146-159

Driedger, P. E., and Blumberg, P. M. (1977). The effect of phorbol diesters on chicken embryo fibroblasts. Cancer Res. 37:3257-3265.

Dunkel, V. C., Wolff, J. S., and Pienta, R. J. (1977). In vitro transformation as a presumptive test for detecting chemical carcinogens. In The Cancer Bulletin, R. L. Clark (Ed.). Medical Arts Publishing Foundation, Houston, Tex., 29:167-174.

Duran-Reynals, F. (1952). Studies on the combined effects of fowl pox virus and methylcholanthrene in chickens. Ann. NY Acad. Sci. 54:977-991.

Duran-Reynals, M. L. (1962). Carcinogenesis in cortisone-treated mice following vaccinia dermal infection and application of methylcholanthrene. J. Natl. Cancer Inst. 29:635-651.

Durston, W. E., and Ames, B. N. (1974). A simple method for the detection of mutagens in urine: Studies with the carcinogen 2-acetylaminofluorene. Proc. Natl. Acad. Sci. USA 71:737-740.

Epstein, S. S., Arnold, E., Andrea, J., Bass, W., and Bishop, Y. (1972). Detection of chemical mutagens by the dominant lethal assay in the mouse. Toxicol. Appl. Pharmacol. 23:288-325.

Evans, C. H., and DiPaolo, J. A. (1975). Neoplastic transformation of guinea pig fetal cells in culture induced by chemical carcinogens. Cancer Res. 35:1035-1044

Evans, C. H., and DiPaolo, J. A. (1976). A comparison of nude mice with the host species for evaluation of the tumorigenicity of guinea pig and hamster cells transformed in vitro by chemical carcinogens. Cancer Res. 36:128-131.

Evans, C. H., Rabin, E. S., and DiPaolo, J. A. (1977). The susceptibility of guinea pig cells to the colony-inhibitory activity of lymphotoxin during carcinogenesis. Cancer Res. 37: 898-903.

Evans, H. J., and O'Riordan, M. L. (1975). Human peripheral blood lymphocytes for the analysis of chromosome aberrations in mutagen tests. Mutat. Res. 31: 135-148.

Fahmy, O. G., and Fahmy, M. J. (1970). Gene elimination in carcinogenesis: reinterpretation of the somatic mutation theory. Cancer Res. 30: 195-205.

Fahrig, R. (1977). The mammalian spot test (fellfleckentest) with mice. Arch. Toxicol. 38: 87-98.

Fischer, G. A., Lee, S. Y., and Calabresi, P. (1974). Detection of chemical mutagens using a host-mediated assay (L-5178Y) mutagenesis system. Mutat. Res. 26: 501-511.

Fishbein, L., Flamm, W. G., and Falk, H. L. (1970). Chemical Mutagens, Environmental Effects on Biological Systems. Academic Press, New York.

Fisher, P. B. (1980). The multifactor and multistep nature of viral transformation. Guidelines to Metabolic Therapy, in press.

Fisher, P. B., Bozzone, J. H., and Weinstein, I. B. (1979d). Tumor promoters and epidermal growth factor stimulate anchorage-independent growth of adenovirus transformed rat embryo cells. Cell 18: 695-705.

Fisher, P. B., Dorsch-Häsler, K., Weinstein, I. B., and Ginsberg, H. S. (1979c). Tumor promoters enhance anchorage-independent growth of adenovirus-transformed cells without altering the integration pattern of viral sequences. Nature 281: 591-594.

Fisher, P. B., Dorsch-Häsler, K., Weinstein, I. B., and Ginsberg, H. S. (1981). Interactions between initiating chemical carcinogens, tumor promoters and adenovirus in cell transformation. Teratogenesis, Carcinogenesis and Mutagenesis, in press.

Fisher, P. B., Goldstein, N. I., and Weinstein, I. B. (1979b). Phenotypic properties and tumor promoter induced alterations in rat embryo cells transformed by adenovirus. Cancer. Res. 39: 3051-3057.

Fisher, P. B., Schachter, D., Flamm, M., and Weinstein, I. B. (1979a). Tumor promoters induce membrane changes detected by fluorescence polarization. Biochem. Biophys. Res. Commun. 86: 1063-1068.

Fisher, P. B., and Weinstein, I. B. (1980). Chemical-viral interactions and multistep aspects of cell transformation. In: Molecular and Cellular Aspects of Carcinogen Screening Tests, R. Montesano, H. Bartsch, and L. Tomatis (Eds.). IARC Scientific Publication, No. 37. Lyon France, pp. 113-131.

Fisher, P. B., Weinstein, I. B., Eisenberg, D., and Ginsberg, H. S. (1978). Interactions between adenovirus, a tumor promoter, and chemical carcinogens in transformation of rat embryo cell cultures. Proc. Natl. Acad. Sci. USA 75: 2311-2314.

Foulds, L. (1969). Neoplastic Development. Academic Press, New York.

Freedman, V. H., and Shin, S. (1974). Cellular tumorigenicity in nude mice: correlation with cell growth in semi-solid medium. Cell 3: 355-359.

Freeman, A. E. (1978). In vitro testing of chemical carcinogens: an overview. In Short Term In Vitro Testing for Carcinogenesis, Mutagenesis and Toxicity, J. Berky and P. C. Sherrod (Eds.). The Franklin Institute Press, Philadelphia, pp. 8-22.

Freeman, A. E., Igel, H. J., and Price, P. J. (1975). Carcinogenesis in vitro I. In vitro transformation of rat embryo cells: correlations with the known tumorigenic activities of chemicals in rodents. In Vitro 11: 107-113.

Freeman, A. E., Price, P. J., Igel, H. J., Young, J. C., Maryak, J. M., and Huebner, R. J. (1970). Morphological transformation of rat embryo cells induced by diethylnitrosamine and murine leukemia viruses. J. Natl. Cancer Inst. 44: 65-78.

Freeman, A. E., Weisburger, E. K., Weisburger, J. H., Wolford, R. G., Maryak, J. M., and Huebner, R. J. (1973). Transformation of cell cultures as an indication of the cancinogenic potential of chemicals. J. Natl. Cancer Inst. 51: 799-808.

Gelboin, H. V. (1969). A microsome-dependent binding of benzo(a)pyrene to DNA. Cancer Res. 29: 1272-1276.

Generoso, W. M. (1973). Evaluation of chromosome aberration effects of chemicals on mouse germ cells. Environ. Health Perspect. 6: 13-22.

Ginsberg, H. S., Ensinger, M. J., Kauffman, R. S., Mayer, A. J., and Lundholm, U. (1974). Cell transformation: a study of regulation with types 5 and 12 adenovirus temperature-sensitive mutants. Cold Spring Harbor Symposium 39: 419-426.

Goldstein, N. I., and Fisher, P. B. (1980). Surface properties of normal and adenovirus transformed rat embryo cells. J. Cell Sci., 45: 87-97.

Green, M. H., and Muriel, W. J. (1976). Mutagen testing using try$^+$ reversion in Escherichia coli. Mutat. Res. 38: 3-32.

Grover, P. L., Sims, P., Huberman, E., Marquardt, H., Kuroki, T., and Heidelberger, C. (1971). In vitro transformation of rodent cells by K-region derivatives of polycyclic hydrocarbons. Proc. Natl. Acad. Sci. USA 68: 1098-1101.

Haenszel, W. (1961). Cancer mortality among the foreign-born in the United States. J. Natl. Cancer Inst. 26: 37-132.

Haenszel, W., and Kurihara, M. (1968). Mortality from cancer and other diseases among Japanese in the United States. J. Natl. Cancer Inst. 40: 43-68.

Hatch, G. G., Balwierz, P. J., Casto, B. C., and DiPaolo, J. A. (1978). Characteristics of hamster cells transformed by the combined action of chemical and virus. Int. J. Cancer 21: 121-127.

Hawkes, S. P., and Bartholomew, J. C. (1977). Quantitative determination of transformed cells in a mixed population by simultaneous fluorescence analysis of cell surface and DNA in individual cells. Proc. Natl. Acad. Sci. USA 74: 1626-1630.

Hecker, E. (1975). Cocarcinogens and cocarcinogenesis. In Handbuch der Allgemeinen Pathologie, Vol. IV, 16, E. Grundman (Ed.). Springer-Verlag, Berlin, pp. 651-676.

Heidelberger, C. (1973). Chemical oncogenesis in culture. Adv. Cancer Res. 18: 317-366.

Higginson, J. and Muir, C. S. (1973). Epidemiology. In Cancer Medicine, J. F. Holland and E. Frei, III (Ed.). Lea and Febringer, Philadelphia, pp. 241-306.

Hirai, K., Defendi, V., and Diamond, L. (1974). Enhancement of simian virus 40 transformation and integration by 4-Nitroquinoline 1-oxide. Cancer Res. 34: 3497-3500.

Hollstein, M. J., McCann, J., Angelosanto, F., and Nichols, W. (1979). Short-term tests for carcinogens and mutagens. Mutat. Res. 65: 133-226.

Hsie, A. W., Brimer, P. A., Mitchell, T. J., and Gosslee, D. G. (1975a). The dose-response relationship for ethyl methanesulfonate-induced mutations at the hypoxanthine-guanine phosphoribosyl transferase locus in Chinese hamster ovary cells. Somatic Cell Genet. 1: 247-261.

Hsie, A. W., Brimer, P. A., Mitchell, T. J., and Gosslee, D. G. (1975b). The dose-response relationship for ultraviolet light-induced mutations at the hypoxanthine-guanine phosphoribosyl transferase locus in Chinese hamster ovary cells. Somatic Cell Genet. 1: 383-389.

Hsu, I. C., Stoner, G. D., Autrup, H., Trump, B. F., Selkirk, J. K., and Harris, C. C. (1978). Human bronchus-mediated mutagenesis of mammalian cells by carcinogenic polynuclear aromatic hydrocarbons. Proc. Natl. Acad. Sci. USA 75: 2003-2007.

Huberman, E. (1975). Mammalian cell transformation and cell-mediated mutagenesis by carcinogenic polycyclic hydrocarbons. Mutat. Res. 29: 285-291.

Huberman, E. (1976). Cell-mediated mutagenicity of different genetic loci in mammalian cells by polycyclic hydrocarbons. In Screening Tests in Chemical Carcinogenesis, R. Montesano, H. Bartsch, and L. Tomatis (Eds.). IARC Scientific Publication No. 12, Lyon, France, pp. 521-532.

Huberman, E., Aspiras, L., Heidelberger, C., Grover, P. L., and Sims, P. (1971a). Mutagenicity to mammalian cells of epoxides and other derivatives of polycyclic hydrocarbons. Proc. Natl. Acad. Sci. USA 68: 3195-3199.

Huberman, E., Kuroki, T., Marquardt, H., Selkirk, J. K., Heidelberger, C., Grover, P. L., and Sims, P. (1972). Transformation of hamster embryo cells by epoxides and other derivatives of polycyclic hydrocarbons. Cancer Res. 32: 1391-1396.

Huberman, E., Mager, R., and Sachs, L. (1976). Mutagenesis and transformation of normal cells by chemical carcinogens. Nature 264: 360-361.

Huberman, E., and Sachs, L. (1966). Cell susceptibility to transformation and cytotoxicity by the carcinogenic hydrocarbon benzo(a)pyrene. Proc. Natl. Acad. Sci. USA 56: 1123-1129.

Huberman, E., and Sachs, L. (1973). Metabolism of the carcinogenic hydrocarbon benzo(a)pyrene in human fibroblast and epithelial cells. Int. J. Cancer 11: 412-418.

Huberman, E., and Sachs, L. (1974). Cell-mediated mutagenesis with chemical carcinogens. Int. J. Cancer 13: 326-333.

Huberman, E., and Sachs, L. (1976). Mutability of different genetic loci in mammalian cells by metabotically activated carcinogenic polycyclic hydrocarbons. Proc. Natl. Acad. Sci. USA 73: 188-192.

Huberman, E., Selkirk, J. K., Heidelberger, C. (1971b). Metabolism of polycyclic aromatic hydrocarbons in cell culture. Cancer Res. 31: 2161-2167.

Ichinotsubo, D., Mower, H. F., Setliff, J., and Mandel, M. (1977). The use of rec$^-$ bacteria for testing of carcinogenic substances. Mutat. Res. 46: 53-62.

Ishidate, M., Jr., and Odashima, S. (1977). Chromosome tests with 134 compounds on Chinese hamster cells in vitro—a screening for chemical carcinogens. Mutat. Res. 48: 337-354.

Ishii, D. N., Fibach, E., Yamasaki, H., and Weinstein, I. B. (1978). Tumor promoters inhibit morphological differentiation in cultured mouse neuroblastoma cells. Science 200: 556-559.

Ishii, Y., Elliot, J. A., Mishra, N. K., and Lieberman, M. W. (1977). Quantitative studies of transformation by chemical carcinogens and ultraviolet radiation using a subclone of BHK 21 clone 13 Syrian hamster cells. Cancer Res. 37: 2023-2029.

Ivanovic, V., Geacintov, N. E., and Weinstein, I. B. (1976). Cellular binding of benzo(a)pyrene to DNA characterized by low temperature fluorescence. Biochem. Biophys. Res. Commun. 70: 1172-1179.

Ivanovic, V., Geacintov, N. E., Jeffrey, A. M., Fu, P. P., Harvey, R. G., and Weinstein, I. B. (1978a). Cell and microsome mediated binding of 7, 12-dimethylbenz(a)anthracene to DNA studied by fluorescence spectroscopy. Cancer Lett. 4: 131-140.

Ivanovic, V., Geacintov, N. E., Yamasaki, H., and Weinstein, I. B. (1978b). DNA and RNA adducts formed in hamster embryos cell cultures exposed to benzo(a)pyrene. Biochemistry 17: 1597-1603.

Jeffrey, A. M., Blobstein, S. H., Weinstein, I. B., and Harvey, R. (1976). High pressure liquid chromatography of carcinogen nucleoside conjugates: separation of 7, 12-dimethylbenz(a)anthracene derivatives. Anal. Biochem. 73: 378-385.

Jeffrey, A. M., Weinstein, I. B., Jennette, K. W., Gojeskowiak, V., and Nakanishi, K. (1977). Structures of BP-nucleic adducts formed in human and bovine bronchial explants. Nature 269: 348-350.

Jennette, K. W., Jeffrey, A. M., Blobstein, S. H., Beland, F., Harvey, R. G., and Weinstein, I. B. (1977). Characterization of nucleoside adducts from the in vitro reaction of benzo(a)pyrene 4, 5-oxide with nucleic acids. Biochemistry 16: 932-938.

Jones, P. A., Benedict, W. F., Baker, M. S., Mondal, S., Rapp, U., and Heidelberger, C. (1976). Oncogenic transformation of C3H/10T1/2 clone 8 mouse embryo cells by halogenated pyrimidine nucleosides. Cancer Res. 36: 101-107.

Kafer, E., Marshall, P., and Cohen, G. (1976). Well-marked strains of _Aspergillus_ for tests of environmental mutagens: identification of induced mitotic recombination and mutation. Mutat. Res. 38: 141-146.

Kakunaga, T. (1973). A quantitative system for assay of malignant transformation by chemical carcinogens using a clone derived from Balb/3T3. Int. J. Cancer 12: 463-473.

Kakunaga, T. (1977). The transformation of human diploid cells by chemical carcinogens. In The Origins of Human Cancer, H. H. Hiatt, J. D. Watson, and J. A. Winston (Eds.). Cold Spring Harbor Conference on Cell Proliferation, IV, Cold Spring Harbor, N.Y., pp. 1537-1548.

Kakunaga, T. (1978). Neoplastic transformation of human diploid fibroblast cells by chemical carcinogens. Proc. Natl. Acad. Sci. USA 75: 1334-1338.

Kakunaga, T., and Kamahora, J. (1968). Properties of hamster embryonic cells transformed by 4-nitroquinoline-1-oxide in vitro and their correlations with the malignant properties of the cells. Biken J. 11: 313-332.

Kamahora, J., and Kakunaga, T. (1966). In vitro carcinogenesis of 4-nitroquinoline-1-oxide with golden hamster embryonic cells. Proc. Jap. Acad. 42: 1079-1081.

Kao, F. T., and Puck, T. T. (1967). Genetics of somatic mammalian cells. IV. Properties of Chinese hamster cell mutants with respect to the requirement for proline. Genetics 55: 513-518.

Kao, F. T., and Puck, T. T. (1969). Genetics of somatic mammalian cells. IX. Quantitation of mutagenesis by physical and chemical agents. J. Cell Physiol. 74: 245-250.

Kato, R., Bruze, M., and Tegner, Y. (1969). Chromosome breakage induced in vivo by a carcinogenic hydrocarbon in the bone marrow cells of the Chinese hamster. Heriditas 61: 1-8.

Katsuta, H., and Takaoka, T. (1968). Transformation of epithelial cultures of rat liver by 4NQO. Proc. Jap. Cancer Assoc. p. 95.

Katsuta, H., and Takaoka, T. (1972). Carcinogenesis in tissue culture. XIV. Malignant transformation of rat liver parenchymal cells treated with 4-nitroquinoline-1-oxide in tissue culture. J. Natl. Cancer Inst. 49: 1563-1576.

Kennedy, A. R., Mondal, S., Heidelberger, C., and Little, J. B. (1978). Enhancement of X-ray transformation by 12-O-tetradecanoyl-phorbol-13-acetate in a cloned line of C3H mouse embryo cells. Cancer Res. 38: 439-443.

Knudson, A. G., Jr. (1971). Mutation and cancer: statistical study of retinoblastoma. Proc. Natl. Acad. Sci. USA 68: 820-823.

Krahn, D. F., and Heidelberger, C. (1977). Liver homogenate-mediated mutagenesis in Chinese hamster V79 cells by polycyclic aromatic hydrocarbons and aflatoxins. Mutat. Res. 46: 27-44.

Kuroki, T., Goto, M., and Sato, H. (1967). Malignant transformation of hamster embryonic cells by 4-hydroxyaminoquinoline-N-oxide in tissue culture. Tohoku J. Exp. Med. 91: 109-118.

Kuroki, T., and Sato, H. (1968). Transformation and neoplastic development in vitro of hamster embryonic cells by 4-nitroquinoline-1-oxide and its derivatives. J. Natl. Cancer Inst. 41: 53-71.

Langenbach, R., Freed, H. J., and Huberman, E. (1978). Liver cell-mediated mutagenesis of mammalian cells by liver carcinogens. Proc. Natl. Acad. Sci. USA 75: 2864-2867.

Laishes, B. A., and Stich, H. F. (1973a). Repair synthesis and sedimentation analysis of DNA of human cells exposed to dimethylnitrosamine and activated dimethylnitrosamine. Biochem. Biophys. Res. Commun. 52: 827-833.

Laishes, B. A., and Stich, H. F. (1973b). Relative DNA damage induced in cultured human fibroblasts by the precarcinogen 2-acetylaminofluorene, the proximate carcinogen N-hydroxy-2-acetylaminofluorene and the ultimate carcinogen N-acetoxy-2-acetylaminofluorene. Can. J. Biochem. 51: 990-994.

Lambert, B., Lindblad, A., Nordenskyjold, M., and Wereliuss, B. (1978). Increased frequency of sister chromatid exchanges in cigarette smokers. Heriditas 88: 147-149.

Lasne, C., Gentil, A., and Chouroulinkov, I. (1974). Two-stage malignant transformation of rat fibroblasts in tissue culture. Nature 247: 490-491.

Latt, S. A. (1974). Sister chromatid exchanges, indices of human chromosome damage and repair: detection by fluorescence and induction by mitomycin-C. Proc. Natl. Acad. Sci. USA 71: 3162-3166.

Lee, L. S., and Weinstein, I. B. (1978). Tumor promoting phorbol esters inhibit binding of epidermal growth factor to cellular receptors. Science 202:313-315.

Legator, M. S., and Malling, H. V. (1971). The host-mediated assay. A practical procedure for evaluating potential mutagenic agents in mammals. In Chemical Mutagens: Principles and Methods for Their Detection, Vol. 2, A. Hollaender (Ed.). Plenum Press, New York, pp. 569-589.

Levin, W., Lu, A. Y., Yagi, H., Hernandez, O., Jerina, D. M., and Conney, A. H. (1976). Metabolism of benzo(a)pyrene derivatives to mutagenic products by highly purified hepatic microsome enzymes. J. Biol. Chem. 251:4882-4890.

Levine, L. (1977). Chemical carcinogens stimulate canine kidney (MDCK) cells to produce prostaglandins. Nature 268:447-448.

Lieberman, M. W., Baney, R. N., Lee, R. E., Sell, S., and Farber, E. (1971). Studies on DNA repair in human lymphocytes treated with proximate carcinogens and alkylating agents. Cancer Res. 31:1297-1306.

Lieberman, M. W., and Poirier, M. C. (1973). Deoxyribonucleoside incorporation during DNA repair of carcinogen-induced damage in human diploid fibroblasts. Cancer Res. 33:2097-2103.

Lin, R. C., and Snodgrass, P. J. (1975). Primary culture of normal adult rat liver cells which maintain stable urea cycle enzymes. Biochem. Biophys. Res. Commun. 64:725-734.

Lubs, H. A., and Samuelson, J. (1967). Chromosome abnormalities in lymphocytes from normal human subjects. Cytogenetics 6:402-411.

MacGregor, J. T., and Sacks, L. E. (1976). The sporulation system of Bacillus subtilis as the basis of a multigene mutagen screening test. Mutat. Res. 38:271-286.

Mager, R., Huberman, E., Yang, S. K., Gelboin, H. V., and Sachs, L. (1977). Transformation of normal hamster cells by benzo(a)pyrene diolepoxide. Int. J. Cancer 19: 814-817.

Maher, V. M., Lesko, J. A., Straat, P. A., and Ts'o, P. O. (1971). Mutagenic action, loss of transforming activity, and inhibition of deoxyribonucleic acid template activity in vitro caused by chemical linkage of carcinogenic polycyclic hydrocarbons to deoxyribonucleic acid. J. Bacteriol. 108:202-212.

Maher, V. M., McCormick, J. J., Grover, P. L., and Sims, P. (1977). Effect of DNA repair on the cytotoxicity and mutagenicity of polycyclic hydrocarbon derivatives in normal and Xeroderma pigmentosum human fibroblasts. Mutat. Res. 43:117-138.

Maher, V. M., Miller, J. A., Miller, E. C., and Summers, W. C. (1970). Mutations and loss of transforming activity of Bacillus subtilis DNA after reaction with esters of carcinogenic N-hydroxy aromatic amides. Cancer Res. 30:1473-1480.

Maher, V. M., Miller, E. C., Miller, J. A., and Szybalski, W. (1968). Mutations and decreases in density of transforming DNA produced by derivatives of the carcinogens 2-acetylaminofluorene and N-methyl-4-aminoazobenzene. Mol. Pharmacol. 4:411-426.

Maher, V. M., and Summers, W. C. (1970). Mutagenic action of aflatoxin B1 on transforming DNA and inhibition of DNA template activity in vitro. Nature 225:68-70.

Malling, H. V., and de Serres, F. J. (1969). Mutagenicity of alkylating carcinogens. Ann. NY Acad. Sci. 163:788-800.

Marquardt, H. (1974). Cell cycle dependence of chemically induced malignant transformation in vitro. Cancer Res. 34:1612-1615.

Marquardt, H., Kuroki, T., Huberman, E., Selkirk, J. K., Heidelberger, C., Grover, P. L., and Sims, P. (1972). Malignant transformation of cells derived from mouse prostate by epoxides and other derivatives of polycyclic hydrocarbons. Cancer Res. 32:716-720.

McCann, J. (1978). Mutagenesis, carcinogenesis, and the Salmonella test. In Short Term In Vitro Testing for Carcinogenesis, Mutagenesis and Toxicity, J. Berky, and P. C. Sherrod (Eds.). The Franklin Institute Press, Philadelphia, pp. 280-292.

McCann, J., and Ames, B. N. (1976a). Detection of carcinogens as mutagens in the Salmonella/microsome test: assay of 300 chemicals: discussion. Proc. Natl. Acad. Sci. USA 73:950-954.

McCann, J., and Ames, B. N. (1976b). A simple method for detecting environmental carcinogens as mutagens. Ann. NY Acad. Sci. 271:5-13.

McCann, J., and Ames, B. N. (1977). The Salmonella/microsome mutagenicity test: predictive value for animal carcinogenicity. In The Origins of Human Cancer, H. H. Hiatt, J. D. Watson, and J. A. Winston (Eds.). Cold Spring Harbor Conferences on Cell Proliferation, IV, Cold Spring Harbor, N.Y., pp. 1431-1450.

McCann, J., Choi, E., Yamasaki, E., and Ames, B. N. (1975a). Detection of carcinogens as mutagen in the Salmonella/microsome test: Assay of 300 chemicals. Proc. Natl. Acad. Sci. USA 72:5135-5139.

McCann, J., Spingarn, N. E., Kobori, J., and Ames, B. N. (1975b). The detection of carcinogens as mutagens: bacterial tester strains with R factor plasmids. Proc. Natl. Acad. Sci. USA 72:979-983.

McMahon, R. E., Cline, J. C., and Thompson, C. Z. (1979). Assay of 855 test chemicals in ten tester strains using a new modification of the Ames test for bacterial mutagens. Cancer Res. 39:682-693.

Meselson, M., and Russell, K. (1977). Comparisons of carcinogenic and mutagenic potency. In The Origins of Human Cancer, H. H. Hiatt, J. D. Watson, and J. A. Winston (Eds.). Cold Spring Harbor Conference on Cell Proliferation, IV, Cold Spring Harbor, N.Y., pp. 1473-1481.

Michalopoulos, G., and Pitot, H. C. (1975). Primary culture of parenchymal liver cells on collagen membranes. Exp. Cell. Res. 94:70-78.

Miller, E. C. (1978). Some current perspectives on chemical carcinogenesis in human and experimental animals: presidential address. Cancer Res. 38:1479-1496.

Miller, E. C., and Miller, J. A. (1967). Low carcinogenicity of the K-region epoxides of 7-methylbenz(a)anthracene and benz(a)anthracene in the mouse and rat. Proc. Soc. Exp. Biol. Med. 124:915-919.

Miller, E. C. and Miller, J. A. (1969). Studies on the mechanism of activation of aromatic amine and amide carcinogens to ultimate carcinogenic electrophilic reactants. Ann. NY Acad. Sci. 163:731-750.

Miller, E. C., and Miller, J. A. (1971). The mutagenicity of chemical carcinogens: correlations, problems and interpretations. In Chemical Mutagens: Principles and Methods for Their Detection, A. Hollaender (Ed.). Plenum Press, New York, pp. 83-119.

Miller, J. A. (1970). Carcinogenesis by chemicals: an overview. GHA Clowes Memorial Lecture. Cancer Res. 30:559-576.

Milo, G. E., and DiPaolo, J. A. (1978). Neoplastic transformation of human diploid cells in vitro after chemical carcinogen treatment. Nature 275:130-132.

Mishra, N. K., and diMayorca, G. (1974). In vitro malignant transformation of cells by chemical carcinogens. Biochim. Biophys. Acta 355:205-219.

Mohn, G., Ellenberger, J., and McGregor, D. (1974). Development of mutagenicity tests using Escherichia coli K-12 as an indicator organism. Mutat. Res. 23:187-196.

Mollet, P., and Weilenmann, W. (1976). Characteristics of a new mutagenicity test-induction of somatic recombination and mutation in drosophilia by different chemicals. Mutat. Res. 38:131-132.

Mollet, P., and Wurgler, F. E. (1974). Detection of somatic recombination and mutation in drosophila. A method for testing genetic activity of chemical compounds. Mutat. Res. 25:421-424.

Mondal, S., Brankow, D. W., and Heidelberger, C. (1976). Two-stage chemical oncogenesis in cultures of C3H/10T½ cells. Cancer Res. 36:2254-2260.

Mondal, S., and Heidelberger, C. (1976). Transformation of C3H/10T½ C1 8 mouse embryo fibroblasts by ultraviolet irradiation and a phorbol ester. Nature 260:710-711.

Montesano, R. (1978). The use of mutagenicity tests in screening chemical carcinogens. Prog. Biochem. Pharmacol. 14:157-162.

Montesano, R., Bartsch, H., and Tomatis, L. (1980). Molecular and Cellular Aspects of Carcinogen Screening Tests. IARC Publications No. 27, Lyon, France, pp. 1-370.

Montesano, R., Drevon, C., Kuroki, T., Saint Vincent, L., Handleman, S., Sanford, K. K., DeFeo, D., and Weinstein, I. B. (1977). Test for malignant transformation of rat liver cells in culture: Cytology, growth in soft agar, and production of plasminogen activator. J. Natl. Cancer Inst. 59:1651-1658.

Montesano, R., Saint-Vincent, L., and Tomatis, L. (1973). Malignant transformation in vitro of rat liver cells by dimethylnitrosamine and N-methyl-N'-nitro-N-nitrosoguanidine. Br. J. Cancer 28:215-220.

Moreau, P., Bailone, A., and Devoret, R. (1976). Prophage induction in Escherichia coli K12 env A uvr B: A highly sensitive test for potential carcinogens. Proc. Natl. Acad. Sci. USA 73:3700-3704.

Moreau, P., and Devoret, R. (1977). Potential carcinogens tested by induction and mutagenesis of prophage λ in Escherichia coli K12. In The Origins of Human Cancer, H. H. Hiatt, J. D. Watson, and J. A. Winston (Eds.). Cold Spring Harbor Conferences on Cell Proliferation, IV, Cold Spring Harbor, N.Y., pp. 1451-1472.

Moutschen, J., and Colizzi, A. (1975). Absence of acrosome: an efficient tool in mammalian mutation research. Mutat. Res. 30:267-272.

Mufson, R. A., Fisher, P. B., and Weinstein, I. B. (1979). Effect of phorbol ester tumor promoters on the expression of melanogenesis in B-16 melanoma cells. Cancer Res. 39:3915-3919.

Mukai, F., and Troll, W. (1969). The mutagenicity and initiating activity of some aromatic amine metabolites. Ann. NY Acad. Sci. 163:828-836.

Müller, R., and Rajewsky, M. F. (1980). Immunological quantitation by high-affinity antibodies of O^6-ethyldeoxyguanosine in DNA exposed to N-ethyl-N-nitrosourea. Cancer Res. 40:887-896.

Nagao, M. and Sugimura, T. (1978). Environmental mutagens and carcinogens. Ann. Rev. Genet. 12:117-159.

Nakamura, J., Suzuki, N., and Okada, S. (1977). Mutagenicity of furylfuramide, a food preservative, tested by using alanine-requiring mouse L5178Y cells in vitro and in vivo. Mutat. Res. 46:355-364.

Namba, M., Masuji, H., and Sato, J. (1969). Carcinogenesis in tissue culture. IV. Malignant transformation of cultured rat cells treated with 4-nitroquinoline-1-oxide. Jap. J. Exp. Med. 39:253-265.

Natarajan, A. T., Tates, A. D., Van Buul, P. P., Meijers, M., and de Vogel, N. (1976). Cytogenetic effects of mutagens/carcinogens after activation in a microsomal system in vitro. I. Induction of chromosome aberrations and siter chromatid exchanges by diethylnitrosamine (DEN) and dimethylnitrosamine (DMN) in CHO cells in the presence of rat liver microsomes. Mutat. Res. 37:83-90.

Neish, W. J., Parry, E. W., and Ghadially, F. N. (1967). Tumor induction in the rat by a mixture of two noncarcinogenic aminoazo dyes. Oncology 21:229-240.

O'Brien, T. G., and Diamond, L. (1978). Ornithine decarboxylase, polyamines, and tumor promoters. In Mechanisms of Tumor Promotion and Cocarcinogenesis, Carcinogenesis, Vol. 2, T. J. Slaga, A. Sivak, and R. K. Boutwell (Eds.). Raven Press, New York, pp. 273-287.

O'Brien, T. G., Simsiman, R. C., and Boutwell, R. K. (1975). Induction of the polyamine-biosynthetic enzymes in mouse epidermis and their specificity for tumor promotion. Cancer Res. 35:2426-2433.

O'Neill, J. P., Brimer, P. A., Machanoff, R., Hirsch, G. P., and Hsie, A. W. (1977a). Quantitative assay of mutation induction at the hypoxanthine-guanine phosphoribosyl transferase locus in Chinese hamster ovary cells: development and definition of the system. Mutat. Res. 45:91-101.

O'Neill, J. P., Couch, D. B., Machanoff, R., San Sebastian, J. R., Brimer, P. A., and Hsie, A. W. (1977b). A quantitative assay of mutation induction at the hypoxanthine-guanine phosphoribosyl transferase locus in Chinese hamster ovary cells (CHO/HGPRT system): utilization with a variety of mutagenic agents. Mutat. Res. 45:103-109.

O'Neill, J. P., Fuscoe, J. C., and Hsie, A. W. (1978). Mutagenicity of heterocyclic nitrogen mustards (ICR compounds) in cultured mammalian cells. Cancer Res. 38: 506-509.

O'Neill, J. P., and Hsie, A. W. (1977). Chemical mutagenesis of mammalian cells can be quantified. Nature 269:815-817.

Ong, T-M., and de Serres, F. J. (1972). Mutagenicity of chemical carcinogens in Neurospora crassa. Cancer Res. 32:1890-1893.

Pacifici, M. and Holtzer, H. (1977). Effects of a tumor-promoting agent on chondrogenesis. Am. J. Anat. 150:207-212.

Painter, R. B. (1977). Rapid test to detect agents that damage human DNA. Nature 265: 650-651.

Painter, R. B., and Howard, R. (1978). A comparison of the Hela DNA synthesis inhibition test and the Ames test for screening mutagenic carcinogens. Mutat. Res. 54:113-115.

Peraino, C., Fry, R. J., and Grube, D. D. (1978). Drug induced enhancement of hepatic tumorigenesis. In Mechanisms of Tumor Promotion and Carcinogenesis, Carcinogenesis, Vol. 2, T. J. Slaga, A. Sivak, and R. K. Boutwell (Eds.). Raven Press, New York, pp. 421-432.

Perry, P., and Evans, H. J. (1975). Cytological detection of mutagen-carcinogen exposure by sister chromatid exchange. Nature 258:121-125.

Peterson, A. R., Bertram, J. S., and Heidelberger, C. (1974). Cell cycle dependency of DNA damage and repair in transformable mouse fibroblasts treated with N-methyl-N'-nitro-N-nitrosoguanidine. Cancer Res. 34:1600-1607.

Pienta, R. J., Poiley, J. A., and Lebherz, W. B., III. (1977). Morphological transformation of early passage golden Syrian hamster embryo cells derived from cryopreserved primary cultures as a reliable in vitro bioassay for identifying diverse carcinogens. Int. J. Cancer 19:642-655.

Pietropaolo, C., Yamaguchi, N., Weinstein, I. B., and Glick, M. C. (1977). Glycopeptides from epithelial cell mutants: Temperature sensitive for the transformation phenotype. Int. J. Cancer 20:738-747.

Poirier, L. A. (1976). Mutagenic screening tests for carcinogenicity. In Screening Tests in Chemical Carcinogenesis, R. Montesano, H. Bartsch, and L. Tomatis (Eds.). IARC Scientific Publication No. 12, Lyon, France, pp. 15-24.

Poirier, M. C., Yuspa, S. H., Weinstein, I. B., and Blobstein, S. (1977). Detection of carcinogen-DNA adducts by radioimmunoassay. Nature 270:186-188.

Poirier, M. C., Santella, R. S., Weinstein, I. B., Grunberger, D., and Yuspa, S. H. (1980). Quantitation of benzo(a)pyrene-deoxyguanosine adducts by radioimmunoassay. Cancer Res. 40:412-416.

Popescu, N. C., Turnbull, D., and DiPaolo, J. A. (1977). Sister chromatid exchange and chromosome aberration analysis with the use of several carcinogens and noncarcinogens: brief communication. J. Natl. Cancer Inst. 59:289-293.

Price, P. J., Freeman, A. E., Lane, W. T., and Huebner, R. J. (1971). Morphological transformation of rat embryo cells by the combined action of 3-methylcholantrene and Rauscher leukemia virus. Nature New Biol. 230:144-145.

Puck, T. T., Ciecuira, S., and Robinson, A. (1958). Genetics of somatic mammalian cells. III. Long term cultivation of euploid cells from human and animal subjects. J. Exp. Med. 108:945-948.

Purchase, I. F., Longstaff, E., Ashby, J., Styles, J. A., Anderson, D., Lefevre, P. A., and Westwood, F. R. (1976). Evaluation of six short term tests for detecting organic chemical carcinogens and recommendations for their use. Nature 264:624-627.

Regan, J. D., Setlow, R. B., and Ley, R. D. (1971). Normal and defective repair of damaged DNA in human cells: a sensitive assay utilizing photolysis of bromodeoxyuridine. Proc. Natl. Acad. Sci. USA 68:708-712.

Reznikoff, C. A., Bertram, J. S., Brankow, D. W., and Heidelberger, C. (1973a). Quantitative and qualitative studies of chemical transformation of cloned C3H mouse embryo cells sensitive to postconfluence inhibition of cell division. Cancer Res. 33:3239-3249.

Reznikoff, C. A., Brankow, D. W., and Heidelberger, C. (1973b). Establishment and characterization of a cloned line of C3H mouse embryo cells sensitive to postconfluence inhibition of division. Cancer Res. 33:3231-3238.

Rheinwald, J. G., and Green, H. (1975). Serial cultivation of strains of human epidermal keratinocytes: the formation of keratinizing colonies from single cells. Cell 6:331-344.

Rhim, J. S., and Huebner, R. J. (1973). Transformation of rat embryo cells in vitro by chemical carcinogens. Cancer Res. 33:695-700.

Rhim, J. S., Park, D. K., Weisburger, E. K., and Weisburger, J. H. (1974). Evaluation of an in vitro assay system for carcinogens based on prior infection of rodent cells with nontransforming RNA tumor virus. J. Natl. Cancer Inst. 52:1167-1173.

Rhim, J. S., Vass, W., Cho, H. Y., and Heubner, R. J. (1971). Malignant transformation induced by 7,12-dimethylbenz(a)anthracene in rat embryo cells infected with Rauscher leukemia virus. Int. J. Cancer 7:65-74.

Risser, R., and Pollack, R. (1974). A nonselective analysis of SV_{40} transformation of mouse 3T3 cells. Virology 59:477-489.

Rous, P., and Kidd, J. G. (1938). The carcinogenic effect of papilloma virus on the tarred skin of rabbits. I. Description of the phenomenon. J. Exp. Med. 67:399-428.

Rovera, G., O'Brien, T. A., and Diamond, L. (1977). Tumor promoters inhibit spontaneous differentiation of Friend erythroleukemia cells in culture. Proc. Natl. Acad. Sci. USA 74:2894-2898.

Russell, L. B. (1977). Validation of the in vivo somatic mutation method in the mouse as a prescreen for germinal point mutation. Arch. Toxicol. 38:75-85.

Salaman, M. H., Rowson, K. E., Roe, F. J., Ball, J. K., Harvey, J. J., and deBenedictus, G. (1963). The combined action of viruses and other carcinogens. In Viruses, Nucleic Acids and Cancer, 17th Annual Symposium on Fundamental Cancer Research, M. D. Anderson Tumor Institute, Univ. of Texas. Williams and Wilkins, Baltimore, Md., pp. 544-558.

San, R. H., and Stich, H. F. (1975). DNA repair synthesis of cultured human cells as a rapid bioassay for chemical carcinogens. Int. J. Cancer 16:284-291.

San, R. H., and Williams, G. M. (1977). Rat hepatocyte primary cell culture-mediated mutagenesis of adult rat liver epithelial cells by procarcinogens. Proc. Soc. Exp. Biol. Med. 156:534-538.

Sanford, K. K. (1974). Biologic manifestation of oncogenesis in vitro: a critique. J. Natl. Cancer Inst. 53:1481-1485.

Sarma, D. S., Rajalakshmi, S., and Farber, E. (1975). Chemical carcinogenesis: interactions of carcinogens with nucleic acids. In Cancer, A Comprehensive Treatise, Etiology: Chemical and Physical Carcinogenesis, Vol. 1, F. F. Becker (Ed.). Plenum Press, New York, pp. 235-287.

Sato, H., and Kuroki, T. (1966). Malignization in vitro of hamster embryonic cells by chemical carcinogens. Proc. Jap. Acad. 42:1211-1216.

Sato, K., Slesinski, R. S., and Littlefield, J. W. (1972). Chemical mutagenesis at the phosphoribosyltransferase locus in cultured human lymphocytes. Proc. Natl. Acad. Sci. 69:1244-1248.

Schmid, W. (1975). The micronucleus test. Mutat. Res. 31:9-15.

Searle, A. G. (1975). The specific locus test in the mouse. Mutat. Res. 31:277-290.

Selby, P. B., and Selby, P. R. (1977). Gamma-ray-induced dominant mutations that cause skeletal abnormalities in mice. Mutat. Res. 43:357-375.

Setlow, R. B., Ahmed, F. E., and Grist, E. (1977). Xeroderma pigmentosum: damage to DNA is involved in carcinogenesis. In The Origins of Human Cancer, H. H. Hiatt,

J. D. Watson, and J. A. Winston (Eds.). Cold Spring Harbor Conference on Cell Proliferation, IV, Cold Spring Harbor, N.Y., pp. 889-902.

Shearman, C. W., and Loeb, L. A. (1977). Depurination decreases fidelity of DNA synthesis in vitro. Nature 270:537-538.

Shields, R. (1976). Transformation and tumorigenicity. Nature 262:348.

Shimkin, M. B., and Stoner, G. D. (1975). Lung tumors in mice: application to carcinogenesis bioassay. Adv. Cancer Res. 21:1-58.

Shimkin, M. B., Weisburger, J. H., Weisburger, E. K., Gabareff, N., and Suntzeff, V. (1966). Bioassay of 29 alkylating chemicals by pulmonary-tumor response in strain A mice. J. Natl. Cancer Inst. 36:915-935.

Shin, S., Freedman, V. H., Risser, R., and Pollack, R. (1975). Tumorigenicity of virus-transformed cells in nude mice is correlated specifically with anchorage independent growth in vitro. Proc. Natl. Acad. Sci. USA 72:4435-4439.

Shopek, T. R., Liber, J. L., Krolewski, J. J., and Thilly, W. G. (1978). Quantitative forward mutation assay in Salmonella typhimurium using 8-azaguanine resistance as a genetic marker. Proc. Natl. Acad. Sci. USA 75:410-414.

Siminovitch, L. (1976). On the nature of hereditable variation in cultured somatic cells. Cell 7:1-11.

Sirover, M. A., and Loeb, L. A. (1974). Erroneous base-pairing induced by a chemical carcinogen during DNA synthesis. Nature 252:414-416.

Sirover, M. A. and Loeb, L. A. (1976). Infidelity of DNA synthesis in vitro: screening for potential metal mutagens or carcinogens. Science 194:1434-1436.

Sivak, A., and Van Duuren, B. L. (1971). Cellular interactions of phorbol myristate acetate in tumor promotion. Chem. Biol. Interact. 3:401-411.

Slaga, T. J., Sivak, A., and Boutwell, R. K. (Eds.). Carcinogenesis, Mechanisms of Tumor Promotion and Cocarcinogenesis, Vol. 2. Raven Press, New York, 1978.

Slater, E. E., Anderson, M. D., and Rosenkranz, H. (1971). Rapid detection of mutagens and carcinogens. Cancer Res. 31:970-973.

Stanbridge, E. J. and Wilkinson, J. (1978). Analysis of malignancy in human cells: Malignant and transformed phenotypes are under separate genetic control. Proc. Natl. Acad. Sci. USA 75:1466-1469.

Stetka, D. G., and Wolff, S. (1976). Sister chromatid exchange as an assay for genetic damage induced by mutagen-carcinogens. Part I. In vivo test for compounds requiring metabolic activation. Mutat. Res. 41:333-342.

Stich, H. F., Kieser, D., Laishes, B. A., and San, R. H. (1973). The use of DNA repair in the identification of carcinogens, precarcinogens and target tissue. In Canadian Cancer Conference: Proceedings of the Tenth Canadian Cancer Conference, Vol. 10, P. G. Scholefield (Ed.). University of Toronto Press, Toronto, pp. 83-110.

Stich, H. F., and San, R. H. (1970). DNA repair and chromatid anomalies in mammalian cells exposed to 4-nitroquinoline-1-oxide. Mutat. Res. 10:389-404.

Stich, H. F., and San, R. H. (1973). DNA repair synthesis and cell survival of repair-deficient human cells exposed to the K-region epoxide of benz(a)anthracene. Proc. Soc. Exp. Biol. Med. 142:155-158.

Stich, H. F., San, R. H., Lam, P. P., Koropatrick, D. J., Lo, L. W., and Laishes, B. A. cells exposed to a series of oncogenic and non-oncogenic derivatives of 4-nitroquinoline-1-oxide. Nature 229:416-419.

Stich, J. F., San, R. H., Lam, P. P., Koropatnick, D. J., Lo, L. W., and Laishes, B. A. (1976). DNA fragmentation and DNA repair as an in vitro and in vivo assay for chemical procarcinogens, carcinogens and carcinogenic nitrosation products. In Screening Tests in Chemical Carcinogenesis, R. Montesano, H. Bartsch, and L. Tomatis (Eds.). IARC Scientific Publication No. 12, Lyon, France, pp. 617-636.

Stich, H. F., San, R. H., Lam, P., Koropatrick, D. J., and Lo, L. (1977). Unscheduled DNA synthesis of human cells as a short-term assay for chemical carcinogens. In The Origins of Human Cancer, H. H. Hiatt, J. D. Watson, and J. A. Winston (Eds.). Cold Spring Harbor Conference on Cell Proliferation, IV, Cold Spring Harbor, N.Y., pp. 1499-1512.

Stiles, C. D., Desmond, W., Sato, G., and Saier, M. H. (1975). Failure of human cells transformed by simian virus 40 to form tumors in athymic nude mice. Proc. Natl. Acad. Sci. USA 72:4971-4975.

Stoltz, D. R., Poirier, L. A., Irving, C. C., Stich, H. F., Weisburger, E. K., and Grice, H. C. (1974). Evaluation of short-term tests for carcinogenicity. Toxicol. Appl. Pharmacol. 29:157-180.

Stoner, G. D., Shimkin, M. B., Kniazeff, A. J., Weisburger, J. H., Weisburger, E. K., and Gorgi, G. B. (1973). Test for carcinogenicity of food additive and chemotherapeutic agents by the pulmonary tumor response in strain A mice. Cancer Res. 33:3069-3085.

Styles, J. A. (1977). A method for detecting carcinogenic organic chemicals using mammalian cells in culture. Br. J. Cancer 36:558-563.

Sumner, A. T., Evans, H. J., and Buckland, R. A. (1971). New technique for distinguishing between human chromosomes. Nature New Biol. 232:31-32.

Süss, R., Kreibich, G., and Kinzel, V. (1972). Phorbol esters as a tool in cell research. Eur. J. Cancer 8:299-304.

Swenberg, J. A., Petzold, G. L., and Harbach, P. R. (1976). In vitro DNA damage/alkaline elution assay for predicting carcinogenic potential. Biochem. Biophys. Res. Commun. 72:732-738.

Takayama, S., Hirakawa, T., and Sugimura, T. (1978). Malignant transformation in vitro by tryptophan pyrolysis products. Proc. Jap. Acad. 54:418-422.

Tanaka, S., and Southam, C. M. (1962). Joint action of West Nile virus and chemical carcinogens on production of papillomas in mice. J. Natl. Cancer Inst. 29:711-722.

Tanooka, J. (1977). Development and applications of Bacillus subtilis test systems for mutagens, involving DNA-repair deficiency and suppressible auxotrophic mutations. Mutat. Res. 42:19-32.

Tatematsu, M., Shirai, T., Tsuda, H., Miyata, Y., Shinohara, Y., and Ito, N. (1977). Rapid production of hyperplastic liver nodules in rats tested with carcinogenic chemicals: a new approach for an in vivo short-term screening test for hepatocarcinogens. Gan. 68:499-507.

Terzaghi, M., and Little, J. B. (1975). Repair of potentially lethal radiation damage in mammalian cells is associated with enhancement of malignant transformation. Nature 253:548-549.

Thilly, W. G., De Luca, J. G., Hoppe, H., and Penman, B. W. (1976). Mutation of human lymphoblasts by methylnitrosourea. Chem. Biol. Interact. 15:33-50.

Tomatis, L. (1977). The value of long-term testing for the implementation of primary prevention. In The Origins of Human Cancer, H. H. Hiatt, J. D. Watson, and J. A. Winston (Eds.). Cold Spring Harbor Conference on Cell Proliferation, IV, Cold Spring Harbor, N.Y., pp. 1339-1357.

Tomatis, L., Agthe, C., Bartsch, H., Huff, J., Montesano, R., Saracci, R., Walter, E., and Wilbourn, J. (1978). Evaluation of the carcinogenicity of chemicals: a review of the monograph program of the International Agency for Research on Cancer. Cancer Res. 38:877-885.

Tooze, J. (1973). The Molecular Biology of Tumour Viruses, Cold Spring Harbor Monograph Series, Cold Spring Harbor, N.Y., pp. 1-743.

Ueda, N., Uenaka, H., Akematsu, T., and Sugiyama, T. (1976). Parallel distribution of sister chromatid exchanges and chromosome aberrations. Nature 262:581-583.

Van Duuren, B. L. (1969). Tumor promoting agents in two-stage carcinogenesis. Prog. Exp. Tumor Res. 11:31-68.

Vigny, P., Duquesne, M., Coulomb, H., Lacombe, C., Tierney, B., Grover, P. L., and Sims, P. (1977). Fluorescence spectral evidence is consistent with metabolism at the 1,2- and 3,4- double bonds of 7-methylbenz(a)anthracene. FEBS Lett. 75:9-12.

Vogel, E. (1977). Identification of carcinogens by mutagen testing in drosophilia: The relative reliability for the kinds of genetic damage measured. In The Origins of Human Cancer, H. H. Hiatt, J. D. Watson, and J. A. Winston (Eds.). Cold Spring Harbor Conferences on Cell Proliferation, IV, Cold Spring Harbor, N.Y., pp. 1483-1497.

Warwick, G. P. (1967). The covalent binding of metabolites of tritiated 2-methyl-4-dimethylaminoazobenzene to rat liver nucleic acids and proteins, and the carcinogenicity of the unlabelled compound in partially hepatectomized rats. Eur. J. Cancer 3:227-233.

Weinhouse, S. (1977). Problems in the assessment of human risk of carcinogenesis from chemicals. In The Origins of Human Cancer, H. H. Hiatt, J. D. Watson, and J. A. Winston (Eds.). Cold Spring Harbor Conferences on Cell Proliferation, IV, Cold Spring Harbor, N.Y., pp. 1307-1309.

Weinstein, I. B. (1979). Molecular events in chemical carcinogenesis. In Advances in Pathobiology, Vol. 4, Cancer Biology II, Etiology and Therapy, C. M. Fenoglio and D. W. King (Eds.). Stratton Intercontinental Medical Book Corp., New York, pp. 106-117.

Weinstein, I. B. (1978). Current concepts on mechanisms of chemical carcinogenesis. Bull. N.Y. Acad. Sci. 54:366-383.

Weinstein, I. B., and Wigler, M. (1977). Cell culture studies provide new information on tumor promoters. Nature 270:669-670.

Weinstein, I. B., Jeffrey, A. M., Leffler, S., Pulkrabek, P., Yamasaki, H., and Grunberger, D. (1978a). Interactions between polycyclic aromatic hydrocarbons and cellular macromolecules. In Polycyclic Hydrocarbons and Cancer, P.O.P. Ts'o and H. Gelboin (Eds.). Academic Press, New York, pp. 4-36.

Weinstein, I. B., Wigler, M., Fisher, P. B., Sisskin, E., and Pietropaolo, C. (1978b). Cell culture studies on the biologic effects of tumor promoters. In Mechanisms of Tumor Promotion and Cocarcinogenesis, Carcinogenesis, Vol. 2, T. J. Slaga, A. Sivak, and R. K. Boutwell (Eds.). Raven Press, New York, pp. 313-333.

Weinstein, I. B., Wigler, M., and Pietropaolo, C. (1977). The action of tumor-promoting agents in cell culture. In The Origins of Human Cancer, Cold Spring Harbor Conference on Cell Proliferation, IV, H. H. Hiatt, J. D. Watson, and J. A. Winston (Eds.). Cold Spring Harbor, N.Y., pp. 751-772.

Weinstein, I. B., Wigler, M., and Stadler, U. (1976). Analysis of the mechanism of chemical carcinogenesis in epithelial cell cultures. In Screening Tests in Chemical Carcinogenesis, R. Montesano, H. Bartsch, and L. Tomatis (Eds.). IARC Scientific Publication No. 12, Lyon, France, pp. 355-381.

Weinstein, I. B., Wigler, M., Yamasaki, H., Lee, L. S., Fisher, P. B., and Mufson, R. A. (1978c). Regulation of the expression of certain biologic markers of neoplasia. In Biological Markers of Neoplasia: Basic and Applied Aspects, R. W. Ruddon (Ed.). Elsevier North-Holland, New York, pp. 451-471.

Weinstein, I. B., Yamasaki, H., Wigler, M., Lee, L. S., Fisher, P. B., Jeffrey, A. M., and Grunberger, D. (1979). Molecular and cellular events associated with the action of initiating carcinogens and tumor promoters. In Carcinogens, Identification and Mechanisms of Action. A. C. Griffin and C. R. Shaw (Eds.). Raven Press, New York, pp. 399-418.

Wenner, C. E., Moroney, J., and Porter, C. W. (1978). Early membrane effects of phorbol esters in 3T3 cells. In Mechanisms of Tumor Promotion and Cocarcinogenesis, Carcinogenesis, Vol 2, T. J. Slaga, A. Sivak, and R. K. Boutwell (Eds.). Raven Press, New York, pp. 363-378.

Wigler, M., DeFeo, D., and Weinstein, I. B. (1978). Induction of plasminogen activator in cultured cells by macrocyclic plant diterpene esters and other agents related to tumor promotion. Cancer Res. 38:1434-1437.

Wigler, M., and Weinstein, I. B. (1976). Tumor promoter induces plasminogen activator. Nature 259:232-233.

Williams, G. C., Elliott, J. M., and Weisburger, J. H. (1973). Carcinoma after malignant conversion in vitro of epithelial-like cells from rat liver following exposure to chemical carcinogens. Cancer Res. 33:606-612.

Williams, G. M. (1977). Detection of chemical carcinogens by unscheduled DNA synthesis in rat liver primary cell cultures. Cancer Res. 37:1845-1851.

Wolff, S. (1977). Sister chromatid exchange. Ann. Rev. Genet. 11:183-201.

Wolff, S., Rodin, B., and Cleaver, J. E. (1977). Sister chromatid exchanges induced by mutagenic carcinogens in normal and Xeroderma pigmentosum cells. Nature 265:347-349.

Wood, A. W., Levin, W., Lu, A. Y., Yagi, H., Hernandez, O., Jerina, D. M., and Conney, A. H. (1976). Metabolism of BP and BP derivatives to mutagenic products by highly purified hepatic microsomal enzymes. J. Biol. Chem. 257:4882-4890.

Wyrobek, A. J., and Bruce, W. R. (1975). Chemical induction of sperm abnormalities in mice. Proc. Natl. Acad. Sci. USA 72:4425-4429.

Yamaguchi, N., and Weinstein, I. B. (1975). Temperature sensitive (TS) mutants of chemically transformed rat liver epithelial cells. Proc. Natl. Acad. Sci. USA 72: 214-218.

Yamamoto, N., and zur Hausen, H. (1979). Tumour promoter TPA enhances transformation of human leukocytes by Epstein-Barr virus. Nature 280:244-245.

Yamasaki, E., and Ames, B. N. (1977). Concentration of mutagens from urine by adsorption with the nonpolar resin XAD-2: Cigarette smokers have mutagenic urine. Proc. Natl. Acad. Sci. USA 74:3555-3559.

Yamasaki, H., Fibach, E., Nudel, U., Weinstein, I. B., Rifkind, R. A., and Marks, P. A. (1977). Tumor promoters inhibit spontaneous and induced differentiation of murine erythroleukemia cells in culture. Proc. Natl. Acad. Sci. USA 74:3451-3455.

Yamasaki, H., Fibach, E., Weinstein, I. B., Nudel, U., Rifkind, R. A., and Marks, P. A. (1979). Inhibition of Friend leukemia cell differentiation by tumor promoters. In Oncogenic Viruses and Host Cell Genes, Y. Ikawa and T. Odaka (Eds.). Academic Press, New York, pp. 365-376.

Yamasaki, H., Huberman, E., and Sachs, L. (1975). Regulation of aryl hydrocarbon (benzo(a)pyrene) hydroxylase activity in mammalian cells. Induction of hydroxylase activity in mammalian cells. Induction of hydroxylase activity by dibutyryl-cyclic AMP and aminophylline. J. Biol. Chem. 250:7766-7770.

Yuspa, S. H., Lichti, U., Ben, T., Patterson, E., Hennings, H., Slaga, T. J., Colburn, N., and Kelsey, W. (1976). Phorbol esters stimulate DNA synthesis and ornithine decarboxylase activity in mouse epidermal cell cultures. Nature 262:402-404.

Zimmermann, F. K. (1975). Procedures used in the induction of mitotic recombination and mutation in the yeast Saccharomyces cerevisiae. Mutat. Res. 31:71-86.

7

Environmental Chemicals

YIN-TAK WOO* and JOSEPH C. ARCOS† / Tulane University School of Medicine, and U.S. Public Health Service Hospital, New Orleans, Louisiana

---

Present affiliations:

*JRB Associates, Inc., McLean, Virginia

†Environmental Protection Agency TS-792, Washington, D.C.

The restriction of the scope of this chapter to polycyclic aromatic hydrocarbons, nitrosamines, and inorganic carcinogens does not imply the total absence in the environment of other carcinogens, which have escaped their original settings of use (e.g., polychlorinated biphenyls, chlorinated aliphatic hydrocarbons, and pesticides). Also, carcinogens of exclusively industrial significance, which do not as yet represent a hazard in the environment at large (such as nickel), as well as radioactive elements (such as plutonium), are not covered in this article.

I. GENERAL INTRODUCTION

Chemical carcinogenesis, the induction of cancer by chemicals, has long been recognized as an occupational hazard. Already in the eighteenth century a British surgeon, Percivall Pott (1775), reported his astute observation that the high incidence of scrotal cancer in chimney sweeps was related to their chronic exposure to soot. The significance of this finding was, however, not fully appreciated until the late nineteenth century. With the rapid advancement of industrial and agricultural technology and the proliferation of new chemicals, the problem of environmental pollution by chemical carcinogens has since escalated. During the past several decades, a large number of industrial chemicals have been found to be carcinogenic, and extensive progress has been made in identifying these occupational carcinogens and, in a number of cases, in developing protective measures (Saffiotti and Wagoner, 1976).

In a much less conspicuous way, while the runaway development of modern technology has brought us an affluent way of life, it has also presented us with potential health hazards. Smoking, urban and industrial environmental pollution, and the indiscriminate introduction of inadequately tested chemicals into various products, all contribute to the spread of chemical carcinogens in the general population. Hence, it is becoming apparent that the problem of chemical carcinogens has escaped its traditional setting as an occupational hazard, to advance to the stage of a potential threat to the population at large. Nowadays it is not necessary to crawl into chimneys to be exposed to substantial levels of carcinogens, such as benzo(a)pyrene, the principal carcinogen in soot. Benzo(a)pyrene can now be found in well measurable amounts in the air, the water, and the food. It is the consensus from epidemiological studies that 75-90% of cancers are due to environmental factors, mainly to environmental chemicals (WHO, 1964; UICC, 1970; Higginson and Muir, 1973). Hence, the problem of environmental carcinogenesis must receive greater attention, and proper preventive measures must be developed and instituted. The public must be made more aware of the life-styles that lead to unnecessary exposure to carcinogens. Governmental regulatory agencies must closely monitor, reduce, and eliminate carcinogens from the environment. Moreover, beyond formal compliance with regulatory requirements, industries must develop a greater sense of responsibility for their waste treatment as well as a searching attitude toward the safety of consumer products manufactured. More research must be devoted to the development of sensitive and unequivocal detection methods, to the elucidation of the mechanism of action of carcinogens, and to the designing of protective and preventive measures.

This chapter summarizes three major groups of environmental chemical carcinogens: (1) aromatic hydrocarbons, (2) nitrosamines, and (3) inorganic carcinogens (metals and asbestos). The emphasis is placed on the formation, occurrence, and human exposure to these chemicals. However, metabolism, mechanism of action, and factors modifying the carcinogenicity of these chemicals are also discussed.

II. AROMATIC HYDROCARBON CARCINOGENS

A. Introduction

1. Historical Note

Aromatic hydrocarbons are the class of chemicals in which carcinogens were first identified. Most of the more potent carcinogens in this group have more than three benzene rings, hence, the name, polycyclic (or polynuclear) aromatic hydrocarbons. The saga of the discovery, separation, and identification of polycyclic aromatic hydrocarbons (PAHs) as carcinogens has been eloquently portrayed by many authors (Haddow and Kon, 1946/47; Wolf, 1952; Shimkin and Triolo, 1969). The history of chemical carcinogenesis can be traced back to 1775 when Pott published his report attributing exposure to soot as the cause of scrotal cancer in chimney sweeps. A century later von Volkmann, a German physician, noted the high incidence of skin cancer among tar workers and recognized that tar itself is carcinogenic. A flurry of research activity ensued in order to obtain experimental confirmation, but it was not until 1915 that two Japanese investigators, Yamagiwa and Ichikawa, succeeded in inducing skin cancer in the rabbit's ear by repeatedly painting coal tar for several months. The carcinogenic substance in the tar could be concentrated in the higher-boiling fractions as a neutral compound and was recognized as a probable cyclic hydrocarbon by Bloch and Dreifuss in Switzerland. In 1925 Kennaway succeeded in producing carcinogenic tars by the pyrolysis of petroleum, coal, and organic matter. Since the carcinogenic tars and oils usually showed a pronounced fluorescence, Mayneord examined their fluorescence spectra and discovered several characteristic bands. This groundwork finally led Cook, Hewett, and Hieger to make the needed breakthrough in 1933. Guided by the fluorescent nature of the carcinogenic compound, these investigators isolated from two tons of coal tar minute amounts of the pure carcinogen, which was eventually identified as benzo(a)pyrene (B(a)P). This work, along with the earlier discovery that synthetic dibenz(a,h)anthracene is also carcinogenic, led Cook and then Fieser and others to undertake a large-scale synthetic program to study the structure-activity relationship of aromatic hydrocarbons. To date, hundreds of aromatic hydrocarbons have been synthesized and tested for carcinogenicity. The most potent carcinogens in this group include B(a)P, 7,12-dimethylbenz(a)anthracene, and 3-methylcholanthrene. Polycyclic aromatic hydrocarbons are known to be widely distributed in the environment. Many PAHs are formed by incomplete combustion or pyrolysis (treatment with high heat) of virtually any kind of organic matter, principally fuel (especially coal), food, and refuse. Benzo(a)pyrene, the most ubiquitous carcinogen, has been found in the air, water, and food, and is one of the major carcinogens in tobacco smoke.

2. Nomenclature

The complexity of the structure of aromatic hydrocarbons has caused considerable confusion in the naming of the compounds. To date, there are still two systems of nomenclature used in the literature: the currently accepted system formulated by the International Union of Pure and Applied Chemistry (IUPAC, also known as the Chemical Abstract system) and the old but still extensively used Richter system. The details of the rules of these systems have been clearly described (Stelzner, 1921; IUPAC, 1958; Cohn, 1959; Chemical Society, 1960). Briefly, in both systems the name of an aromatic hydrocarbon is built up by (1) choosing from the structural formula the largest possible structural unit with a trivial name, (2) numbering the carbon atoms of that unit and in the IUPAC system, assigning letters to all faces of the unit, and (3) defining the position(s) and the type(s) of substituent(s) or fused ring(s) on the unit. Three of the most commonly used basic structural units are phenanthrene,

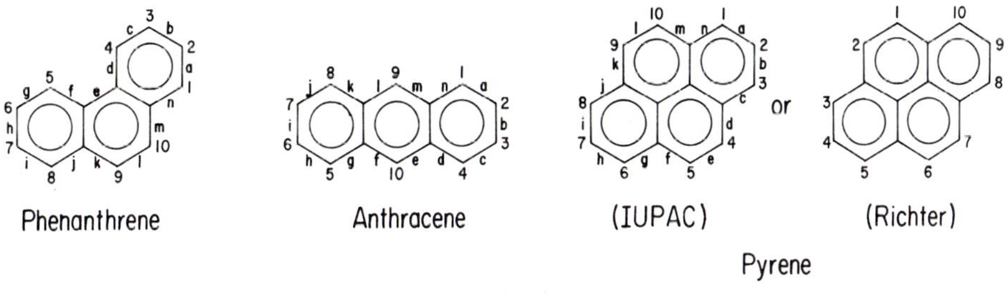

FIGURE 1 The basic structural units of carcinogenic polycyclic aromatic hydrocarbons (PAHs).

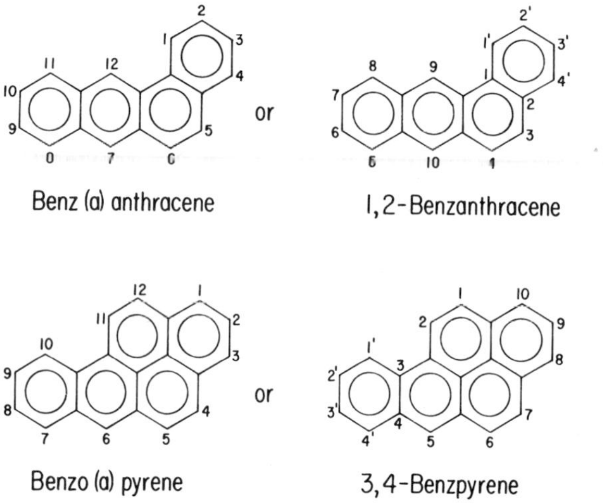

FIGURE 2 The numbering of benz(a)anthracene and benzo(a)pyrene (B(a)P).

anthracene, and pyrene, as shown in Fig. 1. Fusion of a benzene ring to face "a" of anthracene and pyrene gives rise to two of the most extensively studied aromatic hydrocarbons: benz(a)anthracne and benzo(a)pyrene, respectively. As shown in Fig. 2, the numbering of carbon atoms in these two compounds is completely different in the two systems. In the IUPAC system the numbering is carried out by placing the formula in such a way that (1) the maximum number of rings lies in a horizontal row, and (2) as many rings as possible are above and to the right of the horizontal row with as few rings as possible below and to the left of the horizontal row. The carbon atoms are then numbered in a clockwise direction starting with the carbon atom not engaged in ring fusion in the most counterclockwise position of the uppermost ring, or the uppermost ring which is farthest to the right. In the Richter system the numbering of the trivial-named unit remains unchanged, whereas the fused benzo ring is numbered 1', 2', . . . starting from the first carbon atom, next to the lower-numbered carbon atom of the two atoms of the trivial-named unit (to which the benzo ring is fused). In this chapter the IUPAC names are used throughout with the Richter names shown in brackets.

3. Polycyclic Aromatic Hydrocarbons in the Environment and Their General Properties

The formulae of PAHs encountered in the environment and their structural interrelationships are depicted in Fig. 3. Polycyclic aromatic hydrocarbons are sparingly soluble or practically insoluble in water. The solubility of B(a)P in water is of the order of 10^{-8} to 10^{-7} mol/liter; surfactants such as detergents can substantially increase its solubility by formation of micelles. Most organic solvents such as benzene, acetone, hexane, and tetrahydrofuran readily dissolve PAHs. Carcinogenic PAHs of environmental interest readily vaporize at high temperatures and have boiling points over 300°C. They have a high tendency to adsorb to particulate matter such as dust particles. Most of the PAHs in the atmosphere are thus adsorbed, and these particles play an essential role in the uptake of the hydrocarbons into the lung. Most of the PAHs are fluorescent in ultraviolet light and are photosensitive, forming endoperoxides which then undergo ring cleavage and dealkylation. Ozone readily reacts with PAHs, yielding oxidized products. There is some evidence that PAHs adsorbed to particles have a greater susceptibility to photooxidation; this subject is of great interest in view of its potential as a means of reducing the airborne aromatics (NAS, 1972). There is also evidence that some PAHs may be biodegradable; this subject has been reviewed by Harrison et al. (1975).

4. Analytical Methods

The methodology for collection, extraction, separation, identification, and quantification of PAHs in environmental samples has been described in detail (NAS, 1972; Micure and Dietrich, 1973). Extensive progress has been made in the past several years. Essentially, the procedure includes: (1) collection of PAHs from environmental samples by glass fiber filters, or adsorbents such as XAD-2 resin or Tenas porous polymer beads, or carbon filter; (2) extraction of the aromatics by organic solvents, followed by evaporation of the solvent or freeze-drying or concentration by further adsorption on resin; (3) separation of compounds by various chromatographic techniques; and (4) identification by various criteria such as gas chromatographic or high-performance liquid chromatographic retention time, cochromatography, ultraviolet, fluorescent, and mass spectrometry, and quantitation by analysis of peak area or absorbency. The current method of choice is the computerized combination gas chromatography-mass spectrometry (GC/MS) method, which is capable of analyzing a hundred or more compounds within several hours. Polycyclic aromatic hydrocarbons are separated by gas chromatography and identified by comparison of their mass spectra with those of known compounds compiled in the computer. The use of high-performance liquid chromatography (HPLC) is also rapidly gaining popularity, especially for separating PAHs present in complex samples such as fossil fuels, soil, and recent sediments. The extremely active development in this analytical field has prompted a number of excellent recent reviews and symposia by Alford (1975, 1977) and Burlingame et al. (1976) (mass spectrometry), Cram and Juvet (1976) (gas chromatography), Majors (1977) (high-performance liquid chromatography), Keith (1976) and Fishman and Erdmann (1975) (water analysis), and Freudenthal and Jones (1976) (various analytical techniques).

B. Carcinogenicity, Metabolism, and Mechanism of Action

1. Carcinogenicity

A complete survey of the carcinogenicity of various carcinogens including PAHs has been published (see Hartwell, 1951, for the first volume of this ongoing series). The potency of a carcinogen is reflected by two parameters: the Iball index and the curve of dose-response relationship. The Iball index is defined as the ratio: tumor incidence (percent animals with tumor) over latent period (number of days for the induction), multiplied by 100. A strong carcinogen causes high tumor incidence in a short period of time. A list of the Iball indexes of environmental PAHs has been included in the legend to Fig. 3. On the other hand, the dose-response curve shows the relationship between the tumor incidence and the dose administered. Table 1 presents one such study using B(a)P.

Polycyclic aromatic hydrocarbons generally induce tumors at the site of application. They have been predominantly tested on the skin of mice, and, thus, the impression has been created that they are mainly skin carcinogens. However, induction of tumors at other sites, such as lung, kidney, stomach, and so on, has also been reported. On oral administration high doses are necessary; concentrations of at least 30-100 ppm (mg/kg) in food are needed for the induction of a low incidence of stomach tumors in mice, hamsters, and rats. The capability of PAHs to induce lung cancer has been unequivocally proven by intrabronchial pellet implantation experiments, in which implantation of 0.3-3 mg of B(a)P has been shown to induce cancer in a dose-dependent fashion. Inhalation of PAHs along with an irritant, such as sulfur dioxide, or inert particles such as iron oxide, induces tumors of the respiratory tract in rats, hamsters, mice, and monkeys. The doses range from 1.4 μg B(a)P/liter air for mouse inhalation studies, to 10 μg/liter for 1 hr daily in the presence of sulfur dioxide in rat inhalation studies; weekly intratracheal instillation of 0.25 mg B(a)P has been used in hamsters and 3-15 mg B(a)P (adsorbed to iron oxide particles) in monkeys. There is considerable species difference regarding the carcinogenicity of PAHs, and the difference in metabolism among these compounds has been suggested as one of the main reasons. Furthermore, age can play a major role in determining the carcinogenicity of PAHs in living organisms. There is substantial evidence indicating that fetal and newborn animals are particularly

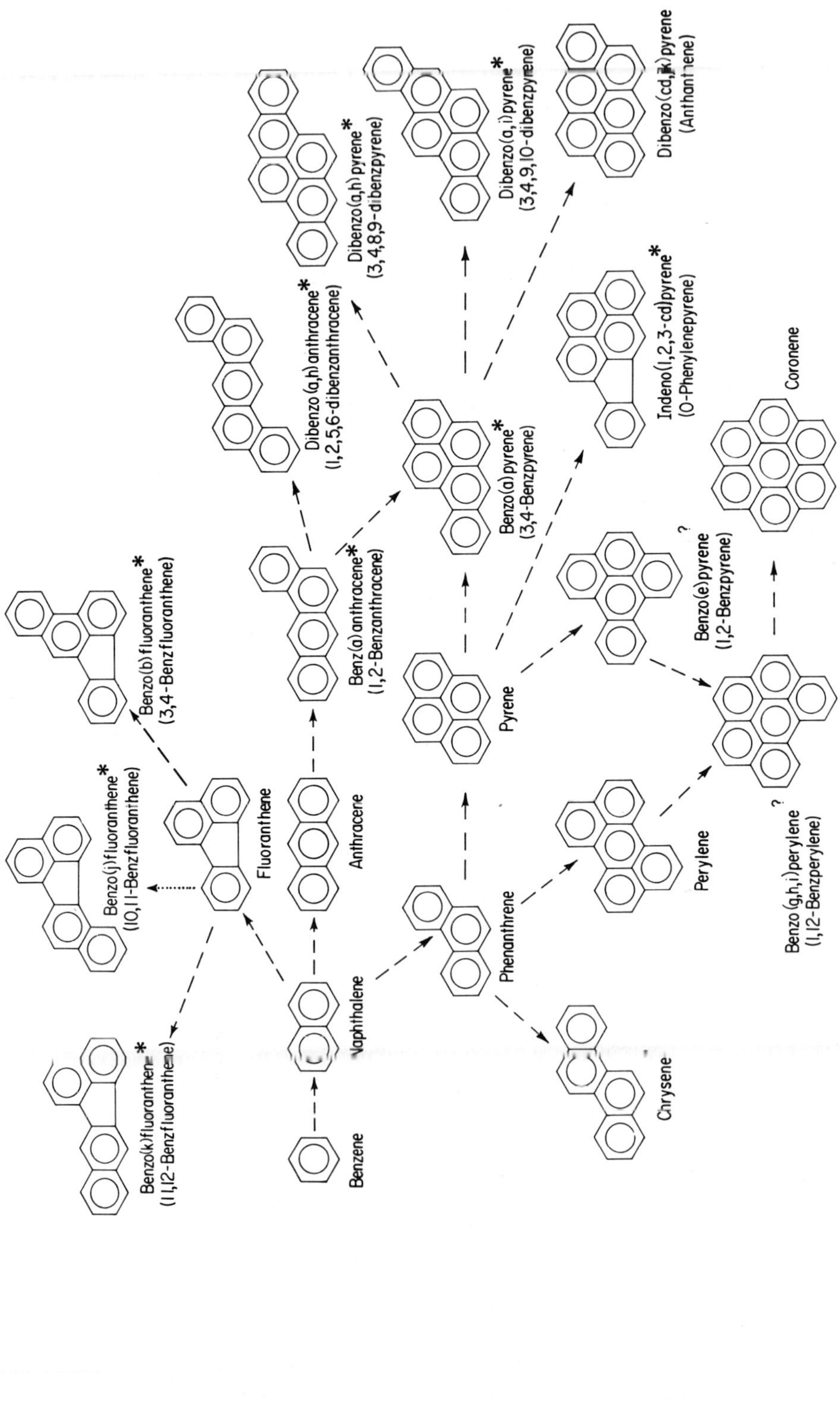
Benzene
Naphthalene
Phenanthrene
Chrysene
Anthracene
Fluoranthene
Pyrene
Perylene
Benzo(k)fluoranthene*
(11,12-Benzfluoranthene)
Benzo(j)fluoranthene*
(10,11-Benzfluoranthene)
Benzo(b)fluoranthene*
(3,4-Benzfluoranthene)
Benz(a)anthracene*
(1,2-Benzanthracene)
Dibenzo(a,h)anthracene*
(1,2,5,6-dibenzanthracene)
Benzo(a)pyrene*
(3,4-Benzpyrene)
Benzo(e)pyrene ?
(1,2-Benzpyrene)
Benzo(g,h,i)perylene ?
(1,12-Benzperylene)
Coronene
Indeno(1,2,3-cd)pyrene*
(O-Phenylenepyrene)
Dibenzo(a,h)pyrene*
(3,4,8,9-dibenzpyrene)
Dibenzo(a,i)pyrene*
(3,4,9,10-dibenzpyrene)
Dibenzo(cd,jk)pyrene
(Anthanthrene)

FIGURE 3 Structural interrelationship of PAHs encountered in the environment. Compounds with asterisks have been clearly demonstrated to be carcinogenic, while those with question marks are marginally active. The Iball indexes (sarcoma and/or epithelioma) are as follows: dibenzo(a, i)pyrene, 78; benzo(a)pyrene, 72; benzo(b)fluoranthene, 68; dibenzo(a,h)pyrene, 60; benzo(j)fluoranthene, 59; dibenz(a,h)anthracene, 25; dibenzo(cd, jk)pyrene, 21; ideno(1, 2, 3-cd)pyrene, 16; benzo(k)fluoranthene, 15; benz(a)anthracene, 5; benzo(e)pyrene, 2; chrysene, 1; benzo(g, h, i)perylene, marginal; anthracene, 0; benzene, 0; coronene, 0; fluoranthene, 0; naphthalene, 0; perylene, 0; phenanthrene, 0; pyrene, 0. The Iball carcinogenicity index of dibenzo(cd, jk)pyrene (also known as anthanthrene) was calculated from the recent data of Cavalieri et al. (1977); previously, this hydrocarbon was regarded as noncarcinogenic. Kennaway (cited in Cooper and Lindsey, 1955) found benzo(g, h, i)perylene to be marginally carcinogenic; however, Lijinsky and Saffiotti (1965) reported this compound to be inactive by skin painting in the mouse. In animal bioassays benzene was not found to be carcinogenic; however, industrial epidemiological data indicate that extensive exposure to benzene leads to leukemia (Vigliani, 1976).

TABLE 1 Subcutaneous Tumor Incidence in Mice Treated with Different Doses of Benzo(a)pyrene

Benzo(a)pyrene injected (mg)	Number of mice	% tumor incidence			
		At 4 months	At 6 months	At 9 months	At 12 months
0.2	120	34	57	67	68
0.1	194	19	56	65	65
0.08	50	32	52	54	56
0.065	270	5	32	43	45
0.05	121	6	25	36	38

Source: Adapted from Leiter and Shear, 1942/43.

susceptible to carcinogens (Della Porta and Terracini, 1969; Schoental, 1974). Transplacental transport of carcinogens (including PAHs) has also been observed (Bulay and Wattenberg, 1970; Tomatis and Mohr, 1973). Furthermore, since the young have longer life expectancy and since the induction of cancer generally requires long latent periods, the relative carcinogenic risk after exposure to a certain amount of carcinogens is expected to be greater for the young. Hence, special considerations must be given in assessing the human risk of the exposure of the young and the fetus to carcinogens.

2. Structure-Activity Relationships

The study of the structure-activity relationships was initiated in the 1930s in an attempt to delineate the structural features of chemical compounds responsible for their carcinogenic activity. Although thousands of compounds have been tested for carcinogenicity to date, it is evident that the structure-activity relationships remain largely unresolved and are meaningful only within a class of chemical agents. For example, some general structural features common to carcinogenic PAHs are known. Carcinogenic PAHs are essentially planar molecules. Unsubstituted PAHs with only three rings are inactive, and a few with more than six rings still show some activity; there is a correlation between the molecular size and the carcinogenicity of these compounds. Carcinogenic activity is greatest for PAHs with a molecular area between 100 and 140 Å^2, and peak activity was observed at 120 Å^2 (Arcos and Argus, 1974). In general, the presence of an angular ring pattern (phenanthrene) in the molecule is necessary for carcinogenicity.

The angular ring structure is of particular interest because the central ring contains a bond (e.g., 9,10 of phenanthrene, 5,6 of benz(a)anthracene, 4,5 of benzo(a)pyrene) with the highest double bond character (i.e., is more reactive than ordinary aromatic double bonds). Osmium tetroxide readily and exclusively reacts with such a bond, and the reactivity of a series of typical unsubstituted PAHs toward osmium tetroxide has been correlated with the carcinogenicity of these compounds. This bond was termed the K-region (K for "Krebs," German for cancer). In addition to the K-region, some PAHs have another region (L-region) of high reactivity (e.g., 9,10 of anthracene, and 7,12 of benz(a)anthracene). These carbon atoms are the most reactive sites for substitution reactions. Using wave mechanical calculations, Pullman and Pullman (1955) postulated an electronic theory of chemical carcinogenesis (the K- and L-region theory). For a PAH to be carcinogenic, it must have a reactive K-region and an inactive L-region (inactivated by substitution or ring fusion); the K-region was concluded to be the site of critical reaction between the carcinogen and the cell constituents

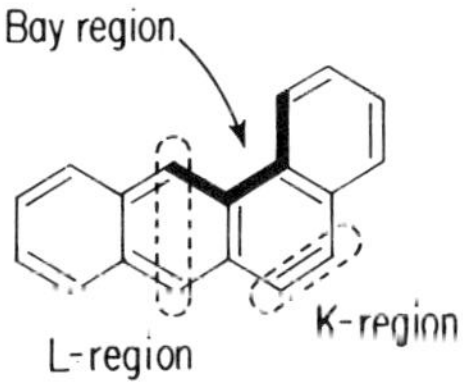

involved in carcinogenesis. With a number of exceptions, this theory enjoyed considerable acceptance until recently. It has been known for many years that carcinogenic PAHs must be metabolically activated to reactive intermediates (proximate or ultimate carcinogens) to exert their action (see Sec. II.B.3). Boyland (1950) had conceived that the reactive intermediates of PAHs might be epoxides. However, it is only recently that a substantial body of evidence has been gathered in its support (Sims and Grover, 1974; Jerina and Daly, 1974). Numerous investigations have been carried out to study the carcinogenicity, mutagenicity, and reactivity of epoxides of PAHs. The majority of the results, however, consistently indicate that K-region epoxides are not more carcinogenic than their parent compounds, suggesting that the K-region is not involved in the reactions leading to carcinogenesis. Instead, a new region (the "bay" region) is now considered to be the critical molecular site. A bay region in a PAH exists when two nonadjacent benzene rings, one of which is a benzo-ring, are in close proximity. The prototype of a bay region is the sterically hindered area between the 4- and 5-positions of the phenanthrene molecule. Thus, the regions between the 10- and 11-positions of benzo(a)pyrene, the 1- and 12-positions of benz(a)anthracene, and both the 4- and 5-positions and 10- and 11-positions of chrysene are also bay regions. Using benzo(a)-pyrene as a model compound, several groups of investigators have independently arrived at the same conclusion that 7,8-dihydrodiol-9,10-oxide of benzo(a)pyrene, a bay region epoxide, is the ultimate carcinogen of benzo(a)pyrene (Slaga et al., 1976; Wislocki et al., 1976; Mar-

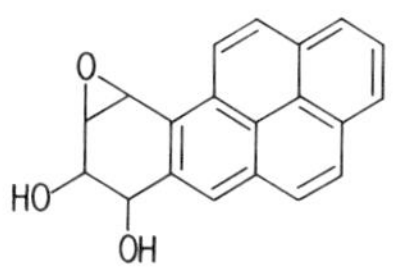

quardt et al., 1977; Yang et al., 1977; see also Lehr and Jerina, 1977). Based on perturbational molecular orbital calculation, it can be predicted that diol epoxides are more reactive than K-region epoxides and that bay region epoxides on saturated, angular benzo-rings of unsubstituted PAHs are ultimate carcinogens. This theory has gained considerable support from experimental work; studies on benz(a)anthracene (Wood et al., 1977a; Lehr and Jerina, 1977), chrysene (Wood et al., 1977b), and 7,12-dimethylbenz(a)anthracene (Moschel et al., 1977) are all consistent with and supportive of the theory. A detailed description of the bay region theory has been published (Jerina et al., 1976; Jerina and Daly, 1977; Lehr and Jerina, 1977).

Substitution of ring hydrogen of PAHs by substituent groups such as alkyl, hydroxyl, halogen, and so on can yield compounds of enhanced or reduced carcinogenicity, depending on the nature of the substituent group and the position of substitution. The classical example is the transformation of the relatively weak benz(a)anthracene to one of the strongest carcinogens by methyl substitution at the 7- and 12-positions. The literature on the effect of various substitutions has been extensively reviewed (Arcos and Argus, 1974; Dipple, 1976). It is of interest to mention several types of substitutions of PAHs of environmental importance. Chrysene has been found to be marginally active as a carcinogen. Recent investigations have indicated that methyl substitution at the 5-position yields a potent carcinogen, comparable to B(a)P in activity. 3-Methylchrysene is slightly more active in initiating carcinogenesis than the parent compound, whereas methyl substitution at other positions has little or no effect. Methylchrysenes (including 5-methylchrysene) are present in tobacco smoke and are suspected to contribute to the carcinogenicity of this inhalant (Hecht et al., 1974, 1976; Hoffmann et al., 1974). Hydroxylations of PAHs have long been considered as pathways of detoxification. Recently, however, an extensive study (Wislocki et al., 1977) of the various hydroxylated (phenolic) derivatives of B(a)P has revealed that 2-hydroxybenzo(a)pyrene is an exception; it is as potent as B(a)P and represents the first example of a phenolic derivative of a PAH that possesses strong carcinogenic activity. Hydroxylation of PAHs in the atmosphere by photooxidation is known to occur. The effect of halogenation on the carcinogenicity of condensed PAHs is still a virtually unexplored area despite the fact that chlorination of the inactive compound, biphenyl, yields polychlorinated biphenyls which are known to display carcinogenic activity (Ito et al., 1974; Kimbrough and Linder, 1974; Kimbrough et al., 1975). More research is needed in this area in view of the concern over the safety of the general practice of chlorinating drinking water.

3. Metabolism

It is now well documented that the majority of carcinogens are not carcinogenic as such (i.e., they are procarcinogens); they must be metabolically activated to reactive intermediates (proximate carcinogens) to initiate carcinogenesis. The mixed-function oxidases, which are cytochrome P-450 containing enzymes present in the endoplasmic reticulum (microsomes) of cells, are the principal enzyme systems responsible for the metabolism of these compounds. Mixed-function oxidases are adaptive enzymes, that is, their activities can be increased (induced) or decreased (repressed) by treatment of animals with specific chemicals (inducers or repressors). Whereas the metabolic processes leading to the generation of the proximate carcinogens of aromatic amines are now reasonably well established (Miller and Miller, 1969), the exact mechanism of the metabolic activation of various PAHs still remains to be elucidated. Much of the difficulty lies in the complexity of the metabolism of PAHs involving a variety of enzyme pathways. The reactive intermediates are in a dynamic state with their amounts (pool sizes) regulated by various activating and detoxifying pathways. The established pathways of PAH metabolism, based mainly on studies with B(a)P, are summarized in Fig. 4. Epoxides of PAHs are formed by the action of the activating enzymes, epoxidases. The reactive intermediates (epoxides) can, in turn, be inactivated by a variety of enzymes, including glutathione-S-epoxide transferase(s), UDP-glucuronic acid epoxide transferase(s), and epoxide reductase(s), or by spontaneous chemical reaction (an isomerization known as the "NIH shift") to yield less reactive products. The enzyme, epoxide hydrase, appears to play a dual role: on the one hand, it hydrates the reactive epoxide to the relatively noncarcinogenic dihydrodiol metabolite; yet, on the other hand, the dihydrodiol metabolite may become the substrate of epoxidase to give rise to dihydrodiol epoxide which is more reactive and more biologically active than the original epoxide. Extensive discussion of the role of metabolism in PAH carcinogenesis has been given in a number of excellent reviews (Sims and Grover, 1974; Jerina and Daly, 1974, 1977; Jerina et al., 1976; Magee et al., 1975; Dipple, 1976; Miller and Miller, 1976; DePierre and Ernster, 1978; Lehr and Jerina, 1977).

As mentioned in Sec. II.B.2, recent investigations have provided increasing support for the theory that bay region dihydrodiol epoxides of unsubstituted PAHs may be the ultimate carcinogens. Studies on B(a)P have led several groups of investigators to conclude that the 7,8-dihydrodiol-9,10-oxide of B(a)P is the ultimate carcinogen of B(a)P. Some of the earlier important studies leading to this discovery have been described by Lehr and Jerina (1977). This bay region diol epoxide of B(a)P has now been shown to be markedly more carcinogenic and mutagenic than the parent compound (Slaga et al., 1976; Wislocki et al., 1976; Marquardt et al., 1977; Kapitulnik et al., 1978). There are two diastercoisomers, one of which appears to play a more significant role in vivo in initiating tumor induction (Kapitulnik et al., 1978) or interacting with cellular macromolecules (Koreeda et al., 1978). In addition to B(a)P, there is some evidence that the bay region epoxides—3,4-dihydrodiol-1,2-oxide of benz(a)-

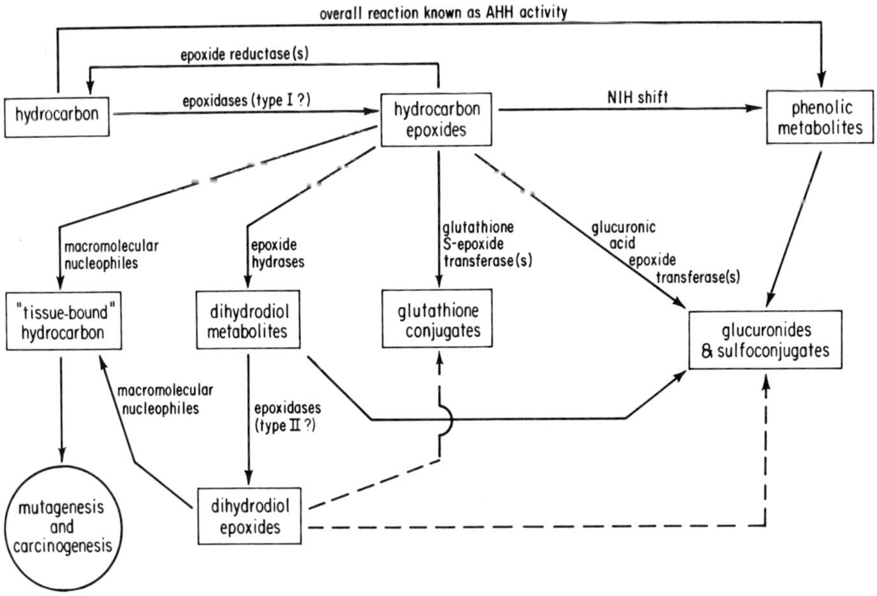

FIGURE 4 The metabolic pathways of PAHs.

anthracene (Wood et al., 1977a; Lehr and Jerina, 1977) and 1,2-dihydrodiol-3,4-oxide of chrysene (Wood et al., 1977b)—may be the proximate or ultimate carcinogens. Whether or not the bay region dihydrodiol epoxides are the only proximate or ultimate carcinogens of PAHs is not known at the present time and a number of other possibilities have been suggested (Miller and Miller, 1976; Cavalieri et al., 1978).

4. Mechanism of Action

The study of the mechanism of carcinogenic action of chemicals is one of the most fascinating areas in cancer research. Many theories have been proposed. It is possible that because of the extreme complexity of carcinogenesis, no single theory may account for the phenomenon. Thus, whereas much experimental evidence supports the mutation theory of carcinogenesis, other theories, such as selection of preexisting cancer cells, isolation of cells from growth regulation, and dedifferentiation (genetic "reprogramming") of somatic cells also appear to have some validity.

There is now ample evidence to suggest that the metabolically activated intermediates of carcinogenic hydrocarbons initiate carcinogenesis by binding covalently to DNA in the target tissue. The infidelity of the subsequent DNA replication results in mutations leading to carcinogenesis. Covalent binding of carcinogenic hydrocarbons to DNA has been demonstrated under both in vitro and in vivo conditions. With a few exceptions, there is good correlation between the carcinogenic potency of a hydrocarbon and binding to DNA. The binding is persistent and may last for a long period of time, but whether this persistent binding is truly relevant to the carcinogenic process still remains to be elucidated. The exact nature of the critical interaction of carcinogenic hydrocarbon with DNA is also not clear. Moreover, it is well established that complete carcinogenesis involves two stages: initiation and promotion. In the stage of initiation latent tumor cells are formed; these latent cells are then promoted in order to bring about the emergence of a tumor. Promoter agents are known as cocarcinogens (e.g., croton oil and its cocarcinogenic principal, phorbol ester).

C. Formation

Three different mechanisms have been proposed for the generation of PAHs: pyrolytic, geochemical, and biochemical formation. Of these, pyrolytic formation is the most important mechanism and has been extensively studied.

1. Mechanism of Pyrolytic Formation of Aromatic Hydrocarbons

The discovery of the presence of carcinogenic hydrocarbons in coal tar (the pyrolytic degradation product of soft coal) and the production by Kennaway (1925, 1930) of carcinogenic tars by pyrolysis of petroleum, skin, hair, yeast, cholesterol, and common triglycerides led to the early recognition that incomplete combustion confers carcinogenic activity to various types of organic materials. Nevertheless, for many years, this subject remained highly controversial because many of the early studies by others were oriented toward confirming or refuting the carcinogenic activity of overheated cholesterol. Oral administration was used as the testing method which is now known to be not very appropriate for studies with PAHs, and the temperature used in many experiments was not sufficiently high. Owing to the extensive studies by Badger and others (1960, 1962, 1964), there is now a vast body of evidence indicating that PAHs are formed during incomplete combustion or pyrogenation of virtually any kind of organic material.

It was known for a number of decades that high temperatures produce the cracking of carbon compounds (breaking up of a molecule into small molecules and fragments, as the result of heat and pressure) and repolymerization of the resulting molecular fragments; loss of hydrogen also occurs leading to the aromatization of the polycyclic carbon skeletons formed. Extensive studies on the conditions governing the formation of PAHs at high temperatures have been carried out by Badger and co-workers. They found that B(a)P, benzo(b)fluoranthene, benzo(j)fluoranthene, and a number of other aromatic hydrocarbons are formed by the pyrolysis of simple hydrocarbons such as acetylene, butadiene, ethylbenzene, styrene, vinylcyclohexene, n-butylbenzene, 1-phenyl-butadiene, and tetralin at 700° C. The alkylbenzene having a C_6-C_4 structure, namely n-butyl benzene, gave the highest yield of B(a)P.

These studies, carried out with radioactively labeled ^{14}C-hydrocarbons (as a tracer), led Badger and his co-workers to propose the reaction mechanism shown in Fig. 5. At the temperature of pyrolysis (about 700° C), aromatic ring systems are the most stable among the structural types present, while aliphatic carbon-carbon bonds and carbon-hydrogen bonds readily break down to yield molecular fragments of free radical character which then undergo recombinations. The relatively greater stability of the aromatic rings thus allows the gradual accumulation of condensed ring structures as the duration of pyrolysis progresses. Under these conditions acetylene and butadiene undergo chain-lengthening leading first to vinylcyclohexene and then to tetralin. The saturated carbon-carbon bonds in tetralin readily undergo cleavage to yield the n-butylbenzene radical. A molecule of n-butylbenzene radical can then join a molecule of tetralin to form 1-phenyl-4-(1,2,3,4-tetrahydro-5-naphthyl)butane, which in turn yields B(a)P and benzo(j)fluoranthene following ring closure and dehydrogenation. Acetylene is actually formed during the thermal decomposition of many organic materials. However, it is not necessary to assume that the pyrolytic formation of B(a)P invariably involves initial cracking down to acetylene. Long-chain alkanes may be split to C_{10} units which then undergo cyclization to form the C_6-C_4 units. Dimerization of two vinylcyclohexene to dodecahydropyrene also occurs, which, followed by the addition of a molecule of butadiene and aromatization, yields B(a)P. Benzo(a)pyrene is probably formed by both mechanisms as shown in Fig. 5.

The importance of temperature dependence of the formation of PAHs is exemplified by the study of Badger et al. (1964) using n-butylbenzene as the starting molecule. As shown in Fig. 6, it appears that for most PAHs, in particular for B(a)P, benzo(b)fluoranthene and benzo(j)fluoranthene, there is an optimum temperature around 700° C beyond which the yield rapidly decreases.

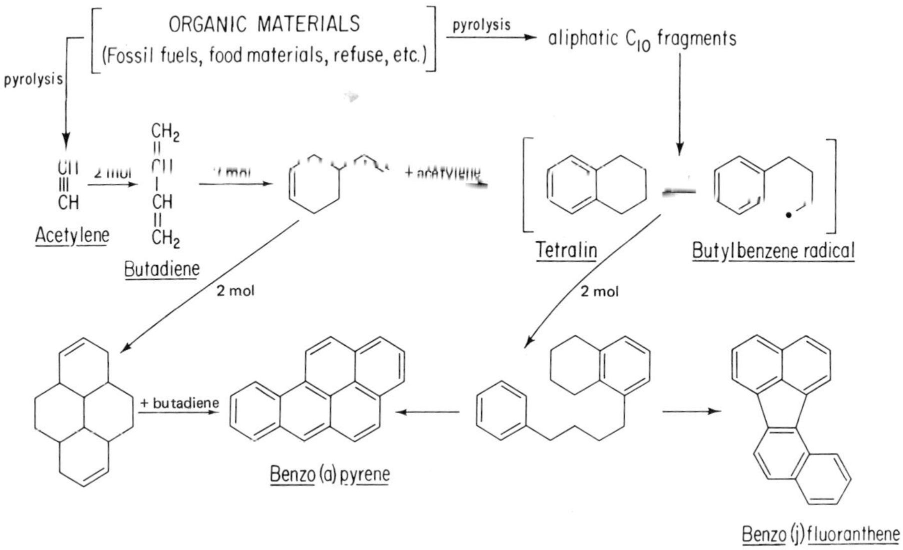

FIGURE 5 Mechanism of pyrolytic formation of benzo(a)pyrene and benzo(j)fluoranthene from organic materials. (Adapted from Badger, 1962; Badger et al., 1964).

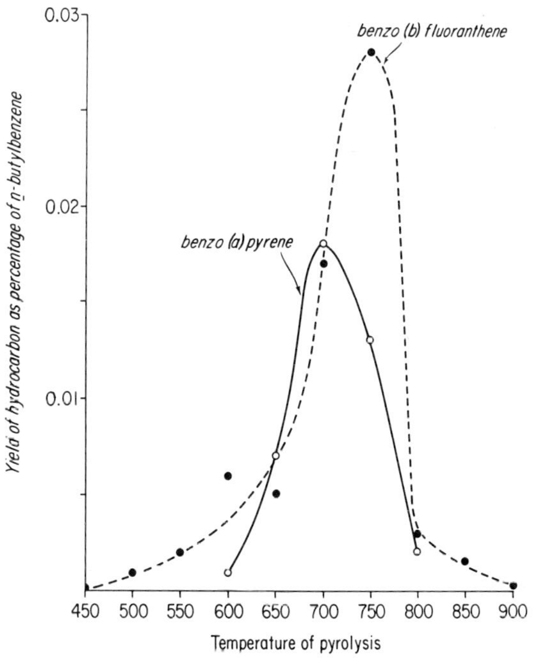

FIGURE 6 The effect of temperature on the formation of benzo(a)pyrene and benzo(b)fluoranthene in the pyrolysis of n-butylbenzene (adapted from Badger, 1962; Badger et al., 1964).

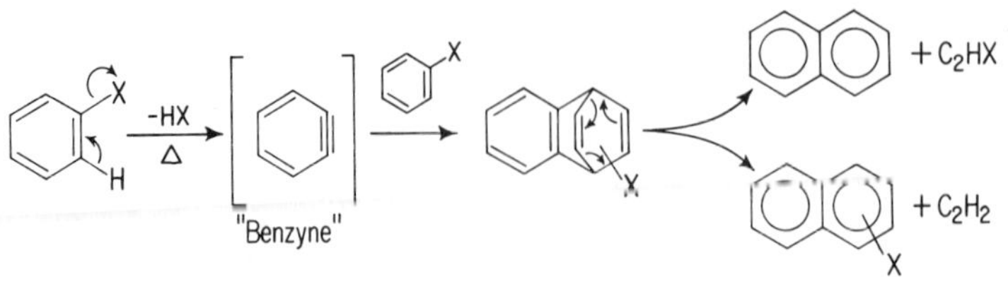

FIGURE 7 Hypothetical mechanism of pyrolytic formation of naphthalene from benzene (adapted from Schmeltz and Hoffmann, 1976).

Crittenden and Long (1976) have summarized their study on the mechanism of formation of PAHs during the pyrolysis of molecules of simple aliphatic fuels. Batch and continuous samples were withdrawn from the different reaction zones of oxyacetylene and oxyethylene flames and analyzed. The concentration of ethylene in oxyethylene flame falls rapidly with concomitant rise in the concentration of acetylene and hydrogen, suggesting conversion of ethylene to acetylene. The blue reaction zone favors both decomposition and dehydrogenation of hydrocarbon species, providing acetylenic radicals for the formation of polyacetylene. The combination of branched or straight-chain polymeric radicals could yield indene, styrene, and phenylacetylene. It was concluded that C_6-C_2 units (styrene or phenylacetylene) may be of importance for the formation of PAHs.

The possibility that there may be more than one general pathway for the formation of PAHs has been suggested by Schmeltz and Hoffman (1976). These authors have extensively investigated the pyrolysis of simple aromatic compounds such as benzene, toluene, and phenol in nitrogen and in air. Pyrolysis of benzene in nitrogen (at 800° C) gives predominantly one product, biphenyl, by free radical reaction. Pyrolysis of benzene in air, however, produces relatively high yields of phenol in addition to a complex mixture of PAHs. To explain the formation of the products observed, these authors postulated that the pyrolysis of benzene in air could involve a "benzyne" intermediate. Thus, benzene exposed to high temperatures in the presence of air would first be converted to phenol, which upon loss of water, would transform to "benzyne." The latter, via 1,4-addition across benzene, gives rise to benzobicyclo(2,2,2)-octatriene, which spontaneously decomposes to acetylene and naphthalene (see Fig. 7). Similarly, naphthalene could give rise to "naphthalynes" and ultimately to higher PAHs.

2. Geochemical Formation

Some refined petroleum fractions are known to contain carcinogenic PAHs because the very nature of the refining processes involves treatment at high temperature. However, the fact that crude, untreated oils are also carcinogenic suggests the natural geochemical formation of PAHs. An extensive study on the carcinogenic activity of crude oils was initiated in the late 1950s by Cook, Carruthers, and Woodhouse and concluded in 1968 (MRC, 1968). Representative crude oils were obtained from fields in Kuwait, Langunillas (Venezuela) and Oklahoma (United States). Low-pressure distillation, steam distillation, chromatography on alumina, and crystallization of polycyclic aromatic components as picrates were used to fractionate these crude oils. Carcinogens were found to be associated with the fraction boiling, under normal pressure, at 300-400° C. Using both mice and rabbits as test animals, fractions of oil from Langunillas (a naphthenic-type oil) were found to be more carcinogenic than those of the asphaltic-paraffinic type from Kuwait, whereas the paraffinic type from Oklahoma had little carcinogenic activity. The Kuwait oil, which had been extensively investigated, contained, in addition to sulfur-containing aromatic hydrocarbons, several PAHs, including methyl derivatives of benz(a)anthracene.

The presence of PAHs in the soil has been reported by investigators in various countries. Blumer (1961) found concentrations of B(a)P between 40 and 1300 μg/kg dried soil samples obtained from forests and fields where contamination by urban pollution was unlikely (but cannot be excluded). The origin of B(a)P in these rural soils is not clear. One possibility is by geochemical formation, the same low-temperature processes that bring about the transformation of organic matter to peat and lignite. Alternatively, PAHs may also be the biosynthetic products of microorganisms present in the soil.

3. Biosynthesis

The biosynthesis of PAHs is a subject of considerable interest and controversy. Possible environmental contamination is the main concern in establishing the validity of biosynthesis. Presence of PAHs in various forms of plant life has been reported. Borneff and Fischer (1962) identified several PAHs, including B(a)P, in phytoplanktons—microscopic organisms upon which small fish depend as their major source of food. Knorr and Schenk (1968) reported the production of B(a)P, benz(a)anthracene, benzo(b)fluoranthene, and benzo(j)fluoranthene in several strains of human saprophytic or pathogenic bacteria such as *Escherichia coli* and *Mycobacterium smegmatis*. The possibility of environmental contamination in these experiments cannot be completely ruled out. The evidence is much more convincing for the synthesis of PAHs by the alga, *Chlorella vulgaris*, as reported by Borneff et al. (1968a, b). The algae were grown in neutral media with acetate as the sole carbon source. Radioactively labeled PAHs were obtained when the algae were grown in the presence of radioactively labeled ^{14}C-acetate. Gräf and Diehl (1966) showed that PAHs were synthesized during the germination and growth of rye, wheat, and lentils. An increase of up to fivefold in the content of PAHs was observed in leaves during yellowing and in seeds soon after germination. Contamination from the environment or soil to this extent was thought to be unlikely. Wagner and Siddiqi (1970), however, were unable to detect synthesis of PAHs in wheat plant. More recently Hase and Hites (1976) have reported their study on the biosynthesis of PAHs by plants and anaerobic bacteria. Under conditions in which precautions have been taken to exclude or monitor outside contamination, no biosynthesis of PAHs could be demonstrated. Instead, they have shown that the bioaccumulation effect is quite strong and suggested that differential accumulating ability may account for the different content of PAHs in plants. Thus, the role, if any, of biosynthesis in the formation of PAHs remains to be elucidated.

D. Sources, Occurrence, and Exposure

Aromatic hydrocarbons are ubiquitously found in the environment and the level of these compounds parallels industrial and urban development. B(a)P has generally been used as an indicator of the environmental presence of PAHs. However, the use of B(a)P level as a "barometer" of the entire class of PAHs is not entirely justifiable, and the use of benzanthrone (7H-benz(d,e)anthracen-7-one) as an additional indicator has been proposed by the U.S. Environmental Protection Agency (NAS, 1972). Nevertheless, the fact that B(a)P is a potent carcinogen stresses the importance of a close surveillance of this hydrocarbon. Benzo(a)-pyrene has been found in the air, water, and food, implicating the presence of other PAHs as well. Exposure of the general population to these hydrocarbons is mainly via inhalation and ingestion.

1. Air

Cancer of the respiratory tract is one of the commonest causes of cancer mortality in the technologically developed countries. Epidemiological studies indicate that environmental factors play a crucial role in the induction of lung cancer. The incidence of lung cancer, especially in men, has been steadily increasing at an alarming rate in the past 2 decades. Pollutants in the air, as well as tobacco (especially cigarette) smoking, have been implicated as the main factors. Polycyclic aromatic hydrocarbons are among the main carcinogenic agents in polluted air and tobacco smoke. Most of the PAHs in the air are adsorbed to particulate matter.

a. Sources of polycyclic aromatic hydrocarbons in the air

Recognition of the source of emission of PAHs is the first important step toward regulating and reducing their environmental concentration. Although accurate information is not available, the Committee on Biologic Effects of Atmospheric Pollutants (NAS, 1972) has recently estimated and categorized the contribution of a number of known sources of PAH emission in the United States. Combustion of fossil fuels or, more generally, compounds containing carbon and hydrogen, is the principal source. The amount of PAH emission varies widely; inefficient, uncontrolled burning favors high emission. The main sources of PAHs, expressed in terms of B(a)P emission, are: heat and power generation (500 tons/year), refuse burning (600 tons/year), coke production (200 tons/year), and motor vehicles (20 tons/year). These values are only crude nationwide estimates and do not apply to individual areas.

Heat and power generation Coal, oil, gas, and wood are used as fuel in a variety of installations. Table 2 shows a summary of the Committee on the estimation of B(a)P emission from heat and power generation sources in the United States. That the efficiency of combustion rather than the fuel used is the main controlling parameter, is emphasized by the low B(a)P emission factor found in power plants burning crushed or pulverized coal. No firm data are available on the extent of PAH emission from wood-burning combustion units. The growing popularity of home fireplaces, as well as rural heating demands call for further evaluation of this factor. Total B(a)P emissions of the order of 500 tons/year were estimated for heat and power generation sources (Table 2).

Refuse burning The intentional burning of solid wastes, as well as accidental or naturally occurring uncontrolled combustion processes, contribute significantly to the overall

TABLE 2 Estimated Benzo(a)pyrene Emission from Heat and Power Generation Sources in the United States

Type of unit	Gross heat (Btu/hr)	Benzo(a)pyrene emission factor ($\mu g/10^6$ Btu)	Benzo(a)pyrene emission (tons/year)
Coal			
Hand-stoked residential furnaces	0.1×10^6	1,700,000-3,300,000	420
Intermediate units (chain-grate and spreader stokers)	$60\text{-}250 \times 10^6$	15-40	10
Coal-fired steam power plants	$1000\text{-}2000 \times 10^6$	20-400	1
Oil			
Low-pressure air-atomized	0.7×10^6	900	2
Other	$0.02\text{-}21 \times 10^6$	100	
Gas			
Premix burners	$0.01\text{-}9 \times 10^6$	20-200	2
Wood		50,000	40

Source: From NAS, 1972.

TABLE 3 Estimated Benzo(a)pyrene Emission from Refuse-Burning in the United States

Source of benzo(a)pyrene	Benzo(a)pyrene emission (tons/year)
Enclosed incineration	
Municipal	< 1
Commercial and industrial	23
Institutional	2
Apartment	8
Open burning	
Municipal	4
Commercial and industrial	10
Domestic	10
Forest and agricultural	140
Vehicle disposal	50
Coal refuse fires	340

Source: From NAS, 1972.

emission of PAHs. Such sources should come under closer scrutiny in view of the increasing solid-waste disposal problem in the United States today. Table 3 shows an estimate of B(a)P emission from refuse burning. Again the importance of efficient combustion in reducing PAH emission is emphasized. Large municipal incinerators had B(a)P emission factors of 0.1-6 μg/lb of charged refuse, compared to 50-260 μg/lb for their industrial and commercial counterparts. The B(a)P emission factor is much higher for open burning; combustion of automobile components such as used tires, yielded a B(a)P emission factor of 1.3×10^4 μg/lb. The spontaneous burning of coal refuse is the major source of emission. Coal refuse, consisting of heaps of rocks and shale intermixed with small pieces of coal, is a major by-product of the coal-mining industry. Proper treatment and new application of this by-product must be sought by the industry. The total B(a)P emission from refuse burning was estimated to be 600 tons/year.

Coke production and other industrial activities The most obvious sources of PAH emission in the petroleum industry are catalytic cracking of petroleum in the refineries and air-blowing of asphalt. In the catalytic cracking process organic molecules in the crude oil are broken down into lighter components and used in the manufacture of gasoline, heating oil, aviation fuel, and so on. The cracking takes place in the presence of a catalyst, which can become deactivated through deposition of carbon or coke on the active sites. It is in the regeneration of the catalyst, through combustion of the coke on the catalyst surface, that PAHs are formed. The eventual emission of PAHs into the atmosphere depends on whether or not the effluent is passed through a carbon monoxide waste-heat boiler, which removes most of the PAHs present. The increasing use of the carbon monoxide burners in the industry has reduced the emission in recent years. Nevertheless, the annual emission of B(a)P due to the catalytic cracking in the refineries was estimated to be around 6 tons/year. Air-blowing of asphalt is a procedure designed to yield materials of higher softening point for roofing applications. The effluent from air-blowing of asphalt may contain many PAHs, and the annual emission of B(a)P due to this process was estimated to be 0.03 tons (NAS, 1972).

Estimation of PAH emission from other industrial activities is more indirect (by sampling the air in the vicinity of the emission source) and often imprecise. Some of the processes considered include coke production in the iron and steel industry, processes involving the use of carbon black, coal-tar pitch, asphalt-hot-road mix, and general chemical processes. Except for coke production, none of the industrial processes mentioned above can be clearly

TABLE 4 Estimated Benzo(a)pyrene Emission from Motor Vehicles in the United States

Vehicle type	Fuel consumed (gal/year)	Benzo(a)pyrene emission factor (μg/gal)	Benzo(a)pyrene emission (tons/year)
Gasoline-powered			
Automobiles	56.4×10^9	170	10
Trucks	24.2×10^9	~500	~12
Diesel-fuel-powered			
Trucks and buses	5.8×10^9	62	0.4
Total			~22

Source: From NAS, 1972.

shown to contribute significantly to the emission of PAHs into the atmosphere. Higher atmospheric B(a)P concentrations in the areas surrounding coke production sites have, however, been demonstrated. The Committee estimated the annual production of B(a)P emission due to coke production to be around 200 tons/year.

Transportation sources A significant mobile source of atmospheric PAHs are the conventional automobiles, powered by spark-ignited internal combustion engines. Table 4 shows an assessment by the Committee of the vehicular B(a)P contribution, compiled from nationwide fuel-consumption data. The emission of PAHs by gasoline-powered vehicles can be affected by two factors: the characteristics of the vehicle and the composition of the fuel. The characteristics of the vehicle include the nature of emission control devices, operating modes, deterioration, combustion chamber deposits, and the setting of carburetion (e.g., "leaner" fuel-air mixture—that is higher air : fuel ratio—favors more complete combustion and, thus, less emission). The composition of the fuel includes such variables as the aromaticity, fuel PAH level, additive(s), and lubricants. Table 5 shows the B(a)P emission factors of automobiles manufactured at various years. Moran (see Bridbord et al., 1976) has recently estimated that the emission factor of 1975 cars has been reduced to 3-4% of that of pre-1968 cars. Hoffman and Wynder (1976) have summarized their data on the effect of aromaticity of fuel on the emission of PAHs. The increasing concern with the emission of lead from gasoline engines prompted the introduction of low lead fuels. The increase of aromatic portion (benzene, toluene, and xylene) for keeping the antiknock number high in low-lead fuels can increase the emission of PAHs (Table 6). The recent practice of adding the aliphatic isooctane (2,2,4-trimethylpentane) to replace or reduce the aromatic portion is regarded with favor.

TABLE 5 Automotive Benzo(a)pyrene Emission Factors

Source	Benzo(a)pyrene emission factors (μg/gal of fuel consumed)
Uncontrolled car (1956-1964)	170
1966 Uncontrolled car	45-70
1968 Emission-controlled vehicle	20-30
Advanced systems	<10

Source: From NAS, 1972.

TABLE 6 Fuel Types, Benzo(a)pyrene, Benz(a)anthracene, and Phenol Emission Rates with Gasoline and Hydrocarbon Fuels (1-Min Run)

Fuel	B(a)P (μg)	B(a)A (μg)	Phenol (mg)
Gasoline	9.6	17.3	1.4
2,2,4-Trimethylpentane	2.6	0.8	0.013
2,4,4-Trimethyl-1-pentene	0.7	0.4	0.059
50% O-xylene-50% benzene	25.8	56.3	5.56
25% 2,2,4-Trimethylpentane + +25% 2-Methylbutane +50% o-xylene	9.0	32.3	0.46

Source: From Hoffmann and Wynder, 1976, p. 348.

Although automobile exhausts (estimated B(a)P emission: 20 tons/year) contributed less than 2% of the nationwide overall B(a)P emission (about 1300 tons/year), in many cities and their outlying suburbs, automobile exhausts may be the major contributors. It was estimated in 1971 that 42% of the particulate emission in Los Angeles County was caused by motor vehicles, and that in downtown Los Angeles virtually all the B(a)P in the air was from this source (Gordon and Bryan, 1973). Similarly, it was estimated that motor vehicles contributed 5% of total B(a)P in the Detroit downtown area, 18% of B(a)P in the freeway area, and 42% in the suburbs (Collucci and Begemen, 1965).

Quantitative data are not generally available for the other mobile sources, such as aircraft engines, and various nondiesel two-cycle engines (lawnmowers, outboard motors, and motorcycles). The B(a)P emission factor was estimated to be 11 mg/gal for two-cycle engines. High concentrations of B(a)P were found in airplane engine soot (Linnik et al., 1971); values as high as 25 and 35 mg B(a)P/kg soot from airplane turbines and piston engines, respectively, were reported. This is consistent with the report of Shabad and Smirnov (1969), who estimated that an aircraft engine ejects 2-10 mg B(a)P/min. The overall contribution from these mobile sources remains to be elucidated.

The major noncombustion transportation source of PAHs is probably the degradation of automobile tires in use. Emission of 4.3 tons of rubber particles/day/million people in the U.S. was estimated; the resulting B(a)P emission was, however, relatively low with the figure of 0.3 lb/day/million people projected. The contribution due to the degradation of bituminous (asphaltic) road surfaces is virtually unexplored.

Tobacco smoke Tobacco smoke is the major nonindustrial source of PAHs in indoor environments. Investigators at the Naylor Dana Institute for Disease Prevention and others have carried out an extensive study on the formation and presence of PAHs in tobacco smoke (Schmeltz and Hoffmann, 1976; Brunnemann and Hoffmann, 1976; Hoffmann and Wynder, 1976; Severson et al., 1976). Polycyclic aromatic hydrocarbons are almost exclusively associated with the particulate phase (in contrast to the gaseous phase) of the smoke. Table 7 shows the concentration of various carcinogenic PAHs in the particulate phase of the mainstream of cigarette smoke. During smoking the mainstream is inhaled, and, in the interval between puffs while the cigarette smoulders, the sidestream smoke escapes into the environment. The sidestream is the major contributor to indoor pollution. Schmeltz et al. (1975) have reviewed the literature on the comparison of concentrations of various constituents in the sidestream and mainstream smoke; the sidestream smoke generally contains greater concentrations of smoke constituents (the ratio of sidestream to mainstream concentration for B(a)P is between 2 and 3), and sidestream also represents a greater portion of tobacco consumed during burning. In addition to carcinogenic PAHs, high concentrations of tumor promotors of cocarcinogens such as phenol and catechol are also present. The impact of tobacco smoking on indoor pollution is dependent on the extent of smoking activity and the condition of the indoor environment; this subject is considered in Sec. II.D.1.d.

TABLE 7 Carcinogenic Polycyclic Aromatic Hydrocarbons Identified in the Particulate Phase of Tobacco Smoke

Hydrocarbon	Relative activity	μg/100 cigarettes
Benzo(a)pyrene	+++	3.0-4.0
5-Methylchrysene	+++	0.06
Dibenz(a,h)anthracene	++	0.4
Dibenzo(a,i)pyrene	++	Traces
Dibenzo(a,l)pyrene	++	Traces
Benzo(b)fluoranthene	++	0.3
Benzo(j)fluoranthene	++	0.6
Indeno(1,2,3-cd)pyrene	+	0.4
Benz(a)anthracene	+	6.0-8.0
Benzo(c)phenanthrene	+	Traces
2-Methylfluoranthene	+	0.2
3-Methylfluoranthene	+	0.2
Chrysene	+	4.0
1-, 2-, 3-, and 6-Methylchrysenes	+	2.0

Source: Adapted from Hoffmann and Wynder, 1976.

b. Effect of particulate matter

As mentioned above, PAHs in the air are predominantly adsorbed to particulate matter such as dust particles. To be effectively carcinogenic, carcinogens must be adsorbed to such particles that can penetrate into the bronchiolar or alveolar wall where the particles are phagocytized by macrophages. The carcinogens are then eluted out by plasma and diffuse around to impregnate the lung tissues reaching up to the bronchial mucosa. The nature and the size of particles play a crucial role in determining the carcinogenicity of the adsorbed PAHs by affecting their passage, deposition, retention, and elution in the respiratory tract.

Commercial carbon black may contain carcinogenic amounts of B(a)P, yet it is apparently noncarcinogenic; in contrast, B(a)P adsorbed to soot is highly carcinogenic. The different surface structure of the carbon granules in soot and carbon black could account for the difference; PAHs are apparently more strongly adsorbed to the colloidal surface of carbon black. Other "inert" dust particles such as iron oxide (hematin) particles have also been successfully used as carrier particles for various carcinogens in inhalation carcinogenesis studies (Saffiotti, 1969, 1970).

The effect of particle size has been discussed in a symposium on inhalation carcinogenesis (Hanna et al., 1970) and has recently been reviewed by Hoffmann and Wynder (1976). Particles with diameters ranging from 0.25 to 10 μm are considered as "lung damaging." Particles less than 0.25 μm are seldom retained in the lung and if so, they remain located in the alveolar regions. Particles greater than 10 μm are lodged in the upper tract and do not reach the bronchi. Various pollution sources produce particles of "lung-damaging" size range. The effect of carbon particles and particle size on the retention and elution of B(a)P in the respiratory tract of mice has recently been studied by Creasia et al. (1976). Carbon particles increased the retention time of B(a)P in the lung more than 20 times over that for unadsorbed B(a)P. Larger particles (15-30 μm) are retained longer than smaller particles (0.5-1 μm); however, the elution of B(a)P is more effective in the smaller particles. Thus, B(a)P adsorbed to small particles (0.5-5 μm) is the most carcinogenic.

The retention of particles in the lung can also be affected by the mucus flow in the tracheobronchial tract. The constant upward propelling action of the mucus layer by ciliated cells can significantly reduce the retention time of the particles so that particulate-bound carcinogens may be cleared before sufficient amounts of carcinogens could be eluted. This is part of the natural defense mechanism of the respiratory tract. However, a variety of chemicals or irritants can impede the mucus flow by poisoning the cilia or thickening the mucus; these chemicals include some aromatic hydrocarbons, phenols and inorganic chemicals, and so on, which are commonly encountered in urban pollution and in cigarette smoke (Hoffmann and Wynder, 1976).

c. Polycyclic aromatic hydrocarbons in the atmosphere

A summary of the concentrations of PAHs in urban atmospheres is presented in Table 8. It should be emphasized that regional industrial activities, seasonal demand for heat and power generation, local traffic, and meteorological conditions can all significantly alter the atmospheric PAH concentrations in individual areas. These variations are shown by the study of Sawicki et al. (1960). Table 9 lists the average values for B(a)P concentrations in the air of some U.S. cities in 1959. The range was from 0.4 to 61 μg/1000 m^3 of air. The average B(a)P concentration in nonurban areas was less than 1 μg/1000 m^3. The seasonal variations of B(a)P concentrations are illustrated by Fig. 8; apparently, the greater demand for heat and power generation could account for the higher B(a)P concentrations in the winter months. It has been estimated that under adverse weather conditions, the atmospheric concentration of B(a)P in the vicinity of highways could be as much as 18 times higher than the concentration under typical weather (Bridbord et al., 1976). An extreme case was reported from London in 1957; during smog an atmospheric B(a)P concentration of 2200 μg/1000 m^3 was observed.

d. Indoor atmosphere

The majority of the general population spends most of its time indoors—in domestic premises, public buildings, or transport vehicles. The overwhelming evidence linking cigarette smoking to lung cancer and other diseases has drawn increasingly the attention of the general public, the scientific community, and the public health authorities to the pollution of the indoor atmosphere. Schmeltz et al. (1975), Noonan (1976), and Sterling and Kobayashi (1977) have recently reviewed the literature concerning indoor pollution. The major sources of indoor pollution are tobacco smoke, improperly vented furnaces, incinerators, leakage from outdoors, and cooking. The major factors regulating the concentrations of indoor

TABLE 8 Concentrations of Polycyclic Aromatic Hydrocarbons Found in U.S. Urban Atmosphere

Hydrocarbon	Carcinogenicity index	Concentration (μg/1000 m^3)[a]
Benzo(a)pyrene	72	0.05-74 (av. 6)
Benzo(b)fluoranthene	68	2.3-7.4
Benzo(j)fluoranthene	59	0.8-4.4
Dibenzo(cd, jk)pyrene	21	av. 0.26
Ideno(1, 2, 3-cd)pyrene	16	1.5-8.2
Benz(a)anthracene	5	0.1-21.6 (av. 4)
Benzo(c)pyrene	2	1-25 (av. 5)
Chrysene	1	1.3-13.3
Benzo(g, h, i)perylene	Marginal	2-35
Corenene	0	av. 2
Fluoranthene	0	av. 4
Perylene	0	av. 0.7
Pyrene	0	0-35

[a]Adapted from compilation of Hoffmann and Wynder, 1976.

TABLE 9 Benzo(a)pyrene Concentrations in Air at Urban Sampling Sites for January-March 1959

High B(a)P		Low B(a)P	
Location	Concentration (μg/1000 m^3)	Location	Concentration (μg/1000 m^3)
Montgomery, Ala	24	Little Rock, Ark.	1.5
Indianapolis, Ind.	26	Glendale, Calif.	0.8
Des Moines, Iowa	23	San Jose, Calif.	0.6
Portland, Maine	21	Miami, Fla.	1.9
St. Louis, Mo.	54	Shreveport, La.	0.7
Charlotte, N.C.	39	Jackson, Miss.	1.2
Cleveland, Ohio	24	Las Vegas, Nev.	1.4
Youngstown, Ohio	28	Bismarck, N. Dak.	0.4
Altoona, Pa.	61	Tulsa, Okla.	1.0
Columbia, S.C.	24	Dallas, Tex.	1.4
Chattanooga, Tenn.	31	Houston, Tex.	1.6
Knoxville, Tenn.	24	Salt Lake City, Utah	0.5
Richmond, Va.	45	Burlington, Vt.	1.0
Wheeling, W. Va.	21	Cheyenne, Wy.	1.2

Source: From Sawicki et al., 1965.

pollutants include the activity of the emission source (e.g., the frequency of smoking), the ventilation (air turnover rate), and the size of the room. It has been estimated (NAS, 1972) that the smoking of one unfiltered cigarette (85 mm long) releases 30-50 mg of tar, which contains 0.10-0.15 μg of B(a)P, 0.20-0.30 μg of pyrene, and 0.25 μg of chrysene. In a medium-size room (40 m^3), three smokers can pollute the air with 2-4 μg of B(a)P, 5-8 μg of pyrene, and 6 μg of chrysene per 1000 m^3 of air. Depending on ventilation and the smoking activities, the indoor pollution by cigarette sidestream can be significantly higher.

Stocks et al. (1961) reported that offices have 25-70% lower PAH concentrations than those found in the immediate outdoor atmosphere. Under certain circumstances, however, the indoor PAH concentrations may be substantially higher than those outside. Table 10 lists the available data on indoor B(a)P concentrations. The extent that tobacco smoke may pollute the indoor air is indicated by the high concentrations of B(a)P found in a beer hall and restau-

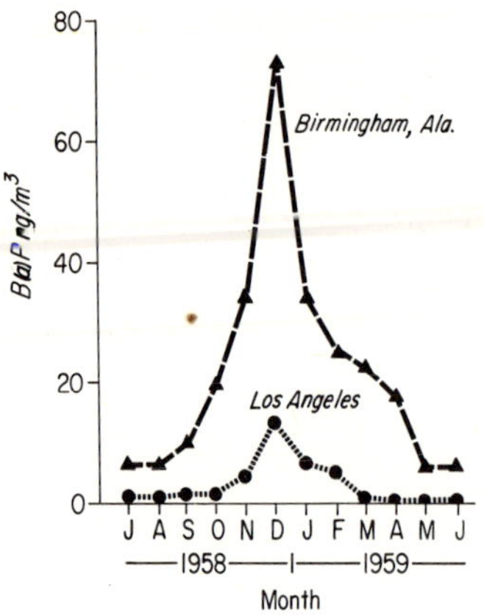

FIGURE 8 Average monthly benzo(a)pyrene concentrations in the air of Birmingham, Alabama and Los Angeles, California: July 1958 to June 1959 (adapted from Sawicki et al., 1960).

TABLE 10 Benzo(a)pyrene Concentrations in Polluted Indoor Atmosphere

Location	B(a)P concentration ($\mu g/1000\ m^3$)	Suspected cause
Beer hall and restaurant in Prague[a]	28–144	Smoking and possibly cooking
Kenyan huts[b]		
Coastal region	0–24	Very poor ventilation, heating with open wood or cow manure fire, and cooking
Mountain region	85–291	
Inside aircrafts[c]		
Transatlantic flights	85	Smoking
Domestic flights	150	Smoking
Sport arenas[d]	12.5	Smoking

[a]Galuškinová, 1964.

[b]Hoffmann and Wynder, 1976.

[c]Cited in Bridbord et al., 1976; data compiled by National Institute for Occupational Safety and Health prior to the establishment of smoking and nonsmoking sections.

[d]Elliott and Rowe, 1975.

rant in the city of Prague, and inside aircrafts and sport arenas. It is evident from these data that considerable exposure of nonsmokers to PAHs may occur under similar circumstances. The importance of ventilation is stressed by the finding of high atmospheric PAH concentrations in the dwellings of some Kenyan mountain tribes; the very poor ventilation coupled with the constant emission of PAHs from heating and cooking made the Kenyan huts notorious examples of indoor pollution. The higher incidence of nasopharyngeal cancer among natives of certain Kenyan tribes in the mountains (as compared to those in the coastal region) may be related to their higher indoor exposure.

The extent that nonsmokers may be affected by PAHs in indoor air polluted by smokers remains to be assessed systematically. There is little doubt that passive smokers (nonsmokers who are compelled by certain circumstances to inhale cigarette smoke generated by smokers) also inhale carbon monoxide and nicotine. Increases in the carboxyhemoglobin (carbon monoxide-hemoglobin complex) levels in the blood and nicotine concentrations in the urine of passive smokers have been reported by various investigators; their potential negative health consequences have been discussed (Schmeltz et al., 1975; Sterling and Kobayashi, 1977). There is very little information available on the exposure of nonsmokers to PAHs in polluted indoor air. Increase in urinary PAH level in passive smokers has been reported in one such study (Malý, 1971). Using paper chromatographic separation and UV quantitation, Malý measured the PAH levels in the urine of an active smoker and a passive smoker, both sitting 8 hr a day in a closed room of 35 m^3. Increases in urinary PAH levels were observed; in particular, the dibenzo(a,l)pyrene (1,2,3,4-dibenzpyrene) was 1.1 μg/liter urine in the active smoker and 0.3 μg/liter in the passive smoker. The urinary dibenzo(a,l)pyrene level of the passive smoker dropped to zero 2 weeks after removal from exposure. Dibenzo(a,l)-pyrene was chosen because it is metabolized to a lesser extent than lower PAHs such as B(a)P. Although the details of the study were not presented, the results suggest that passive smokers inhale PAHs generated by smokers. Thus, it is evident from available information that the indoor pollution problem must receive more attention. The very nature of confinement of indoor environment makes indoor pollution potentially more harmful than that encountered outside.

e. Assessment of exposure via inhalation

Assessment of human exposure to carcinogenic PAHs is of vital importance for evaluating the environmental impact of these compounds as a potential health hazard. Unfortunately, most of the information needed for the assessment are only rough estimates, and it is obvious that only semiquantitative estimates can at best be made out of the available information. To convert atmospheric concentrations of B(a)P (μg/1000 m^3) to amounts of B(a)P the lung is in contact with per day, we need to know the volume of air a person inhales per day, the proportion of B(a)P adsorbed onto particles that will actually reach the lung, and the retention characteristics of the inhaled B(a)P. Information on the latter two parameters is lacking and depends on individual cases; the volume of air a person inhales per day is of the order of 10 to 20 m^3 (NAS, 1972; Pike et al., 1975) or 30 m^3 (Bridbord et al., 1976). Assuming that all B(a)P inhaled will effectively reach the lung, the amount of B(a)P in contact can be calculated by simply multiplying the atmospheric concentrations of B(a)P per m^3 by 20 (the average number of m^3 of air inhaled daily). Thus, depending on where we live, we could inhale anywhere from 0.001 to 1.5 μg B(a)P/day from outdoor urban air (concentration 0.05-74 μg/1,000 m^3), or 0.4 to 550 μg/year. Similar estimates have been made by investigators in various countries (Pike et al., 1975; Bridbord et al., 1976; Preussmann, 1976). In some studies, the effect of B(a)P in air has been compared to cigarette smoking. Bridbord et al. (1976) listed several groups of persons at high risk of cancer due to PAH exposure in terms of B(a)P intake and cigarette equivalents (Table 11). The relative effect of increase of B(a)P in the air, and of cigarette smoking, on the increase in male lung cancer death rate in the United States and United Kingdom has been discussed (Pike et al., 1975).

It should be stressed that except for occupational exposure, cigarette smoking is the major source of B(a)P exposure for smokers. Smokers of one pack of cigarettes/day inhale about 0.4 μg B(a)P from filtered cigarettes and 0.7 μg from unfiltered cigarettes (NAS, 1972).

TABLE 11 Influence of Occupational and Other Factors on Benzo(a)pyrene Intake

Factor	B(a)P intake (μg/day)	Cigarette equivalents (packs/day)
Smoking one pack of cigarettes each day	0.4	1
Coke oven worker		
Top side exposures	180	450
Side and bench exposure	70	175
Coal tar pitch worker	750	1875
Airplane pilot		
Transatlantic flights	0.93	2.3
Domestic cross-country	1.38	3.5
Employee in restaurant	0.8	2
Person living near expressway 24 hr/day (adverse meteorology)	0.02	0.05
Commuter on an expressway 2 hr/day (adverse meteorology)	0.04	0.10
Exposure to ambient B(a)P levels 8 hr/day	0.02	0.05

Source: From Bridbord et al., 1976.

The evidence linking cigarette smoking to high incidence of lung cancer is overwhelming (Hammond, 1975; Pike et al., 1975; Hoffmann and Wynder, 1976). The cancer risk of smokers is roughly proportional to the number of cigarettes smoked per day and the degree of inhalation. The effect of duration of smoking is even more dramatic, as the lung cancer rate is approximately proportional to the duration of smoking to the fourth power. Thus, at age 65 a smoker of a certain number of cigarettes who started smoking at age 15 will have a death rate of 2.4 (i.e., $50^4/40^4$) times the rate of a smoker who smoked the same number of cigarettes but started at age 25 (Peto, 1974, cited in Pike et al., 1975). In addition to lung cancer, the incidence of cancer of buccal cavity, larynx, esophagus, bladder, and pancreas is also higher in smokers. It should be noted that exposure of smokers to carcinogens is not limited to B(a)P. Other carcinogenic PAHs, carcinogenic nitrosamines, and inorganic chemicals have also been found in the cigarette smoke. Furthermore, the presence of large amounts of promotors (cocarcinogens) are believed to be almost as important as the carcinogenic compounds themselves. While carcinogens initiate the induction of latent cancer cells, the eventual transformation of the latent to actively proliferating cancer cells is brought about by promotors. The reduction of cancer risk of exsmokers is believed to be related in part to the cessation of cocarcinogen intake from the smoke.

2. Water

The earth's aqueous environment has long been neglected. It has been generally assumed that the aqueous environment, by virtue of its vastness, is endowed with unlimited buffering capacity to handle pollutants generated by human activities. This assumption, however, may soon reach its limitations. With the proliferation of industrial technology and a worldwide population increase, the increased waste disposal and sewage could soon lead to contaminated waterways unless effective control procedures are instituted. Considerable increases have already been observed in the concentrations of organic and inorganic chemical pollutants in the oceans and in the waterways of various countries; the carcinogenic activity of these pollutants is reflected in the increase in the incidence of tumors in fish (Stich and Acton, 1976; Kraybill, 1976; Kraybill et al., 1977). Polycyclic aromatic hydrocarbons constitute an important part of the organic chemical carcinogens in the aqueous environment.

a. Sources and occurrence

The PAHs in the aqueous environment originate from a variety of sources. Quantitative data on the relative contribution of these sources are not generally available and in some cases, probably not obtainable. Harrison et al. (1975), Shabad (1975), Kraybill (1976), and Hase and Hites (1976) have extensively reviewed the literature pertaining to the sources of PAHs in the aqueous environment. The sources include: (1) industrial sewage, (2) domestic sewage, (3) atmospheric fallout, (4) leaching or infiltration from soil, (5) roadway runoff, (6) exhausts from internal combustion engine of motorboats and ships, (7) oil spillage from tankers, (8) natural marine oil seepage, and possibly, (9) biosynthesis by marine organisms. The major sources of PAHs in inland and coastal waters are industrial and domestic sewage (including atmospheric fallout, soil leaching, and road runoff) and motorboat engine exhausts. The major source of PAHs in marine and oceanic environment is from oil spillage and seepage; atmospheric fallout could also play a role.

Industrial sewage effluents As would be expected, most of the industries responsible for the emission of PAHs into the atmosphere are also the major contributors of these chemicals in industrial sewage. Table 12 shows the major contributors. Even after treatment (such as filtration, pond settling, biochemical treatment, or dephenolization) designed to remove most of the PAHs in the raw sewage, substantial amounts of B(a)P can still be found in the effluents. In addition to these industries, aromatic hydrocarbons are also detected in the sewage from wood preserving, plastics and dyestuff manufacture plants (EPA, 1975).

The extent that water may be polluted is shown by a study of Borneff and Kunte (1964) on the level of B(a)P in various waters (Table 13). The pollution of rivers and lakes by industrial sewage is a well-known phenomenon in industrialized countries. In the United

TABLE 12 Benzo(a)pyrene Concentrations in Industrial Sewage

Industry	Concentration (μg/l)
Shale oil	
After dephenolization	2-312
Coke by-product	
After biochemical treatment	12-16
Gasworks	
After filtration through coke beds	20
After dephenolization	130-290
Oil refineries	
Coking of residues after direct distillation of oil	0.48-5.0
Catalytic cracking	0.07-0.29
Thermal cracking	0.09-3.0
Pyrolysis of ethane-ethylene fractions	3.6
After settling ponds of various refineries	Up to 0.22

Source: Adapted from compilation of Harrison et al., 1975.

States the 10 most polluted waterways are: Ohio River, Houston Ship Canal (Texas), Cuyahoga River (Ohio), River Rouge (Michigan), Buffalo River (New York), Merrimack River (New Hampshire), Androscoggin River (Maine), Escambia River (Florida) and the Passaic and Arthur Kill Rivers (New Jersey) (Geraghty et al., 1973).

Domestic sewage Domestic sewage may contain light to moderately high amounts of PAHs depending on the weather. Benzo(a)pyrene and its metabolites have been found in mammalian urine and feces, but it is unlikely that they can play a major role in contributing PAHs to domestic sewage. The majority of PAHs in domestic sewage is most likely from atmospheric fallout, soil leaching, and road runoff. Borneff and Kunte (1965) have compared the PAH levels in domestic sewage during dry and wet weather (Table 14). The dramatic increase during heavy rain substantiates the importance of atmospheric precipitation.

Atmospheric fallout, soil leaching, and roadway runoff As mentioned above, precipitation can wash down PAHs in the atmosphere, soil, and roadway into the domestic sewage. The source of atmospheric PAHs has been discussed. The presence of PAHs in soil is also well documented; even in the apparent absence of urban pollution, B(a)P concentrations of 40-1300 μg/kg can be detected (Blumer, 1961). High levels of B(a)P in soil samples near oil refinery and coke production plants were reported; the B(a)P concentrations were as high as 200 mg/kg soil (Shabad, 1975). Polycyclic aromatic hydrocarbons in roadway runoff can

TABLE 13 Benzo(a)pyrene Concentrations in Various Types of Water

Type of water	Concentration (μg/m^3)
Groundwater	1-10
Clean or sparingly polluted river or lake water	10-50
Moderately polluted surface water	50-100
Highly polluted surface water	100-1,000
Waste water	<100,000 or >100,000

Source: Adapted from Borneff and Kunte, 1964.

TABLE 14 Polycyclic Aromatic Hydrocarbons in Domestic Sewage During Dry and Wet Weather

Hydrocarbon	Concentration during dry weather (ng/liter)	Concentration during heavy rain (ng/liter)
Fluoranthene	352	16,350
Pyrene	254	16,050
Benzo(a)anthracene	25	10,360
Benzo(b)fluoranthene	39	9,910
Benzo(j)fluoranthene	57	10,790
Benzo(k)fluoranthene	22	4,180
Benzo(a)pyrene	1	1,840
Benzo(ghi)perylene	4	3,840
Indeno(1,2,3-cd)pyrene	17	4,980

Source: Adapted from Borneff and Kunte, 1965.

arise from automobile exhausts deposited on the road surface and the "wearing-off" of bituminous (asphaltic) road surfaces and of automobile tires.

Exhausts from motorboat engines Motorboats play an important role in the pollution of bodies of water with carcinogenic PAHs formed by incomplete combustion of fuel. Investigators in the laboratory of Shabad (1975) have measured the output of B(a)P present in motorboat exhausts; during one hour of running, a hanging boat engine emitted 500 μg of B(a)P into the water. A diesel engine emitted only one-tenth as much B(a)P as a gasoline engine.

Oil spillage and natural oil seepage The majority of PAHs in marine and oceanic environment are believed to originate from oil spillage. Quantitative data on the oil spillage from tankers (intentional or accidental) are not available. Natural marine oil seepage is also a source of PAH pollution of bodies of water. Wilson et al. (1974) have calculated that the probable range of such seepage is of the order of 0.2 to 6 million metric tons per year. The Pacific Ocean appears to have more areas of high seepage potential; South California is among one of the few seepage-prone areas of the world.

Biosynthesis by marine organisms As discussed in Sec. II.C.3, biosynthesis plays an as yet undetermined role as PAH contributor. The evidence suggesting biosynthesis by marine organisms is based on the observation that aquatic algae and mollusks in Greenland contain exceptionally high concentrations of B(a)P (60 μg/kg). The lack of urban pollution in Greenland can be substantiated by the very low concentrations of B(a)P (5 μg/kg) in marine sediments in the same area (Harrison et al., 1975). Whether the high B(a)P concentration in these aquatic organisms represents biosynthesis or bioaccumulation remains to be resolved.

The presence of PAHs in marine sediments has been reported by various investigators (Harrison et al., 1975). Recent discovery that the PAH mixtures in various recent New England sediments are extremely complex and have different composition from those in the air has stirred some interest in studying the origin of these PAHs (Giger and Blumer, 1974; Blumer and Youngblood, 1975; Hites and Biemann, 1975). Various suggestions have been made and the possible geochemical, analytical and environmental significance has been discussed (Blumer and Youngblood, 1975; Hase and Hites, 1976).

b. Environmental impact of polycyclic aromatic hydrocarbons in water

Drinking water Of immediate and direct concern to the general population is the safety of the drinking water. A survey conducted by the World Health Organization in 1970 on 90 selected developing countries indicated that only 23% of the total population surveyed had a safe water supply. Fortunately, however, following proper treatment the extent of contamination of drinking water by PAHs found thus far is not known to be hazardous. The B(a)P concentration in treated drinking water was reported to be between 0.1 and 23.4 ng/l in Germany (Preussmann, 1976). In the United States, the "safety quality" of treated drinking water is closely monitored by the Environmental Protection Agency. Analysis and identification of organic compounds present in the treated drinking water of 13 U.S. cities failed to detect the presence of PAHs. The source of water supply in these cities ranges from uncontaminated upland or groundwater to water from rivers contaminated by industrial or municipal wastes or agricultural runoff (EPA, 1975; Keith et al., 1976).

Polycyclic aromatic hydrocarbons in polluted water are present in three forms: (1) associated with solid particles, (2) in dispersed form, and (3) in dissolved form. The relative proportion of these three forms is dependent on the concentration of PAH and presence of other chemicals. At high PAH concentrations, due to the very low solubility of most PAHs in water, a large proportion of PAHs are particulate-bound. Presence of surfactants such as detergent increases the solubility of PAHs by forming micelles. The various methods designed to remove PAHs in polluted water have been extensively reviewed by Harrison et al. (1975). The treatments include settling, filtration, biochemical treatment, dephenolization, filtration through activated carbon, coagulation, and flocculation. Filtration through beds of activated carbon is considered to be the most effective means of removing PAHs from water. Chlorination of water can also destroy PAHs through oxidation (Harrison et al., 1976). However, further investigations are necessary to establish the nature of the products resulting from chlorination in view of the possible health hazard of halogenated organic compounds. The importance of considering the extraction efficiency achieved in the removal of PAHs from water prior to analysis has been stressed by Harrison et al. (1975). It has been pointed out that efficiency data obtained from laboratory studies using unrealistically high concentration of PAHs do not necessarily apply to the consequences of actual water treatment.

Effect of polycyclic aromatic hydrocarbons in water on aquatic life Aquatic life, both fish and plants, are the direct victims of pollution of the aqueous environment. The carcinogenic activity of pollutants is readily reflected by the high incidence of tumors in fish in polluted areas. High frequencies of tumors: up to 58% for skin papilloma in several flatfish species, up to 55% for melanoma in *Agryosomus argentatus*, and up to 44% for tumors of the parabranchial body of cod, have been reported (Stich and Acton, 1976; Kraybill et al., 1977). The possibility of using fish as indicator organisms in monitoring carcinogens in the aqueous environment has been discussed. Clearly, the current pollution control leaves much to be desired; unless the situation improves, it is not inconceivable that fish will become "endangered species" in polluted areas. Although the role of PAHs in the causation of fish tumors has not been clearly established, the fact that high amounts of PAHs can be found in aquatic life in polluted areas indicates their involvement.

The negative health consequences of PAHs in water is not limited to aquatic life. Polycyclic aromatic hydrocarbons in polluted water can circulate from microscopic aquatic organisms (such as phytoplanktons) to crustaceans (such as shrimp) to fish and eventually to humans through the food chain. Table 15 lists the concentrations of B(a)P detected in marine animals in the various parts of the world. It is obvious that the safety of seafood from polluted areas for human consumption is questionable. The human population may become the eventual victim of its own uncontrolled pollution of the aqueous environment.

3. Polycyclic Aromatic Hydrocarbons in Foods: Sources, Occurrence, and Exposure

Food intake is another major route of human exposure to carcinogenic PAHs. It has been estimated (Fritz, 1971) that the annual oral intake of B(a)P may amount to 0.35-1.5 mg/year/person in Western countries. Benzo(a)pyrene, dibenz(a,h)anthracene, benz(a)anthracene, and other PAHs at concentrations up to 98 μg/kg have been found in various foods; high levels of PAHs are generally found in smoked foods. Whether the levels of PAHs in food present any risk to the general population is still not clear. The strongest evidence linking dietary

TABLE 15 Benzo(a)pyrene Concentrations in Marine Animals at Different Geographic Locations

Marine organism	Location	Concentration (μg/kg)
Oysters	Norfolk, Va.	10-20
Oysters	French coast	1-70
Mussels	Toulon roads, France	2-30
Holothurians	Villefranche Bay, France	Up to 2,000
Holothurians	West coast of Greenland	Nil
Codfish and shellfish	West coast of Greenland	16-60
Fish and shellfish	Saint-Malo Bay, France	3-125
Fish and crustaceans	Villefranche Bay, France	Nil-400
Crustaceans	Arctic Ocean	Nil-230
Isopod crustaceans	Clipperton Lagoon	Up to 530
Various fishes	Adriatic Coast, Italy	Nil-900
Invertebrates	Adriatic Coast, Italy	Nil-2,200

Source: From Zobell, 1971.

PAHs to human cancer is that all populations consuming high amounts of smoked fish seem to be at high risk for stomach (gastric) cancer (Sigurjonsson, 1967). The converse is, however, not necessarily true; smoked foods cannot account for all high-risk stomach cancer. Bowel cancer is also apparently associated with beef intake (Haenszel et al., 1973); PAHs produced in grilling of beef may be a factor in this association (Berg, 1975).

Polycyclic aromatic hydrocarbons in foods may originate from three major sources: (1) pyrolytic formation due to cooking or processing, (2) possible biosynthesis in plants, and (3) environmental contamination. High temperature, open flame, and high fat content in food are some of the major conditions favoring the pyrolytic formation of PAHs. Environmental contamination may occur via contamination of food products by atmospheric fallout, accumulation of PAHs in seafood from polluted water, and uptake of PAHs by plants from contaminated soil. Some of the data on PAHs in foods have been compiled by Grasso and O'Hare (1976), as shown in Table 16. Polycyclic aromatic hydrocarbons can be found in processed or cooked foods and raw or unprocessed foods.

a. Polycyclic aromatic hydrocarbons in raw or unprocessed foods

The presence of PAHs in fresh vegetables has been demonstrated by a number of investigators. Grimmer and Hildebrandt (1965a) identified 13 PAHs (including B(a)P and dibenz(a,h)-anthracene) in lettuce, tomatoes, leek, cabbage, and spinach from various parts of Germany. The B(a)P concentration in these vegetables ranged from 2.85 to 24.5 μg/kg; cabbage and spinach were especially rich in PAHs. This finding has been confirmed by Gräf and Diehl (1966); in addition, presence of PAHs in food products manufactured or derived from plants has also been demonstrated. The source of PAHs in plants is not clear; biosynthesis, uptake from contaminated soil, and atmospheric fallout have all been suggested (see Sec. II.C.3). Despite the fairly widespread distribution of PAHs in vegetables, there is no indication that vegetarians have a higher cancer incidence that the rest of the population. However, in our view, such correlation, even if it exists, is unlikely to be demonstrated under nonlaboratory conditions. The increased intake of PAHs from vegetables by vegetarians is likely to be more than offset by their decreased intake of PAHs from cooked (especially smoked or grilled) meat products.

The contamination of seafood by polluted water has been discussed in the previous section (see also Table 15). The negative health consequences of polluted seafood on the general

TABLE 16 Polycyclic Aromatic Hydrocarbons in Foods

Foodstuff	Benzo(a)pyrene (μg/kg)	Benz(a)anthracene (μg/kg)
Fresh vegetables	2.85-24.5	0.3-43.6
Vegetable oils	0.4-1.4	0.8-1.1
Coconut oil	43.7	98.0
Margarine	0.4-0.5	1.4-3.0
Mayonnaise	0.4	2.2
Coffee	0.3-1.3	1.3-3.0
Tea	3.9	2.9-4.6
Grain	0.19-4.13	0.40-6.85
Oysters and mussels	1.5-9.0	—
Smoked ham	3.2	2.8
Smoked fish	0.83-8.5	1.9
Smoked bonito	37	189
Cooked sausage	12.5-18.8	17.5-26.2
Singed meat	35-99	28-79
Broiled meat	0.17-0.63	0.2-0.4
Charcoal-broiled steak	8.0	4.5
Broiled mackerel	0.9	2.9
Barbecued beef	3.3	13.2
Barbecued ribs	10.5	3.6

Source: Adapted from Grasso and O'Hare, 1976.

population have not been studied. However, it is likely that individuals on high seafood diet in polluted areas may be exposed to high amounts of PAHs.

Contamination of unprocessed cereal grains by PAHs has also been reported (Grimmer and Hildebrandt, 1965b; Tilgner, 1970); their origin may again be diverse. However, the finding of Tilgner that the PAH content of grain freshly harvested from fields close to industrial sites was about 10 times higher than that from rural areas suggests that atmospheric fallout of pollutants may be the major source of crop contamination in certain areas. Crop contamination is probably one of the chief contributors of PAHs in flour reported by various investigators.

b. Polycyclic aromatic hydrocarbons in processed foods

Food processing, especially those involving smoke, may give rise to PAHs through pyrolytic formation. In some cases the increase may be substantial.

Food products derived from plants may also contain carcinogenic PAHs. They have been detected in refined vegetable oils derived from soybean, cottonseed, corn, olive, and peanut. Crude coconut oil derived from smoke-dried copra contained B(a)P as high as 43.7 μg/kg (Grimmer and Hildebrandt, 1968); the high content of B(a)P may be partly caused by smoke-drying. The widespread presence of PAHs in vegetable oils helps to explain the presence of these chemicals in margarine and mayonnaise (Table 16).

Polycyclic aromatic hydrocarbons, including carcinogenic hydrocarbons, have been detected in the "coffee soots," a by-product in commercial roasting of coffee beans (Kuratsune and Hueper, 1958). An investigation of the PAH contents in four different commercial brands of roasted coffee beans has been carried out (Kuratsune and Hueper, 1960). In one of these brands (the most darkly roasted brand), small but measurable amounts of nine PAHs including B(a)P were detected. In two other brands of moderately dark roasted coffee, only pyrene and fluoranthene were identified, whereas no appreciable amounts of PAHs could be detected in another brand of darkly roasted coffee. The roasting procedure of the most darkly roasted brand was not described. The conditions favoring the formation of PAHs during roasting of coffee beans remains to be studied. Roasting of chicory-based coffee substitutes may also yield PAHs. Maier and Stender (1969) studied the effect of temperature on the production of B(a)P from chicory mixtures. When chicory mixtures were roasted for 30 min at temperatures from 50° to 240°C, the B(a)P content increased from 100°C on, with a sharp increase at 175°C and above. This finding is of particular interest in view of the fact that much higher temperatures are generally required for the pyrolytic formation of PAHs (see Sec. II.C.1); it is possible that some raw materials in the coffee substitutes may act as catalyst for PAH formation.

The effect of different drying methods on the B(a)P content in dried prunes was the subject of a study by Ruchkovskii et al. (1969). The use of California hot-air driers or tunnel driers yielded products containing the lowest amounts of B(a)P (1.1-1.5 μg/kg) which could be further reduced to 0.2 μg/kg by washing with a 0.03% detergent solution. In contrast, the B(a)P content was 15.5-16 μg/kg in prunes dried in an oven in which the fruit was exposed to smoke from wood burned in an open combustion chamber.

Native Japanese have an unusually high mortality rate from stomach cancer (50,000 deaths in 1976). In analyzing the dietary habits of the Japanese, Masuda and Kuratsune (1971) found that Japanese smoked fish (katsuobushi) contained high concentrations of B(a)P and other PAHs. They described the usual commercial preparation of katsuobushi as follows:

> A large piece of fresh meat of bonito is boiled, unboned, smoked by exposing to wood smoke intermittently for one or two weeks, cleaned, if necessary, by scraping the superficial tissue, dried carefully in the sun, and then stored in wooden boxes for about one week to let mold grow on the surface. These drying and molding processes are alternatively repeated a few times, yielding the final product, katsuobushi.

Of interest is that while katsuobushi may contain as high as 37 μg B(a)P/kg product, two other fish products, sababushi and urumebushi (which are prepared from mackerel or sardines by a similar but simplified process, shortening the smoking process and omitting the molding) contained only 7 and 2 μg/kg B(a)P, respectively. The possible biosynthesis of PAH by microorganisms during the molding process of katsuobushi should be explored. Katsuobushi is consumed frequently, and used for the flavoring of soups by the Japanese. A relatively high mortality rate from esophageal cancer has been recorded for males in the Kagoshima Prefecture where katsuobushi and similar products are produced and consumed in a large amount.

c. Polycyclic aromatic hydrocarbons in cooked foods

Cooking, especially grilling or smoking, may give rise to carcinogenic PAHs. A change in cooking habits could significantly reduce human exposure to PAHs in foods. Various reports on PAHs in cooked foods are summarized in Table 16. Lijinsky and Ross (1967) have extensively studied the conditions leading to the pyrolytic formation of PAHs during cooking. High temperatures, open flame, and high fat content of the food are the main conditions favoring PAH formation. Thus, after broiling, a hamburger with a high fat content could contain about 43 μg/kg of total PAHs including 2.6 μg/kg B(a)P. In contrast, lean hamburgers contained only 2.8 μg/kg total PAHs with no B(a)P. Cooking close to the flame gave rise to a higher content of PAHs than slow cooking away from heat sources. Separation of dripping fat from the flame is also effective in reducing PAH formation. Lijinsky and Shubik (1964, 1965) detected the presence of B(a)P and other PAHs in charcoal-broiled steak, especially in the outer surfaces of the steak with B(a)P concentrations of 5-50 μg/kg. These authors concluded that the pyrolysis of the fat dripping onto the hot coals led to the formation of PAHs. It is of interest to note that substantially lesser amounts of B(a)P could be detected in oven-broiled steaks. Thus, to minimize carcinogen formation due to cooking, Lijinsky and Ross (1967) concluded that "the method of cooking should be such as to avoid contact of the food with cooking flames, to cook for a longer period at lower temperatures and to use meat with a minimum of fat." In agreement with these conclusions, Rhee and Bratzler (1970) showed that wrapping meat in cellulose sheets prior to smoking could reduce the B(a)P concentrations in the final product from 11-12 μg/kg to 4.5 μg/kg. A similar reduction in B(a)P could also be achieved by discarding the fat released during the cooking of smoked bacon.

The effect of different methods of cooking on the formation of PAHs in German sausages has been studied by Fabian (1968). The total carcinogenic PAH level was 1.5 μg/kg before cooking. After pan frying, charcoal grilling, grilling over pine cones, and infrared grilling, the total carcinogenic PAH level was 7.4, 54.8, 88.5, and 0.17 μg/kg, respectively. The carcinogenic PAHs included B(a)P, benzo(b)fluoranthene, indeno(1,2,3-cd)pyrene, and benz(a)anthracene. It was concluded that the carcinogenic PAHs are formed pyrolytically and enter the sausages with smoke. In a similar study, Fritz (1973) measured the B(a)P contents in roast beef, pork chops, and sausages grilled on a conventional or camping grill over charcoal, paper, or pine cones. After grilling over charcoal, the B(a)P content was 8-12 μg/kg in sausages, 6-8 μg/kg in fat pork chops, 4.2-4.5 μg/kg in lean pork chops and 0.6-0.8 μg/kg in roast beef. Paper and pine cones caused considerably more contamination with B(a)P (between 18 and 140 μg/kg).

The effect of repeatedly heating cooking oil on the formation of carcinogenic compounds has been studied by Vysheslavova (1968) and O'Gara et al. (1969). The carcinogenicity of heated oil was tested by various routes of administration. The data were inconclusive; nevertheless the results "do suggest the advisability of avoiding the excessive reuse of cooking fats in the preparation of food for human consumption."

d. Polycyclic aromatic hydrocarbons due to packaging

Packaging of food may also be a potential source of food contamination by PAHs. Paraffin wax was used at one time for the coating of pasteboard food containers. Falk et al. (1958, 1959) showed that PAH contaminants present in the paraffin wax used for coating of milk containers can be eluted into the milk. Apparently, milk proteins can form complex with PAHs, thus facilitating the elution of PAH contaminants from paraffin. The use of paraffin for coating of milk containers was discontinued in the 1960s. However, paraffin coating is used presently for preventing cheeses from drying out.

E. Heterocyclic Aromatic Compounds

Replacement of carbon atom(s) of carcinogenic PAHs by heteroatoms such as nitrogen or sulfur gives rise to heterocyclic aromatic compounds; in many instances the heteroaromatics may retain most or all of the carcinogenic activity. In a few cases the carcinogenicity of the heteroaromatics may even be higher than that of the hydrocarbon analogs. Most of the

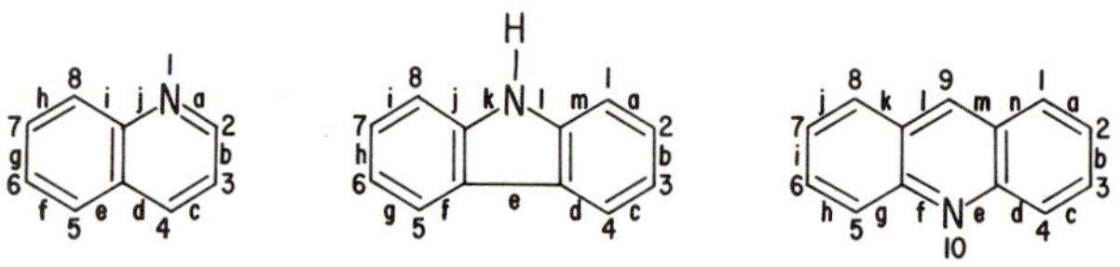

Quinoline Carbazole Acridine

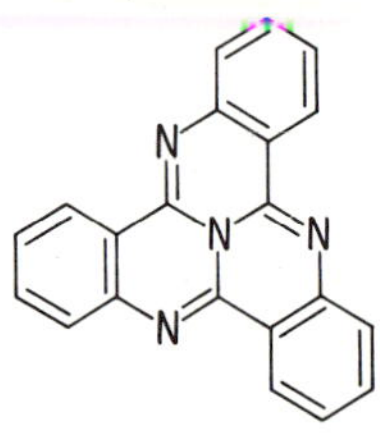

Tricycloquinazoline

FIGURE 9 Basic structural units of some aza-arenes.

TABLE 17 Concentration of the Major Aza-Arenes Present in the Suspended Particulate Matter of New York City's Atmosphere

Compound	Concentration ($ng/1000\ m^3$)	
	Sample 1	Sample 2
Quinoline	69	22
Methylquinolines	35	33
Dimethylquinolines	48	44
Isoquinoline	180	140
5- or 8-Methylisoquinoline	310	170
Other methylisoquinolines	76	70
Ethylisoquinolines	160	68
Benzo(f)quinoline	11	10
Benzo(h)quinoline	10	13
Benzo(f)isoquinoline	110	34
11 H-indeno(1,2-b)quinoline	Trace	Trace
Acridine	41	40

Source: Summarized from Dong et al., 1977.

heteroaromatics of environmental interest are nitrogen-containing compounds; they are known as aza-arenes. Several of the basic structural units of aza-arenes are shown in Fig. 9.

Aza-arenes are very similar to PAHs in many respects; pyrolytic formation of these compounds has also been observed. Sawicki et al. (1965) reported the presence of benzoquinolines in American urban atmosphere; the concentration was of the order of 0.2, 0.3, and 0.1 $\mu g/1000\ m^3$ for benzo(f)quinoline, benzo(h)quinoline, and 11 H-ideno(1,2-b)quinoline, respectively. Quinoline could not be detected in this study. A more recent investigation by Dong et al. (1977), however, found that quinoline, isoquinoline, and their alkyl derivatives were present at higher concentrations in urban atmosphere than benzoquinolines. Using newer techniques, Dong et al. (1977) were able to detect the presence of over 20 aza-arenes in the suspended particulate matter of New York City's atmosphere. Table 17 shows some of the quantitative data on atmospheric aza-arenes. The highest concentration was found to be associated with a methyl derivative of isoquinoline, identified as either 5-methyl or 8-methylisoquinoline. Quinoline has recently been found to be a liver carcinogen (Hirao et al., 1976).

Benzo- and dibenzo-derivatives of acridine were reported to be present in the American urban atmosphere. The concentrations ranged from 0.04 to 0.6 $\mu g/1000\ m^3$ air (Sawicki et al., 1965). Of these acridine compounds, only dibenz(a,h)acridine and dibenz(a,j)acridine have been clearly demonstrated to be carcinogenic by skin painting and s.c. injection; the Iball indexes are 11 and 29, respectively. Dibenzacridines are also present in tobacco smoke. The amount of dibenz(a,j)acridine present is of the order of 1 $\mu g/100$ cigarettes and trace amounts of dibenz(a,h)acridine can also be detected (Hoffmann and Wynder, 1976).

Trace amounts of dibenzo(c,g)carbazole are present in the cigarette smoke. Dibenzo-(c,g)carbazole has been found to be a strong carcinogen with Iball indexes (sarcoma and epithelioma) ranging from 25 to 73. The strong carcinogenicity of dibenzo(c,g)carbazole toward the respiratory system has also been demonstrated. High incidences (up to 89% of tumors of the respiratory tract can be induced by intratracheal instillations of the compound along with inert iron oxide particles. In fact, in some cases, the carcinogenicity of dibenzo-(c,g)carbazole is even higher than that of B(a)P emphasizing the fact that B(a)P is not the only strong carcinogen in the tobacco smoke (Sellakumar and Shubik, 1972).

Aza-arenes have also been found in recent marine sediments. Using mass spectrometric analysis, Blumer et al. (1977) have recently discovered complex series of aza-arenes with three- to eight-membered rings and with homologs containing alkyl substituents up to eight carbons. Their composition resembles that of the PAHs found in the same sediments. The authors postulated that these heteroaromatics are formed pyrolytically in forest and prairie fires, dispersed and mixed by air transport, and eventually deposited in the sediments. The environmental impact of these newly discovered series of aza-arenes remains to be elucidated.

Tricycloquinazoline is another aza-arene of environmental interest. Baldwin and associates (1959, 1965) have extensively studied the carcinogenicity and formation of this compound. Tricycloquinazoline is a moderately strong carcinogen with an Iball index of 40 (epithelioma). It can be readily formed by pyrolysis of derivatives of anthranilic acid, including methyl anthranilate, which has a wide occurrence in plants. The exceptional chemical stability of this compound and its sublimation temperature of 500-600°C suggest that substantial amounts of this compound could escape into the environment during combustion of plants.

III. NITROSAMINE CARCINOGENS

A. Introduction

1. Historical Note

N-Nitrosamines are secondary amines with the amino hydrogen replaced by a nitroso group. The first recognition that nitrosamines have an adverse effect in man is due to Freund (1937), who recorded the case histories of two chemists who became ill after heavy exposure to dimethylnitrosamine (DMN). One died shortly after the exposure. The findings at autopsy indicated liver necrosis and intense regenerative proliferation of cells in some areas of the liver. Experiments with mice and dogs exposed to DMN vapor confirmed these effects. However, the hepatotoxicity of DMN was not fully appreciated until the mid-fifties when severe liver damage occurred in several workers involved in the production of 1,1-dimethylhydrazine, a liquid rocket propellant. These toxic effects were again traced to DMN, an intermediate in the production of the propellant. Further investigations by Magee and Barnes (1956) revealed that DMN is not only toxic but also strongly carcinogenic in the rat, and a high incidence of liver tumors was induced by feeding low doses of the compound. The environmental significance of nitrosamines remained, however, unrecognized until the early sixties when an outbreak of poisoning occurred in sheep fed nitrite-preserved fish meal. A Norwegian report (Ender et al., 1964) identified DMN as the toxic substance and exemplified the ease of nitrosamine formation from its precursors, that is, secondary amines such as dimethylamine (abundant in fish meal) and nitrosating agents, such as nitrite. These findings stimulated intensive research and led to an important development in the field of chemical carcinogenesis. To date over a hundred N-nitrosamines, N-nitrosamides, and N-nitrosamidines (collectively called N-nitroso compounds) have been tested for carcinogenicity. The majority (over 75%) of these compounds have been found to be carcinogenic, inducing a variety of tumors in rats and many other species, including monkeys. The recent development of new analytical methods has enabled investigators to determine low levels of N-nitroso compounds more reliably. Measurable amounts of nitrosamines can be detected in a variety of foods, especially nitrite-preserved fish products and cured meats. Furthermore, N-nitroso compounds can be readily formed, both chemically and inside the human body, from precursors that are widely distributed in the environment. Despite the apparent lack of unequivocal epidemiological evidence of N-nitroso compounds as human carcinogens, the high potency of these compounds as experimental carcinogens, and their wide occurrence in the environment have prompted many investigators to assess their potential health hazard. The concern over nitrosamines as environmental carcinogens is reflected by the large number of recent reviews and symposia (Bogovski and Walker, 1975; Fiddler, 1975; Scanlan, 1975; Wogan and Tannenbaum, 1975; Issenberg, 1976; Preussmann, 1976; Chambon and Chambon, 1976; Magee et al., 1976; Fishbein, 1977; Mirvish, 1977).

2. Environmental Nitrosamines and Their General Properties

The principal types of carcinogenic nitrosamines encountered in the environment are depicted in Table 18. It is of interest to note that, in sharp contrast to PAHs, nitrosamines have very simple chemical structures.

The chemistry of N-nitroso compounds has been reviewed by Feuer (1970) and more recently by Magee et al. (1976). N-Nitrosamines are relatively stable in solution whereas N-nitrosamides readily decompose. Except for the dimethyl and diethyl derivatives, nitrosamines are quite insoluble in water, but soluble in many organic solvents. Most nitrosamines of environmental interest are volatile; however, little information is available on nonvolatile nitrosamines in the environment. The volatility of nitrosamines decreases with increasing alkyl carbon chain length. Nitrosamines are photosensitive, yielding secondary amines and nitrous acid. Reduction of nitrosamines gives rise to the corresponding hydrazine ($R_1R_2NNH_2$) or amines, whereas oxidation results in the formation of aldehyde and nitro compounds. Denitrosation of nitrosamines may take place in the presence of strong acids.

3. Analytical Methods

Accurate determination of minute amounts of nitrosamines (of the order of ng/kg or parts per billion, ppb) in environmental samples has proved to be a difficult task. Although a variety of methods has been developed, few can provide unambiguous identification and quantitative assay in the ppb range. Most of the methods either lack specificity or are susceptible to interference by extraneous materials. Thus, some of the data obtained by older methods, especially those prior to 1970, may be erroneous. The methodology for the determination of N-nitroso compounds was the subject of two symposia sponsored by the International Agency for Research on Cancer (IARC) (Bogovski et al., 1972b; Bogovski and Walker, 1975), and has been reviewed since then (Fiddler, 1975; Scanlan, 1975; Chambon and Chambon, 1976; Issenberg, 1976).

Nitrosamines present in environmental samples (mostly food products) can be separated from the bulk of the sample by solvent extraction or distillation. Dichloromethane has been used as the standard solvent. Samples may be extracted directly or digested in alkali-methanol before extraction. The distillation techniques used include steam, fractional, and vacuum distillation. Further purification and separation may be achieved by thin-layer, column, and gas or gas-liquid chromatography. A wide range of methods has been developed for the detection and estimation of nitrosamines. They may be divided into direct methods for the determination of intact nitrosamines and indirect methods for the determination of derivatives prepared from nitrosamines. The direct methods include: (1) quantitation of purified nitrosamines by polarography, and (2) gas or gas-liquid chromatographic separation followed by detection by conventional flame-ionization detector, or the more sensitive, nitrogen-specific thermionic or alkali flame-ionization detector, or Coulson electrolytic-conductivity detector, or the nitroso-compound-specific thermal energy analyzer (TEA), or mass spectrometry (MS). Gas chromatography-coupled MS and TEA have emerged as the current methods of choice. The indirect methods include: (1) separation of nitrosamines by thin-layer chromatography followed by hydrolysis (catalyzed by UV light or HBr) of nitrosamines to yield nitrous acid and secondary amines, which can be detected colorimetrically by spray reagents such as Griess reagent, ninhydrin, and so on, (2) oxidation of nitrosamines with trifluoroperacetic acid to yield nitramines which can be detected with a gas chromatography-electron capture detector, (3) reduction of nitrosamines to hydrazines and subsequent reaction with aromatic aldehydes to form hydrazones which can be separated and detected by various methods, and (4) reaction of the secondary amine (obtained by hydrolysis of nitrosamine) with 1-fluoro-2,4-dinitrobenzene, followed by separation of the derivative by liquid chromatography and detection. Systematic study of nonvolatile nitrosamines is still lacking; recent methods for the analysis of nonvolatile nitrosamines have been described (Walters et al., 1975; Fine and Rufeh, 1975).

TABLE 18 Carcinogenic N-Nitrosamines Encountered in the Environment

	Dialkylnitrosamines	Cycloalkylnitrosamines (cyclic nitrosamines)	Alkylacylnitrosamines (N-nitrosamides)
General formula:	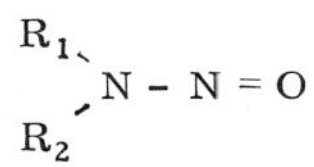	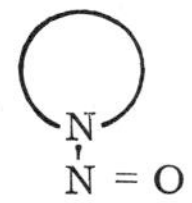	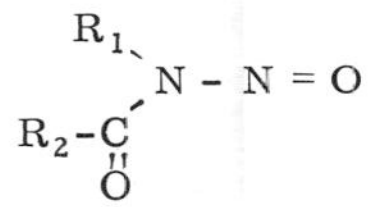
	N-nitrosodimethylamine (dimethylnitrosamine, DMN) $R_1 = R_2 = CH_3$	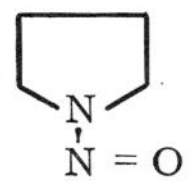 N-nitrosopyrrolidine	N-methyl-N-nitrosourea (methylnitrosourea) $R_1 = CH_3$; $R_2 = NH_2$
	N-nitrosodiethylamine (diethylnitrosamine, DEN) $R_1 = R_2 = C_2H_5$		N-ethyl-N-nitrosourea (ethylnitrosourea) $R_1 = C_2H_5$; $R_2 = NH_2$
	N-nitroso-di-n-propylamine (di-n-propylnitrosamine) $R_1 = R_2 = C_3H_7$	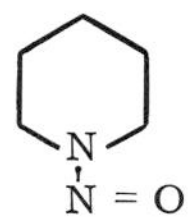 N-nitrosopiperidine	
	N-nitroso-di-n-butylamine (di-n-butylnitrosamine) $R_1 = R_2 = C_4H_9$		
	N-nitrosomethylethylamine (ethylmethylnitrosamine) $R_1 = CH_3$; $R_2 = C_2H_5$	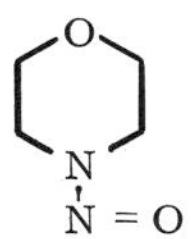 N-nitrosomorpholine	
	N-nitrosomethyl-n-butylamine (methyl-n-butylnitrosamine) $R_1 = CH_3$; $R_2 = C_4H_9$		

B. Carcinogenicity, Metabolism, and Mechanism of Action

1. Carcinogenicity

Nitrosamines are among the most potent and versatile carcinogens in experimental animals. They induce tumors in a wide variety of organs and tissues in a large number of animal species. The tissue(s) affected depend on (1) the structure of the compound, (2) the dosage, (3) the route of administration, and (4) the animal species. Druckrey (1973b) and Magee et al. (1976) have extensively reviewed the subject. The main organs affected are: the liver, kidney, lung, bladder, esophagus, stomach, intestine, nose, skin, tongue, brain, and the nervous system. In systematic studies with 65 nitrosamines, striking organotropic effects (i.e., selective induction of tumor in specific organ) dependent on the structure of the compound have been observed (Druckrey et al. 1967), especially toward the esophagus, the olfactory bulbs, and the urinary bladder. Dimethylnitrosamine, diethylnitrosamine (DEN), di-n-butylnitrosamine, methyl-alkyl-nitrosamines, N-nitrosopiperidine (NPiP), and alkylnitrosoureas are "model" compounds for the selective induction of tumors in kidney, liver, bladder, esophagus, ethmoturbinalia, and nervous system, respectively (Druckrey, 1973b). The doses administered range from 0.5 mg/kg for i.v. injection to 400 mg/kg for subcutaneous injection. The effect of dosage may be exemplified by DMN which induces kidney tumors in the rat, when given in single large doses (30 mg/kg), but induces predominantly liver tumors when given in small doses over an extended period of time. Oral administration of DEN to Syrian golden hamsters induces mainly liver tumors, whereas subcutaneous injections induce mainly respiratory tumors (Montesano and Saffiotti, 1970). An interesting example of species specificity is the cyclic nitrosamine, N-nitrosoazetidine, which induces tumors of the liver and other organs in rats and mice but does not have any carcinogenic effect in hamsters (Lijinsky et al., 1970).

N-Nitroso compounds have been extensively used in studies of transplacental carcinogenesis. N-Nitrosamides have been shown to be potent transplacental carcinogens inducing predominantly neurogenic tumors in the offspring and rendering the offspring more susceptible to the carcinogens in subsequent postnatal exposure. Using ethylnitrosourea, Ivankovic and Druckrey (1968) have demonstrated that the time of exposure during gestation is the critical factor in transplacental carcinogenesis. In BD rats neurogenic tumors could be observed in the offspring if the fetuses are exposed to a single dose of the carcinogen at the 15th day of gestation, with high incidence among those exposed at the 18th day of gestation and shortly before birth. The dose sufficient to show carcinogenic response may be as low as 2 mg/kg, which is about 50 times lower than that for adult rats (Druckrey et al., 1969). Sprague-Dawley and Long-Evans rats are even more susceptible than BD rats. Dimethylnitrosamine and DEN have also been shown to display transplacental carcinogenic effects in a number of animal species; the period of administration is usually limited to the last days of gestation for obtaining a positive response. As we discuss in the next section, nitrosamines must be metabolically activated to exert their carcinogenic action; presumably, the enzymes required for activation are not fully developed until the last days of gestation. The transplacental carcinogenesis by N-nitroso compounds has been extensively discussed by Druckrey (1973a,b) and Magee et al. (1976).

The structure-activity relationship of nitroso compounds is much simpler than that of PAHs. The majority of the compounds tested have proved to be carcinogenic. As mentioned earlier, there is striking organotropic effect dependent on chemical structure (Druckrey et al., 1967). All symmetrically substituted dialkylnitrosamines tested so far produce liver tumors. The di-n-butyl and di-n-amyl derivatives also produce bladder tumors and pulmonary tumors, respectively. Asymmetric dialkylnitrosamines, especially those with a methyl group as one of the alkyl groups, induce predominantly cancer of the esophagus. Of the cyclic nitrosamines N-nitrosopyrrolidine (NPy) induces mainly liver tumors, whereas NPiP shows organotropic effect toward the esophagus in the rat. Several nitrosamines in Druckrey's studies were found to be noncarcinogenic. They include the methyl-tert-butyl, ethyl-tert-butyl, diallyl, dicyclohexyl, dibenzyl, and diphenyl derivatives, and two cyclic nitrosamines, which may be derived from proline ethylester and trimethylene triamine. The lack of carcinogenic activity of these compounds may be due to electronic factors unfavorable for hydroxylation at the carbon atom, which is adjacent to the nitrogen atom of the nitroso group (α-carbon). Hydroxylation at the α-carbon has been postulated to be the first step for the bioactivation of nitrosamines. Systematic studies on the carcinogenicity of cyclic nitrosamines have been carried out by Lijinsky and others. In general, their findings are consistent with the α-hydroxylation requirement: for example, α-deuterium substitution of 4-nitrosomorpholine leads to the reduction of carcinogenicity of the compound (Lijinsky et al., 1976); also, all the methylated dinitrosopiperazine derivatives are carcinogenic, except the tetramethylated derivative, which has no hydrogen atom on the α-carbon (Lijinsky and Taylor, 1977).

2. Metabolism and Mechanism of Action

The metabolism and possible mechanisms of action of N-nitroso compounds have been extensively discussed by various authors (Magee and Barnes, 1967; Krüger, 1972; Magee, 1972; Lawley, 1972; Druckrey, 1973b; Magee et al., 1976). Both nitrosamines and nitrosamides are believed to initiate carcinogenesis by binding covalently to cellular macromolecules such as DNA, RNA, and proteins. The processes leading to the generation of reactive intermediates (believed to be carbonium ions) are, however, different. Nitrosamides spontaneously decompose in aqueous solution to yield carbonium ions, as exemplified with methylnitrosourea in Fig. 10. The rate of decomposition is substantially higher in the presence of alkali or a number of heavy metal ions such as Cu^{2+} or Ni^{2+} (Preussmann et al., 1975). On the other hand, nitrosamines must first be metabolically activated. The postulated metabolic pathway of DMN is depicted in Fig. 10. Hydroxylation at the α-carbon is believed to be the critical first step. The putative α-hydroxylated DMN is extremely unstable and yields, upon hydrolysis, formaldehyde, and monomethylnitrosamine. The overall reaction is N-demethylation. Monomethylnitrosamine, in turn, undergoes rearrangement to give rise to methyldiazonium hydroxide and eventually to the reactive carbonium ion (methonium ion). The metabolic activation of DEN is also believed to proceed via α-hydroxylation, leading eventually to the formation of ethonium ion as the alkylating species.

However, an alternative mechanism involving β-oxidation of DEN has been suggested (Fahmy and Fahmy, 1976). Indeed, di-n-propylnitrosamine appeared to be metabolized mainly via β-oxidation in in vivo studies (Krüger, 1972; Krüger and Bertram, 1973); yet, carcinogenicity studies of putative β-oxidized metabolites could not establish β-oxidation as the activating pathway for di-n-propylnitrosamine (Althoff et al., 1977). Under in vitro conditions, α-hydroxylation was found to be the predominant pathway for the metabolism of di-n-propylnitrosamine (Park et al., 1977; cf., Arcos et al., 1976). The extent of in vitro dealkylation of DMN, DEN, and di-n-propylnitrosamine, via α-oxidation, increases with the alkyl chain length (Arcos et al., 1976). The in vivo metabolism of di-n-butylnitrosamine may occur at the terminal carbon (ω-oxidation) as well as at the α- or β-carbon. There is some evidence that ω-oxidation leads to reactive intermediate(s) responsible for tumor induction in the urinary bladder, whereas α-oxidation may generate metabolites for the induction of liver tumors (Okada et al., 1976). The metabolic activation of cyclic nitrosamine is not clearly understood. The first step may involve hydroxylation either at the α- or the β-carbon (Krüger and Bertram, 1975; Krüger et al., 1976; Ross and Mirvish, 1977), and there is some evidence that the ring may be opened during metabolism.

It has been known for some years that the enzymes involved in the metabolism of DMN (DMN-demethylase(s)) and other nitrosamines are present in the endoplasmic reticulum (microsomes) of mammalian cells. In vitro studies have firmly established that the metabolism of DMN requires the presence of microsomes, NADPH, and oxygen, and may be inhibited by carbon monoxide. These and some other characteristics have led many investigators to conclude that microsomal mixed-function oxidases (MFOs) are solely responsible for the metabolic activation of DMN. Recently, however, there is increasing evidence that DMN demethylase(s) may differ from typical MFOs in several aspects and that the metabolic activation of DMN may be more complex than has hitherto been postulated. Studies by Lake

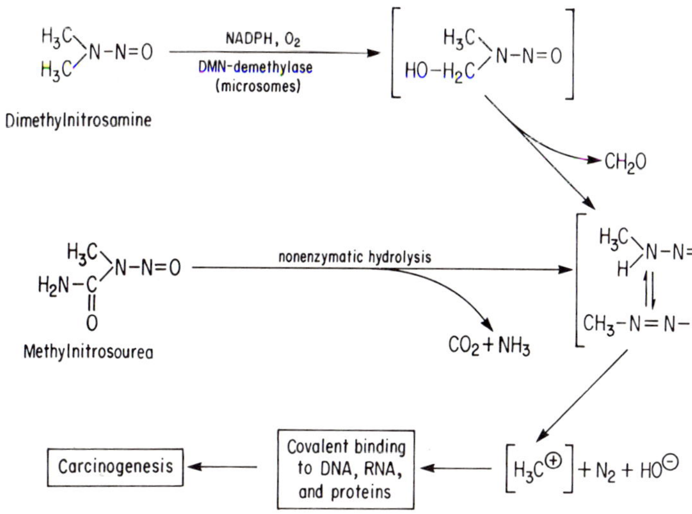

FIGURE 10 Postulated mechanism of formation of carbonium ion proximate carcinogen from dimethylnitrosamine and methylnitrosourea.

et al. (1974), Arcos et al. (1977), and Sipes et al. (1978) have revealed that there are apparently two or more enzymic forms of DMN demethylase with different kinetic properties (K_m and V_{max}) in the rat liver. Pretreatment of rats with classical inducers of MFOs (e.g., Aroclor 1254, 3-methylcholanthrene, phenobarbital) repress the enzyme activity at low substrate concentrations but enhance the activity at high concentrations (Arcos et al., 1977; Sipes et al., 1978). A number of typical inhibitors of MFOs (e.g., SKF 525A, metapyrone) appear to have little or no effect on DMN demethylase; however, a wide variety of compounds (e.g., pyrazole, disulfiram, alcohols) that have no effect on MFOs may significantly inhibit DMN demethylation (Phillips et al., 1977). Furthermore, a number of recent findings have seriously questioned the validity of the hypothesis that DMN demethylase(s) may be solely responsible for the generation of carcinogenic and/or toxic reactive intermediates. Friedman and Sanders (1976) found that piperonyl butoxide significantly inhibits the demethylation of DMN without affecting its acute toxicity or covalent binding to nucleic acids. The investigations of Sipes et al. (1978) suggest that the extent of binding of DMN to macromolecules may not be directly related to activity of DMN demethylase. Argus et al. (1978) demonstrated that β-naphthoflavone substantially inhibits DMN demethylase activity but markedly enhances (rather than decreases) the hepatocarcinogenicity of DMN in the rat. These findings have led various investigators (Lake et al., 1974; Phillips et al., 1977; Argus et al., 1978) to conclude that the metabolic activation of nitrosamines is more complex than has hitherto been postulated. Further investigations are needed to delineate the mechanism.

Covalent binding of reactive intermediates of carcinogens to cellular macromolecules has generally been considered as the mechanism of initiating carcinogenesis by most chemical agents. Covalent binding of DMN to nucleic acids of rat liver was first demonstrated in vivo by Magee and Farber (1962). Since then, a variety of reports has appeared showing the covalent binding of various nitrosamides and dialkylnitrosamines to macromolecules under both in vivo and in vitro conditions. Magee (1972), Magee et al., (1976), and Lawley (1972) have extensively reviewed the literature on binding of nitroso compounds and discussed its significance. The main site of alkylation in nucleic acids by alkylnitroso compounds is the N-7 position of guanine. Alkylation at other sites has also been observed; they include the O-6 and N-3 positions of guanine, N-1, N-3, and N-7 positions of adenine, and N-3 position of cytosine, thymine, and uracil. Alkylation at the O-6 position of guanine has been considered as the reaction most likely to be involved in carcinogenesis and mutagenesis (Loveless, 1969; Lawley, 1972). An alternative to the alkylation hypothesis has been proposed by Schoental (1973) who suggested that the reactive intermediate of dialkylnitrosamines may be their oxidation product. Oxidation products which still retain the alkylnitrosamino moiety but have become multifunctional (e.g., with carbonyl group at one end and nitroso group at the other end) may be formed by β- or ω-oxidation of an alkyl group. Schoental (1973) postulated that such an intermediate may form a cross linking bridge between an amino group of nucleic acid base and a thiol group of a protein chain in vicinity, to lead eventually to infidelity of nucleic acid replication.

C. Formation

Nitrosamines are normally present in trace amounts in the environment; however, the precursors capable of forming nitrosamines and other nitroso compounds are ubiquitous and abundant in the environment. Nitrosamines may readily arise in a wide variety of conditions: in preserved foods, inside the mammalian body, in sewage and soil, and so on. The rate of formation may be affected by a variety of chemicals and microorganisms. A clear understanding of the mechanisms underlying the formation of these compounds is of the utmost importance for assessing the extent of human exposure.

1. Chemistry of Nitrosamine Formation

The literature on the chemistry of nitrosamine formation is voluminous. A number of recent symposia (Bogovski et al., 1972b; Bogovski and Walker, 1975) and reviews (Mirvish, 1972, 1975, 1977; Sander et al., 1975c; Wogan and Tannenbaum, 1975; Magee et al., 1976) have dealt extensively with this subject. Essentially, the overall nitrosation reaction may be represented by the following equation:

$$\underset{(\text{e.g., } HNO_2)}{\text{Nitrosating agent}} + \underset{(\text{e.g., } R_2NH)}{\text{nitrosatable amino compound}} \rightarrow \underset{(\text{e.g., } R_2NNO)}{\text{nitroso compound}} + \underset{(H_2O)}{\text{water}}$$

a. The nitrosating agents

A variety of chemical agents that are related to nitrous acid and have the structure NOX (where X = halogen, NO_2, NO_3, tetrafluoroborate, O-alkyl, or OH_2^+, etc.) is capable of serving as nitrosating agent. The actual nitrosating species may, however, be different and is dependent on the experimental conditions and the type of substrate involved. In aqueous solution, the nitrosating species generated from nitrous acid may appear as NO^+ (nitrosyl cation), $H_2NO_2^+$ (nitrous acidium ion), or N_2O_3 (nitrous anhydride or dinitrogen trioxide), depending on the acidity of the solution (Sander et al., 1975c). Under the most widely studied, mildly acidic conditions (pH 1-5), N_2O_3 has been generally accepted to be the nitrosating species in nitrosamine formation.

The nitrosation reaction in aqueous solution is not limited to acidic conditions, however. Challis and Kyrtopoulos (1977) have recently found that substantial amount of nitrosamines can be formed in alkaline solutions containing secondary amines by injecting nitrogen oxide gas. A free radical mechanism with NO and NO_2 radicals as reactive species has been proposed. Formation of nitrosamines by reaction of dialkylamines with nitrogen oxides in the gas phase has been observed and the reactive species has been considered to be N_2O_3 (Neurath, 1972) or NO_2 (Gehlert and Rolle, 1977).

b. The nitrosatable amino compounds

A variety of nitrogenous compounds may be nitrosated to yield nitroso compounds. In chemical terms, they include amines, amides, guanidines, polyamines, and amino acids. In terms of their occurrence and usage, they include drugs (Lijinsky, 1974; Rao and Krishna, 1975), pesticides (Sen et al., 1975), agricultural chemicals (Eisenbrand et al., 1975), natural substances of foodstuffs and tobacco (Singer and Lijinsky, 1976a, b), and constituents and metabolites of the human body.

Amines are the most extensively studied nitrosatable compounds. Secondary amines readily react with nitrosating agents under acidic conditions to yield nitrosamines; tertiary and quaternary amines, following dealkylation, may also serve as substrates for nitrosation. Since the nitrosation reaction involves an electrophilic attack by the nitrosating species on the lone pair of electrons of the nitrogen atom, only unprotonated amine molecules may serve as substrates. The reactivity of the secondary amine toward nitrosation is therefore inversely correlated with its basicity (Mirvish, 1975). Strongly basic amines (with high pK_a) have less tendency to be nitrosated than weakly basic amines. Steric hindrance may also play a role in the nitrosation; for example, Jones et al. (1974) showed that methyl substitutions of piperidine at the carbon atom α to the nitrogen substantially decreases the rate of nitrosation.

c. The kinetics of nitrosation reactions

Most of the kinetic studies of nitrosation reactions in aqueous solutions have been carried out under mildly acidic conditions using nitrite as the nitrosating agent. The details of the findings have been reviewed by Mirvish (1975) and Sander et al. (1975c). Secondary amines are nitrosated according to the equations:

$$2NO_2^- + 2H^+ \rightleftarrows 2HNO_2 \rightleftarrows N_2O_3 + H_2O \quad (1)$$

$$R_2NH + N_2O_3 \rightarrow R_2NNO + HNO_2 \quad (2)$$

The rate of nitrosation is therefore proportional to the concentration of the amine and the square of the concentration of nitrite, and can be expressed by the equation: rate = k(amine)(nitrite)^2. The rate constant k is pH dependent and is maximal at the optimum pH of nitrosation. The optimum pH and the rate constant of a number of amines are shown in Table 19. Amides appear to be nitrosated by nitrous acidium ions and the rate follows the equation: rate = k(amide)(nitrite)(H^+).

d. Catalysis of nitrosation

A large number of chemicals, including anions, aldehydes, surfactants, and nitrosophenols, are capable of catalyzing the nitrosation of amino compounds.

Anions It has been known for years that various anions catalyze nitrosation (Ridd, 1961). This subject is receiving increasing attention since thiocyanate, an anion of physiological significance, has been clearly shown to be a potent catalyst (Boyland et al., 1971). Thiocyanate is found in the human saliva and its concentration is affected by smoking and diet. Thiocyanate is believed to play an important role in the in vivo formation of nitrosamines (Boyland and Walker, 1975). The mechanism and kinetics of anion catalysis have been extensively studied by Fan and Tannenbaum (1973a), Mirvish et al. (1973), Boyland and Walker

TABLE 19 Rate Constants for the Nitrosation of Amines at the Optimum pH and 25° C

Amine	pK_a	Optimum pH	k (M/sec)
Piperidine	11.2	3.0	0.00045
Dimethylamine	10.7	3.4	0.0017
Pyrrolidine	11.3	3.0	0.0053
N-methylethanolamine	9.5	3.2	0.01
N-methylbenzylamine	9.5	3.0	0.013
Morpholine	8.7	3.4	0.42
Mononitrosopiperazine	6.8	3.0	6.7
Aminopyrine	5.0	2.0	80
Piperazine	5.6	3.0	83

Source: Adapted from Mirvish, 1975.

(1975), and Schweinsberg (1975). Anions catalyze nitrosation by reacting with nitrous acid to form an active nitrosating intermediate, NOX, where X = SCN^-, halides, acetate, or other anions. The pH optimum of nitrosation is generally lowered in the presence of thiocyanate. The effectiveness of anion as catalyst follows the order: $I^- > SCN^- >> Br^- > Cl^-$ (Ridd, 1961; Boyland et al., 1971).

Aldehydes It has been generally accepted that nitrite must be protonated to nitrous acid to generate active nitrosating species. Keefer and Roller (1973), however, have demonstrated that under certain conditions, nitrite itself can serve as nitrosating species. These authors showed that, in the presence of formaldehyde (HCHO) or chloral (CCl_3CHO), nitrosamines can be formed from amine and nitrite in neutral or basic aqueous solutions. It has been proposed that formaldehyde catalyzes nitrosation by reacting with amine to form an unstable cation [e.g., $(R_2N - CH_2)^+$] intermediate, which can then be directly nitrosated by nitrite ions. The significance of this finding is that formaldehyde can be found in the environment. It is used as a germicide and fungicide for plants, and in combination with nitrite, as a preservative for fish. Furthermore, it is formed during incomplete combustion of many organic substances and is especially abundant in smoke used for smoking ham and fish.

Surfactants Surfactants are among the recently discovered catalysts of nitrosation. Okun and Archer (1977) showed that the nitrosation of dialkylamines can be enhanced in the presence of surfactants such as decyltrimethylammonium bromide (a cationic surfactant), Triton X-100, or lecithin. The nitrosation of dihexylamine can be enhanced up to 800-fold by the cationic surfactant under optimal condition. It has been suggested that amine molecules form micelles with their hydrophobic hydrocarbon chains buried in the interior of the micelles. Electrostatic interactions between the positive groups at the micellar surface would then lead to destabilization of protonated amine molecules and increase in nitrosatable unprotonated amine. This finding is intriguing in view of the fact that many micelle-forming surfactants, especially lecithin, are present in various biological systems including food materials and the human alimentary tract. Their possible effect on nitrosamine formation during food processing, storage, and digestion remains to be elucidated.

Nitrosophenols Nitrosophenols are also potent catalysts of nitrosation (Davies and McWeeny, 1977). This subject is further discussed in Sec. III.C.1.f.

In addition to chemicals, temperature may have a significant effect on nitrosamine formation. The formation of N-nitrosomorpholine from morpholine and nitrite is increased by freezing, due to concentration of reactants (Fan and Tannenbaum, 1973b). High temperatures, especially in the pyrolytic range, may also promote nitrosamine formation; for example, the formation of nitrosopyrrolidine in fried bacon is dependent on the temperature of frying (see Sec. III.D.3.b).

e. Inhibition of nitrosation

Chemicals capable of reacting with nitrosating agents at a faster rate than amines are potential inhibitors of the nitrosation of amines. A number of physiologically important chemicals are potent inhibitors.

Ascorbic acid (vitamin C) has long been used as an antioxidant in foodstuffs. The finding by Mirvish et al. (1972b) and Fiddler et al. (1973) that ascorbate inhibits the formation of nitroso compounds has stirred considerable interest in incorporating the vitamin into foodstuffs and drugs so as to minimize possible nitrosamine formation. The mechanism of inhibition by ascorbate is believed to be a competition with amines or amides for the available nitrosating agent; an excess of ascorbate is usually needed for effective blocking (Mirvish et al., 1972b; Fan and Tannenbaum, 1973c; Sen and Donaldson, 1975). The effectiveness of ascorbate to inhibit nitrosamine formation is dependent on (1) the pH, (2) the reactivity of amine towards nitrosation, and (3) the extent of oxygenation of the system. Ascorbate anion is nitrosated about 240 times more rapidly than ascorbic acid. Highly reactive amines (e.g., N-methylaniline) successfully compete with ascorbate for the nitrosating agent. Oxygen depletes ascorbate by oxidation and, thus, the blocking effect of ascorbate is substantially diminished by oxygenation (Archer et al., 1975).

In addition to ascorbate and its derivatives, glutathione (Sen and Donaldson, 1975), urea and ammonium sulfamate (Mirvish et al., 1972b), an unidentified component of milk (Fan and Tannenbaum, 1973c), sodium sulfite and cysteine (Mirvish, 1975), and some phenolic compounds have been shown to inhibit nitrosation by competing for the available nitrosating agent.

f. Phenolic compounds

Phenolic compounds have a wide occurrence in the environment; they include some common constituents of the human body (e.g., epinephrine, tyrosine) and are present in human foods and beverages. Phenolic compounds are very reactive toward nitrosating agents. For example, phenol reacts with nitrite 10,000 times faster than dimethylamine (Challis, 1973). Thus, phenolic compounds are expected to be strong inhibitors of nitrosamine formation; this is in fact the case for tannins, which is a family of phenolic compounds commonly found in tea, beer, and apple juice. Tannins markedly inhibit the nitrosation of dimethylamine and diethylamine (Bogovski et al., 1972a), and morpholine and piperazine (Mirvish, 1975). Similarly, gallic acid, which is a hydrolysis product of tannins, is also inhibitory (Mirvish, 1975). However, under some conditions gallic acid may catalyze nitrosation rather than inhibit it (Walker et al., 1975). Chlorogenic acid and 4-methylcatechol are also catalysts rather than inhibitors (Challis and Bartlett, 1975). These apparently conflicting results can probably be explained by a recent finding of Davies and McWeeny (1977). These authors showed that the initial nitrosation product of phenol is nitrosophenol. This relatively unstable intermediate, nitrosophenol (which can be further oxidized to the final stable product, nitrophenol), has been found to be a potent catalyst of nitrosamine formation. It has been proposed that in a system containing nitrite, a phenol, and a secondary amine, the rate of nitrosamine formation will be retarded by the phenol but enhanced by the unstable nitrosophenol. The overall effect is dependent on the steady-state concentration of the nitrosophenol and the relative degrees of retardation and enhancement exerted by the phenol and the nitrosophenol, respectively.

2. In Vivo Formation of Nitrosamines

The ease of nitrosamine formation in in vitro systems has caused considerable concern over the potential health hazard of human exposure to nitrosamine precursors widely present in the environment. Druckrey et al. (1963) and Sander (1967) first suggested that nitroso compounds might be formed from precursors under the acidic conditions of the human stomach. Since then a variety of reports has appeared supporting the hypothesis. In addition, with the finding by Sander (1968) that bacteria could catalyze nitrosation of amines at neutral pH, the potential site of in vivo formation of nitrosamines has been extended to include any site where secondary amines, nitrate/nitrite, and bacteria can coexist. There is now little doubt that nitroso compounds can be formed inside the mammalian body. The formation is nonenzymatic in the normal stomach and may be catalyzed by bacteria in other sites such as the urinary bladder, intestines, and vagina (Mirvish, 1975, 1977; Sander et al., 1975c).

Studies on the formation of nitroso compounds in the mammalian stomach include (1) in vitro formation under simulated stomach conditions, (2) analysis of the stomach contents, and (3) carcinogenic or toxic effects of concurrent administration of nitrites and amines or amides.

The demonstration of nitrosamine formation from precursors under simulated stomach conditions was first achieved by Sander (1967) using human gastric juice. A more detailed study by Sen et al. (1969) confirmed the finding; in addition, they found that rabbits and cats may be more suitable test species because of the pH of their gastric juice closely matches that of humans. The optimum pH for nitrosation of dimethylamine in human gastric juice is 2.5 (instead of 3.4 in an in vitro system), and the presence of thiocyanate is the apparent cause of the lower pH (Lane and Bailey, 1973).

The in vivo formation of nitroso compounds can also be demonstrated by analyzing the stomach contents of animals fed precursors. Mirvish and Chu (1973), for example, detected nitrosoalkylureas in the stomach contents of rats given nitrite and alkylureas. In vivo formation of nitrosamines in rat stomach has also been observed (Sander et al., 1975a). However, these authors pointed out that the amount of nitroso compound detected in the stomach contents merely represented the difference between its formation and its disappearance from the stomach (through absorption and degradation) and was subject to substantial variations caused by a number of factors such as differences in local concentrations of precursors, acid secretion, and the presence of catalysts or inhibitors in the stomach.

Carcinogenesis and liver necrosis are the biological responses of experimental animals to chronic and acute administration of precursors, respectively. In most cases, the biological effect observed may be attributed to the formation of nitroso compounds in the stomach. The literature on carcinogenesis by long-term feeding of precursors has been reviewed (Sander et al., 1975c; Mirvish, 1975), and some correlation between the in vitro and in vivo formation may be seen. Of the many amino compounds tested, secondary amines of low or moderate basicity, which react well in vitro, were shown to induce tumors when fed concurrently with nitrite to rodents. These amine compounds include morpholine, piperazine, N-methylaniline (Greenblatt et al., 1971; Sander et al., 1975c), N-methylbenzylamine (Sander et al., 1975c), aminopyrine and oxytetracycline (Taylor and Lijinsky, 1975). A variety of alkylureas are also carcinogenic when given together with nitrite, inducing tumors in both adult animals (Mirvish et al., 1972a; Rustia, 1974) and offspring (Druckrey, 1973a, b; Magee et al., 1976). With some exceptions, the in vivo formation of nitroso compounds, as measured by tumor yield, is roughly in qualitative agreement with the kinetic data (Mirvish, 1972, 1975). Dose-response studies of the carcinogenicity of nitrite plus piperazine (Greenblatt et al., 1972) or morpholine (Shank and Newberne, 1976) showed that the tumor yield was affected to a greater extent by the concentration of nitrite than by the concentration of the amine, consistent with the in vitro nitrosation kinetics.

In addition to the stomach, in vivo nitrosation at three other sites has been proposed: the intestine (Alam et al., 1971; Hashimoto et al., 1976), the infected urinary bladder (Hawksworth and Hill, 1971, 1974), and the infected vagina (Harrington et al., 1973; Allsobrook et al., 1975). At all these sites bacteria may play an important role in the nitrosation by generating precursors and possibly by catalyzing the nitrosation reaction. This subject is further discussed in the next section. Another potential site of in vivo nitrosation that has been virtually unexplored is the lung. It is well known that nitrogen dioxide, a potential nitrosating agent, can be found in cigarette smoke and in polluted urban air. The possible link between nitrogen dioxide and lung cancer through nitrosamine formation remains to be studied.

3. Bacterial Catalysis of Nitrosamine Formation

Bacteria may play an important role in the in vivo formation of nitrosamines as well as in foodstuffs, sewage, and soil. Bacteria contribute to the formation of nitrosamines in nature by (1) producing nitrite by reduction of nitrate or oxidation of ammonia, (2) converting tertiary amines to secondary amines, and (3) catalyzing nitrosation of amines by nitrite.

Evidence implicating bacterial involvement in nitrosamine formation was first provided by Sander (1968). He demonstrated that several genera of nitrate-reducing bacteria catalyzed the nitrosation of some amines by nitrite under conditions (neutral solutions) that did not permit spontaneous chemical reaction to any significant extent. This finding has since been confirmed in many laboratories using various intestinal bacteria (e.g., Klubes et al., 1972; Hill and Hawksworth, 1972). In vitro formation of DMN from dimethylamine and nitrate has also been demonstrated using some intestinal bacteria (Thacker and Brooks, 1974; Hashimoto et al., 1975). Bacteria in the infected urinary bladder (*Escherichia coli*) were shown to catalyze nitrosamine formation (Hill et al., 1973; Hawksworth and Hill, 1974), whereas *Trichomonas vaginalis* was the prime suspect responsible for the presence of nitrosamines in the human vaginal vault (Allsobrook et al., 1975). The exact in vivo implication of bacterial involvement in nitrosamine formation is not clear. Considering the possibility of coexistence of nitrate, amine, and bacteria, Hill and Hawksworth (1972) have proposed that in humans bacterial involvement may be significant in infected urinary bladder and the stomach of achlorhydric patients. The hypoacidity of achlorhydric stomachs allows the growth of bacteria that could generate nitrites from dietary nitrates. The possible relationship between dietary nitrate and gastric cancer has been discussed (Hill et al., 1973; Hawksworth et al., 1975).

Bacteria in foodstuffs may also be involved in nitrosamine production. Collins-Thompson et al. (1972), for example, showed that several Streptococcus species (which may be isolated from some meat products) catalyze nitrosation. The catalysis is probably due to bacterial metabolites. Fong and Chan (1973b) found that innoculation of fish broth with Staphylococcus aureus (present in contaminated salted fish) substantially increases the production of DMN. Storage conditions, the degree of bacterial contamination, and the amount of precursors present are key factors in determining the contamination of foodstuffs by nitrosamines.

The possible microbial contribution to nitrosamine formation in sewage and soil has been studied by Ayanaba et al. (1973a). Microorganisms in sewage convert trimethylamine to dimethylamine, reduce nitrate to nitrite, and catalyze the formation of DMN. Within the pH range of 4-7, both the dealkylation and nitrosation reactions are higher at neutral pH than acidic pH, strongly suggesting that microorganisms catalyze DMN formation not only by producing the precursors, but also by catalyzing the nitrosation reaction itself.

D. Sources, Occurrence, and Exposure

Nitroso compounds and their precursors are widely distributed in the environment. There is now sufficient evidence to indicate that nitroso compounds represent a serious potential health hazard, although the magnitude of this hazard remains to be established. Exposure of the general population to nitroso compounds and their precursors is mainly via ingestion; however, in some cases inhalation may become the major route of exposure.

1. Nitrosamines and Nitrogen Oxides in the Air

The incidence of "urban cancer," especially that of lung cancer, has been increasing at an alarming rate in the past two decades. As discussed in the previous section, PAHs have been strongly implicated as the causative agents. However, existing evidence indicates that it is unlikely that PAHs can be solely responsible for these increases. A number of other environmental chemical carcinogens have been considered and nitrosamines have emerged as a prime suspect (Shapley, 1976). The general population may be directly or indirectly exposed to nitrosamines via (1) nitrosamines in the air, (2) nitrogen oxides in the air, and (3) both nitrosamines and nitrogen oxides in tobacco smoke.

a. Nitrosamines in ambient air

It has been generally assumed earlier that insignificant amounts of nitrosamines (which are photosensitive) are present in the air. Recently, however, careful studies by Fine et al. (1976a, b) have revealed that exceptionally high atmospheric concentrations of DMN can be detected in at least some areas of two U.S. cities, Baltimore, Md. and Bell, W. Va. In the immediate vicinity of a chemical factory at Baltimore which manufactures rocket fuel, for which DMN is an intermediate, atmospheric DMN concentrations as high as 1000-36,000 ng/m^3 air were detected. Atmospheric DMN was also detected in the Baltimore area (3-320 ng/m^3) upwind of the rocket fuel factory and in the Belle area (5-170 ng/m^3). The potential DMN sources in these areas included industrial users of amines and combustion products of stationary and nonstationary sources. Detection of DMN in the ambient air (0.001 to 0.43 ppb) of a German amine factory has also been reported (Bretschneider and Matz, 1973). The peak DMN value was dependent on the concentration of ambient nitrogen dioxide. Nitrosation of the amine in the air was the most likely mechanism. Formation of DEN by reaction of diethylamine with nitrogen dioxide can be demonstrated experimentally (Gehlert and Rolle, 1977). No significant amounts of DMN could be detected in air samples from other U.S. cities: Philadelphia, Pa., Wilmington, Del., and Waltham, Mass.

The finding of the presence of DMN in the ambient air of some U.S. cities has caused considerable concern, especially because the amount of DMN was quite large when compared to other airborne carcinogens such as B(a)P. Apparently, DMN and possibly some other volatile carcinogenic nitrosamines may remain undegraded in the air for some time. Thus, residents in the polluted areas may be exposed to substantial amounts of nitrosamine via inhalation. Fine et al. (1976b) calculated that an adult, breathing air containing 1000 ng/m^3 of DMN for 24 hr, would inhale about 10,000-14,000 ng of DMN. By comparison, the estimated intake of DMN from four slices of bacon and 20 cigarettes would be only about 500 ng and 1000 ng, respectively. The carcinogenic risk of human exposure to atmospheric DMN levels of 50-30,000 ng/m^3 is not known; more data are needed before realistic assessment can be made. Dimethylnitrosamine has been shown to be carcinogenic in inhalation studies using rats and mice; the lowest carcinogenic level so far tested was 200,000 ng/m^3 (Moiseev and Bonemonskii, 1975).

b. Nitrogen oxides in the ambient air

A variety of nitrogen oxides (NO_X), such as nitrous oxide (N_2O), nitric oxide (NO), and nitrogen dioxide (NO_2), are present in the atmosphere. They may arise either from natural sources through biological action and organic decomposition in the soil and ocean (mainly N_2O) or from human activities through combustion (mainly NO and NO_2). In recent years epidemiologists have been baffled by the observed statistical correlation between the high level of NO_2 in the air and the high incidence of cancer in many urban areas. Neither NO_2 nor NO has been demonstrated to be carcinogenic in experimental animals (Shapley, 1976). The possibility that there may be a "nitrogen oxide-nitrosamine-cancer link" has been proposed (Fine et al., 1974; Shapley, 1976). Nitrogen oxides (NO_2 and NO) may generate nitrosamines by directly nitrosating amines in gaseous phase (Neurath, 1972; Gehlert and Rolle, 1977) or aqueous systems (Challis and Kyrtopoulos, 1977) or indirectly reacting with amines in solution via forming nitrous acid. The possibility of in vivo formation of nitrosamines from inhaled nitrogen oxides remains to be tested and additional studies are needed before the "nitrogen oxide-nitrosamine-cancer link" can be established.

The literature on the sources and occurrence of atmospheric nitrogen oxides has been recently reviewed by Fishbein (1976). In the United States the estimated NO_X emissions (in millions of tons) were: traffic, 8.1; fuel consumption, 10.0; industry, 0.2; and miscellaneous, 2.3 (DHEW, 1968). Automobile exhaust has been a major contributor of human-made NO_X. Most of the emission is initially in the form of NO, which can then be readily oxidized to NO_2 (Berry and Lehman, 1971). Emissions from aircraft represent another polluting source of NO_X; it was estimated that 16,000 tons of NO_X were released by civil aircraft in the United States in 1967. Excessive pollution can occur in localized areas around major airports. It is envisaged that the NO_X emission of newer and larger aircraft engines would cause an even greater problem in the future (Hendel, 1973). The average atmospheric concentration of NO_X in seven major U.S. cities is of the order of 0.03-0.10 ppm for NO, and 0.03-0.06 ppm for NO_2. During days of high pollution the atmospheric concentrations may reach as high as 0.68-1.35 ppm and 0.24-0.79 ppm for NO and NO_2, respectively (Tebbens, 1968).

c. Nitrosamines and nitrogen oxides in tobacco smoke

The evidence linking cigarette smoking to high incidence of lung cancer and cancers of the oral cavity is overwhelming; in addition to PAHs, the presence of nitrogen oxides and carcinogenic nitrosamines in tobacco and tobacco smoke has been demonstrated.

The nitrogen oxide present in fresh tobacco smoke is almost exclusively in the form of NO. Nitrogen dioxide is formed as a result of oxidation by oxygen as the smoke ages. Various investigators have shown that the NO content in the tobacco smoke is dependent on the nitrate content of the tobacco. Broaddus et al. (1965), for example, demonstrated that cigarettes of uniform quality with nitrate contents varying from 0.2 to 1.0% nitrate nitrogen produced corresponding amounts of NO in the range of 1000 to 3500 ppm in the smoke. Similarly, high NO contents have been found in the smoke of air-cured burley and cigar types of tobacco which contain up to 6% of nitrate nitrogen, whereas low values were obtained with Virginia and oriental types of tobacco (nitrate nitrogen content: 0.0–0.5%) (Neurath, 1972; Neurath and Dünger, 1975). The nitrate content of the tobacco is dependent on the environmental conditions during growing (especially the nitrogen content in the soil), as well as the type of tobacco. The amount of NO and NO_2 in tobacco smoke has been determined by several investigators. Tada (1962) reported that the concentration of NO varies between 72 and 271 mg/kg, whereas that of NO_2 is between 19 and 118 mg/kg. Only 0.25 mg/kg NO_2 but 442–1008 mg/kg NO were found by Norman and Keith (1965). Apparently, NO_2 in the cigarette smoke can be formed by oxidation of NO as the smoke ages; therefore, special care must be exercised for the accurate determination of the NO_2 content (Neurath and Dünger, 1975). These nitrogen oxides, NO and NO_2, are believed to combine to N_2O_3 which is regarded to be responsible for the formation of some carcinogenic nitrosamines during smoking, by nitrosating the amines in the gaseous phase (Neurath, 1972).

A variety of nitrosamines can be found in tobacco and tobacco smoke (Schmeltz and Hoffmann, 1977); they are either present in the unburned processed tobacco (e.g., nitrosodiethanolamine, N'-nitrosonornicotine) or may be formed during smoking. The possible

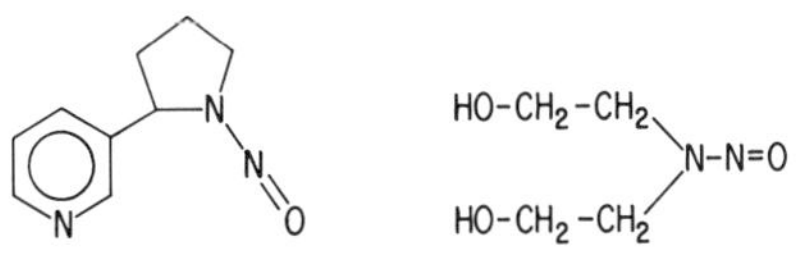

N'-Nitrosonornicotine N-Nitrosodiethanolamine

presence of nitrosamines in cigarette smoke was first proposed by Druckrey and Preussmann (1962); however, the lack of analytical methodology prevented testing of this postulate until recently. Rhoades and Johnson (1972) reported that DMN may be found in the condensate of tobacco smoke in the amounts of 0–140 ng/cigarette. The highest value was obtained using a burley-type tobacco grown in soil with high nitrogen content. This finding was confirmed by McCormick et al. (1973), who have extended the study to include several other nitrosamines. The results are summarized in Table 20. It is evident from the table that the nitrosamine levels positively correlate with the nitrate content and the total volatile base of the tobacco. Agronomic factors affecting the DMN content in cigarette smoke have been studied by Tso et al. (1975). The DMN content in the smoke generally increases with the rate of nitrogen fertilization of the soil. However, there are also some wide seasonal, cultural, and varietal effects. Burley-type tobacco yields a much higher level of DMN than bright-type tobacco. The DMN content is positively related to the total nitrogen, total alkaloids, total volatile bases, and nitrate nitrogen of the leaf, but it is negatively related to reducing sugars. In the mainstream smoke of a typical blended U.S. cigarette (85 mm; 0.9% nitrate; 2.05% nicotine), Hoffmann et al. (1975) have detected an average of 84 ng DMN, 30 ng nitrosoethylmethylamine, traces of DEN (less than 5 ng), and 137 ng N'-nitrosonornicotine. The volatile nitrosamines in the smoke are believed to be formed by reaction of nitrogen oxides with amines in the gaseous phase. It has been proposed that an equimolar mixture of NO and NO_2 is needed for the nitrosation of amines in the gaseous phase according to the equation: $2\ R_2NH + NO + NO_2 \rightarrow 2\ R_2NNO + H_2O$. In a model experiment with dimethylamine, NO or NO_2 alone failed to produce any DMN (Neurath, 1972). A more recent study by Gehlert and Rolle (1977) has, however, revealed that the nitrosation of diethylamine by nitrogen oxides in the gaseous phase appears to follow the equation:

$$2\ NO_2 + 2\ R_2NH \rightarrow R_2NNO + (R_2NH_2)NO_3$$

The presence of N'-nitrosonornicotine has also been detected in unburned tobacco (Hoffmann et al., 1974). The amount in commercial U.S. tobacco products is between 1.9 and 88.6 ppm, one of the highest levels of an environmental nitrosamine yet reported. The highest value for N'-nitrosonornicotine was obtained using fine-cut chewing tobacco and it has been proposed that the correlation between chewing tobacco and induction of oral cancer may be

TABLE 20 Nitrosamines in Smoke Condensate Extracts

Tobacco type or blend	Tobacco analysis		Delivery of nitrosamine (ng/cigarette)[a]				
	Total volatile bases, % N	Total nitrate, % NH_3	DMN	DEN	NPy	NPiP	MEN
Flue-cured	0.25	0.06	5	nd	6	nd	nd
French	0.56	0.27	143	6	110	nd	12
German	0.30	0.19	10	1	26	1	1
Swiss	0.42	0.24	17	1	16	3	2
Cigar	0.64	0.31	160	28	42	nd	40
Catterton (low)[b]	0.38	0.11	19	nd	5	nd	nd
Catterton (high)	0.49	0.54	120	2	55	7	9
Robinson (low)	0.22	0.07	9	nd	6	nd	nd
Robinson (high)	0.46	0.53	110	2	68	5	nd
Burley (low)	0.44	0.13	11	nd	1	nd	nd
Burley (high)	0.85	1.02	180	4	76	9	13

[a]The abbreviations used are: DMN = dimethylnitrosamine, DEN = diethylnitrosamine, NPy = N-nitrosopyrrolidine, NPiP = N-nitrosopiperidine, MEN = methylethylnitrosamine, and nd = not detected.

[b]"Low" and "high" denote the nitrogen content of the soil in which the tobacco was grown.

Source: Adapted from McCormick et al., 1973.

related to this compound. N'-Nitrosonornicotine administered in drinking water induces esophageal tumors in rats and tracheal tumors in Syrian golden hamsters (Schmeltz and Hoffmann, 1977). N'-Nitrosonornicotine has been shown to arise during processing either from nicotine or nornicotine in the leaf, but because of the abundance of the former alkaloid in the leaf, nicotine is probably the major precursor (Hoffmann et al., 1975). Hecht et al. (1975) have suggested that N'-nitrosonornicotine in the leaf may be produced by bacterial or enzymatic nitrosation of nicotine (or nornicotine), probably during curing and fermentation. At least part of the N'-nitrosonornicotine in the leaf may be transferred to the smoke (Hoffmann et al., 1975). Another carcinogenic nitrosamine recently isolated from unburned processed tobacco is nitrosodiethanolamine (Schmeltz et al., 1977); the amount detected ranges from 0.1-173 ppb. The highest value was obtained using burley-type tobacco, whereas commercial blended tobacco contains 104 ppb of the nitrosamine. The source of the nitrosamine in tobacco leaf was traced to the use of the herbicide MH-30 (maleic hydrazine), which is commonly formulated as the diethanolamine salt. Nitrosodiethanolamine is nonvolatile and is expected to have significance principally for tobacco chewers; whether it contributes to the carcinogenicity of the smoke remains to be elucidated.

2. Nitrosamines in Water

The ease of nitrosamine formation from precursors in aqueous systems has caused concern about their possible formation in fresh waters, polluted waters, and soil. Nitrosamine precursors are widely present in the aqueous environment. Nitrite can be generated from ammonium or nitrate fertilizers and may sometimes accumulate to high concentrations. Secondary amines are present in pesticides and industrial wastes, as normal constituents of plants, and may be formed during decomposition of pesticides and natural products. Recent studies by Ayanaba et al. (1973a) have revealed that microorganisms present in the sewage and soil are capable of promoting nitrosamine formation by (1) converting tertiary amines to secondary amines, (2) reducing nitrate to nitrite, and (3) catalyzing the formation of nitrosamine. Formation of nitrosamines from simple amines and nitrate or nitrite added to samples of soil (Ayanaba et al., 1973b), and sewage and lake water (Ayanaba and Alexander, 1974) has been demonstrated. Furthermore, in contrast to the common assumption that nitrosamines would be readily degraded in natural aqueous ecosystems due to their photochemical lability, Tate and Alexander (1975) have shown that nitrosamines added to lake water may persist up to 3 1/2 months without significant loss. A lag of nearly 30 days occurred before their slow disappearance from soil, and over 50% of the added nitrosamines still remained in the sewage after 14 days. The stability of nitrosamines in samples of natural ecosystems has prompted these authors to suggest that great care should be exercised in the use and disposal of materials that may provide amine precursors for nitrosamine formation.

The demonstration that nitrosamines could indeed be detected in the aqueous environment was recently reported by Fine and Rounbehler (1976). Using a nitroso-compound-specific thermal energy analyzer, they showed that DMN may be detected in the sewage effluents and the ocean water near Baltimore. The amount detected ranged from 0.08 to nearly 3 μg DMN/liter water, the latter value being obtained from samples taken near a sewage treatment facility. Apparently, the sewage effluent and/or runoff water from the factory are the prime sources. The sewage from several chemical companies has been found to contain DMN of the order of 2-4 μg/liter (Fine et al., 1976b). Precipitation of DMN from the air could be a potential source of DMN in the ocean (Fine and Rounbehler, 1976), since DMN is manufactured as a synthetic intermediate in a nearby chemical plant and can be detected in the ambient air (Fine et al., 1976a). The finding of Fine and Rounbehler (1976) represents the first confirmed report of the presence of a volatile nitrosamine in water and establishes that nitrosamines can exist for considerable periods of time in nature. Further studies are needed before the environmental impact of water pollution by nitrosamines can be assessed.

Nitrate in drinking water has been considered a potential source of nitrosating agent, as nitrates may be reduced to nitrites by bacterial action in a number of in vivo sites. Possible correlation between high nitrate content in drinking water and high incidence of cancer has been suggested (Zaldivar, 1970; Hill et al., 1973; Hawksworth et al., 1975). The role of nitrate is discussed in Sec. III.D.3.c.

3. Nitrosamines and Their Precursors in Food

The discovery of DMN as the toxic substance responsible for the epidemic poisoning of sheep fed nitrite-preserved fish meal (Ender et al., 1964) has stimulated intensive investigations on the possible presence of nitrosamines in food for human consumption. It is now well established that trace amounts of nitrosamines are present in a variety of foodstuffs, especially marine fish and cured meat products. The possible presence of nitrosamines in the diet has been postulated by various investigators to be related to the high incidence of cancer in some population groups. Of equal if not greater importance is the common occurrence of nitrosamine precursors in food. Secondary amines and some other nitrosatable amino compounds are common constituents of food, whereas the use of nitrite as a food preservative or additive has been a common practice (Scanlan, 1975).

The confirmed reports of nitrosamine occurrence in food materials are summarized in Table 21. As mentioned in Sec. III.A.3, some of the analytical methods used for nitrosamine detection prior to 1970 are not sufficiently specific and sensitive. The values obtained using those methods may therefore be erroneous and the identity questionable; confirmation by mass spectrometry is now generally adopted for positive identification. Thus, trace amounts of nitrosamines can be found in many processed or cooked food products and in some raw or unprocessed foods. It is important to note that large variation in nitrosamine content among various samples or brands of the same type of product may be observed. Evidently, the nature of the food, the amount of ingredients or additives, and the conditions of storage, processing, and cooking are key factors in determining the extent of food contamination by nitrosamines. A clear delineation of these factors is imperative in future attempts to implement preventive measures to minimize nitrosamine formation in food.

a. Nitrosamines in raw or unprocessed food

The discovery of DMN in nitrite-preserved fish meal has led many investigators to study the possible occurrence of nitrosamines in edible plants, especially those grown in soil enriched with nitrogen-containing fertilizers and those known to have high nitrate content. Marquardt and Hedler (1966) reported the occurrence of what they regarded to be "DEN" in wheat flour; the identification was made using thin-layer chromatography. Studies by Ender and Čeh (1968) indicated the presence of volatile nitrosamines in various kinds of mushrooms; the amount detected ranged from 0.4 to 30 μg/kg. The nitrosamine seemed to be identical with DMN as shown by thin-layer chromatography. Another interesting observation of possible occurrence of nitrosamines in edible plants was made during a search for possible factors responsible for the high incidence of esophageal cancer among Bantu tribes in Transkei, South Africa. It was noted that areas of high cancer incidence coincided with areas of molybdenum deficiency in the leaves of many edible plants. Molybdenum deficiency is known to cause a disturbance in nitrogen metabolism, thus leading to the accumulation of nitrate in these plants. This prompted DuPlessis et al. (1969) to test the possibility that nitrosamines in nitrate-rich plant food consumed by the natives may be related to their high incidence of cancer. They selected the fruit of a solanaceous bush (Solanum incanum) and succeeded in isolating from the extract of the fruit a nitrosamine that was identified to be DMN by thin-layer chromatography, infrared and nuclear magnetic spectrometry, and gas chromatography. The juice of the fruit has been used by the natives to curdle milk which is their principal protein food in their young and adolescent years. It is not certain whether the nitrosamines detected in these early studies are indeed authentic nitrosamines; confirmation by mass spectrometry appears necessary. In a more recent study by Sander et al. (1973), the possible presence of nitrosamines in wheat, grown in soil fertilized with a mixture of nitrate and secondary amines was investigated. No nitrosamine could be detected at the 0.3-2 μg/kg level. The possible accumulation in edible plants of nitrosamines present in the soil has been studied by Sander et al. (1975b). Using cress plants in a model experiment, it was found that various nitrosamines added to the cultivation media are readily taken up into the plants. However, it appears that the plant can degrade the nitrosamines because the concentration of these compounds in the plant falls to trace levels after 3-4 days. Further studies are needed before the role of edible plants as a potential source of human exposure to nitrosamines can be established.

Presence of nitrosamines in fresh or raw fish has been sporadically detected (Fazio et al., 1971a; Crosby et al., 1972). The possible source of these nitrosamines is not clear.

b. Nitrosamines in processed or cooked food

Processed fish products and cured meat products are the main categories of food materials in which trace amounts of nitrosamines may be found (Table 21). Since fish and meat are a rich source of nitrosatable amino compounds (amines, amino acids), whereas nitrite has been commonly used as an additive or preservative (the legally permitted level in the United States is 200 mg/kg), it is not surprising that nitrosamines can be detected.

The conditions conducive to nitrosamine formation in food have been extensively studied by various investigators. Using a model system containing large amounts of fish or meat product and nitrite, Ender and Čeh (1971) showed that the formation of nitrosamine depended mainly on (1) the presence of nitrite and nitrosatable amines, (2) pH and temperature, (3) time of reaction, and (4) the presence of a protecting colloid—such as starch or other glutineous substances—which prevents the evaporation of the formed nitrosamines at high temperatures. The effect of temperature is particularly intriguing; a large increase in the nitrosamine yield was observed if the temperature was raised from 130°C to 150°C. Apparently, high temperatures caused the breakdown of proteins yielding more nitrosatable amino compounds.

Under conditions closer to the normal dietary situations Fiddler et al. (1972) found that processing with 1500 mg/kg sodium nitrite consistently produced frankfurters containing approximately 10 μg/kg of DMN; this did not occur when 156 mg/kg sodium nitrite was used. Increasing the processing time from 2 to 4 hr produced more DMN. Inclusion of ascorbic acid during processing substantially decreased the nitrosamine formation, whereas glucono-delta-lactone, a cure component, significantly increased nitrosamine yield (Wasserman and Fiddler, 1975).

The demonstration that curing components can contribute to the presence of nitrosamines in food has also been shown by Sen et al. (1973b). Substantial amounts of nitrosopyrrolidine (2500-6000 μg/kg) and nitrosopiperidine (7000-25,000 μg/kg) may be formed in the curing mixture of Mettwurst sausages. The spices added, black pepper and paprika, are capable of reacting with nitrite to yield mainly nitrosopiperidine and nitrosopyrrolidine, respectively. The presence of DMN in souse and similar products has also been reported (Fiddler et al., 1975).

Bacteria may play an important role in the formation of nitrosamine in foodstuffs during storage or processing. Fong and Chan (1973b), for example, showed that innoculation of fish broth with bacteria (Staphylococcus aureus) isolated from commercially available Chinese salted marine fish substantially increases the formation of DMN. Bacterial involvement was proposed to be responsible for the presence of DMN in the salted fish found earlier by the same group (Fong and Chan, 1973a). Methods designed to limit DMN formation in salted fish have been proposed (Fong and Chan, 1976); they include: (1) use of benzoic acid to inhibit bacterial growth, (2) salting with pure sodium chloride instead of the crude salt which contains nitrate, and (3) use of freshwater fish, which contains less nitrosatable amines.

Cooking is known to be conducive to nitrosamine formation in foodstuffs. This is best illustrated by the frying of bacon (Fazio et al., 1973; Sen et al., 1973a; Wasserman and Fiddler, 1975). Fiddler and co-workers (reported in Wasserman and Fiddler, 1975) have studied the effect of frying conditions on the formation of nitrosopyrrolidine in bacon. The results have been summarized in Table 22. The amount of nitrosopyrrolidine formed was

TABLE 21 Confirmed Reports of Nitrosamine Occurrence in Foodstuffs

Substance	Nitrosamine (μg/kg)[a,b]				Reference
	DMN	DEN	NPy	NPiP	
Various fish products					
Processed sable, salmon, shad	4–26				Fazio et al., 1971a
Raw sable	0–4				Fazio et al., 1971a
Various fish samples	1–9 (15/35)				Crosby et al., 1972
fresh fish	1–4 (3/15)				Crosby et al., 1972
salted fish	1–4 (2/2)				Crosby et al., 1972
baked fish	5–9 (1/1)				Crosby et al., 1972
fried fish	1–9 (9/11)				Crosby et al., 1972
Salt-dried fish	10–1000 (16/17)				Fong and Chan, 1973a
Dried shrimp	2–10 (7/13)		10–37 (10/13)		Fong and Chan, 1977
Cured meat and related products					
Ham	5 (1/5)				Fazio et al., 1971b

Pork, chopped Danish	1-4 (1/1)	1-4 (1/1)			Crosby et al., 1972
Sausages					
Smoked Sausage and salami	10-80 (5/36)				Sen (1972)
Salami	1-4 (1/6)	nd			Crosby et al., 1972
Mettwurst sausage			13-105 (3/6)	Trace-60 (2/6)	Sen et al. (1973b
Chinese sausage	3-15 (6/10)		nd		Fong and Chan, 1977
Bacon					
Fried bacon	Trace-4 (13/24)	< 1 (1/24)	Trace-40 (13/24)	< 1 (1/24)	Crosby et al., 1972
Raw bacon			nd (8/8)		Fazio et al., 1973
Fried bacon			10-108 (8/8)		Fazio et al., 1973
Fat cooked out of bacon			45-207 (8/8)		Fazio et al., 1973
Fried or uncooked bacon	2-30 (6/16)		4-25 (7/16)		Sen et al., 1973a
Souse and similar gelatin products	3-63 (8/10)		19 (1/10)		Fiddler et al , 1975
Other foodstuffs					
Cheese	1-4 (6/12)	nd			Crosby et al., 1972

[a]Numbers in parentheses indicate the number of positive samples/total number of samples analyzed.

[b]The abbreviations used are: DMN = dimethylnitrosamine, DEN = diethylnitrosamine, NPy = N-nitrosopyrrolidine, NPiP = N-nitrosopiperidine, and nd = not detected.

TABLE 22 Effect of Frying Conditions on Nitrosopyrrolidine Formation in Bacon

Temperature (°F)	Frying conditions: Time (min)	Frying conditions: Degree of cooking	Nitrosopyrrolidine (μg/kg)
210	105	Medium well	0
275	30	Medium well	8
350	6	Medium well	10
400	4	Medium well	17
210	10	Raw	0
275	10	Very light	0
350	10	Well	15
400	10	Burned	19

Source: Adapted from Wasserman and Fiddler, 1975.

primarily dependent on the frying temperature rather than the duration of frying. A study of other cooking methods, including microwave cooking, baking, broiling, and a "baconer," showed that the smallest amount of nitrosopyrrolidine was formed by microwave cooking (Pensabene et al., 1974). Nitrosopyrrolidine was mainly formed in the adipose tissue but not the lean tissue of fried bacon (Fiddler et al., 1974). It has been suggested that nitrosopyrrolidine may be formed by decarboxylation of nitrosoproline at temperatures of frying (Pensabene et al., 1974). Nitrosoproline has been identified in uncooked bacon (Kushnir et al., 1975), where it may be formed from the collagen. Cooking may also increase nitrosamine formation by increasing the amount of nitrosatable amino compounds. For example, Lijinsky and Epstein (1970) suggested that cooking of protein foods might produce free amino acids (such as proline, hydroxyproline, and arginine), yielding secondary amines such as pyrrolidine and piperidine.

c. Secondary amines, nitrites, and nitrates in the diet

As discussed in Sec. III.C.2, nitrosamine formation readily occurs in vivo inside the human body, as well as in in vitro systems. The potential in vivo sites of nitrosamine formation include the stomach, intestine, and urinary bladder. Assessment of human exposure to nitrosamines should therefore include consideration of exposure to reactants capable of forming nitroso compounds. Of these reactants, secondary amines, nitrites, and nitrates have received the most attention.

Studies on the occurrence of secondary amines in the food for human consumption have recently been carried out by several investigators (Ishidate et al., 1972; Neurath and Schreiber, 1975; Fong and Chan, 1976; Singer and Lijinsky, 1976a). The results of some of these findings are summarized in Table 23. It appears that dimethylamine and morpholine are almost ubiquitously present in various foodstuffs, whereas pyrrolidine and piperidine are mainly associated with plant-derived materials. Fish samples consistently show the presence of dimethylamine, although large variations in amine content are observed. These variations have been attributed mainly to species differences (Singer and Lijinsky, 1976a). Freshwater fish contain much lower amounts of nitrosatable amines than marine fish (Fong and Chan, 1976). Dimethylamine in fish is believed to originate from trimethylamine oxide, which is abundant in marine fish. The natural source of morpholine in the food is not known, whereas pyrrolidine and piperidine probably derive from plant alkaloids. The level of secondary amines in food may be affected by storage conditions and cooking. Free dimethylamine may be formed during storage (Reay and Shewan, 1949), especially under conditions favoring bacterial growth. Roasting of mackerel, pike, and sardines (widely consumed foods in Japan) may lead to a more than 10-fold increase in dimethylamine content. Processing (such as drying, smoking, canning) may also result in large increase in the amine content in fish (Ishidate et al., 1972).

TABLE 23 Secondary Amines in Foodstuffs

Substance	Secondary amine (mg/kg)			
	Dimethylamine	Morpholine	Pyrrolidine	Piperidine
Fish				
Canned tuna[a]	23	<0.6		
Frozen ocean-perch[a]	180	9		
Frozen cod[a]	740	Trace		
Spotted trout[a,c]	7	6		
Smallmouth bass[a,c]	110	<0.7		
Salmon[a]	82	1.0		
Herring in oil (preserve)[b,d]	45			
Salted herring[b]	3			
Meats				
Baked ham[a,c]	2	0.5	Trace	0.2
Frankfurters[a]	1	0.4		
Beverages				
Evaporated milk[a]	3	0.2	0.7	0.3
Whole milk[a]	0.2			0.11
Coffee[a]	2	1	6	1
Coffee extract[b,d]	4		10	2
Coffee (freeze-dried)[b]	3-6		7-11	1-2
Tea[a]	0.7	Trace		
Cocoa (defatted)[b]			0.5	9
Beer (canned)[a]	0.6	0.4		
Beer (bottled)[a]	0.7	<0.2	Trace	
Wine[a]	0.07	<0.7	0.06	

[a]Data summarized from Singer and Lijinsky, 1976a.

[b]Data summarized from Neurath and Schreiber, 1975.

[c]Traces of di-n-propylamine (<1 mg/kg) have also been detected.

[d]Traces of ethylmethylamine (1 mg/kg) have also been detected.

TABLE 24 Estimated Average Daily Ingestion of Nitrate and Nitrite for U.S. Resident

Source	Nitrate		Nitrite	
	(mg)	%	(mg)	%
Vegetables	86.1	86.3	0.20	1.8
Fruits, juices	1.4	1.4	0.00	0
Milk and products	0.2	0.2	0.00	0
Bread	2.0	2.0	0.02	0.2
Water	0.7	0.7	0.00	0
Cured meats	9.4	9.4	2.38	21.2
Saliva	30.0[a]	—	8.62	76.8
Total	99.8	100.0	11.22	100.0

[a]Not included in the total.

Source: Adapted from White, 1975. The values for cured meat were erroneous in the original article and were corrected in errata added subsequently.

Nitrites and the precursor nitrates are nitrosating agents under appropriate conditions. Assessment of potential in vivo nitrosamine formation is impossible without knowledge of nitrite and nitrate intake. White (1975) has recently gathered information on the dietary sources of nitrites and nitrates and estimated the average daily ingestion of these anions by U.S. residents (Table 24). The major intake (86.3%) of nitrates comes from vegetables. A variety of vegetables has been found to be particularly rich in nitrate: beets (average content 2.76 g/kg), celery (2.34 g/kg), spinach (1.86 g/kg), lettuce (0.85 g/kg), and broccoli (0.78 g/kg). The nitrate content of vegetables may be even higher under some conditions, such as (1) high levels of fertilization, especially during the ripening period, (2) plant nutrient (e.g., molybdenum) deficiency, (3) conditions of reduced light intensity during maturation, (4) lack of water, and (5) plant damage from chemical treatments (Wolff and Wasserman, 1972). The second major source (9.4%) of nitrates is cured meats. Nitrate is commonly used as an additive; the legally permitted residual level is 500 mg/kg. High nitrate content is usually found in ham and related products. The origin of salivary nitrate is not clear, and it is assumed that salivary nitrate originates from the food (White, 1975).

The major concern over human exposure to nitrates stems from the fact that nitrates are readily reduced to nitrites by bacterial action. This may occur in vivo as well as in food materials. In vivo reduction of nitrates may occur in the oral cavity, stomach, intestine, and urinary bladder, especially when the conditions permit bacterial growth. In this respect, infants and the elderly are particularly susceptible. Infants under about 4 months of age and achlorhydric patients (often found among the elderly) produce less acid in the stomach and therefore may permit bacterial growth. It has been suggested that the high nitrate content in drinking water may be related to the high incidence of cancer in some areas of the world (Table 25). The formation of nitrites from nitrates during storage is well known (e.g., Weisburger and Raineri, 1975). It has been postulated that the observed decrease in the incidence of gastric cancer in the United States may be partly attributable to the increased availability of refrigerators in the homes, preventing bacterial growth that would reduce nitrate to nitrite (Weisburger and Raineri, 1975).

The major source of nitrites comes from saliva. Nitrite is produced from nitrate by oral microorganisms (Tannenbaum et al., 1974); the amount produced is relatively constant for an individual and does not seem to be strongly influenced by the diet. Cured meats represent the major (almost exclusive) dietary source of nitrite. Nitrite has been commonly used as a food additive and preservative. The action of nitrite in the curing process is threefold: (1) to give characteristic color by reacting with myoglobin to form the red-pink nitrosylmyoglobin, (2) to produce cured flavor by reacting with meat components, and (3) to inhibit bacterial growth, particularly against <u>Clostridium botulinum</u> (Wolff and Wasserman, 1972; Scanlan, 1975).

In addition to nitrosamine precursors, ingestion of catalysts or inhibitors of nitrosamine formation may have profound effects on the in vivo formation of nitrosamines (Secs. III.C.1. d.-f). In particular, ingestion of ascorbic acid may be expected to reduce the in vivo formation of nitroso compounds, whereas ingestion of thiocyanate-related compounds may do the reverse. Thiocyanate is secreted in human saliva, and its content may be increased by foods containing cyanogenetic glucosides which can be found in bitter almonds, bitter cassava, bamboo, and lima beans. Smoking also increases thiocyanate secretion in saliva (Boyland and Walker, 1975).

4. Assessment of Potential Health Hazard

Assessment of the potential health hazard of human exposure to nitrosamines and their precursors present in the environment has been the subject of intensive discussion and debate in the recent years (Lijinsky and Epstein, 1970; Wogan and Tannenbaum, 1975; Weisburger and Raineri, 1975; Shapley, 1976; Preussmann, 1976; Issenberg, 1976; Mirvish, 1977; Archer and Wishnok, 1977). The opinions are divided on the magnitude of the health hazard that environmental nitrosamines may pose because realistic assessment at this stage is impossible due to lack of sufficient data.

TABLE 25 Possible Nitrosamine Involvement in the Induction of Cancer in Some High-Risk Groups

Population group or geographic location	Type of cancer	Suspected cause	Reference
Bantu tribes in Transkei, S. Africa	Esophageal	Possible presence of DMN in food additive	DuPlessis et al., 1969
Northern Iran	Esophageal	Nitrosamines (?) in diet	McGlashan, 1970
Chile	Stomach		Zaldivar, 1970
English borough of Worshop	Stomach	Nitrate in drinking water	Hill et al., 1973
Southwest Colombia	Stomach		Hawksworth et al., 1975
Japanese in Hawaii	Stomach	Nitrosamines in salted/dried fish	Haenszel et al., 1972 Haenszel, 1975
Southern China	Nasopharyngeal	DMN in salted/dried fish	Ho, 1976

The literature on the possible involvement of nitrosamines in the induction of cancer in a number of high-risk population groups has been summarized in Table 25. Unequivocal association has yet to be established. The difficulty arises mainly because of the lack of clearly identifiable, unusual types of cancer that the nitrosamines induce, and in none of the studies mentioned has nitrosamine been clearly identified as the principal agent. Evidently, more epidemiological data are needed before the role of nitrosamines as human carcinogens can be established. In this respect, it must be noted that a recent study by Fan et al. (1977) has revealed that extremely high concentrations (up to 30 g/kg) of a carcinogenic nitrosamine nitrosodiethanolamine are found in some synthetic cutting fluids. Users of these products (e.g., machine operators) must be cautioned, preventive regulations enacted, and prospective epidemiological studies initiated.

Since nitrosamines are among the highly potent experimental carcinogens and every species of animals tested so far was found susceptible to one or more types of nitrosamines, it is not unreasonable to assume that humans are also susceptible to the carcinogenic action of nitrosamines. Realistic assessment of carcinogenic risk of human exposure to environmental levels of nitrosamines still awaits further study. The finding of relatively high concentrations of atmospheric DMN in some areas of two U.S. cities (Fine et al., 1976a, b) is alarming. It indicates that residents in the polluted areas are exposed to substantial amounts of nitrosamines via inhalation. Considering the trace levels and somewhat sporadic occurrence of nitrosamines in foodstuffs, it has been suggested that nitrosamines in food do not appear to represent an imminent hazard to public health in the United States (Issenberg, 1976). Archer and Wishnok (1977) have calculated the estimated daily intake of nitrosamines in terms of molecules/cell/day and arrived at the conclusion that the levels of nitrosamines in food are not significantly hazardous. This conclusion was reached, however, on the assumption that a threshold dose of 10^4 molecules per cell is needed for carcinogenesis. The possible existence of threshold dose has been one of the most hotly disputed concepts in the field of chemical carcinogenesis (Claus et al., 1974; Kotin, 1976; Preussmann, 1976). Based on a recent study of the absorption and metabolism in rats of small oral doses of DMN, Gomez et al. (1977) have suggested that DMN present in food may be absorbed and transformed into a methylating agent even at the lowest dose tested (1 μg/kg body weight). Thus, even the smallest dose is potentially of some consequence. However, the metabolism and activation of dietary levels of DMN would probably be confined to the liver because the DMN in the portal blood would be metabolized before reaching other organs.

It must be stressed that the present knowledge on environmental nitrosamines is limited to the relatively more easily detected volatile nitrosamines. Very little is known about nonvolatile nitrosamines, which could play an important role as environmental carcinogens. Recently N-nitrosodiethanolamine, a nonvolatile carcinogenic nitrosamine, has been detected in cutting fluids (Fan et al., 1977), processed tobacco leaf (Schmeltz et al., 1977), and cosmetic products (Chem. Eng. News, 1977) at levels up to 30 g/kg, 137 μg/kg, and 48 mg/kg, respectively. The total extent of environmental nitrosamine hazard cannot be appreciated without knowing the occurrence and level of human exposure to nonvolatile nitrosamines.

Human exposure to precursors of nitrosamines and other nitroso compounds is probably of equal (if not greater) importance to that of preformed nitrosamines. Assessment of carcinogenic risk is rendered more difficult because of the complexity of the problem. In vivo formation of nitroso compounds from precursors is affected not only by the precursors themselves, but also by the condition and physiology of the host and the presence of modifying factors. Relatively few experiments have been carried out thus far to assess the carcinogenic risk of concurrent administration of trace levels of precursors. A recent study by Shank and Newberne (1976) has shown that, at least for morpholine, concentrations as low as 5 ppm each of nitrite and morpholine are capable of inducing liver tumors in the rat. Morpholine is ubiquitously present in various foods. Further substantial limitation of the use of nitrite as food additive, and inclusion of ascorbate to minimize nitrosation, should be implemented as preventive measures.

The central problem of environmental carcinogenesis probably lies in the fact that humans are exposed to a wide variety of carcinogens rather than to a single carcinogen.

Synergism among various carcinogens may result in substantially greater carcinogenic risk. The possible mechanisms of combination effects in chemical carcinogenesis have been discussed by Falk (1976). Synergism between PAHs and nitrosamines was first reported by Hoch-Ligeti et al. (1968) who showed that a combined administration of low doses of DMN and 3-methylcholanthrene brought about a 15% pulmonary tumor incidence in the rat. At the doses given, neither DMN nor 3-methylcholanthrene alone was carcinogenic in the lung. Similar synergistic effects have been reported by Cardesa et al. (1973) and Montesano et al. (1974). Argus and Arcos (1976) have suggested that synergism between nitrosamines and PAHs may play an important role in lung tumorigenesis in tobacco smokers. Whether nitrosamines could also act synergistically with other carcinogens is not known; it is obvious that the assessment of health hazard of environmental nitrosamines cannot be complete without further studies in this area.

IV. INORGANIC CARCINOGENS

A. Asbestos

1. Historical Note and Scope of the Problem

The use of asbestos in some form or another is older than recorded history (Brodeur, 1972). Archeological evidence indicates that asbestos was used in pottery, mixed with clay, already in the Stone Age. The Greeks and Romans knew well the fire-resistant properties of asbestos fibers, and in many societies during Antiquity asbestos cloth was used for tailoring the costly "funeral dress of kings" used in cremations. Although the use of asbestos appeared to decrease considerably during the Middle Ages, it was regarded as a treasured novelty in the households of high nobles and the courts of kings. Emperor Charlemagne is said to have possessed asbestos tablecloths, and in the thirteenth century the Venetian traveler Marco Polo recorded the use of fire-resistant cloth made from woollike mineral fibers in the Great Empire of Tartary (now a part of Siberia).

The first attempt to revive the use of asbestos in the modern era was made in 1720 when asbestos deposits were discovered in the Ural Mountains and a factory was established for manufacturing asbestos products. This attempt was, however, doomed to failure because of the limited demand for and few known uses of the mineral at that time.

The commercial mining of asbestos was first undertaken in 1879 at Thetford in Quebec. In 1890 an asbestos weaving mill was built near Calvados in Normandy. From then on asbestos has achieved enormous economic importance. The first mining operations at Thetford produced only 300 tons of the mineral. However, by 1910 the annual world production was up to 30,000 tons, increasing to 500,000 tons by about 1935; the total world production is over 5 million tons today.

Asbestos possesses unique physical properties which explain its ubiquitous use in industry and its enormous commercial success (Hendry, 1965). Asbestos has been termed "the magic mineral," "the mineral of unparalleled properties," "the mineral of a thousand uses." Liberated from the ore, it appears as a feathery, fluffy mass which can be carded, spun, and woven just as cotton or wool. Since asbestos consists of various types of magnesium silicates, it is incombustible. Its microscopic fibers have a very high tensile strength and great flexibility. Yet, despite the fluffiness of a mass of asbestos, the individual fibers have a high density; hence, the multitude of uses of asbestos for fashioning heat-resistant friction facings. Moreover, the fibers of asbestos possess a highly adsorbent surface which makes it a material of choice for manufacturing different filters, as active "filler" component in such products as asbestos cement, asbestos tiles, paints, caulking compounds, and for combining with asphalt and plastics. In these products the individual fibers serve the function of tiny reinforcing rods, owing to chemical interaction of the hydroxyl group-studded surface of the fibers with the main component in the finished products.

Because of its unique properties, the applications of asbestos have soared. It is estimated that the mineral has over 3000 different kinds of uses. Since its use parallels indus-

TABLE 26 Scope of Distribution of and Exposure to Asbestos

Operations and products with contact to asbestos for producers, processors, users, consumers, residents	Population groups with occupational and environmental exposure to asbestos
Asbestos rock mining, leading, shipping, crushing, milling; asbestos spinning, weaving, mixing, cutting, pressing, molding, plastering, cementing, spraying of steel construction, undercoating of automobiles, insulating pipes, etc.; safety clothing, cloths, sheets, blankets, draperies and curtains, lagging, pot holders, ironing-board covers, rugs, motion picture screens, gas mask filters, mailbags, prison-cell padding, airplane fittings, stove and lamp wicks, spark plugs, fire hose, textiles used in the processing of fruit juices, acids, beer and medicine, brake linings, clutch facings, and other woven asbestos friction materials, asbestos cloth packings, seals and gaskets, yarns, tape, cords, ropes, twines, ribbons, artificial snow, filter pads, filter paper, artificial wood, tiles, shingles, card boards, wall boards, sheets for interior and exterior walls, insulation board, casings for electric motors, partitions, panels, paper, roofing, piano padding, stove lining, heaters, filing cabinets, military helmets, automobile mufflers and hoods, armored cars, carpets, cartridges, boiler jackets, radiator covers, clapboard, fireproof wallboard, acoustical ceilings, plasterboard, filler in rubber goods, plastics and roof coatings, filter cloths, electrical switch boxes, safes, table pads, stove mats, ovens, dry kilns, pipe coverings, pipes, insulation blocks, insulation jackets, pump packings, electric wire insulation, structural heat insulation, facings of acoustical building materials, catalyst supports in sulfuric acid production, putties, sealants, paints, roof-coating and road-building compounds, caulking, other crack-fillers, plaster and stucco, clays used for pottery and sculpture	Occupational groups: Asbestos rock miners, loaders, truckers, crushers, millers; asbestos spinners, weavers; electrical appliance and wire manufacturers, masons, carpenters, heating equipment workers, rubber workers, shingle and tile manufacturers, building material manufacturers, filtering material manufacturers, molders of asbestos products, asbestos-asphalt makers, putty manufacturers, asbestos cement makers, asbestos paper cardboard and brake-lining producers, asbestos felt insulation workers, asbestos sound insulation workers, asbestos insulators, pipe coverers, asbestos tube wrappers, asbestos cork insulation workers, construction workers, automobile makers, garage attendants Nonoccupational groups: Predominantly residents in vicinity of asbestos processing, asbestos cement and textile mills, inhaling plant effluents polluted with asbestos dust, and individuals living and working along roads on which asbestos is trucked; inhabitants of houses with asbestos insulation; increasingly the general population at large

Source: Patterned after Hueper, 1966a.

TABLE 27 Chrysotile Asbestos Content of Ambient Air in New York City by Borrough

Sampling locations	Asbestos level (10^{-9} g/m^3 air) Range	Average
Manhattan	8-65	30
Brooklyn	6-39	19
Bronx	2-25	12
Queens	3-18	9
Staten Island	5-14	8

Source: From Nicholson and Pundsack, 1973.

trialization, the United States is by far the largest consumer of asbestos in the world. There is not an automobile, train, airplane, or ship which does not contain asbestos. Asbestos is used in the construction of virtually every building in the country. Table 26 illustrates the ubiquity of asbestos in the environment and the exposure of population groups. Asbestos is a component of a multitude of industrial products which are not specified as containing asbestos.

It was not anticipated that asbestos pollution may pose any health hazard to the general population. However, there are now several reports that the typical asbestos-induced lung cancer, mesothelioma, occurs not only in family contacts of asbestos workers but also in individuals whose only identified asbestos exposure was that of living within 1/2 mile of an asbestos products plant (cited in Anderson et al., 1976). Increasingly, the foci of asbestos pollution are not limited to industrial sources. Because of the gradual wear and disintegration of products containing asbestos, such as roofing materials, pipes, floor tiles, asbestos-containing coatings, brake linings, and so on, and the dust produced in the demolition of buildings, the asbestos level in the environment will keep on increasing (Nicholson and Pundsack, 1973). Recently, attention has been drawn to an instance of considerable air pollution with asbestos due to the use of crushed asbestos minerals for paving roads and resurfacing highways and parking lots (Rohl et al., 1977). Environmental pollution with asbestos in the United States is illustrated by the data shown in Tables 27, 28, and 29.

As a mineral, asbestos, once released in the environment, will never dissolve or decay, and will become an everlasting contaminant. It has been predicted that in the next few decades asbestos-induced neoplasms will rival cigarette smoking-induced lung cancer (Thomson et al., 1963, 1966). A brief, intense exposure to asbestos can be as dangerous as prolonged contact (Selikoff, 1976). The scope and gravity of the problem of asbestos pollution is put in an even sharper focus by a combination of two circumstances: (1) the

TABLE 28 Chrysotile Asbestos Content in Ambient Air near Spray Fireproofing Sites

Sampling location from site (miles)	Asbestos level (10^{-9} g/m^3 air) Range	Average
1/8-1/4	9-375	60
1/4-1/2	8-54	25
1/2-1	0.5-36	18

Source: From Nicholson and Pundsack, 1973.

TABLE 29 Chrysotile Asbestos Content of Eastern U.S. River Waters

Sample source	Range (μg/gal)	Average (μg/gal)
Juniata River		
Breezewood, Pa.	0-9.2	2.2
Newton-Hamilton, Pa.	0-6.2	2.2
Lewistown, Pa.	0-15.0	4.7
Amity Hall, Pa.	0-14.8	3.5
Connecticut River		
Canaan, Vt.	0-13.9	2.6
Littleton, N.H.	0-13.8	2.6
Lebanon, N.H.	0-2.6	1.3
Greenfield, Mass.	0-23.5	5.1
Middletown, Conn.	0-14.5	5.9

Source: From Nicholson and Pundsack, 1973.

statistic of industrial epidemiology that asbestos workers who smoke have 92 times the risk of lung cancer than people who neither work with asbestos nor smoke (Selikoff et al., 1968; Selikoff and Hammond, 1975), and (2) the continued increase in the habit of cigarette smoking. The combined effect of asbestos exposure and smoking on mortality from lung cancer in factory workers has been confirmed (Berry et al., 1972), and the synergistic effect of chrysotile asbestos and benzo(a)pyrene (the principal hydrocarbon carcinogen in tobacco smoke) has been shown in hamsters (Miller et al., 1965).

2. Types and Chemical Nature of Asbestos

Asbestos is a generic term describing a variety of silicates; there are six distinct types of asbestiform minerals (Table 30). Only three of these types are produced in commercial quantities; about 95% of the total production is chrysotile (white asbestos) with the rest divided between amosite (brown asbestos) and crocidolite (blue asbestos). All are silicates containing various amounts of calcium, magnesium, and iron.

Electron microscopic study of chrysotile revealed that the fibrils are not solid but cylindrical, hollow tubes. The fibrils themselves and the interfibril spaces are filled with an amorphous solid of similar composition to the crystalline tube wall. Chrysotile asbestos consists of bundles of these tubes tightly packed together (Gaze, 1965; Atkinson et al., 1971). The chemical structure of a segment of the crystalline tube wall is diagrammatically represented in Fig. 11 (Daykin, 1971). In addition to magnesium, which forms a part of the crystal lattice, chrysotile asbestos usually contains the impurities iron, chromium, cobalt, nickel, and scandium. These cations, as well as the magnesium, can be extracted from chrysotile fibers by mild acid treatment (Harris and Grimshaw, 1971; Atkinson and Rickards, 1971). As Fig. 11 illustrates, the outer surface of the chrysotile fibril consists of a layer of magnesium ion-linked hydroxyl ions, which confer to the fibril strong basic properties and chemical reactivity. Removal of the magnesium ions by acid brings about loss of the hydroxyl content and collapse of the original crystal lattice (Monkman, 1971).

As Table 30 shows, all other asbestos minerals belong in the amphibole group. The structure of amphibole asbestos is quite different from that of chrysotile. It consists of octahedral cation-oxide units arranged in narrow strips and sandwiched between corresponding strips made up of hexagonally arranged silica tetrahedra. The strips are loosely bonded to each other, and cleavage to fibers readily occurs (Gaze, 1965).

TABLE 30 Varieties of Asbestos Minerals

	Serpentine	Amphiboles				
	Chrysotile	Actinolite	Tremolite	Anthophyllite	Amosite	Crocidolite
Composition	$3MgO \cdot 2SiO_2 \cdot 2H_2O$	$2CaO \cdot 4MgO \cdot FeO \cdot 8SiO_2 \cdot H_2O$	$2CaO \cdot 5MgO \cdot 8SiO_2 \cdot H_2O$	$7MgO \cdot 8SiO_2 \cdot H_2O$	$5.5FeO \cdot 1.5MgO \cdot 8SiO_2 \cdot H_2O$	$Na_2O \cdot Fe_2O_3 \cdot 3FeO \cdot 8SiO \cdot H_2O$
Smallest fiber diameter[a]	0.01	—	0.08–0.1	0.1	0.1	0.08
Crystal system	Monoclinic	Monoclinic	Monoclinic	Orthorhombic	Monoclinic	Monoclinic
Specific gravity	2.36–2.5	3.03–3.5	2.9–3.2	2.85–3.5	2.6–3.0	3.0–3.45
Refractive index	1.49–1.57	1.62–1.68	1.60–1.65	1.60–1.66	1.66–1.70	1.69–1.71

[a]Approximate diameter in μ. Data from Gaze, 1965 and Arthur M. Langer, 1977, personal communication.

Source: Adapted from McCrone and Stewart, 1974.

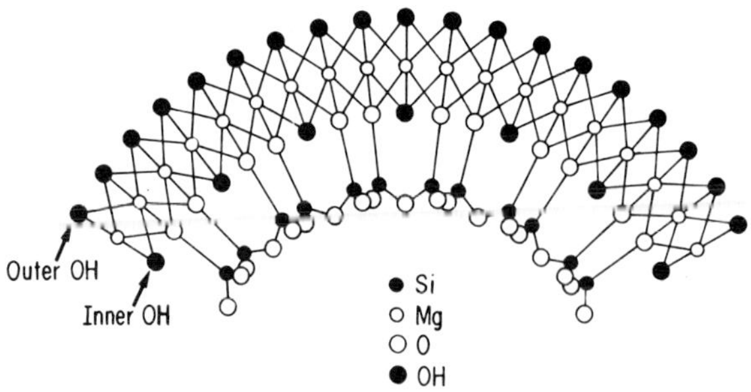

FIGURE 11 Diagrammatic representation of the crystalline structure of chrysotile fibril tube wall, showing the two main types of hydroxyls (after Daykin, 1971).

3. Tissue Distribution and Pulmonary Fibrogenic Effect. Carcinogenic Activity

The common and biologically critical characteristic shared by the different types of asbestos is that once separated from the ore, they appear in the form of microscopic fibers. These fibers readily cleave to submicroscopic fibrils, detectable only by electron microscopy. Chrysotile fibrils have a soft, wavy appearance, whereas fibrils of crocidolite and amosite are much more rigid, straight, and have a larger diameter (Table 30). Because of their shape (i.e., long needles of submicroscopic dimensions) asbestos fibrils readily penetrate and migrate through tissue linings and cell membranes, and circulate throughout the body (e.g., Smith et al., 1965b; Westlake et al., 1965; Kanazawa et al., 1970; Cunningham and Pontefract, 1973; Pontefract and Cunningham, 1973; Allison, 1973). There is also evidence for the placental transfer of asbestos fibrils (Cunningham and Pontefract, 1974). The possibility that asbestos may be teratogenic has not been investigated.

That exposure to asbestos would lead to the development of a disabling respiratory disease was known in Antiquity. In the first century the Greek geographer Strabo and the Roman naturalist Pliny the Elder recorded briefly the sickness of the lungs in slaves assigned to weaving asbestos into cloth (Brodeur, 1972). However, in the modern era it was relatively recently that the pneumoconiotic hazard due to asbestos inhalation was recognized (Murray, 1907). ("Pneumoconiosis" is the general term describing fibrosis of the lung due to inhalation of irritating dusts. The fine scarring of functional lung tissue by the dust particles brings about gradual replacement by fibrous tissue, leading to difficulty in breathing, poor oxygen absorption, and poor carbon dioxide removal.)

Asbestos-dust-induced pneumoconiosis, called asbestosis, is accompanied by the typical presence in the lungs of yellowish-brown particles called "asbestos bodies." It was in the late thirties that the presence of asbestos bodies in the lung was first correlated with exposure to asbestos (e.g., Cooke, 1929; Stewart and Haddow, 1929). The incidence and number of asbestos bodies are thought to be proportional with the length and severity of exposure (e.g., Oldham, 1973). In individuals who received heavy and continued exposure, asbestos bodies are readily seen in the sputum (e.g., Planteyd, 1968; Greenberg et al., 1976); "asbestos warts" on the skin of fingers is another manifestation of continued, direct contact. However, asbestos bodies are now also found with increasing regularity at autopsy in the lungs of deceased individuals of the population at large, with no verifiable contact with asbestos; this indicates a rising general pollution of the urban environment with asbestos (e.g., Thomson and Graves, 1966; Selikoff et al., 1967; Selikoff et al., 1972b; Oldham, 1973). Oldham (1973) estimated that the number of individuals in whom asbestos bodies can be found in the lungs postmortem increases by about 1%/year (in persons over 30 years of age) in the London area. There is growing concern as the "threat of asbestos disease widens" (Med. World News, 1976).

Extensive studies have been carried out on the structure and development of asbestos bodies (Bryson and Bischoff, 1967; Botham and Holt, 1968; Suzuki and Churg, 1969). Asbestos bodies consist of fibers heavily coated with what is regarded to be a ferroprotein (probably ferritin) or a combination of protein and an iron-containing pigment (hemosiderin); the coating material may contain as much as 40% iron, as oxide (Bryson and Bischoff, 1967; see also Haley, 1975). Coating with ferroprotein begins following phagocytosis of the fibers by alveolar macrophages. The phagocytizing cells appear to attempt at first to digest the fibers. This is suggested by studies on the chemical characterization of the cores of asbestos bodies; chrysotile asbestos cores are markedly degraded, whereas amosite cores show no significant chemical degradation even after prolonged stay in the cells (Suzuki and Churg, 1969; Langer et al., 1972). However, many fibers are not transformed into asbestos bodies, and it is these uncoated submicroscopic fibers that are believed to be responsible for the biologic (Suzuki and Churg, 1969) and especially carcinogenic (Maroudas et al., 1973) effects.

The first reports suggesting that a causal relationship exists between asbestosis and lung cancer are due to Merewether (1930), Lynch and Smith (1935), and Gloyne (1935). Since then, vast epidemiological evidence has accumulated showing that if the individuals with asbestosis survive long enough, malignant tumors of the lung will arise (Bonser et al., 1955; Doll, 1955; Wagner et al., 1960; Selikoff et al., 1964; McEwen et al., 1971; Selikoff et al., 1972a; Enterline et al., 1973; Dohner et al., 1975; IARC, 1977). Cancer of the lung affects over 50% of people with asbestosis (Buchanan, 1965). The tumors always arise in the lower lobes which are also the initial sites of fibrotic involvement. Moreover, there is increasing realization that the carcinogenic potential of asbestos is not limited to the induction of lung carcinoma and to pleural mesothelioma, the typical asbestos cancer. It has been established that exposure to asbestos also leads to mesothelioma of the peritoneum and carcinoma of the larynx, esophagus, and stomach (Enticknap and Smither, 1964; Selikoff et al., 1964; Masson et al., 1974; Stell and McGill, 1975; Shettigara and Morgan, 1975). The carcinogenicity of asbestos has been amply confirmed in animal experiments (Smith et al., 1965a; Pott et al., 1972; Shabad et al., 1974; Wagner et al., 1974; Davis, 1974; Pylev, 1974; Haley, 1975; IARC, 1977). Review of the literature (Desbordes et al., 1968) indicates that the latent period for asbestos-induced cancer in humans is 20-40 years; in rats and hamsters the latent period for tumor induction ranges from 8 to 15 months (Selikoff et al., 1967).

4. Significance of Critical Fiber Size. Nonasbestos Fibers

An extensively pursued investigative approach followed up the working hypothesis that the carcinogenicity of asbestos minerals is due either to carcinogenic heavy metal ions, such as chromium or nickel, present in the fibers as impurities, or to oils present in the fibers "naturally" or adsorbed to them during processing from the ore (Harrington, 1973). However, various types of evidence accumulating since about 1970 increasingly lend credence to the notion that carcinogenicity of asbestos fibers is due to their submicroscopic-needlelike shape, rather than to their chemical composition, physico-chemical properties, or impurities introduced during extractive processing from the ore. It is now established that for carcinogenic activity submicroscopic fibers must have diameters < 1.5 μm and lengths > 8 μm, and that tumorigenicity increases with the decrease of fiber diameter and increase of the length (Stanton et al., 1977). Excessive milling of asbestos, which decreases the length of the fibers, also reduces the carcinogenicity (Pott et al., 1972; Pott and Friedrichs, 1972; Stanton and Wrench, 1972; Stanton, 1973) and fibrogenicity (quoted in Gorski et al., 1976) of the material.

Mesotheliomas have been induced experimentally with nonasbestos substances occurring naturally as fibrous materials or processed to critical fiber dimensions. They include the fibrous $Mg(OH)_2$ minerals, brucite (Wagner and Berry, 1972) and nemalith (Pott and Friedrichs, 1972), various types of fibrous glass (Pott and Friedrichs, 1972; Stanton and Wrench, 1972; Stanton et al., 1977), and different fibrous aluminium oxide preparations (Stanton, 1973). Nonfibrous samples of the same materials are not carcinogenic. Testing of vermiculite (a type of laminar, rather than fibrous, Al-Fe-Mg-silicate appearing as thin, flat flakes) produced no tumors under conditions in which chrysotile induced a 48% incidence of mesotheliomas (Hunter and Thomson, 1973).

Despite the fact that epidemiological data analyzed to date do not substantiate health hazard to fibrous glass production workers (Gross et al., 1971; Hill et al., 1973; Enterline and Henderson, 1975), it is disquieting to note that in the 1960s several plants began manufacturing glass fibers of small diameter (most <3 μm and many <1 μm). Industrial hygiene surveys conducted in six plants that produce or make use of this material revealed that a large majority of the airborne fibers were <0.5 μm in diameter and >5 μm in length (Bayliss et al., 1976). These facilities have not been in operation sufficiently long to allow epidemiologic evaluation of the effect of small diameter glass fibers on humans, since the latent period of cancer induction by fibers of asbestos ranges from 20 to 40 years. Nonetheless, animal studies with nonasbestos materials clearly indicate that all fibrous materials of critical fiber size are suspect and should be handled with great caution and adequate safeguards. It is the writers' view that all newly developed fibrous materials, destined for industrial use or for commercial distribution, should be tested for carcinogenic activity because of the possibility that critical fiber dimensions have been reached.

5. Hypothesis of the Mechanism of Fiber Carcinogenesis

The observations of Stanton et al. (1977) that fibers <8 μm in length are inactivated by phagocytosis and that increasing length correlates with increased carcinogenicity of the fibers suggest a hypothesis of the mechanism of action. Since asbestos fibers travel through tissues and cell organelles including the nucleus, it is possible that these long, durable, submicroscopic needles—impervious to metabolic degradation—may mechanically interfere in the chromatin with the precisely timed sequence of transport and conformational rearrangements of macromolecules involved in template replication. Given enough time, the probability will arise that a fibril may be in such a position in the chromatin that, by its very presence, it will mechanically "force out" some nucleotide(s) from DNA and this will result in mutation; alternatively, the interference by fibrils may result in faulty transcription. Hence, a fibril of critical carcinogenic dimensions may be regarded, colloquially speaking, as a molecular "monkey wrench." It may be readily perceived that the longer and more rigid the fibrils are, the greater is their expectable effectiveness to bring about template alterations. Of possible significance in this regard is that crocidolite, which has straighter and much more rigid fibrils than chrysotile, appears to be more potent in inducing mesotheliomas in humans (Wagner, 1972; Enterline and Henderson, 1973). Consistent with its neoplastic properties, asbestos has been shown to induce chromosomal changes in cultured hamster ovary cells (Sincock and Seabright, 1975) and hamster embryo cells (Lavappa et al., 1975), and cell proliferation in organ culture (Rajan and Evans, 1973). A correlation has been drawn between the length of asbestos and other mineral fibers, which induce mesothelioma in the rat, and the length of glass fibers which support "anchorage-dependent" growth of fibroblasts in culture (Maroudas et al., 1973).

6. Asbestos Dust Control and Fiber Identification

The standard set for asbestos dust control in the workplace is based on the concept of "threshold limit values" (TLV). The concept of the TLV has been originally proposed "to limit exposure of workers to toxic substances" which "would produce short-term acute effects such as irritation, narcosis, or alteration of body functions" (Nicholson, 1976). The flexible concept of the TLV standard to limit exposure to asbestos was originally proposed by Dreessen et al. (1938) when no massive evidence existed as yet linking asbestos exposure with any cancer. There is now growing recognition that in dealing with carcinogens no truly meaningful TLV can be set (Nicholson, 1976), especially in the light of the overwhelming evidence that many cancers have a multifactorial etiology. The considerably increased lung cancer risk incurred by asbestos workers who smoke (Selikoff et al., 1968) is a case to the point.

Since for carcinogenic agents any exposure above zero level may be assumed to be associated with some risk, the TLV for such substances more correctly represents "risk limitation values" (Nicholson, 1976); Nicholson notes that "in the case of asbestos, the information we have is that an extraordinary rate of cancer occurs at asbestos concentrations considerably above the TLV." This of course leaves the open-ended question as to what is an acceptable risk versus economic benefits for the workers and a society increasingly exposed to asbestos.

The problem is compounded by the fact that enforcement to the adherence of the TLV values has been limited, frequently absent, and often ineffective. In many situations workers are exposed to levels well above the standard (Nicholson, 1976). Nonetheless, the concept of the TLV has been useful in stimulating the development and application of dust control procedures. From 1938 to 1975 the TLV has been gradually reduced from 5×10^6 fibers/ft^3 to $5 \times 10^5/\text{m}^3$.

Different methods have been used to measure asbestos dust concentration in the air. Past U.S. studies were based mainly on the impinger method. In this method the air sample passes through a shallow cell used as a trap, containing, in general, water or alcohol. After a definite sampling period the number of particles that have settled in the cell are counted using a light microscope. A shortcoming of this method is that it is not sensitive enough to detect submicroscopic asbestos fibrils present in the air of asbestos textile plants, which do not settle and are not seen by light microscopy (Ayer et al., 1965).

The medium for dust sampling that has come into wide use in recent years is the Millipore membrane filter; these filters collect particles as small as 0.1 μm in diameter with practically 100% efficiency. Following sampling, the filters are treated (with a mixture of dimethylphthalate and diethyloxalate) to render them transparent and are examined by light or electron microscopy. Comparative studies of the impinger and membrane filter techniques have been carried out by Ayer et al. (1965) and Roach (1965).

In England the thermal precipitator was the standard air sampling instrument for many years. The dust deposit was collected directly on glass cover slips, which could be incinerated before counting to remove any organic fiber. However, the thermal precipitator could not detect fibers longer than about 10 μm and was gradually abandoned in favor of the membrane filter technique (Holmes, 1965, 1973). Another instrument in use is the Royco automatic particle counter based on the light-scattering of dust particles (Addingley, 1965; Roach, 1965; Holmes, 1973). Dust measurement methods and protective equipment have been reviewed by Haley (1975).

Light microscopy is ideal for rapid identification of asbestos in powdered samples of various materials: dust, mortar, insulation or wallboard, mineral samples such as talc, and so on. Identification is based on the measurement of refractive index using a polarizing microscope. The samples are mounted in appropriate Cargille refractive index media for fiber identification by use of the dispersion colors. Under these conditions each type of asbestos shows two characteristic dispersion colors, one for the plane of polarization parallel and another perpendicular to the longitudinal axis of the fiber, as summarized in Table 31 (McCrone and Stewart, 1974). By this method fibers >0.5 μm in diameter may be detected. Electron microscopy must be used for detection of fibers too fine to observe by light micros-

TABLE 31 Dispersion Staining Colors for Asbestos

Asbestos type	Refractive index liquid	Dispersion staining color: Parallel	Dispersion staining color: Perpendicular
Chrysotile	1.560	Light blue	Magenta
Anthophyllite	1.610	Blue-green	Golden yellow
Amosite	1.670	Red magenta	Golden yellow
Crocidolite	1.700	Magenta	Blue magenta

Source: From McCrone and Stewart, 1974.

copy, such as those present in water supplies, soft drinks, beer, fruit juices, or injectable parenteral drugs.

The count of asbestos bodies in sputum specimens is a recommended method for measuring the severity of industrial exposure of individuals to asbestos (Greenberg et al., 1976). A promising and potentially important new method is based on the analysis of feces for asbestos as an indicator of the quantitative exposure to ingested as well as inhaled fibers (Cunningham et al., 1976). In fact, due to the mobility of asbestos fibers throughout the body, up to 75% of inhaled asbestos may appear in the feces within 30 days (Evans et al., 1973).

B. Metal and Metalloid Carcinogens

1. Introduction. Nature, Reactions, and Scope of Carcinogenic Elements

Toxic metals and metalloids represent a long-term threat in the environment. Perhaps because of inherent familiarity with these inorganic toxicants, stemming from the fact that they originate from the crust of the earth, and because of the known physiologic roles of trace amounts of certain heavy metals, their dangerous environmental potentials have been largely overlooked until recent years. It was not until after the resolution of the causes of the "Minamata disaster" in the early sixties and an exactly similar occurrence in Niigata in 1965, both due to mercury poisoning of an entire region of Japan (Tucker, 1972a), as well as the official recognition in 1968 by the Japanese Ministry of Health and Welfare of the extremely painful terminal disease, itai-itai, as being due to chronic cadmium poisoning (Tsuchiya, 1969, 1976a), that awareness of the toxic effects of metals started to take root in the environmental consciousness of the public.

The term "heavy metals" is often used, meaning toxic elements having a density greater than 5 (Passow et al., 1961). However, they are more correctly designated by the term "toxic metals and metalloids," since this category includes the light metal beryllium, as well as the metalloids arsenic and selenium. The toxic metals and arsenic share the characteristic of reacting with -SH groups and the ability to form coordination complexes and chelates with various compounds and structures in the cell. Examples of biological ligands which may be of importance in these reactions are amino, carboxyl, phosphoryl, and imidazole groupings. The -SH and coordination complexes and chelates formed in living organisms have been termed "biocomplexes" (Clarkson, 1977). The relative stabilities of complexes of some typical coordinating metals decrease in the order: Hg > Be > Cu > Ni > Co > Pb > Zn > Cd > Fe > Mn (Martin and Martin, 1964). The reaction products of mercury with sulfhydryl compounds are extremely stable; for example, the stability constant for dissociation of the glutathione adduct is 1×10^{-41} (Stricks and Kolthoff, 1953). Moreover, the -SH adducts of mercury are stable over the entire pH range. The very high stability of these adducts provides a rationale for the considerable toxicity of mercury.

An important endogenous heavy metal acceptor is metallothionein, a low-molecular-weight protein, rich in -SH groups (26 -SH/mol). The exact cellular function of metallothionein is not yet understood, and it has been proposed to be a heavy metal "scavenger protein" (Sandstead and Klevay, 1975). Metal-bound metallothionein contains 59,500 ppm cadmium, 16,900 ppm zinc, 1500 ppm copper, and 310 ppm iron (quoted in Sandstead and Klevay, 1975). It has been hypothesized that this protein may also play a major role in cadmium transport in the body (Friberg et al., 1974). There is evidence that cadmium (Nordberg, 1971; Piotrowski et al., 1974; Cempel and Webb, 1976), mercury (Piotrowski et al., 1974), and zinc (Chen et al., 1974) induce the synthesis of metallothionein in the liver. Kidney cells can also synthesize metallothionein in response to cadmium and mercury (Piotrowski et al., 1974; Webb and Daniel, 1975; Cherian and Clarkson, 1976). The protein does not appear to be an exclusive binding trap and/or binding carrier for heavy metals, since no in vivo binding of Mn^{2+}, Ni^{2+} (Webb, 1972a; Sabbioni and Malafante, 1975), and Co^{2+} (Webb, 1972a) to metallothionein has been detected.

The metals that were confirmed to display strong-to-moderate carcinogenic activity in experimental animals are beryllium, cadmium, chromium, cobalt, nickel, and lead. There is very substantial epidemiological evidence indicating that arsenic is markedly carcinogenic principally toward the lung and skin in humans; however, all experimental attempts to confirm this in animals—or to unequivocally demonstrate the carcinogenic activity of arsenic in animals—have consistently failed (Pelfrene, 1976). In addition to these elements, copper, manganese, molybdenum, silver, titanium, and zinc are weakly-to-marginally carcinogenic at high dose levels. The carcinogenic metals and metalloids that are probably the most important from the standpoint of general environmental exposure are arsenic, beryllium, cadmium, chromium, and lead; these are reviewed in the following section. Reported evidence for the carcinogenicity of Co, Cu, Mn, Mo, Ni, Ag, Ti, and Zn are presented in tabular form (Table 32). A number of articles summarized the field of metal and metalloid carcinogenesis (Roe and Lancaster, 1964; Hueper, 1966b; Furst and Haro, 1969a, 1969b; Kanisawa, 1971; Furst, 1971; Sunderman, 1971; Williams, 1972; IARC, 1973a; Fishbein, 1976; Sunderman, 1977).

Despite the considerable toxicity of mercury, there is so far only one unrepeated study suggesting that this element is carcinogenic in rats when injected i.p. in the metallic form (Druckrey et al., 1957); there is no evidence that exposure to mercury leads to excess cancer mortality in humans. It remains that methylmercury, to which inorganic mercury is metabolized by microorganisms in the environment, has been found to increase the frequency of chromosome breaks in lymphocytes from Swedish fishermen and their families who were exposed through consumption of environmentally contaminated fish (Skerfving et al., 1974). Moreover, mutagenic effects of methylmercury have been reported in rats, drosophila, and certain plant cells (cited in Clarkson et al., 1976). Inorganic mercury was found mutagenic in a bacterial system (Nisioka, 1975).

Although initial reports indicated hepatic cirrhogenic and neoplastic effects of selenium (Nelson et al., 1943; Tscherkes et al., 1963), the total evidence is conflicting whether this element is truly carcinogenic or not (Shapiro, 1972). Selenium also has a reputation as a cancer-preventive and antineoplastic agent (Shapiro, 1972), and it has been shown that selenium and organoselenium compounds in μg quantities protect rats against dietary liver necrosis (Schwarz and Porter, 1972). In trace amounts selenium is a biologically indispensable element (Stadtman, 1974; Leach and Fuller, 1975). The nutritional requirement was approximated to lie between 0.1 and 0.3 ppm; however, even in moderately excessive quantities (3-4 ppm in the diet of humans and animals) it can be extremely toxic (Coles, 1974; see also West, 1967; and Frost and West, 1967). Actually, selenium first attracted attention as being the etiologic agent of "alkali disease," chronic poisoning of the livestock that fed on plants, concentrating large amounts of Se from the soil, in certain areas of the Great Plains in the United States (Levander, 1972). Sourcebooks on detailed biological aspects of selenium have appeared (Rosenfeld and Beath, 1964; Muth, 1967).

2. Environmentally Significant Metal and Metalloid Carcinogens

a. Arsenic

The carcinogenicity of arsenic to humans was first recognized by the English physician Paris (1820), who recorded that copper smelters were occasionally affected by ". . . a cancerous disease of the scrotum, similar to that which infests the chimney sweeps. . . ." The next 120 years saw a variety of novel applications (metallurgical, chemical, agricultural, and medicinal) of inorganic and organic arsenicals, and by about 1930 the relationship between the exposure to arsenicals and the development of skin cancer in the affected individuals was generally accepted. A series of epidemiological studies beginning with Hill and Faning (1948) revealed substantial excess mortality in arsenic-exposed individuals due to cancers of the lung, larynx, nasal sinuses, and lymphatics, in addition to cancers of the skin; the development of epitheliomatous proliferative ulcerations of the skin is characteristically preceded by pigmentation and keratosis (Bowen's disease). Many of these epidemiological studies have

TABLE 32 Carcinogenicity of Metals with the Exception of Beryllium, Cadmium, Chromium, and Lead[a,b]

Element	Form administered	Species	Route	Histological type of tumor	Reference
Cobalt	Metal powder, cobalt oxide, and sulfide	Rat and rabbit	s.c., i.m., intrathoracic, and intraosseous	Various types of sarcomas	Summarized in Table IV of Sunderman, 1977
	Cobalt oxide and sulfide	Mouse	i.m.	No tumors	Gilman, 1962; Gilman and Ruckerbauer, 1962
	Cobaltic acetate	Mouse	i.p.	No tumors	Stoner et al., 1976
Copper[c]	Copper sulfate	Fowl	Intratesticular	Teratomas	Falin and Anissimora, 1940a, b
	Copper chloride	Mouse	Intratesticular	Teratomas	Bresler, 1964
	Copper sulfide	Rat	i.m.	No tumors	Gilman, 1962
	Industrial exposure	Human epidemiological data		Lung tumors	Agnese et al., 1959; Newman et al., 1976
Manganese	Manganous sulfate	Mouse	i.p.	Lung adenomas	Stoner et al., 1976
Molybdenum	Molybdenum trioxide	Mouse	i.p.	Lung adenomas	Stoner et al., 1976
Nickel	Metal dust, nickel sulfide, nickeltetracarbonyl, and nickelocene	Rat, mouse, hamster, guinea pig, and rabbit	Parenteral routes and inhalation	Diverse tumors	Summarized in Table X of Sunderman, 1977
	Industrial exposure	Human epidemiological data		Tumors of lung and nasal passage	Hueper, 1966b; Sunderman, 1977
Silver[d]	Colloidal metal	Rat (BD strain)	s.c. + i.v.	Spindle cell sarcomas (at s.c. site)	Schmähl and Steinhoff, 1960
Titanium	Titanocene	Rat	i.m.	Fibrosarcomas and lymphomas	
	Titanocene	Mouse	On skin	No tumors	Furst and Haro, 1970
	Titanocene	Mouse	Oral	No tumors	

Zinc[c]	Zinc chloride and zinc sulfate	Fowl, rat, and hamster	Intratesticular	Teratomas	Summarized in Table VII of Sunderman, 1977
	Zinc acetate	Mouse (A strain)	i.p.	No tumors	Stoner et al., 1976
	Metal powder	Rat	i.m.	No tumors	Furst and Cassetta, 1972

[a]Inorganic aluminum compounds have been noted to induce nonmalignant granulomas at the site of s.c. or i.m. injection (White et al., 1955; Voss and Tolki, 1960; Diezel, 1961; Erdohazi and Newman, 1971). There is no evidence for increased cancer mortality associated with bauxite mining or the aluminum production industry.

[b]Although metallic iron and its inorganic salts are not known to be carcinogenic (e.g., Hueper and Payne, 1962; Stoner et al., 1976), medicinally used iron-dextran complex ("Imferon") has been shown in many laboratories to induce sarcomas in mice, rats and rabbits at the site of parenteral administration at high doses (Roe and Lancaster, 1964; Furst and Haro, 1969b; Sunderman, 1977), as well as distant tumors (Langvad, 1968). The metal appears to be necessary for the carcinogenicity, since the polysaccharide moiety by itself is not carcinogenic (Haddow and Horning, 1960; Kunz et al., 1963; Neukomm, 1969). However, this does not necessarily imply that iron, per se, has some degree of carcinogenicity, since whereas dextran alone has a molecular weight of about 2500, the molecular weight of iron-dextran complex is many times higher (Roe and Lancaster, 1964). Thus, the carcinogenicity of iron-dextran may represent a special instance of carcinogenesis by soluble high-polymers (Hueper, 1964). Nonetheless, the findings caution that medicinal iron preparations should be given orally rather than parenterally whenever possible (Roe and Lancaster, 1964).

[c]There is no evidence so far that copper and zinc are carcinogenic in experimental animals by any other route except by intratesticular injection. Copper but not zinc is potentially mutagenic in that it decreases the fidelity of DNA synthesis (Sirover and Loeb, 1976).

[d]Furst and Schlauder (1977) found silver to be not carcinogenic by i.m. injection into Fisher rats.

been tabulated by Hueper (1966b; in Table 27) and Blejer and Wagner (1976; in Table 1), as well as reviewed by Fishbein (1976), Pelfrene (1976), Pinto and Nelson (1976), and Sunderman (1977); several case histories are reviewed in detail by Buchanan (1962).

Blejer and Wagner (1976) concluded that excess mortality from skin cancer was observed only in workers of veterinary arsenical pesticide ("sheep-dip" and "cattle-dip") manufacturing; on the other hand, inhalation of arsenical fumes, dust, and insecticide sprays has been generally blamed for causing respiratory cancer of vineyard and metal smelter workers. The carcinogenicity of medicinally used arsenical preparations has been reviewed by Neubauer (1947), Hueper (1967), and Ehlers (1968). The latent period of medicinal arsenic cancer was estimated to lie between 25 and 75 years and that of occupational arsenic cancers between 35 and 60 years (Hueper, 1959). Excessive cancer rates and typical arsenical dermal keratosis were noted in geographic areas with naturally high arsenic content in the drinking water (Tello, 1963; Yeh, 1963, 1973; Tseng et al., 1968; Hueper, 1966b).

In an attempt to obtain a dose-response relationship of inorganic arsenicals-induced carcinogenesis in humans, Lee and Fraumeni (1969) and Ott et al. (1974) correlated work exposure levels with observed mortality. Lee and Fraumeni (1969) showed that excess mortality due to respiratory cancer was eight times higher among workers who were heavily exposed to arsenic for over 15 years than in the general population. Recalculation and reinterpretation of the data of Ott et al. by Blejer and Wagner (1976) suggest, however, the important possibility that there is no excess mortality due to arsenic up to an atmospheric concentration of 1-1.5 $\mu g/m^3$ (as a time-weighted-average concentration for an 8-hr day, projected for a 40-year working life), as shown in Table 33. Epidemiologic studies indicate that both the trivalent arsenicals (arsenic trioxide) and the pentavelent arsenicals (arsenates) are carcinogenic toward the same tissue targets (Hueper, 1966b; Fishbein, 1976).

Pelfrene (1976) has exhaustively reviewed the inconclusive bioassay studies attempting to induce tumors with arsenic in experimental animals. The only investigation to date that recorded positive results is that of Osswald and Goerttler (1971); these authors obtained a significant increase in the incidence of lymphomas in Swiss mice following s.c. or i.v. administration of sodium arsenate.

Probably of much greater practical importance are other experimental findings reviewed by Pelfrene (1976) that arsenic displays potent teratogenic properties in a high incidence of the offspring of pretreated mothers. Moreover, the mutagenicity of both trivalent and pentavalent arsenicals in a bacterial assay system was recently reported by Nisioka (1975). The

TABLE 33 Ratio of Observed to Expected Respiratory Cancer Death by 40-Year Dosage and Daily Arsenic Exposure Categories

40-Year dosage (Log_e mg)	Daily TWA dose[a] ($\mu g/m^3$)	Respiratory cancer deaths (observed/expected)
3.74	1	0.6
4.84	3	2.0
5.53	6	2.9
6.04	10	2.2
6.68	20	1.8
7.35	40	2.1
8.17	90	3.9
8.78	160	6.3
10.30	740	7.0

[a]TWA = time-weighted average.

Source: From Blejer and Wagner, 1976.

TABLE 34 Souces of Potential Nonoccupational Exposure to Arsenic

Paints and inks (as pigment); colored paper and wallpaper (as pigment); colored crayons; sealing wax; wood, pelts and furs (as preservative); textile (as mordant and pigment); poison bait for rodents; chemicals for horticulture; hair lotion (traces in some); arsenic-containing tonics and pharmaceuticals; residues on fruit and vegetables and in tobacco sprayed with arsenical insecticide
Hobby and repair activities in the home: pottery glazing; gardening; use of arsenical pigment containing paints and enamels; dust-producing grinding of colored rubber; inhaling fumes from fluxes during soldering and welding
Living in the vicinity of copper, zinc, or lead smelters, of orchards, fields and woods dusted and sprayed with arsenical pesticides, and of large, coal-burning power plants; smoking tobacco high in arsenical residues; consuming drinking water naturally high in or polluted with arsenic; consuming unpeeled fruit treated with arsenical insecticides; prolonged consumption of arsenic-containing medicinal preparations

significance of these findings lies in the facts themselves, as well as in the well-known correlation between teratogenicity and mutagenicity, on one hand, and carcinogenic activity in laboratory animals, on the other hand (DiPaolo and Kotin, 1966).

A searching review of the environmental forms of arsenic and of the arsenical pollution sources and exposure levels has been given by Fishbein (1976). He concluded that "in most areas other than the vicinity of smelters, arsenic concentration in the air is very low and often below detectable limits." Air quality data from the National Air Surveillance Networks show that the average daily concentration for 133 locations in the United States was 0.02 $\mu g/m^3$ in 1964, with occasional values as high as 0.8 $\mu g/m^3$ (NASN, 1964). Vallee (1973) lists the major sources of arsenical air pollution as: combustion of coal, metal smelters, pesticides, and cotton gin dust. Coal contains 0.08-16 μg As/g. Copper smelters also contribute substantially to arsenical pollution as these ores may contain as much as 3% of As (Vallee, 1973). To date, the epidemiologically identifiable health consequences of environmental arsenic in the United States remain isolated in the areas of high air pollution density; this is suggested by the study of Blot and Fraumeni (1975) that among the 3021 counties lung cancer mortality rates were significantly higher in the 36 counties primarily involved in the smelting and refining of copper, zinc, and lead, which are the ores yielding arsenic as a by-product. Potential nonoccupational contacts with arsenic are summarized in Table 34.

There is little arsenical pollution in the rivers and lakes in the United States; arsenic was found in < 6% of the samples surveyed, with levels ranging from 0.035 to 0.068 ppm (Vallee, 1973). This is close to the arsenic content of seawater (0.0006-0.03 ppm) as determined around 1960. In the proximity of industrial effluent drainage points, however, the arsenic concentration may be as high as 1.0 ppm (Vallee et al., 1960).

In fruits and vegetables arsenic derives from pesticide residues and, in the vicinity of industrial pollution sources, from atmospheric fallout. In the United States the maximum allowed concentration of arsenic in fruits and vegetables is 1.4 ppm (Hueper, 1966b). In dairy products a survey conducted in 28 U.S. cities in 1969-1970 indicated that the arsenical levels were not higher than 0.1 ppm; in meat, fish, and poultry the level was between 0.1 to 2.6 ppm (Corneliussen, 1972). Shellfish is high in arsenic from natural sources, with levels ranging from 3 ppm for oysters to as much as 174 ppm for prawns (Hueper, 1966b).

Discontinuation in the early 1950s of the use of arsenical insecticide sprays on tobacco crops in the United States brought about a notable decline of the arsenic content of cigarettes to an average of 7.7 μg As/g tobacco (Lee and Murphy, 1969). Arsenic in tobacco has been considered by some investigators as an important contributing factor in the causation of lung cancer in smokers.

TABLE 35 Sources of Contact with Beryllium: Typical Industries and Uses

Primary: Mining and milling of ore. Beryllium extraction plants. Production and processing of beryllium-containing alloys.

Secondary: Production of aircraft and spacecraft engines. Production and use as high-energy rocket solid-propellant. Nuclear energy industry: Coal-burning utilities (effluent from). Production of electrical contacts and other precision metal parts of switchboards and computers. Machine shops involved in the production of metal parts of various precision instruments, high tolerance engines and pumps. Production of radio tubes, cathode-, and x-ray tubes. Ceramics industry. Manufacture of space vehicle reentry cones. Production of crucibles, refractories, and beryllium glass. Production of beryllium-containing artificial semiprecious stones. Production and use of gas lantern mantles.

Duggan and Lipscome (1969) calculated the average daily intake of arsenic in the United States to be 0.137-0.330 mg/individual. Recently the National Institute of Occupational Safety and Health (NIOSH) proposed to set the permissible atmospheric exposure limit to 0.004 mg As/m^3 per 8-hr period (DOL, 1975a). Fishbein (1976) lists the Maximum Allowable Concentrations in other countries: 0.5 mg As/m^3 in England, Federal Republic of Germany, and Yugoslavia; 0.3 mg As/m^3 in Czechoslovakia, German Democratic Republic, Hungary; 0.15 mg As/m^3 in Poland; 0.003 mg As/m^3 (per 24-hr period) in the USSR.

Arsenicals are biomethylated to the volatile gaseous derivatives, dimethylarsine, trimethylarsine, cacodylic acid (hydroxydimethylarsine), and methyl- and dimethylarsinic acid in anaerobic sediments, such as in lakes and ponds (Braman and Foreback, 1973). Biomethylated derivatives of arsenic have not been detected so far in the oceans (Braman, 1975). Arsines are highly toxic but are rapidly oxidized in the air. Their possible role in the cycling of arsenic between ecological compartments of the environment is not clearly understood.

b. Beryllium

A metal lighter and stronger than aluminum, beryllium has become a quasi indispensable material in modern industry. The extent to which it is now ubiquitous in various applications of high technology is illustrated in Table 35. This gives a perspective of the potential magnitude of beryllium dissemination in the environment.

Pulmonary berylliosis was first described as an occupational disease by Weber and Engelhard (1933) and confirmed in two further reports (Marradi-Fabroni, 1935; Gelman, 1936). However, these early reports were generally disregarded until the enormously increased use of the metal beginning with World War II brought about a great upsurge of beryllium disease. Reeves (1977) notes that the production of the first atomic bombs (Manhattan Project) alone required more beryllium than the world consumption of the metal until 1940. Beryl, the ore from which beryllium is extracted, is mined in the United States, Brazil, India, and the Malagasy Republic.

Rediscovery of the beryllium syndrome began with observations on workers of the fluorescent tube industry in Massachusetts, which started to use, in the early 1940s, traces of zinc-beryllium silicates as phosphors in order to bring about the desired light emission. However, the etiology of the disease, as due to chronic exposure to the dust of beryllium or insoluble beryllium compounds, was not generally recognized or accepted until the 1950s, and a Beryllium Case Registry was established at the Massachusetts General Hospital. Reeves (1977) gives an interesting discussion of the conflicting observations on the two types of clinical courses of beryllium disease. The acute form of the disease, encountered mainly in the beryllium extraction industry and caused by inhalation of relatively high doses of soluble beryllium compounds, represents a type of "chemical pneumonia" (acute inflammation of the lung), which is generally followed by recovery. On the other hand, exposure to very much smaller amounts but <u>insoluble</u> forms beryllium is, in a seemingly contradictory fashion, more hazardous and leads to the debilitating and often fatal chronic form of the disease. The biological reason for the two courses of the disease is unknown (Reeves, 1977).

Chronic berylliosis is a slow but progressive multifocal granulomatous inflammation of lung tissue resembling sarcoidosis (Boech's sarcoidosis is an idiopathic disease characterized by granulomatous tubercular lesions principally of the skin, lungs, eyes, and lymph nodes.) Granulomatous lesions due to beryllium may also develop in other tissues, such as the skin (De Nardi et al., 1949; McCord, 1951). Chronic exposure to beryllium leads to the development of cutaneous hypersensitivity to the metal or its compounds, which phenomenon is used as a diagnostic tool (Curtis's test) for the early recognition of chronic berylliosis (Waksman, 1959; Niemöller, 1962). Besides Curtis's skin test, other immunological tests were explored for the recognition of berylliosis. The various types of immunological responses support the hypothesis (Sterner and Eisenbud, 1951) that berylliosis is an autoimmune disease. Partial immunization against pulmonary berylliosis has been obtained in the guinea pig (Reeves, 1977).

As of early 1974, 837 cases of chronic berylliosis had been filed in the Beryllium Case Registry (Stoeckle and Mancuso, 1974). Recent cases in the United States and abroad involve workers in a variety of industries, such as electronics and neon tube (Izumi and Kobara, 1966), nuclear energy (DHEW, 1972; Hasan and Kazemi, 1974), and ceramics (Izumi et al., 1976). Cases were observed also in the general population surrounding beryllium plants (Machle, 1948; Eisenbud et al., 1949; Chesner, 1950; Perry, 1955; Campbell, 1961; Metzner and Lieben, 1961). Beryllium hazards may be transferred into the environment when contaminated work clothes are laundered in commercial laundries (Cohen, 1963). Women appear to be more sensitive to chronic berylliosis than men (De Nardi, 1959). Several articles and books have reviewed the toxic properties of beryllium and its compounds (Tepper et al., 1961; Stokinger, 1966; Hueper, 1966b; Kimmerle, 1966; Tepper, 1972a, b; IARC, 1972a). Various preventive and control procedures have been introduced in the 1950s to minimize beryllium hazards (Hueper, 1966b).

Principal evidence for the carcinogenic activity of beryllium comes from animal experiments. Intravenous injection of suspensions of beryllium oxide, phosphate, and zinc-beryllium silicate induced osteogenic sarcomas in mice and rabbits, and intratracheal instillation or inhalation of aerosols of beryllium oxide, hydroxide, sulfate, or phosphate produced pulmonary carcinomas in rats and monkeys (summarized through 1968 in Table I of Sunderman, 1977; Tapp, 1969; Groth and MacKay, 1971). Beryllium metal powder (Barnes, 1950), the beryllium ore, beryl (Wagner et al., 1969), and beryllium-containing exhaust products from rocket motors (Spencer et al., 1968) are also effective carcinogens in animals. In contrast to beryl, bertrandite ore dust did not induce malignant pulmonary tumors in rats, and only occasional atypical proliferations were observed (Wagner et al., 1969). As compared to rats, hamsters appear to be relatively resistant to the pulmonary neoplastic effect of beryllium-containing materials (Spencer et al., 1968; Wagner et al., 1969). The histopathology of beryllium-induced tumors has been extensively discussed by Schepers (1961) and Komitowski (1968). The pathogenicity of beryllium oxide depends on the firing temperature during its production; "low-fired" dusts, calcined at about 500° C, show marked biological activity (Spencer et al., 1968; Sanders et al, 1974) while "high-fired" dusts produced at 1400-1500° C are much less toxic (Conradi et al., 1971; Sanders et al., 1974). The firing temperature possibly determines the crystal structure (Crossmon and Vandemark, 1954) and, hence, the chemical reactivity of the surface of the particles toward cell constituents.

Most interestingly, guinea pigs are resistant to induction of malignant tumors by beryllium compounds either by injection or inhalation (Vorwald, 1950; Reeves and Krivanek, 1974); on the other hand, guinea pigs—just as humans, but unlike other rodents—develop the typical symptoms of chronic berylliosis (Reeves and Krivanek, 1974). Whether monkeys—which are susceptible to the carcinogenic effects of beryllium—are also susceptible to chronic berylliosis does not appear to have been reported.

Consensus appears to be lacking on the carcinogenicity of beryllium to humans. Hueper (1966b) reviewed a total of seven cases of lung cancer attributable to exposure to beryllium dust or fumes that have been described in the literature up to 1966. It is important to note the observations of Niemöller (1963) that lung cancer may develop in exposed individuals lacking the typical radiologic signs of berylliosis, yet their lung tissues contain spectrographically identifiable beryllium. The argument presented in support of the new exposure limit proposed in 1975 by NIOSH recognizes the definite carcinogenic potential of beryllium to humans (Fed. Reg., 1975). Yet, Reeves (1977) concluded in his review that "the sum of evidence, at least thus far, favors the view that humans, like the guinea pigs, are susceptible to berylliosis but resistant to beryllium cancer." In 1977 a struggle developed between the Occupational Safety and Health Administration (OSHA) and the beryllium industry over the question of whether epidemiological evidence is strong enough to warrant declaring beryllium a "carcinogen" and to enforce the exposure limit proposed in 1975 (Shapley, 1977).

The pulmonary granulomatous reaction to beryllium may take years to become manifest (Hueper, 1966b; Reeves, 1977). Hueper (1966b) estimated that the latent period for beryllium-induced cancer of the lung in humans is between 20 and 30 years and for beryllium cancers in animals between 11 and 24 months.

Even if the view is accepted that beryllium, singly, does not represent an as yet demonstrably substantial cancer hazard to humans, another consideration suggests that the setting of low exposure limits (2 $\mu g/m^3$ on the TLV list and 0.01 $\mu g/m^3$ on the air quality standard list) was the better part of wisdom; the question is, rather, whether even the new exposure limit of 1 $\mu g/m^3$, as recently proposed by NIOSH, is stringent enough. Indeed, synergistic interactions among beryllium and other metallic and organic carcinogens, as well as asbestos, are a definite possibility. An even more worrisome prospect follows from the well-known immune-suppressant effect of many organic carcinogens. If resistance to beryllium-induced neoplasia and susceptibility to berylliosis are due to the same immunological mechanism, then carcinogens and other immune-suppressant agents may synergize the latent carcinogenic effect of beryllium while decreasing or abolishing the granolomatous tissue response (Niemöller, 1963). This would render it particularly difficult to assign an etiological or participatory role to beryllium in human cancer. Yet, a spectrographic study by Tietz et al. (1957) indicates that already 20 years ago a large sector of the general population harbored in their pulmonary tissues significant amounts of beryllium. The metal is not known to have a physiological role as an indispensable trace element. Sources of environmental beryllium pollution have been briefly reviewed by Fishbein (1976).

c. Cadmium

Cadmium is a low-melting-point, ductile metal, which is universally used in the electroplating industry because of its marked resistance to corrosion and the pleasing silvery finish it gives to metal surfaces. Cadmium is used in the fabrication of household objects, such as ice-cube trays, cooking utensils, and metal pitchers, in the metallurgy of copper alloys, in nickel-cadmium batteries, as a component of soldering-brazing alloys, in sleeve bearings of engines operating at high temperatures (automobile, aircraft, marine), in colored pigment used in paints, soap, and glass, in wood finishes (such as varnish), as a stabilizer in plastics, and in fungicides. Approximately 100 times as much cadmium is used today as was used 70 years ago. In 1970 the world production of the metal was 16,000 tons, and according to the present trend over 50,000 tons/year will be produced by 1980. It has been estimated (Heindl, 1970; Ashley, 1972) that the U.S. consumption of the metal—6300 tons in 1972—will increase two- to three-fold by the year 2000.

Christensen and Olsen (1957) stated that "cadmium has probably more lethal possibilities than any of the metals." The consequences of cadmium toxicity include retardation of growth, anemia, heart abnormalities, hypertension, damage principally to the kidneys and liver, and cancer of the lung and prostate. However, by far the most widely known and appalling affliction is the cadmium-induced osteoporosis/osteomalacia, itai-itai disease, which is endemic in an area of northern Japan, the Toyama Prefecture. (Osteoporosis represents loss of the principal inorganic constituents of bone, calcium and phosphate, whereas osteomalacia represents loss of these inorganics together with loss of organic matrix from bone.)

Tucker (1972b) gives an impressive description of the disease

> which, beginning with simple symptoms such as "lumbago" or "joint pains" . . . leads to bone porosity and to the total inhibition of bone repair mechanism so that, stage by stage as the disease progresses, the load-bearing bones of the skeleton suffer deformation, fracture and collapse. The agony accompanying such a process defies description and . . . long before death, sufferers . . . "characteristically reveal a decreased stature." The Japanese term for the disease, "itai-itai-byo" . . . mimics the cries of sufferers, and has been humorously translated as "Ouchi-Ouchi Disease." There is nothing humorous about it.

There have been notable efforts recently by apologists to exonerate cadmium from being the etiologic agent of itai-itai-byo and to classify the disease "as a nutritional osteomalacia caused by vitamin D deficiency and other nutritional factors" (Tsuchiya, 1976a). However, as Tsuchiya (1976a) himself recognizes "the question remains, nevertheless, why itai-itai disease is confined to that particular area where cadmium pollution exists." The occurrence of this occupational osteoporotic disease is not limited to any particular area, but is clearly associated with exposure to cadmium, irrespective of geography (Adams et al., 1969).

The toxicity of cadmium encompasses a wide gamut of effects. An acute effect of the inhalation of toxic fumes from smelting and brazing operations is the "metal fume fever"; however, this has also been observed as a result of exposure to fume-emitting industrial processes involving zinc, copper, and magnesium (Flick et al., 1971). Chronic effects of inhaled cadmium include total or partial loss of smell, coughing, difficulty in breathing, loss of appetite, weight loss, often a yellow staining of the teeth, and general irritability (Arena, 1963).

Chronic administration of cadmium to rats, rabbits, and calves leads to loss of body weight, skin changes, loss of hair, anemia, and enlargement of and damage to the heart, kidneys, and testes (Decker et al., 1958; Schroeder et al., 1963; Powell et al., 1964); the same pathological effects are seen in humans chronically exposed to cadmium. Moreover, Itokawa et al. (1974) and Yoshiki et al. (1975) found that cadmium-fed rats develop osteomalacia/osteoporosis, reproducing the characteristic bone lesions of the itai-itai disease.

The major part of the cadmium intake accumulates, bound to metallothionein (see Sec. IV.B.1) in the kidneys and the liver, and the accumulation is dose dependent in mice (Probst et al., 1975), rats (Colucci et al., 1975; Loeser and Lorke, 1977a), and dogs (Loeser and Lorke, 1977b). The kidneys and the liver are also the tissues of cadmium storage in humans (Syversen, 1975).

Organ-bound cadmium is retained very efficiently and only very small amounts are excreted (Berlin and Ullberg, 1963; Lucis et al., 1969). It has been estimated that during the life span humans accumulate at least 30 mg metallothionein-bound cadmium (Webb, 1975), which is believed to be released with a half-life of 10-40 years (Nordberg, 1974; Tsuchiya et al., 1974; Kjellstrom and Friberg, 1974). In rats the small amount released is excreted through the bile, bound to glutathione (Cherian and Vostal, 1977).

Because of the relative biological inertness of bound cadmium while in the storage organs, probably critical tissue concentrations must be reached before toxic effects become manifest (Friberg et al., 1974; Colucci et al., 1975). Sudden release of large amounts of cadmium from storage organs under some circumstances may have toxic consequences, just as a new, large intake (Bremner, 1974; Webb, 1975).

Cadmium poisoning causes hepatic (Faeder et al., 1977) and renal (Axelsson et al., 1968; Nomiyama et al., 1973) damage in experimental animals, and the proteinuria seen as a consequence of the renal damage is also a typical manifestation of chronic cadmium exposure in humans (Lauwerys et al., 1974; Tsuchiya, 1976b). The toxic effects of cadmium toward the liver and kidneys, as well as the testicles, cardiovascular system, and bone (and the dose-response relationships of these effects) have been reviewed by Friberg et al. (1974). Considerable effort has been devoted to epidemiological studies of the cardiovascular and hypertensive effects of environmental cadmium in humans; some of these studies were reviewed by Flick et al. (1971). Manifestations of the testicular toxic effects of cadmium involve degeneration of the interstitial cells (Leydig cells) and of the seminiferous tubules, followed by regeneration (Donnelly and Monty, 1977); these tissue manifestations generally precede the emergence of cadmium-induced malignant tumors of the testes in animals.

Epidemiologic investigations in the United States and abroad show an excessive number of bronchogenic and prostatic cancers among workers exposed to cadmium (Kipling and Waterhouse, 1967; Potts, 1965; Adams et al., 1969; Blejer and Caplan, 1971; Lemen et al., 1976; Friberg et al., 1974, 1975). Consistent with the neoplastic effects, severe chromosomal aberrations (dicentric and ring chromosomes) have been observed in peripheral blood leukocytes of workers occupationally exposed to cadmium (Léonard et al., 1974; Deknudt and Léonard, 1975) and in leucocytes of itai-itai patients (Shiraishi and Yoshida, 1972).

Experimental studies provide strong confirmation of the carcinogenicity of cadmium. Administration of cadmium metal powder, cadmium oxide, chloride, sulfide, and sulfate by various parenteral routes to mice, rats, and chickens induced local sarcomas and tumors of the Leydig cells ("Leydigiomas"); on the other hand, intratesticular injection of cadmium chloride into chickens produced teratomas. Several reviews cover these studies (Roe and Lancaster, 1964; Furst and Haro, 1969a; Lacassagne, 1971; Flick et al., 1971; Sunderman, 1977, summarized in Table II). Stoner et al. (1976) obtained no tumors in strain A mice by 23 weekly i.p. injections of cadmium acetate (total dose 14 mg/kg). Despite the fact that the testis is a target tissue of cadmium-induced carcinogenesis, i.p. injection of cadmium chloride to male mice did not increase the number of dominant lethal mutants; neither were chromosome rearrangements observed in the treated males (Gilliavod and Léonard, 1975). This is surprising in view of the marked chromosomal aberrations in cadmium-exposed humans already noted. However, in an in vitro system cadmium salts brought about a decrease in the fidelity of DNA synthesis, indicating their potential mutagenicity (Sirover and Loeb, 1976). The genetic effects have been reviewed by Friberg et al. (1974). Teratogenic effects of cadmium in rats (Chernoff, 1973) and chickens (Ribas and Schmidt, 1973) were described. The various toxic effects of cadmium have been covered in comprehensive reviews (Flick et al., 1971; IARC, 1973c; Friberg et al., 1974, 1975; Fassett, 1975; Jugo, 1977).

There is growing evidence that cadmium (and other toxic metals) in the air occur mainly in the form of aerosol particulates, minute solid particles, or liquid droplets ranging in size from 0.005 to 50 microns (Fennelly, 1976). Cadmium in the particulates is probably in the form of oxide (Nordberg, 1974). Aerosol particulates of less than several microns in diameter are suspected to be of prime importance to the etiology of pollution-related diseases, as they are capable of bypassing the filtering systems of the respiratory passage and penetrating deep into the lungs.

Davis (1970) estimated that because of the vapor pressure of cadmium metal (b.p. 767°C), about 90% of the cadmium emission into the atmosphere in the United States in 1968 was due to the smelting of ores and the manufacturing and reprocessing of cadmium alloys and cadmium-plated metals. From this estimate and the known secondary sources of cadmium emission, as well as from the cadmium consumption of the United States in 1968, Fishbein (1976) concluded that "the atmospheric emissions of cadmium amounted to approximately 34% of the cadmium consumption for that year." Notwithstanding the estimated emission of over 2000 metric tons of cadmium into the atmosphere in 1968, the average concentration of cadmium in the air of U.S. cities was at 0.006-0.36 μg/m^3 (NASN, 1968); these figures are low compared to the mean values (0.01-0.53 μg/m^3) measured in Tokyo air during several months of 1969-1971 (Nordberg, 1974).

In unpolluted natural waters the cadmium concentrations are < 1 μg/kg (Kopp and Kroner, 1970; Nordberg, 1974). In the United States and Sweden the concentration in the drinking water is generally below 5 μg/kg (Fishbein, 1976). Nonetheless, the quality of the drinking water in several U.S. cities, in terms of cadmium content, raised concern because of the association between cadmium intake and cardiovascular diseases (Punsar, 1973).

Little is known of the ecological cycling of cadmium among compartments of the environment. However, it appears that most of the atmospheric input eventually concentrates in the soil, and in the sediments of rivers and lakes. Even in areas believed to be unpolluted, cadmium concentrations in the soil in the United States approach 1 mg/kg. In certain polluted agricultural areas of Japan concentrations ranged between 1 and 69 mg/kg soil (Nordberg, 1974). In the neighborhood of cadmium-emitting plants as much as several milligrams per square meter of ground surface are deposited monthly (Friberg et al., 1974).

Plants, cereals, and bread grains grown on polluted soils take up and accumulate cadmium (Flick et al., 1971; Nordberg, 1974; Friberg et al., 1974). The concentration of cadmium present in vegetation grown in polluted soils is directly proportional to the extent of pollution (Flick et al., 1971). Itai-itai disease in the Toyama area has been traced to the contamination of agricultural land, from which cadmium concentrates in rice and other vegetables (Tucker, 1972b). Cadmium is present at high levels in phosphate fertilizers (Schroeder and Balassa, 1961).

Expectedly, then, the principal sources of cadmium intake for individuals in the general population are food and smoking (Fishbein, 1976). The concentration of cadmium in various food materials show wide variations, with an approximate median of 0.05 mg/kg (Nordberg, 1974). High concentrations were found in shellfish (in particular oysters and lobsters), in beef and pork kidney and liver, apple cider, various vegetables, roasted peanuts, and sugar beet pulp (Schroeder and Balassa, 1961). In cadmium-polluted areas of Japan concentrations of 1 mg/kg or higher were found in rice (Nordberg, 1974).

Regarding the intake from smoking, a pack of 20 cigarettes contains about 30 μg of cadmium (quoted in Fishbein, 1976), and about 70% of it passes into the smoke (Nandi et al., 1969). Thus, cigarette smoking represents a significant contribution to cadmium accumulation in the body (Lewis et al., 1972). Moreover, cadmium is a potent inhibitor of ciliary activity in the trachea (Adalis et al., 1977), which represents the clearing mechanism for inhaled particulates; this effect may be an important contributor to the susceptibility of smokers to pollution-related respiratory diseases.

Estimates of the daily intake of cadmium in industrialized countries (United States, England, West Germany, Japan, Canada, Czechoslovakia, and Roumania) in the period of 1969-1973 ranged between 15 and 80 μg/day (Friberg et al., 1974; Webb, 1975). The cadmium content of the main storage organs (kidney and liver) can serve as an index of the cadmium pollution in different regions. Thus, Schroeder (1960) and Schroeder and Balassa (1961) determined the cadmium content of ash from autopsy specimens of kidney tissue from different countries. Their studies gave the following distribution in terms of ppm cadmium in the ash: Japan, 6030 ± 800; Hong Kong, 5620 ± 950; Thailand (Bangkok), 4910 ± 1470; Taiwan, 4150 ± 1160; United States, 2910 ± 110; England, >1000 (?); Switzerland (Bern), 2260 ± 480; India (Delhi and Lucknow), 2120 ± 310; Nigeria, 1700 ± 150; Ruanda-Urundi, 710 ± 150. The cadmium levels in the liver (about one-tenth of the renal levels) showed a similar pattern. The considerable accumulation of cadmium in the storage organs is best illustrated by the high concentration found in the liver of shellfish (420 mg/kg wet weight) (Nordberg, 1974), the highest level found in any food material.

Several excellent reviews summarize the cadmium pollution sources, emission and exposure levels, and their trends (Flick et al., 1971; Friberg et al., 1974, 1975; Nordberg, 1974; Webb, 1975; Fishbein, 1976).

In view of the various health dangers represented by cadmium, singly, or in combination with other metals, the levels recommended as "tolerable" or set as "threshold" are probably too high and should be lowered. The Commission of European Communities (CEC, 1974) accepted an average intake of 20-50 μg/day as "tolerable," while a World Health Organization Committee (WHO, 1972) set the "tolerable" intake at 70 μg/day. As of 1973 the industrial threshold limit values listed in the United States were 100 $\mu g/m^3$ for cadmium fumes and at 200 $\mu g/m^3$ for metal dust and soluble salts (ACGIH, 1973). A comparison of standards set for chemicals in other countries (USSR, West Germany, Japan) shows comparably high values (Winnell, 1975).

d. Chromium

Principally because of its metallurgical use in alloys, the production of chromium in the form of metal and its compounds is the highest among the environmentally significant carcinogenic elements. The realization that exposure to dusts and fumes of chromium compounds represents a substantial cancer hazard to humans emerged in the period 1937-1946 (Hueper, 1966b). Overwhelming epidemiological evidence shows a considerable excess of chromium-compounds-induced occupational cancers, with a predilection to the lung, nasal cavity, sinuses, and larynx (Hueper, 1966b; Enterline, 1974; Baetjer et al., 1974); Hueper (1966b) estimated that 70% of the cases had latent periods between 11 and 30 years. Table 36 presents data of Hueper and Conway (1964), illustrating the degree of cancer hazard of chromate exposure to humans. Dermatitis is an often-occurring stigmata of exposure.

Animal experiments fully confirm the carcinogenic activity of chromates and establish the carcinogenicity of chromium metal powder as well; administration by intraosseous, i.m., s.c., i.p., and intrapleural route to mice, rats, and rabbits produced local sarcomas (summarized in Table III of Sunderman, 1977). By intrabronchial implantation of pellets of calcium chromate into rats, Laskin et al. (1970) and Kuschner and Laskin (1971) obtained a high incidence of squamous cell carcinomas and adenocarcinomas of the lung. Exposure of mice to inhalation of chromate dust induced alveologenic adenomas and adenocarcinomas (Nettesheim et al., 1971); however, no squamous cell carcinomas were obtained by inhalation (Baetjer et al., 1959; Steffee and Baetjer, 1965). Lead chromate displays the tissue target specificity of both chromate and lead, since local sarcomas and renal carcinomas were obtained upon i.m. injection to rats (Furst et al., 1976). The carcinogenicity of chromium carbonyl [$Cr(CO)_6$] has been shown in an assay system of tracheal grafts (Lane and Mass, 1977).

Chromium may be bi-, tri-, and hexavalent in its compounds. The overwhelming majority of epidemiological reports are based on data from workers in industries using soluble chromates, and there is a belief that only hexavalent chromium compounds represent cancer hazard to humans. Attempts to demonstrate the carcinogenicity of chromite ore (Shimkin and Leiter, 1940/1941) or chromium (II) sulfate (Stoner et al., 1976) in the strain A mouse pulmonary tumorigenesis assay system were unsuccessful. Also, Ivankovic and Preussman (1975) reported that rats fed Cr_2O_3 at 1%, 2%, and 5% level for 2 years tolerated the compound well and no teratogenic effect in the offspring were observed; this green compound (known as C-green 9 or pigment green 17) is used industrially and is incorporated into eye makeup, particularly as eye shadow. It remains that Hueper (1966b) observed the development of ulcerative squamous cell carcinomas of the skin of the snout in rats exposed to chromite ore dust. Moreover, both chromium (II) chloride and chromium (III) chloride are potentially mutagenic according to Sirover and Loeb (1976), in that they induced infidelity of DNA synthesis in triple-blind studies. On the other hand, Nisioka (1975) found chromate but not chromite to be mutagenic in a bacterial system. The carcinogenic activity of parenterally administered chromium metal powder itself has already been stated. Clearly, further studies are urgently needed to definitively establish the role of the valence state of chromium in the carcinogenicity of its compounds.

TABLE 36 Lung Cancer in Chromate Workers in the United States, England, and Germany

Country	Morbidity ratio		Lung cancers/100,000	
	Expected	Observed	General population	Chromate workers
United States	1.9	31.9	16.7	470.8
England	1.3	7	—	—
Germany	1	43	—	—

Source: From Hueper and Conway, 1964.

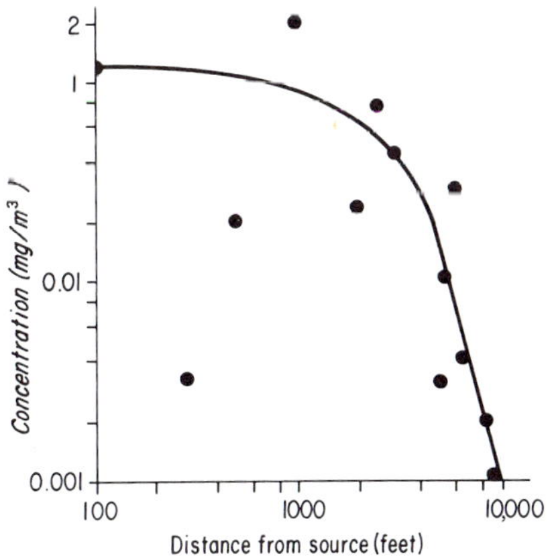

FIGURE 12 Chromium content of the air in the environment of a chromate plant (from Bourne and Rushin, 1950).

Chromium is a typical example of indispensable trace elements which at higher concentrations display toxic and/or carcinogenic properties. Animal studies show that in trace amounts chromium is needed for growth, longevity, and resistance to disease. It is considered essential for the maintenance of normal glucose tolerance in experimental animals and probably in humans (Mertz et al., 1974; Anderson and Mertz, 1977).

The prospect has been raised early that the accumulation of chromium in the environment may represent a spillover of cancer hazard from the industries to the population at large. The extent of this spillover from industries to the neighborhoods, as a function of the distance from the source, has been studied by Bourne and Rushin (1950); their findings are summarized in Fig. 12. Atmospheric neighborhood pollution has been reviewed by Hueper (1966b).

Besides industries producing or using chromium-containing products, other sources add to the chromium burden of the environment. For example, the burning of coal is probably responsible for much of the chromium in the urban atmospheres (Sullivan, 1969). Plants producing portland cement is an additional source of atmospheric chromium because of the presence of the metal in limestone (Denton et al., 1954). Effluents of domestic and industrial incinerators represent another potential source with the increase of wastes resulting from the manufacture and use of chromium-containing products. Fishbein (1976) reviewed the contribution of different sources to environmental chromium pollution. Table 37 presents the spectrum of contacts of nonoccupational chromium exposure.

TABLE 37 Sources of Potential Nonoccupational Exposure to Chromium

Paints, inks, and woodstains (as pigment); colored prints (in printing inks as pigment); colored crayons, colored candles and other wax products (as pigment); traces in blueprints and linoleum; textiles (as mordant for dying and color printing); leather (as tanning agent); wood (as preservative); match heads (as ingredient); fabrics, felt hats, and drapes (water-repellent treatment of); cosmetics (eye shadow); antirusting agent in steam-heating circuits
Hobby and repair activities in the home: pottery glazing; photographic developing; use of chromate pigment containing paints and enamels; dust-producing grinding of chromium-alloys (stainless steel), leather, colored rubber, fiberglass
Living in the vicinity of chromate plants, oil refineries, scrap metal smelters, incinerators, and large, coal-burning power plants

Atmospheric chromium levels in the United States range from <0.01 μg/m^3 in nonurban areas to 0.01-0.03 μg/m^3 in typical metropolitan areas (National Research Council, 1974). Stocks (1960) reported considerably higher levels in England based on sampling in 23 localities (0.9-21.5 μg/m^3). Concentration in United States river waters ranges between 1 and 10 μg/kg (National Research Council, 1974). The average daily chromium intake of individuals in the United States was estimated by Schroeder (1970) to be 0.28, 4, and 280 μg from air, water, and food, respectively.

e. Lead

Although lead is a naturally occurring element in the environment, it is also a most ubiquitous contaminant. The global mean natural lead content of lakes and rivers has been estimated (Fishbein, 1976) to be between 1 and 10 μg/liter. Most of the lead of natural origin concentrates in the soil. The principal source of lead pollution in the industrialized countries is the combustion of lead alkyl additives of gasoline (Hicks, 1972). In the United States 184,000 tons of lead aerosol are released in the atmosphere yearly (quoted in Fishbein, 1976) of which over 95% is attributable to motor vehicle exhausts. However, on a worldwide scale, the amount of atmospheric lead originating from combustion of coal approximately equals that originating from combusted gasoline. Atmospheric lead has been detected in the air of even the most remote areas of the globe. Airborne lead is mainly concentrated in aerosol particulates (Fennelly, 1976).

Atmospheric lead does not appear to increase significantly the average lead content of water in the major rivers in North America beyond the estimated natural level. In fact, the average lead content of samples of 33 major rivers was 6.6 μg/liter (National Research Council, 1971). The stability of the level of lead is probably due to the rapid clearing from the water by sediments and soils. There is evidence that in the deep anaerobic sediments lead is microbially transformed to volatile tetramethyl-lead (Wong et al., 1975; Jarvie et al., 1975) and is then recycled into the atmosphere.

The diet is the major source of lead intake. Estimates of daily intake in different industrialized countries (Table 38) range from 70 to about 520 μg (Boppel, 1975). King (1971) has estimated that the level of lead that may be ingested without clinical symptoms is 300-400 μg/day for adults and half as much for children between 2 and 3 years old. Principal sources of lead contamination accessible to young children range from city dust and dirt, through paint chips and toothpaste, to printed matter (quoted in Bogden et al., 1975).

Evidence for the carcinogenicity of lead in mammals originates exclusively from animal bioassay experiments. There is no indication from epidemiological data so far that exposure to lead would bring about an increase in the incidence in any type of cancer in humans (Dingwall-Fordyce and Lane, 1963; Hammond et al., 1972; Cooper, 1976). On the other hand, a number of reports show that administration of lead (as acetate or basic acetate) to rats and mice by oral, i.p., or s.c. route induces renal adenomas and adenocarcinomas (summarized in Table VI of Sunderman, 1977); hamsters were refractory to renal tumor induction by feeding basic lead acetate (Van Esch and Kroes, 1969). Renal tumors were also found in wild rats that were living and feeding on burning refuse dumps; analysis of their tissues revealed that these animals had chronic lead poisoning (Kilham et al., 1962). Deviating from the generality of lead-induced renal tumors in rats, Coogan et al. (1971) obtained an over 30% incidence of fibrosarcomas at the site of s.c. administration of lead subacetate to Sprague-Dawley rats. Stoner et al. (1976) found lead subacetate to be weakly carcinogenic toward the mouse lung when tested in the strain A mouse lung bioassay system. Epstein and Mantel (1968) tested the carcinogenicity of tetraethyl lead by s.c. injection to newborn mice; although their results are not unequivocal, they may be regarded as suggestive of the weak carcinogenicity (lymphosarcomas) of the compound. Lead is also potentially mutagenic as it decreases the fidelity of DNA synthesis (Sirover and Loeb, 1976). Lead carcinogenesis is discussed in detail in two volumes of IARC (1972b, 1973b) monographs.

The problem of environmental and occupational lead toxicity was the subject of several symposia and books (AMA, 1971; Goyer, 1974; Waldron and Stöfen, 1974). A very readable account of the environmental impact of lead toxicity is given by Tucker (1972c). Environmental exposure levels have been reviewed by Fishbein (1976). The recently proposed new maximum occupational exposure limit of lead is 100 μg/m^3 in the air (DOL, 1975b).

3. Cross-Reactions Between Effects of Metals

Beyond the toxicity and/or carcinogenicity of metals tested singly, antagonistic and synergistic effects of combinations of metals have been described. The antagonistic effects are probably due to competition for essential -SH groups (Clarkson, 1977) and/or coordination ligands in the tissues. Metal-metal cross-reactions involving cadmium have been studied the most extensively.

Daniel and Webb (1964) reported the protection of cell cultures by zinc against the toxic effects of cadmium, cobalt, and nickel. Interestingly, the protective effect holds only in a relatively narrow zinc concentration range, which is different for the three metals. With cadmium, the most toxic of these metals to the cultures, protection is essentially total at zinc concentrations between 4 and 6×10^{-5} M, and there is lesser protection against cobalt and nickel toxicity. In contrast, at higher concentrations zinc strongly potentiates the toxic effects of cobalt and nickel, suggesting the possibly critical significance of the relative levels of heavy metals in vivo.

Zinc in vivo protects against the acute toxicity of cadmium (Webb, 1972b) and against cadmium-induced vascular injury to and destruction of the mouse testis (Parizek, 1957; Gunn et al., 1968a). Sandstead and Klevay (1975) have reviewed the health implications of cadmium-zinc interactions. The protective effect of selenium against cadmium-induced testicular damage, when administered simultaneously in equimolar amounts (Gunn et al., 1968a, b), may be attributed to the stability of topically formed CdSe preventing cadmium from engaging in the formation of biocomplexes in the tissue. When both elements are administered simultaneously, but in different parts of the body, there is a dramatic rise of both the cadmium and selenium levels in the blood plasma (Clarkson, 1977).

Consistent with the protective effects of zinc against cadmium, zinc acetate inhibits the induction of interstitial cell tumors of the testis in rodents by cadmium chloride (Gunn et al., 1963, 1964). However, the induction of sarcomas by i.m. injection of cadmium metal powder is not inhibited by simultaneous injection of zinc metal powder (Furst and Casetta, 1972).

TABLE 38 Lead Uptake in the Daily Diet

Country	μg Pb/day
West Germany (1969)	518
West Germany (1969–1971)	75–86
United States (1943)	Approx. 300
United States (1947)	Approx. 300
United States (1961)	Approx. 330
United States (1965)	Approx. 300
United States (1968)	100–500
United States (1966–1967)	285
United States (1968–1969)	70–80
United States (1970–1971)	70–80
Japan (1965)	230–320
England (1949)	100
England (1972)	200
Canada (1974)	138

Source: Adapted from the compilation by Boppel, 1975 of published estimates by different authors.

When cadmium, mercury, and zinc are administered s.c. together in a single injection the retention of mercury and cadmium affects the retention of zinc at the injection site more than zinc affects the retention of the other two heavy metals (Magos and Webb, 1976). This follows the ranking of stability constants of the respective -SH adducts of the metals: 1×10^{-41} for Hg, 2.8×10^{-30} for Cd, and 4×10^{-28} for Zn (based on combination with glutathione). Competition for different binding or carrier compounds in the blood might explain why cadmium accumulates mainly in the liver and mercury in the kidneys. As expected, mercury decreases the uptake of cadmium in the kidneys; however, it increases the uptake of zinc. Also, contrary to expectation, cadmium enhances the uptake of both zinc and mercury by the liver, its principal storage organ. The complexity of these changes indicates that despite the fact that all three metals induce the synthesis of metallothionein, their interaction cannot be explained by a single mechanism (Magos and Webb, 1976).

Manganese is rather specific in inhibiting the induction of local sarcomas by i.m. administration of nickel subsulfide (Ni_3S_2) dust in suspension, whereas admixture of dusts of aluminum, copper, or chromium does not inhibit sarcomatogenesis by Ni_3S_2 (Sunderman et al., 1974, 1976). The 1976 study revealed that admixture of manganese dust lowers the rate of in vitro solubilization of Ni_3S_2 in blood serum. However, manganese dust did not affect the in vivo uptake of nickel in the tissue, but after several months a significant reduction was found in the concentration of tissue-bound nickel at the injection sites of manganese-coadministered rats (Sunderman et al., 1976).

An instance of antagonism of environmental importance is the one between arsenic and selenium (Levander, 1972; Tucker, 1972d), the general mammalian acute toxicity of selenium being in some circumstances about 10,000 higher than that of arsenic. The protective effect of arsenic consists in displacing selenium from the liver and stimulating its excretion through the bile (Levander, 1972).

In contrast to the antagonistic effects reviewed above, evidence is accumulating on synergism of toxic and teratogenic effects in man and animals of certain combinations of metals and metalloids, such as arsenic and lead (USSR Ministry of Health, 1969, cited in Tucker, 1972e), cadmium and lead (Ferm, 1969; Der et al., 1976), cadmium and mercury (Magos et al., 1974), and mercury and copper (quoted in Tucker, 1972c). Subclinical lead toxicity is promoted to manifest lead toxicity by reduced dietary calcium (Six and Grover, 1970). Challop (1971) considered the possible role of cadmium-lead synergism in children with clinical manifestations of lead poisoning.

ACKNOWLEDGMENTS

The authors wish to express their gratitude to Dr. Mary F. Argus for scientific reviewing of the entire manuscript, for helpful critical comments on substance, style and form, as well as for helping with the logistics of organization of the material. We also wish to record here our sincere appreciation and indebtedness to Mrs. Barbara J. Baxter for the excellent and painstakingly accurate typing of the manuscript, for a number of useful and pertinent comments regarding form and organization of the material, as well as for her faithful and efficient devotion to the multifaceted secretarial duties of the laboratory. This writing was carried out during periods of support by the following grants: 922 A from the Council for Tobacco Research, CA-15111 from the National Cancer Institute, and LM-03036 from the National Library of Medicine.

REFERENCES

Sections I and II

Alford, A. (1975). Environmental applications of mass spectrometry. Biomed. Mass Spectrom. 2:229-253.

Alford, A. (1977). Environmental applications of mass spectrometry. Biomed. Mass Spectrom. 4:1-22.

Arcos, J. C., and Argus, M. F. (1974). Chemical Induction of Cancer. Structural Bases and Biological Mechanisms, Vol. IIA. Academic Press, New York.

Badger, G. M. (1962). The Chemical Basis of Carcinogenic Activity. Thomas, Springfield, Ill.

Badger, G. M., Kimber, R. W., and Novotny, J. (1964). Formation of aromatic hydrocarbons at high temperatures. XXI. Pyrolysis of n-butylbenzene over a range of temperatures from 300° to 900° at 50° intervals. Aust. J. Chem. 17:778-786.

Badger, G. M., Kimber, R. W., and Spotwood, T. M. (1960). Mode of formation of 3,4-benzpyrene in human environment. Nature 187:663-665.

Baldwin, R. W., Cunningham, G. J., Dean, H. G., Patridge, M. W., Surtees, S. J., and Vipond, H. J. (1965). Further studies on the influence of peripheral ring substitution on the carcinogenicity of tricycloquinazoline. Biochem. Pharmacol. 14:323-331.

Baldwin, R. W., Cunningham, G. J., and Patridge, M. W. (1959). Studies of the carcinogenic action of tricycloquinazoline. Br. J. Cancer 13:94-98.

Berg, J. W. (1975). Diet. In Persons at High Risk of Cancer. An Approach to Cancer Etiology and Control, J. F. Fraumeni, Jr. (Ed.). Academic Press, New York, pp. 201-224.

Blumer, M. (1961). Benzopyrenes in soil. Science 134:474-475.

Blumer, M., Dorsey, T., and Sass, J. (1977). Azaarenes in recent marine sediments. Science 195:283-285.

Blumer, M., and Youngblood, W. W. (1975). Polycyclic aromatic hydrocarbons in soils and recent sediments. Science 188:53-55.

Borneff, J., and Fischer, R. (1962). Carcinogenic substances in water and soil. X: Investigation on phyto-plankton of an inland-lake for PAH. Arch. Hyg. Bakteriol. 146:334-345.

Borneff, J., and Kunte, H. (1964). Carcinogenic substances in water and soil XVI: Evidence of PAH in water samples through direct extraction. Arch. Hyg. Bakteriol. 148:585-597.

Borneff, J., and Kunte, H. (1965). Carcinogenic substances in water and soil. XVII: About the origin and evaluation of the PAH in water. Arch. Hyg. Bakteriol. 149:226-243.

Borneff, J., Selenka, F., Kunte, H., and Maximos, A. (1968a). Experimental studies on the formation of polycyclic aromatic hydrocarbons in plants. Environ. Res. 2:22-29.

Borneff, J., Selenka, F., Kunte, H., and Maximos, A. (1968b). Synthesis of 3,4-benzpyrene and other polycyclic aromatic hydrocarbons in plants. Arch. Hyg. Bakteriol. 152:279-282.

Boyland, E. (1950). The biological significance of metabolism of polycyclic compounds. Biochem. Soc. Symp. 5:40-54.

Bridbord, K., Finklea, J. F., Wagoner, J. K., Moran, J. B., and Caplan, P. (1976). Human exposure to polynuclear aromatic hydrocarbons. In Carcinogenesis: A Comprehensive Survey, Vol. I, Polynuclear Aromatic Hydrocarbons. Chemistry, Metabolism, and Carcinogenesis, R. Freudenthal and P. W. Jones (Eds.). Raven Press, New York, pp. 319-324.

Brunnenmann, K. D., and Hoffmann, D. (1976). Analysis of polynuclear aromatic hydrocarbons in the respiratory environment. In Carcinogenesis: A Comprehensive Survey, Vol. I, Polynuclear Aromatic Hydrocarbons. Chemistry, Metabolism, and Carcinogenesis, R. Freudenthal and P. W. Jones (Eds.). Raven Press, New York, pp. 283-297.

Bulay, O. M., and Wattenberg, L. W. (1970). Carcinogenic effects of subcutaneous administration of benzo(a)pyrene during pregnancy on the progeny. Proc. Soc. Exp. Biol. Med. 135:84-86.

Burlingame, A. L., Kimblo, B. J., and Derrick, P. J. (1976). Mass spectrometry. Anal. Chem. 48:368R-403R.

Cavalieri, E., Mailander, P., and Pelfrene, A. (1977). Carcinogenic activity of anthanthrene on mouse skin. Z. Krebsforsch. 89:113-118.

Cavalieri, E., Roth, R., Rogan, E., Grandjean, C., and Althoff, J. (1978). Mechanisms of tumor initiation by polycyclic aromatic hydrocarbons. In Proceedings of the 2nd International Symposium on Polycyclic Aromatic Hydrocarbons. Battelle Columbus Laboratories, Columbus, Ohio, September 1977. (in press)

Chemical Society (1960). The Chemical Society Special Publication No. 14, Handbook for Chemical Society Authors. The Chemical Society, London.

Cohn, R. S. (1959). An Introduction to Chemical Nomenclature. Buterworths, London.

Collucci, J. M., and Begeman, C. R. (1965). The automotive contribution to air-borne polynuclear aromatic hydrocarbons in Detroit. J. Air Pollut. Control Assoc. 15:113-122

Cooper, R. L., and Lindsey, A. J. (1955). 3,4-Benzpyrene and other polycyclic hydrocarbons in cigarette smoke. Br. J. Cancer 9:304-309.

Cram, S. P., and Juvĕt, R. S., Jr. (1976). Gas chromatography. Anal. Chem. 48:411R-442R.

Creasia, D. A., Poggenburg, J. K., and Nettesheim, P. (1976). Elution of benzo(a)pyrene from carbon particles in the respiratory tract of mice. J. Toxicol. Environ. Health 1:967-975.

Crittenden, B. D., and Long, R. (1976). The mechanisms of formation of polynuclear aromatic compounds in combustion systems. In Carcinogenesis: A Comprehensive Survey, Vol. I, Polynuclear Aromatic Hydrocarbons: Chemistry, Metabolism, and Carcinogenesis, R. Freudenthal and P. W. Jones (Eds.). Raven Press, New York, pp. 209-223.

Della Porta, G., and Terracini, B. (1969). Chemical carcinogenesis in infant animals. Prog. Exp. Tumor Res. 11:334-363.

DePierre, J. W., and Ernster, L. (1978). The metabolism of polycyclic hydrocarbons and its relationship to cancer. Biochim. Biophys. Acta 473:149-186.

Dipple, A. (1976). Polynuclear aromatic hydrocarbons. In Chemical Carcinogens, ACS Monograph 173, C. E. Searle (Ed.). American Chemical Society, Washington, D.C., pp. 245-314.

Dong, M. W., Locke, D. C., and Hoffmann, D. (1977). Characterization of azaarenes in basic organic portion of suspended particulate matter. Environ. Sci. Tech. 11:612-618.

Elliott, L. P., and Rowe, D. R. (1975). Air quality during public gatherings. J. Air Pollut. Control Assoc. 25:635-636.

EPA (1975). Preliminary Assessment of Suspected Carcinogens in Drinking Water and Appendices. Interim Report to Congress, Office of Toxic Substances, U.S. Environmental Protection Agency, Washington, D.C.

Fábián, B. (1968). Carcinogenic substances in edible fats and oils. V. Studies of sausage after different methods of cooking. Arch. Hyg. Bakteriol. 152:251-254.

Falk, H. L., Kotin, P., and Miller, A. (1959). Milk as an eluant of polycyclic aromatic hydrocarbons added to wax. Nature 183:1184-1185.

Falk, H. L., Miller, A., and Kotin, P. (1958). Elution of 3,4-benzpyrene and related hydrocarbons from soots by plasma proteins. Science 127:474-475.

Fishman, M. J., and Erdmann, D. E. (1975). Water analysis. Anal. Chem. 47:334R-361R.

Freudenthal, R., and Jones, P. W. (Eds.) (1976). Carcinogenesis: A Comprehensive Survey, Vol. I, Polynuclear Aromatic Hydrocarbons. Chemistry, Metabolism, and Carcinogenesis. Raven Press, New York.

Fritz, W. (1971). Umfang und Quellen der Kontamination unserer Lebensmittel mit krebserregenden Kohlenwasserstoffen. Ernährungsforschung 16:547-557.

Fritz, W. (1973). The formation of carcinogenic hydrocarbons during heating of foods. 5. Contamination on grills over charcoal. Deut. Lebensm. Rundschau. 69:119-122.

Galuškinová, V. (1964). 3,4-Benzpyrene determination in the smoky atmosphere of social meeting rooms and restaurants. Neoplasm 11:465-468.

Geraghty, J. J., Miller, D. W., van der Leeden, F., and Troise, F. L. (1973). Water Atlas of the United States. Water Information Center, Port Washington, N.Y.

Giger, W., and Blumer, M. (1974). Polycyclic aromatic hydrocarbons in the environment: isolation and characterization by chromatography, visible, ultraviolet and mass spectrometry. Anal. Chem. 46:1663-1671.

Gordon, R. J., and Bryan, R. J. (1973). Patterns in airborne polynuclear hydrocarbon concentrations at four Los Angeles sites. Environ. Sci. Tech. 7:1050-1053.

Gräf, W., and Diehl, H. (1966). About the natural background of carcinogenic polycyclic aromatics and its cause. Arch. Hyg. Bakteriol. 150:49-59.

Grasso, P., and O'Hare, C. (1976). Carcinogens in food. In Chemical Carcinogens, ACS Monograph 173, C. E. Searle (Ed.). American Chemical Society, Washington, D.C., pp. 701-728.

Grimmer, G., and Hildebrandt, A. (1965a). Hydrocarbons in the human environment. III. Content of polycyclic hydrocarbons in different vegetables. Deut. Lebensm. Rundschau. 61:237-239.

Grimmer, G., and Hildebrandt, A. (1965b). Kohlenwasserstoffe in der Umgebung des Menschen. II. Der Gehalt polycyclischer Kohlenwasserstoffe in Brotgetreide verschiedener Standorte. Z. Krebsforsch. 67:272-277.

Grimmer, G., and Hildebrandt, A. (1968). Hydrocarbons in the human environment. VI. The content of polycyclic hydrocarbons in crude vegetable oils. Arch. Hyg. Bakteriol. 152:255-259.

Haddow, A., and Kon, G. A. (1946/47). Chemistry of carcinogenic compounds. Br. Med. Bull. 4:314-325.

Haenszel, W., Berg, J. W., Segi, M., Kurihara, M., and Locke, F. (1973). Large-bowel cancer in Hawaiian Japanese. J. Natl. Cancer Inst. 51:1765-1779.

Hammond, E. C. (1975). Tobacco. In Persons at High Risk of Cancer. An Approach to Cancer Etiology and Control, J. F. Fraumeni, Jr. (Ed.). Academic Press, New York, pp. 131-138.

Hanna, M. G., Jr., Nettesheim, P., and Gilbert, J. R. (Eds.) (1970). Inhalation Carcinogenesis, AEC Symposium Series 18, U.S. Atomic Energy Commission, Oak Ridge, Tenn.

Harrison, R. M., Perry, R., and Wellings, R. A. (1975). Polynuclear aromatic hydrocarbons in raw, potable and waste waters. Water Res. 9:331-346.

Harrison, R. M., Perry, R., and Wellings, R. A. (1976). Effect of water chlorination upon levels of some polynuclear aromatic hydrocarbons in water. Environ. Sci. Tech. 10:1151-1156.

Hartwell, J. L. (1951). Survey of Compounds Which Have Been Tested for Carcinogenic Activity, USPHS Publication 149. U.S. Public Health Service, Washington. Shubik, P., and Hartwell, J. L. (1957) Ibid., Supplement I; (1969) Ibid., Supplement II. This series has been continued by U.S. Public Health Service: 1961-1967 volume, Section I and II; 1968-1969 volume; 1970-1971 volume; 1972-1973 volume.

Hase, A., and Hites, R. A. (1976). On the origin of polycyclic aromatic hydrocarbons in the aqueous environment. In Identification and Analysis of Organic Pollutants in Water, L. H. Keith (Ed.). Ann Arbor Science Publishers, Ann Arbor, Mich., pp. 205-214.

Hecht, S. S., Bondinell, W. E., and Hoffmann, D. (1974). Chrysene and methylchrysenes: presence in tobacco smoke and carcinogenicity. J. Natl. Cancer Inst. 53:1121-1133.

Hecht, S. S., Loy, M., and Hoffmann, D. (1976). On the structure and carcinogenicity of the methylchrysenes. In Carcinogenesis—A Comprehensive Survey, Vol. I, Polynuclear Aromatic Hydrocarbons. Chemistry, Metabolism, and Carcinogenesis, R. Freudenthal and P. W. Jones (Eds.). Raven Press, New York, pp. 325-329.

Higginson, J., and Muir, C. S. (1973). Epidemiology. In Cancer Medicine, J. F. Holland and E. Frei (Eds.). Lee and Febiger, Philadelphia, pp. 241-306.

Hirao, K., Shinohara, Y., Tsuda, H., Fukushima, S., Takahashi, M., and Ito, N. (1976). Carcinogenic activity of quinoline on rat liver. Cancer Res. 36:329-335.

Hites, R. A., and Biemann, W. G. (1975). Identification of specific organic compounds in a highly anoxic sediment by gas chromatographic-mass spectrometry and high resolution mass spectrometry. Adv. Chem. 147:188-201.

Hoffmann, D., Bondinell, W. E., and Wynder, E. L. (1974). Carcinogenicity of methylchrysenes. Science 183:215-216.

Hoffmann, D., and Wynder, E. L. (1976). Environmental respiratory carcinogenesis. In Chemical Carcinogens, ACS Monograph 173, C. E. Searle (Ed.). American Chemical Society, Washington, D.C., pp. 324-365.

Ito, N., Nagasaki, H., Makiura, S., and Arai, M. (1974). Histopathological studies on liver tumorigenesis in rats treated with polychlorinated biphenyls. Gann. 65:545-549.

IUPAC (1958). IUPAC Nomenclature of Organic Chemistry, 1957. Buttersworth, London.

Jerina, D. M., and Daly, J. W. (1974). Arene oxides: a new aspect of drug metabolism. Science 185:573-582.

Jerina, D. M., and Daly, J. W. (1977). Oxidation at carbon. In Drug Metabolism, D. V. Parke and R. L. Smith (Eds.). Taylor and Francis, London, pp. 13-32.

Jerina, D. M., Lehr, R. E., Yagi, H., Hernandez, O., Dansette, P. M., Wislocki, P. G., Wood, A. W., Chang, R. L., Levin, W., and Conney, A. H. (1976). Mutagenicity of benzo(a)pyrene derivatives and the description of a quantum mechanical model which predicts the ease of carbonium ion formation from diol epoxides. In In Vitro Metabolic Activation in Mutagenesis Testing, F. J. de Serres, J. R. Fouts, J. R. Bend, and R. M. Philpott (Eds.). Elsevier-North Holland, Amsterdam, pp. 159-179.

Kapitulnik, J., Wislocki, P. G., Levin, W., Yagi, H., Jerina, D. M., and Conney, A. H. (1978). Tumorigenicity studies with diol-epoxides of benzo(a)pyrene which indicate that (±)-trans-7β, 8α-dihydroxy-9α, 10α-epoxy-7,8,9,10-tetrahydrobenzo(a)pyrene is an ultimate carcinogen in newborn mice. Cancer Res. 38:354-358.

Keith, L. H. (Ed.) (1976). Identification and Analysis of Organic Pollutants in Water. Ann Arbor Science Publishers, Ann Arbor, Mich.

Keith, L. H., Garrison, A. W., Allen, F. R., Carter, M. H., Floyd, T. L., Pope, J. D., and Thruston, A. D., Jr. (1976). Identification of organic compounds in drinking water from thirteen U.S. cities. In Identification and Analysis of Organic Pollutants in Water, L. H. Keith (Ed.). Ann Arbor Science Publishers, Ann Arbor, Mich., pp. 329-373.

Kennaway, E. L. (1925). Experiments on cancer-producing substances. Br. Med. J. 2: 1-4.

Kennaway, E. L. (1930). Further experiments on cancer-producing substances. Biochem. J. 24:497-504.

Kimbrough, R. D., and Linder, R. E. (1974). Induction of adenofibrosis and hepatomas of the liver in BALB-cJ mice by polychlorinated biphenyls (Aroclor 1254). J. Natl. Cancer Inst. 53:547-552.

Kimbrough, R. D., Squire, R. A., Linder, R. E., Strandberg, J. D., Montali, R. J., and Burse, V. W. (1975). Induction of liver tumors in Sherman strain female rats by polychlorinated biphenyl Aroclor 1260. J. Natl. Cancer Inst. 55:1453-1459.

Knorr, M., and Schenk, D. (1968). Synthesis of polycyclic aromatic compounds by bacteria. Arch. Hyg. Bakteriol. 152:282-284.

Koreeda, M., Moore, P. D., Wislocki, P. G., Levin, W., Conney, A. H., Yagi, H., and Jerina, D. M. (1978). Binding of benzo(a)pyrene 7,8-diol-9,10-epoxides to DNA, RNA, and protein of mouse skin occurs with high stereoselectivity. Science 199:778-781.

Kraybill, H. F. (1976). Distribution of chemical carcinogens in aquatic environments. Prog. Exp. Tumor Res. 20:3-34.

Kraybill, H. F., Dawe, C. J., Harshbarger, J. C., and Tardiff, R. J. (Eds.) (1977). Ann. NY Acad. Sci., Vol. 298, Aquatic Pollutants and Biologic Effects with Emphasis on Neoplasia. N.Y. Academy of Sciences, New York.

Kuratsune, M., and Hueper, W. C. (1958). Polycyclic aromatic hydrocarbons in coffee soots. J. Natl. Cancer Inst. 20:37-51.

Kuratsune, M., and Hueper, W. C. (1960). Polycyclic aromatic hydrocarbons in roasted coffee. J. Natl. Cancer Inst. 24:463-469.

Lacassagne, A., Buu-Hoi, N. P., and Zajdela, F. (1957). Sur l'activite cancerogene de derives methyles du peryline et du 1, 12-benzoperyline. C. R. Acad. Sci. [D] (Paris) 245:991-994.

Lehr, R. E., and Jerina, D. M. (1977). Relationships of quantum mechanical calculations, relative mutagenicity of benzo(a)anthracene diol epoxides, and "Bay Region" concept of aromatic hydrocarbon carcinogenicity. J. Toxicol. Environ. Health 2:1259-1267.

Leiter, J., and Shear, M. G. (1942/43). Quantitative experiments on production of subcutaneous tumors in strain A mice with marginal doses of 3,4-benzpyrene. J. Natl. Cancer Inst. 3:455-477.

Lijinsky, W., and Ross, A. E. (1967). Production of carcinogenic polynuclear hydrocarbons in the cooking of food. Food Cosmet. Toxicol. 5:343-347.

Lijinsky, W., and Saffiotti, U. (1965). Relationships between structure and skin tumorigenic activity among hydrogenated derivatives of several polycyclic aromatic hydrocarbons. Ann. Ital. Derm. Clin. Sper. 19:34-44.

Lijinsky, W., and Shubik, P. (1964). Benzo(a)pyrene and other polynuclear hydrocarbons in charcoal-broiled meat. Science 145:53-55.

Lijinsky, W., and Shubik, P. (1965). Polynuclear hydrocarbon carcinogens in cooked meat and smoked food. Ind. Med. Surg. 34:152-154.

Linnik, A. B., Smirnov, G. A., and Shabad, L. M. (1971). Carcinogenicity of airplane engine soot in experimental animals. Biull. Eksp. Biol. Med. 71:83-87.

Magee, P. N., Pegg, A. E., and Swann, P. F. (1975). Molecular mechanisms of chemical carcinogenesis. In Handbook of General Pathology, Vol. 6, Tumors II, Part 6, H.-W. Altmann, F. Buchner, H. Cottier, E. Grundmann, G. Holle, E. Letterer, W. Masshoff, H. Meesen, F. Roulet, G. Seifert, and G. Siebert (Eds.). Springer-Verlag, Berlin-Heidelberg, pp. 329-419.

Maier, H. G., and Stender, W. (1969). Carcinogenic hydrocarbons in coffee substitutes. Deut. Lebensm. Rundsch. 65:341-343.

Majors, R. E. (1977). Recent advances in high performance liquid chromatography packings and columns. J. Chromatog. Sci. 15:344-351.

Malý, E. (1971). A simple test for exposure to polycyclic hydrocarbons. Bull. Environ. Contam. Toxicol. 6:422-425.

Marquardt, H., Baker, S., Grover, P. L., and Sims, P. (1977). Malignant transformation and mutagenesis in mammalian cells induced by vicinal diol-epoxides derived from benzo(a)pyrene. Cancer Lett. 3:31-36.

Masuda, Y., and Kuratsune, M. (1971). Polycyclic aromatic hydrocarbons in smoked fish, "katsuobushi." Gann. 62:27-30.

Mieure, J. P., and Dietrich, M. W. (1973). Determination of trace organics in air and water. J. Chromatogr. Sci. 11:559-570.

Miller, E. C., and Miller, J. A. (1976). The metabolism of chemical carcinogens to reactive electrophiles and their possible mechanisms of action in carcinogenesis. In Chemical Carcinogens, ACS Monograph 173, C. E. Searle (Ed.). American Chemical Society, Washington, D.C., pp. 737-762.

Miller, J. A., and Miller, E. C. (1969). Metabolic activation of carcinogenic aromatic amines and amides via N-hydroxylation and N-hydroxy-esterification and its relationship to ultimate carcinogens as electrophilic reactants. In The Jerusalem Symposia on Quantum Chemistry and Biochemistry, Vol. I, Physico-Chemical Mechanisms of Carcinogenesis, E. D. Bergmann and B. Pullman (Eds.). Israel Academy of Sciences and Humanities, Jerusalem, pp. 237-261.

Moschel, R. C., Baird, W. M., and Dipple, A. (1977). Metabolic activation of the carcinogen 7,12-dimethylbenz(a)anthracene for DNA binding. Biochem. Biophys. Res. Commun. 76:1092-1098.

MRC (1968). The Carcinogenic Action of Mineral Oils: A Chemical and Biological Study. Medical Research Council Carcinogenic Action of Mineral Oils Committee. Her Majesty's Stationery Office, London.

NAS (1972). Particulate Polycyclic Organic Matter. Committee on Biologic Effects of Atmospheric Pollutants, National Academy of Sciences (NAS), Washington, D.C.

Noonan, G. (1976). Passive smoking in enclosed public places. Med. J. Aust. 2:68-70.

O'Gara, R. W., Stewart, L., Brown, J., and Hueper, W. C. (1969). Carcinogenicity of heated fats and fat fractions. J. Natl. Cancer Inst. 42:275-287.

Pike, M. C., Gordon, R. J., Henderson, B. E., Menck, H. R., and SooHoo, J. (1975). Air pollution. In Persons at High Risk of Cancer. An Approach to Cancer Etiology and Control, J. F. Fraumeni, Jr. (Ed.). Academic Press, New York, pp. 225-239.

Pott, P. (1775). Chirurgical Observations. Hawes, Clarke & Collings, London.

Preussmann, R. (1976). Chemical carcinogens in the human environment. Problems and quantitative aspects. Oncology 33:51-57.

Pullman, A., and Pullman, B. (1955). Electronic structure and carcinogenic activity of aromatic molecules: new developments. Adv. Cancer Res. 3:117-167.

Rhee, K. S., and Bratzler, L. J. (1970). Benzo(a)pyrene in smoked meat products. J. Food Sci. 35:146-149.

Ruchkovskii, B. S., Borisiuk, I. P., Tiktin, L. A., Popovskii, V. G., Mordkovich, M. S., and Silich, A. A. (1969). 3,4-Benzpyrene content of prunes dried by different methods. Gig. Sanit. 34:134-135.

Saffiotti, U. (1969). Experimental respiratory tract carcinogenesis. Prog. Exp. Tumor Res. 11:302-333.

Saffiotti, U. (1970). Experimental respiratory tract carcinogenesis and its relation to inhalation exposure. In Inhalation Carcinogenesis, AEC Symposium Series 18, M. G. Hanna, Jr., P. Nettesheim, and J. R. Gilbert (Eds.). U.S. Atomic Energy Commission, Oak Ridge, Tenn., pp. 27-54.

Saffiotti, U., and Wagoner, J. K. (Eds.) (1976). Ann NY Acad. Sci., Vol. 271, Occupational Carcinogenesis. N.Y. Academy of Sciences, New York.

Sawicki, E., Elbert, W. C., Hauser, T. R., Fox, F. T., and Stanley, T. W. (1960). Benzo(a)pyrene content of the air of American communities. Am. Ind. Hyg. Assoc. J. 21:443-451.

Sawicki, E., McPherson, S. P., Stanley, T. M., Meeker, J., and Elbert, W. C. (1965). Quantitative composition of the urban atmosphere in terms of polynuclear aza heterocyclic compounds and hydrocarbons. Int. J. Air Water Pollut. 9:515-524.

Schmeltz, I., and Hoffmann, D. (1976). Formation of polynuclear aromatic hydrocarbons from combustion of organic matter. In Carcinogenesis: A Comprehensive Survey, Vol. I, Polynuclear Aromatic Hydrocarbons. Chemistry, Metabolism, and Carcinogenesis, R. Freudenthal and P. W. Jones (Eds.). Raven Press, New York, pp. 225-239.

Schmeltz, I., Hoffmann, D., and Wynder, E. L. (1975). The influence of tobacco smoke on indoor atmospheres. I. An overview. Prev. Med. 4:66-82.

Schoental, R. (1974). Carcinogenicity as related to age. Annu. Rev. Pharmacol. Toxicol. 14:185-204.

Sellakumar, A., and Shubik, P. (1972). Carcinogenicity of 7H-dibenzo(c,g)carbazole in the respiratory tract of hamsters. J. Natl. Cancer Inst. 48:1641-1646.

Severson, R. F., Snook, M. E., Higman, H. C., Chortyk, O. T., and Akin, F. J. (1976). Isolation, identification, and quantitation of the polynuclear aromatic hydrocarbons in tobacco smoke. In Carcinogenesis: A Comprehensive Survey, Vol. I, Polynuclear Aromatic Hydrocarbons. Chemistry, Metabolism, and Carcinogenesis, R. Freudenthal and P. W. Jones (Eds.). Raven Press, New York, pp. 253-270.

Shabad, L. M. (1975). Circulation of carcinogenic substances in the environment: From laboratory experiments to field investigations. In Recent Topics in Chemical Carcinogenesis, GANN Monograph on Cancer Research No. 17, S. Odashima, S. Takayama, and H. Sato (Eds.). University of Tokyo Press, Tokyo, pp. 179-187.

Shabad, L. M., and Smirnov, G. A. (1969). 3,4-Benzpyrene containing in the soot and exhaust gases of turbo jet and turbo-prop engines. Gig. Sanit. 2:98-99 (in Russian).

Shimkin, M. B., and Triolo, V. A. (1969). History of chemical carcinogenesis: some prospective remarks. Prog. Exp. Tumor Res. 11:1-20.

Sigurjonsson, J. (1967). Occupational variations in mortality from gastric cancer in relation to dietary differences. Br. J. Cancer 21:651-656.

Sims, P., and Grover, P. L. (1974). Epoxides in polycyclic aromatic hydrocarbon metabolism and carcinogenesis. Adv. Cancer Res. 20:165-274.

Slaga, T. J., Viaje, A., Berry, D. L., Bracken, W., Buty, S. G., and Scribner, J. D. (1976). Skin tumor initiating ability of benzo(a)pyrene 4,5-, 7,8-, and 7,8-diol-9,10-epoxides and 7,8-diol. Cancer Lett. 2:115-121.

Stelzner, R. (1921). *Literatur-Register der organischen Chemie: 1914-1915*, Vol. III. Springer-Verlag, Berlin, pp. 21-24.

Sterling, T. D., and Kobayashi, D. M. (1977). Exposure to pollutants in enclosed "living spaces." Environ. Res. 13:1-35.

Stich, H. F., and Acton, A. B. (1976). The possible use of fish tumors in monitoring for carcinogens in the marine environment. Prog. Exp. Tumor Res. 20:44-54.

Stocks, P., Commins, B. T., and Aubrey, K. V. (1961). A study of polycyclic hydrocarbons and trace elements in smoke in Menseyside and other northern localities. Int. J. Air Water Pollut. 4:141-153.

Tilgner, D. J. (1970). Food in a carcinogenic environment. Food Manuf. 48:47-50.

Tomatis, L., and Mohr, U. (Eds.) (1973). *Transplacental Carcinogenesis*, IARC Scientific Publication No. 4, Lyon.

UICC (1970). *UICC Technical Report Series*, Vol. 4, *The Quantification of Environmental Carcinogenesis*. International Union against Cancer (UICC), Geneva, Switzerland.

Vigliani, E. C. (1976). Leukemia associated with benzene exposure. Ann. NY Acad. Sci. 271:143-151.

Vysheslavova, M. I. (1968). Carcinogenic effects of overheated fats. Vopr. Pitan. 27:63-68.

Wagner, K. H., and Siddiqi, I. (1970). Der Stoffwechsel von 3,4 Benzpyren und 3,4 Benzfluoranthen im Sommerweizen. Z. Pflanzenernahrung Bodenkunde 127:211-218.

WHO (1964). *Prevention of Cancer*, WHO Technical Report Series No. 276, World Health Organization, Geneva, Switzerland.

Wilson, R. D., Monoghan, P. H., Osanik, A., Price, L. C., and Rogers, M. A. (1974). Natural marine oil seepage. Science 184:857-865.

Wislocki, P. G., Wood, A. W., Chang, R. L., Levin, W., Yagi, H., Hernandez, O., Jerina, D. M., and Conney, A. H. (1976). High mutagenicity and toxicity of a diol epoxide derived from benzo(a)pyrene. Biochem. Biophys. Res. Commun. 68:1006-1012.

Wislocki, P. G., Chang, R. L., Wood, A. W., Levin, W., Yagi, H., Hernandez, O., Mah, H. D., Dansette, P. M., Jerina, D. M., and Conney, A. H. (1977). High carcinogenicity of 2-hydroxybenzo(a)pyrene on mouse skin. Cancer Res. 37:2608-2611.

Wolf, G. (1952). *Chemical Induction of Cancer*. Cassel, London.

Wood, A. W., Levin, W., Chang, R. L., Lehr, R. E., Schaefer-Ridder, M., Karle, J. M., Jerina, D. M., and Conney, A. H. (1977a). Tumorigenicity of five dihydrodiols of benz(a)anthracene on mouse skin: exceptional activity of benz(a)anthracene 3,4-dihydrodiol. Proc. Natl. Acad. Sci. USA 74:3176-3179.

Wood, A. W., Levin, W., Ryan, D., Thomas, P. E., Yagi, H., Mah, H. D., Thakker, D. R., Jerina, D. M., and Conney, A. H. (1977b). High mutagenicity of metabolically activated chrysene 1,2 dihydrodiol: evidence for bay region activation of chrysene. Biochem. Biophys. Res. Commun. 78:847-854.

Yang, S. K., Gelboin, H. V., Trump, B. F., Autrup, H., and Harris, C. C. (1977). Metabolic activation of benzo(a)pyrene and binding to DNA in cultured human bronchus. Cancer Res. 37:1210-1215.

Zobell, C. E. (1971). Sources and biodegradation of carcinogenic hydrocarbons. In *Proc. of Convention on Prevention and Control of Oil Spills*. U.S. Coast Guard, American

Petroleum Institute, and the Environmental Protection Agency. American Petroleum Institute, Washington, D.C.

Section III

Alam, B. S., Saporoschetz, I. D., and Epstein, S. S. (1971). Synthesis of nitrosopiperidine from nitrate and piperidine in the gastro-intestinal tract of the rat. Nature 232:199-200.

Allsobrook, A. J., du Plessis, L. S., Harrington, J. S., Nunn, A. J., and Nunn, J. R. (1975). Nitrosamines in the human vaginal vault. In N-Nitroso Compounds in the Environment, P. Bogovski and E. A. Walker (Eds.). IARC Scientific Publication No. 9, Lyon, France, pp. 197-199.

Althoff, J., Grandjean, C., Pour, P., and Bertram, B. (1977). Comparison of the effect of β-oxidized dipropylnitrosamine metabolites administered at equimolar doses to Syrian hamsters. Z. Krebsforsch. 90:141-148.

Archer, M. C., Tannenbaum, S. R., Fan, T.-Y., and Weisman, M. (1975). Reaction of nitrite with ascorbate and its relation to nitrosamine formation. J. Natl. Cancer Inst. 54:1203-1205.

Archer, M. C., and Wishnok, J. S. (1977). Quantitative aspects of human exposure to nitrosamines. Food Cosmet. Toxicol. 15:233-235.

Arcos, J. C., Bryant, G. M., Pastor, K. M., and Argus, M. F. (1976). Structural limits of specificity of methylcholanthrene-repressible nitrosamine N-dealkylases. Inhibition by analog substrates. Z. Krebsforsch. 86:171-183.

Arcos, J. C., Davies, D. L., Brown, C. E., and Argus, M. F. (1977). Repressible and inducible enzymic forms of dimethylnitrosamine-demethylase. Z. Krebsforsch. 89: 181-199.

Argus, M. F., and Arcos, J. C. (1976). Hydrocarbon-nitrosamine synergism as a possible amplifying factor in lung tumorigenesis by tobacco smoke. J. Theor. Biol. 56:491-498.

Argus, M. F., Hoch-Ligeti, C., Arcos, J. C., and Conney, A. H. (1978). Differential effects of β-naphthoflavone and pregnenolone-16α-carbonitrile on dimethylnitrosamine hepatocarcinogenesis. J. Natl. Cancer Inst. 61:441-449.

Ayanaba, A., and Alexander, M. (1974). Transformations of methylamines and formation of a hazardous product, dimethylnitrosamine, in samples of treated sewage and lake water. J. Environ. Qual. 3:83-89.

Ayanaba, A., Verstraete, W., and Alexander, M. (1973a). Possible nicrobial contribution to nitrosamine formation in sewage and soil. J. Natl. Cancer Inst. 50:811-813.

Ayanaba, A., Verstraete, W., and Alexander, M. (1973b). Formation of dimethylnitrosamine, a carcinogen and mutagen, in soils treated with nitrogen compounds. Soil Sci. Soc. Am. Proc. 37:565-568.

Berry, R. S., and Lehman, P. A. (1971). Aerochemistry of air pollution. Annu. Rev. Phys. Chem. 22:47-84.

Bogovski, P., Castegnaro, M., Pignatelli, B., and Walker, E. A. (1972a). The inhibiting effect of tannins on the formation of nitrosamines. In N-Nitroso Compounds Analysis and Formation, P. Bogovski, R. Preussmann, and E. A. Walker (Eds.). IARC Scientific Publication No. 3, Lyon, France, pp. 127-129.

Bogovski, P., Preussmann, R., and Walker, E. A. (Eds.) (1972b). N-Nitroso Compounds Analysis and Formation. IARC Scientific Publication No. 3, Lyon, France.

Bogovski, P., and Walker, E. A. (Eds.) (1975). N-Nitroso Compounds in the Environment. IARC Scientific Publication No. 9, Lyon, France.

Boyland, E., Nice, E., and Williams, K. (1971). The catalysis of nitrosation by thiocyanate from saliva. Food Cosmet. Toxicol. 9:639-643.

Boyland, E., and Walker, S. A. (1975). Thiocyanate catalysis of nitrosamine formation and some dietary implications. In N-Nitroso Compounds in the Environment, P. Bogovski and E. A. Walker (Eds.). IARC Scientific Publication No. 9, Lyon, France, pp. 132-136.

Bretschneider, K., and Matz, J. (1973). Nitrosamine (NA) in der atmospharischen und in der Luft am Arbeitsplatz. Arch. Geschwulstforsch. 42:36-41.

Broaddus, G. M., York, J. E., Jr., and Moseley, J. M. (1965). Factors affecting the levels of nitrate nitrogen in cured tobacco leaves. Tobacco Sci. 9:149-157.

Cardesa, A., Pour, P., Rustia, M., Althoff, J., and Mohr, U. (1973). The syncarcinogenic effect of methylcholanthrene and dimethylnitrosamine in Swiss mice. Z. Krebsforsch. 79:98-107.

Challis, B. C. (1973). Rapid nitrosation of phenols and its implications for health hazards from dietary nitrites. Nature 244:466.

Challis, B. C., and Bartlett, C. D. (1975). Possible cocarcinogenic effects of coffee constituents. Nature 254:532-533.

Challis, B. C., and Kyrtopoulos, S. A. (1977). Rapid formation of carcinogenic N-nitrosamines in aqueous alkaline solutions. Br. J. Cancer 35:693-696.

Chambon, P., and Chambon, R. (1976). Cancerogénèse et environement: les N-nitrosamines. Lyon Pharmaceutique 27:259-265.

Chem. Eng. News (1977). N-Nitrosamines found in toiletry products. 55(13):7-8.

Claus, G., Krisko, I., and Bolander, K. (1974). Chemical carcinogens in the environment and in the human diet: Can a threshold be established? Food Cosmet. Toxicol. 12: 737-746.

Collins-Thompson, D. L., Sen, N. P., Aris, B., and Schwinghamer, L. (1972). Non-enzymic in vitro formation of nitrosamines by bacteria isolated from meat products. Can. J. Microbiol. 18:1968-1971.

Crosby, N. T., Foreman, J. K., Palframan, J. F., and Sawyer, J. R. (1972). Estimation of steam-volatile N-nitrosamines in foods at the 1 μg/kg level. Nature 238:342-343.

Davies, R., and McWeeny, D. J. (1977). Catalytic effect of nitrosophenols on N-nitrosamine formation. Nature 266:657-658.

DHEW (1968). Nationwide Inventory of Air Pollutant Emissions. APGA Publication No. AP-73. U.S. Dept. of Health, Education, and Welfare, Washington, D.C.

Druckrey, H. (1973a). Chemical structure and action in transplacental carcinogenesis and teratogenesis. In Transplacental Carcinogenesis, L. Tomatis and U. Mohr (Eds.). IARC Scientific Publication No. 4, Lyon, France, pp. 45-58.

Druckrey, H. (1973b). Specific carcinogenic and teratogenic effects of 'indirect' alkylating methyl and ethyl compounds, and their dependency on stages of ontogenic development. Xenobiotica 3:271-303.

Druckrey, H., and Preussmann, R. (1962). Zur Entstehung carcinogener Nitrosamine am Beispiel des Tabakrauchs. Naturwissenschaften 49:498-499.

Druckrey, H., Preussmann, R., and Ivankovic, S. (1969). N-Nitrosocompounds in organotropic and transplacental carcinogenesis. Ann. NY Acad. Sci. 163:676-696.

Druckrey, H., Preussmann, R., Ivankovic, S., and Schmähl, D. (1967). Organotrope carcinogene Wirkungen bei 65 verschiedenen N-Nitroso-Verbindungen an BD-Ratten. Z. Krebsforsch. 69:103-201.

Druckrey, H., Steinhoff, D., Beuthner, H., Schneider, H., and Klarner, P. (1963). Prufung von Nitrit auf chronisch toxische Wirkung an Ratten. Arzneim. Forsch. 13: 320-323.

DuPlessis, L. S., Nunn, J. R., and Roach, W. A. (1969). Carcinogen in a Transkeian Bantu food additive. Nature 222:1198-1199.

Eisenbrand, G., Ungerer, O., and Preussmann, R. (1975). Formation of N-nitroso compounds from agricultural chemicals and nitrite. In N-Nitroso Compounds in the Environment, P. Bogovski and E. A. Walker (Eds.). IARC Scientific Publication No. 9, Lyon, France, pp. 71-74.

Ender, F., and Čeh, L. (1968). Occurrence of nitrosamines in foodstuffs for human and animal consumption. Food Cosmet. Toxicol. 6:569-571.

Ender, F., and Čeh, L. (1971). Conditions and chemical reaction mechanisms by which nitrosamines may be formed in biological products with reference to their possible occurrence in food products. Z. Lebensm. Unters Forsch. 145:133-142.

Ender, F., Havre, C., Helgebostad, A., Koppang, N., Madsen, R., and Čeh, L. (1964). Isolation and identification of a hepatotoxic factor in herring meal produced from sodium nitrite preserved herring. Naturwissenchaften 51: 637-638.

Fahmy, O. G., and Fahmy, M. J. (1976). Mutagenicity of N-α-acetoxy-N-ethylnitrosamine and N, N-diethylnitrosamine in relation to the mechanisms of metabolic activation of dialkylnitrosamines. Cancer Res. 36:4504-4512.

Falk, H. L. (1976). Possible mechanisms of combination effects in chemical carcinogenesis. Oncology 33: 77-85.

Fan, T.-Y., Morrison, J., Rounbehler, D. P., Ross, R., Fine, D. H., Miles, W., and Sen, N. P. (1977). N-Nitrosodiethanolamine in synthetic cutting fluids: A part-per-hundred impurity. Science 196: 70-71.

Fan, T.-Y., and Tannenbaum, S. R. (1973a). Factors influencing the rate of formation of nitrosomorpholine from morpholine and nitrite: Acceleration by thiocyanate and other anions. J. Agric. Food Chem. 21: 237-240.

Fan, T.-Y., and Tannenbaum, S. R. (1973b). Factors influencing the rate of formation of nitrosomorpholine from morpholine and nitrite. II. Rate enhancement in frozen solution. J. Agric. Food Chem. 21: 967-969.

Fan, T.-Y., and Tannenbaum, S. R. (1973c). Natural inhibitors of nitrosation reactions: concept of available nitrite. J. Food Sci. 38: 1067-1068.

Fazio, T., Damico, J. N., Howard, J. W., White, R. H., and Watts, J. O. (1971a). Gas chromatographic determination and mass spectrometric confirmation of N-nitrosodimethylamine in smoke-processed marine fish. J. Agric. Food Chem. 19: 250-253.

Fazio, T., White, R. H., Dusold, L. R., and Howard, J. W. (1973). Nitrosopyrrolidine in cooked bacon. J. Assoc. Off. Anal. Chem. 56: 919-921.

Fazio, T., White, R. H., and Howard, J. W. (1971b). Analysis of nitrite- and/or nitrate-processed meats for N-nitrosodimethylamine. J. Assoc. Off. Anal. Chem. 54: 1157-1159.

Feuer, H. (Ed.) (1970). The Chemistry of the Nitro and Nitroso Compounds, Part 2, Wiley Interscience, New York.

Fiddler, W. (1975). The occurrence and determination of N-nitroso compounds. Toxicol. Appl. Pharmacol. 31: 352-360.

Fiddler, W., Feinberg, J. I., Pensabene, J. W., Williams, A. C., and Dooley, C. J. (1975). Dimethylnitrosamine in souse and similar jellied cured-meat products. Food Cosmet. Toxicol. 13: 653-654.

Fiddler, W., Pensabene, J. W., Fagan, J. C., Thorne, E. J., Piotrowski, E. G., and Wasserman, A. E. (1974). The role of lean and adipose tissue in the formation of nitrosopyrrolidine in fried bacon. J. Food Sci. 39: 1070-1071.

Fiddler, W., Pensabene, J. W., Piotrowski, E. G., Doerr, R. C., and Wasserman, A. E. (1973). Use of sodium ascorbate or erythorbate to inhibit formation of N-nitrosodimethylamine in frankfurters. J. Food Sci. 38: 1084-1085.

Fiddler, W., Piotrowski, E. G., Pensabene, J. W., Doerr, R. C., and Wasserman, A. E. (1972). Effect of sodium nitrite concentration on N-nitrosodimethylamine formation in frankfurters. J. Food Sci. 37: 668-670.

Fine, D. H., and Rounbehler, D. P. (1976). N-Nitroso compounds in water. In Identification and Analysis of Organic Pollutants in Water, L. H. Keith (Ed.). Ann Arbor Science Publishers, Ann Arbor, Mich., pp. 255-263.

Fine, D. H., Rounbehler, D. P., Belcher, N. M., and Epstein, S. S. (1976a). N-Nitroso compounds: detection in ambient air. Science 192: 1328-1330.

Fine, D. H., Rounbehler, D. P., Pellizzari, E. D., Bunch, J. E., Berkley, R. W., McCrae, J., Bursey, J. T., Sawicki, E., Krost, K., and DeMarrais, G. A. (1976b). N-Nitrosodimethylamine in air. Bull. Environ. Contam. Toxicol. 15: 739-746.

Fine, D. H., and Rufeh, F. (1975). Analysis of μg/kg levels of non-volatile and volatile N-nitroso compounds in foodstuffs. In N-Nitroso Compounds in the Environment,

P. Bogovski and E. A. Walker (Eds.). IARC Scientific Publication No. 9, Lyon, France, pp. 53-56.

Fine, D. H., Rufeh, F., Lieb, D., and Epstein, S. S. (1974). A possible nitrogen oxide-nitrosamine-cancer link. Bull. Environ. Contam. Toxicol. 11:18-19.

Fishbein, L. (1976). Atmospheric mutagens. I. Sulfur oxides and nitrogen oxides. Mutat. Res. 32:309-330.

Fishbein, L. (1977). Nitrosamines. In Potential Industrial Carcinogens and Mutagens. Office of Toxic Substances, Environmental Protection Agency, Washington, D.C., pp. 225-244.

Fong, Y. Y., and Chan, W. C. (1973a). Dimethylnitrosamine in Chinese marine salt fish. Food Cosmet. Toxicol. 11:841-845.

Fong, Y. Y., and Chan, W. C. (1973b). Bacterial production of dimethylnitrosamine in salted fish. Nature 243:421-422.

Fong, Y. Y., and Chan, W. C. (1976). Methods for limiting the content of dimethylnitrosamine in Chinese marine salt fish. Food Cosmet. Toxicol. 14:95-98.

Fong, Y. Y., and Chan, W. C. (1977). Nitrate, nitrite, dimethylnitrosamine and N-nitrosopyrrolidine in some Chinese food products. Food Cosmet. Toxicol. 15:143-145.

Freund, H. A. (1937). Clinical manifestations and studies in parenchymatous hepatitis. Ann. Intern. Med. 10:1144-1155.

Friedman, M. A., and Sanders, V. (1976). Effects of piperonyl butoxide on dimethylnitrosamine metabolism and toxicity in Swiss mice. J. Toxicol. Environ. Health 2:67-75.

Gehlert, P., and Rolle, W. (1977). Uber die Bildung von Diäthylnitrosamin durch Reaktion von Diäthylamin mit Stickstoffdioxid in der Gasphase. Experientia 33:579-581.

Gomez, M. I., Swann, P. F., and Magee, P. N. (1977). The absorption and metabolism in rats of small oral doses of dimethylnitrosamine. Implication for the possible hazard of dimethylnitrosamine in human food. Biochem. J. 164:497-500.

Greenblatt, M., and Mirvish, S. S. (1972). Dose-response studies with concurrent administration of piperazine and sodium nitrite to strain A mice. J. Natl. Cancer Inst. 49: 119-124.

Greenblatt, M., Mirvish, S. S., and So, B. T. (1971). Nitrosamine studies: induction of lung adenomas by concurrent administration of sodium nitrite and secondary amines in Swiss mice. J. Natl. Cancer Inst. 46:1029-1034.

Haenszel, W. (1975). Migrant studies. In Persons at High Risk of Cancer, J. F. Fraumeni, Jr. (Ed.). Academic Press, New York, pp. 361-371.

Haenszel, W., Kurihara, M., Segi, M., and Lee, R. K. (1972). Stomach cancer among Japanese in Hawaii. J. Natl. Cancer Inst. 49:969-988.

Harrington, J. S., Nunn, J. R., and Irwig, L. (1973). Dimethylnitrosamine in the human vaginal vault. Nature 241:49-50.

Hashimoto, S., Kawai, Y., and Mutai, M. (1975). In vitro N-nitrosodimethylamine formation by some bacteria. Infect. Immun. 11:1405-1406.

Hashimoto, S., Yokokura, T., Kawai, Y., and Mutai, M. (1976). Dimethylnitrosamine formation in the gastro-intestinal tract of rats. Food Cosmet. Toxicol. 14:553-556.

Hawksworth, G. M., and Hill, M. J. (1971). Bacteria and the N-nitrosation of secondary amines. Br. J. Cancer 25:520-526.

Hawksworth, G., and Hill, M. J. (1974). The in vivo formation of N-nitrosamines in the rat bladder and their subsequent absorption. Br. J. Cancer 29:353-358.

Hawksworth, G., Hill, M. J., Gordillo, G., and Cuello, C. (1975). Possible relationship between nitrates, nitrosamines and gastric cancer in southwest Colombia. In N-Nitroso Compounds in the Environment, P. Bogovski and E. A. Walker (Eds.). IARC Scientific Publication No. 9, Lyon, France, pp. 229-234.

Hecht, S. S., Ornaf, R. M., and Hoffmann, D. (1975). Chemical studies on tobacco smoke. XXXIII. N'-Nitrosonornicotine in tobacco: analysis of possible contributing factors and biologic implications. J. Natl. Cancer Inst. 54:1237-1244.

Hendel, F. J. (1973). Aerothermochemistry of the terrestial atmosphere. Crit. Rev. Environ. Control 3:129-152.

Hill, M. J., and Hawksworth, G. (1972). Bacterial production of nitrosamines in vitro and in vivo. In N-Nitroso Compounds Analysis and Formation, P. Bogovski, R. Preussmann, and E. A. Walker (Eds.). IARC Scientific Publication No. 3, Lyon, France, pp. 116-121.

Hill, M. J., Hawksworth, G., and Tattersall, G. (1973). Bacteria, nitrosamines and cancer of the stomach. Br. J. Cancer 28:562-567.

Ho, H. C. (1976). Epidemiology of nasopharyngeal carcinoma. Gann. Monogr. Cancer Res. 18:49-61.

Hoch-Ligeti, C., Argus, M. F., and Arcos, J. C. (1968). Combined carcinogenic effects of dimethylnitrosamine and 3-methylcholanthrene in the rat. J. Natl. Cancer Inst. 40: 535-549.

Hoffmann, D., Hecht, S. S., Ornaf, R. M., and Wynder, E. L. (1974). N'-Nitrosonornicotine in tobacco. Science 186:265-267.

Hoffmann, D., Rathkamp, G., and Liu, Y. Y. (1975). Chemical studies on tobacco smoke. XXVI. On the isolation and identification of volatile and non-volatile N-nitrosamines and hydrazines in cigarette smoke. In N-Nitroso Compounds in the Environment, P. Bogovski and E. A. Walker (Eds.). IARC Scientific Publication No. 9, Lyon, France, pp. 159-165.

Ishidate, M., Tanimura, A., Ito, Y., Sakai, A., Sakuta, H., Kawamura, T., Saki, K., Miyazawa, F., and Wada, H. (1972). Secondary amines, nitrites and nitrosamines in Japanese foods. In Topics in Chemical Carcinogenesis, W. Nakahara, S. Takayama, T. Sugimura, and S. Odashima (Eds.). University Park Press, Baltimore, pp. 313-322.

Issenberg, P. (1976). Nitrite, nitrosamines, and cancer. Fed. Proc. 35:1322-1326.

Ivankovic, S., and Druckrey, H. (1968). Transplazentare Erzeugung maligner Tumoren des Nervensystems. I. Athylnitrosoharnstoff (ANH) an BD IX-Ratten. Z. Krebsforsch. 71:320-360.

Jones, A. R., Lijinsky, W., and Singer, G. M. (1974). Steric effects in the nitrosation of piperidines. Cancer Res. 34:1079-1081.

Keefer, L. K., and Roller, P. P. (1973). N-Nitrosation by nitrite ion in neutral and basic medium. Science 181:1245-1247.

Klubes, P., Cerna, I., Rabinowitz, A. D., and Jondorf, W. R. (1972). Factors affecting dimethylnitrosamine formation from simple precursors by rat intestinal bacteria. Food Cosmet. Toxicol. 10:757-767.

Kotin, P. (1976). Dose-response relationship and threshold concepts. Ann. NY Acad. Sci. 271:22-28.

Kruger, F. W. (1972). New aspects in metabolism of carcinogenic nitrosamines. In Topics in Chemical Carcinogenesis, W. Nakahara, S. Takayama, T. Sugimura, and S. Odashima (Eds.). University Park Press, Baltimore, pp. 213-235.

Kruger, F. W., and Bertram, B. (1973). Metabolism of nitrosamines in vivo. III. On the methylation of nucleic acids by aliphatic di-n-alkylnitrosamines in vivo resulting from β-oxidation: the formation of 7-methylguanine after application of 2-oxopropyl-propyl-nitrosamine and methyl-propyl-nitrosamine. Z. Krebsforsch. 80:189-196.

Kruger, F. W., and Bertram, B. (1975). Metabolism of nitrosamines in vivo. IV. Isolation of 3-hydroxy-1-nitrosopyrrolidine from rat urine after application of 1-nitrosopyrrolidine. Z. Krebsforsch. 83:255-260.

Kruger, F. W., Bertram, B., and Eisenbrand, G. (1976). Metabolism of nitrosamines in vivo. V. Investigation on $^{14}CO_2$ exhalation, liver RNA labelling and isolation of two metabolites from urine after administration of (2,5-^{14}C)dinitrosopiperazine to rats. Z. Krebsforsch. 85:125-134.

Kushnir, I., Feinberg, J. I., Pensabene, J. W., Piotrowski, E. G., Fiddler, W., and Wasserman, A. E. (1975). The isolation and identification of nitrosoproline in uncooked bacon. J. Food Sci. 40:427-428.

Lake, B. G., Heading, C. E., Phillips, J. C., Gangolli, S. D., and Lloyd, A. G. (1974). Some studies on the metabolism in vitro of dimethylnitrosamine by rat liver. Biochem. Soc. Trans. 2:610-612.

Lane, R. P., and Bailey, M. E. (1973). The effect of pH on dimethylnitrosamine formation in human gastric juice. Food Cosmet. Toxicol. 11:851-854.

Lawley, P. D. (1972). The action of alkylating mutagens and carcinogens on nucleic acids: N-Methyl-N-nitroso compounds as methylating agents. In Topics in Chemical Carcinogenesis, W. Nakahara, S. Takayama, T. Sugimura, and S. Odashima (Eds.). University Park Press, Baltimore, pp. 237-258.

Lijinsky, W. (1974). Reaction of drugs with nitrous acid as a source of carcinogenic nitrosamines. Cancer Res. 34:255-258.

Lijinsky, W., and Epstein, S. S. (1970). Nitrosamines as environmental carcinogens. Nature 225:21-23.

Lijinsky, W., Ferrero, A., Montesano, R., and Wenyon, C. E. (1970). Tumorigenicity of cyclic nitrosamines in Syrian golden hamsters. Z. Krebsforsch. 74:185-189.

Lijinsky, W., and Taylor, H. W. (1977). Carcinogenic tests of nitroso-N-methylpiperazine, 2,3,5,6-tetramethyldinitrosopiperazine, nitrosoisonipecotic acid and nitrosomethoxymethylamine in rats. Z. Krebsforsch. 89:31-36.

Lijinsky, W., Taylor, H. W., and Keefer, L. K. (1976). Reduction of rat liver carcinogenicity of 4-nitrosomorpholine by α-deuterium substitution. J. Natl. Cancer Inst. 57:1311-1313.

Loveless, A. (1969). Possible relevance of O-6 alkylation of deoxyguanosine to mutagenicity and carcinogenicity of nitrosamines and nitrosamides. Nature 223:206-207.

Magee, P. N. (1972). Possible mechanisms of carcinogenesis and mutagenesis by nitrosamines. In Topics in Chemical Carcinogenesis, W. Nakahara, S. Takayama, T. Sugimura, and S. Odashima (Eds.). University Park Press, Baltimore, pp. 259-278.

Magee, P. N., and Barnes, J. M. (1956). The production of malignant primary hepatic tumors in the rat by feeding dimethylnitrosamine. Br. J. Cancer 10:114-122.

Magee, P. N., and Barnes, J. M. (1967). Carcinogenic nitroso compounds. Adv. Cancer Res. 10:163-246.

Magee, P. N., and Farber, E. (1962). Methylation of rat liver nucleic acids by dimethylnitrosamine in vivo. Biochem. J. 83:114-124.

Magee, P. N., Montesano, R., and Preussmann, R. (1976). N-Nitroso compounds and related carcinogens. In Chemical Carcinogens. ACS Monograph 173, C. E. Searle (Ed.). American Chemical Society, Washington, D.C., pp. 491-625.

Marquardt, P., and Hedler, L. (1966). Über das Vorkommen von Nitrosaminen in Weizenmehl. Arzneim. Forsch. 16:778-779.

McCormick, A., Nicholson, M. J., Baylis, M. A., and Underwood, J. G. (1973). Nitrosamines in cigarette smoke condensate. Nature 244:237-238

McGlashan, N. D. (1970). Oesophaegeal cancer in Northern Iran. Bull. Int. Acad. Pathol. 11:5-53.

Mirvish, S. S. (1972). Studies on N-nitrosation reactions: kinetics of nitrosation, correlation with mouse feeding experiments, and natural occurrence of nitrosatable compounds (ureides and guanidines). In Topics in Chemical Carcinogenesis, W. Nakahara, S. Takayama, T. Sugimura, and S. Odashima (Eds.). University Park Press, Baltimore, pp. 279-295.

Mirvish, S. S. (1975). Formation of N-nitroso compounds: chemistry, kinetics, and in vivo occurrence. Toxicol. Appl. Pharmacol. 31:325-351.

Mirvish, S. S. (1977). N-Nitroso compounds: their chemical and in vivo formation and possible importance as environmental carcinogens. J. Toxicol. Environ. Health 2: 1267-1277.

Mirvish, S. S., and Chu, C. (1973). Chemical determination of methylnitrosourea and ethylnitrosourea in stomach contents of rats, after intubation of the alkylureas plus sodium nitrite. J. Natl. Cancer Inst. 50:745-750.

Mirvish, S. S., Greenblatt, M., and Kommineni, V. R. (1972a). Nitrosamide formation in vivo: induction of lung adenomas in Swiss mice by concurrent feeding of nitrite and methylurea or ethylurea. J. Natl. Cancer Inst. 48:1311-1315.

Mirvish, S. S., Sams, J., Fan, T.-Y., and Tannenbaum, S. R. (1973). Kinetics of nitrosation of the amino acids proline, hydroxyproline, and sarcosine. J. Natl. Cancer Inst. 51:1833-1840.

Mirvish, S. S., Wallcave, L., Eagen, M., and Shubik, P. (1972b). Ascorbate-nitrite reaction: possible means of blocking the formation of carcinogenic N-nitroso compounds. Science 177:65-68.

Moiseev, G. E., and Bonemonskii, V. V. (1975). On carcinogenic activity of low concentrations of N-nitrosodimethylamine in inhalation. Vopr. Onkol. 21:107-109.

Montesano, R., and Saffiotti, U. (1970). Carcinogenic response of the hamster respiratory tract to single subcutaneous administration of diethylnitrosamine at birth. J. Natl. Cancer Inst. 44:413-417.

Montesano, R., Saffiotti, U., Ferrero, A., and Kaufman, D. G. (1974). Synergistic effects of benzo(a)pyrene and diethylnitrosamine on respiratory carcinogenesis in hamsters. J. Natl. Cancer Inst. 53:1395-1397.

Neurath, G. B. (1972). Nitrosamine formation from precursors in tobacco smoke. In N-Nitroso Compounds Analysis and Formation, P. Bogovski, R. Preussmann, and E. A. Walker (Eds.). IARC Scientific Publication No. 3, Lyon, France, pp. 134-136.

Neurath, G. B., and Dunger, M. (1975). Measurement of nitrogen oxides in tobacco smoke by means of the chemiluminescence method. In N-Nitroso Compounds in the Environment, P. Bogovski and E. A. Walker (Eds.). IARC Scientific Publication No. 9, Lyon, France, pp. 177-179.

Neurath, G. B., and Schreiber, O. (1975). Investigations on amines in the human environment. In N-Nitroso Compounds in the Environment, P. Bogovski and E. A. Walker (Eds.). IARC Scientific Publications No. 9, International Agency for Research on Cancer, Lyon, France, pp. 211-214.

Norman, V., and Keith, C. H. (1965). Nitrogen oxides in tobacco smoke. Nature 205: 915-916.

Okada, M., Suzuki, E., and Hashimoto, Y. (1976). Carcinogenicity of N-nitrosamines related to N-butyl-N-(4-hydroxybutyl)nitrosamine and N,N-dibutylnitrosamine in ACI/N rats. Gan. 67:825-834.

Okun, J. D., and Archer, M. C. (1977). Kinetics of nitrosamine formation in the presence of micelle-forming surfactants. J. Natl. Cancer Inst. 58:409-411.

Park, K. K., Wishnok, J. S., and Archer, M. C. (1977). Mechanism of alkylation by N-nitroso compounds: detection of rearranged alcohol in the microsomal metabolism of N-nitroso-di-n-propylamine and base-catalyzed decomposition of N-n-propyl-N-nitrosourea. Chem. Biol. Interac. 18:349-354.

Pensabene, J. W., Fiddler, W., Gates, R. A., Fagan, J. C., and Wasserman, A. E. (1974). Effect of frying and other cooking conditions on nitrosopyrrolidine formation in bacon. J. Food Sci. 39:314-316.

Phillips, J. C., Lake, B. G., Gangolli, S. D., Grasso, P., and Lloyd, A. G. (1977). Effects of pyrazole and 3-amino-1,2,4-triazole on the metabolism and toxicity of dimethylnitrosamine in the rat. J. Natl. Cancer Inst. 58:629-633.

Preussmann, R. (1976). Chemical carcinogens in the human environment. Problems and quantitative aspects. Oncology 33:51-57.

Preussmann, R., Deutsch-Wenzel, R., and Eisenbrand, G. (1975). The effect of heavy metal ions on the rate of decomposition of N-ethyl-N-nitrosourea and other carcinogenic N-nitrosamides. Z. Krebsforsch. 84:75-80.

Rao, G. S., and Krishna, G. (1975). Drug-nitrite interactions: formation of N-nitroso, C-nitroso, and nitro compounds from sodium nitrite and various drugs under physiological conditions. J. Pharm. Sci. 64:1579-1581.

Reay, G. A., and Shewan, J. M. (1949). The spoilage of fish and its preservation by chilling. Adv. Food Res. 2:343-398.

Rhoades, J. W., and Johnson, D. E. (1972). N-Dimethylnitrosamine in tobacco smoke condensate. Nature 236:307-308.

Ridd, J. H. (1961). Nitrosation, diazotisation and deamination. Q. Rev. Chem. Soc. 15: 418-441.

Ross, A. E., and Mirvish, S. S. (1977). Metabolism of N-nitrosohexamethyleneimine to give 1,6-hexanediol bound to rat liver nucleic acids. J. Natl. Cancer Inst. 58:651-655.

Rustia, M. (1974). Multiple carcinogenic effects of the ethylnitrosourea precursors ethylurea and sodium nitrite in hamster. Cancer Res. 34:3232-3244.

Sander, J. (1967). Kann Nitrit in der menschlichen Nahrung Ursache einer Krebsentstehung durch Nitrosaminbildung sein? Arch. Hyg. Bakteriol. 151:22-28.

Sander, J. (1968). Nitrosaminsynthese durch Bakterien. Hoppe Seylers Z. Physiol. Chem. 349:429-432.

Sander, J., Aeikens, B., Schweinsberg, F., and Eisenbrand, G. (1973). Untersuchungen zur Frage einer Akkumulation mit Nitrosaminen in Weizen nach gleichzeitiger Dungung mit Nitrat und sekundaren Aminen. Z. Krebsforsch. 80:11-15.

Sander, J., LaBar, J., Ladenstein, M., and Schweinsberg, F. (1975a). Quantitative measurement of in vivo nitrosamine formation. In N-Nitroso Compounds in the Environment, P. Bogovski and E. A. Walker (Eds.). IARC Scientific Publications No. 9, Lyon, France, pp. 123-131.

Sander, J., Ladenstein, M., LaBar, J., and Schweinsberg, F. (1975b). Experiments on the degradation of nitrosamines by plants. In N-Nitroso Compounds in the Environment, P. Bogovski and E. A. Walker (Eds.). IARC Scientific Publications No. 9, Lyon, France, pp. 205-210.

Sander, J., Schweinsberg, F., LaBar, J., Burkle, G., and Schweinsberg, E. (1975c). Nitrite and nitrosable amino compounds in carcinogenesis. In Recent Topics in Chemical Carcinogenesis, S. Odashima, S. Takayama, and H. Sato (Eds.). University Park Press, Baltimore, pp. 145-160.

Scanlan, R. A. (1975). N-Nitrosamines in foods. Crit. Rev. Food Tech. 5:357-402.

Schmeltz, I., Abidi, S., and Hoffmann, D. (1977). Tumorigenic agents in unburned processed tobacco: N-Nitrosodiethanolamine and 1,1-dimethylhydrazine. Cancer Lett. 2:125-132.

Schmeltz, I., and Hoffmann, D. (1977). Nitrogen-containing compounds in tobacco and tobacco smoke. Chem. Rev. 77:295-311.

Schoental, R. (1973). The mechanisms of action of the carcinogenic nitroso and related compounds. Br. J. Cancer 28:436-439.

Schweinsberg, F. (1975). Catalysis of nitrosamine synthesis. In N-Nitroso Compounds in the Environment, P. Bogovski and E. A. Walker (Eds.). IARC Scientific Publication No. 9, Lyon, France, pp. 80-85.

Sen, N. P. (1972). The evidence for the presence of dimethylnitrosamine in meat products. Food Cosmet. Toxicol. 10:219-223.

Sen, N. P., and Donaldson, B. (1975). The effect of ascorbic acid and glutathione on the formation of nitrosopiperazines from piperazine adipate and nitrite. In N-Nitroso Compounds in the Environment, P. Bogovski and E. A. Walker (Eds.). IARC Scientific Publication No. 9, Lyon, France, pp. 103-106.

Sen, N. P., Donaldson, B. A., and Charbonneau, C. (1975). Formation of nitrosodimethylamine from the interaction of certain pesticides and nitrite. In N-Nitroso Compounds in the Environment, P. Bogovski and E. A. Walker (Eds.). IARC Scientific Publication No. 9, Lyon, France, pp. 75-79.

Sen, N. P., Donaldson, B., Iyengar, J. R., and Panalaks, T. (1973a). Nitrosopyrrolidine and dimethylnitrosamine in bacon. Nature 241:473-474.

Sen, N. P., Miles, W. F., Donaldson, B., Panalaks, T., and Iyengar, J. R. (1973b). Formation of nitrosamines in a meat curing mixture. Nature 245:104-105.

Sen, N. P., Smith, D. C., and Schwinghamer, L. (1969). Formation of N-nitrosamines from secondary amines and nitrite in human and animal gastric juice. Food. Cosmet. Toxicol. 7:301-307.

Shank, R. C., and Newberne, P. M. (1976). Dose-response study of the carcinogenicity of dietary sodium nitrite and morpholine in rats and hamsters. Food Cosmet. Toxicol. 14:1-8.

Shapley, D. (1976). Nitrosamines: scientists on the trail of prime suspect in urban cancer. Science 191:268-270.

Singer, G. M., and Lijinsky, W. (1976a). Naturally occurring nitrosatable compounds. I. Secondary amines in foodstuffs. J. Agric. Food Chem. 24:550-552.

Singer, G. M., and Lijinsky, W. (1976b). Naturally occurring nitrosatable amines. II. Secondary amines in tobacco and cigarette smoke condensate. J. Agric. Food Chem. 24:553-555.

Sipes, I. G., Slocumb, M. L., and Holtzman, G. (1978). Stimulation of microsomal dimethylnitrosamine-demethylase by pretreatment of mice with aceton. Chem.-Biol. Interact. 21:155-166.

Tada, O. (1962). Nitrogen oxides in cigarette smoke. Rep. Inst. Sci. Lab. Kurashiki 60: 7-10.

Tannenbaum, S. R., Sinskey, A. J., Weisman, M., and Bishop, W. (1974). Nitrite in human saliva. Its possible relationship to nitrosamine formation. J. Natl. Cancer Inst. 53:79-84.

Tate, R. L., III, and Alexander, M. (1975). Stability of nitrosamines in samples of lake water, soil, and sewage. J. Natl. Cancer Inst. 54:327-330.

Taylor, H. W., and Lijinsky, W. (1975). Tumor induction in rats by feeding aminopyrine or oxytetracycline with nitrite. Int. J. Cancer 16:211-215.

Tebbens, B. D. (1968). Gaseous pollutants in the air. In Air Pollution, 2nd Ed., Vol. 1, Air Pollution and Its Effects, A. C. Stern (Ed.). Academic Press, New York, pp. 23-46.

Thacker, L., and Brooks, J. B. (1974). In vitro production of N-nitrosodimethylamine and other amines by Proteus species. Infect. Immun. 9:648-653.

Tso, T. C., Sims, J. L., and Johnson, D. E. (1975). Some agronomic factors affecting N-dimethylnitrosamine content in cigarette smoke. Beitrage zur Tabakforschung 8: 34-38.

Walker, E. A., Pignatelli, B., and Castegnaro, M. (1975). Effects of gallic acid on nitrosamine formation. Nature 258:176.

Walters, C. L., Fueggle, D. G., and Lunt, T. G. (1975). The determination of total non-volatile nitrosamines in microgram amounts. In N-Nitroso Compounds in the Environment, P. Bogovski and E. A. Walker (Eds.). IARC Scientific Publication No. 9, Lyon, France, pp. 22-25.

Wasserman, A. E., and Fiddler, W. (1975). Nitrosamines in cured meat products. In N-Nitroso Compounds in the Environment, P. Bovogski and E. A. Walker (Eds.). IARC Scientific Publication No. 9, Lyon, France, pp. 147-150.

Weisburger, J. H., and Raineri, R. (1975). Assessment of human exposure and response to N-nitroso compounds: a new view on the etiology of digestive tract cancers. Toxicol. Appl. Pharmacol. 31:369-374.

White, J. W. (1975). Relative significance of dietary sources of nitrate and nitrite. J. Agric. Food Chem. 23:886-891.

Wogan, G. N., and Tannenbaum, S. R. (1975). Environmental N-nitroso compounds: implications for public health. Toxicol. Appl. Pharmacol. 31:375-383.

Wolff, I. A., and Wasserman, A. E. (1972). Nitrates, nitrites, and nitrosamines. Science 177:15-19.

Zaldivar, R. (1970). Geographic pathology of oral, esophageal, gastric, and intestinal cancer in Chile. Z. Krebsforsch. 75:1-13.

Section IV

ACGIH (1973). Threshold limit values for chemical substances and physical agents in the unknown environment with intended changes for 1973. American Conference of Governmental and Industrial Hygienists. J. Occup. Med. 16:39-49.

Adalis, D., Gardner, D. E., Miller, F. J., and Coffin, D. L. (1977). Toxic effects of cadmium on ciliary activity using a tracheal ring model system. Environ. Res. 13: 111-120.

Adams, R. G., Harrison, J. F., and Scott, P. (1969). The development of cadmium-induced proteinuria, impaired renal function, and osteomalacia in alkaline battery workers. Q. J. Med. 38:425-443.

Addingley, C. G. (1965). Dust measurement and monitoring in the asbestos industry. In Biological Effects of Asbestos, I. J. Selikoff and J. Churg (Eds.). Ann. NY Acad. Sci. 132:298-305.

Agnese, T., Veris, B. D., and Santolini, B. (1959). Incidence of lung cancer in relation to occupation in Genoa. Igiene Mod. 52:149-160.

Allison, A. C. (1973). Cell and tissue culture: effects of asbestos particles on macrophages, mesothelial cells and fibroblasts. In Biological Effects of Asbestos, P. Bogovski, J. C. Gilson, V. Timbrell, and J. C. Wagner (Eds.). IARC, Lyon, France, pp. 89-93.

AMA (1971). Conference on inorganic lead. Arch. Environ. Health 23:245-311.

Anderson, H. A., Lilis, R., Daum, S. M., Fischbein, A. S., and Selikoff, I. J. (1976). Household-contact asbestos neoplastic risk. In Occupational Carcinogenesis, U. Saffiotti and J. K. Wagoner (Eds.). Ann. NY Acad. Sci. 271:311-323.

Anderson, R. A., and Mertz, W. (1977). Glucose tolerance factor: an essential dietary agent. Trends Biochem. Sci. 2:277-279.

Arena, J. M. (1963). Poisoning—Chemistry, Symptoms, Treatment. Thomas, Springfield, Ill., pp. 92 and 127.

Ashley, B. E. (1972). Cadmium. In Minerals Yearbook, Vol. I, Metals, Minerals, and Fuels. Bureau of Mines, U.S. Dept. of Interior. U.S. Government Printing Office, Washington, D.C., pp. 227-233.

Atkinson, A. W., Gettins, R. B., and Rickards, A. L. (1971). Morphology of chrysotile. In 2nd Int. Conf. on "The Physics and Chemistry of Asbestos Minerals." Louvain Univ., Sept. 6-9, 1971. Abstracts of Papers, No. 2:4.

Axelsson, B., Dahlgreen, S. E., and Piscator, M. (1968). Renal lesions in the rabbit after long-term exposure to cadmium. Arch. Environ. Health 17:24-28.

Ayer, H. E., Lynch, J. R., and Fanney, J. H. (1965). A comparison of impinger and membrane filter techniques for evaluating air samples in asbestos plants. In Biological Effects of Asbestos, I. J. Selikoff and J. Churg (Eds.). Ann NY Acad. Sci. 132: 274-287.

Baetjer, A. M., Birmingham, D. J., Enterline, P. E., Mertz, W., and Pierce, J. V. (1974). Chromium. NAS, Washington, D.C., pp. 1-155.

Baetjer, A. M., Lowney, J. F., Steffee, H., and Budacz, V. (1959). The effect of chromium on incidence of lung tumors in mice and rats. Arch. Ind. Health 20:124-135.

Barnes, J. M. (1950). Experimental production of malignant tumours by beryllium. Lancet 1:463.

Bayliss, D. L., Dement, J. M., Wagoner, J. K., and Blejer, H. P. (1976). Mortality patterns among fibrous glass production workers. In Occupational Carcinogenesis, U. Saffiotti and J. K. Wagoner (Eds.). Ann. NY Acad. Sci. 271:324-335.

Berlin, M., and Ullberg, S. (1963). The fate of ^{109}Cd in the mouse. An autographic study after a single intravenous injection of $^{109}CdCl_2$. Arch. Environ. Health 7:686-693.

Berry, G., Newhouse, M. L., and Turok, L. (1972). Combined effect of asbestos exposure and smoking on mortality from lung cancer in factory workers. Lancet 2:476-479.

Blejer, H. P., and Caplan, P. E. (1971). Cadmium Inhalation Poisoning—Occupational Health Aspects with Special Reference to Welding and Silver Brazing, 2nd Ed. California State Dept. Public Health, Berkeley, Calif.

Blejer, H. P., and Wagner, W. (1976). Inorganic arsenic—ambient level approach to the control of occupational cancerigenic exposures. In Occupational Carcinogenesis, U. Saffiotti and J. K. Wagoner (Eds.). Ann. NY Acad. Sci. 271:179-186.

Blot, W. J., and Fraumeni, J. F. (1975). Arsenical air pollution and lung cancer. Lancet 2:142-144.

Bogden, J. D., Joselow, M. M., and Singh, N. P. (1975). Extraction of lead from printed matter at physiological values of pH. Arch. Environ. Health 31:442-444.

Bonser, G. M., Faulds, J. S., and Stewart, M. J. (1955). Occupational cancer of the urinary bladder in dyestuffs operatives and of the lung in asbestos textile workers and iron ore miners. Am. J. Clin. Pathol. 25:126-134.

Boppel, B. (1975). Bleigehalte von Lebensmitteln. 3. Blei-Aufnahme durch tägliche Nahrung. Z. Lebensm. Unters. Forsch. 158:287-290.

Botham, S. K., and Holt, P. F. (1968). The mechanism of formation of asbestos bodies. J. Pathol. Bact. 96:443-453.

Bourne, H. G., and Rushin, W. R. (1950). Atmospheric pollution in the vicinity of a chromate plant. Ind. Med. Surg. 19:568-569.

Braman, R. S. (1975). Arsenic in the environment. In Arsenical Pesticides Symposium, 1974. ACS Symposium Series 7, American Chemical Society, Washington, D.C., pp. 108-123.

Braman, R. S., and Foreback, C. C. (1973). Methylated forms of arsenic in the environment. Science 182:1247-1249.

Bremner, I. (1974). Heavy metal toxicities. Q. Rev. Biophys. 7:75-124.

Bresler, W. M. (1964). On the dynamics of blastomogenesis in the testis. Acta Un. Intern. Contra Cancrum 20:1501-1503.

Brodeur, P. (1972). Asbestos and Enzymes. Ballantine, New York, pp. 3-52.

Bryson, G., and Bischoff, F. (1967). Silicate-induced neoplasms. Prog. Exp. Tumor Res. 9:77-164.

Buchanan, W. D. (1962). Toxicity of Arsenic Compounds. Elsevier, Amsterdam, pp. 103-126.

Buchanan, W. D. (1965). Asbestosis and primary intrathoracic neoplasms. In Biological Effects of Asbestos, I. J. Selikoff and J. Churg (Eds.). Ann. NY Acad. Sci. 132: 507-518.

Campbell, R. O. (1961). A study of beryllium exposures at a high explosive test assembly facility. Am. Ind. Hyg. Assoc. J. 22:385-391.

CEC (1974). Problems of the contamination of man and his environment by cadmium and mercury. In Proc. Int. Symp. Luxembourg, July 3-5, 1973. Commission of the European Communities, Luxembourg.

Cempel, M., and Webb, M. (1976). The time-course of cadmium-thionein synthesis in the rat. Biochem. Pharmacol. 25:2067-2071.

Challop, R. S. (1971). Role of cadmium in lead poisoning. N. Engl. J. Med. 285:970-971.

Chen, R. W., Eakin, D. J., and Whanger, P. D. (1974). Biological function of metallothionein. II. Its role in zinc metabolism in the rat. Nutr. Rep. Intern. 10:195-200.

Cherian, M. G., and Clarkson, T. W. (1976). Biochemical changes in rat kidney on exposure to elemental mercury vapor: effect on biosynthesis of metallothionein induced nephropathy. Chem. Biol. Interac. 12:109-120.

Cherian, M. G., and Vostal, J. J. (1977). Biliary excretion of cadmium in rat. I. Dose-dependent biliary excretion and the form of cadmium in the bile. J. Toxicol. Environ. Health 2:945-954.

Chernoff, N. (1973). Teratogenic effects of cadmium in rats. Teratology 8:29-32.

Chesner, C. (1950). Chronic pulmonary granulomatosis in residents of community near beryllium plant. Ann. Intern. Med. 32:1028-1048.

Christensen, F. C., and Olsen, E. C. (1957). Cadmium poisoning. Arch. Ind. Health 16:8-13.

Clarkson, T. W. (1977). Factors involved in heavy metal poisoning. Fed. Proc. 36:1634-1639.

Clarkson, T. W., Amin-Zaki, L., and Al-Tikriti, S. K. (1976). An outbreak of methylmercury poisoning due to contaminated grain. Fed. Proc. 35:2395-2399.

Cohen, J. J. (1963). Methods of handling and laundering beryllium-contaminated garments. Am. Ind. Hyg. Assoc. J. 24:576-583.

Coles, L. E. (1974). Selenium: a review. J. Assoc. Pub. Anal. 12:68-72.

Colucci, A. V., Winge, D., and Krasno, J. (1975). Cadmium accumulation in rat liver. Arch. Environ. Health 30:153-157.

Conradi, C., Burri, P. H., Kapanci, Y., Robinson, F. R., and Weibel, E. R. (1971). Lung changes after beryllium inhalation—ultrastructural and morphometric study. Arch. Environ. Health 23:348-358.

Coogan, P., Hsu, G., Frank, L., and Stein, L. (1971). Parenteral lead subacetate induced sarcomas in rats. Fed. Proc. 30:289.

Cooke, J. W. (1929). Asbestos dust and the curious bodies found in pulmonary asbestosis. Br. Med. J. 2:578-580.

Cooper, W. C. (1976). Cancer mortality patterns in the lead industry. In Occupational Carcinogenesis, U. Saffiotti and J. K. Wagoner (Eds.). Ann. NY Acad. Sci. 271: 250-259.

Corneliussen, P. A. (1972). Residues in food and feed. Pestic. Monit. J. 5:313-330.

Crossmon, G. C., and Vandemark, W. C. (1954). Microscopic observations correlating toxicity of beryllium oxide with crystal structure. Arch. Ind. Hyg. Occup. Med. 9: 481-487.

Cunningham, H. M., and Pontefract, R. D. (1973). Asbestos fibers in beverages, drinking water, and tissues: their passage through the intestinal wall and movement through the body. J. Assoc. Off. Anal. Chem. 56:976-986.

Cunningham, H. M., and Pontefract, R. D. (1974). Placental transfer of asbestos. Nature 249:177-178.

Cunningham, H. M., Pontefract, R. D., and O'Brien, R. C. (1976). Quantitative relationship of fecal asbestos to asbestos exposure. J. Toxicol. Environ Health 1:377-379.

Daniel, M., and Webb, M. (1964). Protection of cell-cultures by Zn^{2+} against the toxic action of carcinogenic metals. Rep. Br. Emp. Cancer Campaign 42:376-378.

Davis, J. M. (1974). Histogenesis and fine structure of peritoneal tumors produced in animals by injection of asbestos. J. Natl. Cancer Inst. 52:1823-1837.

Davis, W. E. (1970). National Inventory of Sources and Emissions, 1964. Cadmium: Report to National Air Pollution Control Administration. February, pp. 1-44. Rep. PB 192250, U.S. Dept. of Commerce, Nat. Tech. Info. Serv., Springfield, Va., Natl. Air Sampling Network, DHEW, unpublished data quoted in Nordberg (1974).

Daykin, C. W. (1971). A study of the infra-red spectra of chrysotile and related minerals. In 2nd Int. Conf. on "The Physics and Chemistry of Asbestos Minerals." Louvain Univ., Sept. 6-9, 1971. Abstracts of Papers, No. 2:6.

Decker, L. E., Byerrum, R. U., Decker, C. F., Hoppert, C. A., and Langham, R. F. (1958). Chronic toxicity studies. I. Cadmium administered in drinking water to rats. Arch. Ind. Health 18:228-231.

Deknudt, G., and Léonard, A. (1975). Cytogenetic investigations on leucocytes of workers from a cadmium plant. Environ. Physiol. Biochem. 5:319-327.

De Nardi, J. M. (1959). Long-term experience with beryllium disease. Arch. Ind. Health 19:110-116.

De Nardi, J. M., Van Ordstrand, H. S., and Carmody, M. G. (1949). Acute dermatitis and pneumonitis in beryllium workers: review of 406 cases in eight-year period with follow-up on recoveries. Ohio State Med. J. 45:567-575.

Denton, C. R., Keenan, R. G., and Birmingham, D. J. (1954). The chromium content of cement and its significance in cement dermatitis. J. Invest. Dermatol. 23: 189-192.

Der, R., Fahim, Z., Yousef, M., and Fahim, M. (1976). Environmental interaction of lead and cadmium on reproduction and metabolism of male rats. Res. Commun. Chem. Pathol. Pharmacol. 14: 689-713.

Desbordes, J., Tayot, J., and Dousset, G. (1968). Reflections on the carcinogenic effect of asbestos. Poumon Coeur 24: 607-623.

DHEW (1972). Occupational Exposure to Beryllium. U.S. Dept. of Health, Education and Welfare, Washington, D.C., No. 72-10268.

Diezel, P. B. (1961). Gewebsreaktion nach Injektion von Al_2O_3-Impfstoff. Arzneim. Forsch. 11: 905-908.

Dingwall-Fordyce, I., and Lane, R. E. (1963). A follow-up study of lead workers. Br. J. Ind. Med. 20: 313-315.

DiPaolo, J. A., and Kotin, P. (1966). Teratogenesis-oncogenesis: a study of possible relationship. Arch. Pathol. 81: 3-23.

Dohner, V. A., Beegle, R. G., and Miller, W. T. (1975). Asbestos exposure and multiple primary tumors. Annu. Rev. Resp. Dis. 112: 181-199.

DOL (1975a). Inorganic arsenic: proposed exposure standard. Department of Labor, Fed. Reg. 40: 3392-3404.

DOL (1975b). Lead, occupational exposure, proposed standard. Department of Labor, Fed. Reg. 40: 45934-45948.

Doll, R. (1955). Mortality from lung cancer in asbestos workers. Br. J. Ind. Med. 12: 81-86.

Donnelly, P. A., and Monty, D. E. (1977). Toxicological effects of cadmium chloride on the canine testis following various routes of administration. Toxicol. Lett. 1: 53-58.

Dreessen, W. C., Dallavalle, J. M., Edwards, T. I., Miller, J. W., and Sayers, R. R. (1938). A Study of Asbestosis in the Asbestos Textile Industry, U.S. Public Health Bulletin, No. 241 (Aug. 1938), pp. 1-126.

Druckrey, H., Hamperl, H., and Schmähl, D. (1957). Cancerogene Wirkung von metallischen Quecksilber nach intraperitonealer Gabe bei Ratten. Z. Krebsforsch. 61: 511-519.

Duggan, R. E., and Lipscome, G. Q. (1969). Dietary intake of pesticide chemicals in the United States. II. June 1966-April 1968. Pestic. Monit. J. 2: 153-160.

Ehlers, G. (1968). Clinical and histological studies of drug-induced arsenic tumors. Z. HautKr. 22: 763-774.

Eisenbud, M., Wanta, R. C., Dustan, C., Steadman, L. T., Harris, W. B., and Wolfe, B. S. (1949). Non-occupational berylliosis. J. Ind. Hyg. Toxicol. 31: 282-294.

Enterline, P. E. (1974). Respiratory cancer among chromate workers. J. Occup. Med. 16: 523-526.

Enterline, P., De Coufle, P., and Henderson, V. (1973). Respiratory cancer in relation to occupational exposures among retired asbestos workers. Br. J. Ind. Med. 30: 162-166.

Enterline, P. E., and Henderson, V. (1973). Type of asbestos and respiratory cancer in the asbestos industry. Arch. Environ. Health 27: 312-317.

Enterline, P. E., and Henderson, V. (1975). The health of retired fibrous glass workers. Arch. Environ. Health 30: 113-116.

Enticknap, J. B., and Smither, W. J. (1964). Peritoneal tumours in asbestosis. Br. J. Ind. Med. 21: 20-31.

EPA (1975). Interim Report to Congress, Preliminary Assessment of Suspected Carcinogens in Drinking Water and Appendices. Office of Toxic Substances, U.S. Environmental Protection Agency, Washington, D.C.

Epstein, S. S., and Mantel, N. (1968). Carcinogenicity of tetraethyl lead. Experientia 24: 580-581.

Erdohazi, M., and Newman, R. L. (1971). Aluminium hydroxyde granuloma. Br. Med. J. 3:621-623.

Evans, J. C., Evans, R. J., Holmes, A., Hounam, R. F., Jones, D. M., Morgan, A., and Walsh, M. (1973). Studies on the deposition of inhaled fibrous material in the respiratory tract of the rat and its subsequent clearance using radioactive tracer techniques. 1. UICC crocidolite asbestos. Environ. Res. 6:180-201.

Faeder, E. J., Chaney, S. Q., King, L. C., Hinners, T. A., Bruce, R., and Fowler, B. A. (1977). Biochemical and ultrastructural changes in livers of cadmium-treated rats. Toxicol. Appl. Pharmacol. 39:473-487.

Falin, L. I., and Anissimora, W. W. (1940a). Zur Pathogenese der experimentellen teratoiden Geschwülste der Geschlechtsdrüsen Teratoide Hodengeschwulst beim Hahn, erzeugt durch Einführung von $CuSO_4$-Lösung. Z. Krebsforsch. 50:339-351.

Falin, L. I., and Anissimora, V. (1940b). De la pathogénie des tumeurs experimentales teratoides des glandes génitales: tumeur tératoide du coq causée par l'injection d'une solution de sulfate de cuivre. Bull. Biol. Med. Exp. 9:519-520.

Fassett, D. W. (1975). Cadmium: biological effects and occurrence in the environment. Annu. Rev. Pharmacol. Toxicol. 15:425-436.

Fed. Reg. (1975). Beryllium: proposed occupational safety and health standard. 42:48814-48827.

Fennelly, P. F. (1976). The origin and influence of airborne particulates. Am. Sci. 64: 46-56.

Ferm, V. H. (1969). The synergistic effects of lead and cadmium. Experientia 25:56-57.

Fishbein, L. (1976). Environmental metallic carcinogens. An overview of exposure levels. J. Toxicol. Environ. Health 2:77-109.

Flick, D. F., Kraybill, H. F., and Dimitroff, J. M. (1971). Toxic effects of cadmium: a review. Environ. Res. 4:71-85.

Friberg, L., Kjellstrom, T., Nordberg, G., and Piscator, M. (1975). Cadmium in the Environment—III. Office of Research and Monitoring, U.S. Environmental Protection Agency, Washington, D.C.

Friberg, L., Piscator, M., Nordberg, G. F., and Kjellstrom, T. (1974). Cadmium in the Environment, 2nd Ed. CRC, Cleveland, Ohio.

Frost, D. V., and West, P. W. (1967). Selenium and cancer. In "Letters," Chem. Eng. News 45:6-7.

Furst, A. (1971). Trace elements related to specific chronic diseases: cancer. In Environmental Geochemistry, H. L. Cannon and H. C. Hops (Eds.). Geological Society of America, Boulder, Col., pp. 109-129.

Furst, A., and Cassetta, D. (1972). Failure of zinc to negate cadmium carcinogenesis. Proc. Am. Assoc. Cancer Res. 13:62.

Furst, A., and Haro, R. T. (1969a). A survey of metal carcinogenesis. Prog. Exp. Tumor Res. 12:102-133.

Furst, A., and Haro, R. T. (1969b). Possible mechanisms of metal ion carcinogenesis. In Jerusalem Symposium on Quantum Chemistry and Biochemistry, Vol. I, E. D. Bergman and B. Pullman (Eds.). Israel Academy Sciences and Humanities, Jerusalem, pp. 310-320.

Furst, A., and Haro, R. T. (1970). Carcinogenicity of metal pi-complex compounds: metallocenes. In 10th Int. Cancer Cong., Houston. Abstracts, p. 28 (Abstr. #42).

Furst, A., and Schlauder, M. C. (1977). Inactivity of two noble metals as carcinogens. J. Environ. Pathol. Toxicol. 1:51-57.

Furst, A., Schlauder, M., and Sasmore, D. P. (1976). Tumorigenic activity of lead chromate. Cancer Res. 36:1779-1783.

Gaze, R. (1965). The physical and molecular structure of asbestos. In Biological Effects of Asbestos, I. J. Selikoff and J. Churg (Eds.). Ann. NY Acad. Sci. 132:23-30.

Gelman, I. (1936). Poisoning by vapors of beryllium oxyfluoride. J. Ind. Hyg. 18:371-379.

Gilliavod, N., and Léonard, A. (1975). Mutagenicity tests with cadmium in the mouse. Toxicology 5:43-47.

Gilman, J. P. (1962). Metal carcinogenesis. II. A study of the carcinogenic activity of cobalt, copper, iron, and nickel compounds. Cancer Res. 22:158-165.

Gilman, J. P., and Ruckerbauer, G. M. (1962). Metal carcinogenesis. I. Observations on the carcinogenicity of a refinery dust, cobalt oxide, and colloidal thorium dioxide. Cancer Res. 22:152-157.

Gloyne, S. R. (1935). Squamous carcinoma of the lung occurring in asbestosis. Tubercle 17:5-10.

Gorski, C. H., Stettler, L. E., and Lempert, B. L. (1976). The porosity of amosite and chrysotile asbestos. Am. Ind. Hyg. Assoc. J. 37:117-122.

Goyer, R. A. (1974). Low level of lead toxicity and the environmental impact of cadmium. Environ. Health Perspect., Experimental Issue No. 7, pp. 3-252.

Greenberg, S. D., Hurst, G. A., Matlage, W. T., Miller, J. M., Hurst, I. J., and Mabry, L. C. (1976). Tyler asbestos workers program. In Occupational Carcinogenesis, U. Saffiotti and J. K. Wagoner (Eds.). Ann. NY Acad. Sci. 271:353-364.

Groetenbriel, C., Van Ganse, W. F., and Oleffe, J. (1970). A propos d'un cas d'intoxication chronique au béryllium: considérations pathogéniques et valeur due "patch-test" pour le diagnostic. Acta Tuberc. Pneumol. Belg. 61:363-376.

Gross, P., Tuma, J., and de Treville, R. T. (1971). Lungs of workers exposed to fiber glass. Arch. Environ. Health 23:67-76.

Groth, D. H., and MacKay, G. R. (1971). Chronic pulmonary pathology in rats after the the intratracheal injection of 0.4, 4, and 40 μg of beryllium as beryllium hydroxide. Toxicol. Appl. Pharmacol. 19:392.

Gunn, S. A., Gould, T. C., and Anderson, W. A. (1963). Cadmium-induced interstitial cell tumors in rats and mice and their prevention by zinc. J. Natl. Cancer Inst. 31: 745-759.

Gunn, S. A., Gould, T. C., and Anderson, W. A. (1964). Effect of zinc on cancerogenesis by cadmium. Proc. Soc. Exp. Biol. Med. 115:653-657.

Gunn, S. A., Gould, T. C., and Anderson, W. A. (1968a). Mechanisms of zinc, cystein and selenium protection against cadmium-induced vascular injury to mouse testis. J. Reprod. Fertil. 15:65-70.

Gunn, S. A., Gould, T. C., and Anderson, W. A. (1968b). Selectivity of organ response to cadmium injury and various protective measures. J. Path. Bact. 96:89-96.

Haddow, A., and Horning, E. S. (1960). On the carcinogenicity of an iron-dextran complex. J. Natl. Cancer Inst. 24:109-147.

Haley, T. J. (1975). Asbestosis: a reassessment of the overall problem. J. Pharm. Sci. 64:1435-1449.

Hammond, P. B., Aronson, A. L., Chisolm, J. J., Falk, J. L., Keenan, R. G., and Sandstead, H. H. (1972). Airborne Lead in Perspective. NAS, Washington, D.C.

Harrington, J. S. (1973). Chemical factors (including trace elements) as etiological mechanisms. In Biological Effects of Asbestos, P. Bogovski, J. C. Gilson, V. Timbrell, and J. C. Wagner (Eds.). IARC, Lyon, France, pp. 304-311.

Harris, A. M., and Grimshaw, R. W. (1971). The leaching of ground chrysotile. In 2nd Intern. Conf. on "The Physics and Chemistry of Asbestos Minerals." Louvain Univ., Louvain, Belgium. Sept. 6-9, 1971. Abstracts of Papers, No. 3:2B.

Hasan, F. M., and Kazemi, H. (1974). Chronic beryllium disease: a continuing epidemiological hazard. Chest 65:289-293.

Heindl, R. A. (1970). Cadmium. In Mineral Facts and Problems. Bureau of Mines Bulletin No. 650. U.S. Dept. of Interior, U.S. Government Printing Office, Washington, D.C., pp. 515-526.

Hendry, N. W. (1965). The geology, occurrences and major uses of asbestos. In Biological Effects of Asbestos, I. J. Selikoff and J. Churg (Eds.). Ann. NY Acad. Sci. 132: 12-22.

Hicks, R. M. (1972). Air-borne lead as environmental toxin: a review. Chem. Biol. Interact. 5:361-390.

Hill, A. B., and Faning, E. L. (1948). Cancer from inorganic arsenic compounds. I. Mortality experience in the factory. Br. J. Ind. Med. 5:2-6.

Hill, J. W., Whitehead, W. S., Cameron, J. D., and Hedgecock, G. A. (1973). Glass fibers: absence of pulmonary hazard in production workers. Br. J. Ind. Med. 30: 174-179.

Holmes, S. (1965). Developments in dust sampling and counting techniques in the asbestos industry. In Biological Effects of Asbestos, I. J. Selikoff and J. Churg (Eds.). Ann. NY Acad. Sci. 132:288-297.

Holmes, S. (1973). Sampling methods. In Biological Effects of Asbestos, P. Bogovski, V. Timbrell, J. C. Gilson, and J. C. Wagner (Eds.). IARC, Lyon, France, pp. 109-112.

Hueper, W. C. (1959). Environmental cancer. In Physiopathology of Cancer, F. Homburger (Ed.). Hoeber-Harper, New York, pp. 919-970.

Hueper, W. C. (1964). Macromolecular agents as benign and malignant cell proliferants. Natl. Cancer Inst. Monogr. 14:357-377.

Hueper, W. C. (1966a). Occupational and Environmental Cancers of the Respiratory System. Springer-Verlag, New York, p. 40.

Hueper, W. C. (1966b). Occupational and Environmental Cancers of the Respiratory System. Springer-Verlag, New York, pp. 30-38 and 56-103.

Hueper, W. C. (1967). Carcinogenic hazards for arsenic and metal containing drugs. In Potential Carcinogenic Hazards from Drugs, R. Truhaut (Ed.). UICC Monographs Vol. 7. Springer-Verlag, Berlin, pp. 79-104.

Hueper, W. C., and Conway, W. D. (1964). Chemical Carcinogenesis and Cancers. Thomas, Springfield, Ill., p. 133.

Hueper, W. C., and Payne, W. W. (1962). Experimental studies in metal carcinogenesis. Arch. Environ. Health 5:445-462.

Hunter, B., and Thomson, C. (1973). Evaluation of tumorigenic potential of vermiculite by intrapleural injection in rats. Br. J. Ind. Med. 30:167-173.

IARC (1972a). Beryllium and beryllium compounds. In Evaluation of Carcinogenic Risk of Chemicals to Man, IARC Monographs, Vol. 1. Lyon, France, pp. 17-28.

IARC (1972b). Lead salts. In Evaluation of Carcinogenic Risk of Chemicals to Man, IARC Monographs, Vol. 1. Lyon, France, pp. 40-50.

IARC (1973a). Evaluation of Carcinogenic Risk of Chemicals to Man—Some Inorganic and Organometallic Compounds, IARC Monographs, Vol. 2. Lyon, France.

IARC (1973b). Chromium and inorganic chromium compounds. In Evaluation of Carcinogenic Risk of Chemicals to Man—Some Inorganic and Organometallic Compounds, IARC Monographs, Vol. 2. Lyon, France, pp. 100-125.

IARC (1973c). Cadmium and inorganic cadmium compounds. In Evaluation of Carcinogenic Risk of Chemicals to Man—Some Inorganic and Organometallic Compounds, IARC Monographs, Vol. 2. Lyon, France, pp. 74-99.

IARC (1977). Asbestos. In Evaluation of the Carcinogenic Risk of Chemicals to Man, IARC Monographs, Vol. 14. Lyon, France.

Itokawa, Y., Abe, T., Tabei, R., and Tanaka, S. (1974). Renal and skeletal lesions in experimental cadmium poisoning. Arch. Environ. Health 28:149-154.

Ivankovic, S., and Preussman, R. (1975). Absence of toxic and carcinogenic effects after administration of high doses of chromic oxide pigment in subacute and long-term feeding experiments in rats. Food Cosmet. Toxicol. 13:347-351.

Izumi, T., and Kobara, Y. (1966). Beryllium poisoning. Lancet 2:152-154.

Izumi, T., Kobara, Y., Inui, S., Tokunaga, R., Orita, Y., Kitano, M., and Williams, W. J. (1976). The first seven cases of chronic beryllium disease in ceramic factory workers in Japan. Ann. NY Acad. Sci. 278:636-653.

Jarvie, A. W., Markall, R. N., and Patter, H. R. (1975). Chemical alkylation of lead. Nature 225: 217-218.

Jugo, S. (1977). Metabolism of toxic heavy metals in growing organisms: a review. Environ Res. 13:36-46.

Kanazawa, K., Birbeck, M. S., Carter, R. L., and Roe, F. J. (1970). Migration of asbestos fibers from subcutaneous injection sites in mice. Br. J. Cancer 24: 96-106.

Kanisawa, M. (1971). Aspects of metal carcinogenesis. Chiba Daigaku Kogakubu Kenkyn Hokuku 24: 1-35.

Kilham, L., Row, R. J., Conti, S. F., and Dallenbach, F. D. (1962). Intranuclear inclusions and neoplasms in the kidneys of wild rat. J. Natl. Cancer Inst. 29: 863-885.

Kimmerle, G. (1966). Beryllium. (Handbuch der experimentellen Pharmakologie, Vol. 21). Springer-Verlag, Berlin.

King, C. V. (1971). Maximum daily intake of lead without excessive body lead-burden. Am. J. Dis. Child 122: 337-340.

Kipling, M. D., and Waterhouse, J. A. (1967). Cadmium and prostatic carcinoma. Lancet 1: 730-731.

Kjellstrom, T., and Friberg, L. (1974). Interpretation of empirically documented body burdens by age, of metals with long biological half times, with special reference to past changes in exposure. In Proc. 17th Intern. Cong. Occup. Health, Buenos Aires, (Abst.).

Komitowski, D. (1968). Pathodynamics of the neoplastic process in experimental berylliosis. Med. Dosw. Mikrobiol. 38:57-91 (in Polish).

Kopp, J. F., and Kromer, R. C. (1970). Trace Metals in Waters of the United States, Oct. 1, 1962-Sept. 30, 1967. Dept. of Interior, Federal Water Pollution Control Administration, Div. of Pollution Surveillance, Cincinnati.

Kunz, J., Shahab, L., Henze, K., and David, H. (1963). Experimentelle Untersuchungen zur cancerogenen Wirkung von Eisendextran (Ursoferran). Acta Biol. Med. Germ. 10: 602-614.

Kuschner, M., and Laskin, S. (1971). Experimental models in environmental carcinogenesis. Am. J. Pathol. 64: 183-191.

Lacassagne, A. (1971). Revue critique des tumeurs expérimentales des cellules Leydig, plus particulièrement chez le rat. Bull. Cancer 58: 235-276.

Lane, B. P., and Mass, M. J. (1977). Carcinogenicity and cocarcinogenicity of chromium carbonyl in heterotopic tracheal grafts. Cancer Res. 37: 1476-1479.

Langer, A. M., Rubin, I. B., and Selikoff, I. J. (1972). Chemical characterization of asbestos body cores by electron microprobe analysis. J. Histochem. Cytochem. 20: 723-734.

Langvad, E. (1968). Iron-dextran induction of distant tumours in mice. Int. J. Cancer 3: 415-423.

Laskin, S., Kuschner, M., and Drew, R. T. (1970). Studies in pulmonary carcinogenesis. In Inhalation Carcinogenesis, M. G. Hanna, P. Nesheim, and J. R. Gilbert (Eds.). U.S. Atomic Energy Commission, Washington, D.C., pp. 321-351.

Lauwerys, R. R., Buchet, J. P., Roels, H. A., Brouwers, J., and Stanescu, D. (1974). Epidemiological survey of workers exposed to cadmium—effect on lung, kidney and several biological indices. Arch. Environ. Health 28: 145-148.

Lavappa, K. S., Fu, M. M., and Epstein, S. S. (1975). Cytogenetic studies on chrysotile asbestos. Environ. Res. 10: 165-173.

Leach, R. M., and Fuller, H. L. (Eds.) (1975). Symposium on "Biochemical function of selenium and its interrelationship with other trace elements and vitamin E." Fed. Proc. 34: 2082-2100.

Lee, A. M., and Fraumeni, J. F. (1969). Arsenic and respiratory cancer in man: an occupational study. J. Natl. Cancer Inst. 42: 1045-1052.

Lee, B. K., and Murphy, G. (1969). Determination of arsenic content of American cigarettes by neutron activation analysis. Cancer 23: 1315-1317.

Lemen, R. A., Lee, J. S., Wagoner, J. K., and Blejer, H. P. (1976). Cancer mortality among cadmium production workers. In Occupational Carcinogenesis, U. Saffiotti and J. K. Wagoner (Eds.). Ann. NY Acad. Sci. 271:273-279.

Léonard, A., Deknudt, G., and Gilliavod, N. (1974). Les dangers génétiques du cadmium. Ann. Gembloux 80:87-93.

Levander, O. A. (1972). Metabolic interrelationships and adaptations in selenium toxicity. Ann. NY Acad. Sci. 192:181-192.

Lewis, G. P., Jusko, W. J., Coughlin, L. L., and Hartz, S. (1972). Contribution of cigarette smoking to cadmium accumulation in man. Lancet 1:291-292.

Loeser, E., and Lorke, D. (1977a). Semichronic oral toxicity of cadmium. 1. Studies on rats. Toxicology 7:215-224.

Loeser, E., and Lorke, D. (1977b). Semichronic oral toxicity of cadmium. 2. Studies on dogs. Toxicology 7:225-232.

Lucis, O. J., Lynk, M. E., and Lucis, R. (1969). Turnover of ^{109}Cd in rats. Arch. Environ. Health 18:307-310.

Lynch, K. M., and Smith, W. A. (1935). Pulmonary asbestosis. III. Carcinoma in the lung in asbestosilicosis. Am. J. Cancer 24:56-64.

Machle, W. (1948). "Discussion," Symposium on Industrial Diseases. Radiology 50:785.

Magos, L., and Webb, M. (1976). The interaction between cadmium, mercury and zinc—administered subcutaneously in a single injection. Arch. Toxicol. 36:53-61.

Magos, L., Webb, M., and Butler, W. H. (1974). The effect of cadmium pretreatment on the nephrotoxic action and kidney uptake of mercury in male and female rats. Br. J. Exp. Pathol. 55:589-594.

Maroudas, N. G., O'Neil, C. H., and Stanton, M. F. (1973). Fibroblast anchorage and carcinogenesis by fibres. Lancet 1:807-809.

Marradi-Fabroni, S. (1935). Patologia polmonare da polveri di berillio. Med. Lav. 26: 297-303.

Martin, D. F., and Martin, B. B. (1964). Coordination Compounds. McGraw-Hill, New York, p. 81.

Masson, T. J., McKay, F. W., and Miller, R. W. (1974). Asbestos-like fibers in Duluth water supply. Relation to cancer mortality. JAMA 228:1019-1020.

McCord, C. P. (1951). Beryllium as a sensitizing agent. Ind. Med. Surg. 20:336.

McCrone, W. C., and Stewart, I. M. (1974). Asbestos. Am. Lab. 6:13-18.

McEwen, J., Finlayson, A., Mair, A., and Gibson, A. A. (1971). Asbestos and mesothelioma in Scotland—an epidemiological study. Int. Arch. Arbeitsmed. 28:301-311.

Med. World News (1976). Threat of asbestos disease widens. 17:41-48.

Merewether, E. R. (1930). The occurrence of pulmonary fibrosis and other pulmonary affections in asbestos workers. J. Ind. Hyg. Toxicol. 12:198-222 and 239-257.

Mertz, W., Toepfer, E. W., Roginski, E. E., and Polansky, M. M. (1974). Present knowledge of the role of chromium. Fed. Proc. 33:2275-2280.

Metzner, F. N., and Lieben, J. (1961). Respiratory disease associated beryllium refining and alloy fabrication. J. Occup. Med. 3:341-345.

Miller, L., Smith, W. E., and Berliner, S. W. (1965). Tests for effect of asbestos on benzo(a)pyrene carcinogenesis in the respiratory tract. In Biological Effect of Asbestos, I. J. Selikoff and J. Churg (Eds.). Ann NY Acad. Sci. 132:489-500.

Monkman, L. J. (1971). Some chemical and mineralogical aspects of the acid decomposition of chrysotile. In 2nd Int. Conf. on "The Physics and Chemistry of Asbestos Minerals." Louvain Univ., Louvain, Belgium. Sept. 6-9, 1971. Abstracts of Papers, No. 3:2.

Murray, H. M. (1907). In Report of the Departmental Committee on Compensation for Industrial Diseases. H. M. Stationary Office, London, pp. 3495-3496.

Muth, O. H. (1967). Selenium in Biomedicine. AVI, Westport, Conn.

Nandi, M., Jick, H., Slone, D., Shapiro, S., and Lewis, G. P. (1969). Cadmium content of cigarettes. Lancet 2:1329-1330.

NASN (1964). Air Quality Data. (National Air Surveillance Networks). U.S. Dept. of Health, Education, and Welfare, National Air Pollution Control Administration, Cincinnati, Ohio.

NASN (1968). Air Quality Data from the National Air Surveillance Networks and Contributing State and Local Networks. 1966 Ed., Publication No. APTD 68-9. U.S. Dept. of Health, Education, and Welfare, Durham, N.C., p. 157.

National Research Council (1971). Airborne Lead in Perspective. NAS, Washington, D.C.

National Research Council (1974). Chromium. NAS, Washington, D.C.

Nelson, A. A., Fitzhugh, O. G., and Calvery, H. O. (1943). Liver tumors following cirrhosis caused by selenium in rats. Cancer Res. 3:230-236.

Nettesheim, P., Hanna, M. G., Dohertz, D. G., Newell, R. F., and Hellman, A. (1971). Effect of calcium chromate dust, influenza virus and 100-γ whole-body x-radiation on lung tumor incidence in mice. J. Natl. Cancer Inst. 47:1129-1144.

Neubauer, O. (1947). Arsenical cancer: a review. Br. J. Cancer 1:192-251.

Neukomm, S. (1969). Recherches sur le pouvoir cancerigene et co-cancerigene de diverses preparations à base de fer. Proc. Eur. Soc. Drug Toxic. 2:174-177.

Newman, J. A., Archer, V. E., Saccomanno, G., Kuschner, M., Auerbach, O., Grondahl, R. D., and Wilson, J. C. (1976). Histologic types of bronchogenic carcinoma among members of copper-mining and smelting communities. In Occupational Carcinogenesis, U. Saffiotti and J. K. Wagoner (Eds.). Ann. NY Acad. Sci. 271:260-268.

Nicholson, W. J. (1976). Asbestos—the TLV approach. In Occupational Carcinogenesis U. Saffiotti and J. K. Wagoner (Eds.). Ann. NY Acad. Sci. 271:152-169.

Nicholson, W. J., and Pundsack, F. L. (1973). Asbestos in the environment. In Biological Effects of Asbestos, P. Bogovski, J. C. Gilson, V. Timbrell, and J. C. Wagner (Eds.). IARC, Lyon, France, pp. 126-130.

Niemöller, H. K. (1962). Skin test for beryllium according to Curtis and its modifications. Int. Arch. Gewerbepathol. 19:27-34.

Niemöller, H. K. (1963). Spätcarcinome durch Berylliumaerosole beim Menschen. Int. Arch. Gewerbepathol. 20:180-186.

Nisioka, H. (1975). Mutagenic activities of metal compounds in bacteria. Mutat. Res. 31: 185-189.

Nomiyama, K., Sato, C., and Yamamoto, A. (1973). Early signs of cadmium intoxication in rabbits. Toxicol. Appl. Pharmacol. 24:625-635.

Nordberg, G. F. (1971). Effects of acute and chronic cadmium exposure on the testicles of mice and special reference to the protective effect of metallothionein. Exp. Physiol. 1:171-187.

Nordberg, G. F. (1974). Health hazards of environmental cadmium pollution. Ambio 3: 55-66.

Oldham, P. D. (1973). Asbestos in lung tissue. In Biological Effects of Asbestos, P. Bogovski, J. C. Gilson, V. Timbrell, and J. C. Wagner (Eds.). IARC, Lyon, pp. 231-235.

Osswald, H., and Goerttler, K. (1971). Leukosen bei der Maus nach diaplazentare und postnatale Arsenic Applikation. Verh. Dtsch. Ges. Pathol. 55:289-293.

Ott, M., Holder, B., and Gordon, H. (1974). Respiratory cancer and occupational exposure to arsenicals. Arch. Environ. Health 29:250-255.

Paris, J. A. (1820). Pharmacologia or the History of Medicinal Substances with a View of Establishing the Art of Prescribing, 4th Ed. Phillips, London.

Parizek, J. (1957). The destructive effect of cadmium ion on testicular tissue and its prevention by zinc. J. Endocrinol. 15:56-63.

Passow, H., Rothstein, A., and Clarkson, T. W. (1961). The general pharmacology of the heavy metals. Pharmacol. Rev. 13:185-224.

Pelfrene, A. (1976). Arsenic and cancer: the still unanswered question. J. Toxicol. Environ. Health 1:1003-1016.

Perry, K. M. (1955). Pulmonary disease in relation to metallic oxide. Lancet 2:463-468.

Pinto, S. S., and Nelson, K. W. (1976). Arsenic toxicology and industrial exposure. Annu. Rev. Pharmacol. Toxicol. 16:95-100.

Piotrowski, J. K., Trojanowska, B., Wisniewska-Knype, J. M., and Bolanorska, W. (1974). Mercury binding in the kidney and liver of rats repeatedly exposed to mercuric chloride: induction of metallothionein by mercury and cadmium. Toxicol. Appl. Pharmacol. 27:11-19.

Planteyd, H. T. (1968). Mesothelioma and asbestos bodies in sputum of workers in a shipyard. Poumon Coeur 24:545-548.

Pontefract, R. D., and Cunningham, H. M. (1973). Penetration of asbestos through the digestive tract of rats. Nature 243:352-353.

Pott, F., and Friedrichs, K. H. (1972). Tumoren der Ratte nach i.p.-Injektion faserförmiger Staube. Naturwissenschaften 59:318.

Pott, F., Huth, F., and Friedrichs, K. H. (1972). Tumoren der Ratte nach i.p. Injektion von gemahlenen Chrysotil und Benzo(a)pyren. Zentralbl. Bakteriol. [Segment 1, series B] 155:463-469.

Potts, C. L. (1965). Cadmium proteinuria—the health of battery workers exposed to cadmium oxide dust. Ann. Occup. Hyg. 8:55-61.

Powell, G. W., Miller, W. J., Morton, J. D., and Clifton, C. M. (1964). Influence of dietary cadmium level and supplemental zinc on cadmium toxicity in the bovine. J. Nutr. 84:205-214.

Probst, G. S., Bousquet, W. F., and Miya, T. S. (1975). Metallothionein: correlation of hepatic levels with acute cadmium toxicity in the mouse. The Pharmacologist 17:213.

Punsar, S. (1973). Cardiovascular mortality and quality of drinking water: an evaluation of the literature from an epidemiological point of view. Work Environ. Health 10: 107-125.

Pylev, L. N. (1974). Carcinogenic activity of serpentine asbestos after intrapleural administration in rats. Vopr. Onkol. 20:47-53.

Rajan, K. T., and Evans, P. H. (1973). Experimental methods—organ culture. In Biological Effects of Asbestos, P. Bogovski, J. C. Gilson, V. Timbrell, and J. C. Wagner (Eds.). IARC, Lyon, France, pp. 94-98.

Reeves, A. L. (1977). Beryllium in the environment. Clin. Toxicol. 10:37-48.

Reeves, A. L., and Krivanek, N. D. (1974). The influence of cutaneous hypersensitivity to beryllium on the development of experimental pulmonary berylliosis. Trans. NY Acad. Sci. Ser. II. 36:78-93.

Ribas, B., and Schmidt, W. (1973). Der Einfluss von Cadmium auf die Entwicklung von Hühnerembryos. Gegenbaurs Morphol. Jahrb. 119:358-366.

Roach, S. A. (1965). Measurement of airborne asbestos dust by instruments measuring different parameters. In Biological Effects of Asbestos, I. J. Selikoff and J. Churg (Eds.). Ann. NY Acad. Sci. 132:306-315.

Roe, F. J., and Lancaster, M. C. (1964). Natural, metallic and other substances as carcinogens. In Mechanisms of Carcinogenesis: Chemical, Physical and Viral, E. Boyland (Ed.). Br. Med. Bull. 19:127-133.

Rohl, A. N., Langer, A. M., and Selikoff, I. J. (1977). Environmental asbestos pollution related to the use of quarried serpentine rock. Science 196:1319-1322.

Rosenfeld, I., and Beath, O. A. (1964). Selenium—Geobotany, Biochemistry, Toxicity, Nutrition. Academic Press, New York.

Sabbioni, E., and Malafante, E. (1975). Heavy metals in rat liver cadmium binding protein. Environ. Physiol. Biochem. 5:132-141.

Sanders, C. L., Cannon, W. C., Powers, G. J., and Adee, R. R. (1974). Toxicology of Inhaled Low-Fired and High-Fired Beryllium Oxides in Rat and Hamster. Battelle NW Lab. Rep. No. 1818, Richland.

Sandstead, H. H., and Klevay, L. M. (1975). Cadmium-zinc interactions: implications for health. In Trace Element Geochemistry in Health and Disease, J. Freedman (Ed.). Geology Society of America, Boulder, Col., pp. 73-81.

Schepers, G. W. (1961). Neoplasia experimentally induced by beryllium compounds. Prog. Exp. Tumor Res. 2:203-244.

Schmähl, D., and Steinhoff, D. (1960). Versuche zur Krebserzeugung mit kolloidalen Silber- und Goldlösungen an Ratten. Z. Krebsforsch. 63:586-591.

Schroeder, H. A. (1960). Possible relationship between trace metals and chronic diseases. In Metal Binding in Medicine, M. J. Seven (Ed.). Lippincott, Philadelphia, pp. 59-67.

Schroeder, H. A. (1970). Chromium Air Quality. Monograph No. 70-15, American Petroleum Institute, Washington, D.C.

Schroeder, H. A., and Balassa, J. J. (1961). Abnormal trace metals in man: Cadmium. J. Chronic Dis. 14:236-258.

Schroeder, H. A., Vinton, W. H., and Balassa, J. J. (1963). Effect of chromium, cadmium and lead on the growth and survival of rats. J. Nutr. 80:48-54.

Schwarz, K., and Porter, L. A. (1972). Some regularities in the structure-function relationship of organoselenium compounds effective against dietary liver necrosis. Ann. NY Acad. Sci. 192:200-214.

Selikoff, I. J. (1976). Asbestos disease in the United States 1918-1975. Rev. Mal. Resp. 4 (Suppl. 1):7-24.

Selikoff, I. J., Bader, R. A., Bader, M. E., Churg, J., and Hammond, E. C. (1967). Editorial—asbestos and neoplasia. Am. J. Med. 42:487-496.

Selikoff, I. J., Churg, J., and Hammond, E. C. (1964). Asbestos exposure and neoplasia. JAMA 188:22-26.

Selikoff, I. J., and Hammond, C. E. (1975). Multiple risk factors in environmental cancer. In Persons at High Risk of Cancer—An Approach to Cancer Etiology and Control, J. F. Fraumeni (Ed.). Academic Press, New York, pp. 467-483.

Selikoff, I. J., Hammond, E. C., and Churg, J. (1968). Asbestos exposure, smoking and neoplasia. JAMA 204:106-112.

Selikoff, I. J., Hammond, E. C., and Churg, J. (1972a). Carcinogenicity of amosite asbestos. Arch. Environ. Health 25:183-186.

Selikoff, I. J., Nicholson, W. J., and Langer, A. M. (1972b). Asbestos air pollution. Arch. Environ. Health 25:1-13.

Shabad, L. M., Pylev, L. N., Krivosheeva, L. V., Kulagina, T. F., and Nemenko, B. A. (1974). Experimental studies on asbestos carcinogenicity. J. Natl. Cancer Inst. 52: 1175-1187.

Shapiro, J. R. (1972). Selenium and carcinogenesis: a review. Ann. NY Acad. Sci. 192: 215-219.

Shapley, D. (1977). Occupational cancer: government challenged in beryllium proceeding. Science 198:898-901.

Shettigara, P. T., and Morgan, R. W. (1975). Asbestos, smoking and laryngeal carcinoma. Arch. Environ. Health 30:517-519.

Shimkin, M. D., and Leiter, J. (1940/41). Induction of pulmonary tumors in mice. III. The role of chronic irritation in the production of pulmonary tumors in strain A mice. J. Natl. Cancer Inst. 1:241-254.

Shiraishi, Y., and Yoshida, T. H. (1972). Chromosomal abnormalities in cultured leucocyte cells from itai-itai disease patients. Proc. Jap. Acad. 48:248-251.

Sincock, A. M., and Seabright, M. (1975). Induction of chromosome changes in Chinese hamster cells by exposure to asbestos fibers. Nature 257:56-58.

Sirover, M. A., and Loeb, L. A. (1976). Infidelity of DNA synthesis in vitro: screening for potential metal mutagens or carcinogens. Science 194:1434-1436.

Six, K. M., and Gover, R. A. (1970). Enhancement of subclinical lead toxicity by low calcium diet. Fed. Proc. 29:568.

Skerfving, S., Hansson, K., Mangs, C., Lindsten, J., and Ryman, N. (1974). Methylmercury-induced chromosome damage in man. Environ. Res. 7:83-98.

Smith, W. E., Miller, L., Churg, J., and Selikoff, I. J. (1965a). Mesotheliomas in hamsters following intrapleural injection of asbestos. J. Mt. Sinai Hosp. 32:1-8.

Smith, W. E., Miller, L., Elsasser, R. E., and Hubert, D. D. (1965b). Test for carcinogenicity of asbestos. In Biological Effects of Asbestos, I. J. Selikoff and J. Churg (Eds.). Ann. NY Acad. Sci. 132:456-488.

Spencer, H. C., Hook, R. H., Blumenshine, J. A., McCollister, S. B., Sadek, S. E., and Jones, J. C. (1968). Toxicological studies on beryllium oxides and beryllium-containing exhaust products. Aerospace Med. Res. Lab. (AMRL-TR) 68-148:1-236.

Stadtman, T. C. (1974). Selenium biochemistry. Science 183:915-922.

Stanton, M. F. (1973). Some etiological considerations of fibre carcinogenesis. In Biological Effects of Asbestos, P. Bogovski, J. C. Gilson, V. Timbrell, and J. C. Wagner (Eds.). IARC, Lyon, France, pp. 289-294.

Stanton, M. F., Layard, M., Tegeris, A., Miller, E., May, M., and Kent, E. (1977). Carcinogenicity of fibrous glass: pleural response in the rat in relation to fiber dimension. J. Natl. Cancer Inst. 58:587-603.

Stanton, M. F., and Wrench, C. (1972). Mechanism of mesothelioma induction with asbestos and fibrous glass. J. Natl. Cancer Inst. 48:797-821.

Steffee, C. H., and Baetjer, A. M. (1965). Histopathologic effects of chromate chemicals. Report of studies in rabbits, guinea pigs, rats and mice. Arch. Environ. Health 11: 66-75.

Stell, P. M., and McGill, T. (1975). Exposure to asbestos and laryngeal carcinoma. J. Laryngol. Otol. 89:513-517.

Sterner, J. H., and Eisenbud, M. (1951). Epidemiology of beryllium intoxication. Arch. Ind. Hyg. Occup. Med. 4:123-151.

Stewart, M. J., and Haddow, A. C. (1929). Demonstration of the peculiar bodies of pulmonary asbestosis (asbestos bodies) in material obtained by lung puncture and in the sputum. J. Path. Bact. 32:172.

Stocks, P. (1960). On the relation between atmospheric pollution in urban and rural localities and mortality from cancer, bronchitis and pneumonia, with particular reference to 3,4-benzopyrene, beryllium, molybdenum, vanadium and arsenic. Br. J. Cancer 14:397-418.

Stoeckle, J. D., and Mancuso, T. (1974). Beryllium disease (meeting report). Science 183:449.

Stokinger, H. E. (Ed.) (1966). Beryllium: Its Industrial Hygiene Aspects. Academic Press, New York.

Stoner, G. D., Shimkin, M. B., Troxell, M. C., Thompson, T. L., and Terry, L. S. (1976). Test for carcinogenicity of metallic compounds by the pulmonary tumor response in strain A mice. Cancer Res. 36:1744-1747.

Stricks, W., and Kolthoff, I. M. (1953). Reactions between mercuric mercury and cysteine and glutathione. J. Am. Chem. Soc. 75:5673-5681.

Sullivan. (1969). Preliminary Air Pollution Survey of Chromium and its Compounds. A Literature Review. Natl. Air Pollution Administration, Raleigh, N.C., APTD 69-34.

Sunderman, F. W. (1971). Metal carcinogenesis in experimental animals. Food Cosmet. Toxicol. 9:105-120.

Sunderman, F. W. (1977). Metal Carcinogenesis. In Advances in Modern Toxicology, Vol. 2, Toxicology of Trace Elements, R. A. Goyer and M. A. Mehlman (Eds.). Hemisphere, Washington, D.C., pp. 257-295.

Sunderman, F. W., Kasprzak, K. S., Lau, T. J., Minghetti, P. P., Maenza, R. M., Becker, N., Onkelinx, C., and Goldblatt, P. J. (1976). Effects of manganese on carcinogenicity and metabolism of nickel subsulfide. Cancer Res. 36:1790-1800.

Sunderman, F. W., Lau, T. J., and Cralley, L. J. (1974). Inhibitory effect of manganese upon muscle tumorigenesis by nickel subsulfide. Cancer Res. 34:92-95.

Suzuki, Y., and Churg, J. (1969). Structure and development of the asbestos body. Am. J. Pathol. 55:79-107.

Syversen, T. L. (1975). Cadmium-binding in human liver and kidney. Arch. Environ. Health 30:158-161.

Tapp, E. (1969). Osteogenic sarcoma in rabbits following subperiostal implantation of beryllium. Arch. Pathol. 88:89-95.

Tello, E. E. (1963). Epitheliomas of arsenical origin. Rev. Fac. Cienc. Med. Cordoba 20:197-206.

Tepper, L. B. (1972a). Beryllium. CRC Crit. Rev. Toxicol. 1:235-256.

Tepper, L. B. (1972b). Beryllium. In Metallic Contaminants and Human Health, D. H. Lee (Ed.). Academic Press, New York, pp. 127-137.

Tepper, L. B., Hardy, H. L., and Chamberlin, R. I. (1961). Toxicity of Beryllium Compounds. Elsevier, Amsterdam.

Thomson, J. G., and Graves, W. M. (1966). Asbestos as an urban air contaminant. Arch. Pathol. 81:458-464.

Thomson, J. G., Kaschula, R. O., and MacDonald, R. R. (1963). Asbestos as a modern urban hazard. S. Afr. Med. J. 27:77-81.

Tietz, N. W., Hirsch, E. F., and Neyman, B. (1957). Spectrographic study of trace elements in cancerous and noncancerous human tissue. JAMA 65:2187-2192.

Tscherkes, A. A., Volgarev, M. N., and Aptekar, S. G. (1963). Selenium-caused tumours. Acta Un. Intern. Contra Cancrum 19:632-633.

Tseng, W. P., Chu, H. M., How, S. W., Fong, J. M., Lin, C. S., and Yeh, S. (1968). Prevalence of skin cancer in an endemic area of chronic arsenicism in Taiwan. J. Natl. Cancer Inst. 40:453-463.

Tsuchiya, K. (1969). Causation of ouch-ouch disease (itai-itai-byo). An introductory review. Keio J. Med. 18:181-211.

Tsuchiya, K. (1976a). Epidemiological studies on cadmium in the environment in Japan: etiology of itai-itai disease. Fed. Proc. 35:2412-2418.

Tsuchiya, K. (1976b). Proteinuria of cadmium workers. J. Occup. Med. 18:463-466.

Tsuchiya, K., Sugita, M., and Seki, Y. A. (1974). A mathematical approach to deriving biological half time of cadmium in some organs calculated from accumulation of metals in organs. In Proc. 17th Int. Cong. Occup. Health, Buenos Aires, Abstracts.

Tucker, A. (1972a). The Toxic Metals. Ballantine, New York, pp. 15-46.

Tucker, A. (1972b). The Toxic Metals. Ballantine, New York, pp. 174-207.

Tucker, A. (1972c). The Toxic Metals. Ballantine, New York, pp. 88-137.

Tucker, A. (1972d). The Toxic Metals. Ballantine, New York, pp. 162-163.

Tucker, A. (1972e). The Toxic Metals. Ballantine, New York, p. 163.

USSR Ministry of Health. (1969). Arsenic-lead synergism. Hyg. Sanit. 34:123 (transl. Gigiena i Sanitariia).

Vallee, B. L. (1973). Arsenic. Air Quality Monograph No. 73-18, American Petroleum Institute, Washington, D.C.

Vallee, B. L., Ulmer, D. D., and Wacker, W. E. (1960). Arsenic toxicology and biochemistry. Arch. Ind. Health 21:132-151.

Van Esch, G. J., and Kroes, R. (1969). The induction of renal tumours by feeding basic lead acetate to mice and hamsters. Br. J. Cancer 23:765-771.

Vorwald, A. J. (1950). The beryllium problem—experimental aspects: animal methods. In Pneumoconoisis—Leroy U. Gardner Memorial Volume, A. J. Vorwald (Ed.). Hoeber, New York, pp. 391-425.

Voss, H., and Tolki, V. (1960). On a vaccine granuloma in man, after approximately 1 year. Zentralbl. Bakteriol. 178:291-299.

Wagner, J. C. (1972). Current opinions on the asbestos cancer problem. Ann. Occup. Hyg. 15:61-64.

Wagner, J. C., and Berry, G. (1972). Considerations of aetiological mechanisms and other factors—information obtained from animal experiments. In Conf. on "Biological Effect of Asbestos," IARC, Lyon, Oct. 2-5. Paper No. 43, conf. preprint, p. 10.

Wagner, J. C., Berry, G., Skidmore, J. W., and Timbrell, V. (1974). The effects of the inhalation of asbestos in rats. Br. J. Cancer 29:252-269.

Wagner, J. C., Sleggs, C. A., and Marchand, P. (1960). Diffuse pleural mesothelioma and asbestos exposure in the Northwestern Cape province. Br. J. Ind. Med. 17:260-271.

Wagner, W. D., Groth, D. H., Holtz, J. L., Madden, G. E., and Stokinger, H. E. (1969). Comparative chronic inhalation toxicity of beryllium ores, bertrandite and beryl, with production of pulmonary tumors by beryl. Toxicol. Appl. Pharmacol. 15:10-29.

Waksman, B. H. (1959). The diagnosis of beryllium disease with special reference to the patch test. Arch. Ind. Health 19:154-156.

Waldron, H. A., and Stöfer, D. (1974). Sub-Clinical Lead Poisoning. Academic Press, New York.

Webb, M. (1972a). Binding of cadmium ions by rat liver and kidney. Biochem. Pharmacol. 21:2751-2765.

Webb, M. (1972b). Protection by zinc against cadmium toxicity. Biochem. Pharmacol. 21: 2767-2771.

Webb, M. (1975). Cadmium. Br. Med. Bull. 31:246-250.

Webb, M., and Daniel, M. (1975). Induced synthesis of metallothionein by pig kidney cells in vitro in response to cadmium. Chem. Biol. Interact. 10:269-276.

Weber, H. H., and Engelhard, W. E. (1933). Apparatus for producing low dust concentrations of high constancy and the microgalvimetric determination of dust. Dusts in the production of beryllium. Zentralbl. Gewerbehyg. 20:41-47.

West, P. W. (1967). Selenium-containing inorganics in paper may play cancer role. Chem. Eng. News 45:12.

Westlake, G. E., Spjut, H. J., and Smith, M. N. (1965). Penetration of colonic mucosa by asbestos particles. An electron microscopic study in rats fed asbestos dust. Lab. Invest. 14:2029-2033.

White, R. G., Coons, A. H., and Connolly, J. M. (1955). Studies on antibody production. III. The alum granuloma. J. Exp. Med. 102:73-82.

WHO (1972). Evaluation of certain food additives and the contaminants mercury, lead and cadmium. World Health Organization Technical Reports, Series 505.

Williams, D. R. (1972). Metals, ligands and cancer. Chem. Rev. 72:203-213.

Winnell, M. (1975). An international comparison of hygienic standards for chemicals in the work environment. Ambio 4:34-36.

Wong, P. T., Chan, Y. K., and Luxon, P. L. (1975). Methylation of lead in the environment. Nature 253:263-264.

Yeh, S. (1963). Relative incidence of skin cancer in Chinese in Taiwan: with special reference to arsenical cancer. Natl. Cancer Inst. Monogr. 10:81-107.

Yeh, S. (1973). Skin cancer in chronic arsenicalism. Hum. Pathol. 4:469-485.

Yoshiki, S., Yanagisawa, T., Kimura, M., Otaki, N., Suzuki, M., and Suda, T. (1975). Bone and kidney lesions in experimental cadmium intoxication. Arch. Environ. Health 30:559-562.

8

Nonnitrogenous Carcinogenic Industrial Chemicals

BERNARD M. GOLDSCHMIDT / New York University Medical Center, New York, New York

I. INTRODUCTION

In this chapter data on the carcinogenicity of nonnitrogenous industrial compounds are presented. The omission of nitrogenous compounds from this chapter has no relationship to their cancer-induction properties or their presence as environmental contaminants. The term "industrial compound" is used to denote a compound that is produced and used in industry. Although many of the compounds discussed in this chapter have limited production and uses, it is important to list such substances, since it is obvious that the future uses of specific organic compounds are not exactly predictable. Other listed compounds are not exclusively used in industry, but have agricultural, medicinal, and other nonindustrial uses. Thus, some compounds are discussed in this chapter, and closely related substances are examined in other chapters. In addition, substances that have been shown not to be carcinogenic by any criteria will be mentioned. The reason for including noncarcinogenic compounds is to emphasize the structural features of inactive compounds compared with the corresponding active compounds. Structural formulas of the compounds discussed are included for the same reason.

A reader who is seeking information pertaining to a particular compound should realize that the majority of chemical compounds have not been tested for carcinogenicity. If compounds have been tested and have shown no carcinogenic activity, they are probably not listed in this chapter. A complete listing of all substances tested for carcinogenicity and the results of such tests may be found in Natl. Cancer Inst. Monogr. 149. This monograph is a series of volumes published by the National Cancer Institute, which is periodically updated, and which describes how substances were tested for carcinogenic activity and the results of the tests. If a compound is not found in this chapter, it may still have some structural relationship to compounds discussed in this chapter. Thus, some idea of the carcinogenic potential of a compound, it is hoped, may be obtained by comparing its structure with those of the biologically active and inactive compounds described herein.

In the discussion of each compound, the reader finds experiments with animals used to determine the carcinogenicity of the substance in question. In a few cases, data with respect to human exposure are presented. This is detailed when such data are available. A brief description of the rationale for animal testing of industrial compounds for carcinogenicity is provided below.

Chemicals are tested for one or more of four types of carcinogenic potential: whole carcinogen, initiating agent, promoting agent, and cocarcinogen. A whole carcinogen may be defined as a substance which when given to an animal by itself once or repeatedly will ultimately lead to tumors (benign and/or malignant). When a chemical is said to cause cancer, the understood concept is that <u>one</u> substance induces tumors. However, it has long been noted that cancer is a complex disease and exposure to combinations of substances simultaneously or sequentially may lead to higher incidences of cancer than exposure to any one of the substances singularly. An initiating agent is a substance which when given to a test subject once at a certain dose level will not cause any tumors unless another agent, the promoting agent, is given subsequently. Thus, a promoting agent is a compound which will elicit tumors when given subsequent to an initiator. No tumors will be caused by promoting agents unless the animal had prior exposure to an initiating agent. A cocarcinogen is a substance which when given simultaneously with a carcinogen will exert a synergistic effect.

In the animal experiments described there are a number of substances used which have pronounced initiating or promoting or cocarcinogenic properties, but few of the other properties. These substances are used in conjunction with the substances to be tested. Carcinogenic aromatic hydrocarbons such as 7,12-dimethylbenz(a)anthracene and benzo(a)pyrene are given to animals at a low dose as initiating agents and are followed by repeated applications of various compounds such as hydrocarbons, petroleum fractions, esters, and so on, being tested as promoting agents. The animal groups receiving only the initiating agent or only the promoter are compared to the group of animals receiving both the initiator and the promoter.

Other widely used experimental substances are the phorbol ester promoters. These compounds, which are natural products found in a tropical plant, are used as tumor-promoting agents to test other substances for initiating ability. These natural products are diesters of the diterpene pentaol called phorbol. Phorbol myristate acetate is one such ester and is the most potent known tumor promoter. Earlier workers used mixtures of phorbol esters often containing other chemicals for tumor promotion studies. These mixtures were called croton oils or croton resins since they were extracts from the plant <u>Croton tiglium L</u>. Experiments are usually carried out by applying the compound whose carcinogenic initiating ability is being determined to mouse skin once or several times for a short span of the animal's lifetime. After a period of days to several weeks of treatment with the compound in question, repeated low doses of the phorbol ester promoting agent are applied for some months up to the lifetime of the animals. Tumor yields of the animals treated with the two agents are then compared with those of animals only initiated with the test compound or only promoted with the phorbol ester. Some initiation promotion assays have been carried out in which repeated sequential treatment of the phorbol esters and the substance being tested for carcinogenicity were applied to mouse skin.

Catechol, the most prevalent phenol in cigarette smoke condensate, has been found to be a good cocarcinogen. This was determined as follows: one group of animals repeatedly received a low dose of the carcinogenic aromatic hydrocarbon benzo(a)pyrene simultaneously with catechol, while another group of animals only received the carcinogenic aromatic hydrocarbon and another group only catechol. At the end of the experiment the benign and malignant tumors in the three groups were compared. Although catechol applied alone induced no tumors, the animals that received catechol with benzo(a)pyrene had far more tumors than the animals that received only benzo(a)pyrene. A number of other substances are known which in themselves may or may not be carcinogenic, but when given with another compound, are cocarcinogens—that is, they result in an increased tumor incidence compared with the same dose of either substance given alone to animals under the same conditions.

The literature reveals that chemicals are tested for carcinogenicity not only by a number of different protocols, as described above, but are given to the animals by a variety of routes. Substances are applied to mouse skin or injected subcutaneously (s.c.), intraperitoneally (i.p.), or intravenously (i.v.) to mice, rats, and other animals. Animals can receive chemicals by inhalation, intubation into the respiratory tract, mixed in their food or water, and by gavage. In addition to these routes, direct injections or implantation in specific organs, for example, breast, bladder, and so on, have been carried out. Why is there such a diversity of routes? One reason is that cancer occurs in a variety of organs and humans come in contact with carcinogens by a number of routes. In addition, scientists determining the carcinogenicity of a substance often have hypotheses in mind when they plan an experiment, and it is also for this reason that one encounters so many different protocols for testing substances for tumor-induction properties. To study the mode of action of carcinogens, different types of rodents are used in these experiments: fetuses, newborn, young, and mature animals of inbred, outbred, and crossbred strains. It is understandable why a substance like vinyl chloride, which is gas at room temperature and normal pressure, is tested for carcinogenicity by inhalation exposure. Some workers in the petroleum industry are known to have a high incidence of skin cancer, thus petroleum fractions are tested for carcinogenicity on mouse skin. Why are so many substances given s.c. and i.p.?: because these are convenient ways of introducing a high concentration of a test substance into an animal. Experience has shown that substances that can induce local sarcomas by the s.c. route or a high incidence of lung, kidney, or liver tumors by i.p. injection are likely to be carcinogens when tested by other routes. However, mouse skin, for good reason, is still the most-used target organ. Papillomas and squamous carcinomas of mouse skin are tumors originating from epithelial cells, and most human tumors are of epithelial cell origin, and some chemicals, for example, urethane and 1,2-dibromo-3-chloropropane, have been shown to cause internal tumors after skin application. There is some incidence of human skin cancer due to exposure to certain chemicals. From the experimentalists' point of view, mice are inexpensive, take up little space, are easy to handle, the test substances are easy to apply, and the skin is always observable! Hence for this combination of reasons there are so many mouse skin carcinogenesis experiments. Rat skin is generally not used because it is relatively resistant to cancer induction by chemicals.

The most difficult question to answer is how one can extrapolate animal data to human exposure. There is little problem when one discovers that an industrial chemical such as bis(chloromethyl) ether causes a high incidence of tumors in rodents by a variety of routes at relatively low doses. If there were no federal regulations with respect to this chemical (and there currently are) most individuals would conclude that the less exposure to bis(chloromethyl)ether the better, and best would be zero exposure. However, most of the substances which have been tested for carcinogenicity are not as potent as this ether, and approximately 80% of the known organic chemicals have never induced a tumor. What does one do in these cases? Ideally there should be zero exposure to foreign chemicals because deleterious effects of a given chemical may be discovered in the future. True, beneficial effects such as the cancer-inhibitory properties of certain antioxidants have been found.

However, one substance with one deleterious effect is all that is necessary to cause morbidity and mortality. Benzene is a good example of a dangerous weakly tumorigenic industrial compound; it induces a few skin tumors on mouse skin and appears to have a cocarcinogenic effect with a number of industrial compounds. More significantly benzene itself causes a high incidence of anemia and subsequently leukemia in humans exposed to it. Thus, one may conclude that the ideal goal should be zero exposure to foreign chemicals. However, in the real world one would have to settle for decisions on human exposure based on a risk-versus-benefits relationship.

II. ALIPHATIC HYDROCARBONS, ALKYL-AROMATICS, PETROLEUM FRACTIONS, AND CUTTING OILS

Octane

$H_3C(CH_2)_6CH_3$

Mice treated first with benzo(a)pyrene and then octane (100 mg, 3 times/week) on the skin did not have an accelerated rate of tumor formation (Horton et al., 1957).

Female Swiss mice receiving repeated doses of octane in cyclohexane after an initiating dose of 7,12-dimethylbenz(a)anthracene on the skin failed to develop tumors (Sicé, 1966).

Decane

$H_3C(CH_2)_8CH_3$

C3H mice, when first treated with benzo(a)pyrene and then with 50 mg of decane 3 times/week on the skin showed an average tumor-free life of about 17 weeks. Using the same protocol mice receiving 100 mg of octane had an average tumor-free life of 27 weeks (Horton et al. 1957). In another experiment male C3H/HeJ mice received repeated applications of decane (50 μl, 3 times/week) on their backs followed by irradiation with ultraviolet light at one of three wavelengths—254 nm, 290-320 nm, and >350 nm. The tumor incidence of animals treated with decane and light was greater at each wavelength than that obtained when the animals were treated with light alone. The shorter the wavelength of irradiation, the greater the number of tumors. Decane alone induced no tumors (Bingham and Nord, 1977).

In a skin cocarcinogenesis experiment, 50 female ICR/Ha Swiss mice received 25 mg of decane 3 times/week, while a second group received 2.5 μg of benzo(a)pyrene along with decane. In the group treated with the aromatic hydrocarbon alone 16 mice had a total of 26 papillomas and 12 squamous carcinomas after 1 year. In the group that received decane simultaneously with the aromatic hydrocarbon, 38 mice had a total of 73 papillomas and 34 squamous carcinomas (Van Duuren and Goldschmidt, 1976).

When female Swiss mice received an initiating dose of 7,12-dimethylbenz(a)anthracene on the skin, promotion with decane in cyclohexane for 60 weeks gave rise to two tumors in a colony of 30 mice (Sicé, 1966).

Undecane

$H_3C(CH_2)_9CH_3$

In one experiment 50 female ICR/Ha Swiss mice were treated with undecane, 25 mg, 3 times/week applied to the dorsal skin area for more than 1 year, and no skin tumors were observed. A comparable group of animals had the same treatment on the skin but concurrently received 5 μg of benzo(a)pyrene. Forty-four of these animals had 105 papillomas and 11 squamous carcinomas. In the control group, which received the aromatic hydrocarbon alone, 16 animals had 26 papillomas and 12 squamous carcinomas (Van Duuren and Goldschmidt, 1976).

Dodecane

$H_3C(CH_2)_{10}CH_3$

When dodecane was applied to the backs of male and female mice repeatedly, a few papillomas were observed (Saffiotti and Shubik, 1963). However, when tested as a promoting agent by repeated application started 1 week after mice were initiated with a 1% 7,12-dimethylbenz(a)anthracene in mineral oil solution, 12 mice of 30 bore 26 tumors (Saffiotti and Shubik, 1963). Similarly, when C3H mice were treated on the skin with benzo(a)pyrene followed by 50 mg of dodecane 3 times/week, the "average duration of tumor-free life" was considerably reduced (Horton et al., 1957). A later experiment using female Swiss mice confirmed the fact that after initiation with 7,12-dimethylbenz(a)anthracene, repeated applications of dodecane elicit a high tumor response (Sicé, 1966).

When tested for cocarcinogenicity with 0.14% benzo(a)pyrene in decalin, dodecane showed some activity (Horton et al., 1976). In another series of experiments male C3H/HeJ mice received (3 times/week) 50 µl of dodecane first followed immediately by irradiation with short-, medium-, or long-wavelength ultraviolet light. The highest tumor incidence, 49 benign and 12 malignant tumors in 24 mice, was observed at the medium wavelength (290-320 nm). In contrast, animals which were irradiated only had 10 benign and six malignant tumors. The cocarcinogenic effect of ultraviolet light and dodecane was also evident for long-wavelength (>350 nm) and short-wavelength (254 nm) irradiation (Bingham and Nord, 1977).

Tetradecane

$H_3C(CH_2)_{12}CH_3$

C3H/HeJ mice receiving 50 µl application of the compound alone 3 times/week on the dorsal skin developed no tumors. When the mice were irradiated after application of the chemical, few tumors above that inducible by the light itself appeared only at irradiation with short wavelength light. At the middle and longer wavelengths no cocarcinogenic effect was observed (Bingham and Nord, 1977). In another cocarcinogenic experiment, one group of 50 female ICR/Ha Swiss mice received 25 mg of tetradecane 3 times/week containing 5 µg benzo(a)pyrene on the dorsal skin, another group tetradecane alone, and a third group received the aromatic hydrocarbon alone. Tetradecane given by itself caused no tumors. Of 50 mice that received the aromatic hydrocarbon alone, 16 had 26 papillomas and 12 squamous carcinomas. The 50 mice that received tetradecane simultaneously with benzo(a)pyrene 32 had 58 papillomas and 19 squamous carcinomas (Van Duuren and Goldschmidt, 1976).

Tetradecane shows some potency as a tumor-promoting agent. Female Swiss mice which were treated with an initiating dose of 7,12-dimethylbenz(a)anthracene on the skin and then received applications 3 times/week of tetradecane in cyclohexane for 60 weeks developed five tumors in 30 animals (Sicé, 1966).

Hexadecane

$H_3C(CH_2)_{14}CH_3$

In a cocarcinogenesis experiment 25 mg aliquots of n-hexadecane were applied to the dorsal skin of female ICR/Ha mice either alone or with 5 µg of benzo(a)pyrene. The animals that received hexadecane alone had no tumors. Animals that received the hydrocarbon along with benzo(a)pyrene had fewer benign and malignant tumors than those that only received benzo(a)pyrene. Thus, hexadecane is a partial inhibitor of benzo(a)pyrene induced skin cancer. This is in contrast to the lower molecular weight hydrocarbons (e.g., tetradecane, undecane, and decane), which in the same set of experiments (already described) acted as cocarcinogens (Van Duuren and Goldschmidt, 1976). However, in an earlier experiment hexadecane applied with benzo(a)pyrene to C3H mice was reported to have tumor-accelerating properties (Horton et al., 1957). In a tumor-promotion experiment, female mice initiated with 7,12-dimethylbenz(a)anthracene followed by repeated treatment with hexadecane in cyclohexane developed one tumor among 50 initiated animals (Sicé, 1966).

Octadecane

$H_3C(CH_2)_{16}CH_3$

When tested as a cocarcinogen with benzo(a)pyrene on the skin of C3H male mice, octadecane showed some activity (Horton, et al., 1976). The compound was tested for tumor-promoting activity in mouse skin, using 0.4% 7,12-dimethylbenz(a)anthracene in decalin as the initiating dose. Octadecane was shown to be a tumor promoter since the number of malignant tumors increased as the concentration of the admixed decalin decreased and the octadecane concentration increased (Horton et al., 1976). In an earlier tumor-promotion experiment, octadecane showed weak promoting ability in female Swiss mice initiated with 7,12-dimethylbenz(a)anthracene (Sicé, 1966).

Eicosane

$H_3C(CH_2)_{18}CH_3$

When tested on mouse skin for cocarcinogenic activity with benzo(a)pyrene in decalin, eicosane was positive. It also showed promoting activity in mice initiated with 7,12-dimethylbenz(a)anthracene (Horton et al., 1976). An earlier investigator who applied the material in cyclohexane to female Swiss mice, after an initiating treatment of 7,12-dimethylbenz(a)anthracene, observed one tumor after 52 weeks in a group of 30 treated animals (Sicé, 1966).

Tetracosane and Octacosane

$H_3C(CH_2)_{22}CH_3$ and $H_3C(CH_2)_{26}CH_3$

Tests for tumor-promoting activity in mice initiated with 7,12-dimethylbenz(a)anthracene showed that tetracosane had marginal activity. The investigators suspected that traces of impurities may have inhibited its tumorigenic properties (Horton, et al., 1976). When tested as a tumor promoter in mice treated with 0.4% 7,12-dimethylbenz(a)anthracene in benzene, octacosane showed some activity (Horton et al., 1976).

Miscellaneous Saturated Aliphatic Hydrocarbons

Decahydronaphthalene (decalin) is not a tumor promoter, but 1-cyclohexyldecane, 7-cyclohexltridecane, and 7-n-hexyltridecane have tumor-promoting activity on the skin of C3H mice (Horton et al., 1957).

Hexadecene-1

$H_3C(CH_2)_{13}CH{=}CH_2$

Hexadecene-1 was reported to be a tumor promoter based on experiments in which C3H mice received a repeated dose of a carcinogenic aromatic hydrocarbon alone with hexadecene on skin (Horton et al., 1957).

Squalene

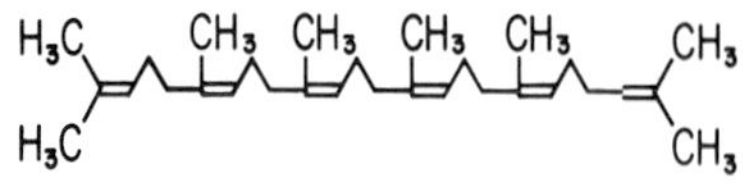

The natural product squalene was tested for tumor-promoting ability by topical application as a 20% solution in decalin to mice that had received an initiating treatment of 7,12-dimethylbenz(a)anthracene in benzene. This procedure caused two malignant tumors in 12 animals (Horton et al., 1976). Wnen applied to the dorsal skin of female ICR/Ha Swiss mice along with benzo(a)pyrene, it inhibited the tumorigenic properties of the aromatic hydrocarbon (Van Duuren and Goldschmidt, 1976). It had previously shown tumor-inhibition properties when mice initiated with 7,12-dimethylbenz(a)anthracene and then treated repeatedly with croton resin and squalene developed fewer tumors than mice that received the initiation treatment followed by croton resin alone (Shamberger, 1971).

Styrene

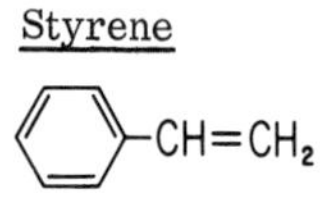

Styrene is prepared on a large scale throughout the industrial world since it is the monomeric unit used to synthesize polystryene plastics and resins. A report (Chem. Eng. News, 1978a) stated that 2-year inhalation studies of male and female rats at 0, 600, and 1000 ppm of styrene suggested that an increased incidence of lymphoid and hematopoietic tumors may be due to styrene exposure. Pregnant rats and rabbits exposed to 0, 300, and 600 ppm had a decreased weight gain. No teratogenic effect was seen.

Alkyl Benzenes and Alkyl Naphthalenes

A series of alkyl benzenes and alkyl naphthalenes were tested for tumor promotion on C3H mice, which were initially treated with 20-methylcholanthrene or benzo(a)pyrene (Horton et al., 1957). Sec-amylbenzene (2-phenylpentane) did not accelerate skin tumor formation of 20-methylcholanthrene-treated mice, whereas t-dodecylbenzene (2,4,6-trimethyl-2-phenylnonane, a compound formed by the alkylation of benzene with a tetramer of propylene) greatly enhanced tumor formation. For mice initiated with benzo(a)pyrene, t-dodecylbenzene was also shown to be a strong tumor promoter. Using the same experimental protocol, diisopropylbenzene, 85% 2-methylnaphthalene (15% benzene), and dinonylnaphthalene showed little if any tumor-promoting ability. 1,3,5-triisopropylbenzene, t-octyltoluene, 1-phenyldecane, 7-phenyltridecane, butyldimethylnaphthalene, 2-sec-amylnaphthalene, di-sec-amylnaphthalene showed varying degrees of tumor-promotion ability, 7-phenyltridecane being the most potent.

A long-term series of experiments involving cancer induction in rhesus monkeys (Macaca mulatta), galagos (Galago crassicaudatus), and pottos (Perodicticus potto) was carried out (Palotay et al., 1976). The animals received repeated doses of 7,12-dimethylbenz(a)anthracene on the dorsal skin followed by dodecylbenzene and sometimes irradiation with ultraviolet light. One group of each species was painted with the aromatic hydrocarbon followed by dodecylbenzene for 15 months and another group for 6.5 years. Ten years after the cutaneous applications were started the rhesus monkeys had dermal melanosis, papillomas, basal cell tumors, and mesodermal sarcomas. The galagos also had skin cancers. The pottos had no survivors because of a high early mortality. Unfortunately, there were no primate groups that received the 7,12-dimethylbenz(a)anthracene, dodecylbenzene or UV (ultraviolet) light only. Thus it is difficult to interpret the results with respect to which substance(s) caused skin cancer in these primates.

Petroleum Fractions

In a series of experiments by Horton et al. (1957) oil samples containing 0.16% benzo(a)pyrene were applied to the dorsal skin of C3H mice. A fraction boiling at 282-315°C of a previously cracked oil showed some acceleration of tumor formation, and two fractions boiling at 288-345°C and 345-365°C showed some promoting ability. An uncracked oil showed no tumor-promoting ability.

In an investigation by Saffiotti and Shubik (1963) male and female mice were treated once with 0.1% 7,12-dimethylbenz(a)anthracene in mineral oil and fractions of a catalytically cracked petroleum oil were applied to the skin 2 times/week. The highest fraction used boiled at 800-750°F and the lowest at 650-600°F. The tumor-promoting ability increased markedly with increasing boiling point. It was noted that the activity of the oils decreased with storage. The most active oils were tested alone (repeated applications) and produced tumors on rabbit flanks and ears. Similarly, fractions of a steam cracked oil, when applied to rabbit skin after initiation with 7,12-dimethylbenz(a)anthracene, yielded a remarkably increased tumor incidence and a shorter latent period compared with that in uninitiated animals treated with the same oils. Again, the highest boiling fractions were the most active in tumor promotion.

The recent Toxic Substances Control Act (Fed. Reg., 1978) requires chemical producers to report on the toxic properties of their products. A report from the Sun Petroleum Products Company (a division of the Sun Oil Company of Pennsylvania) to the EPA (Winch, 1978) described the results of a mouse skin painting experiment with seven of their oils. These oils caused a statistically significant increase in the incidence of benign and malignant tumors in CD_1 mice. Table 1 describes the oils tested, control groups used, and the tumor yields obtained in this study.

TABLE 1 Results of Skin Application of Petroleum Oils[a]

Oil description, viscosity	Percentage of males with skin tumors[b]	Percentage of females with skin tumors[b]
Heavy paraffinic distillate solvent extract, 160 SUS at 100°F	48	40
Heavy paraffinic distillate solvent extract, 470 SUS at 100°F	4	48
Heavy catalytic cracked distillate, 224 SUS at 100°F	80	80
Heavy naphthenic distillate, 115 SUS at 100°F	8	16
White mineral oil (control group, 150 mice)	1.3	0
Untreated mice (200 animals)	—	0.5

[a] 20 mg/application, 3 times/week for 18 months to test groups of 25 CD_1 mice.

[b] Benign and malignant tumors.

Cutting Oils

It is known that the oil used on spindles is responsible for the mule spinners' cancer of workers in the cotton industry. Early in this century it was observed that of 35 cases of carcinoma of the scrotum recorded at the Manchester Royal Infirmary, 27 were mule spinners (Southam and Wilson, 1922). Mule-spinning has virtually disappeared from the cotton industry, but the use of oils in other occupations is still widespread (Waterhouse, 1971).

It has also been known for some time that workers continuously exposed to cutting oil while working with manual and automatic machinery have a higher incidence of skin cancer than workers with no cutting oil exposure (Decoufle, 1976). An example of such an incidence is one where six histologically verified cases of squamous cell carcinoma occurred in one machine plant (Mastromatteo, 1955). The average period of exposure was 21 years, and the average age of tumor onset was 51. This plant had a calculated incidence rate for skin cancer of 87.5/100,000 which is well above any reported national incidence rate.

A more recent study of workers in a single U.S. plant who had at least 5 years exposure to cutting oil mists showed that for most cancer sites (including respiratory) there was no significant difference in the observed and expected deaths by all comparisons. However, a twofold greater risk of stomach and large intestine cancer was seen in workers who started being exposed to cutting oil mist more than 20 years ago (Decoufle, 1978).

A laboratory study using three strains of mice—C3H, C57BL, and a strain called Rockland Farm was carried out with oils (Gilman and Vesselinovitch, 1955). Used and unused oil and used and unused oil diluted in water emulsions (as utilized in industrial practice) were applied to the animals' skin for over 300 days. The responses varied, but a tumor incidence of 19-61% was found. Dilution increased the induction time for tumor formation.

III. ALCOHOLS, DIHYDROXYBENZENES, QUINONES, ACIDS, ANHYDRIDES, ESTERS, AND PEROXIDES

n-Propyl Alcohol

$CH_3CH_2CH_2OH$

n-Propyl alcohol (1-propanol) was given to male and female Wistar rats twice a week s.c. (0.06 ml/kg) or via stomach tube (0.3 ml/kg) for their lifetime. In 31 animals receiving the s.c. dose 15 malignant and 7 benign tumors were found, in contrast to the saline controls (25 animals) which had no malignant tumors and two benign tumors. The 18 animals receiving the oral dose of n-propyl alcohol had five malignant and 10 benign tumors. A control group (25 animals) had three benign and no malignant tumors (Gibel et al., 1975).

n-Propyl alcohol is used as a solvent for drugs and cosmetics and is found, for example, in hair, face, and shaving lotions. It is also used as a solvent for cellulose, paints, oils, and plastics. More than 134 million lb of n-propyl alcohol were produced in the United States in 1976. It is found in scotch, cognac, and bourbon at >10 mg/100 ml (Murphee et al., 1967).

Isobutyl Alcohol

$(H_3C)_2CHCH_2OH$

In a lifetime study of Wistar rats given isobutyl alcohol (2-methyl-1-propanol) s.c. or via stomach tube twice weekly, 12 tumors were found in 19 treated animals versus three tumors in 25 animals in the controls via the oral route. In the s.c. study 11 animals in a group of 24 had tumors, versus two in 25 animals in the controls (Gibel et al., 1975).

Large quantities of isobutyl alcohol are prepared for commercial use. It is used as a solvent in paints and lacquers and as an intermediate in the preparation of resins. In 1976 about 175 million lb were produced in the United States. Isobutyl alcohol has been found at >15 mg/100 ml in scotch, cognac, and bourbon (Murphee et al., 1967).

Isoamyl Alcohol

$(H_3C)_2CHCH_2CH_2OH$

Groups of Wistar rats received a biweekly oral dose (0.2 mg/kg) or s.c. injections (0.05 mg/kg) of isoamyl alcohol (3-methyl-1-butanol) for their lifetimes. The group that received the alcohol orally had seven tumors in 15 animals, versus the saline controls in which three out of 25 animals had tumors. Those animals that had injections of the alcohol s.c. had 15 tumors in 24 animals versus two tumors in 25 animals in the control group (Gibel et al., 1975).

Isoamyl alcohol is a common minor component of alcoholic beverages. Canadian whiskey was found to have 16 mg/100 ml of isoamyl alcohol; scotch, 26 mg/100 ml; cognac, 98 mg/100 ml; and bourbon 120 mg/100 ml (Murphee et al., 1967).

Hexanol, Octanol, and Decanol

$H_3C(CH_2)_4CH_2OH$, $H_3C(CH_2)_6CH_2OH$, and $H_3C(CH_2)_8CH_2OH$

Hexanol applied to the backs of female Swiss mice in tumor promotion tests after 7,12-dimethylbenz(a)anthracene initiation induced no tumors. When octanol was tested using the same protocol, one tumor developed after 24 weeks in 40 animals which progressed into a squamous cell carcinoma (Sicé, 1966). When decanol (20%) in cyclohexane was applied 3 times/week to a group of 30 female Swiss mice which had previously been initiated with 7,12-dimethylbenz(a)anthracene six tumors appeared, two of which developed into squamous carcinomas (Sicé, 1966).

Dodecanol

$CH_3(CH_2)_{10}CH_2OH$

When dodecanol (lauryl alcohol) was applied 3 times/week in cyclohexane to female Swiss mice previously initiated with 7,12-dimethylbenz(a)anthracene (Sicé, 1966), two papillomas in a group of 30 animals appeared. In a cocarcinogenesis experiment, when 10 mg of lauryl alcohol were applied simultaneously with 5 μg of benzo(a)pyrene, the number of tumors and cancers after 440 days was slightly greater than that in the animal group which had received the aromatic hydrocarbon alone (Van Duuren and Goldschmidt, 1976).

Tetradecanol, Hexadecanol, and Octadecanol

$H_3C(CH_2)_{12}CH_2OH$, $H_3C(CH_2)_{14}CH_2OH$, and $H_3C(CH_2)_{16}CH_2OH$

In a tumor-promotion experiment with 7,12-dimethylbenz(a)anthracene-initiated mice, tetradecanol caused two tumors in a group of 50 Swiss mice (Sicé, 1966). Hexadecanol produced one tumor in 40 animals after 53 weeks and octadecanol caused one tumor in 30 animals using the same protocol.

A number of research workers investigated the induction of bladder cancer in rodents by implanting pellets containing the potential carcinogen into the bladder. One of the goals was to find a suitable inert material which by itself would not yield tumors when implanted. Cholesterol by itself in Chester Beatty Research Institute stock mice induced up to 12% tumors (Boyland et al., 1964), and stearic acid induced about the same percentage of tumors in stock albino mice (Bonser et al., 1963). n-Octadecanol however, produced a 26% tumor incidence in Chester Beatty Research Institute stock mice (Boyland et al., 1964), while n-hexadecanol produced the same percentage of tumors in these mice as cholesterol.

Dihydroxybenzenes

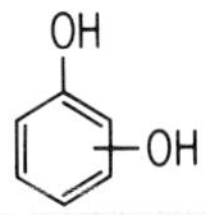

Catechol (pyrocatechol, 1,2-dihydroxybenzene, ortho-dihydroxybenzene) is an important commercial chemical. Worldwide use in 1973 was estimated to be 1.4-2.3 million kg. Its major use is in the preparation of 4-t-butylcatechol, a chemical that inhibits the polymerization of styrene. Catechol is also used in photographic developing agents, dyes, and metal plating. It and its esters are found in plants, and it is the most prevalent phenol in cigarette smoke condensate.

In female ICR/Ha Swiss mice, catechol showed potent cocarcinogenic properties. When 50 mice received 2.0 mg topical applications 3 times/week for 368 days, one animal developed a papilloma which became a carcinoma. Similar groups of animals received 5 μg benzo(a)pyrene or a mixture of 5 μg benzo(a)pyrene and 2.0 mg catechol. In the phenol plus hydrocarbon group, 36 animals had 90 papillomas and 31 carcinomas, while in the group treated with the hydrocarbon only, 14 animals had 16 papillomas and 10 carcinomas. When tested as a tumor promoter in ICR/Ha Swiss mice initiated with 150 μg of benzo(a)pyrene, catechol showed no activity, in contrast to phorbol myristate acetate, the positive control, which elicited 155 papillomas and 18 carcinomas in the 40 animals that were initiated with benzo(a)pyrene (Van Duuren et al., 1973; Van Duuren and Goldschmidt, 1976).

About 16 million kg of resorcinol (1,3-dihydroxybenzene, meta-dihydroxybenzene) were produced in the United States in 1974. It was estimated that 67% of this was used in rubber products, 20% in wood adhesives, and the rest in miscellaneous uses. Resorcinol-formaldehyde resins are added to rubber to improve its adhesive and physical properties.

Using the same protocol as in the cocarcinogenesis experiments already described (Van Duuren et al., 1973; Van Duuren and Goldschmidt, 1976), resorcinol, when applied to mouse skin, 10 mg, 3 times/week for 368 days, produced no tumors in a group of 50 mice. Resorcinol applied at this dose level with 5 μg of the carcinogen benzo(a)pyrene yielded fewer tumors than benzo(a)pyrene alone. Thus, in contrast to catechol, which is a good cocarcinogen for benzo(a)pyrene on mouse skin, resorcinol is a cocarcinogenic inhibitor for this aromatic hydrocarbon. When tested for promoting ability in ICR/Ha mice with benzo(a)pyrene as the initiator, resorcinol showed no activity. In another study (Stenbäck and Shubik, 1974) in which resorcinol solutions were applied to the backs of female Swiss mice, no more tumors were induced than in the solvent control group.

Hydroquinone (1,4-dihydroxybenzene, para-dihydroxybenzene) is used as a developer in black and white photography. It is also used as an antioxidant and polymerization inhibitor. In 1975 7.5 million kg were produced in the United States.

In a bladder-implantation experiment, 10-mg cholesterol pellets containing 20% hydroquinone were given to mice. After 25 weeks six of 19 mice had carcinomas. In the cholesterol control group, four adenomas or papillomas and five carcinomas were found after 25 weeks in the 77 mice receiving the implant (Boyland et al., 1964).

When tested as an initiating agent on mouse skin, one 0.3-ml application of a 6.7% solution in acetone followed by 18 weekly applications of croton oil on 22 mice, resulted in one papilloma (Roe and Salaman, 1955).

In our study hydroquinone also did not show any initiating properties (Van Duuren and Goldschmidt, 1976). Hydroquinone was also not a cocarcinogen when applied with benzo(a)pyrene to the backs of Swiss mice (Van Duuren and Goldschmidt, 1976). Hydroquinone, like resorcinol, inhibited the carcinogenicity of the aromatic hydrocarbon.

para-Quinone

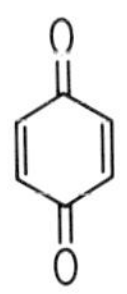

para-Quinone (benzoquinone) is found naturally in a variety of arthropods and has been used in the chemical industry since the nineteenth century. Its major present use is for the production of hydroquinone.

An early experiment by Takizawa (1940) involved topical application of 0.10 or 0.25% benzene solutions of para-quinone to mice. After more than 200 days, six of the 41 animals had papillomas, two had cancer, and 10 developed lung adenocarcinomas in the low-dose group. The higher dose group had a slightly lower incidence of the same malignancies. The benzene controls had one papilloma and two lung adenocarcinomas in 46 animals.

When 24 rats received s.c. injections of para-quinone in propylene glycol, the 17 survivors had received 81 mg of quinone and 16.5 ml of propylene glycol after 394 days. Two fibrosarcomas were found in this group (Umeda, 1957).

In an inhalation experiment, mice exposed to para-quinone vapor did not develop a statistically significant greater number of lung adenomas than the controls (Kishizawa, 1956).

Lauric Acid

$CH_3(CH_2)_{10}CO_2H$

Lauric acid is used in alkyl resins, wetting agents, soaps, detergents, and cosmetics.

Mice initiated with 7,12-dimethylbenz(a)anthracene and then painted with a 20% lauric acid (dodecanoic acid) solution in chloroform had a tumor incidence of 33% (30 tumors in 14 animals in a test group of 42) at the end of 31 weeks. The control group (i.e., animals receiving only the solvent or only lauric acid solution) had no tumors (Holsti, 1959).

Stearic Acid

$CH_3(CH_2)_{16}CO_2H$

Stearic acid is used mainly to prepare stearate esters. These are used in lubricants, soaps, pharmaceuticals, cosmetics, and as dispersing agents in shoe and metal polishes and in rubber compounds. Male and female white mice of a noninbred strain initiated on the dorsal skin with 7,12-dimethylbenz(a)anthracene and then treated repeatedly (6 times/week) for 31 weeks with a 20% stearic acid (octadecanoic acid) solution in chloroform had no tumors. This is in contrast to oleic and lauric acid, which were shown to be potent tumor promoters in mouse skin when the same protocol was used (Holsti, 1959).

When tested for cocarcinogenic activity in female Swiss mice with the aromatic hydrocarbon carcinogen benzo(a)pyrene the results were inconclusive. After 440 days animals that received a 3 times/week dose of 4 mg of stearic acid, along with 5 μg of the benzo(a)pyrene on the dorsal skin had more papillomas but fewer carcinomas than the group receiving only the benzo(a)pyrene. Animals treated with stearic acid alone had no tumors (Van Duuren and Goldschmidt, 1976).

Stearic Acid Derivatives

A rigorous study on the biological activity of stearic acid and derivatives of stearic acid was carried out by Swern et al. (1970). They tested these compounds for carcinogenicity by s.c. injections 3 times/week for 4 weeks in the inguinal area of female CFW (Swiss-Webster)

TABLE 2 Carcinogenicity of Stearic Acid Derivatives

Compound	No. of mice alive at 6 months	SC sarcomas	Pulmonary tumors	Breast cancer	Lymphomas	Other tumors
Stearic acid	83	4	3	0	1	1
4-Ketostearic acid	13	2	0	0	0	0
2-Hydroxystearic acid	14	0	2	0	0	0
12-Hydroxystearic acid	28	9	2	0	2	0
9 and 10-Monohydroxystearic acid	13	1	1	0	0	0
Methyl stearate	32	2	2	0	0	0
Methyl 12-hydroxystearate	27	8	2	1	0	0
Stearohydroxamic acid	14	3	5	0	2	0
γ-Stearolactone	117	15	11	0	0	3
cis-9, 10-Epoxystearic acid	70	6	5	1	1	4
trans-9, 10-Epoxystearic acid	14	1	0	0	0	0
Tricaprylin (solvent)	104	1	5	2	0	4
No treatment	202	1	11	14	4	2

and/or BALB/c (mammary tumor virus-free) mice. The results, adapted from the original report, are summarized in Table 2.

9,10-Epoxystearic acid and 9,10,12,13-diepoxystearic acid were tested earlier by Van Duuren et al. (1963) in male Swiss-Millerton mice. Skin application of a 10% acetone solution of each compound to 30 male Swiss-Millerton mice per group resulted in three papillomas after treatment with the monepoxide and four with the diepoxide.

As seen in Table 2, 12-hydroxystearic acid and its methyl ester induce a relatively high number of sarcomas. One investigation showed that the acid and its methyl ester disrupted oxidative phosphorylation in rat liver mitochondria, and it was suggested that this can lead to tumor formation (Hadler and Mueller, 1977).

Oleic Acid

$H_3C(CH_2)_7CH{=}CH(CH_2)_7CO_2H$

Oleic acid is found in vegetable oils and is used as a soap base and in the preparation of esters (oleates). These esters and oleic acid are used in ointments, cosmetics, polishing compounds, and lubricants.

Random-bred male and female white mice that had received an initiating dose of 7,12-dimethylbenz(a)anthracene on the dorsal skin were treated with repeated applications (6 times/week) of oleic acid (cis-9-octadecenoic acid) neat or with a 20% chloroform solution of this compound. Noninitiated animals that were treated with oleic acid for 31 weeks had no tumors. However, 61% of the animals which received the 20% solution had tumors at the end of 31 weeks (Holsti, 1959). Using the same protocol, palmitic acid (hexadecanoic acid) caused no tumors.

In contrast, when oleic acid was tested for cocarcinogenicity with benzo(a)pyrene on the skin of female Swiss mice, it completely inhibited the aromatic hydrocarbon carcinogenesis. The dose applied was high—25 mg 3 times/week—and the test was continued for 440 days (Van Duuren and Goldschmidt, 1976).

β-Bromopropionic Acid

$BrCH_2CH_2CO_2H$

Searle (1966) investigated the carcinogenicity of this compound and several other halogenated compounds, some of which are used in agriculture. Using male and female outbred stock albino mice they treated groups of 10 on the dorsal skin with a 2.5% acetone solution of β-bromopropionic acid 2 times/week for 12 weeks. For the following 20 weeks the animals were treated with croton oil. The number of tumors was reported at 10-week periods after the start of the croton oil treatment. For example, at the 20th week eight male mice had 69 tumors, while seven female mice had 16 tumors. The male mice were more susceptible than the female mice; however, even the less susceptible female mice had more tumors than the croton oil controls.

It is interesting to note that this compound could be metabolized or spontaneously cyclized to the more well-known carcinogen β-propiolactone. Acids with good leaving groups on the β- or γ-carbon are frequently used as precursors of the corresponding lactones in organic synthesis. A recent paper showed that repeated intraperitoneal injections of 3-chloropropionic acid (the chloro-analogue of 3-bromopropionic acid) in 0.9% sodium chloride solutions, led to a significant number of lung tumors in strain A mice. At the highest dose used, 12 injections each of 0.56 mmol/kg, resulted in an average of 0.90 tumors/mouse. At the lower doses used animal survival was better, but the tumor incidence was not significant (Theiss et al., 1979).

Cyclic Anhydrides

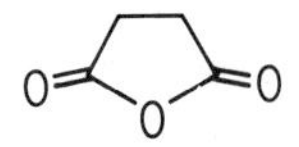

A number of saturated and unsaturated five-membered cyclic anhydrides were tested for carcinogenicity in male Wistar rats by repeated s.c. injections (Dickens and Jones, 1963, 1965). Maleic anhydride caused two local fibrosarcomas in three rats. The saturated analogue succinic anhydride caused three local sarcomas in three rats and α, β-dimethyl maleic anhydride caused three local sarcomas in five rats.

Linalyl Esters

```
                      OCOR
                      |
(H3C)2C=CHCH2CH  CCH=CH
                      |
                      CH3
```

The acetate, laurate, and oleate esters of linalol were tested for cocarcinogenicity. The esters were applied to the dorsal skin of groups of 20 female ICR/Ha Swiss mice, 10 mg, 3 times/week for 1 year. The applied acetone solution also contained 5 μg of benzo(a)pyrene. The acetate and oleate esters applied with the carcinogenic aromatic hydrocarbon caused more papillomas and carcinomas than the aromatic hydrocarbon applied alone: 10 (4), 11 (4), versus 8 (1), papillomas and (carcinomas) respectively, and hence can be classified as weak cocarcinogens. The animal group treated with linalyl laurate and benzo(a)pyrene had fewer tumors than the group receiving only benzo(a)pyrene, and hence, linalyl laurate may be considered a cocarcinogenic inhibitor. Another group of 20 animals was initiated with 7,12-dimethylbenz(a)anthracene and then received repeated skin applications of linalyl oleate. Only one papilloma developed among the 20 animals. From the data for these experiments, it was concluded that linalyl oleate was not a whole carcinogen or a tumor promoter (Van Duuren, et al., 1971a).

Glycidyl Esters

```
  O
 / \
CH2-CHCH2OCOR
```

The glycidyl esters of caproic, lauric, stearic, and oleic acid were tested for carcinogenicity by s.c. injections in albino rats. The compounds were dissolved in arachis oil, and injections were given to young animals. Sarcomas appeared after 1 or 2 years. The caproic acid ester gave seven tumors in 12 animals, the lauric acid ester six in 12, the stearic acid ester four in 12, and the oleic acid ester zero tumors in 12 animals (Walpole, 1958).

When glycidyl laurate, oleate, and stearate were given s.c. to female Swiss-Webster and BALB/c mice, the laurate ester led to 15 subcutaneous and seven pulmonary tumors in three test groups which started with 18 mice/group. The oleate ester was also active, for one group of 16 had five sarcomas, four pulmonary tumors, and one lymphoma. Glycidyl stearate by comparison would be regarded as inactive, as three groups of 16 mice, a total of 48 mice, had an incidence of three sarcomas, five pulmonary tumors, and one breast cancer. This represented a somewhat different distribution but a similar tumor incidence compared with various control groups (Swern et al., 1970).

Bornyl Esters

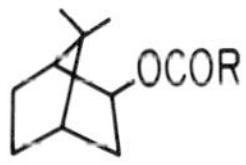

Three esters of the alcohol borneol (acetate, laurate, and oleate) were tested for cocarcinogenicity on mouse skin using groups of 25 female ICR/Ha mice. The esters were applied to mouse skin 3 times/week at a dose of 10 mg mixed with 5 μg of benzo(a)pyrene. After 460 days the animals that received the three bornyl esters and the aromatic hydrocarbons had about the same number of papillomas and fewer cancers as the animals that received the aromatic hydrocarbon alone. Bornyl oleate applied alone to the dorsal skin of animals of the same strain caused no tumors. However, animals initiated with 7,12-dimethylbenz(a)anthracene and then treated repeatedly with this ester had five papillomas out of 20 animals after 360 days of testing. A control group that received only the initiating dose of the hydrocarbon had no tumors (Van Duuren et al., 1971a).

Ethyl Bromoacetate

$BrCH_2CO_2CH_2CH_3$

Ethyl bromoacetate, a highly reactive α-bromoester, was tested for carcinogenicity by a number of routes. When tested as a whole carcinogen in female ICR/Ha Swiss mice by repeated skin application, it elicited no tumors. However, when tested as an initiating agent in female mice of the same strain with phorbol myristate acetate as the promoting agent, it yielded eight papillomas and one carcinoma in 30 mice. Given s.c. to 50 female mice of this strain it evoked nine local sarcomas. When administered i.p., ethyl bromoacetate gave no local sarcomas and no more lung tumors than the solvent control (Van Duuren et al., 1974).

t-Butyl Hydroperoxide

$(H_3C)_3CCOOH$

When tested as a whole carcinogen on the backs of female ddN mice, a 16.6% solution of t-butyl hydroperoxide in benzene applied 6 times/week for 450 days yielded no tumors. Female mice of the same strain treated with 4-nitroquinoline-1-oxide (20 treatments of 0.05 mg) followed by treatment with the hydroperoxide had four papillomas and nine malignant skin tumors in 38 mice (Hoshino et al., 1970). Using the same protocol, initiation with 4-nitroquinoline oxide and promotion with t-butanol yielded no tumors in 50 mice. An earlier study reported that mice (groups of 30) treated 3 times/week with a 3% benzene solution of t-butyl hydroperoxide for 522 days developed no tumors, although there was some skin damage (Van Duuren et al., 1967a).

The dialkyl peroxide di-t-butylperoxide is prepared in large quantities in this country. In 1976 2,600,000 lb of this compound were synthesized.

IV. PHOSPHATES, PHOSPHONATES, ALDEHYDES, AND KETONES

Trimethylphosphate

$(CH_3O)_3P=O$

Trimethylphosphate is used as a chemical intermediate, as a flame retardant in paints, and as an additive in gasoline.

Groups of 50 Fischer 344 rats and B6C3F1 mice of each sex were administered this compound in water 3 times/week by gavage at 50 or 100 mg/kg for the rats and 250 or 500 mg/kg for the mice (NCI, 1978e). After over 100 weeks female rats and male mice showed no effects. In the male rats fibromas of the subcutaneous tissue occurred 2/50, 9/49, and 0/20, tumors/animals on test in the low-dose, high-dose, and control groups, respectively. In the female mice the incidence of adenocarcinomas of the endometrium was 7/40, 13/37, and 0/16 in the low-dose, high-dose, and control groups, respectively.

Tris(2,3-Dibromopropyl)phosphate

$$\overset{O}{\overset{\|}{P}}(OCH_2CHBrCH_2Br)_3$$

Tris(2,3-dibromopropyl)phosphate (Tris) has been used to make children's sleepwear and other apparel more fire retardant. It has usually been applied to garments made of pure polyester or blends of polyester and acetate or triacetate. After application to fabrics, a certain low concentration of Tris is present as monomer. The assumption was made that a certain amount of skin absorption of Tris could take place and infant mouthing habits being what they are, the child's saliva could also extract the Tris. Weisburger (NCI, 1978c) carried out a study in which 50 and 100 ppm of Tris in the diet were fed daily to male and female Charles River rats and 500 and 1000 ppm to B6C3F1 mice. At the end of 2 years the animals were sacrificed. Male rats had a 45 and 52% incidence of kidney tumors at the low and high doses, respectively. Female rats were not as susceptible, since their tumor incidence was 7 and 18% at the low and high doses of Tris, respectively. None of the 108 control rats had kidney tumors. Mice fed Tris had an increased tumor incidence at multiple sites. Again, male mice were more susceptible than female mice to kidney tumor induction. However, female mice were more susceptible to liver tumor induction, and mice of both sexes had high incidences of squamous cell tumors of the stomach; females had a 29 and 45% incidence at the low and high doses, respectively, versus 4.0% in the controls, while males had 21 and 26% incidence, versus none in the controls.

In a study at our institute, we wished to determine whether Tris is carcinogenic on mouse skin. Groups of 30 female ICR/Ha Swiss Madison mice were given 10 mg or 30 mg applications of Tris in acetone on their shaven backs 3 times/week for more than 1 year. In the high-dose group, five animals had tumors and one a skin cancer. In both the high-dose and low-dose groups there was a high incidence of papillary lung tumors, in addition to papillomas and squamous carcinomas of the forestomach, that is, 13 and seven in the high-dose group and seven and three in the low-dose group, respectively. Since the animals could ingest the applied Tris by licking the skin, several animals actually developed tumors of the tongue and gums, a most unusual finding in any type of cancer bioassay. At present, it is not clear whether the exposure route for these internal tumors involved either or both ingestion and adsorption through the skin (Van Duuren et al., 1978).

Diethyl-β-γ-Epoxypropylphosphonate

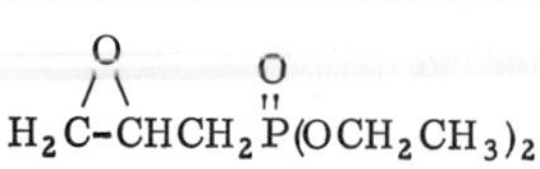

When tested as a whole carcinogen or initiating agent on the backs of female ICR/Ha Swiss mice, this epoxyphosphonate elicited no tumors. When given i.p. to mice, it induced two local sarcomas in 30 animals and more papillary lung tumors than the solvent or the no-treatment controls. Its sarcomengenic properties were noted again, since 30 animals that received 5.0 mg 3 times/week s.c. for 580 days had four sarcomas and two squamous cell carcinomas (Van Duuren et al., 1974).

Malonaldehyde

$OHCCH_2CHO$

Malonaldehyde is a reactive electrophile and is formed in animal tissues from peroxidative fat metabolism, especially in animals whose diet is deficient in antioxidants. Groups of 30 female Swiss mice were administered 12 or 0.36 mg of malonaldehyde on their shaven backs daily for 9 weeks and 36 weeks, respectively. The mortality in the high-dose group was severe, but a number of animals lived long enough to develop liver carcinomas. In another experiment animals of the same strain and sex received one skin application of 12 mg of the dialdehyde and after 3 weeks, treatments 5 times/week with 0.25 ml of 0.1% croton oil for 30 weeks. The skin tumors that developed were keratoacanthomas. The percentage of animals with tumors was less than the group initiated with 0.125 mg of 7,12-dimethylbenz(a)anthracene, the potent aromatic hydrocarbon carcinogen, but more than the groups initiated with 0.3 mg of β-propiolactone or 2.5 mg of glycidaldehyde, two direct-acting carcinogenic alkylating agents (Shamberger et al., 1974).

Some recent work by Hamburger and Goldstein (1978) suggests a possible molecular basis for malonaldehyde's biological activity. Incubation of calf-thymus DNA, calf-thymus histone, and malonaldehyde resulted in cross-linking of amino groups as evidenced by increased fluorescence and greater stability to deproteinization. In addition, incubation of Chinese hamster V79 cells in culture with malonaldehyde resulted in cell death, interference with growth and cessation of DNA synthesis.

Chloroacetone

$ClCH_2\overset{O}{\overset{\|}{C}}CH_3$

Searle (1966) determined the carcinogenicity of a number of chlorocompounds. Ten male and ten female outbred stock albino mice received a 0.3% acetone solution 2 times/week of chloroacetone (MgO stabilized) for 12 weeks. For the next 20 weeks the same animals were treated with croton oil. Chloroacetone caused tumors in both male and female mice. A plot of the average number of skin tumors/surviving mice showed that chloroacetone under these conditions is more carcinogenic than croton oil alone, but less carcinogenic than β-bromopropionic acid.

V. SATURATED HALOGENATED COMPOUNDS

Methyl Iodide

CH_3I

Methyl iodide was tested as a whole carcinogen by Druckrey and co-workers (1970a) in BD rats by s.c. injections at three dose levels: 10, 20, and 50 mg/kg body weight. The highest dose was given once, and the lower two doses were given weekly for 50 and 45 weeks, respectively. At the lowest dose nine out of 12 rats had local sarcomas and two other tumors, while the animals that received the middle dose had six sarcomas out of eight animals. The single treatment with the highest dose resulted in four sarcomas in 14 animals and two tumors in other organs.

In another experiment groups of 20 A/He mice received i.p. injections 3 times/week of methyl iodide in tricaprylin. Three dose levels were used, 8.5, 21.3, and 44.0 mg/kg body weight. After 6 months the animals were sacrificed, and the lung tumor incidence was found to be 0.21, 0.30, and 0.55 tumors/mouse going from the lowest to the highest dose, respectively. The no-treatment animals had 0.21 and the tricaprylin controls 0.22 tumors/mouse (Poirier et al., 1975).

Chloroform

$CHCl_3$

In 1976 approximately 291 million lb of chloroform were produced in the United States. Most of this, 230 million lb, was used to produce the refrigerant aerosol chlorodifluormethane. The remainder was used in pharmaceuticals, toiletries, as a laboratory and industrial solvent, and for some miscellaneous uses. That it is present throughout the environment is shown, for example, by the fact that when it was assayed in the air at Liverpool, England, and at sea, it was found at concentrations of 18 and 8 ng/m^3, respectively (Murray and Riley, 1973). Chloroform has been found in foodstuffs—cheshire cheese, butter, and tea—at concentrations of 33, 22, and 18 μg/kg, respectively (McConnell et al., 1975).

An oral feeding study of chloroform was conducted with Osborne-Mendel rats and B6C3F1 mice. This was one of a series of careful, thorough investigations of the carcinogenicity of various haloalkanes directed by Dr. E. Weisburger of the National Cancer Institute. The animals received the chloroform in corn oil 5 times/week for a period of 78 weeks. One group of rodents of each sex received the maximum tolerated dose and the other group approximately half that dose. For male and female rats the low-dose range was 90-120 mg/kg body weight, and the high-dose range was 180-200 mg/kg body weight. For male mice the low dose was 140 mg/kg body weight, and for female mice it was 240 mg/kg body weight. At the high dose 20% of the male rats and 2% of the female rats developed kidney tumors after these oral doses. In mice 63% of the males and 87% of the females developed hepatocellular carcinomas. The control animals that received the solvent only had a lower tumor incidence or no tumors in all cases (Powers and Voelker, 1976; Weisburger, 1977).

In an inhalation exposure experiment, pregnant Sprague-Dawley rats were exposed to chloroform at 300 ppm, 7 hr/day on days 6 through 15 of gestation. This caused a significant reduction in viable concepti, 15% versus 88% in the controls. The fetuses of rats exposed to 100 or 30 ppm of chloroform during gestation showed a significant number of abnormalities—absence of tails, imperforate anus, subcutaneous edema, delayed ossification of bones, and so on. It was concluded that chloroform has some maternal toxicity but greater embryo and fetotoxicity (Schwetz et al., 1974).

In a teratology study on rabbits, the dams were given two doses on day 6-15 of gestation. Among those animals given 100 mg/kg body weight, three out of five died of toxic hepatitis and nephrosis. The two surviving dams had four resorption sites and no viable concepti (Thompson et al., 1974).

A recent paper described in vitro experiments in which chloroform in the presence of microsomes, oxygen, and a NADPH-system-generated phosgene. The phosgene reacted with cysteine to yield 4-carboxythiazolidine-2-one. The in vivo generated phosgene is a likely candidate for the proximal carcinogen of chloroform (Mansuy et al., 1977).

Bromoform

$CHBr_3$

The induction of lung adenomas in strain A mice following multiple i.p. injections of bromoform, a drinking water contaminant, was investigated. Three dose levels—4, 48, and 100 mg/kg body weight per injection—were used with 20 animals/dose level. The injections were continued for almost 20 weeks. Twenty-four weeks after the first injection the animals were sacrificed, and 0.53, 1.13, and 0.67 lung tumors/mouse were found in the three different dose groups, respectively. The tricaprylin solvent control group had 0.27 lung tumors/mouse. It should be noted that in this same study several weak hepatocarcinogens, that is, chloroform and tetrachloroethylene, induced no more lung tumors than the solvent alone. Urethane was used as a positive control in these experiments. A single 1000 mg/kg body weight i.p. injection of urethane caused about 20 lung tumors/mouse (Theiss et al., 1977).

Iodoform

CHI_3

Using Osborne-Mendel rats and B6C3F1 mice of both sexes, iodoform was tested for carcinogenicity by oral intubation. The male and female mice that received 100 mg/kg body weight in corn oil 6 times/week for 78 weeks showed no notable difference in tumor incidence from the controls. In rats for which the high dose was 120 mg/kg body weight for the males and 60 mg/kg body weight for the females, the males had an elevated incidence of thyroid adenomas and carcinomas, while the females had more mammary fibromas or fibroadenomas and adenocarcinomas than the controls (Weisburger, 1977).

Carbon Tetrachloride

CCl_4

Over 428,000 tons of carbon tetrachloride were produced in the United States in 1976. Most of this was used to make the refrigerants dichlorodifluoromethane and trichlorofluoromethane. The remainder is mixed with other chemicals, used as a grain fumigant, used in industrial fire extinguishers, and used as a solvent and degreasing agent. Carbon tetrachloride is found in the atmosphere and in fresh and salt water. Photoreactions of chloroalkanes may account for its presence in the air (Lillian et al., 1975). In one survey it was found in 10% of 80 city drinking water supplies at low ppb levels (EPA, 1975).

Because of the enormous toxic hazard associated with carbon tetrachloride, the Food and Drug Administration (FDA) has placed a ban on its uses in the home. The human oral lethal dose is 5-10 ml. The threshold limit value is 10 ppm. Poisoning by carbon tetrachloride is enhanced by contemporaneous use of alcohol, poor nutrition, a calcium deficiency, and preexisting liver impairment (Gosselin et al., 1976). The principal toxic effects of carbon tetrachloride are central nervous system depression and necrosis of the liver and kidney. Three persons were reported to have developed aplastic anemia after chronic exposure to carbon tetrachloride (Straus, 1954). A case of a man is recorded who developed a primary hepatoma 7 years after he was hospitalized for an incidence of carbon tetrachloride poisoning (Tracey and Sherlock, 1968).

As of 1960 at least 13 studies confirmed the fact that repeated oral doses of carbon tetrachloride in mice leads to the formation of hepatomas (IARC, 1972). Rainbow trout and hamsters are also susceptible to liver cancer because of ingestion of carbon tetrachloride in contrast to dogs and rats, which are more resistant (IARC, 1972). In an inhalation study with albino rats a high incidence of liver nodules and early or established liver carcinomas was found (Costa et al., 1963). A variety of other studies—subcutaneous and intrarectal in mice and rats—established that carbon tetrachloride is a potent hepatocarcinogen. In fact, carbon tetrachloride is often used as a positive control in experiments in which the carcinogenicity of a substance is being determined by a feeding regimen (Weisburger, 1977). Evidence indicates that carbon tetrachloride is not a proximal carcinogen. Detoxification in the liver gives rise to reactive radicals which cause cellular destruction and probably initiate the neoplastic process (Gallagher, 1962).

1,1-Dichloroethane

Cl_2CHCH_3

1,1-Dichloroethane was tested for carcinogenicity by oral intubation in Osborne-Mendel rats and B6C3F1 mice of both sexes. Animals received a high and low dose in corn oil 5 times/week for 78 weeks. The compound was relatively nontoxic for a halogenated alkane, as the high dose for all rats was 900 mg/kg and 3600 mg/kg body weight for female mice and 3000 mg/kg body weight for male mice. The male rats showed no effects while the female rats had few additional tumors compared with the controls. The female mice showed little effect but the male mice had some liver hepatocellular carcinomas, eight tumors out of 47 animals and eight tumors out of 79 animals at the high and low dose, respectively, versus one tumor out of 19 animals in the controls (Weisburger, 1977).

1,2-Dichloroethane

$ClCH_2CH_2Cl$

Groups of 50 Osborne-Mendel rats and B6C3F1 mice of both sexes at two dose levels were used to determine the carcinogenicity of 1,2-dichloroethane by oral intubation. Animals received the compound in corn oil 5 times/week for 78 weeks. The male mice received 200 mg/kg body weight and the female mice 300 mg/kg body weight at the high-dose level. All groups except the low-dose male mice had an increased level of lung tumors. The male and female rats received 100 mg/kg body weight at the high-dose level. The male rats had an increased incidence of hemangiosarcomas and a few stomach cancers, while the female rats had hemangiosarcomas and mammary fibroadenomas (Weisburger, 1977).

In our study we tested 1,2-dichloroethane on mouse skin. Using 30 animals/group topical applications at two dose levels 3 times/week, 42 mg and 126 mg, for more than 1 year yielded no skin tumors. Nor was 1,2-dichloroethane active as an initiating agent with phorbol myristate acetate as the promoter (Van Duuren et al., 1979).

1,2-Dichloroethane is a weak mutagen when tested on *Salmonella typhimurium* TA 1535 (Brem et al., 1974). Its activity can be increased by the addition of postmitochondrial liver fraction (S-9). Glutathione, but not cysteine or mercaptoethanol, can further enhance its activation (Rannug et al., 1978).

1,1,2-Trichloroethane

Cl_2CHCH_2Cl

This compound was administered orally to Osborne-Mendel rats and B6C3F1 mice of both sexes. The compound was relatively toxic, and the high dose was 100 mg/kg body weight for all the animal groups. After oral intubation 5 times/week for 78 weeks, the mice showed a high incidence of liver cancer in the males, 18 tumors out of 79 animals at the low dose, and 37 tumors out of 50 animals at the high dose, versus two tumors out of 20 animals in the controls. The female mice had a comparable tumor incidence. The female rats had a high incidence of mammary tumors nine out of 50, 18 out of 50, and two out of 50 in the high-dose, low-dose, and solvent-control groups, respectively (Weisburger, 1977).

1,1,2,2-Tetrachloroethane

$Cl_2CHCHCl_2$

It is estimated that 40 million lb of 1,1,2,2-tetrachloroethane were produced in the United States in 1975. Most of this is used in the preparation of trichloroethylene and tetrachloroethylene.

Male and female Osborne-Mendel rats and B6C3F1 mice were used in a chronic oral feeding study to determine the carcinogenic potential of this halohydrocarbon. The compound was administered in 5% corn oil by gastric intubation 5 times/week for most of 78 weeks to groups of 50 animals at a high dose and to 50 animals at a low dose. The time-weighted average dosages were 108 and 62 mg/kg body weight/day for male rats, 76 and 43 mg/kg body weight/day for female rats and 282 and 142 mg/kg body weight/day for male and female mice. No statistically significant incidence of neoplastic lesions was observed in the male or female rats. In the mice, however, 1,1,2,2-tetrachloroethane was shown to be a liver cancinogen. In male mice 44 out of 49 animals with carcinomas were seen at the high dose, 13 out of 50 animals at the low, versus one animal out of 18 in the vehicle controls and two out of 16 animals in the no-treatment controls. The incidence of liver cancer in female mice was comparable to that of male mice (NCI, 1978a).

Hexachloroethane

Cl_3CCCl_3

Hexachloroethane was one of a series of halogenated compounds tested by oral intubation in Osborne-Mendel rats and B6C3F1 mice of both sexes. All the animals received a high dose of 300 mg/kg body weight 5 times/week for 78 weeks. Little effect was seen in the rats. The male and female mice showed an increased liver cancer incidence—29 out of 49 with cancer in the male, versus three out of 20 in the control male group, while 15 animals out of of 49 had cancer in the female test group, compared to two out of 20 in the corresponding control group (Weisburger, 1977).

1,2-Dibromoethane

$BrCH_2CH_2Br$

When tested for mutagenicity on various strains of Salmonella, 1,2-dibromoethane (ethylene dibromide) showed many more revertants than 1,1-dibromoethane or 1,1,2,2-tetrabromoethane (Olson et al., 1973).

When administered by intragastric tube 5 times/week to female and male Osborne-Mendel rats and B6C3F1 mice at a maximally tolerated dose, 40 mg/kg body weight for rats and 120 mg/kg body weight for mice, and at a lower dose level the rats had a >90% incidence of stomach squamous carcinoma after 62 weeks of treatments (Powers et al., 1975). The treated mice also developed stomach tumors (Weisburger, 1977) somewhat slower, but nonetheless, nearly all mice eventually developed stomach cancer with numerous metastases. In contrast, no control animals developed stomach cancer.

It was reported (Chem. Eng. News, 1978b) that a Dow Chemical Company study of its own employees working with 1,2-dibromoethane over the past 50 years revealed that out of 156 employees eight had tumors. This was the normal medical expectation. If they had used the EPA's projection from the rat-feeding data, there should have been 85 tumors.

In our study groups of 30 female ICR/Ha Swiss mice received skin applications of dibromoethane 3 times/week at three dose levels: 75, 50, and 25 mg/application. After more than 1 year of treatment no skin papillomas or cancers were evident. The alkyl halide also was not active as an initiating agent when the mice were promoted with phorbol myristate acetate (Van Duuren et al., 1979).

Groups of 16 pregnant Charles River CD rats and 20 CD-1 mice inhaled dibromoethane at 20, 38, and 80 ppm for 23 hr/day for a total of 10 days starting on day 6 of gestation. Adverse effects on maternal welfare were noted which probably caused some of the morphological changes noted in the fetuses. It was concluded that dibromoethane is not a teratogen in these rats or mice (Short et al., 1978).

Interestingly, although this substance is a reactive electrophilic alkylating agent, in rodent liver and stomach, covalent binding with endogenous protein is mostly—and binding with exogenous DNA is entirely—dependent on metabolism by the cellular microsomes (Banerjee and Van Duuren, 1978). A potential metabolite of dibromethane, bromoethanol, was recently shown to induce lung tumors in strain A mice. Groups of 20 animals received 24 weekly intraperitoneal injections. The lowest dose group received 1.2 mmol/kg total dose and had the highest tumor incidence, 0.79 tumors/mouse, while the 2.4 and 4.8 mmol/kg dosed groups had 0.55 and 0.42 tumors/mouse, respectively (Theiss et al., 1979).

1, 2-Dibromo-3-Chloropropane

$BrCH_2BrCHCH_2Cl$

This polyhaloalkane is widely used as a soil fumigant and nematocide. According to the U.S. Department of Agriculture 1.6 million kg were used on crops on U.S. farms in 1971.

When given to male and female C57BLxC3H-F mice and Osborne-Mendel rats in corn oil by intragastric feeding 5 times/week, 1, 2-dibromo-3-chloropropane gave rise to stomach tumors with numerous metastases in both sexes and species (Olson and co-workers, 1973; Powers and co-workers, 1975; Weisburger, 1977).

Although the overall dosage that the animals received was large, animal survival was good in spite of the toxic nephropathy caused by the haloalkane. What was most striking was the near 100% incidence of squamous cell carcinoma of the stomach in the treated animals and the total absence of this tumor in the control animals.

In our study groups of 30 female ICR/Ha Swiss mice received topical applications of 35 mg or 12 mg of 1, 2-dibromo-3-chloropropane 3 times/week in acetone. At the end of 1 year no papillomas or carcinomas were present on the treated dorsal skin area; however, a significant number of papillary lung tumors, papillary hyperplasia and papillomas of the forestomach, and squamous carcinomas of the forestomach were found (Van Duuren et al., 1979).

During the summer of 1977 it was discovered that workers with repeated exposure to 1, 2-dibromo-3-chloropropane had reduced sperm counts or none at all (Chem. Eng. News, 1977). An earlier study indicated that a variety of laboratory animals exposed to 1, 2-dibromo-3-chloropropane vapor experienced atrophy and degeneration of the testes (Torkelson et al., 1961).

Benzyl Chloride

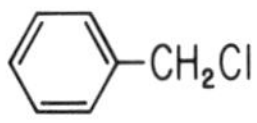

According to the U.S. Tariff Commission report of 1974, 36 million kg of benzyl chloride were produced in the United States in 1972. Most of this was used to synthesize butyl benzoyl phthalate, a vinyl resin plasticizer.

When tested in animals, benzyl chloride showed carcinogenic potential. Druckrey et al. (1970a) and Preussmann (1968) tested it in BD rats. Given at 40 mg/kg body weight s.c. weekly, three of 14 animals developed local sarcomas. At 80 mg/kg body weight, six of eight animals developed sarcomas.

Using strain A mice of both sexes, i.p. injections at three dose levels (total doses of 0.6, 1.5, and 2 g/kg body weight) led to a lung tumor incidence comparable to that of the untreated controls (Poirier et al., 1975).

VI. UNSATURATED HALOGENATED COMPOUNDS AND NITRILES

Vinyl Chloride

$H_2C{=}CHCl$

Vinyl chloride is the monomer used to prepare the polymer polyvinyl chloride and a copolymer of Saran and other plastics. The monomer and polymer are typical of many such substances which were developed in the last 30-40 years by industrial countries. The halogenated substances are inexpensive to make and chemically relatively inert. The assumption was that their "unreactivity" would render them nonharmful to humans. Now we know that via metabolic activation many so-called unreactive chemical substances can become toxins, teratogens, mutagens, and carcinogens. For example, a recent report (Capurro and Eldridge, 1978) described an unusually high incidence of malignant lymphomas and pancreatic cancer among a small population living near a chemical recycling plant. A variety of chemicals had been detected in the atmosphere near the plant, including aromatic hydrocarbons and chlorinated aliphatic hydrocarbons. Vinyl chloride and polyvinyl chloride are still major industrial chemicals. In the United States over 2,800,000 tons of vinyl chloride were produced in 1976.

It is now known that vinyl chloride is able to cause cancer. It has been established for a long time that vinyl chloride is responsible for a variety of ailments incurred by workers producing and polymerizing it. Vinyl chloride affected the nervous system (dizziness, headache, paresthesia of the limbs), the digestive system (anorexia and pain in the hypochondrium), the liver and spleen, respiratory system, and skeletal system (Lilis et al., 1975).

In 1971 it was reported that Wistar rats exposed for 4 hr/day, 5 days/week for 1 year to 30,000 ppm of vinyl chloride developed tumors of the skin and lungs in almost all the surviving animals (Viola et al., 1971). At this level of exposure (30,000 ppm = 3% vol/vol) a meaningful extrapolation to the industrial worker's exposure was questionable.

A more extensive study of the effects of vinyl chloride on rats was undertaken by Maltoni and Lefemine (1974). Animals were exposed to vinyl chloride at a variety of concentrations. Sprague-Dawley rats after 131 weeks of exposure for 4 hr/day, 5 days/week, had a tumor incidence of 39% at 10,000 ppm, 29% at 6000-2500 ppm, 24% at 500 ppm, and 16% at 250 ppm. At 50 ppm no tumors were found. The tumors were predominantly zymbal gland carcinomas, nephroblastomas, and liver angiosarcomas. Swiss mice were exposed to the same range of concentrations of vinyl chloride as the rats. After 61 weeks 36, 39, 31, 42, and 38% neoplasms were found in the 10,000, 6000, 2500, 500, and 250 ppm exposure groups, respectively. At 50 ppm a 16% incidence of tumors was found, compared with 5% in the treatment group. Not unexpectedly more pulmonary and mammary tumors were seen in the mice, but a few liver angiosarcomas were also found. Another species of animal, the golden hamster, was also found to be susceptible to tumor induction by vinyl chloride vapor (Maltoni, 1975). Differences in strain susceptibility to vinyl chloride were noted in a recent paper by Maltoni (1977). Sprague-Dawley rats incurred far more zymbal gland carcinomas than Wistar rats when exposed to vinyl chloride under identical conditions. It was also noted that younger Sprague-Dawley rats, 1 day old, incurred far more angiosarcomas and hepatomas when exposed to vinyl chloride than rats which were older, 13 weeks, at the start of the treatment.

The molecular mechanism of tumor induction by vinyl chloride probably involves the metabolic activation of the haloalkene followed by a reaction of the electrophiles formed with cellular targets. Recent investigations by Hathway (1977), Henschler (1977) and Bolt and Filser (1977) present chemical data to support this view.

Creech and Johnson (1974), the plant physician and Director of Environmental Health, respectively, of the B. F. Goodrich Chemical Company, published a special communication that stated that three employees of a plant manufacturing polyvinyl chloride and copolymers died of angiosarcomas of the liver. A further search indicated that 5 years earlier another worker may have died from the same disease. Since this is a rare tumor and all three persons worked in the same plant and had a similar type of chemical exposure, the conclusion (Viola's work from 1971 was already known) was evident: vinyl chloride causes human angiosarcomas.

A careful epidemiological study was carried out at a plant in western New York State, where vinyl chloride was concerted to polyvinyl chloride. The workers were classified in production (which included operating the reactor to make polyvinyl chloride, cleaning it, and bagging the product), maintenance, shipping, and laboratory. Only workers with a minimum of 5 years of exposure were considered at risk in the study. Age-adjusted cancer deaths expected, 3.9, were compared to the found, 90, three of which were hemangiosarcomas, all among the production workers (Nicholson et al., 1975).

Another study (Heath et al., 1975), which was described at the N.Y. Academy of Sciences meeting on the hazards of vinyl chloride and polyvinyl chloride, summarized the reported human angiosarcoma deaths among vinyl chloride workers in the United States until 1975. Thirteen cases were reported. The mean age at time of diagnosis was 40.2 years, and the mean time of exposure to vinyl chloride was 18.0 years. Since vinyl chloride is produced throughout the world, its toxic and carcinogenic effects will be worldwide. A paper at the N.Y. Academy meeting also described angiosarcoma of the liver in two Swedish vinyl chloride/polyvinyl chloride workers (Byrén and Holmberg, 1975). Finally, a recent case described a 22-year-old man, a nonsmoker and nondrinker, who developed a squamous cell carcinoma of the buccal mucosa. This unusual tumor was explained by the fact that for the past 14 years this patient had chewed plastic materials containing polyvinyl chloride (Casterline et al., 1977).

A more recent report from Canada confirms the earlier epidemiology studies. Ten cases of angiosarcoma of the liver have been diagnosed in Shawinigan Quebec since 1955. All have occurred in men who worked in a vinyl chloride polymerization plant. Cigarettes and alcohol do not seem to be related to tumor incidence (Delorne and Thériault, 1978).

Vinyl Bromide

$H_2C{=}CHBr$

Vinyl bromide in trioctanoin (250 mg/0.5 ml) was fed once a week to 20 male Sprague-Dawley rats. After 600 days no tumors had occurred. Tested on the skin with female ICR/Ha Swiss mice as a whole carcinogen or as an initiating agent, after 419 days no tumors were observed. When tested subcutaneously in the same mice, it induced no local tumors (Van Duuren, 1977). The same research group tested polyvinyl bromide suspensions. When given orally to rats or placed on mouse skin, no tumors resulted. When this aqueous suspension of polyvinyl bromide was given subcutaneously to mice, a high incidence, 19 animals out of 30, of local sarcomas with lipid elements was observed. This was interpreted as tumor induction due to the polymer's physical rather than chemical properties.

Vinylidene Chloride

$H_2C{=}CCl_2$

Vinylidene chloride (1,1-dichloroethylene; 1,1-dichloroethene) is used primarily for the copolymerization of other monomers, such as acrylonitrile, vinyl chloride, etc. The products are referred to as "Saran" and are mainly used for food wraps.

Albino Weston rats exposed to vinylidene chloride at 200 ppm (after 6 months lowered to 100 ppm) for 4 hr/day, 5 days/week after about 2 years had a number of abdominal tumors which did not differ significantly from those of the control animals. Similarly, Sprague-Dawley rats of both sexes exposed to vinylidene chloride at 75 or 100 ppm did not have a tumor incidence greater than the untreated control animals (Viola and Caputo, 1977).

An experiment with Swiss mice of both sexes showed that vinylidene chloride is a carcinogen. The animals were exposed to 25 ppm of vinylidene chloride 4 hr/day, 4-5 days/week for 1 year. After 98 weeks 16% (24 of 150) of the male mice had adenocarcinomas of the kidney. Only one female mouse in 150 had this tumor, and no kidney adenocarcinomas were found in the control animals (Maltoni, 1977). A partial explanation for the higher biological activity of vinylidene chloride in the mouse versus the rat was recently presented (Jones and Hathway, 1978). These investigators found that a greater proportion of an oral dose of radiolabeled vinylidene chloride was metabolized by mice compared to rats. This is consistent with the higher level of cytochrome P-450 activity in mice compared to rats.

Trichloroethylene

$Cl_2C{=}CHCl$

In 1976 over 315 million lb of trichloroethylene were produced in the United States. It has been estimated that about 283,000 U.S. workers are exposed to trichloroethylene (Lloyd et al., 1975). Trichloroethylene's major use is as a degreasing agent. It has been used in dry cleaning, in the preparation of inks and paints, and as an anesthetic. It has also been used in decaffeinating coffee, preparing coffee extract, and in spice oleoresins. Maximum tolerated levels of 2.5, 10, and 30 ppm for these respective food substances have been established by the FDA. Trichloroethylene has been reported to be present in municipal water supplies and in the air over Liverpool, England, at 850 ng/m^3 and in the atmosphere over the ocean at 7 ng/m^3 (Dowty et al., 1975).

Trichloroethylene was tested at two dose levels in both male and female Osborne-Mendel rats and B6C3F1 mice.

Animals received the compound 5 times/week for 78 weeks by oral gavage. For rats the low dose was 549 mg/kg body weight, and the high dose was 1097 mg/kg body weight. For mice the doses were 1169 and 2339 mg/kg body weight for the males and 869 and 1739 mg/kg body weight for females. The treated mice had a high incidence of primary malignant tumors of the liver, that is, hepatocellular carcinoma. The males were more susceptible than the females, since 31 out of 48 male compared to 11 out of 47 female mice developed tumors at the high dose. Osborne-Mendel rats were less sensitive to tumor induction by trichloroethylene since only about 5% developed hepatocellular carcinomas (Weisburger, 1977).

This difference in sex and species susceptibility may be explained as follows. Work in our laboratory showed that trichloroethylene is probably not a proximal carcinogen; it must be metabolically transformed into a carcinogen. The enzyme system that carries out this transformation is more active in the male than the female mouse and in B6C3F1 mice compared to Osborne-Mendel rats (Van Duuren, Banerjee, 1976; Banerjee et al., 1977; Banerjee and Van Duuren, 1978).

Tetrachloroethylene

$Cl_2C{=}CCl_2$

Nearly 670 million lb of tetrachloroethylene (perchloroethylene) were produced in the United States in 1976. It was one of a series of compounds tested by oral intubation for carcinogenicity in Osborne-Mendel rats and B6C3F1 mice of both sexes. The high and low time-weighted average dosages given were 941 and 471 mg/kg body weight/day for male rats, 949 and 474 mg/kg body weight/day for female rats, 1072 and 536 mg/kg body weight/day for male mice, and 772 and 386 mg/kg body weight/day for the female mice (NCI, Report #13, 1977). Fifty animals per group received the compound 5 times/week for about 1-1/2 years. The rats did not show any increased incidence of neoplastic lesions after this treatment, but both sexes of mice had a higher liver cancer incidence. At the high dose 27 out of 47 males and 19 out of 48 females developed tumors compared to two out of 20 and zero out of 20 animals in the vehicle control groups (Weisburger, 1977).

When we tested tetrachloroethylene for skin carcinogenicity in mice, groups of 30 female ICR/Ha mice which received 18 mg or 54 mg 3 times/week for more than 1 year developed no tumors. When tested for initiating ability in the same strain of mouse, one 163-mg dose followed by treatment 3 times/week with 5 μg of phorbol myristate acetate resulted in two mice out of 30 with three papillomas (Van Duuren et al., 1979).

When tested by i.p. injection in strain A mice for the production of lung adenomas, tetrachloroethylene was negative (Theiss et al., 1977).

1-Chloropropene

$CHCl{=}CHCH_3$

We decided to determine the carcinogenicity of the simplest homologue of vinyl chloride, 1-chloropropene. Repeated skin application (3 times/week) of 2.5 mg of the alkene or a single initiator treatment with the same dose followed by promotion with phorbol myristate acetate on the backs of groups of 30 female ICR/Ha Swiss mice failed to yield a significant number of tumors. However, weekly intragastric feeding (1.0 mg) to the same sex and strain of mice led to a statistically significant number of forestomach papillomas (13/30) with three carcinomas ($P < 0.0005$). Interestingly, the male mice were not as susceptible to 1-chloropropene, as only four forestomach papillomas and one carcinoma formed in 30 animals. Subcutaneous weekly injections of the alkene (1 mg) in 30 female ICR/Ha Swiss mice led to only one local sarcoma (Van Duuren et al., 1979). Although the parent alkene failed to react with guanine, two potential metabolites, 1-chloro-1,2-epoxypropane and 2-chloropropanal, did. They yielded a unique substituted eneamine by reacting with the 2-amino of guanine (Goldschmidt et al., 1979).

trans-1,4-Dichlorobutene-2

$ClCH_2CH=CHCH_2Cl$

trans-1,4-Dichlorobutene-2 is used in the chemical industry as a monomer in the manufacture of copolymers and as an intermediate for various syntheses (Suermondt, 1961), such as that of hexamethylenediamine and chloroprene. We tested this haloalkene for carcinogenicity in female ICR/Ha Swiss mice by skin application of 1.0 mg/0.1 ml of cyclohexane 3 times/week for 537 days. No papillomas or carcinomas appeared. Similarly, when tested as an initiating agent in the same strain and sex of mice with phorbol myristate acetate as the promoter, no tumors occurred among the 30 animals so treated. When given s.c. to these Swiss mice, at 0.05 mg/0.05 ml of tricaprylin weekly for 537 days, three of the 30 animals developed local sarcomas and no vehicle control animals developed sarcomas. Given i.p. at the same dose, also weekly, two of 30 animals developed local sarcomas (Van Duuren et al., 1975). We concluded that trans-1,4-dichlorobutene is a weak carcinogen. Because of its industrial use the E. I. duPont de Nemours & Company initiated a long-term inhalation study in rats. A preliminary report of this study submitted by C. F. Reinhardt, M.D. to the EPA showed that at 5.0 ppm, but not at 0.5 ppm, 1,4-dichlorobutene-2 causes a statistically significant incidence of malignant nasal tumors in rats after 11 months of exposure.

Chloroprene

$CH_2=CClCH=CH_2$

Chloroprene is the principal monomer used to make synthetic rubber. The total production of polychloroprene rubber in the United States was estimated to be over 362 million lb in 1976.

Two publications by Khachatryan (1972a, 1972b) from the Soviet Union showed a hazard for chemical workers utilizing this intermediate. One study showed an increased incidence of skin cancer among chloroprene workers, and the other study showed a higher incidence of lung cancer among chloroprene workers.

In the skin cancer study (Khachatryan, 1972a) 24,989 persons over 25 years of age were examined, and 137 cases of primary skin cancer were found. Five groups of workers were compared:

1. Those who never worked in industry
2. Those with extensive industrial experience
3. Those whose only work was the production of chloroprene
4. Those who worked with chloroprene derivatives
5. Those who worked with chemicals unrelated to chloroprene

The greatest frequency of skin cancer was among group 3 (3%), among workers in the chloroprene plants. This cancer incidence was 25-fold more than that of group 1. Group 4 had a tumor incidence 13.3% greater than the control groups 1 and 2. Group 5, chemical workers not producing chloroprene, had a skin cancer incidence 5.5-fold greater than the control groups.

There were also differences in the site of chloroprene-induced skin cancer compared to other chemically induced skin cancers. The latter cancers occurred predominantly at the face, neck, hands, and sites of skin birth defects, while a high percentage of the chloroprene-exposed workers' skin cancers occurred at the nose and ears. Both groups had a high incidence of prior dystrophic or inflammatory skin conditions (eczema, cracks, dyskeratoses).

The second study of Khachatryan (1972b) compared the incidence of primary lung cancer among four populations, (1) a group with prolonged contact with chloroprene and its derivatives; (2) a group with prolonged contact with other chemicals (gasoline, lacquer, acetone, benzene, and acids); (3) workers in nonchemical industry; and (4) workers in nonindustrial occupations.

The following data were compiled in this study:

Group	Number of Workers	Number of Cancers	%
1	2934	34	1.15
2	4780	22	0.46
3	6045	11	0.18
4	6220	4	0.064

These data substantiate that chloroprene is an etiological factor in human lung cancer and that other chemicals also can enhance human lung cancer incidence. It is of interest to note that Khachatryan's study pointed out that 76% of the lung cancer patients previously had chronic bronchitis and that 66% were long-term heavy smokers. Epidemiological studies on asbestos by Selikoff (1968) and Berry (1972) and their co-workers, also clearly show a greater enhanced risk of respiratory cancer among workers who smoke and are exposed to asbestos, compared to those who are just exposed to asbestos.

Hexachlorobutadiene

$Cl_2C{=}CClCCl{=}CCl_2$

Hexachlorobutadiene (1,1,2,3,4,4-hexachloro-1,3-butadiene) is used as a solvent in industry and as a component of agricultural insecticides and nematocides. A Russian report (Krasnyak et al., 1969) stated that vineyard workers exposed to hexachlorobutadiene and polychlorobutane-80 suffered from increased hypertension, myocardial dystrophy, respiratory diseases, diseases of the nervous system, and hepatic disturbances.

Studies with Alderley Park specific-pathogen-free rats indicated that exposure to hexachlorobutandiene vapor leads to kidney damage (Gage, 1970) and a rat-feeding experiment showed that after 6 months the animals had pronounced morphological changes in the liver, kidneys, and myocardium (Murzakaev, 1967).

In a recently reported study by Kociba and co-workers (1977) male and female Sprague-Dawley rats received hexachlorobutadiene at one of three dose levels: 20 mg, 2.0 mg, or 0.2 mg/kg/day in corn oil by oral gavage for their lifetimes. At the highest dose multiple toxicologic effects were observed: increased mortality of male rats, and for both male and female rats decreased body weight gain, increased urinary excretion of coroprophyrin, and increased terminal weights of the kidneys. Most significantly, approximately 23% of the males and 25% of the females at the 20-mg dose had renal tubular neoplasms. These were renal tubular adenomas or adenocarcinomas, some of which metastasized to the lungs. At the 2.0-mg dose increased hyperplasia of the renal tubular epithelium was noted, but no neoplasms related to hexachlorobutadiene treatment were observed. At the 0.2-mg dose, no discernible ill effects were noted.

ortho- and para-Dichlorobenzene

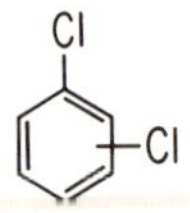

The estimated U.S. production of ortho-dichlorobenzene (1,2-dichlorobenzene) was 32-41 million kg in 1973. Most of this was used to synthesize pesticides. The rest was used in a variety of ways, for example, as a solvent in toluene diisocyanate production, as a component of rustproofing mixtures, in the manufacturing of dyes, and so on. A comparable amount of para-dichlorobenzene is synthesized in the United States. Its major uses are as a space-odorant and for the control of moths.

One early laboratory study sought to determine the carcinogenicity of para-dichlorobenzene (Parsons, 1942). One irradiated mouse that had received one i.p. injection of 0.2 ml of a 0.2% para-dichlorobenzene solution became ill and was sacrificed. It was found to have sarcomatous growth throughout the peritoneum. Upon grafting this growth tissue it yielded tumors. Of 10 nonirradiated mice receiving nine s.c. injections each of 0.2 ml of 2% para-dichlorobenzene in sesame oil, four died within 30 days and one developed a sarcoma with secondary tumor growths.

A number of cases of human exposure to ortho- and para-dichlorobenzene and resulting disease and death have been reported. Hallowell (1959) reported on the case of a 3-year-old child who ingested para-dichlorobenzene mothballs, which resulted in acute haemolytic anaemia. Other cases of serious blood disorders due to exposure of dichlorobenzenes were reported (Girard et al., 1969). These investigators reported two cases of chronic lymphoid leukemia, two cases of acute myeloblastic leukemia, and one case of myeloproliferative syndrome.

Hexachlorobenzene

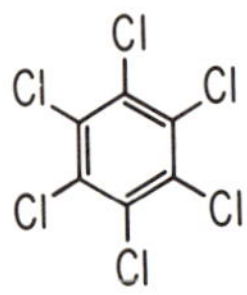

Hexachlorobenzene (HCB) (which should not be confused with the insecticide hexachlorocyclohexane) is used as a fungicide, for producing fire-resistant materials and as a copolymer. In Turkey hexachlorobenzene-treated wheat, which was intended for planting but was then used to prepare food (Cam and Nigogosyan, 1963), caused a severe outbreak of porphyria cutanea tarda symptomatica (Schmid, 1960). In adults this condition begins with bullous lesions which progress to ulceration and heal, leaving pigmented scars. The skin is sensitive to light and mechanical trauma. Hexachlorobenzene is carcinogenic in hamsters (Cabral et al., 1977). Groups of 30-60 animals of both sexes were fed 50, 100, or 200 ppm hexachlorobenzene ad libitum in their regular diet. Overall 10% of control animals had tumors, while 92% of the animals fed 200 ppm hexachlorobenzene had tumors. The treated animals had a significant increase in hepatomas, haemangioendotheliomas, and thyroid adenomas.

In a laboratory experiment designed to determine if the human incidence of porphyria in Turkey is due to hexachlorobenzene, male adult Sprague-Dawley rats were fed diets containing 0.2% hexachlorobenzene. Like the exposed humans, the rats excreted high levels of porphyrins and porphyrin precursors (Ockner and Schmid, 1961). More than one-third of the treated animals (13 of 33) died of neurological complications within the first month. Humans who have ingested hexachlorobenzene also have the porphyrins in the urine, but do not have any neurological complications. The surviving animals had profound disturbances in porphyrin metabolism even after hexachlorobenzene was removed from the diet. In addition to hematological disorders, the surviving rats showed hapatocellular degeneration.

At 100 ppm hexachlorobenzene was found to be mutagenic in <u>Saccharomyces cerevisiae</u> (Guerzoni et al., 1976), but it was shown to be inactive in the Ames test on <u>S. typhimurium</u> (Van Dijek and Van de Voorde, 1976), and failed to induce a significant number of lung adenomas in strain A mice which received weekly i.p. injections for 6 months (Theiss et al., 1977). When given to five adult female rhesus monkeys at daily doses of 128-8.0 mg/kg for 60 days, thymic cortical atrophy occurred, degenerative ovarian changes were noted along with degenerative changes in the liver and kidneys, but no cutaneous or neurological changes were noted (Iatropoulos, 1978).

Polychlorinated Biphenyls

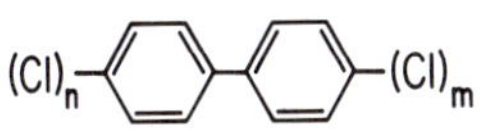

Polychlorinated biphenyls (PCBs) are commercially available as a mixture of chlorinated biphenyls, sometimes containing chlorinated terphenyls (Hutzinger et al., 1974). The composition of a particular commercial batch of PCBs generally consists of a fixed elemental percentage of chlorine and contains certain isomers, for example, five tetrachlorobiphenyls, five pentachlorobiphenyls, totaling 90% of the mixture, with the remainder consisting of trichlorobiphenyls, hexachlorobiphenyls, and so on. The PCBs have a high thermal stability, are resistant to oxidation, and have excellent dielectric properties. Thus, they have been used as fluids in capacitors and transformers, in hydraulic systems, as plasticizers, and in a variety of heat transfer applications.

The PCBs have been dispersed throughout the global ecosystem. Due to their high lipid solubility and resistance to biochemical degradation, they are found in shellfish, fish, animals, and humans (Hammond, 1972). Whether their toxic properties are due to individual chlorinated biphenyls, metabolites of the chlorinated biphenyls such as chlorinated biphenols, chlorodibenzofurans, or chlorodioxane impurities is not known. In Japan an accidental mass poisoning of people who ate a rice oil contaminated with PCBs took place. Neurological disorders persisted years after ingestion of the PCBs.

In a laboratory experiment, Kanechlor-400, a commercial PCB mixture which has six components, five of which were identified as 2,4,3',4'-; 2,5,3',4'-; 2,3,4,4'-; and 3,4,3',4'-tetrachlorobiphenyls and 2,3,4,3',4'-pentachlorobiphenyl, was fed to male and female rats of the Donryu strain. The PCBs were dissolved in olive oil and the oil added to the dry diet (Kimura and Baba, 1973). Unadulterated olive oil was added to the dry diet of the control animals. The total amount of Kanechlor-400 ingested varied from 450 to 1800 mg over a test period of 159 to 560 days. Ten males and 10 females received the PCBs, and five animals of each sex served as controls. All of the rats that ingested more than 700 mg of PCBs showed hypertrophy of the liver. Females ingesting more than 1200 mg of PCBs had nodules on the surface and on the cut surface of the liver, whereas male rats did not have these preneoplastic nodules. It was concluded that PCBs induce a benign neoplastic change, but not malignancy.

A National Cancer Institute study (NCI, 1978b) of Aroclor 1254, a PCB mixture, was carried out with PCBs added to the diet of Fischer rats at doses of 25, 50, and 100 ppm. Although there was a high incidence of hepatocellular proliferative lesions in both male and female treated rats, animals given the medium- and high-dose levels had lower mean body weights, and the male rats showed a decrease in survival time. However, there was not sufficient evidence to implicate Aroclor 1254 as a carcinogen.

There have been at least two studies which show that although PCBs may or may not cause liver tumors in certain strains of rodents when fed at relatively high doses, their real threat to humans may be their cocarcinogenic or tumor-promoting properties. In a paper by Ito and co-workers (1973) the promoting effect of PCBs on the carcinogenicity of benzene hexachloride is described. For example, 26 dd male mice on a diet of 250 ppm of β-benzene hexachloride for 24 weeks incurred no liver tumors, but when a comparable group of 29 mice was fed a PCB mixture in addition to the benzene hexachloride, a 21% incidence of hepatocellular carcinomas occurred. Another experiment (Kimura et al., 1976) showed that PCBs administered after an azo dye caused hepatic tumors. Here seven of 11 female Donryu strain rats had hepatocarcinomas after first receiving 3'-methyl-dimethylaminoazobenzene orally and then had oral feedings with a PCB mixture. In contrast, administration of the PCBs before or together with the azo dye did not induce hepatic tumors.

It is known that PCBs resemble phenobarbital in their effects on the liver, for example, feeding PCBs induces certain detoxifying enzymes in the liver (Litterst and co-workers, 1972; Chen and DuBois, 1973; and Makiura and co-workers, 1974). It has been shown (Makiura and co-workers, 1974) that like phenobarbital, PCB can exert a protective effect against known liver carcinogens such as N-2-fluorenylacetamide and diethylnitrosoamine, probably via their enzyme-induction properties. Thus the PCBs may inhibit certain potential carcinogens in humans, but on the other hand, they may enhance the carcinogenic potential of other agents.

Acrylonitrile

$H_2C{=}CHCN$

Acrylonitrile is the monomeric intermediate used to produce acrylic fibers, synthetic plastics, and rubbers. In 1976 1.5 billion lb were used in the United States. A number of processes have been used to produce the monomer, but the most widely used process currently is the reaction of propylene with ammonia and oxygen.

In May 1977 E. E. duPont de Nemours & Company informed NIOSH of results of a preliminary epidemiological study of its acrylonitrile plants, which revealed that of 470 males who began work during the years 1950-1955, 16 cases of cancer had occurred within this group by 1975. One-half of these had died. Based on national morbidity rates, 6.9 cancers would have been expected. The workers exposed to acrylonitrile, unlike the vinyl chloride workers, did not have cancer predominantly at one specific site. There were six lung cancers, three colon cancers, and one cancer at each of seven other primary sites. Due to the results of this study, the company reduced the threshold exposure limit from 20 ppm (OSHA required) to 2 ppm.

A recent report by the Dow Chemical Company (NIOSH, 1977) described laboratory studies in which acrylonitrile was incorporated into the drinking water of laboratory rats at 35,100 and 300 ppm. After some time toxic symptoms were noted in all of the animals. After 1 year one of 20 rats at 100 ppm, and 12 of 20 rats at 300 ppm exposure had stomach papillomas. Central nervous system tumors were found at all three dose levels—two, six, and three tumors per group of 20 animals, respectively. At the two higher doses two zymbal gland tumors were also found. The controls had no such tumors.

The same laboratory also carried out an inhalation study. Rats were exposed to 20 and 80 ppm acrylonitrile for 6 hr/day, 5 days/week. At the end of 1 year central nervous system tumors, ear canal tumors, and mammary region masses were observed in the high-dose group. Mammary masses were also observed at the lower dose.

VII. ALKYLATING AGENTS

Haloethers

Chloromethyl Methyl Ether

$ClCH_2OCH_3$

Chloromethyl methyl ether (CMME) like bis(chloromethyl)ether (BCME) is mainly used as an intermediate in the production of ion-exchange resins. It is prepared by the reaction of methyl alcohol with formaldehyde and hydrogen chloride.

Its biological activity is related to that of BCME because of their chemical interrelationship. Upon hydrolysis (reaction with water) CMME yields its starting components, methyl alcohol, formaldehyde, and hydrogen chloride.

$$H_3COCH_2Cl + H_2O \rightarrow H_3COH + HCOH + HCl$$

BCME upon hydrolysis also yields its starting components, formaldehyde and hydrogen chloride.

$$ClCH_2OCH_2Cl + H_2O \rightarrow 2HCOH + 2HCl$$

In the case of CMME the hydrolysis products ordinarily are not capable of reforming the starting material. This is not so for BCME, in which depending on the phase (vapor or solution) and the concentration of the ether, some starting material may be reformed from the hydrolysis products formaldehyde and hydrochloric acid (Kallos and Solomon, 1973; Gorrie et al., 1973; Frankel et al., 1974). The relevance of this to the biological activity of CMME is that upon hydrolysis CMME produces formaldehyde and hydrogen chloride, which can recombine to yield BCME. Thus, although the animal studies of CMME described below show that CMME is generally a less potent carcinogen than BCME, the fact is that CMME may in situ generate BCME. In addition, BCME is nearly always an impurity (1-7%) in commercial CMME.

In our studies a 2% solution of CMME in benzene applied 3 times/week for the lifetime of the animals to the shaven dorsal skin of female Swiss mice caused no tumors. However, in another study we showed that CMME can initiate cancer. ICR/Ha female Swiss mice treated once with CMME in benzene and then thrice weekly with the natural product tumor promoter, phorbol myristate acetate, developed papillomas, some of which progressed to carcinomas (Van Duuren et al., 1968; Van Duuren et al., 1969a).

Mice exposed to CMME vapor (6 mg/m^3) for 6 hr/day, 5 days/week for a total of 21 weeks had a higher incidence of lung adenomas (1.5/animal) than the controls (0.9/animal) (Leong et al., 1971). Similarly, newborn mice injected with CMME in a solvent after 6 months had a higher incidence of pulmonary tumors than the animals injected only with the solvent (Gargus et al., 1969).

In an inhalation study with male Sprague-Dawley rats and Syrian golden hamsters, animals were exposed to 1.0 ppm CMME for much of their lifetimes. There was nearly twice as much bronchial hyperplasia in the exposed rats as in the controls. Hamsters showed few differences between exposed and control groups (Laskin et al., 1975; Drew et al., 1975).

The first published report of human lung cancer due to CMME exposure was by Figueroa et al. (1973). They described their preliminary epidemiological investigation of a Rohm & Haas chemical plant located in Bridesburg, Pa. This report listed 12 cases of oat cell carcinoma among workers exposed to CMME for 3-14 years. Most of the workers were nonsmokers. The age at diagnosis was between 33 and 55 years, and nine out of 12 workers were under 50. All these men died within 20 months of diagnosis. The results with respect to the frequency of occurrence, type of tumor, and the age of diagnosis (cancer due to cigarette smoking occurs much more commonly in the sixth and seventh decade of life) lead to the definitive conclusion that CMME (and/or BCME) is a human carcinogen (Nelson, 1973). A full account of chemical workers exposure to these haloethers is vividly described in a book by Randall and Solomon (1975). Since these discoveries, the Rohm & Haas Chemical Company and other producers and users of BCME and CMME have made some effort to minimize the exposure of their workers to these haloethers.

A large-scale epidemiological study of workers exposed to CMME and BCME was published by Albert and co-workers (1975); Pasternack and co-workers (1977). They studied the medical records of about 1800 workers who were exposed to CMME in the period 1948-1972. The control group consisted of about 8000 workers who worked in chemical plants but were not exposed to CMME. Using social security records, they were able to find deceased workers and subsequently obtained copies of their death certificates. The study showed that there is a much higher risk of respiratory cancer among the CMME-exposed workers, which increases with duration and intensity of exposure. The respiratory cancers that did occur had an early age of onset, 77% before age 55. Another epidemiological study of lung cancer related to chloromethyl methyl ether exposure was carried on by Weiss and Boucot (1975) and Weiss (1976). Here the lung cancer victims generally smoked less than their cohorts. A possible explanation for this was the fact that chloromethyl methyl ether is also a bronchial irritant, and thus workers exposed to it may have stopped smoking or smoked less.

Finally, the data in the Soviet Union study show that chemical workers, as a group (see the section on chloroprene)—group 2—have a higher lung cancer incidence than other workers in nonindustrial occupations (group 4). An epidemiological study of bis(chloromethyl)ether and chloromethyl methyl ether (Albert, 1975) also showed a higher incidence of lung cancer among U.S. chemical workers compared to nonindustrial workers. Workers with greater than 5 years exposure had (to date) an age-adjusted cancer death rate of 1.48/1000/year versus 0.59 for the controls. Interestingly, this study pointed out that the controls (other chemical workers) also had a higher probability of death from lung cancer compared to the U.S. white male population. The same result was noted in the Russian study of chloroprene, that is, chemical workers have more lung cancer than nonchemical worker cohorts.

A NIOSH epidemiological study on BCME workers was also carried out (Lemen et al., 1976) which included a sputum cytology survey for a number of the BCME workers. The cytology study of 115 white male current employees found that 34% had abnormal cytology, versus 11% in the control groups. The findings of this study, like those of the NYU group, clearly show that the chloroether workers have an unusually high lung cancer risk. Other epidemiological studies on workers exposed to CMME (and thus to its impurity BCME) substantiated that CMME is a human carcinogen. In the deFonso and Keton study (1976) it was determined that the relative risk of lung cancer was 3.8 times higher in CMME-exposed workers compared to other chemical workers in the same plant. Weiss and Boucot (1975) also noted the usual association between lung cancer and CMME exposure.

Bis(chloromethyl)ether

$ClCH_2OCH_2Cl$

This chloroether can be prepared by the reaction of paraformaldehyde with hydrogen chloride in the presence of sulfuric acid. Its principal use is in the preparation of ion-exchange resins. Bis(chloromethyl)ether (BCME) reacts readily with water to yield hydrochloric acid and formaldehyde; however, an equilibrium can be established between the ether and the acid and aldehyde (Kallos and Solomon, 1973; Gorrie et al., 1973; Frankel et al., 1974). This was discussed in the section on chloromethyl methyl ether. For this reason, it is of some concern that industrial plants in which both components of BCME are present at the same time, that is, hydrochloric acid and formaldehyde, might produce a certain quantity of BCME.

BCME is one of the chemicals subject to the Occupational Safety and Health Administration (OSHA) Emergency Temporary Standard first issued in April 1973, which restricts the usage and handling of these compounds because they are considered human carcinogens.

Historically, many chemicals have been shown to cause cancer in humans and subsequent laboratory investigations showed that they also cause cancer in animals. In the case of BCME, this process was reversed. Van Duuren and I and co-workers (1968, 1969a) first showed that BCME causes tumors on mouse skin. Using female Swiss-Madison mice, we found that upon application of 2 mg of BCME in 0.1 ml of benzene to the backs of mice 3 times/week for nearly 1 year, 12 of 20 mice had papillomas, 12 of which progressed to carcinomas. Other experiments showed that BCME is an initiating agent. After a single application of BCME to the dorsal skin of ICR/Ha Swiss mice followed by applications 3 times/week of phorbol ester promoter, five out of 20 animals had papillomas, while the control group which did not receive the initial BCME treatment had no tumors.

Other laboratories reported similar findings: A/HE mice exposed to 5 mg/m^3 of BCME daily for 82 exposure days had an average 2.9 lung adenomas/mouse after 27 weeks, while a control group had 0.8 lung adenomas/mouse (Leong et al., 1971). Similarly, injection of BCME into newborn mice led to a high incidence of lung adenomas (Gargus et al., 1969).

Kuschner et al. (1975) exposed rats and hamsters to BCME vapor at a variety of dose levels down to 0.1 ppm. Twelve out of 20 rats (60%) which received 100 6 hr/day exposures at 0.1 ppm dose level had cancer. Rats with 80 exposures had a 44% incidence of cancer. The tumor incidence was established as being dose related. In addition, rats and hamsters exposed to 1.0 ppm BCME had a decidedly lower median life span (Drew et al., 1975). Ten 6-hr exposures at 1.0 ppm reduced the life span of rats from 462 days in the controls to 21 days, and in the hamster from 675 days to 137 days. The tumors of the animals exposed to 0.1 ppm BCME were mostly of the nose (esthesioneuroepitheliomas) and the lung (squamous cell carcinomas).

A study of German workers exposed to BCME revealed six cases of lung cancer among 18 men (Thiess et al., 1973). Two other cases were found among 50 production workers. Five of the cases were oat-cell carcinomas. A Japanese report (Sakabe, 1973) also described five cases of lung cancer among workers who synthesized BCME.

Although many alkylating agents were known to be carcinogenic, the finding that bis(chloromethyl)ether (BCME), an alkylating agent, is carcinogenic was unexpected. BCME is an exceptionally reactive alkylating agent; its half-life in aqueous solution is less than a minute. How does it survive in the cell to react with cellular components to induce cancer? The equilibrium between BCME and its hydrolysis products, hydrochloric acid and formaldehyde, could explain its ability to react with critical cellular moieties, since even though it is hydrolyzed so readily, it can be reformed due to the equilibrium. In one study the binding of ^{14}C-labeled BCME with DNA was compared to the binding of ^{14}C-labeled formaldehyde with DNA under the same conditions. BCME bound to the DNA to a greater extent than formaldehyde and the properties of the alkylated DNAs were different (Goldschmidt et al., 1975). This implies that the molecular basis for BCME's cancer induction involves BCME and not formaldehyde, which had no known carcinogenic properties. However, a recent report stated that rats who were chronically exposed to 15 ppm of formaldehyde developed nasal carcinomas (Swenberg et al., 1980).

Other α-Chloroethers

In addition to bis(chloromethyl)ether and chloromethyl methyl ether, a number of other aliphatic α-chloroethers have been shown to be carcinogenic in animals. These ethers are bis(α-chloroethyl)ether, 1,2-bis(chloromethoxy)ethane, 1,2,3-tris(chloromethoxy)propane (II), and 1,4-bis(chloromethoxy)p-xylene.

Bis(α-chloroethyl)ether given to 30 female ICR/Ha mice s.c. weekly for life at a dose level of 0.3 mg/0.05 ml Nujol resulted in four local sarcomas. No sarcomas were found in the Nujol control group. When 1 mg of this haloether in 0.1 ml of benzene was given once to 20 mice of the same strain and sex, followed after a fortnight by 2.5-μg applications of the tumor promoter phorbol myristate acetate 3 times/week for 590 days, seven animals developed nine papillomas, but no cancers. The tumor promoter control group had two animals with two papillomas (Van Duuren et al., 1972).

The data for the bioassays of the three other α-chloroethers, 1,2-bis(chloromethoxy)ethane (I), 1,2,3-tris(chloromethoxy)propane (II), and 1,4-bis(chloromethoxy)p-xylene (III) are shown in Table 3, along with some of the bioassay control groups (Van Duuren et al., 1975).

Epoxides and Sulfides

Diepoxybutane

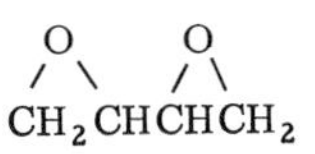

Diepoxybutane has been used to cure polymers, cross-link fibers, and prevent microbial spoilage. In some of the earliest experiments with diepoxybutane (butadiene diepoxide) the toxic action of the diepoxide masked its carcinogenic properties. When male stock mice received 1 drop/day 5 times/week of a 10% solution of arachis oil on their backs for 3 months,

TABLE 3 Carcinogenicity Assay of 1,2-Bis(chloromethoxy)ethane (I), 1,2,3-Tris(chloromethoxy)propane (II), and 1,4-Bis(chloromethoxy)p-xylene (III)

Compound	Dose mg/0.1 ml cyclohexane	Days on test	Median survival time (days)	No. of mice with papillomas (No. of mice with carcinomas)
	3 Mouse skin applications/week, 50 female ICR/Ha Swiss mice/group			
I	1.0	502	>502	4 (4)
II	1.0	502	493	6 (3)
III	1.0	502	484	7 (7)
Cyclohexane	—	504	>504	0 (0)

Compound	Dose mg/0.05 ml tricaprylin	Days on test	Median survival time (days)	No. of mice with local sarcomas
	1 Subcutaneous injection/week, 50 female ICR/Ha Swiss mice/group			
I	0.3	569	362	9
II	0.3	569	349	10
III	0.3	569	401	11
Tricaprylin	0.05 ml	570	436	0
BCME[a]	0.3	371	260	21

[a]BCME is bis(cloromethyl)ether, the positive control.

all the animals were dead at the end of 8 months and no skin tumors were noted. Another experiment by the same research group with a higher dose but shorter treatment time had a similar high mortality, but here the histology indicated that the diepoxide might be carcinogenic. For example, the loss of spermatogenesis in the tubules of the testes of one mouse was noted, as well as pronounced infiltrations with lymphoid cells in the liver of another mouse (Hendry et al., 1951). The same research workers also administered the diepoxide to rats i.p. In 10 male and four female animals so treated only one animal developed a tumor in the peritoneal cavity. Diepoxybutane was subsequently reported to produce sebaceous gland suppression, intense hyperkeratosis, parakeratosis, and epithelial hyperplasia when applied to the shaven skin of mice (McCammon et al., 1957).

Painting a 10% acetone solution of diepoxybutane on C3H mice for 18 months resulted in high mortality, but among the survivors several animals had papillomas and one a carcinoma (Weil et al., 1963).

In a study that compared the activity of the stereoisomers of diepoxybutane, dl-diepoxybutane, and mesodiepoxybutane, it was found that 3% acetone solutions of dl-diepoxybutane applied to mouse skin led to a higher tumor incidence—10 papillomas and six carcinomas in 30 animals—than mesodiepoxybutane, which gave one papilloma and no cancers in 30 animals. Experiments with 10% solutions did not confirm these results because the median survival for animals treated with the dl-stereoisomer was very poor, 165 days, versus 357 days for the meso compound (Van Duuren et al., 1965).

When female ICR/Ha mice, 50 to a group, were given weekly s.c. injections of 0.1 mg of dl-diepoxybutane in tricaprylin, five animals developed fibrosarcomas and two adenocarcinomas. Using Sprague-Dawley rats 50 to a group, s.c. injections of 1 mg/animal/week elicited nine fibrosarcomas and one adenocarcinoma. The same strain fed dl-diepoxybutane (5 mg 1 time/week) developed no tumors (Van Duuren et al., 1966).

In a study by Shimkin and co-workers (1966) A/J mice received 12 i.p. injections of l-diepoxybutane 3 times/week in either water or tricaprylin at a series of dose levels. After 39 weeks the animals were sacrificed and the number of lung tumors determined. In tricaprylin at 2.2 mM/kg total dose, 0.75 lung tumors/mouse were observed, while at 0.56 mM/kg 0.80 lung tumors/mouse occurred. Injections of tricaprylin alone yielded an incidence of 0.47 lung tumors/mouse in males and 0.42 in females. Low doses of l-diepoxybutane caused no more tumors than the solvent alone. Using water as a vehicle comparable results were obtained.

dl-Diepoxybutane is also a carcinogenic initiating agent. When 20 mice received 1 mg in 0.1 ml of benzene once, followed by treatments 3 times/week with croton resin, seven mice had 11 tumors and two had carcinomas after 1 year (Van Duuren et al., 1969b).

Other Aliphatic Diepoxyalkanes and Diepoxyethers

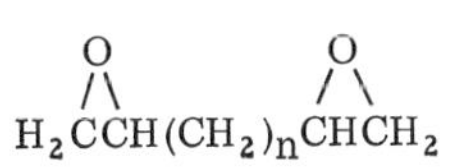

A series of aliphatic diepoxides, in which one epoxide occurs at the first two carbon atoms and the other at the last two carbon atoms in the molecule, was found to be carcinogenic in mice. A 10% acetone solution of 1,2,4,5-diepoxypentane when painted on mouse skin led to 10 papillomas and three carcinomas in 30 female ICR/Ha mice. Similarly, a 5% solution of 1,2,5,6-diepoxyhexane yielded four papillomas but no carcinomas, and a 1% solution of 1,2,6,7-diepoxyheptane gave nine papillomas and one carcinoma in 30 animals (Van Duuren et al., 1965). A later study with 1,2,5,6-diepoxyhexane by the same research group with a lower dose (2.0%) found the compound to be more active, i.e., 13 papillomas and 10 cancers in 30 mice compared to the 5% dose applications. The next higher homologue in this series, 1,2,7,8-diepoxyoctane, when tested in a 1% acetone solution yielded seven keratoacanthomas (instead of the more common papillomas) and four carcinomas (Van Duuren et al., 1967a). Two cyclic analogues of these compounds were also tested for carcinogenicity on mouse skin. Neither 1,2,3,4-diepoxycyclohexane nor 1,2,5,6-diepoxycyclooctane produced any tumors when tested by the same protocol in the same mouse strain. It was concluded that for an aliphatic diepoxide to be carcinogenic, some degree of molecular flexibility, absent in the two cyclic structures, is required.

The diepoxyether bis(2,3-epoxy-2-methylpropyl)ether was tested on mouse skin (Weil et al., 1963). Repeated applications of a 20% acetone solution of this compound to mouse skin yielded seven papillomas, but no carcinomas in the 27 surviving mice. Another diepoxyether, di(2,3-epoxy)propyl ether, when assayed on 20 C57BL mice led to a 40% skin tumor incidence (Kotin and Falk, 1963).

Propylene Oxide

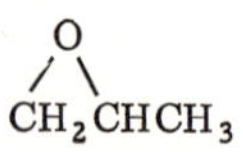

Propylene oxide is produced in sizable quantities in the United States. In 1973 the estimated production was 796 million kg. Most of this (about 64%) is used in the production of polyurethane foams. Another 25% is used to prepare propylene glycol, which in turn is used to prepare polyester resins.

When a cumulative dose of 1500 mg/kg body weight propylene oxide (1,2-epoxypropane) was given to rats s.c. in arachis oil, eight of 12 animals developed local sarcomas. Using the same procedures, ethylene oxide produced no tumors (Walpole, 1958). That the lower homologue ethylene oxide is also not carcinogenic on mouse skin was shown by Van Duuren et al. (1965).

1-Ethyleneoxy-3,4-Epoxycyclohexane

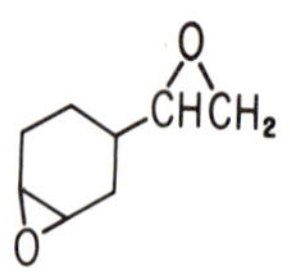

1-Ethyleneoxy-3,4-epoxycyclohexane, also known as vinylcyclohexene diepoxide or vinylcyclohexene dioxide, was shown to be an animal carcinogen in a number of experiments. This diepoxide was first tested as a tumor inhibitor with rats previously given implants of Walker carcinoma. When the diepoxide was given i.p. in oil, it inhibited the growth of the tumor and caused numerous mitotic abnormalities in the tumor cells including the formation of chromosome bridges and fragments. Upon postmortem examination of the treated rats, changes in the testes were noted, including the failure of spermatogenesis and the presence in the tubules of multinucleated giant cells (Rose et al., 1950).

When given i.p. to 10 male and four female stock albino rats at 25 mg/100 g twice weekly for 10 weeks, one male rat had mixed-cell sarcoma tissue disseminated in the peritoneal cavity after 7 months. This sarcoma was maintained after more than 20 successive s.c. transplantations in the same stock rats. Far more tumors were obtained when this diepoxide was applied to the skin of mice. When 20 stock albino male mice were painted with one drop (ca. 16 mg) 5 times/week for 12 months only nine mice died without tumors. Four animals had squamous carcinoma at the site of application, three had sarcomas below the painted area, two animals had both types of tumors, and two others had lung adenomas (Hendry et al., 1951).

Using a group of 30 C3H mice, a brush full of a 10% acetone solution of the diepoxide was applied to the midline of the animals' backs 3 times/week. At the end of 17 months, three papillomas and one carcinoma were observed (Weil et al., 1963). When a 10% benzene solution (100 mg/application) of 1-ethyleneoxy-3,4-epoxycyclohexane was applied to the shaven backs of 30 male ICR/Ha mice 3 times/week for the lifetime of the animals (median survival time 326 days), 14 papillomas and nine cancers formed (Van Duuren et al., 1963).

Other Aliphatic Epoxides

The alkyne diepoxide 2,5-dimethyl-1,2,5,6-diepoxyhex-3-yne when tested on mouse skin at a dosage of 0.25 mg/0.1 ml acetone 3 times/week on 30 female ICR/Ha mice yielded no tumors. When tested by s.c. injection in another group of animals of the same sex and strain at a dosage of 0.5 mg weekly, it caused two local sarcomas and one squamous cell carcinoma in 30 animals (Van Duuren et al., 1974).

The aliphatic triepoxide 1,2,4,5,9,10-triepoxydecane was tested by collaborating investigators at the University of Texas and New York University who both used 0.1 mg applications 3 times/week on mouse skin. Neither group obtained any tumors, but upon s.c. injection (1.0 mg weekly) one group observed four sarcomas and one squamous cell carcinoma in 30 animals, while the other observed five sarcomas and one squamous cell carcinoma (Van Duuren et al., 1974).

Styrene Epoxide

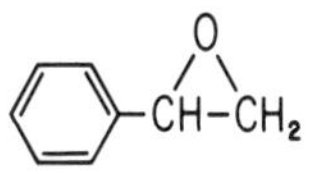

A 10% benzene solution of styrene epoxide (styrene oxide) applied to the back of male ICR/Ha mice 3 times/week caused three papillomas and one cancer among the 30 animals treated. As part of the same study, 150 animals were treated with benzene; of these animals, 6.7% developed tumors, but only one of these was cancer—the others were papillomas (Van Duuren et al., 1963). In another study using C3H mice 10 and 5% acetone solutions of styrene oxide were applied to mouse skin. At the higher dose survival was poor, and treatment with the lower dose resulted in no tumors after 2 years of applications (Weil et al., 1963).

3-4-Epoxy-6-Methylcyclohexylmethyl-3,4-Epoxy-6-Methylcyclohexanecarboxylate

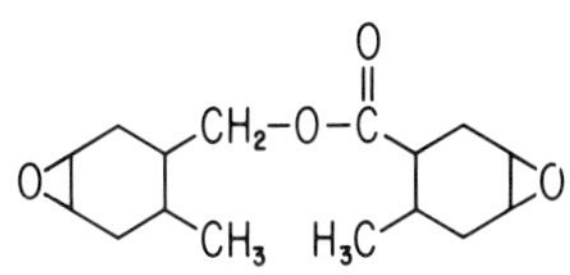

A detailed investigation of the carcinogenicity of this bicyclic diepoxy ester was carried out by Weil et al. (1963). In their studies the authors varied a number of parameters to determine their effect on the carcinogenic activity of this compound. In a skin application protocol they compared the susceptibility of mice of the same age and sex but different strain, C3H versus C57L. The C57L mice had a higher percentage of tumor and cancer incidence than the C3H mice at the dose given. However, since C3H mice had a higher mortality incidence, the number of animals at risk was higher in the C57L strain. When 1-year-old 1C3F1 mice were treated with the undiluted bicyclic diepoxy ester on the skin and the results were compared to C3H mice first treated at a much younger age, the median latent time for tumor formation and the tumor and cancer incidences were not very different. As noted for other carcinogenic epoxides, 5% acetone solutions were inactive, while the undiluted material was active. However, in this study the total dose given undiluted was not equal to the amount given in the dilute solution case. Dodecane was reported to be a potent cocarcinogen with various alkanes and alkyl-substituted aromatic compounds (Horton et al., 1957). The bicyclic diepoxy ester mixed with dodecane showed no cocarcinogenic properties.

In our study of this bicyclic diepoxy ester with female ICR/Ha mice 10% acetone solutions applied to the skin were highly carcinogenic. Lifetime applications (3 times/week) led to 11 keratoacanthomas and 11 carcinomas in a group of 30 animals (Van Duuren et al., 1967a). It is worthy to note for correlations of chemical structure and carcinogenic activity that in the Weil et al. study (1963) and ours already cited (1967a), only this compound is strongly carcinogenic among a number of compounds tested for which the epoxide group is in a cyclic system. Usually aliphatic cyclic epoxides are not carcinogenic, even though the active metabolites of many aromatic hydrocarbons are cyclic epoxides (see Chapter 7).

Glycidaldehyde

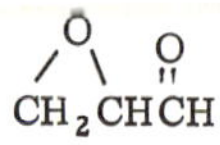

Weekly s.c. injections of glycidaldehyde (epoxyproponal) to mice at a dose of 0.1 mg/injection caused three malignant tumors in 50 animals, and seven malignant tumors in 30 animals when the dose was raised to 3.3 mg. When weekly injections of 1 mg were given s.c. to rats, one fibrosarcoma was found in 50 animals at 33 mg/injection and five sarcomas developed in 20 rats. Upon feeding 33 mg weekly to a small group of rats, no tumors were found (Van Duuren et al., 1966). The result of the feeding experiment is not surprising as the tumorigenic ability of this compound, like that of many carcinogenic diepoxides, is probably dependent on the reaction of the epoxide group with a specific cellular component. The low pH of the stomach facilitates the rapid reaction of the epoxide group with water, thus preventing the critical reactions of the epoxide with the cellular component, which ultimately lead to tumor formation.

When a 3% benzene solution of this compound was applied to the skin of female Swiss mice for life, eight papillomas and eight carcinomas were found in a group of 30 mice (Van Duuren et al., 1965).

Interestingly, when glycidaldehyde reacts with the nucleoside guanosine or guanine moieties in DNA (Goldschmidt et al., 1968a), it reacts with the pyrimidine part of the purine. Usually carcinogenic alkylating agents react predominantly with the imidazole moiety of the purine, particularly at the 7-nitrogen position. In this case, however, the 1-N and 2-amino group of guanine form bonds with two carbons of glycidaldehyde to yield a new fused five-membered ring attached to the original guanine molecule (Goldschmidt et al., 1968b; Van Duuren and Loewengart, 1977).

Glycidaldehyde is also mutagenic to bacteriophage T4, inducing A/T and G/C base-pair transitions and frameshift mutations (Corbett et al., 1970). It induces base-pair mutations in _S. typhimurium_ (McCann et al., 1975) and in _Saccharomyces cerevisiae_ (Izard, 1973).

Epichlorohydrin

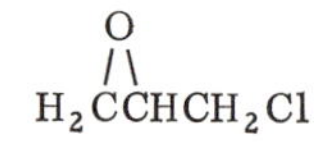

Epichlorohydrin is an important industrial chemical. It is estimated that 156 million kg were produced in the United States in 1973. The United States' consumption pattern for epichlorohydrin in 1973 was 46% for synthetic glycerin, 39% for epoxy resins, 1.7% for elastomers, 9.3% for other products, and export of the remaining 4.0%. The National Institute of Occupational Safety and Health (NIOSH) estimates that 50,000 workers are presently exposed to this compound.

When tested on mouse skin at a level of 2.0 mg/0.1 ml acetone 3 times/week in 50 female ICR/Ha mice, no papillomas or carcinomas were noted after more than 500 days of testing. The median survival time was 506 days (Van Duuren et al., 1974). In the same study, when given s.c., 1.0 mg/0.05 ml tricaprylin given weekly to 50 mice in a 580-day experiment, five sarcomas and one adenocarcinoma were noted, while the solvent control had no tumors. In an initiation-promotion experiment 30 mice received one dose of 2 mg of epichlorohydrin and then promotion with 2.5 μg of phorbol myristate acetate 3 times/week for more than 1 year. Nine papillomas and one cancer developed, versus three papillomas and no cancers in the control group treated with phorbol ester only.

In an inhalation study epichlorohydrin produced reverse mutations in _Neurospora creassa_ (Kolmark and Giles, 1955) in _Escherichia coli_ (Strauss and Okubo, 1960). Epichlorohydrin was also found to be mutagenic when tested on human lymphocytes (Kucerova et al., 1976). Kuschner and co-workers (1980) exposed 100 male Sprague-Dawley rats to epichlorohydrin at levels of 30-100 ppm. Of the survivors, 5-10% had nasal tumors, a type of tumor never seen in control rats.

That epichlorohydrin may indeed be carcinogenic to humans was recently disclosed in a news release (Chem. Eng. News, 1978c). An epidemiological study of 864 Shell chemical employees at Deer Park, Tex. and Norco, La. showed that whereas a 6-7% death rate from respiratory cancer was predicted, a 17% rate was found. The workers' present exposure levels to epichlorohydrin are reportedly lower than those to which some of the older workers were previously exposed.

Ethylene Sulfide

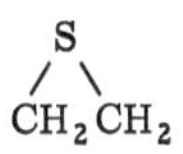

Ethylene sulfide was tested for carcinogenicity in BD rats by s.c. injections (Druckrey et al., 1970a). Groups of 15 animals received 8 or 16 mg/kg body weight weekly in arachis oil. At the high dose four out of 12 animals developed local sarcomas and at the low dose one out of 15.

Lactones and Sultones

β-Propiolactone

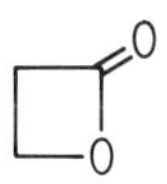

β-Propiolactone is used as an intermediate in the production of acrylic acid and its esters. It is a fairly volatile alkylating agent and has found use as a bactericide in the sterilization of plasma, vaccines, surgical instruments, etc. β-Propiolactone is commercially prepared by the coupling of ketene and formaldehyde.

When this compound is applied to mouse skin, it produces papillomas and squamous cell carcinomas (Roe and Glendenning, 1956; Palmes et al., 1962). Weekly s.c. injections of 0.73 mg of 0.05 ml tricaprylin for 503 days using 30 female ICR/Ha Swiss mice resulted in 18 animals with malignant tumors. No local tumors were observed in 110 control animals which received weekly injections of tricaprylin for 503 days. Given i.p. administration once to both male and female B6AF1 mice less than 2 weeks old, 22 out of 34 males and none of 30 females developed hepatomas; 90% of the males and 20% of the females developed lymphomas (Chernozemski and Warwick, 1970).

The rat is also quite susceptible to cancer induction by β-propiolactone. Male Wistar rats (Dickens and Jones, 1961) or Sprague-Dawley female rats (Van Duuren et al., 1967b), which received the lactone s.c. in arachis oil or tricaprylin, respectively, developed sarcomas at the injection site. After feeding β-propiolactone to female Sprague-Dawley rats, carcinomas of the forestomach formed (Van Duuren et al., 1966). This is in contrast to the results obtained in a feeding study with a carcinogenic diepoxide in which the diepoxide failed to induce stomach tumors, while the β-lactone was carcinogenic. The reason for this probably is that the hydrolysis of epoxides is more susceptible to acid catalysis than the hydrolysis of β-lactones. Thus the epoxide readily becomes a noncarcinogenic diol, while enough β-lactone is present to react with cellular moieties resulting in tumor induction (Goldschmidt, 1965; Van Duuren and Goldschmidt, 1966).

The hydrolysis product of β-propiolactone, β-hydroxypropionic acid, failed to produce sarcomas when given subcutaneously to rats (Dickens and Jones, 1963) or skin tumors when applied to the skin of mice (Searle, 1961). β-Propiolactone is a direct-acting carcinogen. Because of this, β-propiolactone presents a maximum hazard to workers exposed to the pure product and a minimal one to the environment since it hydrolyzes to an inactive product in a matter of hours (Van Duuren and Goldschmidt, 1966).

Early studies showed that β-propiolactone reacts with the 7-nitrogen of guanosine and at the same site in RNA (Roberts and Warwick, (1963). In vivo studies confirmed that the predominant isolated alkylated base from the reaction of DNA or RNA and β-propiolactone was 7-(2-carboxyethyl)guanine (Colburn and Boutwell, 1968; Segal et al., 1974). A more recent study (Maté et al., 1977) showed that β-propiolactone also reacts with the adenine moiety in DNA to yield 1-(2-carboxyethyl)adenine. It has also been shown that the lactone is mutagenic for bacteriophage T4. It causes G/C → A/T base pair transitions (Corbett et al., 1970).

Substituted β-Lactones

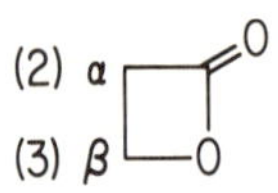

β-Propiolactone, the simplest β-lactone, is a potent monofunctional carcinogenic alkylating agent. Other β-lactones, with substituents at the α- or β-position or at both carbons, have been tested for carcinogenicity. The simplest homologue of β-propiolactone is β-butyrolactone, the former with an additional methyl group on the β-carbon. When 20 female Sprague-Dawley rats were given 100-mg doses of β-butyrolactone s.c., nine animals developed sarcomas. At a 1.0-mg dose no sarcomas developed (Van Duuren et al., 1967b). Female ICR/Ha Swiss mice were painted with 10% solutions of β-butyrolactone in acetone or benzene. The acetone group had one papilloma in 40 mice, while the benzene group had 20 papillomas and 16 carcinomas in 30 mice. Clearly, a strong solvent effect is operating since the benzene controls only had about a 7% incidence of papillomas and no carcinomas. A number of other experiments have confirmed this observation that in general benzene enhances the carcinogenicity of alkylating agents applied to mouse skin compared to acetone, cyclohexane, or dimethylsulfoxide.

An earlier experiment also involved testing of substituted β-lactones by s.c. injection in male rats. α,α-Diphenyl-β-propiolactone and α-carboxy-β-phenyl β-propiolactone given twice weekly at the 1-2 mg level for 19 and 64 weeks, respectively, yielded one tumor each in the five treated rats (Dickens and Jones, 1961). The authors concluded that these substances were weakly carcinogenic. Several other substituted β-lactones—2,2-dimethylbutyric; 2,2-dimethyl-4,4,4-trichlorobutyric, and 2,2,4-trimethylheptanoic—were also tested in acetone solutions on mouse skin. They produced no tumors (Van Duuren et al., 1967a).

One difunctional compound containing both an epoxide moiety and a β-lactone ring structure, 4,5-epoxy-3-hydroxyvaleric acid β-lactone, when tested as a 10% benzene solution applied to mouse skin led to five papillomas and no cancers in 30 mice (Van Duuren et al., 1965).

Substituted αβ-Unsaturated-γ-Lactones

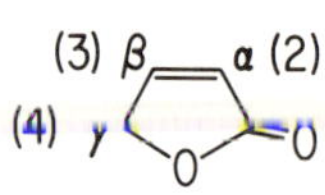

A series of αβ-unsaturated-γ-lactones was tested by Dickens and Jones (1961, 1963, and 1965). Some of these lactones were used as antibiotics or have a chemical structure related to known antibiotics. The compounds were generally tested by repeated twice weekly s.c. injections in male Wistar rats. The compounds were dissolved in arachis oil prior to the injections. The control animals receiving s.c. injections of arachis oil had no sarcomas. Unfortunately, in these experiments the number of animals at risk was small, usually fewer than six rats. The αβ-unsaturated lactones tested which the authors concluded to be carcinogenic, the dose and number of s.c. injections of that dose, and the number of local sarcomas per animals at risk are as follows: α-methyltetronic acid lactone, 2 mg/130 (2/4); 4-hydroxy-2-hexenoic acid lactone, 2 mg/128 (2/4); 4-hydroxy-2,4-hexadienoic acid lactone, 2 mg/128 (3/5); 4-hydroxy-4-hexenoic acid lactone, 1 mg/116 (3/5); 4-hydroxy-2,3-dimethyl-2,4-nonadienoic acid lactone (Bovolide), 2 mg/130 (5/5); 4,4-dihydroxy-3-methoxy-5-methyl 2,5-hexadienoic acid lactone (penicillic acid), 1 mg/128 (4/4); and 0.1 mg/122 (1/4); patulin (clavacin) 0.2 mg/122 (4/4). The authors found that some closely related substances, γ-butyrolactone, 4-hydroxy-3-pentenoic acid lactone (α-angelica lactone) and 4-hydroxy-3-hexenoic acid lactone yielded no tumors when given in the same protocols as just described (Dickens and Jones, 1961).

Dehydroacetic Acid

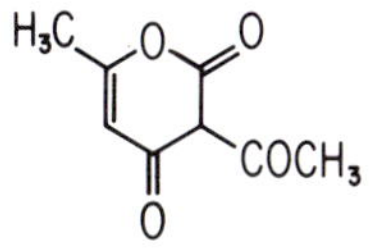

Dehydroacetic acid (2-acetyl-5-hydroxy-3-oxo-4-hexenoic acid δ-lactone) is a polymerization product of diketene, which has found use as a plasticizer compatible with a variety of resins. It has also found use as a fungicide and bactericide. Twice weekly s.c. injections of 2 mg in arachis oil in six male rats for 65 weeks led to five sarcomas at the injection site. When dehydroacetic acid was added to the drinking water of six rats (10 mg/100 ml) for 64 weeks, no tumors were found upon autopsy (Dickens et al., 1966). In an earlier feeding study, rats given 0.02-0.10% dehydroacetic acid in their diets developed no tumors (Spencer et al., 1950).

Coumarin

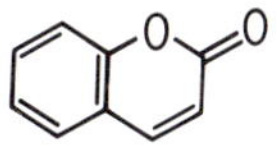

Coumarin is a natural product found in plants and oils. It is usually prepared synthetically for commercial use. Coumarin is used as a stabilizer and odor in perfumes, toilet soaps, tobacco products, and so on.

When given to Osborne-Mendel rats of both sexes at 1.0, 2.5, and 5.0 g/kg of diet for 2 years, bile-duct proliferation, cholangiofibrosis, and focal necrosis were observed at the two highest dose levels (Hagan et al., 1967). When albino rats of both sexes were fed 5.0 g of coumarin/kg diet for 2 years, 11 males and one female of the 24 rats which survived 18 months or more, developed bile-duct carcinomas (Bär and Griepentrog, 1967; Griepentrog, 1973).

Parasorbic Acid

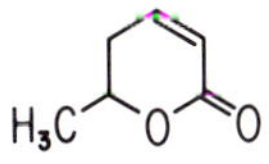

Parasorbic acid (5-hydroxy-2-hexenoic δ-lactone) is a natural product found in ripe mountain ash berries.

In a drinking-water experiment in which groups of six rats received 28 or 198 mg of parasorbic acid over 64 weeks, survival of the animals was poor and one late testicular tumor occurred (Dickens et al., 1966).

When given s.c. to groups of six male rats at 0.2 or 2.0 mg twice weekly for 32 weeks, four of six and four of five rats developed local sarcomas in about 100 weeks at the low and high dose, respectively. The control animals which received only the vehicle arachis oil developed no tumors (Dickens and Jones, 1963).

Propane Sultone

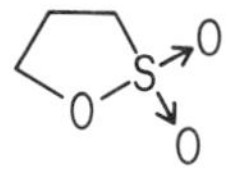

Propane sultone, also known as 3-hydroxy-1-propane sulfonic acid sultone or 1,2-oxathiolane-2,2-dioxide, is prepared by dehydrating the corresponding hydroxy sulfonic acid. Although presently of limited commercial use, it has a variety of possible applications. After alkylating another chemical compound with it, a three-carbon sulfonate group is then present which confers water solubility and simultaneously introduces an acid or ester function into the reacted molecule. In the late 1960s several research groups became cognizant of the similarity in physical and chemical properties of 1,3-propane sultone and β-propiolactone, already a known carcinogen. Thus several studies on the carcinogenicity of propane sultone appeared in the literature at about the same time.

When given to Charles River rats by gavage 3 times/week at doses of 56 mg/kg body weight for 32 weeks and 28 mg/kg body weight for 60 weeks, a high incidence (29 tumors/52 animals and 27 tumors/52 animals, respectively) of brain tumors (gliomas) was found (Ulland et al., 1971). A high percentage of rats given 15 or 30 mg/kg body weight s.c. in arachis oil solutions died of myosarcomas and fibrosarcomas (Druckrey et al., 1968; Druckrey et al., 1970b).

Mice given 0.3 mg of propane sultone in 0.05 ml distilled water by s.c. injection once weekly had a high incidence of tumors at the injection site after 63 weeks. There were 21 out of 30 animals with tumors compared to no tumors in the 30 control animals (Van Duuren et al., 1971b).

The sultone was shown to react irreversibly with DNA and with guanosine to yield the N-7-alkyl nucleoside (Goldschmidt et al., 1974). It is also mutagenic in bacteriophage T4 inducing several types of mutations (Corbett et al., 1970). When bacillus subtilis DNA is alkylated with this sultone or β-propiolactone, changes in its physical properties and transforming activity are observed (Kubinski and Kubinski, 1978).

Butane Sultone

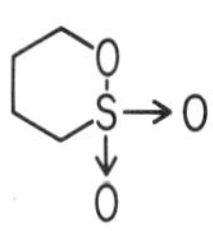

Butane sultone, the next higher homologue of propane sultone, is chemically less active than propane sultone and also less carcinogenic. When given s.c. to BD rats at 30 mg/kg body weight in water weekly for 76 weeks, one rat of the original 12 developed a local sarcoma. Given i.v. at the same dose level to 16 animals of the same strain of rats, no tumors developed (Druckrey et al., 1970b).

When we administered 1.0 mg of butane sultone in 0.05 ml of tricaprylin s.c. to 30 female ICR/Ha Swiss mice weekly for 580 days, three animals developed local sarcomas and one a squamous cell carcinoma (Van Duuren et al., 1974).

Sulfates and Sulfonates

Dimethylsulfate

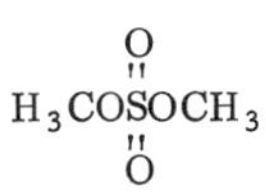

Dimethylsulfate has been produced commercially for at least 50 years. Its major use is to convert active hydrogen compounds, such as acids, phenols, and thiols, to the corresponding methyl derivatives.

Druckrey and his associates (1966, 1970) and Preussmann (1968) carried out an elaborate investigation of the carcinogenicity of dimethylsulfate. BD rats received weekly s.c. injections of 8 or 16 mg/kg body weight of dimethylsulfate for 58 and 48 weeks, respectively. In the low-dose group, seven out of 12 rats developed local sarcomas compared to four out of six in the high-dose group. Survival in the high-dose group was much lower than in the low-dose group with an average lifetime of 330 days versus 500 days, respectively. In a third group of the same rats which received one s.c. injection of 50 mg of dimethylsulfate, seven local tumors occurred among 15 rats. Given i.v. (2 mg/kg body weight) to 12 rats weekly for 4 weeks, dimethylsulfate yielded no tumors. In a transpacental experiment carried out by the Druckrey group, one 20-mg dose given to pregnant rats at the 15th day of gestation resulted in seven of 50 offspring developing malignant tumors, mostly of the nervous system.

Inhalation of 3 or 10 ppm of dimethylsulfate for 1 hr 5 times/week for 130 days produced squamous carcinomas of the nasal cavity or neurogenic tumors in eight out of 27 exposed rats. Another research group (Schlögel and Bannasch, 1970) also carried out an inhalation experiment. Rodents were exposed to 0.5 ppm dimethylsulfate 6 hr/day twice weekly for 15 months or to 2.0 ppm for 6 hr every 2 weeks. The animals were observed for 2.5 years. Benign lung tumors were present in both the control and treated animals. However, the treated animals had six nasal cancers, three lung cancers, one thorax sarcoma, and two lung adenomas.

In our laboratory (Van Duuren et al., 1974) we tested dimethylsulfate on mouse skin. No papillomas or carcinomas appeared when given at 0.1 mg/0.1 ml acetone 3 times/week for 456 days to 20 mice. When tested as an initiating agent, 1.0 mg given once to 30 female ICR/Ha mice followed by applications of phorbol myristate acetate 3 times/week for more than 1 year yielded two papillomas.

An interesting comparison of the relatively weak direct-acting carcinogens dimethylsulfate and methyl methanesulfonate compared with the relatively strong direct-acting carcinogens, 1 methyl-1-nitrosourea and 1-methyl-3-nitro-1-nitrosoguanidine was recently made (Chang and Lee, 1978). Using ^{13}C-enriched alkylating agents the authors allowed the alkylating agents to react with RNA and determined the ^{13}C-NMR spectra of the reaction mixture. The stronger carcinogenic alkylating agents reacted only with the 7-nitrogen of guanine and the phosphate of the nucleotide, while the weaker carcinogens reacted with those sites and the 1-N of guanine and other sites on adenine, cytidine, and uridine.

A study of human workers found that one individual died of oat cell carcinoma of the upper bronchus after 11 years of exposure to dimethylsulfate. Three other workers who worked with this compound also died of bronchial cancer (Druckrey et al., 1966).

Other Alkyl Sulfates

$$RO\overset{\overset{\displaystyle O}{\|}}{\underset{\underset{\displaystyle O}{\|}}{S}}OR$$

Druckrey and co workers (1970a) tested diethyl and di-n-butyl sulfate for carcinogenicity in BD rats. Weekly s.c. injections of the diethyl ester at 25 and 50 mg/kg body weight for 32 weeks resulted in six out of 12 and 11 out of 11 animals with local sarcomas, respectively. The butyl ester was far less toxic and when given at 500 mg/kg body weight weekly for 19 weeks resulted in fewer local sarcomas, that is, two out of seven animals with tumors. In the oral administration of diethyl sulfate, 25 or 50 mg/kg given by gavage for 81 weeks to the same strain of rats led to one carcinoma and six out of 24 animals with papillomas of the forestomach.

In some later experiments from Druckrey's laboratory, diisopropyl sulfate and monomethyl sulfate were tested for carcinogenicity (Druckrey et al., 1973). Using BD rats, diisopropyl sulfate given s.c. at a dosage of 100 mg/kg body weight weekly for 16 weeks produced local sarcomas in 14 of the 15 treated rats. In a single dose (300 mg/kg body weight) experiment, this dialkyl sulfate produced eight sarcomas in 15 rats, two tumors in remote organs, and one pleomorphic glioma of the brain. When monomethyl sulfate was given weekly at a dose level of 100 mg/kg body weight for up to 63 weeks of treatment, it did not yield any tumors. Clearly, the acidity and solubility of the half acid ester is very different from that of the dialkyl diester, and hence the differences in their toxic and carcinogenic properties. Diethyl sulfate also was tested in a transplacental experiment in which one dose of 85 mg/kg body weight was given to rats on the 15th day of gestation. Two out of 30 offspring developed malignant tumors in this study.

The cyclic analogue of dimethyl sulfate, glycol sulfate, is a highly reactive electrophile. However, when tested as a whole carcinogen on mouse skin or as an initiating agent in two-stage carcinogenesis it showed no activity. When tested by s.c. injection in 30 female ICR/Ha Swiss mice at 0.5 mg weekly, 21 sarcomas and one squamous cell carcinoma developed (Van Duuren et al., 1974).

Methyl Methanesulfonate

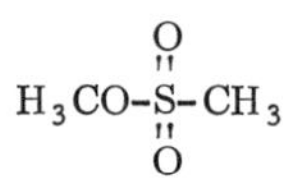

Sixty-three 11-week-old male mice from a noninbred subline of the RF/Un strain were given methyl methanesulfonate in drinking water at 20 mg/100 ml for their lifetime. Autopsies of the dead mice showed that 70% had primary pulmonary tumors compared to 39% of the controls. These tumors were adenomas morphologically indistinguishable from those observed in the untreated animals or those treated with diethylnitrosamine or dimethylnitrosamine. The RF/Un mice treated with methyl methanesulfonate also had a high incidence of thymic lymphomas 14.9% versus 3.7% in the controls (Clapp et al., 1968).

In contrast to the results with the noninbred RF/Un mice, methyl methanesulfonate given to inbred CFW/D mice via i.p. injections (6 mmol/kg body weight) resulted in no greater incidence of lung adenomas or lymphomas than the incidence resulting from the untreated controls. In this same study ethyl methanesulfonate was shown to cause a high incidence of lung adenomas, and methylnitrosourea and ethylnitrosourea led to a significant incidence of lymphomas and lung adenomas compared to the untreated animals (Frei, 1971).

When Wistar albino rats were given i.v. injections of methyl methanesulfonate, the 16 rats that had received 120 mg/kg had no tumors. Among 20 rats that had received 96 mg/kg, there was one tumor (oligodendroglioma) and one nerve tumor (malignant neurofibroma). At a dose of 72 mg/kg body weight there were two brain tumors (astrocytoma) and one spinal cord tumor (meningioma) among 20 treated animals (Swann and Magee, 1968, 1969).

Using 535 BD strain rats, weekly s.c. injections of 4 or 8 mg/kg body weight of methyl methanesulfonate for nearly 1 year resulted in three local sarcomas in 12 rats given the high dose and one nephroblastoma and three local sarcomas in eight rats treated with the low dose (Druckrey et al., 1970a).

Cancer induction is thought to be related to changes in cellular polynucleotides. Thus, a number of investigators using radioactively labeled alkylating agents, have tried to correlate the extent of alkylation of polynucleotides with carcinogenic potential. Methyl methanesulfonate is one of the compounds that has been investigated because of the assumption that its biological potency is related to its ability to transfer the methyl group bound to the oxygen to a cellular target (i.e., alkylation of nucleic acids).

Both methyl methanesulfonate and ethyl methanesulfonate were shown capable of inactivating bacteriophage T2; they alkylated the guanine at the 7-nitrogen and adenine at the 3-nitrogen of the phage DNA. Compared to the difunctional alkylating agents, they were less efficient at inactivating the bacteriophage (Brookes and Lawley, 1963). Methyl methanesulfonate was also shown to alkylate guanine in yeast RNA (Brookes and Lawley, 1961). When albino rats of the Porton strain were given i.p. or i.v. injections of ^{14}C-labeled methyl methanesulfonate, the extent of methylation of rat kidney DNA was greater than that produced by either N-methyl-N-nitrososurea or dimethylnitrosamine at a dose level that the latter two induced a high incidence of kidney tumors (Swann and Magee, 1968). However, as already described, in the case of the albino rats treated with methyl methanesulfonate, tumors occurred (three brain tumors, one nerve tumor, and one spinal cord tumor among 56 treated rats), but there were no kidney tumors. That the situation is rather complex was also shown in another study in which methyl methanesulfonate did not, but ethyl methanesulfonate, N-nitrosos-N-methylurea, and N-ethyl-N-nitrosourea did, react with guanosine to yield O-alkyl derivatives. These derivatives are unstable in strong acid and thus would not be isolated in some of the procedures used to isolate N-alkylated purines and pyrimidines (Loveless, 1969).

Ethyl Methanesulfonate

$$H_3CCH_2O\overset{\overset{\displaystyle O}{\|}}{\underset{\underset{\displaystyle O}{\|}}{S}}CH_3$$

When tested by repeated s.c. injection in 20 mice, a total dose of 145 mg of ethyl methanesulfonate (EMS) produced no local sarcomas; three animals, however, had lymphomas (Haddow et al., 1962). When newborn mice of the BALB/c strain were injected with 100 μg of this alkylating agent in water, 53% (17/32) of the survivors had lung tumors after about 280 days on test. Control groups receiving only solvents, aqueous gelatin, and arachis oil, had a 5-10% incidence of lung tumors (Roe et al., 1962). Five s.c. injection of 0.2 mg of ethyl methanesulfonate once daily for the first 5 days of life induced lung tumors in all surviving BALB/c mice when aqueous gelatin was the vehicle. However, only 15.7% of the animals had lung tumors when arachis oil was used as the vehicle. This lower tumor incidence is comparable to that of the arachis control group. A possible explanation for this suggested by the investigators is that the oil remains at the site of injection longer and does not reach the lungs as readily as the aqueous gelatin (Walters et al., 1967). Another experiment showed that ethyl methanesulfonate in arachis oil could induce tumors in C57B1 mice (Walters et al., 1967).

At approximately half the 30 day LD50 (200 mg/kg body weight) doses of ethyl methanesulfonate were given i.p. in arachis oil weekly for 3 weeks to CBA male mice. The mean animal lifespan was the same as the controls, because the tumors developed slowly. In all, 89% of treated animals had lung and kidney tumors compared to 20% of the controls (Connell, 1961).

Using inbred CFW/D mice bred for more than 50 generations by brother-sister matings, a single i.p. injection of 3 mg/kg of ethyl methanesulfonate was given to adult animals of both sexes. The number of lymphomas produced was insignificant, but a significantly high incidence of lung adenomas was found (Frei, 1971).

Ethyl methanesulfonate induces a high incidence of primary kidney tumors in rats. The tumors are histologically indistinguishable from those induced by dimethylnitrosamine, N-methyl-N-nitrosourea, and the natural product cycasin (Swann and Magee, 1969). In rat experiments 24 100 g female Wistar albino rats of the Porton strain were given three i.p. doses of 27.5 mg in 1 ml of 0.9% aqueous sodium chloride. The first kidney tumor was found 7 months after the first dose, and ultimately 12 rats had kidney tumors. In the same study when 22 rats were given one i.p. dose of 35 mg/kg body weight of EMS, one animal was later found with a brain tumor classified as an ependyoma.

In another study using Sprague-Dawley rats, each animal starting at age 6 weeks had three i.p. injections of 33 mg of the alkylating agent. Male and female animals, intact and nephrectomized, were used. None of the control animals had tumors, but 53% (35 out of 66 animals) of the treated animals developed malignant neoplasms, most of which were anaplastic lung lesions or adenocarcinomas of the abdominal wall. Females were much more susceptible than males, but unilateral nephrectomy did not affect tumor incidence or appearance. Unlike the study of Swann and Magee (1969), no renal tumors developed among these rats (Hrushesky et al., 1972).

Other Alkyl Methanesulfonates

$$RO-\overset{\overset{O}{\|}}{\underset{\underset{O}{\|}}{S}}-CH_3$$

Roe (1957) tested a series of monofunction and difunctional methanesulfonates for carcinogenic properties. The protocol he used consisted of 10 weekly skin applications of the test substance at a specified dosage, in addition to 18 weekly applications of a solution of croton oil. The croton oil treatments began after the first skin application of the test substance and they were continued 8 weeks after the application of the test compound was discontinued. With these procedures, using stock albino male mice of the "S" strain, the croton oil control groups had one tumor-bearing animal in a group of 17 and one in a group of 20 animals, one animal with one and the other with three papillomas. Butyl methanesulfonate at either 8 or 80 mg/application to groups of 10 mice with the concurrent croton oil treatment caused no papillomas. Alkyl methanesulfonate ($R=CH_2-CH=CH_2$) applied at 13.5 mg/application led to 12 tumor bearing animals among 17 survivors. Propargyl methanesulfonate ($R=CH_2-C\equiv CH$) caused four tumors among the 19 surviving animals.

Roe found that the saturated difunctional methanesulfonate Myleran, 1,4-dimethylsufonoxybutane, which is used as a chemotherapeutic agent in myeloid leukemia cases, caused fewer tumors than the croton oil alone. The unsaturated analogue of Myleran, cis- and trans-1,4-dimethylsulfoxy-2-butene, induced papillomas in three out of 17 and 10 out of 18 animals, respectively. The alkyne analogue, 1,4-dimethylsufoxy-3-butyne, caused 14 tumors in five of the 10 surviving animals. 1,8-Dimethanesulfonoxyoctane proved to be inactive.

Esters of p-Toluenesulfonic Acid

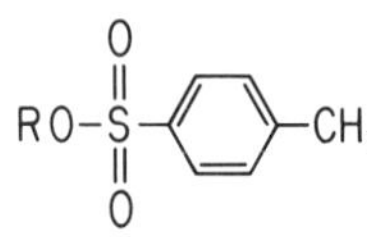

Druckrey and his co-workers (1970a) investigated the carcinogenic potential of a number of esters of p-toluenesulfonic acid. Weekly s.c. injections in groups of 10 BD rats of 15, 50, and 250 mg/kg body weight of the methyl, ethyl, and butyl esters of p-toluenesulfonic acid, respectively, led to seven sarcomas along with three other tumors, three and zero sarcomas, respectively. Of 16 rats that received a 15-mg weekly oral dose of methyl p-toluenesulfonic acid, one developed a fibrosarcoma.

VIII. ACYLATING AGENTS

Dimethylcarbamyl Chloride

$$(H_3C)_2N\overset{\overset{O}{\|}}{C}Cl$$

Dimethylcarbamyl chloride is a reactive acylating agent used as an intermediate in chemical industry and in laboratories. To date, only one other carcinogenic acylating agent, N-acetylimidiazole, is known (Stoner et al., 1975). There are a variety of published patents on the use of dimethylcarbamyl chloride in the preparation of pesticides, fungicides, and medicinal compounds. A present major use of this acylating agent is in the synthesis of the cholinergic agents pyridostigmine, neostigmine bromide, and neostigmine methosulfate, which are used in the treatment of myasthenia graves.

We (Van Duuren et al., 1972a) tested the purified compound by skin application in 50 female ICR/Ha Swiss mice at a dose level of 2 mg (in acetone) 3 times/week. After 385 days on test, 34 mice had a total of 92 papillomas and 11 squamous carcinomas. When given s.c. to the same number and strain of mice, 5 mg weekly, 35 sarcomas developed after 26 weeks of treatment. When 1.0 mg was given i.p. weekly to a third group of 30 mice, eight local sarcomas developed, but the number of papillary lung tumors found was not significantly greater than in the solvent control.

An air inhalation experiment by Laskin and co-workers (1978) using male Sprague-Dawley rats also showed that dimethylcarbamyl chloride is a potent carcinogen. Of 100 rats exposed to 1 ppm of this acylating agent for 6 hr/day, 5 days/week for their lifetimes, 96 of the 98 animals available for examination developed squamous cell carcinoma of the epithelial lining of the nasal cavity. This same research team previously showed that bis(chloromethyl)ether vapor caused nasal tumors, but only one of 17 was a squamous cell carcinoma, while the rest were esthesioneuroepitheliomas (Kuschner et al., 1975). Zapp (1975a) reported that hexamethyl phosphoramide vapor causes squamous cell carcinoma in rats, while nitroso compounds and bis(chloromethyl)ether are known to cause esthesioneuro-epitheliomas (Thomas, 1965).

Benzoyl Chloride

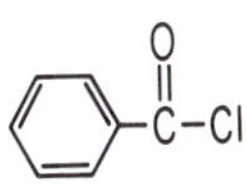

A Japanese chemical plant reported that among 41 workers producing benzoyl chloride over a period of 20 years, four workers developed malignant tumors, three of which were lung tumors and one a lymphoma (Sakabe et al., 1976). Workers at this plant also suffered from a variety of respiratory ailments and skin diseases. The workers had a continued exposure to the major product (benzoyl chloride) and they were also exposed to the starting materials, toluene and chlorine gas, the intermediate (benzotrichloride), and a number of minor chlorinated by-products and various residues and fuels.

IX. MISCELLANEOUS COMPOUNDS

Dioxanes

1,4-Dioxane (p-dioxane) is mainly used as a stabilizer in chlorinated solvents. It is also used as a solvent for cellulose, resins, oils, waxes, and some dyes. In 1976 nearly 15 million lb of dioxane were produced in the United States. Barber (1934) reported that five workers employed in the manufacture of artificial silk who died with central necrosis of the liver and symmetric necrosis of the renal cortex had exposure to dioxane vapor.

When adult male Wistar rats were given 1% p-dioxane in the drinking water for 64 weeks at about 450 days, six of the 26 surviving rats had hepatomas and one had a kidney tumor (Argus et al., 1965). In another study by these investigators male Charles River CD random-bred rats, 30 to a group, received 0.75, 1.0, 1.4, or 1.8% p-dioxane in the drinking water. After 16 months one rat in each of the two lower dose groups and two in each of the two higher dose groups had squamous cell carcinoma of the nasal cavity. No hepatocarcinomas were reported (Hoch-Ligeti et al., 1970).

Groups of 60 Sherman rats were given 0.01, 0.1, or 1.0% p-dioxane in the drinking water for up to 716 days. At the highest dose, 10 hepatocellular carcinomas, two cholargiomas, and three nasal cell carcinomas occurred. No significant number of tumors occurred at the two lower doses (Kociba et al., 1974).

The NIH (NCI, 1978d) recently tested 1,4-dioxane for carcinogenicity by administering it in drinking water at the 0.5% and 1.0% (vol/vol) levels to groups of 35 Osborne-Mendel rats and 60 B6C3F1 mice. Those exposed to the high-dose level drank less water. The rats were dosed for 110 weeks and the mice for 90. In rats a high incidence of squamous cell carcinomas of the nasal turbinates was found: 12/33, 16/34, and 0/33 for male rats at the low, high, and control doses, respectively. Similarly, for the females the incidence was:

10/34, 8/35, and 0/35. Female rats, but not male, also had a significant incidence of hepatocellular adenomas. In both male and female mice 1,4-dioxane induced a high incidence of hepatocellular carcinomas.

The oncogenic activity of 2,6-dimethyl-m-dioxan-4-ol acetate (6-acetoxy-2,4-dimethyl-m-dioxane, also called dimethoxane) was determined in an experiment in which male Wistar rats were given 1% of this dioxane in drinking water for 613 days. The experiment was terminated 3 months later, and 14 tumors were found in 25 rats. Eight of the tumors were hepatomas, and one was a kidney tumor (Hoch-Leğeti et al., 1974).

The commercially available 2,3-dichloro-p-dioxane, which is probably the trans isomer, was tested for carcinogenicity by a number of routes. When applied to the skins of 30 female ICR/Ha mice at a dose of 0.5 mg/0.1 ml acetone 3 times/week for 582 days, it elicited two papillomas and no carcinomas. When tested in the same strain of mice as an initiating agent, one treatment of 0.5 mg, followed by treatments with 2.5 μg of phorbol myristate acetate 3 times/week resulted in eight papillomas and two carcinomas in a group of 30 animals. When given s.c. weekly, 5.0 mg in 0.05 ml of tricaprylin, it induced 14 local sarcomas, one squamous cell carcinoma, and two adenocarcinomas (Van Duuren et al., 1974).

Dioxane may be metabolized to a proximal carcinogen, while the chlorosubstituted p-dioxane is a reactive electrophile and probably is a direct-acting carcinogen; however, the results of a recent biochemical study imply that metabolic activation may not be required for p-dioxane to be a carcinogen. Dioxane given i.p. was found to be distributed among various tissues, especially the liver, spleen, and colon. Pretreatment of male Sprague-Dawley male rats with the monooxygenase enzyme inducers 3-methylcholanthrene, phenobarbital, and polychlorinated biphenyls had no significant effect on the covalent binding of the dioxane to the various liver subcellular fractions (Woo et al., 1977).

Hexamethylphosphoramide

$[(H_3C)_2N]_3PO$

Hexamethylenephosphoramide is used as a processing solvent for aromatic polyamide fibers and as a solvent in chemical laboratories. Haskell Laboratories (Zapp, 1975a, 1975b) using male and female Charles River CD strain rats, 120 per group, exposed the animals 6 hr/day, 5 days/week to 50, 400, and 4000 ppb of the compound. After 6 months those animals that survived in the two high-dose groups had degenerative changes in the convoluted tubules of the kidneys. After 8 months on test animals with enlarged noses and breathing difficulties were noted. Subsequently, many of these animals died of squamous carcinoma of the nasal cavity.

In a previous feeding study, male Sherman rats were kept on daily intakes of 0.78-6.25 mg/kg body weight of hexamethylphosphoramide in their diets. The animals had a poor survival, but the tumor incidence of the survivors was not different from that of the control animals eating the unadulterated diet (Kimbrough and Gaines, 1966). When tested for mutation ability in Salmonella and cell-transforming properties, hexamethylphosphoramide was generally positive, while the unsubstituted compound, phosphoramide, was found to transform a cell line but was not mutagenic. The phenyl-substituted compound, phosphoric trianilide, and N,N',N''-trimethylphosphorothioictriamide were negative in these two assays (Ashby et al., 1977).

X. CONCLUSION

The carcinogenicity of a diverse group of chemical compounds used in industry and sometimes found in the environment has been described in this chapter. Many are direct-acting alkylating or acylating agents, but others are indirect-acting carcinogens, that is, they must be metabolized to yield the proximal carcinogens. Bioassays of all these compounds which are described in this chapter suggest that cancer induction by these chemicals is not a single simple biochemical process. The dose level, route of exposure, species, age, and sex are all relevant in affecting the outcome of a carcinogenesis bioassay. In addition, most animal assays are carried out with single pure substances, whereas the real-world experience with respect to humans is not as simple. Several substances described in this chapter were only carcinogenic when a cocarcinogen was present or if a tumor promoter was used. Humans are undoubtedly exposed to cocarcinogens and tumor promoters in addition to carcinogens. Thus, in the future we must concern ourselves not only with the potential carcinogenicity of a single substance, but with its possible cocarcinogenic and/or tumor-promoting ability as well. We should recognize that chemical carcinogenesis can be a multistep process, and thus, we must concern ourselves with a variety of synergistic agents and effects.

ACKNOWLEDGMENT

The author would like to thank Dr. G. Witz, A. Smith, and S. Melchionne for their helpful comments and editing. The author would also like to thank E. Feigenbaum, D. Gray, and J. Romer for their skilled typing.

REFERENCES

Albert, R. E., Pasternack, B. S., Shore, R. E., Lippmann, M., Nelson, N., and Ferris, B. (1975). Mortality patterns among workers exposed to chloromethyl ethers—a preliminary report. Environ. Health Perspectiv. 11:209-214.

Argus, M. F., Arcos, J. C., and Hoch-Ligeti, C. (1965). Studies on the carcinogenic activity of protein-denaturing agents: Hepatocarcinogenicity of dioxane. J. Natl. Cancer Inst. 35:949-958.

Ashby, J., Styles, J. A., and Anderson, D. (1977). Selection of an in vitro carcinogenicity test for derivatives of the carcinogen hexamethylphosphoramide. Br. J. Cancer 36: 564-571.

Banerjee, S., and Van Duuren, B. L. (1978). Covalent binding of the carcinogen trichloroethylene to hepatic microsomal proteins and to exogenous DNA in vitro. Cancer Res. 38:776-780.

Banerjee, S., Van Duuren, B. L., and Goldschmidt, B. M. (1977). Microsome-dependent covalent binding of the carcinogen trichloroethylene to cellular macromolecules. Proc. Am. Assoc. Cancer Res. 18:34.

Bär, von F., and Griepentrog, F. (1967). The health implications of aromatic substances in food. Med. Evnähr. 8:244-251.

Barber, H. (1934). Haemorrhagic nephritis and necrosis of the liver from dioxan poisoning. Guy's Hosp. Rep. 84:267-280.

Berry, G., Newhouse, M. L., and Turok, M. (1972). Combined effect of asbestos exposure and smoking on mortality from lung cancer in factory workers. Lancet 476-479.

Bingham, E., and Nord, P. J. (1977). Cocarcinogenic effects of n-alkanes and ultraviolet light on mice. J. Natl. Cancer Inst. 58:1099-1101.

Bolt, H. M., and Filser, J. G. (1977). Irreversible binding of chlorinated ethylenes to macromolecules. Environ. Health Perspect. 21:107-112.

Bonser, G. M., Boyland, E., Busby, E. R., Clayson, D. B., Grover, P. L., and Jull, J. W. (1963). Implantation in the mouse as a means of detecting carcinogenic activity: use of crushed paraffin wax or stearic acid as the vehicle. Br. J. Cancer. 17:127-136.

Boyland, E., Busby, E. R., Dukes, C. E., Grover, P. L., and Manson, D. (1964). Further experiments on implantation of materials into the urinary bladder of mice. Br. J. Cancer 18:575-581.

Brem, H., Stein, A. B., and Rosenkranz, H. S. (1974). The mutagenicity and DNA-modifying effect of haloalkanes. Cancer Res. 34:2576-2579.

Brookes, P., and Lawley, P. D. (1961). The reaction of mono- and difunctional alkylating agents with nucleic acids. Biochem. J. 80:496-503.

Brookes, P. B., and Lawley, P. D. (1963). Effects of alkylating agents on T2 and T4 bacteriophages. Biochem. J. 89:138-144.

Byrén, D., and Holmberg, B. (1975). Two possible cases of angiosarcoma of the liver in a group of Swedish vinyl chloride-polyvinyl chloride workers. Ann. NY Acad. Sci. 246:249-250.

Cabral, J. R., Shubik, P., Mollner, T., and Raitano, F. (1977). Carcinogenic activity of hexachlorobenzene in hamsters. Nature 269:510-511.

Cam, C., and Nigogosyan, G. (1963). Acquired toxic prophyria cutanea tarda due to hexachlorobenzene. J. Am. Med. Assoc. 183:88-91.

Capurro, P. U., and Eldridge, J. E. (1978). Solvent exposure and cancer. Lancet 942.

Casterline, C. L., Casterline, P. F., and Jaques, D. A. (1977). Squamous cell carcinoma of the buccal mucosa associated with chronic oral polyvinyl chloride exposure. Cancer 39:1686-1688.

Chang, C.-J., Lee, C.-G. (1978). Direct study of alkylating agent-RNA interaction by ^{13}C nuclear magnetic resonance spectroscopy. Cancer Res. 38:3734-3736.

Chem. Eng. News (1977). 1,2-Dibromo-3-chloropropane. May 30, p. 6.

Chem. Eng. News (1978a). Styrene. Feb. 20, p. 23.

Chem. Eng. News (1978b). Dibromoethane. Feb. 27, p. 17.

Chem. Eng. News (1978c). Epichlorohydrin. Aug. 14, p. 18.

Chen, T. S., and DuBois, K. P. (1973). Studies on the enzyme inducing effect of polychlorinated biphenyls. Toxicol. Appl. Pharmacol. 26:504-512.

Chernozemski, I. N. and Warwick, G. P. (1970). Production of hepatomas in suckling mice after single application of β-propiolactone. J. Natl. Cancer Inst. 45:709-717.

Clapp, N. K., Craig, A. W., and Toya, R. E., Sr. (1968). Oncogenicity by methyl methanesulfonate in male RF mice. Science 161:913-914.

Colburn, N. H. and Boutwell, R. K. (1968). The in vivo binding of β-propiolactone to mouse skin DNA, RNA, and protein. Cancer Res. 28:642-652.

Conncll, D. I. (1961). Carcinogenicity of ethyl methane sulphonate. Br. Emp. Cancer Camp. 39:77.

Corbett, T. H., Heidelberger, C., and Dove, W. F. (1970). Determination of the mutagenic activity to bacteriophage T4 of carcinogenic and noncarcinogenic compounds. Mol. Pharmacol. 6:667-679.

Costa, A., Weber, G., Bartolini St. Omer, F., and Campana, G. (1963). Experimental cancer and cirrhosis induced in the rat by CCl_4. Arch. De Vecchi Anat. Patol. 39: 303-356. Reported in Carcinogenesis Abst. (1963-1964) 1:64-2110.

Creech, J. L., Jr., and Johnson, M. N. (1974). Angiosarcoma of the liver in the manufacture of polyvinyl chloride. J. Occup. Med. 16:150-151.

Decoufle, P. (1976). Occupational carcinogenesis. Cancer mortality among workers exposed to cutting oil mist. Ann. NY Acad. Sci. 271:94-101.

Decoufle, P. (1978). Further analysis of cancer mortality patterns among workers exposed to cutting oil mists. J. Natl. Cancer Inst. 61:1025-1030.

DeFonso, L. R., and Kelton, S. C., Jr. (1976). Lung cancer following exposure to chloromethyl methyl ether. An epidemiological study. Arch. Environ. Health 31: 125-130.

Delorne, F., and Thériault, G. (1978). Ten cases of angiosarcoma of the liver in Shawinigan, Quebec. J. Occup. Med. 20:338-340.

Dickens, F., and Jones, H. E. (1961). Carcinogenic activity of a series of reactive lactones and related substances. Br. J. Cancer 15:85-100.

Dickens, F. and Jones, H. E. (1963). Further studies on the carcinogenic and growth-inhibitory activity of lactones and related substances. Br. J. Cancer 17:100-108.

Dickens, F. and Jones, H. E. (1965). Further studies on the carcinogenic action of certain lactones and related substances in the rat and mouse. Br. J. Cancer 19:392-403.

Dickens, F., Jones, H. E., and Waynforth, H. B. (1966). Oral, subcutaneous and intratracheal administration of carcinogenic lactones and related substances: the intratracheal administration of cigarette tar in the rat. Br. J. Cancer 20:134-144.

Dowty, B., Carlisle, D., Laseter, J., and Stover, J. (1975). Halogenated hydrocarbons in New Orleans drinking water and blood plasma. Science 187:75-77.

Drew, R. T., Laskin, S., Kuschner, M., and Nelson, N. (1975). Inhalation cancinogenicity of alpha halo ethers. I. The acute inhalation toxicity of chloromethyl methyl ether and bis(chloromethyl) ether. Arch. Environ. Health 30:61-69.

Druckrey, H., Gimmy, J., and Landschütz, Ch. (1973). Cancerogenicity of diisopropylsulphate (DIPS) and non-cancerogenicity of monomethylsulphate in BD-rats. Z. Krebsforsch 79:135-140.

Druckrey, H., Kruse, H., and Preussmann, R. (1968). Propanesultone, a potent carcinogen. Naturwissenschaften 55:449.

Druckrey, H., Kruse, H., Preussmann, R., Ivankovic, S., and Landschutz, Ch. (1970a). Cancerogenic alkylating substances. III. Alkyl-halogenides, -sulfates, -sulfonates and strained heterocyclic compounds. Z. Krebsforsch. 74:241-273.

Druckrey, H., Kruse, H., Preussmann, R., Ivankovic, S., Landschutz, Ch., and Gimmy, J. (1970b). Cancerogenic alkylating substances. IV. 1,3-propane sultone and 1,4-butane sultone. Z. Krebsforsch. 75:69-84.

Druckrey, H., Preussmann, R., Nashed, N., and Ivankovic, S. (1966). Carcinogenic alkylating agents. I. Dimethylsulfate, carcinogenic effect in rats and probable cause of occupational cancer. Z. Krebsforsch. 68:103-111.

EPA (1975). Preliminary assessment of suspected carcinogens in drinking water, October Report, Washington, D.C.

Fed. Reg. (1978). Toxic substances control act. 43:No. 52, March 10.

Figueroa, W. G., Raszkowski, R., and Weiss, W. (1973). Lung cancer in chloromethyl ether workers. N. Engl. J. Med. 288:1096-1097.

Frankel, L. S., McCallum, K. S., and Collier, L. (1974). Formation of bis(chloromethyl) ether from formaldehyde and hydrogen chloride. Environ. Sci. Tech. 8:356-359.

Frei, J. V. (1971). Tumour induction by low molecular weight alkylating agents. Chem. Biol. Interact. 3:117-121.

Gage, J. C. (1970). Subacute inhalation toxicity of 109 industrial chemicals. Br. J. Ind. Med. 27:1-18.

Gallagher, C. H. (1962). The effect of antioxidants on poisoning by carbon tetrachloride. Aust. J. Exp. Biol. 40:241-254.

Gargus, J. L., Reese, W. H., Jr., and Rutter, H. A. (1969). Induction of lung adenomas in newborn mice by bis(chloromethyl) ether. Toxicol. Appl. Pharmacol. 15:92-96.

Gibel, W., Lohs, Kh., Wildner, G. P. (1975). Carcinogenic activity of propanol, 2-methyl-1-propanol and 3-methyl-1-butanol. Arch. Geschwulstforsch. 45:19-24.

Gilman, J. P., and Vesselinovitch, S. D. (1955). Cutting oils and squamous-cell carcinoma. Part II: an experimental study of the carcinogenicity of two types of cutting oils. Br. J. Ind. Med. 12:244-248.

Girard, R., Tolot, F., Martin, P., and Bourret, J. (1969). Serious blood disorders due to chlorinated benzene derivatives (relating to seven cases). J. Med. Lyon 50:771-773.

Goldschmidt, B. M. (1965). Carcinogenic epoxides, lactones and hydroperoxides. In <u>Mycotoxins in Foodstuffs</u>, G. N. Wogan (ed.). M.I.T. Press, Cambridge, Mass., pp. 287-288.

Goldschmidt, B. M., Blazej, T. P., Blair, R. D., Langseth, L., and Van Duuren, B. L. (1968a). The reaction of glycidaldehyde with nucleosides and DNA. Proc. Am. Assoc. Cancer Res. 9:25.

Goldschmidt, B. M., Blazej, T. P., and Van Duuren, B. L. (1968b). The reaction of guanosine and deoxyguanosine with glycidaldehyde. Tetrahedron Lett. 13:1583-1586.

Goldschmidt, B. M., Frenkel, K., and Van Duuren, B. L. (1974). The reaction of propane sultone with guanosine, adenosine and related compounds. J. Heterocyclic Chem. 11: 719-722.

Goldschmidt, B. M., Van Duuren, B. L., and Frenkel, K. (1975). The reaction of ^{14}C-labelled bis(chloromethyl)ether with DNA. Proc. Am. Assoc. Cancer Res. 16:66.

Goldschmidt, B. M., Van Duuren, B. L., and Goldstein, R. C. (1979). The reaction of guanine with some potential metabolites of 1-chloropropene. Tetrahedron Lett. No. 14: 1177-1180.

Gorrie, T. M., Raman, S. K., Rouette, H. K., and Zollinger, H. (1973). NMR—investigation of the formaldehyde addition and oligomerisation equilibria in the system formaldehyde/water/acetic acid/hydrochloric acid. Helv. Chim. Acta 56:175-195.

Gosselin, R. E., Hodge, H. C., Smith, R. P., and Gleason, M. N. (1976). <u>Clinical Toxicology of Commercial Products</u>, 4th Ed., Williams and Wilkins, Baltimore.

Griepentrog, F. (1973). Pathological-anatomical findings of the carcinogen coumarin in animal experiments. Toxicology 1:93-102.

Guerzoni, M. E., DelCupolo, L., and Ponti, I. (1976). Mutagenic activity of pesticides. Riv. Sci. Tech. Alimenti Nutr. Un. 6:161-165. Reported in Chem. Abst. (1977), 86:12493b.

Haddow, A., Dukes, C. E., Roe, F. J., Mitchley, B. C., and Everett, J. L. (1962). Carcinogenicity tests. Br. Emp. Cancer Camp. 40:30-34.

Hadler, M. I., and Mueller, K. W. (1977). The disturbance of oxidative phosphorylation in rat liver mitochrondria by the carcinogens 12-hydroxystearic acid and its methyl ester. J. Environ. Pathol. Toxicol. 1:75-85.

Hagan, E. C., Hansen, W. H., Fitzhugh, O. G., Jenner, P. M., Jones, W. I., Taylor, J. M., Long, E. L., Nelson, A. A., and Brouwer, J. B. (1967). Food flavourings and compounds of related structure. II. Subacute and chronic toxicity. Food Cosmet. Toxicol. 5:141-157.

Hallowell, M. (1959). Acute haemolytic anemia following the ingestion of para-dichlorobenzene. Arch. Dis. Child. 34:74-75.

Hamburger, S. J., and Goldstein, B. D. (1978). The cross-linking effects of malonaldehyde on DNA and chromatin protein. Fed. Proc. 37:1641.

Hammond, A. L. (1972). Chemical pollution: polychlorinated biphenyls. Science 175:155-156.

Hathway, D. E. (1977). Comparative mammalian metabolism of vinyl chloride and vinylidene chloride in relation to oncogenic potential. Environ. Health Perspect. 21:55-59.

Heath, C. W., Jr., Falk, H., and Creech, J. L., Jr. (1975). Characteristics of cases of angiosarcoma of the liver among vinyl chloride workers in the United States. Ann. NY Acad. Sci. 246:231-236.

Hendry, J. A., Homer, R. F., Rose, F. L., and Walpole, A. L. (1951). Cytotoxic agents: II, Bis-epoxides and related compounds. Br. J. Pharmacol. 6:235-255.

Henschler, D. (1977). Metabolism and mutagenicity of halogenated olefins—a comparison of structure and activity. Environ. Health Perspect. 21:61-64.

Hoch-Ligeti, C., Argus, M. F., and Arcos, J. C. (1970). Induction of carcinomas in the nasal cavity of rats by dioxane. Br. J. Cancer 24:164-167.

Hoch-Ligeti, C., Argus, M. F., and Arcos, J. C. (1974). Oncogenic activity of an m-dioxane derivative: 2,6-dimethyl-m-dioxan-4-ol acetate (dimethoxane). J. Natl. Cancer Inst. 53:791-794.

Holsti, P. (1959). Tumor promoting effects of some long chain fatty acids in experimental skin carcinogenesis in the mouse. Acta Pathol. Microbiol. Scand. 46:51-58.

Horton, A. W., Denman, D. T., and Trosset, R. P. (1957). Carcinogenesis of the skin. II. The accelerating properties of aliphatic and related hydrocarbons. Cancer Res. 17:758-766.

Horton, A. W., Eshleman, D. N., Schuff, A. R., and Perman, W. H. (1976). Correlation of cocarcinogenic activity among n-alkanes with their physical effects on phospholipid micelles. J. Natl. Cancer Inst. 56:387-391.

Hoshino, H., Chihara, G., and Fukuoka, F. (1970). Detection of potential weak carcinogens and procarcinogens. II. Carcinogenicity of tertiary butyl hydroperoxide. Gan. 61: 121-124.

Hrushesky, W. H., Sampson, D., and Murphy, G. P. (1972). Carcinogenicity of ethylmethanesulfonate. J. Natl. Cancer Inst. 49:1077-1083.

Hutzinger, O., Safe, S., and Zitko, V. (1974). The Chemistry of PCB's. CRC, Cleveland.

Iatropoulos, M. J., Hobson, W., Knauf, V., and Adams, M. P. (1976). Morphological effects of hexachlorobenzene toxicity in female rhesus monkeys. Toxicol. Appl. Pharmacol. 37:433-444.

IARC (1972). Carbon tetrachloride. In Evaluation of Carcinogenic Risk of Chemicals to Man, IARC Monographs, Vol. 1. Lyon, France, pp. 53-60.

Ito, N., Nagasaki, H., Arai, M., Makiura, S., Sugihara, S., and Hirao, K. (1973). Histopathologic studies on liver tumorigenesis induced in mice by technical polychlorinated biphenyls and its promoting effect on liver tumors induced by benzene hexachloride. J. Natl. Cancer Inst. 51:1637-1646.

Izard, M. C. (1973). Research on the effect of the mutagen acrolein and two of its epoxides: glycidol and glycidaldehyde on Saccharomyces cerevisiae. C. R. Acad. Sci. [D] (Paris) 276:3037-3041.

Jones, B. K., and Hathway, D. E. (1978). Differences in metabolism of vinylidene chloride between mice and rats. Br. J. Cancer 37:411-417.

Kallos, G. J., and Solomon, R. A. (1973). Investigations of the formation of bischloromethyl ether in simulated hydrogen chloride-formaldehyde atmospheric environments. Am. Ind. Hyg. Assoc. J. 34:469-473.

Khachatryan, E. A. (1972a). The role of chloroprene compounds in the process of skin neoplasm formation. Gig. Tr. Prof. Zabol. 18:54-55.

Khachatryan, E. A. (1972b). Lung cancer morbidity among persons working with chloroprene. Vopr. Onkol. 18:85-86.

Kimbrough, R. D., and Gaines, T. B. (1966). Toxicity of hexamethylphosphoramide in rats. Nature 211:146-147.

Kimura, N. T., and Baba, T. (1973). Neoplastic changes in the rat liver induced by polychlorinated biphenyl. Gan. 64:105-108.

Kimura, N. T., Kanematsu, T., and Baba, T. (1976). Polychlorinated biphenyls as a promoter in experimental hepatocarcinogenesis in rats. Z. Krebsforsch. 87:257-266.

Kishizawa, F. (1956). Carcinogenic action of para-benzoquinone on the lung of mice by the experimental inhalation. Gan. 47:601-603.

Kociba, R. J., McCollister, S. B., Park, C., Torkelson, T. R., and Gehring, P. J. (1974). 1,4-Dioxane. I. Results of a 2-year ingestion study in rats. Toxicol. Appl. Pharmacol. 30:275-286.

Kociba, R. J., Schwetz, B. A., Keyes, D. G., Jersey, G. C., Ballard, J. J., Dittenbar, D. A., Quast, J. F., Wade, C. E., and Huniston, C. G. (1977). Chronic toxicity and reproduction studies of hexachlorobutadiene in rats. Environ. Health Perspect. 21:49-53.

Kolmark, G., and Giles, N. H. (1955). Comparative studies of monoepoxides as inducers of reverse mutations in Neurospora. Genetics 40:890-902.

Kotin, P., and Falk, H. L. (1963). Organic peroxides, hydrogen peroxide, epoxides and neoplasia. Radiat. Res. (Suppl.) 3:193-211.

Krasnyak, E. P., Zaritskaya, L. A., Boiko, V. G., Voitenko, G. A., and Matokhnyak, L. A. (1969). Health of vineyard workers having contact with the fumigants hexachlorobutadiene and polychlorobutane-80. Vrach. Delo. 7:111-115. Reported in Chem. Abst. (1969), 94514m.

Kubinski, Z. O., and Kubinski, H. (1978). Changes in transforming activity of DNA caused by two carcinogens β-propiolactone and 1,3-propanesultone. Proc. Am. Assoc. Cancer Res. 19:227.

Kucerova, M., Polivkova, Z., Svam, R., and Matousek, V. (1976). Mutagenic effect of epichlorohydrin. I. Testing on human lymphocytes in vitro in comparison with TEPA. Mutat. Res. 34:271-278.

Kuschner, M. (1980). Personal communication.

Kuschner, M., Laskin, S., Drew, R. T., Cappiello, V., and Nelson, N. (1975). Inhalation carcinogenicity of alpha-halo ethers. III. Lifetime and limited period inhalation studies with bis(chloromethyl)ether at 0.1 ppm. Arch. Environ. Health 30:73-77.

Laskin, S., Drew, R. T., Cappiello, V., Kuschner, M., and Nelson, N. (1975). Inhalation carcinogenicity of alpha halo ethers. II. Chronic inhalation studies with chloromethyl methyl ether. Arch. Environ. Health 30:70-72.

Laskin, S., Kuschner, M., Katz, G. V., Sellakumar, A. R., Rusch, G. M., LaMendola, S. L., and Nelson, N. (1980). Upper respiratory tract tumors induced by dimethylcarbamoyl chloride. J. Env. Toxicol. & Path. In Press.

Lemen, R. A., Johnson, W. M., Wagoner, J. K., Archer, V. E., and Saccomanno, G. (1976). Cytologic observations and cancer incidence following exposure to BCME. Ann. NY Acad. Sci. 271:71-80.

Leong, B. K., Macfarland, H. N., and Reese, W. H., Jr. (1971). Induction of lung adenomas by chronic inhalation of bis(chloromethyl) ether. Arch. Environ. Health 22:663-666.

Lilis, R., Anderson, H., Nicholson, W. J., Daum, S., Fischbein, A. S., and Selikoff, I. J. (1975). Prevalence of disease among vinyl chloride and polyvinyl chloride workers. Ann. NY Acad. Sci. 246:22-41.

Lillian, D., Singh, H. B., Appleby, A., Lobban, L., Arnts, R., Gumpert, R., Hague, R., Toomey, J., Kazazis, J., Antell, M., Hansen, D., and Scott, B. (1975). Atmospheric fates of halogenated compounds. Environ. Sci. Tech. 9:1042-1048.

Litterst, C. L., Farber, T. M., Baker, A. M., and Van Loon, E. J. (1972). Effect of polychlorinated biphenyls on hepatic microsomal enzymes in the rat. Toxicol. Appl. Pharmacol. 23:112-122.

Lloyd, J. W., Moore, R. M., and Breslin, P. (1975). Background information on trichloroethylene. J. Occup. Med. 17:603-605.

Loveless, A. (1969). Possible relevance of 0-6 alkylation of deoxyguanosine to the mutagenicity and carcinogenicity of nitrosamines and nitrosamides. Nature 223:206-207.

Makiura, S., Aoe, H., Sugihara, S., Hirao, K., Arai, M., and Ito, N. (1974). Inhibitory effect of polychlorinated biphenyls on liver tumorigenesis in rats treated with 3-methyldimethylaminoazobenzene, N-2-fluorenylacetamide, and diethylnitrosamine. J. Natl. Cancer Inst. 53:1253-1257.

Maltoni, C. (1975). The value of predictive experimental environmental carcinogeneses. An example: vinyl chloride. AMBIO 4:18-23.

Maltoni, C. (1977). Recent findings on the carcinogenicity of chlorinated olefins. Environ. Health Perspect. 21:1-5.

Maltoni, C., and Lefemine, G. (1974). Carcinogenicity bioassays of vinyl chloride. I. Research plans and early results. Environ. Res. 7:387-405.

Mansuy, D., Beaune, P., Cresteil, T., Lange, M., and Leroux, J. P. (1977). Evidence for phosgene formation during liver microsomal oxidation of chloroform. Biochem. Biophys. Res. Commun. 79:513-517.

Mastromatteo, E. (1955). Cutting oils and squamous-cell carcinoma. Part I: incidence in a plant with a report of six cases. Br. J. Ind. Med. 12:240-243.

Maté, U., Solomon, J. J., and Segal, A. (1977). In vitro binding of β-propiolactone to calf thymus DNA and mouse liver DNA to form 1-(2-carboxyethyl)adenine. Chem. Biol. Interact. 18:327-336.

McCammon, C. J., Kotin, P., and Falk, H. L. (1957). The cancerogenic potential of certain diepoxides. Proc. Am. Assoc. Cancer Res. 3:229-230.

McCann, J., Choi, E., Yamasaki, E., and Ames, B. N. (1975). Detection of carcinogens as mutagens in the Salmonella/microsome test. Assay of 300 chemicals. Proc. Natl. Acad. Sci. 72:5135-5139.

McConnell, G., Ferguson, D. M., and Pearson, C. R. (1975). Chlorinated hydrocarbons and the environment. Endeavor 34: 13-18.

Murphree, H. B., Greenberg, L. A., and Carroll, R. G. (1967). Neuropharmacological effects of substances other than ethanol in alcoholic beverages. Fed. Proc. 26: 1468-1473.

Murray, A. J., and Riley, J. P. (1973). Occurrence of some chlorinated aliphatic hydrocarbons in the environment. Nature 242: 37-38.

Murzakaev, F. G. (1967). Action exerted by low hexachlorobutadiene doses on the activity of the central nervous system and morphological changes in animals so poisoned. Gig. Tr. Prof. Zabol. 11: 23-28. Reported in Chem. Abst. (1967), 31040a.

NCI (1977). Carcinogenesis Technical Report Series 13 (Tetrachloroethylene), Washington, D.C.

NCI (1978a). Carcinogenesis Technical Report Series 27 (1, 1, 2, 2-Tetrachloroethane), Washington, D.C.

NCI (1978b). Carcinogenesis Technical Report Series 38 (Aroclor 1254), Washington, D.C.

NCI (1978c). Carcinogenesis Technical Report Series 76 (Tris-(2, 3-dibromopropyl)phosphate), Washington, D.C.

NCI (1978d). Carcinogenesis Technical Report Series 80 (1,4-Dioxane), Washington, D.C.

NCI (1978e). Carcinogenesis Technical Report Series 81 (Trimethylphosphate), Washington, D.C.

Nelson, N. (1973). Carcinogenicity of halo ethers. N. Engl. J. Med. 288: 1123.

Nicholson, W. J., Hammond, E. C., Seidman, H., and Selikoff, I. J. (1975). Mortality experience of a cohort of vinyl chloride-polyvinyl chloride workers. Ann. NY Acad. Sci. 246: 225-230.

NIOSH (1977). Current intelligence bulletin. Acrylonitrile. July 1, Washington, D.C.

Ockner, R. K., and Schmid, R. (1961). Acquired porphyria in man and rat due to hexachlorobenzene intoxication. Nature 189: 499.

Olson, W. A., Habermann, R. T., Weisburger, E. K., Ward, J. M., and Weisburger, J. H. (1973). Brief communication: induction of stomach cancer in rats and mice by halogenated aliphatic fumigants. J. Natl. Cancer Inst. 51: 1993-1995.

Palmes, E. D., Orris, L., and Nelson, N. (1962). Skin irritation and skin tumor production by beta propiolactone (βPL). Am. Ind. Hyg. Assoc. J. 23: 257-264.

Palotay, J. L., Adachi, K., Dobson, R. L., and Pinto, J. S. (1976). Carcinogen-induced cutaneous neoplasms in nonhuman primates. J. Natl. Cancer Inst. 57: 1269-1274.

Parsons, L. D. (1942). On early tumour formation in pure-line mice treated with carcinogenic compounds and the associated blood and tissue changes. J. Pathol. Bact. 54: 321-330.

Pasternack, B. S., Shore, R. E., and Albert, R. E. (1977). Occupational exposure to chloromethyl ethers. J. Occup. Med. 19: 741-746.

Poirier, L. A., Stoner, G. D., and Shimkin, M. B. (1975). Bioassay of alkylhalides and nucleotide base analogs by pulmonary tumor response in strain A mice. Cancer Res. 35: 1411-1415.

Powers, M. B., and Voelker, R. W. (1976). Evaluation of the oncogenic potential of chloroform by long-term oral administration in rodents. Toxicol. Appl. Pharmacol. 37: 179.

Powers, M. B., Voelker, R. W., Page, N. P., Weisburger, E. K., and Kraybill, H. F. (1975). Carcinogenicity of ethylene dibromide (EDB) and 1, 2-dibromo-3-chloropropane (DBCP) after oral administration in rats and mice. Toxicol. Appl. Pharmacol. 33: 171-172.

Preussmann, R. (1968). Direct-acting alkylating agents as carcinogens. Food Cosmet. Toxicol. 6: 567-576.

Randall, W. S., and Solomon, F. D. Building Six. The Tragedy at Bridesburg. Little Brown & Company, Boston, Mass. (1975).

Rannug, V., Sundvall, A., and Ramel, C. (1978). The mutagenic effect of 1, 2-dichloroethane on Salmonella typhimurium I. Activation through conjugation with glutathione in vitro. Chem. Biol. Interact. 20: 1-16.

Roberts, J. J., and Warwick, G. P. (1963). The reaction of β-propiolactone with guanosine, deoxyguanylic acid and RNA. Biochem. Pharmacol. 12:1441-1442.

Roe, F. J. (1957). Tumor initiation in mouse skin by certain esters of methanesulfonic acid. Cancer Res. 17:64-70.

Roe, F. J., and Glendenning, O. M. (1956). The carcinogenicity of β-propiolactone for mouse skin. Br. J. Cancer 10:357-362.

Roe, F. J., and Salaman, M. H. (1955). Further studies on incomplete carcinogenesis: Triethylene melamine (T.E.M.), 1,2-benzanthracene and β-propiolactone as initiators of skin tumour formation in the mouse. Br. J. Cancer 9:177-203.

Roe, F. J., Walters, M., and Mitchley, B. C. (1962). Carcinogenesis tests using newborn mice. Br. Emp. Cancer Camp. 40:42-43.

Rose, F. L., Hendry, J. A., and Walpole, A. L. (1950). New cytotoxic agents with tumour-inhibitory activity. Nature 165:993-996.

Saffiotti, U., and Shubik, P. (1963). Studies on promoting action in skin carcinogenesis. Natl. Cancer Inst. Monogr. 10:489-507.

Sakabe, H. (1973). Lung cancer due to exposure to bis(chloromethyl)ether. Ind. Health 11:145-148.

Sakabe, H., Matsushita, H., and Koshi, S. (1976). Cancer among benzoyl chloride manufacturing workers. Ann. NY Acad. Sci. 271:67-70.

Schlögel, F. A., and Bannasch, P. (1970). Toxicity and carcinogenic properties of inhaled dimethyl sulfate. Naunyn Schmiedebergs Arch. Pharmakol. 266:441.

Schmid, R. (1960). Cutaneous porphyria in Turkey. N. Engl. J. Med. 263:397-398.

Schwetz, B. A., Leong, B. K., and Gehring, P. J. (1974). Embryo- and fetotoxicity of inhaled chloroform in rats. Toxicol. Appl. Pharmacol. 28:442-451.

Searle, C. E. (1961). Experiments on the carcinogenicity and reactivity of β-propiolactone. Br. J. Cancer 15:804-811.

Searle, C. E. (1966). Tumor initiatory activity of some chloromononitrobenzenes and other compounds. Cancer Res. 26:12-17.

Segal, A., Schroeder, M., Barnett, P., and Van Duuren, B. L. (1974). Studies on the effects in vitro of β-propiolactone and β propiolact[^{14}C]one on whole mouse skin chromatin. Biochem. Pharmacol. 23:937-946.

Selikoff, I. J., Hammond, E. C., and Churg, J. (1968). Asbestos exposure, smoking and neoplasia. JAMA 204:106-112.

Shamberger, R. J. (1971). Inhibitory effect of vitamin A on carcinogenesis. J. Natl. Cancer Inst. 47:667-673.

Shamberger, R., Andreane, T. L., and Willis, C. E. (1974). Antioxidants and cancer. IV. Initiating activity of malonaldehyde as a carcinogen. J. Natl. Cancer Inst. 53: 1771-1773.

Shimkin, M. B., Weisburger, J. H., Weisburger, E. K., Gubareff, N., and Suntzeff, V. (1966). Bioassay of 29 alkylating chemicals by the pulmonary-tumor response in strain A mice. J. Natl. Cancer Inst. 36:915-935.

Short, R. D., Minor, J. L., Winston, J. M., Seifter, J., and Lee, C.-C. (1978). Inhalation of ethylene dibromide during gestation by rats and mice. Toxicol. Appl. Pharmacol. 46:173-182.

Sicé, J. (1966). Tumor-promoting activity of n alkanes and 1-alkanols. Toxicol. Appl. Pharmacol. 9:70-74.

Southam, A. H., and Wilson, S. R. (1922). Cancer of the scrotum: the etiology, clinical features, and treatment of the disease. Br. Med. J. (ii):971-973.

Spencer, H. C., Rowe, V. K., and McCollister, D. D. (1950). Dehydroacetic acid (DHA). I. Acute and chronic toxicity. J. Pharmacol. Exp. Ther. 99:57-68.

Stenbäck, F., and Shubik, P. (1974). Lack of toxicity and carcinogenicity of some commonly used cutaneous agents. Toxicol. Appl. Pharmacol. 30:7-13.

Stoner, G. D., Weisburger, E. K., and Shimkin, M. B. (1975). Tumor response in strain A mice exposed to silylating compounds used for gas-liquid chromatography. J. Natl. Cancer Inst. 54:495-497.

Straus, B. (1954). Aplastic anemia following exposure to carbon tetrachloride. JAMA 155:737-739.

Strauss, B., and Okubo, S. (1960). Protein synthesis and the induction of mutations in E. coli by alkylating agents. J. Bacteriol. 79:464-473.

Suermondt, A. A. (1961). Dichlorobutene. Kunstoffe Plastics 3:307-310.

Swann, P. F., and Magee, P. N. (1968). Nitrosamine-induced carcinogenesis. The alkylation of nucleic acids of the rat by N-methyl-N-nitrosourea, dimethylnitrosamine, dimethyl sulfate and methyl methanesulphonate. Biochem. J. 110:39-47.

Swann, P. F., and Magee, P. N. (1969). Induction of rat kidney tumours by ethyl methanesulphonate and nervous tissue tumours by methyl methanesulphonate and ethyl methanesulphonate. Nature 223:947-949.

Swenberg, J. A., Kerns, W. D., Mitchell, R. I., Gralla, E. J., and Parkov, K. L. (1980). Induction of squamous cell carcinomas of the rat nasal cavity by inhalation exposure to formaldehyde vapor. Cancer Res. 40:3398-3402.

Swern, D., Wieder, R., McDonough, M., Meranze, D. R., and Shimkin, M. B. (1970). Investigation of fatty acids and derivatives for carcinogenic activity. Cancer Res. 30:1037-1046.

Takizawa, N. (1940). The experimental induction of skin and lung tumors in the mouse by brush application of quinone. Gan. 34:158-160.

Theiss, J. C., Shimkin, M. B., and Poirier, L. A. (1979). Induction of pulmonary adenomas in strain A mice by substituted organohalides. Cancer Res. 39:391-395.

Theiss, J. C., Stoner, G. D., Shimkin, M. B., and Weisburger, E. K. (1977). Test for carcinogenicity of organic contaminants of United States drinking waters by pulmonary tumor response in strain A mice. Cancer Res. 37:2717-2720.

Thiess, A. M., Hay, W., and Zeller, H. (1973). The toxicology of bis(chloromethyl) ether—a suspected human carcinogen. Zentralbl. Arbeitsmed. Arbeitsschutz Prophyl. 23:97-102.

Thomas, C. (1965). On the morphology of nasal tumors of the rat. Z. Krebsforsch. 67:1-10.

Thompson, D. J., Warner, S. D., and Robinson, V. B. (1974). Teratology studies on orally administered chloroform in the rat and rabbit. Toxicol. Appl. Pharmacol. 29:348-357.

Torkelson, T. R., Sadek, S. E., Rowe, V. K., Kodana, J. K., Anderson, H. H., Loquvan, G. S., and Hine, C. H. (1961). Toxicologic investigations of 1,2-dibromo-3-chloropropane. Toxicol. Appl. Pharmacol. 3:545-549.

Tracey, J. P., and Sherlock, P. (1968). Hepatoma following carbon tetrachloride poisoning. NY State J. Med. 68:2202-2204.

Ulland, B., Finkelstein, M., Weisburger, E. K., Rice, J. M., and Weisburger, J. H. (1971). Carcinogenicity of industrial chemicals propylene imine and propane sultone. Nature 230:460-461.

Umeda, M. (1957). Production of rat sarcoma by injections of propylene glycol solution of p-quinone. Gan. 48:139-144.

Van Dijek, P., and Van de Voorde, H. (1976). Mutagenicity versus carcinogenicity of organochlorine insecticides. Meded. Fac. Landbouwwet. Rijksuniv. Gent. 41:1491-1498. Chem. Abst. (1977) 86, 66590z.

Van Duuren, B. L. (1977). Chemical structure, reactivity and carcinogenicity of halohydrocarbons. Environ. Health Perspect. 21:17-23.

Van Duuren, B. L., and Banerjee, S. (1976). Covalent interaction of metabolites of the carcinogen trichloroethylene in rat hepatic microsomes. Cancer Res. 36:2419-2422.

Van Duuren, B. L., Blazej, T., Goldschmidt, B. M., Katz, C., Melchionne, S., and Sivak, A. (1971a). Cocarcinogenesis studies on mouse skin and inhibition of tumor induction. J. Natl. Cancer Inst. 46:1039-1044.

Van Duuren, B. L., and Goldschmidt, B. M. (1966). Carcinogenicity of epoxides, lactones and peroxy compounds. III. Biological activity and chemical reactivity. J. Med. Chem. 9:77-79.

Van Duuren, B. L., and Goldschmidt, B. M. (1976). Cocarcinogenic and tumor-promoting agents in tobacco carcinogenesis. J. Natl. Cancer Inst. 56:1237-1242.

Van Duuren, B. L., Goldschmidt, B. M., Katz, C., Langseth, L., Mercado, C., and Sivak, A. (1968). Alpha-haloethers: a new type of alkylating carcinogen. Arch. Environ. Health 16:472-476.

Van Duuren, B. L., Goldschmidt, B. M., Katz, C., and Seidman, I. (1972a). Brief communication: dimethylcarbamyl chloride, a multipotential carcinogen. J. Natl. Cancer Inst. 48:1539-1541.

Van Duuren, B. L., Goldschmidt, B. M., Katz, C., Seidman, I., and Paul, J. (1974). Carcinogenic activity of alkylating agents. J. Natl. Cancer Inst. 53:695-700.

Van Duuren, B. L., Goldschmidt, B. M., and Seidman, I. (1975). Carcinogenic activity of di- and trifunctional α-chloro ethers and of 1,4-dichlorobutene-2 in ICR/Ha Swiss mice. Cancer Res. 35:2553-2557.

Van Duuren, B. L., Goldschmidt, B. M., Loewengart, G., Smith, A. C., Melchionne, S., Seidman, I., and Roth, D. (1979). Carcinogenicity of halogenated olefinic and aliphatic hydrocarbons in mice. J. Natl. Cancer Inst. 63:1433-1439.

Van Duuren, B. L., Katz, C., Goldschmidt, B. M. (1973). Brief communication: cocarcinogenic agents in tobacco carcinogenesis. J. Natl. Cancer Inst. 51:703-705.

Van Duuren, B. L., Katz, C., Goldschmidt, B. M., Frenkel, K., and Sivak, A. (1972b). Carcinogenicity of halo-ethers. II. Structure-activity relationships of analogs of bis(chloromethyl) ether. J. Natl. Cancer Inst. 48:1431-1439.

Van Duuren, B. L., Langseth, L., Goldschmidt, B. M., and Orris, L. (1967a). Carcinogenicity of epoxides, lactones and peroxy compounds. VI. Structure and carcinogenic activity. J. Natl. Cancer Inst. 39:1217-1228.

Van Duuren, B. L., Langseth, L., Orris, L., Baden, M., and Kuschner, M. (1967b). Carcinogenicity of epoxides, lactones and peroxy compounds. V. Subcutaneous injections in rats. J. Natl. Cancer Inst. 39:1213-1216.

Van Duuren, B. L., Langseth, L., Orris, L., Teebor, G., Nelson, N., and Kuschner, M. (1966). Carcinogenicity of epoxides, lactones and peroxy compounds. IV. Tumor response in epithelial and connective tissue in mice and rats. J. Natl. Cancer Inst. 37:825-838.

Van Duuren, B. L., and Loewengart, G. (1977). Reaction of DNA with glycidaldehyde. J. Biol. Chem. 252:5370-5371.

Van Duuren, B. L., Loewengart, G., Seidman, I., Smith, A. C., and Melchionne, S. (1978). Mouse skin carcinogenicity tests of the flame retardants tris(2,3-dibromopropyl) phosphate (TRIS), tetrakis(hydroxymethyl)phosphonium chloride (THPC) and polyvinyl bromide (PVBR). Cancer Res. 38:3236-3240.

Van Duuren, B. L., Melchionne, S., Blair, R., Goldschmidt, B. M., and Katz, C. (1971b). Carcinogenicity of isosters of epoxides and lactones: aziridine ethanol, propane sultone, and related compounds. J. Natl. Cancer Inst. 46:143-149.

Van Duuren, B. L., Nelson, N., Orris, L., Palmes, E. D., and Schmitt, F. L. (1963). Carcinogenicity of epoxides, lactones and peroxy compounds. J. Natl. Cancer Inst. 31:41-55.

Van Duuren, B. L., Orris, L., and Nelson, N. (1965). Carcinogenicity of epoxides, lactones and peroxy compounds. Part II. J. Natl. Cancer. Inst. 35:707-717.

Van Duuren, B. L., Sivak, A., Goldschmidt, B. M., Katz, C., and Melchionne, S. (1969a). Carcinogenicity of haloethers. J. Natl. Cancer Inst. 43:481-486.

Van Duuren, B. L., Sivak, A., Katz, C., and Melchionne, S. (1969b). Inhibition of tumor induction in two-stage carcinogenesis on mouse skin. Cancer Res. 29:947-952.

Viola, P. L., Bigotti, A., and Caputo, A. (1971). Oncogenic response of rat skin, lungs and bones to vinyl chloride. Cancer Res. 31:516-519.

Viola, P. L., and Caputo, A. (1977). Carcinogenicity studies on vinylidene chloride. Environ. Health Perspect. 21:45-47.

Walpole, A. L. (1958). Carcinogenic action of alkylating agents. Ann. NY Acad. Sci. 68:750-761.

Walters, M. A., Roe, F. J., Mitchley, B. C., and Walsh, A. (1967). Further tests for carcinogenesis using newborn mice: 2-naphthylamine, 2-naphthylhydroxylamine, 2 acetylaminofluorene and ethyl methanesulphonate. Br. J. Cancer 21:367-372.

Waterhouse, J. A. (1971). Cutting oils and cancer. Ann. Occup. Hyg. 14:161-170.

Weil, C. S., Condra, N., Haun, C., and Striegel, J. A. (1963). Experimental carcinogenicity and acute toxicity of representative epoxides. Am. Ind. Hyg. Assoc. J. 24: 305-325.

Weiss, W. (1976). Chloromethyl ethers, cigarettes, cough and cancer. J. Occup. Med. 18:194-199.

Weiss, W., and Boucot, K. R. (1975). The respiratory effects of chloromethyl methyl ether. JAMA 234:1139-1142.

Weisburger, E. K. (1977). Carcinogenicity studies on halogenated hydrocarbons. Environ. Health Perspect. 21:7-16.

Winch, R. F. (1978). Results of mouse skin painting tests of seven oils. Report to the Document Control Officer, EPA, Washington, D.C.

Woo, Y.-T., Argus, M. F., and Arcos, J. C. (1977). Tissue and subcellular distribution of ^{3}H-dioxane in the rat and apparent lack of microsome-catalyzed covalent binding in the target tissue. Life Sci. 21:1447-1456.

Zapp, J. A., Jr. (1975a). Inhalation toxicity of HMPA. Am. Ind. Hyg. Assoc. J. 36:916.

Zapp, J. A., Jr. (1975b). HMPA: a possible carcinogen. Science 190:422.

9

Nitrogenous Carcinogenic Industrial Chemicals

PRABHAKAR D. LOTLIKAR / Temple University Medical School, Philadelphia, Pennsylvania

---

Research by the author is supported by grants CA-10604 and CA-12227 from the National Cancer Institute, U.S. Public Health Service.

I. INTRODUCTION

It is generally believed that chemicals are largely responsible for the causation of human cancer (Boyland, 1969; Epstein, 1974; Higginson, 1969). There are thousands of chemicals in our environment, most of which are produced and used in various industries. Based on epidemiological data, few of these chemicals, such as benzidine, 4-biphenylamine, and 2-naphthylamine, have been shown to be responsible for the induction of bladder cancer among industrial workers employed in dye-manufacturing plants (Case and Pearson, 1954; Case et al., 1954; Goldblatt, 1947, 1958; Hueper, 1969; Melick et al., 1955, 1971; Scott, 1962; Walpole et al., 1954). It is known that the induction period for chemical carcinogens to exert their carcinogenic effect in humans is usually 2-3 decades. Like humans, the time required for tumor induction in any animal species depends on its total life span. The minimal period required to induce tumors in animals with potent carcinogenic effects ranges from one-eighth to one-fourth of the life span. All chemicals with the exception of arsenic known to produce cancer in humans have also produced cancer in animals by appropriate tests. This does not necessarily mean that all chemicals that are carcinogenic for animals are also carcinogenic for humans. However, such materials ought to be considered as potential carcinogens for humans. Therefore, as soon as a chemical is shown to be carcinogenic in animal tests, appropriate measures must be taken to prevent or reduce human exposure to that particular chemical.

Rats, mice, hamsters, guinea pigs, and rabbits are the animal species generally used for carcinogenicity studies. Age, sex, strain of animals, and diet are some of the important factors that influence the results of carcinogenesis. Since human exposure to many chemicals is by inhalation, skin contact, or ingestion, these are also the preferred routes of administration of chemicals to animals. In addition, many chemicals are given by various injection routes—intravenous (i.v.), intramuscular (i.m.), intraperitoneal (i.p.), or subcutaneous (s.c.)—to detect their carcinogenic effect.

Animal studies for carcinogen testing are usually time consuming and very expensive, hence new screening methods which require only a few days or weeks to provide preliminary results are being developed. One of such rapid screening tests, the Ames test measures the ability of a chemical to modify the DNA of various specially selected bacterial strains of *Salmonella typhimurium* (Ames et al., 1973). Ames test is being used extensively as a first test in screening for human carcinogens, since the great majority of the chemicals (90%) that cause modifications of DNA (mutations) in bacteria also produce cancer in animals (McCann et al., 1975). It should be mentioned now that a positive result on the Ames test does not establish carcinogenicity; rather it identifies a likely candidate for further testing. Detailed results of this test are not presented in this chapter; however, in some cases overall results of this test system for a group of chemicals are presented.

According to the Occupational Safety and Health Administration (OSHA), a chemical is considered to be a carcinogen if properly designed studies show that exposure to the chemical causes cancer in: (1) humans, (2) two different animal (mammalian) species, or (3) one animal species if the results are duplicated in separate studies (Chem. Eng. News, 1978).

In this chapter only nitrogen-containing industrial chemicals are discussed. The list of chemicals to be discussed in this chapter is by no means complete, but it contains many chemicals that have been and/or are currently in use in industry. Many of these chemicals have been found to be carcinogenic in animal studies, whereas some chemicals have shown no carcinogenic activity under the conditions of the testing. In a few cases carcinogenicity data are not conclusive. Some of the chemicals discussed in this chapter are also used in cosmetics, drugs, and agriculture, and are also discussed in other appropriate chapters.

Nitrogen-containing chemicals have been divided into the following five categories:

1. Aromatic amines and related compounds
2. Azo dyes
3. N-Nitroso compounds
4. Hydrazine and related compounds
5. Miscellaneous compounds

These chemicals are discussed separately in terms of their industrial production and use, animal carcinogenicity, and, when data are available, human toxicity. These chemicals are discussed as a group for their metabolism.

II. AROMATIC AMINES AND RELATED COMPOUNDS

Many of the aromatic amines described in this chapter are used not only in the manufacture of dyestuffs, but also in the rubber and cable-making industries, in textile dyeing and printing, and in the manufacture of pigments, paints, and plastics. Excellent reviews on the carcinogenicity of aromatic amines and related compounds and the epidemiology of aromatic amine cancers have recently appeared (Clayson and Garner, 1976; Parkes, 1976). It is known that early evidence of human cancer was attributed to occupational exposure to chemicals. Thus, bladder cancer was shown among workers involved in the manufacture of magenta (Rehn, 1895). At that time these bladder cancers were called "aniline cancer" by Rehn because aniline was used as an intermediate in the production of magenta and these tumors were thought to result from the hemmorrhagic cystitis associated with aniline exposure. Later experimental studies (Bonser et al., 1956a; Hueper et al., 1938; Spitz et al., 1950; Walpole et al., 1954) and epidemiological studies (Case and Pearson, 1954; Case et al., 1954; Goldblatt, 1947, 1958; Hueper, 1969; Walpole et al., 1954; Scott, 1962) indicated that 2-naphthylamine, benzidine, and 4-biphenylamine were the aromatic amines actually responsible for the bladder tumor induction in workers employed in dyestuff industries. It is believed that these three aromatic amines and their derivatives may account for a large proportion of all the known incidence of industrial bladder cancer.

Some aromatic amines, in addition to being used in various industries, are also used in hair-dye formulations. It is estimated that some 20 million people, mainly women, dye their hair in the United States. Ames and co-workers (1975) have shown that 89% of commercial oxidative-type (hydrogen peroxide) hair-dye formulations are mutagenic in the Ames test. In view of their results, many aromatic amines present in these hair dyes are being tested for their carcinogenic potency in animal model systems. There is no epidemiological evidence as yet implicating hair dyes for increased cancer incidence in women using such hair dyes.

A. Aniline and Related Compounds

Aniline

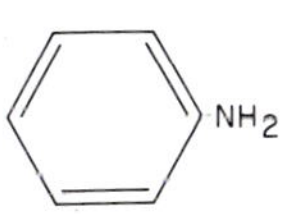

Aniline is a colorless oily liquid that darkens on exposure to air and light. It boils at 184-186°C. It is produced on a commercial scale in the United States. In 1975 the total U.S. production was about 400 million lb (U.S. International Trade Commission, 1977). Aniline is used in the production of at least 150 dyes and dye intermediates. Azo, triphenylmethane, safranine, and anthraquinone are some of the aniline-based dyes. Hydroquinone is one of the most important photographic chemicals derived from aniline. Many pharmaceutical intermediates are also derived from aniline.

Experimental carcinogenesis

In one study rats were given aniline hydrochloride in their drinking water every day over a period of 1-2 years. Under these conditions the total amount of the compound consumed was about 14-16 g/rat. No tumors were seen when bladder, liver, spleen, and kidneys were examined in all rats (Druckrey, 1950). In a recent study, however, aniline hydrochloride was administered in the feed at 0.3 and 0.6% levels to Fischer 344 rats of both sexes for a 2-year period. Under these conditions, aniline was found to be carcinogenic to both sexes, inducing hemangiosarcomas and fibrosarcomas of the spleen. The tumor incidence was much higher in the males than in the females (NCI, 1978f).

Oral administration of aniline hydrochloride in the diet at 0.3 and 0.6% levels to B6C3F1 mice of both sexes for a 2-year period did not induce any tumors in these treated animals (NCI, 1978f). In two separate studies mice were injected s.c. several times with aniline. No tumors were observed in these treated animals (Shear and Stewart, 1941; Hartwell and Andervont, 1951).

Phenylhydroxylamine has not been detected in the urine of animals administered aniline. However, phenylhydroxylamine and nitrosobenzene have been shown to be present in the blood of dogs and cats after these animals have been treated with aniline (Kiese, 1966). No tumors were induced when rats were given repeated i.p. injections of phenylhydroxylamine (Miller et al., 1966; Belman et al., 1968). Tumors did not develop in rats even after repeated s.c. injections of nitrosobenzene (Miller et al., 1965).

Human data

Bladder cancers observed in people involved in the manufacture of fuchsin from commercial aniline were called "aniline bladder cancer" (Rehn, 1895). Later epidemiological studies indicated that 2-naphthylamine, benzidine, and 4-aminobiphenyl were the real etiological agents responsible in the bladder-tumor induction (Walpole et al., 1954; Case and Pearson, 1954; Case et al., 1954; Scott, 1962; Hueper, 1969). These reports appeared to have exonerated aniline as a human carcinogen.

ortho-Toluidine

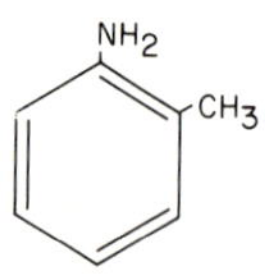

ortho-Toluidine is also known as 2-aminotoluene. It is a light yellow liquid that boils at 200-202°C. According to the International Trade Commission, ortho-toluidine is produced on a commercial scale in the United States (Chem. Eng. News, 1978). A major use of this compound and its hydrochloride (HCl) appears to be as an intermediate in the manufacture of at least 17 dyes that are being produced on a commercial scale in the United States. The most significant dye produced commercially in the United States is CI Vat Red 1. ortho-Aminoazotoluene and a sulfonic acid derivative are also made from ortho-toluidine and its hydrochloride. The last two compounds are used as raw materials for the production of at least 11 dyes in the United States. The most important of these dyes are: CI Acid Red 115, CI Direct Red 72, and CI Solvent Red 26. ortho-Toluidine is also used as an antioxidant in the manufacture of rubber, as an ingredient of a clinical reagent used for blood glucose test, and also to produce special dyes for use in color photography.

Experimental carcinogenesis

Feeding of ortho-toluidine in the diet to male Charles River CD rats for 2 years increased the incidence of s.c. tumors to 83% from the 10% that occurred with the control group. In addition, treated animals developed bladder and liver tumors (Russfield et al., 1973a, b).

Charles River (HA/ICR) CG-1 mice of both sexes given ortho-toluidine in the diet developed vascular tumors (Russfield et al., 1973b).

Human data

ortho-Toluidine is absorbed via the respiratory tract and skin. Acute poisoning with this compound may cause methemoglobinemia and hematuria (ILO, 1971).

According to epidemiological studies carried out among workers in the British chemical industry, there were 812 workers classified as having been exposed to aniline but not to the other suspected carcinogens. Among these, one death certificate indicated bladder tumor, although 0.52 was expected at national rates. Actually, based on the knowledge of aniline production processes, it appears that these workers were actually exposed to ortho-toluidine (Case and Pearson, 1954; Case et al., 1954).

Another study showed two cases of bladder tumors among 75 workers involved in the production of ortho-toluidine and para-toluidine in the Soviet Union during the 1960s. Both workers who had bladder tumors had contact with both isomers (Khlebnikova et al., 1970).

5-Nitro-ortho-Toluidine

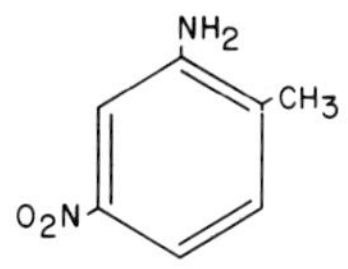

5-Nitro-ortho-toluidine is a yellow crystalline compound that melts at 107-108° C (Weast, 1977-1978). It is also known as 2-methyl-5-nitro-benzenamine. 5-Nitro-ortho-toluidine and its salt are produced commercially in the United States (U.S. International Trade Commission, 1977). According to this report, three companies produced about 1.25×10^5 lb of 5-nitro-ortho-toluidine salt in 1975. It is used as an intermediate in the manufacture of various pigments and azo dyes (Society of Dyers and Colourists, 1971).

Experimental carcinogenesis

In carcinogenicity studies 5-nitro-ortho-toluidine was administered in the diet to Fischer 344 rats and B6C3F1 mice. The concentrations of the compound present in the diet were 0.005 and 0.10% for rats and 0.12 and 0.23% for mice. The test diets were fed for 18 months and the animals were maintained for an additional 6 months. The compound was not carcinogenic to rats; however, it was carcinogenic to mice. The high dose of the compound induced liver tumors in 29/45 males and 20/45 female mice. In control groups liver tumors developed in 12/50 males and 2/47 female mice (NCI, 1978w).

Human data

Symptoms of exposure to 5-nitro-ortho-toluidine include bluish lips and/or fingernails, headache, nausea, and fatigue. Upon dermal contact the compound may irritate the skin, resulting in dermatitis (Synalloy Corporation, 1977). Methemoglobinemia is the major toxic effect observed following excessive absorption of this compound (Hamblin, 1967). The potential for exposure to the compound is greatest for workers at dye-manufacturing facilities. No epidemiological data are yet available.

para-Chloro-ortho-Toluidine

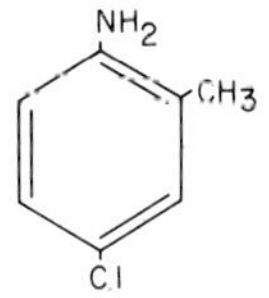

para-Chloro-ortho-toluidine is a greyish-white crystalline compound that melts at 29-30° C. It has been produced on a commercial scale in the United States since 1939. In 1975, both para-chloro-ortho-toluidine and its HCl were produced commercially in the United States (U.S. International Trade Commission, 1977). Both of these compounds are used in the production of various azo dyes for cotton, silk, acetate, and nylon. It is also used as an intermediate in the production of an insecticide used on cotton, fruit and nut trees, and vegetables (IARC, 1978).

Experimental carcinogenesis

Oral lifetime administration of para-chloro-ortho-toluidine HCl to both male and female CD strain mice produced hemangiosarcomas in various organs in these animals. No such tumors developed in control mice (Homburger et al., 1972). No other data are yet available.

Human data

There is one epidemiological study from Switzerland that indicates that among a group of 35 factory workers who were involved in the production of para-chloro-ortho-toluidine during 1924-53, there was no incidence of bladder tumors among these workers (Übelin and Pletscher, 1954). However, it appears that this report did not provide sufficient details on person-years at risk of follow-up to evaluate the significance of their observation (IARC, 1978).

3-Chloro-para-Toluidine

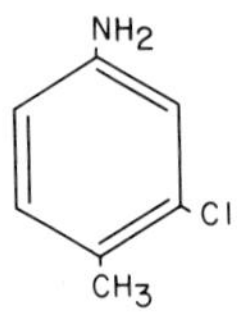

This compound is produced on a commercial scale in the United States (Stanford Research Institute, 1977). 3-Chloro-para-toluidine is used as an intermediate in the production of at least one dye, Palatine Fast Yellow 6GN (Society of Dyers and Colourists, 1956). It is also used as a selective avicide for starling control (Mull and Giri, 1972).

Experimental carcinogenesis

3-Chloro-para-toluidine was tested for carcinogenicity using Fischer 344 strain rats and B6C3F1 mice of both sexes. The dietary concentrations of 3-chloro-para-toluidine administered to rats were 0.16 and 0.33% and to mice were 0.03, 0.06, and 0.12%. The compound was administered in the diet for about 18 months, followed by an observation period of about 6 months. Under these conditions, there was no convincing evidence for the carcinogenicity of 3-chloro-para-toluidine either in rats or mice (NCI, 1978l).

Human data

No case reports or epidemiological data are as yet available.

para-Phenylenediamine

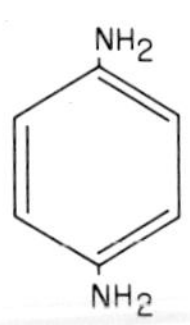

para-Phenylenediamine is a white crystalline compound that darkens on exposure to air; it melts at 145-147°C. The production of para-phenylenediamine on a commercial scale was started in the United States in 1919 (IARC, 1978). The latest report indicates that it was produced commercially in the United States in 1975 (U.S. International Trade Commission, 1977). para-Phenylenediamine has been used in the manufacture of several dyes, accelerating vulcanization, in producing a special fiber used in tires, in hair-dye formulations, in photographic developers, and in a number of antioxidants (IARC, 1978).

Experimental carcinogenesis

In an oral-feeding study daily dose of para-phenylenediamine administered in various concentrations to both male and female rats for an 8-month period did not produce any tumors in these animals. However, daily s.c. administration of this compound at two dose levels for a period of 7 months produced sarcomas at the injection site in 2/5 rats given a low dose. No sarcomas developed in five high-dose-treated and five control rats (Saruta et al., 1958). These investigators failed to indicate the strain of rats used in their studies.

para-Phenylenediamine has been tested in mice by skin-painting technique. In one study this compound was found to be ineffective in producing skin tumors in 19 albino adult mice which survived 20 weeks of treatment (Boutwell and Bosch, 1959). The short duration of the experiment may account for the inability to observe any tumors. In another skin-painting study performed for a longer period (18 months) hair-dye formulations containing other aromatic amines, including para-phenylenediamine, applied on backs of female Webster mice did not show any increase incidence of lung tumors in treated mice compared to the control group (Burnett et al., 1975). It appears that para-phenylenediamine has not been tested adequately to evaluate its carcinogenicity in animals.

Human data

Few cases of para-phenylenediamine fatal poisoning have apparently occurred in women who have used hair dyes containing para-phenylenediamine for several years (Close, 1932; Israels and Susman, 1934; Davison, 1943). Numerous reports of skin allergies to para-phenylenediamine have been reported (Mayer, 1954). No epidemiological data are yet available to implicate involvement of para-phenylenediamine in causing cancer in humans.

meta-Phenylenediamine

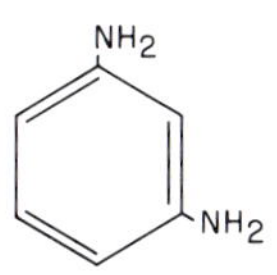

meta-Phenylenediamine is a white crystalline compound that melts at 62-63°C. The commercial production of meta-phenylenediamine was started in the United States in 1919 (IARC, 1978). According to the latest U.S. International Trade Commission Report, this compound was produced on a commercial scale in 1975 (1977). meta-Phenylenediamine is used for the production of various dyes, as a component of hair-dye formulations, as a curing agent for epoxy resins, and for the production of heat-resistant fibers. There are several dyes produced from meta-phenylenediamine which are used to color various textile fibers, leather, paper, polishes, and so on (IARC, 1978).

Experimental carcinogenesis

Wistar-King strain rats were injected s.c. with either meta-phenylenediamine or its hydrochloride at two dose levels on alternate days for 5-11 months. Under these conditions fibrosarcomas were produced in 1/5 animals treated with the lower-dose level of meta-phenylenediamine and 1/5 rats treated with the higher-dose level of its salt. No tumors were observed in the control group (Saruta et al., 1962).

In skin-painting experiments performed with Swiss-Webster mice of both sexes meta-phenylenediamine and other ingredients in a hair-dye formulation did not show any increase incidence of lung tumors compared to their respective controls (Burnett et al., 1975).

It appears that meta-phenylenediamine has not been tested adequately to evaluate its carcinogenicity in animals.

Human data

No information is as yet available.

4-Chloro-meta-Phenylenediamine

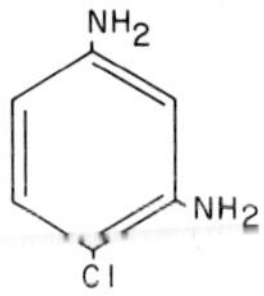

4-Chloro-meta-phenylenediamine is produced on a commercial scale in the United States (Stanford Research Institute, 1977). It is used as an intermediate in the production of several dyes and pigments (Society of Dyers and Colourists, 1956; Mueller, 1976). It can also be used in hair-dye formulations (Corbett, 1973), as a color intensifier in photographic films (Mattor and Price, 1970), and as a cross-linking agent for polyurethane manufacture (Krisnan, 1975).

Experimental carcinogenesis

In this study Fischer 344 rats and B6C3F1 mice of both sexes were administered 4-chloro-meta-phenylenediamine in the diet at concentrations of 0.2 and 0.4% for rats and 0.7 and 1.4% for mice for a period of 18 months. The animals were maintained on a control diet for an additional 6 months. In both species adequate numbers of animals in all groups survived sufficiently long to be at risk from late-developing tumors. Under these conditions 4-chloro-meta-phenylenediamine was carcinogenic to both species, producing liver tumors in female mice and an increased incidence of adrenal tumors in male rats. Liver tumors developed in 8/44 female mice treated with low dose of the compound; no such tumors were observed in 46 control females. Incidences of adrenal tumors in control and high-dose-treated male rats were 9% and 29%, respectively (NCI, 1978j).

Human data

No toxicity or epidemiological data are available.

4-Chloro-ortho-Phenylenediamine

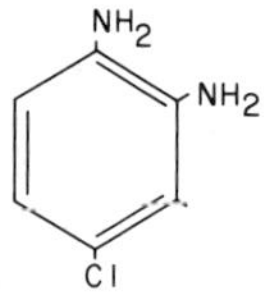

4-Chloro-ortho-phenylenediamine is also known as 4-chloro-1, 2-benzenediamine. It is produced on a commercial scale in the United States (U.S. International Trade Commission, 1977). It is used as an intermediate in the synthesis of dyes for polyester fibers (Kadhim and Peters, 1974). It was used previously in the production of the dye CI Vat Brown 22, which is no longer produced commercially in the United States (U.S. International Trade Commission, 1977).

Experimental carcinogenesis

4-Chloro-ortho-phenylenediamine was administered in the diet to male and female Fischer 344 rats and B6C3F1 mice for a period of 18 months. The concentrations of the test compound in the diet were 0.5 and 1.0% for rats and 0.7 and 1.4% for mice. The animals were maintained on control diet for an additional 6 months. Under these conditions 4-chloro-ortho-phenylenediamine was carcinogenic to both rats and mice. On a high dose of the compound urinary bladder tumors developed in 51 and 71% of surviving male and female rats, respectively. No such tumors developed in control male and female rats. In male mice liver tumors developed in 20% of control and 55% of high-dose-treated animals. Liver tumors also developed in 13% of female mice treated with high dose of the compound. No such tumors were observed in control female mice (NCI, 1978k).

Human data

No data are yet available.

2,4-Xylidine

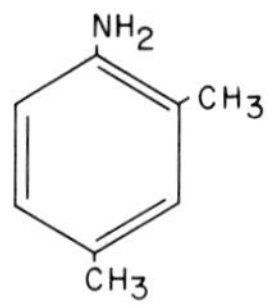

2-4-Xylidine, a colorless liquid that boils at 214°C is also known as 2,4-dimethylaniline. According to the U.S. International Trade Commission (1977), 2,4-xylidine was produced on a commercial scale in 1975. It is used in the production of several dyes, three of which are produced commercially in the United States: CI Acid Red 26, CI Direct Violet 14, and CI Solvent Orange 7.

Experimental carcinogenesis

2,4-Xylidine was administered to 50 male Charles River (Sprague-Dawley) rats in a 2-year feeding study. Subcutaneous tumors occurred in 16% of control animals and 39% of treated animals. The treated animals also developed liver tumors (Russfield et al., 1973a). Experimental details presented in this abstract report are incomplete.

Human data

No data are yet available.

2,5-Xylidine

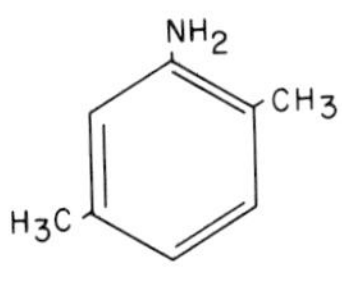

2,5-Xylidine is also known as 2,5-dimethylaniline. It is an almost colorless liquid that boils at 214°C. 2,5-Xylidine is used as an intermediate in the production of at least six dyes, two of which are produced commercially in the United States: CI Direct Violet and Solvent Red 26 (U.S. International Trade Commission, 1977).

Experimental carcinogenesis

Carcinogenicity data on 2,5-xylidine in rats appear to be incomplete. Thus, oral administration of 2,5-xylidine in the diet of male Charles River rats over a 2-year period produced s.c. tumors in 24% of treated rats compared to 16% of control rats. The treated group also developed hepatomas. In this report the number of surviving animals in the treated group and the percentage of animals with hepatomas are not given (Russfield et al., 1973a).

Human data

No data are yet available.

2,4-Diaminotoluene

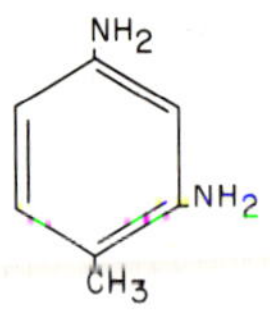

2,4-Diaminotoluene is a colorless crystalline compound that melts at 99°C. It has been produced on a commercial scale in the United States since 1919. According to the U.S. International Trade Commission, 1975 production of 2,4-diaminotoluene in the United States was about 200 million lb (1977). It is used as an intermediate in the production of polyurethane, in hair-dye formulations, and in making dyes for textiles, leather, and furs.

Experimental carcinogenesis

Oral administration of 0.06 or 0.1% of 2,4-diaminotoluene in the diet for 30-36 weeks produced multiple liver tumors in both treated groups of male Wistar rats. In the lower-dose-treated group 7/11 surviving rats had liver tumors, whereas 9/9 rats in the higher-dose group developed liver tumors. Tumors were not observed in any of the six controls (Ito et al., 1969).

Weekly s.c. injection of 2,4-diaminotoluene produced sarcomas at the site of injection in all treated rats that survived. No such tumors developed in control animals (Umeda, 1955).

In skin carcinogenicity study with Swiss-Webster mice of both sexes, a hair-dye formulation containing 2,4-diaminotoluene, 2,5-diaminotoluene sulfate, paraphenylenediamine, and hydrogen peroxide was applied on the shaved skin of these animals for about 19 months. The lung tumor incidence in the treated group was not significantly different from that in the control group (Burnett et al., 1975).

Human data

No information is yet available regarding exposure and toxicity of 2,4-diaminotoluene in humans.

2,5-Diaminotoluene

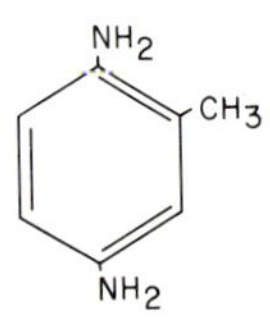

It is a colorless crystalline compound that melts at 64°C. Even though commercial production of 2,5-diaminotoluene was started in the United States in 1920, its commercial production has not been reported in the United States since 1966. Commercial production of its sulfate salt was last reported in the United States in 1970 (IARC, 1978). 2,5-Diaminotoluene has been used as an intermediate in the production of two widely used dyes: CI Basic Red 2 and CI Acid Brown 103. CI Basic Red 2 is produced commercially in the United States (U.S. International Trade Commission, 1977) and is used to dye cotton, leather, wool, silk, and paper, and in pigments. CI Acid Brown 103 is used to dye leather. 2,5-Diaminotoluene and its sulfate are also used in various hair-dye formulations.

Experimental carcinogenesis

Hair-dye formulation containing 2,5-toluenediamine sulfate, paraphenylenediamine with either 2,4-toluenediamine, 2,4-diaminoanisole sulfate, or metaphenylenediamine and hydrogen peroxide was painted twice weekly on the shaved backs of Swiss-Webster mice of either sex for a period of 18 months. Under these conditions the lung tumor incidence was not significantly different from that in control mice (Burnett et al., 1975).

In another skin carcinogenesis study various formulations were applied on the backs of Sprague-Dawley rats of both sexes. One formulation contained 2,5-diaminotoluene sulfate alone; a second formulation contained 2,5-diaminotoluene and 2,4-diaminoanisole. A third formulation without any dyes served as the control. No statistical differences were observed in the tumor incidences between the control and experimental groups (Kinkel and Holzmann, 1973).

In a recent carcinogenicity study Fischer 344 rats and B6C3F1 mice of both sexes were administered 2,5-diaminotoluene as its sulfate salt in the diet at concentrations of 0.06 and 0.2% for rats and 0.06 and 0.1% for mice for a period of 18 months. The animals were maintained on a control diet for an additional 6 months. In both species an adequate number of animals in all groups survived sufficiently long to be at risk from late-developing tumors. A statistically significant incidence of testicular tumors in treated male rats was not considered attributable to administration of the compound, since the spontaneous incidence of these neoplasms in male Fischer 344 rats is both high and variable. In this study there was not sufficient convincing evidence to indicate that 2,5-diaminotoluene sulfate is carcinogenic to either rats or mice (NCI, 1978x).

Human data

2,5-Diaminotoluene is toxic following both ingestion and inhalation. It has a toxic action upon the liver and can cause fatty degeneration of that organ (Sax, 1975). When 2,5-diaminotoluene was applied to the scalp of human volunteers in conjunction with detergents, resorcinol, and hydrogen peroxide, the diacetyl derivative was excreted in the urine for 2 days following application, indicating absorption of this compound through the skin (Kiese and Rauscher, 1968).

Two cases of aplastic anemia have been reported in patients who have been using a new hair dye containing 2,5-diaminotoluene or its sulfate prior to the onset of their symptoms (Hamilton and Sheridan, 1976; Toghill and Wilcox, 1976).

No epidemiological data are yet available to implicate 2,5-diaminotoluene as carcinogenic in humans.

1,2-Diamino-4-Nitrobenzene

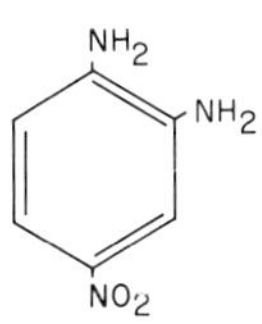

It is a reddish crystalline compound that melts at 199-200°C. Since its first commercial U.S. production in 1936, 1,2-diamino-4-nitrobenzene was reported to be produced commercially in the United States in 1975 (IARC, 1978). It is believed that this chemical is also currently manufactured in the United States. This compound is used primarily in semipermanent and permanent hair-coloring products. It is also reportedly used as a reagent for α-keto acids and as a colorimetric reagent for the determination of ascorbic and dehydroascorbic acids in foods (IARC, 1978).

Experimental carcinogenesis

A hair-dye formulation containing 1,2-diamino-4-nitrobenzene mixed with 1,4-diamino-2-nitrobenzene was tested by repeated applications on skin during carcinogenesis test in adult mice of both sexes of strains DBAf and A. When the experiment was terminated in 80 weeks there were some differences in tumor type and incidence in treated and control groups in DBAf strain mice. Thus, the treated group had five lymphomas and six tumors of the female reproductive tract, whereas one lymphoma, one liver, and one lung tumor developed in control mice. There were no differences in the incidence of tumor between control and treated A strain mice (Searle and Jones, 1977). In this study 1,2-diamino-4-nitrobenzene alone was not tested.

Human data

No data are yet available.

1,4-Diamino-2-Nitrobenzene

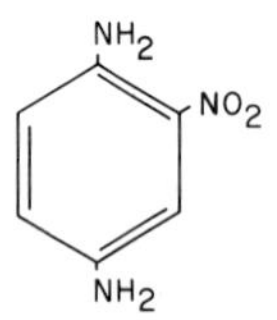

1,4-Diamino-2-nitrobenzene, a black crystalline compound that melts at 137°C, is also known as 2-nitro-p-phenylenediamine. Its latest commercial production in the United States was reported in 1973 (IARC, 1978). It is used in formulations for both permanent and semi-permanent hair-coloring products and in dyeing furs.

Experimental carcinogenesis

Carcinogenicity of 1,4-diamino-2-nitrobenzene was examined using Fischer 344 rats and B6C3F1 mice of both sexes by feeding them the compound in the diet for about 18 months. Two concentrations of the compound were administered. Under these conditions there was no convincing evidence for the carcinogenicity of the compound in Fischer 344 rats or in male mice. However, dietary administration of this compound increased the incidence of liver tumors in female mice. Thus, liver tumors were induced in 1/20 (5%), 10/49 (20%), 17/48 (35%) surviving female mice in control, low-dose, and high-dose groups, respectively (NCI, 1978v).

Another carcinogenicity study has been performed on both DBAf and A strains of mice by repeated application of a mixture of two components on the shaved skin of these animals. The mixture contained 1,4-diamino-2-nitrobenzene and 1,2-diamino-4-nitrobenzene. After the end of the experiment it was noted that there were some differences in both incidence and tumor type in DBAf-treated and control female mice. No differences in tumor incidence were observed between the treated and control groups in A strain mice (Searle and Jones, 1977). In these studies 1,4-diamino-2-nitrobenzene was not tested separately to evaluate its carcinogenic potency.

Human data

No date are yet available regarding the toxicity of 1,4-diamino-2-nitrobenzene in humans.

2,4-Dinitrotoluene

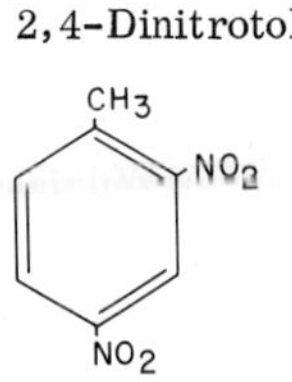

2,4-Dinitrotoluene is a yellow crystalline compound that melts at 70.5°C. According to the U.S. International Trade Commission (1977), 2,4-dinitrotoluene is produced on a commercial scale in the United States. It has been reported that about 272 million lb of 2,4- and 2,6-dinitrotoluene were produced in the United States in 1975. It is used primarily as an intermediate in the production of azo dyes. It is also used by the munitions industry as a modifier for smokeless powders and to a limited extent as a gelatinizing and waterproofing agent in military and commercial explosive compositions (Hawley, 1977; NCI, 1978q).

Experimental carcinogenesis

2,4-Dinitrotoluene was administered in the diet to Fischer rats at 0.008 and 0.02% levels and to B6C3F1 mice at 0.008 and 0.04% levels for a period of 18 months. Under these conditions a significantly increased incidence of fibroma of the skin and s.c. tissue occurred in both low- and high-dose groups of male rats when compared to their respective controls. A statistically significant incidence of fibroadenoma of the mammary gland occurred in the high-dose female rats. Among the mice a variety of tumors was observed, but none were considered to be associated with the dietary administration of 2,4-dinitrotoluene (NCI, 1978q).

Human data

2,4-Dinitrotoluene is rapidly adsorbed through the intact skin; however, toxic levels may also be reached by inhalation or ingestion (Manufacturing Chemists Association, 1966). It can cause anemia, methemoglobinemia, cyanosis, and liver damage (Sax, 1975). No epidemiological data are yet available implicating 2,4-dinitrotoluene in human cancer induction.

4-Amino-2-Nitrophenol

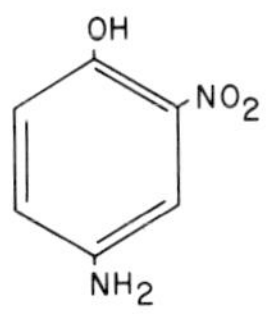

4-Amino-2-nitrophenol, a dark crystalline compound, was first produced commercially in the United States in 1941, and the latest commercial production of this compound was reported in 1972 (U.S. Tariff Commission, 1974). It is used both as an industrial dye intermediate in dyeing furs and as a constituent of hair dyes.

Experimental carcinogenesis

Oral administration of 4-amino-2-nitrophenol at 0.125 and 0.25% levels in the diet for 2 years produced bladder tumors in 13/39 (33%) of surviving male Fischer 344 rats fed the higher-dose level. Females treated in the same manner showed bladder tumors in 1/42 (2%) animals fed the lower dose and 2/46 (4%) animals fed the higher dose. No bladder tumors were found among 220 male and 220 female control rats (NCI, 1978e).

In the same study 4-amino-2-nitrophenol administered to B6C3F1 strain mice of both sexes at two dose levels, 0.125 and 0.25%, in the diet for 2 years produced no tumors in the treated mice (NCI, 1978e). In a skin carcinogenesis study 4-amino-2-nitrophenol mixed with CI Acid Black 107 (an azo-dye metal complex) was tested on adult male and female mice of A and DBAf strains. After the termination of the experiment at 80 weeks few cases of tumors were observed in treated DBAf mice (Searle and Jones, 1977). Since no data on 4-amino-2-nitrophenol alone were available, skin carcinogenicity results cannot be ascribed to 4-amino-2-nitrophenol.

Human data

No studies are yet available.

ortho-Anisidine

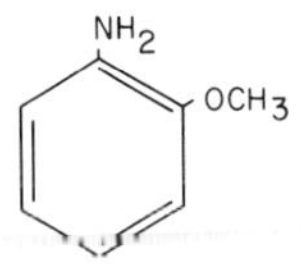

ortho-Anisidine is a yellowish liquid that boils at 225°C. It is used chiefly in the manufacture of a large number of azo dyes. ortho-Anisidine was listed previously as a possible ingredient in hair-dye formulations (Wall, 1972); however, it is not currently used in any hair-dye formulations in the United States (FDA, 1977).

Experimental carcinogenesis

ortho-Anisidine hydrochloride was added in the diet of Fischer 344 strain rats and B6C3F1 mice of both sexes for a period of 2 years. The concentrations of ortho-anisidine HCl in the diet was 0.5 and 1.0% for rats and 0.25 and 0.5% for mice. Under these conditions 52/54 and 52/52 male rats developed bladder tumors in low- and high-dosed groups. No bladder tumors were observed in 51 male and 49 female control rats. In addition, kidney tumors occurred in 3/55 and 7/53 male rats fed the low- and high-dose diet. No kidney tumors were induced in 53 rats in the control group. ortho-Anisidine HCl also induced thyroid tumors in 15-18% of surviving male rats fed low and high dose. Incidence of these tumors was not significant in treated female rats. In mice the significant tumor incidence occurred only in the urinary bladder of both sexes. Thus, tumors developed in 2/55 and 22/53 male mice and 1/51 and 22/50 female mice fed the low and high dose of ortho-anisidine HCl (NCI, 1978g).

Human data

No case report or epidemiological data are as yet available implicating ortho-anisidine in inducing cancer in humans.

5-Nitro-ortho-Anisidine

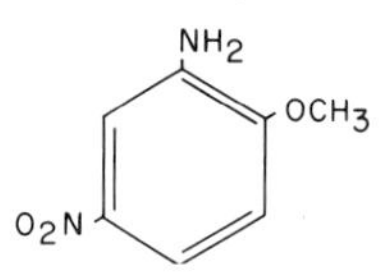

5-Nitro-ortho-anisidine is an orange-red crystalline compound that melts at 118°C (Weast, 1977-1978). It is produced commercially in the United States (Stanford Research Institute, 1977). It is used as an intermediate in the production of CI Pigment Red 23, which is used as a colorant in a wide variety of products, including textiles, paper, rubber, plastics, printing inks, and interior latex paints. It can also be used along with certain coupling components to produce various color hues on cotton, silk, acetate, and nylon (Society of Dyers and Colourists, 1971).

Experimental carcinogenesis

5-Nitro-ortho-anisidine was administered in the diet at two concentrations to male and female rats (Fischer 344) and B6C3F1 mice for a period of 18 months. Under these conditions 5-nitro-ortho-anisidine was found to be carcinogenic to both male and female rats and to female mice. In male rats given high doses of the compound skin carcinoma and ear duct tumors developed in 30/48 and 10/48 animals, respectively. In control male rats only ear duct tumors developed in 1/48 animals. The compound induced clitoral gland and ear duct gland tumors in 20 and 15% of the surviving female rats, respectively. No such tumors appeared in control female rats. Liver tumors were induced in 8/43 female mice fed the high dose of the compound, whereas liver tumors appeared in 1/50 control females (NCI, 1978u).

Human data

No toxicity or epidemiological data are yet available.

para-Anisidine

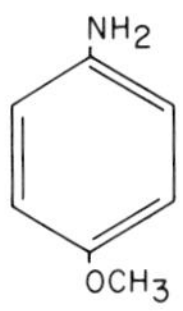

It is a crystalline compound that melts at 57°C. para-Anisidine was produced on a commercial scale in the United States in 1975 (U.S. International Trade Commission, 1977). It is used primarily as an intermediate for the production of several dyes (Society of Dyers and Colourists, 1956).

Experimental carcinogenesis

Carcinogenicity of para-anisidine HCl was examined using Fischer 344 strain rats and B6C3F1 mice of both sexes by feeding the compound in the diet for about 2 years. The concentrations of para-anisidine HCl in the diet were 0.3 and 0.6% for rats and 0.5 and 1.0% for mice. Although there appeared to be an association between chemical administration and the increased incidence of preputial gland tumors in low-dose male rats, the evidence was insufficient to establish the carcinogenicity of para-anisidine HCl in Fischer 344 rats. The compound was not carcinogenic in B6C3F1 mice (NCI, 1978h).

Human data

No case reports or epidemiological data are as yet available.

2,4-Diaminoanisole

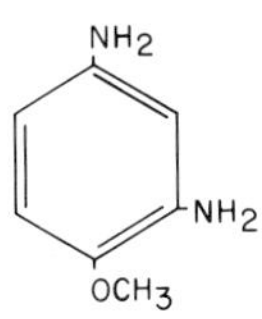

It is a colorless crystalline compound that melts at 67-68°C. 2,4-Diaminoanisole was first produced commercially in the United States in 1933. However, production of this compound as the sulfate salt has not been reported since 1971. 2,4-Diaminoanisole is used as an intermediate for the production of a dye, CI Basic Brown 2 which is used mainly to dye acrylic fibers but is also used to color wool, nylon, polyester, cotton, and leather, as an ingredient of shoe polishes, and in dyeing furs. 2,4-Diaminoanisole is also used in hair colorings (IARC, 1978).

Experimental carcinogenesis

In a recent bioassay of 2,4-diaminoanisole as a sulfate salt it was administered to Fischer 344 strain rats of both sexes at 0.12 and 0.5% levels of the diet for a period of 18 months. Under these conditions 2,4-diaminoanisole sulfate induced increased incidences of malignant tumors of the skin, ear, and thyroid gland in each sex (NCI, 1978o).

In a skin carcinogenesis test a formulation containing 0.75% 2,4-diaminoanisole and 3% 2,5-diaminotoluene both as sulfates and containing 3% hydrogen peroxide was applied repeatedly to the dorsal skin of both male and female Sprague-Dawley rats. No differences were observed in incidences or tumor types between the treated and control groups (Kinkel and Holtzmann, 1973).

2,4-Diaminoanisole sulfate was also administered to B6C3F1 strain male and female mice at 0.12 and 0.24% levels of the diet for a period of 18 months. At the high-dose level 3,4-diaminoanisole sulfate induced thyroid tumors in 11/45 and 8/45 surviving treated male and females, respectively. Under these conditions no thyroid tumors were observed in 40 control male and females (NCI, 1978o).

A hair-dye formulation containing 2,4-diaminoanisole sulfate, diaminotoluene sulfate, para-phenylenediamine, and hydrogen peroxide was applied on the shaved skin of male and female Swiss-Webster mice for 18 months. The lung tumor incidence in the treated groups was not significantly different from that in the control group (Burnett et al., 1975).

Human data

No data are yet available.

meta-Cresidine

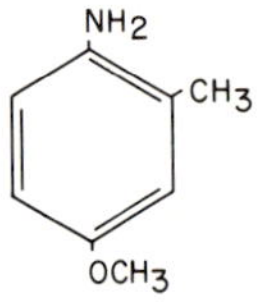

meta-Cresidine is also known as 4-methoxy-2-methylbenzenamine and 2-methyl-para-anisidine. This compound does not appear to be produced on a commercial scale in the United States (Standard Research Institute, 1977). It is presumably used as an intermediate for the synthesis of a diazo-coupling component (Society of Dyers and Colourists, 1956).

Experimental carcinogenesis

meta-Cresidine was administered by gavage to Fischer 344 rats and B6CF1 mice 5 days/week for about an 18-month period. The dosages administered were 0.08 and 0.16 g/kg/day to rats and 0.06 and 0.11 g/kg/day to mice. The urinary bladder and the kidney were the target organs of meta-cresidine toxicity in rats of both sexes. Thus, urinary bladder tumors developed in 5/44 males and 2/44 females in the high-dose group. These tumors occur rarely in the control male and female rats. Actually 1/250 control male and female rats would develop such a urinary bladder tumor. Therefore, even though incidences are low in treated males and females, these bladder carcinomas are considered to be due to the carcinogenic effect of meta-cresidine. Poor survival of male mice receiving meta-cresidine precluded evaluation of the possible carcinogenicity of this compound in these animals. No convincing evidence was provided for carcinogenicity in female mice (NCI, 1978m).

Human data

No data are available.

para-Cresidine

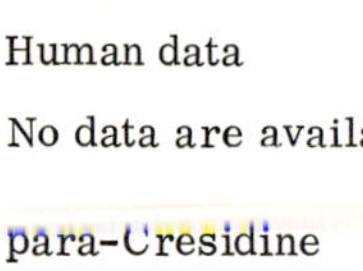

para-Cresidine is also known as 2-methoxy-5-methylbenzenamine and meta-amino-para-cresol methyl ether. It is produced on a commercial scale in the United States, averaging about 600,000 lb/year (NCI, 1978n). It appears to be used primarily as an intermediate for the production of various dyes and pigments. It is believed to be used in the manufacture of at least 11 dyes that are produced commercially in the United States (Society of Dyers and Colourists, 1971).

Experimental carcinogenesis

para-Cresidine was administered in the diet of Fischer 344 rats and B6C3F1 mice of both sexes for a 2-year period. The dietary concentrations of the test compound used in these studies were 0.5 and 1.0% for rats and 0.22 and 0.44% for mice. Under these conditions para-cresidine was found to be carcinogenic to both rats and mice of both sexes. Thus, high doses of the compound induced urinary bladder and nasal cavity tumors in 44/47 and 23/47 males and 43/46 and 11/49 female rats, respectively. In addition, the low dose of the compound produced liver tumors in 13/49 male rats. In mice urinary bladder tumors developed in 40/42 males and 42/46 females on low-dose diets. Liver tumors also developed in 91% of surviving females. No liver, urinary bladder, or nasal cavity tumors developed in any of the 45 to 50 control rats or mice of either sex (NCI, 1978n).

Anthranilic Acid

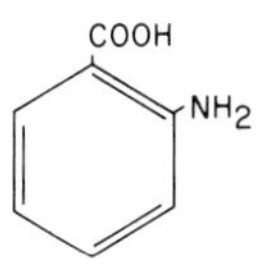

Anthranilic acid is a white to pale yellow crystalline compound that melts at 144-146°C. It has been produced on a commercial scale in the United States for over 50 years. The commercial production of this compound in the United States for 1975 has been reported recently (U.S. International Trade Commission, 1977). Anthranilic acid has been used primarily as an intermediate in the manufacture of several dyes and pigments.

Experimental carcinogenesis

In a recent study anthranilic acid was administered in the diet to Fischer 344 strain rats and B6C3F1 mice of both sexes for a period of 18 months. The concentrations of anthranilic acid in the diet were 1.5 and 3.0% for rats and 2.5 and 5.0% for mice. In rats and mice a variety of neoplasms was observed in both treated and control animals. However, incidences of tumors in treated animals were not statistically significant when compared with controls. Thus, it appears that under the conditions of this bioassay, anthranilic acid was not carcinogenic for either Fischer 344 rats or B6C3F1 mice (NCI, 1978i).

In a previous study, however, anthranilic acid was tested for carcinogenicity by bladder implantation techniques. In this study cholesterol pellets containing 20% anthranilic acid were implanted directly into the bladders of mice. The control mice received implants of cholesterol pellets only. Bladder carcinomas were seen in 10/75 (13%) surviving mice treated with anthranilic acid whereas 4/54 (7%) control mice developed bladder carcinomas (Bryan, 1969). Tumor incidence in treated animals in this study was not statistically significant when compared with controls.

Human data

Anthranilic acid and 3-hydroxyanthranilic acid are metabolites of tryptophan and occur normally in the urine with other tryptophan metabolites. It has been shown that nonoccupational bladder cancer patients excrete larger amounts of 3-hydroxyanthranilic acid and other tryptophan metabolites than normal individuals (Boyland and Williams, 1955). This effect was not observed in occupational bladder cancer patients who were primarily exposed to aromatic amines (Brown et al., 1072). Abnormal tryptophan metabolism occurs not only in bladder cancer patients, but also in patients with other types of neoplasia and a variety of nonneoplastic pathologic conditions (see Arcos and Argus, 1974). No case reports or epidemiological data are yet available.

3-Amino-4-Ethoxyacetanilide

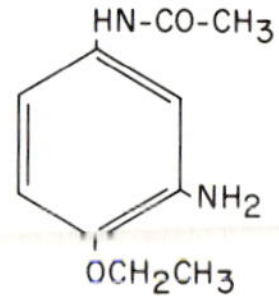

3-Amino-4-ethoxyacetanilide was produced on a commercial scale in the United States in 1975 (Standord Research Institute, 1976). However, its commercial production was not reported in 1976 (Stanford Research Institute, 1977). It is used as an intermediate for the production of azo dyes for synthetic textiles, especially polyesters (Stanley and Farris, 1975).

Experimental carcinogenesis

Both male and female Fischer 344 rats and B6C3F1 mice were fed 3-amino-4-ethoxyacetanilide in the diet for 18 months. The dietary concentrations of the test compound were 0.4 and 1.5% for rats and 0.4 and 0.8% for mice. The experiment was terminated about 2 years after the initiation of the feeding of the test compound. Under these conditions 3-amino-4-ethoxyacetanilide was found to be carcinogenic to male mice inducing carcinomas of the thyroid gland. Evidence was insufficient to establish the carcinogenicity of this compound in female mice or in rats of both sexes (NCI, 1978b).

Human data

Toxicity or epidemiological data are not yet available.

B. Biphenylamine, Benzidine, and Related Compounds

4-Biphenylamine

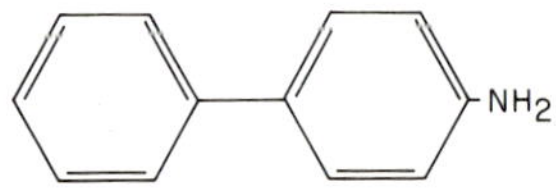

It is a colorless crystalline compound with a melting point (m.p.) of 53°C. It was manufactured on a large scale and was used as a rubber antioxidant and a dye intermediate. However, it is no longer produced commercially (IARC, 1972; Chem. Eng. News, 1978).

Experimental carcinogenesis

Oral administration of this compound in both sexes of C57 × 1F mouse strain produced significantly higher incidence of hepatomas than that in the control group. In addition, this compound induced bladder carcinomas in only one out of 21 surviving male mice (Clayson et al., 1967). Subcutaneous administration of this compound into rats yielded mammary gland and intestinal tumors (Walpole et al., 1952). Bladder papillomas were observed in rabbits given this compound orally (Bonser, 1962). Bladder carcinomas were observed in dogs on oral feeding of this compound (Deichmann et al., 1958b; Walpole et al., 1954).

Human data

The widespread use of this chemical was prevented by excellent epidemiological studies that indicated that out of a population of 171 male workers who were exposed to this chemical during the years between 1935 and 1955, there were 19 cases of bladder cancers among this group (Melick et al., 1955). Recent studies indicate that 53 out of 315 men exposed to this chemical had bladder tumors (Melick et al., 1971). These studies have strongly implicated occurrence of bladder cancer with occupational exposure to 4-biphenylamine.

4-Nitrobiphenyl

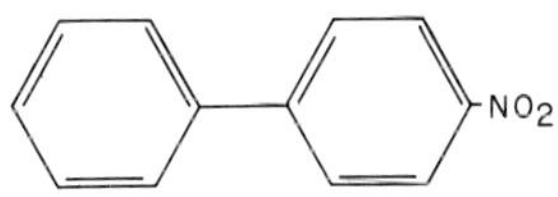

It is a colorless crystalline compound that melts at about 114°C. There is no evidence that 4-nitrobiphenyl is manufactured in the United States (IARC, 1974a; Chem. Eng. News, 1978). It was used as an intermediate in the manufacture of 4-aminobiphenyl, which was used as a rubber antioxidant. Closed systems were used during the reduction of the 4-nitrobiphenyl to 4-aminobiphenyl; therefore, exposure to these chemicals was kept low as possible (Melick et al., 1955, 1971).

Experimental carcinogenesis

It has been shown that oral feeding of a total dose of 4-nitrobiphenyl, 10 g/kg body weight, to four female mongrel dogs induced bladder tumors in two of these animals within 3 years (Deichmann et al., 1958a). However, later studies with this compound indicated that a smaller total dose, 0.77 g/kg gody weight was ineffective in producing bladder tumors in any of six dogs tested (Deichmann et al., 1965).

Human data

Carcinogenicity of 4-nitrobiphenyl among industrial workers is not known. However, since 4-nitrobiphenyl was largely used in the manufacture of 4-aminobiphenyl, it has not been possible to differentiate the exposure of workers to either of these two chemicals. Epidemiological studies have strongly implicated 4-aminobiphenyl as a bladder carcinogen among industrial workers exposed to this chemical (Melick et al., 1955, 1971; IARC, 1972).

2,4'-Biphenyldiamine

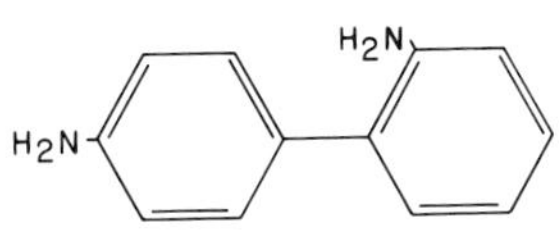

2,4'-Biphenyldiamine is a crystalline compound that melts at 45°C. It is apparently not manufactured commercially in the United States. It was used as an intermediate in the synthesis of azo dyes. It was used as an analytical reagent for the detection of tungsten. Its present use is not known (IARC, 1978).

Experimental carcinogenesis

Oral administration of 2,4'-biphenyldiamine in the diet at a dose level of 2 mg/day for life produced no tumors in male Wistar rats. The average total dose of the compound consumed was about 852 mg. The higher dose was not tested for its carcinogenicity (Marhold et al., 1968).

Oral administration studies with this compound in dogs is not conclusive (Marhold et al., 1968). According to IARC report (1978), 2,4'-biphenyldiamine has not been tested adequately in rats and dogs by oral administration. Therefore, no evaluation of the carcinogenicity of this compound can be made.

Epidemiology

No information is as yet available regarding exposure and toxicity of 2,4'-biphenyldiamine in humans.

Benzidine

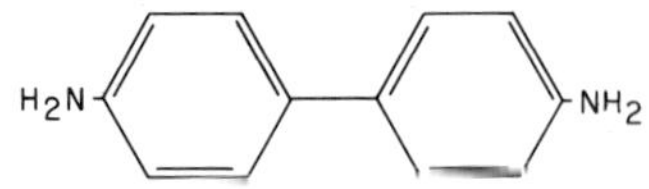

Benzidine is a colorless crystalline compound that melts at 128° C. It has been used as an intermediate in the manufacture of several hundred dyestuffs. Its annual production in the United States amounts to many millions of pounds (IARC, 1972). It is still produced on a commercial scale in the United States (Chem. Eng. News, 1978). It has been used as a hardener in the rubber industry. It is also used in the manufacture of high polymers and heat- and light-resistant fibers. It is used in clinical laboratories for the detection of blood. It is used as a laboratory agent for the quantitative determination of nicotine, as a spray reagent for sugars, and also for the detection of HCN and sulfate. It is also used for the detection of H_2O_2 in milk (IARC, 1972).

Experimental carcinogenesis

Liver tumors have been obtained in rats (Boyland et al., 1954) and hamsters (Saffiotti et al., 1967) on oral administration of benzidine. Subcutaneous injection of this compound in mice has also yielded a significant number of hepatomas (Bonser et al., 1956a). However, when fed to dogs, benzidine produced bladder carcinomas after a long latent period (Bonser et al., 1956a; Spitz et al., 1950).

Human data

The manufacture of benzidine is associated with a high risk of developing bladder cancer. It has been suggested that exposure to benzidine may be by various routes: ingestion, percutaneous absorption, or inhalation (Ehrlicher, 1958; Meigs et al., 1954). However, recent studies demonstrate that the respiratory route is a major port of entry of benzidine (Zavon et al., 1973).

Analyzing a large number of bladder cancer among workers in the dye industry, it has been concluded that benzidine and 2-naphthylamine were chiefly responsible for the induction of bladder tumors (Case et al., 1954; Goldwater et al., 1965; Scott, 1952; Übelin and Pletsher, 1954). In a cohort study of workers exposed to 2-naphthylamine and benzidine it has been shown that benzidine had a lower attack rate than 2-naphthylamine (Mancuso and El-Attar, 1967). However, in a separate study it has been shown that occupancy and exposure to benzidine alone were strongly associated with bladder cancer (Goldwater et al., 1965). Thus, a number of epidemiologic studies from several countries strongly support the relationship between bladder cancer and occupational exposure to benzidine.

N,N'-Diacetylbenzidine

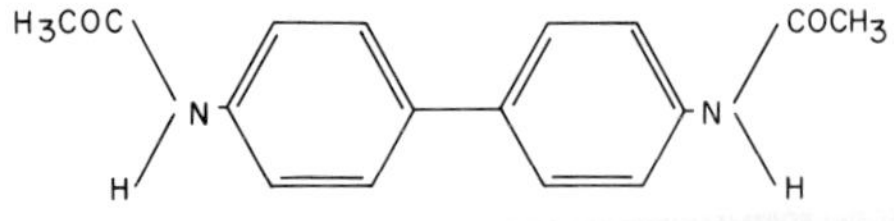

N,N'-Diacetylbenzidine is a white crystalline compound that can be used to prepare 3,3'-dichlorobenzidine, which was used previously as an intermediate in the production of pigments, and 3,3'-dinitrobenzidine, which was used previously in the preparation of CI Sulfur Brown 13. It is not known whether it is now used in the commercial manufacture of these compounds (IARC, 1978).

Experimental carcinogenesis

Oral administration of 0.04% N,N'-diacetylbenzidine in the diet for 8 months produced ear duct tumors in 4/20 male Holtzman rats. No ear duct tumors developed in 45 untreated controls (Miller et al., 1956). In another study weekly s.c. injection of this compound for

9 months induced liver and ear duct tumors in both sexes of Rappolov nursery rats (Pliss, 1962, 1963). In female Wistar rats a single s.c. dose of N,N'-diacetylbenzidine produced mammary gland tumors in 3/6 animals. No tumors were observed in 30 controls used for this study (Bremner and Tange, 1966). Both mammary gland and ear duct gland tumors were induced in female Wistar rats on i.p. administration of this chemical (Bremner and Tange, 1966).

Epidemiology

No information is as yet available regarding exposure and toxicity of N-N'-diacetylbenzidine in humans.

3,3'-Dimethylbenzidine

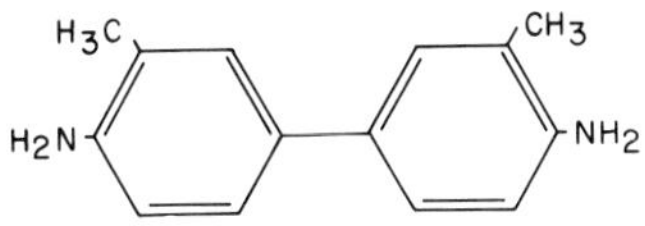

3,3'-Dimethylbenzidine is a white to reddish crystalline powder that melts at 129-131°C. It is used widely in the manufacture of more than 100 dyestuffs and pigments. It is also used as a laboratory agent for the detection of blood and for the colorimetric determination of free chlorine in water and air (IARC, 1972).

Experimental carcinogenesis

Oral feeding of a total dose of 500 mg of 3,3'-dimethylbenzidine by stomach tube to female Sprague-Dawley rats produced mammary carcinomas in three out of 16 surviving animals at the end of 9 months. Among the control group five out of 132 rats had mammary tumors (Griswold et al., 1968). Subcutaneous administration of this compound to random-bred rats yielded tumors of the large sebaceous glands and mammary glands (Pliss and Zabezhinsky, 1970). In feeding experiments with male and female hamsters no tumors were observed when 3,3'-dimethylbenzidine was fed at a dietary level of 0.1% (3.0 g/animal/year) (Saffiotti et al., 1967).

Human data

Like benzidine, 3,3'-dimethylbenzidine may enter the body by ingestion, inhalation, or by percutaneous absorption (Meigs et al., 1954; Zavon et al., 1973). Various metabolites have been detected in the urine of workers manufacturing this compound (Dieteren, 1966). However, epidemiological data implicating this compound as a human carcinogen (Scott, 1962) are not yet available.

3,3'-Dichlorobenzidine

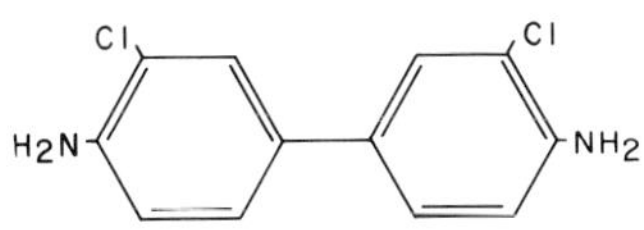

3,3'-Dichlorobenzidine (DCB) is a colorless crystalline compound. Several million pounds of this compound are produced annually in the United States (IARC, 1974a). According to the International Trade Commission, this compound is still being produced on a commercial scale (Chem. Eng. News, 1978) DCB is used as a curing agent for liquid-castable polyurethane elastomers. However, its main use is as an intermediate for the production of at least 13 different dyes and pigments. The DCB-based pigments are used for coloring most plastic resins, rubber, printing inks, metal finishes, and in textile and wallpaper printing (The Society of Dyers and Colourists, 1971).

Experimental carcinogenesis

It has been reported that oral feeding of DCB in the diet for 12 months to rats (total dose 4.5 g/rat) produced a high incidence of tumors in the zymbal gland and other organs, including the bladder (Pliss, 1959). In other studies with rats it has been shown that DCB in the diet yielded tumors in the zymbal gland, mammary gland, and skin of both sexes (Stula et al., 1971, 1975). Subcutaneous administration of this compound in rats produced a high incidence of skin, sebaceous, and mammary gland tumors (Pliss, 1963). Carcinogenicity studies with hamsters performed in Saffiotti's laboratory showed that 0.1% of DCB in the diet did not induce any tumor in this species. However, 0.3% DCB in the diet produced bladder and liver tumors (Saffiotti et al., 1967; Sellakumar et al., 1969).

Human data

Usually 3,3'-dichlorobenzidine and benzidine are manufactured in the same plant. There is no report in which DCB alone has been implicated in cancer induction in humans. Even though no epidemiological data are available, there is a possibility that DCB may have been partly responsible for the bladder cancer attributed to benzidine.

3,3'-Dimethoxybenzidine

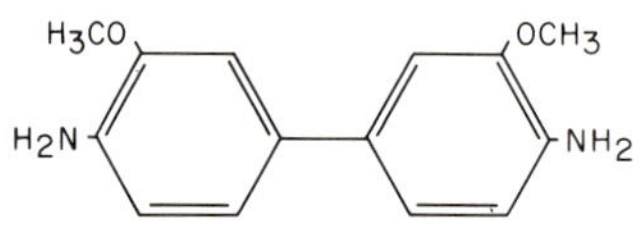

3,3'-Dimethoxybenzidine is a crystalline compound that melts at 137-138°C. According to the International Trade Commission Report, this compound is still produced on a commercial scale in the United States (Che. Eng. News, 1978). It is used as an intermediate in the production of more than 100 dyes and some pigments. These dyes are used for dyeing paper, textiles, plastics, leather, and rubber. The di-isocyanate derivatives of this compound are used in isocyanate-based adhesive systems and as a component of polyurethane elastomers. It is used as a laboratory agent for the detection of the presence of various metals, thiocyanates, and nitrites (IARC, 1974a).

Experimental carcinogenesis

Oral administration of 3,3'-dimethoxybenzidine to rats produced various tumors including those in the zymbal gland, bladder, skin, intestine, and mammary gland (Hadidian et al., 1968; Pliss, 1963, 1965). This compound, when fed to hamsters at 1.0% level, produced forestomach papillomas in 37% of animals. No primary bladder tumors were detected in this group. Only 2% of the control group of hamsters developed stomach papillomas (Saffiotti et al., 1967; Sellakumar et al., 1969).

Human data

Workers exposed to 3,3'-dimethoxybenzidine have been found to excrete this compound in their urine (Meigs et al., 1951, 1954). Most of the workers exposed to this compound have also been exposed to related amines, such as benzidine, which has been strongly associated with the occurrence of human urinary bladder cancer (see the benzidine report this chapter). However, no conclusive epidemiological studies are available which would implicate 3,3'-dimethoxybenzidine alone in any carcinogenicity in humans.

4,4'-Thiodianiline

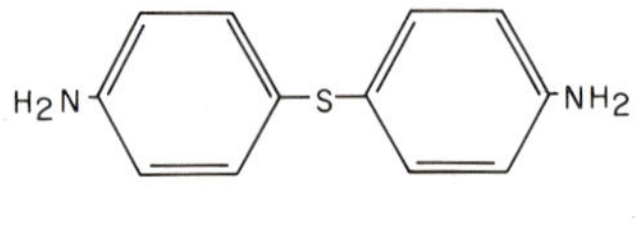

4,4'-Thiodianiline was produced commercially in the United States in 1974 (IARC, 1978). Latest data on commercial production of this compound are not readily available. This compound is used as an intermediate in the commercial production of the dye, CI Mordant Yellow 16 (U.S. International Trade Commission, 1977). It is a crystalline compound that melts at 108° C.

Experimental carcinogenesis

Gastric intubation of 4,4'-thiodiniline in 10 doses of 40 mg/animal every 3 days produced mammary gland tumors in 3/12 surviving female Sprague-Dawley rats 9 months after start of the feeding. In the control group 5/132 animals had mammary tumors. Thus, it appears that the increased incidence of mammary tumors in the treated group was statistically significant compared to the tumor incidence in the control group (Griswold et al., 1968).

No other data on carcinogenicity studies are yet available.

Human data

No information is yet available regarding exposure and toxicity of 4,4'-thiodianiline in humans.

4,4'-Diaminodiphenyl Ether

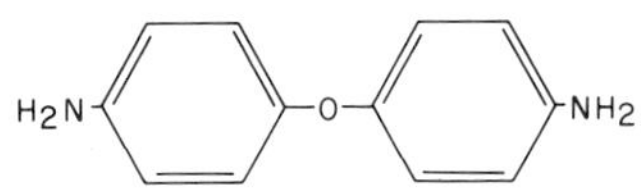

4,4'-Diaminodiphenyl ether, a colorless crystalline compound that melts at 186-187° C is produced in the United States, but amounts of its production are not available. This compound is used as an intermediate in the manufacture of high-temperature resistant resins which are used as a film for insulation tape for various electrical wires and cables, in molding and machine parts, in adhesives, and in coated fabrics and paper (IARC, 1978).

Experimental carcinogenesis

In oral- and s.c.-administration studies performed with rats and mice 4,4'-diaminodiphenyl ether produced tumors at various sites (Dzhioev, 1975). However, in the absence of proper controls the carcinogenic potency of this compound cannot be properly evaluated.

In female Sprague-Dawley rats the compound administered by stomach tube in several doses did not produce mammary tumors in any of the eight surviving animals at 9 months when the experiment was terminated (Griswold et al., 1968).

Epidemiology

No information is as yet available about exposure and toxicity of 4,4'-diaminodiphenyl ether in humans.

4,4'-Methylenedianiline

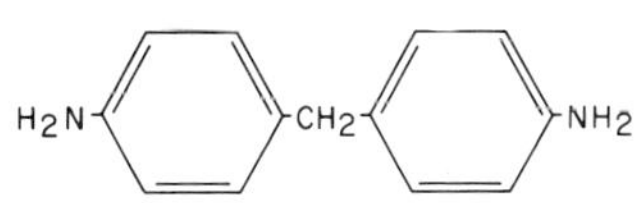

It is also known as 4,4'-diaminodiphenylmethane and DAPM. It is a crystalline compound that melts at 92° C. Several million pounds of 4,4'-methylenedianiline (DAPM) are produced commercially every year. However, only a small amount of DAPM is isolated from the manufactured process. The largest use for unisolated DAPM is in the manufacture of polymethylene polyphenylisocyanate and 4,4'-methylenediphenyl isocyanate. The former isocyanate is used in rigid polyurethane foam, whereas the latter isocyanate is mostly used in the production of spandex fibers.

The most important usage for isolated DAPM is in the production of the corresponding completely hydrogenated diamine, 4,4'-methylene-bis(cyclohexylamine). In the past this hydrogenated diamine has been used almost exclusively to make the corresponding isocyanate which is used in light-stable, high-performance polyurethane coatings. The hydrogenated diamine has also been used as an intermediate in the production of a new nylon yarn. Isolated DAPM is also used as an intermediate in the production of poly(amideimid) resins and fibers, in the synthesis of pararosaniline dye, and as a curing agent for liquid-castable polyurethane elastomers and epoxy resins. It is also used as a corrosion inhibitor and as a laboratory reagent in the determination of tungsten and sulfates (IARC, 1974a).

Experimental carcinogenesis

In one study gastric intubation of maximum tolerated dose of DAPM to rats (total dose 3.3 g/kg body weight) did not produce any tumors for 2 years. All animals, however, showed cirrhosis of the liver (Munn, 1967). In a second study intragastric dosing was continued for about 18 months instead of 10 months used in the previous study (total dose 6 g/kg body weight). Under these conditions several tissue-type tumors including only two liver tumors developed in surviving rats. The same strain of rats when used for testing methylene-bis(2-methylaniline) produced a high incidence of malignant liver tumors, demonstrating that these rats were susceptible to liver carcinogens (Munn, 1967).

Subcutaneous administration of DAPM to both male and female Wistar rats produced higher incidence of benign and malignant tumors in treated compared with control rats (Steinhoff and Grundmann, 1970).

No other animal species has been tested for carcinogenicity with this compound.

Human data

Accidental exposure of 84 persons to DAPM has produced severe hepatotoxic effects in these people (Kopelman et al., 1966a, b). No other human data on this compound are yet available.

4,4'-Methylene-bis(2-Methylaniline)

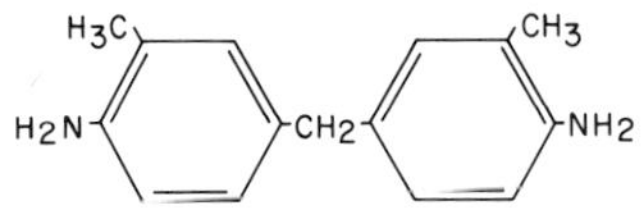

4,4'-Methylene-bis(2-methylaniline), also known as methylenebis(ortho-toluidine), is a white amorphous compound that melts at 149° C. This compound was produced commercially in the United States in the past, but apparently was not produced for sale to others but was used immediately as an unisolated intermediate in the manufacture of the corresponding diisocyanate. 4,4'-Methylene-bis(2-methylaniline) has been investigated experimentally for use as a curing agent for epoxy resins, but there is no indication that it was ever used commercially for this purpose. This compound can be used in the synthesis of the dye CI Basic Violet 2 (IARC, 1974a).

Experimental carcinogenesis

Oral administration of this compound to rats for about 1 year produced liver, lung, and skin tumors in both sexes (Munn, 1967; Stula et al., 1971, 1975).

Human data

No epidemiological data have been reported.

4,4'-Methylene-bis(2-Chloroaniline)

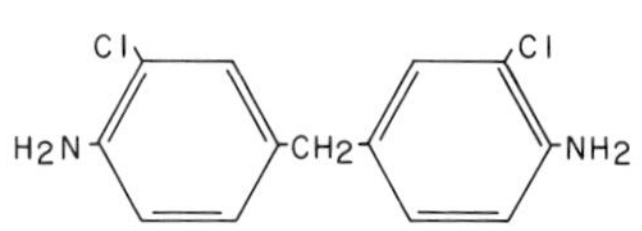

It is also known as 4,4'-diamino-3,3'-dichlorodiphenyl-methane and DACPM. 4,4'-Methylene-bis(2-chloroaniline) (DACPM) is a colorless crystalline compound that melts at 110°C. Almost all of DACPM manufactured in the United States is used as a curing agent for isocyanate-containing polymers. It is a widely used agent for curing liquid-castable polyurethane elastomers suitable for molded mechanical articles and for potting and encapsulating purposes. Less than 1% of total DACPM produced is used as a curing agent for epoxy and epoxy-urethan resin blends. Formulations with other aromatic diamines (e.g., 3,3'-dichlorobenzidine or 4,4'-methylenedianiline) are also made as curing agents (IARC, 1974a).

Experimental carcinogenesis

Oral administration of 0.1% DACPM in the diet of rats produced a very high incidence of lung and liver tumors in both sexes of this species (Grundmann and Steinhoff, 1970; Russfield et al., 1975; Stula, 1971, 1975). In mice the effect of 0.1 and 0.2% DACPM in the diet was examined (Russfield et al., 1975). These experiments showed that at both levels DACPM produced a high incidence of vascular tumors in both sexes. However, in females, in addition to vascular tumors, hepatomas occurred in a large number of animals.

Subcutaneous administration of this compound to rats produced distant tumors in liver and lungs (Steinhoff and Grundmann, 1971).

Human data

Even though DACPM has been detected in the urine of workers exposed to this compound (Linch et al., 1971), no cases of bladder cancer have been found among these workers.

Michler's Ketone

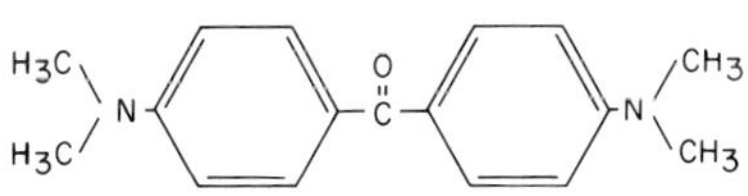

Michler's ketone, a greenish-white crystalline compound is also known as 4,4'-bis(dimethylamino)benzophenone and tetramethyldiaminobenzophenone. It is used in the synthesis of dyestuffs, especially auramine derivatives (Hawley, 1977). Specific production data for Michler's ketone are not available. However, it is known that this compound is produced on a commercial scale in the United States (U.S. International Trade Commission, 1977).

Experimental carcinogenesis

Michler's ketone was administered in the diet at 0.025 and 0.05% levels to male and 0.05 and 0.1% to female Fischer 344 rats and 0.125 and 0.25% levels to both sexes of B6C3F1 mice for an 18-month period. Under these conditions Michler's ketone was found to be carcinogenic to both sexes of rats; and in female mice it caused hepatocellular carcinomas, and in male mice it caused hemangiosarcomas. Thus, incidences of liver cancer were 9/50 and 40/50 in male rats and 41/47 and 44/49 in female rats and 16/49 and 38/50 in female mice in the low dose and high dose, respectively. No liver tumors were observed in the control groups of 20 animals. Among male mice, incidences of hemangiosarcomas were 0/19, 5/50, and 20/50 in the control, low-dose, and high-dose groups, respectively (NCI, 1978s).

Human data

No epidemiological data have yet been reported implicating Michler's ketone in cancer among workers involved in the manufacture of various dyes and pigments.

C. Naphthylamine and Related Compounds

1-Naphthylamine

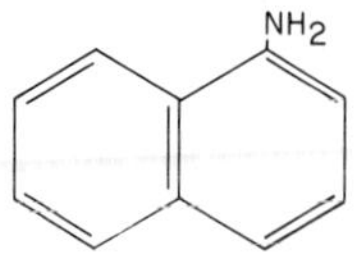

1-Naphthylamine is a colorless crystalline compound that becomes red on exposure to air and melts at 50°C. It is volatile with steam and it sublimes. 1-Naphthylamine is produced on a commercial scale in the United States (Chem. Eng. News, 1978). Its major use is as an intermediate in the manufacture of at least 100 different dyes (Society of Dyers and Colourists, 1971). It has also been used to manufacture the herbicide N-1-naphthylphthalamic acid. N-Phenyl-1-naphthylamine is one of the rubber antioxidants produced from 1-naphthylamine. In the past 1-naphthylamine was used in the production of the rodenticide 1-naphthylthiourea; however, this rodenticide is no longer produced in the United States.

Experimental carcinogenesis

When 1-naphthylamine hydrochloride was given in the drinking water (0.01%) to mice over a period of about 19 months the incidence of hepatoma was 4/18 in treated and 4/24 in the control males. In female mice the hepatoma incidences were 5/43 in the treated and 0/36 in the control (Clayson and Ashton, 1963).

Subcutaneous administration of this compound to newborn male and female Swiss mice gave 5/35 males tumors, which consisted of three pulmonary tumors, one hepatoma, and one lymphosarcoma. In females only 1/26 developed pulmonary tumors (Radomski et al., 1971).

No carcinogenic effect was observed in either male or female Syrian golden hamsters when 1-naphthylamine was administered at either 0.1 or 1% level in the diet (Saffiotti et al., 1967; Sellakumar et al., 1969).

When 1-naphthylamine was fed to five dogs at a dose of about 330 mg 5 times/week for 4.5 years, there was no incidence of bladder tumors in these dogs (Gehrmann et al., 1949). However, in later studies it was found that one out of two mongrel dogs had bladder papilloma after 9 years when 0.5-g dose of 1-naphthylamine was administered to these dogs 3 times/week for life (Bonser et al., 1958).

Human data

Several investigators have implicated 1-naphthylamine as being responsible for a few cases of bladder tumors (Wignall, 1929; Gehrmann et al., 1949; Scott, 1952). In their survey Case et al. (1954) found six deaths due to bladder cancer among 1-naphthylamine workers. Even though these workers had not been engaged in the production of either 2-naphthylamine or benzidine, it is known that commercial 1-naphthylamine was contaminated with 4-10% 2-naphthylamine. Therefore, it is not possible to decide whether 1-naphthylamine free from the 2-isomer is carcinogenic to humans (IARC, 1974a).

2-Naphthylamino

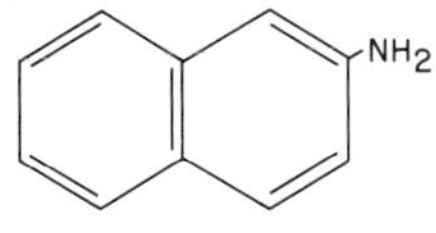

It is a colorless crystalline compound that turns reddish-purple on exposure to air. It melts at 111-113° C and is volatile with steam. Even though 2-naphthylamine was produced commercially in the United States for at least 50 years, its commercial production in the United States has been discontinued since 1972 (IARC, 1974a). However, recent International Trade Commission reports indicate that it is produced on a commercial scale in the United States (Chem. Eng. News, 1978). Several other countries including the United Kingdom have also discontinued its production since 1960 because of very convincing epidemiological evidence linking 2-naphthylamine to bladder cancer among workers exposed to this chemical (Kilner and Samuel, 1960).

The major use for this chemical was to have been as an intermediate in the manufacture of at least 20 different dyes and antioxidants. However, now 2-aminonaphthalene sulfonic acid is substituted for it in the production of various dyes (The Society of Dyers and Colourists, 1971). 2-Naphthylamine was believed to have been used until recently in the synthesis of N-alkyl-2-naphthylamines which were used as dye intermediates.

In recent years antioxidants N-phenyl-2-naphthylamine and its derivative are probably manufactured by the condensation of aniline with 2-naphthol instead of being manufactured directly from 2-naphthylamine.

Experimental carcinogenesis

Oral administration of 2-naphthylamine to rats either in the diet (Bonser et al., 1952) or by gavage (Hadidian et al., 1968) did not produce any bladder tumors.

In two different strains of mice (CBA and IF), 2-naphthylamine administered orally either by gavage or in the diet produced a significant incidence of hepatomas in the treated group (Bonser et al., 1952). Hepatomas and local sarcomas were also obtained when mice were injected with this compound s.c. (Bonser et al., 1956b).

No tumors developed in Syrian golden hamsters when they were fed 0.1% of this compound in their diet. However, 1% of this compound in their diet produced bladder tumors in 50% of these animals of both sexes (Saffiotti et al., 1967; Sellakumar et al., 1969). Only one out of six rabbits developed papilloma of the bladder when 2-naphthylamine was administered orally for a period of 5 years (Bonser et al., 1952).

Several studies with dogs indicate that oral administration of 2-naphthylamine does induce bladder tumors in this species (Bonser, 1943; Bonser et al., 1956b; Conzelman and Moulton, 1972; Hueper et al., 1938). However, direct implantation of 10 mg of this compound in the urinary bladder of dogs did not induce any tumors of the bladder or other tissues of these animals when they were examined at 45 months (Radomski et al., 1971).

Bladder tumors were produced in rhesus monkeys when 2-naphthylamine was given orally (Conzelman et al., 1969).

Human data

Several investigators have implicated 2-naphthylamine in the induction of bladder cancer in workers exposed to this chemical during manufacturing of this compound (Hueper, 1942, Gehrmann et al., 1949; Scott, 1962; Veys, 1969). However, epidemiological studies in England showed that whereas only 0.3 deaths would have been expected due to bladder cancer among whole male population of England and Wales, there were 26 deaths due to bladder cancer among 2-naphthylamine workers (Case et al., 1954). Similarly, a study in a dye factory indicated that 12/48 workers who were exposed to 2-naphthylamine alone developed bladder tumors (Goldwater et al., 1965). In a later study it was pointed out that 2-naphthylamine had an attack rate of 952 per 100,000 which was higher than for benzidine (Mancuso and El-Attar, 1967).

N, N-bis(2-Chloroethyl)-2-Naphthylamine

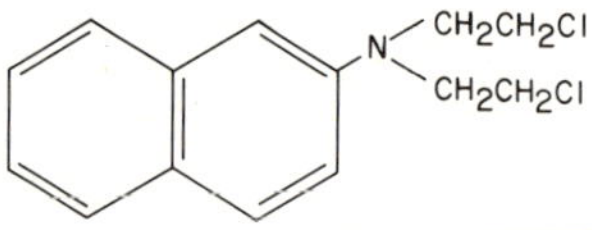

N, N-bis(2-Chloroethyl)-2-naphthylamine is a crystalline compound that melts at 54-50° C; it is also known as naphthylamine mustard and chlornaphazine. There is no evidence that N, N-bis(2-chloroethyl)-2-naphthylamine was ever produced in the United States on a commercial scale (IARC, 1974a). This compound has been used in the past as a chemotherapeutic agent for the treatment of Hodgkin's disease and leukemia and for the control of polycynthaemia vera.

Experimental carcinogenesis

Intraperitoneal administration of chlornaphazine to mice at various dose levels produced a significant increase in incidence and number of pulmonary tumors (Shimkin et al., 1966). In rats, this compound induced local sarcomas on s.c. treatment (Koller, 1953).

Human data

Several investigators have reported a high incidence of bladder cancer among patients who were given chlornaphazine treatment (Videbaek, 1964; Laursen, 1970; Thiede et al., 1964; Thiede and Christensen, 1969). In some of their studies cigarette smoking, occupation, and ^{32}P-sodium phosphate treatment have been ruled out as being responsible for bladder cancer incidence (Thiede et al., 1964; Thiede and Christensen, 1969). These data have shown that chlornaphazine in a total dose as low as 4 g is responsible for bladder cancer incidence.

N-Phenyl-2-Naphthylamine

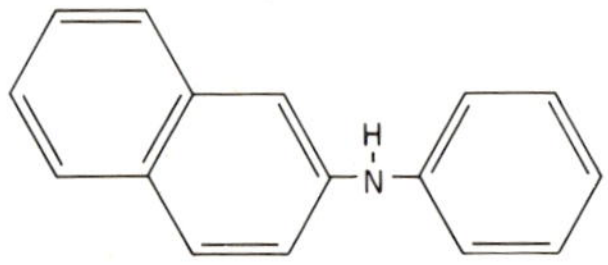

N-Phenyl-2-naphthylamine is also known as phenyl(β-naphthyl)amine and PBNA. It is a greyish powder that melts at 108° C. The commercial production of N-phenyl-2-naphthylamine (PBNA) in the United States was about 1,500,000 lb in 1975 (U.S. International Trade Commission, 1977). It is believed that at present U.S. companies are not producing this chemical commercially because of the pending regulatory action that would limit employees' exposure to it. PBNA is used primarily as an antioxidant in the rubber industry. It is also used as an antioxidant in other polymers, in greases, and in lubricating and transformer oils.

Experimental carcinogenesis

Two strains of mice (C57/BL/6xC3H/AnF)F_1 and (C57BL/6xAKR)F_1 of both sexes were given PBNA by stomach tube for 3 weeks and subsequently in the diet for about 75 weeks. There was a statistically significant increase in hepatoma incidence in males of the first strain. In another study with these two strains of mice the induction of hepatomas by s.c. administration of PBNA was statistically significant in males of the second strain (Innes et al., 1969; NTIS, 1968).

No bladder tumors were observed in three dogs when daily doses of 540 mg of PBNA were administered 5 days/week for 4.5 years (Gehrmann et al., 1949).

Human data

Leucoplakia, acne, and hypersensitivity to sunlight were observed in 36 workers exposed to PBNA for prolonged periods (Sielicka-Zuber, 1961).

Epidemiological studies in the United Kingdom involving 40,000 workers employed in several rubber and cable factories indicated a higher death rate due to bladder cancer in this group (33 compared to 22.7 expected). However, these workers have been exposed to several rubber additives, including PBNA (Fox and Collier, 1976).

According to the National Institute for Occupational Safety and Health (NIOSH), PBNA is metabolized in the human body to 2-naphthylamine, a known human carcinogen. NIOSH estimates that 15,000 workers are potentially exposed to PBNA during its manufacture and use (NIOSH, 1976).

D. Miscellaneous Aromatic Amines

Auramine

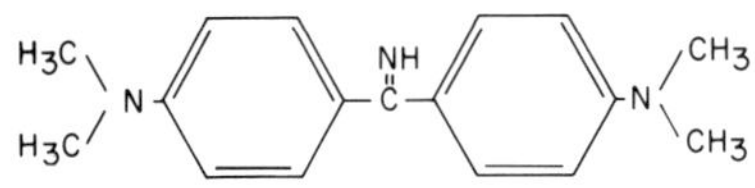

Auramine, a yellow crystalline compound, is used to prepare solvent yellow 34, a solvent soluble yellow dye. Auramine and its hydrochloride are used in large quantities in the coloring of paper and cardboard; they are added during the processing of the raw material prior to manufacture. They are also used in coloring of some textiles and leather (IARC, 1972).

Experimental carcinogenesis

Oral administration of 0.1% auramine in the diet for 52 weeks to both sexes of stock mice produced hepatomas in 57% of the males and 30% of the females. Similar oral doses given to male Wistar rats produced hepatomas in 92% of the animals. No tumors developed in control rats and mice (Williams and Bonser, 1962). When auramine was administered to dogs orally daily for about 7 years no abnormalities were detected (Walpole, 1963). Similarly oral administration of this compound at a tolerated dose level to rabbits indicated metaplasia of the urinary tract epithelium in two out of five rabbits examined.

Human data

Workers engaged in the manufacture of auramine in the British Chemical industry were found to have a relatively high incidence of bladder tumors with latent period ranging between 9 and 28 years (average 19 years) (Case and Pearson, 1954). Overall, there were six deaths, whereas only 0.45 would have been expected from the whole male population of England and Wales ($p < 0.005$). Based on these epidemiological studies, it can be suggested that manufacture of auramine presented an occupational bladder cancer risk.

Magenta

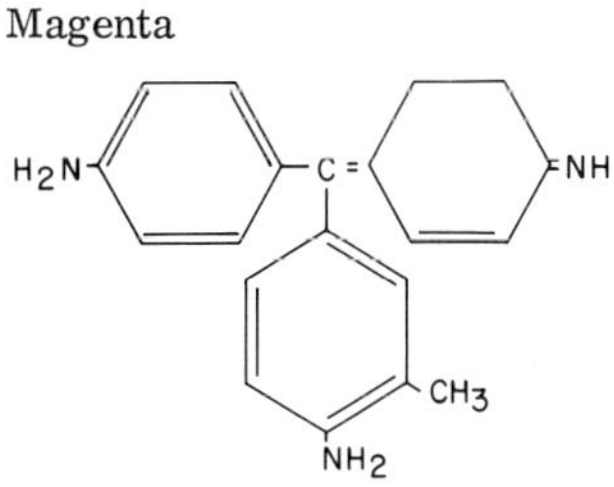

Magenta is a brownish red crystalline compound that decomposes at about 186° C. About a million pounds of magenta are produced annually in the United States (IARC, 1974a). It is used mainly as a dye and to a lesser extent as a dye intermediate. Its main use is in the dyeing of cotton and wool and the coloring of textile fibers, fabrics, and paper products. It is also used in the dyeing of jute fibers, leather, and china clay products, in printing inks, in meat-marking colors, and as a filter dye in photography. In laboratories it is used in microbiological and various biological stains. It is used as an antifungal agent containing phenol and resorcinol. As a dye intermediate, it is used in polishes, carbon paper, and ballpoint pen inks (Society of Dyers and Colourists, 1971).

Experimental carcinogenesis

Magenta was administered to mice by gastric instillation. In these studies some animals in both control and test groups developed lymphomas. These results were not significant (Bonser et al., 1956a). However, significant numbers of local sarcomas in rats were obtained on s.c. administration of paramagenta, one of the components of commercial magenta (Druckrey et al., 1956).

Human data

Bladder cancer in three workers employed in manufacturing magenta was first reported by Rehn (1895). Later it was shown that there was a highly significant risk of contracting bladder cancer among workers involved in manufacturing, but not in purifying or using magenta. This survey indicated that five out of 85 workers who had been involved in manufacturing magenta had developed bladder cancer. According to this report, these 85 workers had not been exposed to either 1- or 2-naphthylamine or benzidine (Case and Pearson, 1954). According to Rehn (1895), these bladder cancers were called as "aniline cancers" because aniline was involved in the manufacture of magenta. However, it is known, that the modern manufacturing process of magenta involves ortho-toluidine instead of aniline. There is therefore a possibility that ortho-toluidine may be one of the chemicals responsible for bladder cancer induction in workers involved in the manufacture of magenta.

2-Aminoanthraquinone

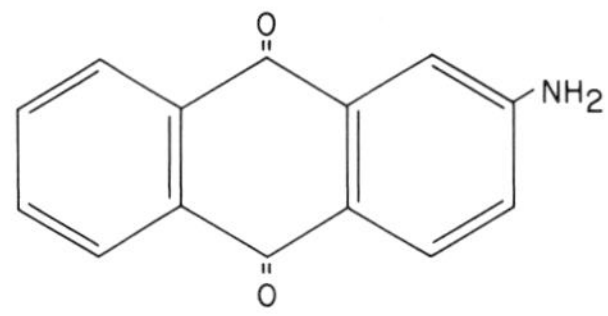

2-Aminoanthraquinone is a red or orange-brown crystalline compound that melts at 302°C (Hawley, 1977). Recent production figures for 2-aminoanthraquinone are considered proprietary and are therefore not available. However, according to U.S. Tariff Commission (1973), about 200,000 lb of the compound and its salts were produced in the United States in 1971, the latest year for which such data were reported. It is used as an intermediate in the manufacture of several dyes and pigments (Society of Dyers and Colourists, 1971; Hawley, 1977).

Experimental carcinogenesis

Oral intubations of 2-aminoanthraquinone to female Sprague-Dawley rats in 10 equal doses of 100 mg each over a period of 30 days did not produce any tumors in these animals when the experiment was terminated approximately 9 months after the administration of the first dose of the test compound (Griswold et al., 1968). In a recent study 2-aminoanthraquinone was administered in the diet of Fischer 344 rats and B6C3F1 mice of both sexes. The dietary concentrations of the compound were 0.35 and 0.69% for male rats, 0.2% for female rats, and 0.5 and 1.0% for male and female mice. The animals were kept for about an additional 6 months after 18 months of feeding of the test compound. Under these conditions 2-aminoanthraquinone was found to be carcinogenic to male rats producing liver tumors. The survival among treated females was poor, and, as a result, no conclusions could be drawn regarding the carcinogenicity of this compound in these animals. The compound was found to be carcinogenic in mice producing liver tumors in both sexes and malignant hematopoietic lymphomas in female mice (NCI, 1978a).

Human data

No data are yet available.

1-Amino-2-Methylanthraquinone

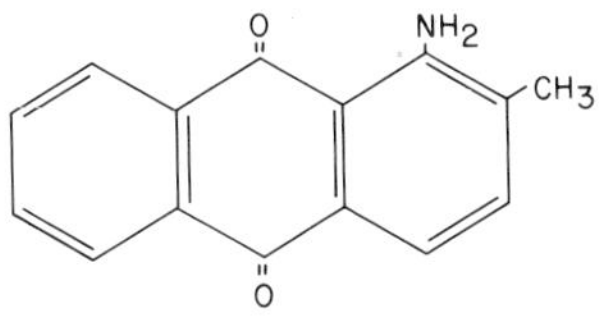

Although 1-amino-2-methylanthraquinone has not been commercially produced in the United States since 1970, significant quantities of this chemical are believed to be imported to the United States annually (NCI, 1978d). It is used as a dye for a variety of synthetic fibers, as well as wool, sheepskins, and furs, and for the surface dyeing of thermoplastics (Society of Dyers and Colourists, 1971). It was also used as an intermediate in the production of a variety of dyes; however, none of these dyes is produced commercially at present in the United States (Society of Dyers and Colourists, 1971; U.S. International Trade Commission, 1977).

Experimental carcinogenesis

A bioassay for possible carcinogenicity of 1-amino-2-methylanthraquinone was conducted using Fischer 344 rats and B6C3F1 mice. The compound was administered in the diet at 0.10 and 0.20% for rats of both sexes and 0.06% for mice. After 18 months of feeding with the test compound the animals were kept for an additional 6-month period. Under these conditions the high dose of the compound induced liver and kidney tumors in 24/48 and 10/48 male rats, respectively. Liver and kidney tumors developed in 3/48 and 0/48 control males, respectively. In female rats liver tumors developed in 11/44 and 2/49 animals in treated and control groups, respectively. The compound was carcinogenic in female mice producing an increased incidence of liver tumors in 12/43 animals compared to 4/44 controls. Tumor incidence in treated male mice was not statistically significant (NCI, 1978d).

Human data

No human data are yet available.

3-Amino-9-Ethylcarbazole

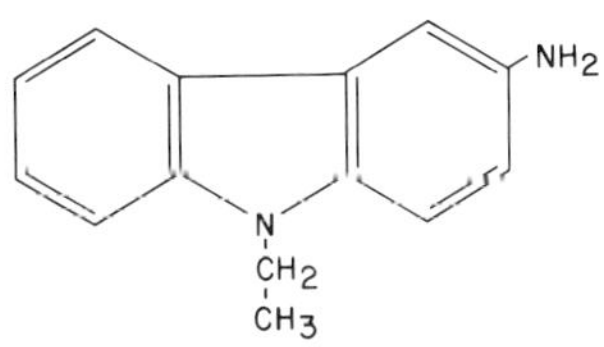

3-Amino-9-ethylcarbazole is produced on a commercial scale in the United States (Stanford Research Institute, 1977). It is used as an intermediate in the manufacture of several dyes (Society of Dyers and Colourists, 1971). It is also used as a laboratory reagent in a colorimetric assay for the enzyme peroxidase (Feinstein and Lindahl, 1973) and as a substitute for benzidine in myeloperoxidase stains (Kaplow, 1975).

Experimental carcinogenesis

Fischer 344 rats and B6C3F1 mice were fed in the diet 3-amino-9-ethylcarbazole at concentrations of 0.08 and 0.20% for rats and 0.08 and 0.12% for mice for a period of about 18 months. The animals were observed for an additional 4-6 months. Under these conditions

3-amino-9-ethylcarbazole was carcinogenic to both rats and mice inducing liver tumors. Thus, the high dose of the compound induced liver tumors in 22/48 male and 6/48 female rats, and in 41/49 male and 43/49 female mice. In the control group liver tumors developed in 1/48 males and 0/50 female rats and 6/48 males and 1/50 female mice. Other tumors in the rats induced by the compound were in the integumentary system in males, in ear duct glands in males and females, and in the uterus (NCI, 1978c).

Human data

No toxicity or epidemiological data are yet available.

5-Nitroacenaphthene

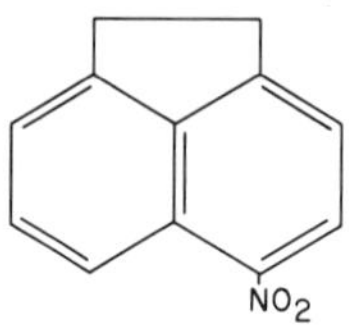

There is no evidence that 5-nitroacenaphthene has ever been produced on a commercial scale in the United States. In Japan, however, it is produced on a commercial scale and it is used as an intermediate in the production of naphthalimide dyes, which are used as fluorescent whitening agents. A small amount of this compound is used to produce a paper dye (IARC, 1978).

Experimental carcinogenesis

Oral feeding of 1% 5-nitroacenaphthene in the diet for about 4 months induced intestinal and mammary gland tumors in female Wistar rats between 9 and 18 months after the initiation of the feeding. In another study it was observed that similar feeding regimen to male Wistar rats did not produce any tumors (Takemura et al., 1974).

In a recent carcinogenesis study 5-nitroacenaphthene was administered in the diet of Fischer 344 strain rats of both sexes at concentrations of 0.12 and 0.24%. Mice, B6C3F1 strain of both sexes were fed this compound at concentrations of 0.06 and 0.12%. After 18 months of feeding 5-nitroacenaphthene was found to be carcinogenic to rats, causing increased incidences of malignant tumors of the ear canal and lung in both sexes and of the clitoral gland and mammary gland in females. In this study 5-nitroacenaphthene was also carcinogenic to female but not male mice, causing liver and ovarian tumors. Thus, in female mice liver tumors developed in 23/47 (49%) and 18/19 (95%) surviving animals on low- and high-dose levels. Liver tumors appeared in only 2/47 (4%) female control mice. The incidence of ovarian tumors was 10 and 19% of surviving mice on low- and high-dose levels and 0% in untreated controls (NCI, 1978t).

Administration of several doses of 5-nitroacenaphthene by i.p. route produced leukemia and reticulum-cell sarcoma in 4/15 and 2/15 surviving female dd strain mice, respectively (Takemura, 1970).

With Syrian hamsters of both sexes 1% 5-nitroacenaphthene in their diet for 6 months produced cholangiomas in 7/13 surviving females 9 months after the start of the feeding. Tumors were not seen in 7 treated male hamsters or in 20 females used as controls (Takemura et al., 1974).

Human data

No information is as yet available regarding the exposure and toxicity of 5-nitroacenaphthene in humans.

E. Metabolism of Aromatic Amines and Related Compounds

Several reviews on the metabolism of carcinogenic aromatic amines have appeared recently (Clayson and Garner, 1976; Irving, 1970, 1971; Kriek, 1974; Miller, 1970; Miller and Miller, 1967, 1969; Kiese, 1966; Weisburger and Weisburger, 1973). It has been known that aromatic amines need to be metabolized in any animal species before they are carcinogenic in that species, because large amounts of compounds are required for tumor induction, and that these tumors appear at sites distant from the sites of administration (Miller and Miller, 1967).

Aromatic amines are usually converted to their ring-hydroxy derivatives, which are excreted in the urine as glucuronides and sulfates (Clayson, 1962; Clayson and Garner, 1976; Kiese, 1966; Weisburger and Weisburger, 1973). Based on the formation of these metabolites, an "ortho-hydroxyamine hypothesis" was proposed to explain the carcinogenic activity of these compounds (Clayson, 1962). However, this hypothesis was shown to be incorrect because several ortho-hydroxyaromatic amines were found to be less carcinogenic than the original compounds (Clayson and Garner, 1976). Several excellent pioneering studies on the mechanism of activation of chemical carcinogens have been carried out in the laboratories of James and Elizabeth Miller at the McArdle Laboratory for Cancer Research, University of Wisconsin in Madison. Like others, Millers' laboratory has also used 2-acetylaminofluorene (AAF) as a model compound in studying chemical carcinogenesis. This chemical is discussed in detail in chapter 14. Like other aromatic amines and amides, AAF was also converted to ring-hydroxylated metabolites which were excreted in the urine as conjugates of glucuronic and sulfuric acids. These ring-hydroxylated metabolites were tested for carcinogenicity and were found to have less or no carcinogenic activity, compared to the parent amide (Miller et al., 1961a; Morris et al., 1960). However, a new metabolite was discovered in the urine of rats fed AAF continuously (Cramer et al., 1960; Miller et al., 1960). This new metabolite was characterized as the glucuronide of N-hydroxy-AAF (Cramer et al., 1960). Unlike ring-hydroxy derivatives, N-hydroxy-AAF was found to be more carcinogenic than the parent amide in the rat (Miller et al., 1961a). All species susceptible to AAF carcinogenesis excreted N-hydroxy-AAF in their urine (Miller et al., 1964; Miller and Miller, 1967). No glucuronide of N-hydroxy-AAF could be detected in the urine of guinea pigs administered AAF. This species is known to be resistant to AAF carcinogenesis (Miller et al., 1964). It was later shown that N-hydroxy-AAF was more carcinogenic than AAF in several species including the guinea pig (Miller et al., 1964; Irving et al., 1967).

Several other aromatic amines, such as 1-naphthylamine, 2-naphthylamine, 4-biphenylamine, 4-stilbenylamine, have each been shown to be N-hydroxylated by animals exposed to the parent arylamines (Andersen et al., 1964; Baldwin et al., 1963; Boyland et al., 1963; Brill and Radomski, 1971; Jagow et al., 1966; Miller et al., 1961b; Radomski and Brill, 1970, 1971; Troll and Nelson, 1961). Radomski and Brill (1970) have demonstrated a correlation of degree of carcinogenicity of 1-naphthylamine, 2-naphthylamine, and 4-biphenylamine with both methemoglobin production in the blood and concentration of N-oxidation products in the urine of dogs. The concentration of N-oxidation products was dependent on the dose administered. No significant difference was observed in N-oxidation products excreted in the urine of dogs between 1-naphthylamine and 2-naphthylamine when these animals were given the maximum acute dose of these amines that they could tolerate (70 mg/kg body weight). However, when the dose was reduced to 5 mg/kg, a dose at which 2-naphthylamine is carcinogenic and 1-naphthylamine is not, negligible quantities of N-oxidation products were found in dogs given 1-naphthylamine, and considerable quantities of N-oxidation products (0.2% of administered dose) were found in dogs given 2-naphthylamine. The same dogs given 5 mg of 4-biphenylamine per kg of body weight produced yet higher amounts of N-oxidation products averaging about 1.5% of the administered dose. Unlike the parent amines, the N-hydroxy-derivatives of 1- and 2-naphthylamine and 4-biphenylamine when introduced into the urinary bladder of mice and dogs induce bladder tumors in these species (Boyland et al., 1964; Clayson and Cooper, 1970; Radomski and Brill, 1970; Radomski et al.,

1971). These N-hydroxy-derivatives are also carcinogenic at injection sites (s.c. or i.p.) (Belman et al., 1968; Boyland et al., 1963; Radomski et al., 1971). It should be emphasized here that these aromatic amines are also N-hydroxylated in humans. Thus, patients dosed with benzidine and 2-naphthylamine excreted N-hydroxylated-derivatives of these compounds in their urine (Troll et al., 1963).

Based on these and several other studies, there is unequivocal evidence that N-hydroxylation is an activation step, whereas ring-hydroxylation is an inactivation step in the carcinogenesis by AAF and several other aromatic amines and amides (Kiese, 1966; Miller and Miller, 1967; Weisburger and Weisburger, 1973).

Kiese's laboratory has also observed N-hydroxylation products in the blood of dogs and cats after i.v. administration of aromatic amines such as aniline, N-methylaniline, N-ethylaniline, meta-toluidine, and para-toluidine (Kiese, 1966).

Since the first direct in vitro demonstration of AAF N-hydroxylation by rabbit liver microsomes in the presence of NADPH and O_2 (Irving, 1964), N-hydroxylation of AAF has also been demonstrated with liver microsomes from several species except the guinea pig (Irving, 1964; Lotlikar et al., 1967). Recent studies by Gutmann and Bell (1977) however have shown trace amounts of AAF N-hydroxylation with liver microsomes from the guinea pig.

Inhibition studies by CO and NADPH-cytochrome c reductase antibodies have shown that AAF N-hydroxylation is mediated via cytochrome P-450 mixed function oxidase system (Gutmann and Bell, 1977; Thorgeirsson et al., 1973). Moreover, differences in inhibition of AAF N- and ring-hydroxylation by CO suggest involvement of multiple forms of cytochrome P-450 (Lotlikar and Zaleski, 1974).

N-Hydroxylation has also been demonstrated in vitro with liver microsomes with various aromatic amines such as aniline, and 4-stilbenylamine (Booth and Boyland, 1964; Brill and Radomski, 1971; Kiese et al., 1966; Uehleke, 1963).

Aniline was not considered to be carcinogenic until recent studies demonstrated its carcinogenicity in rats producing hemangiosarcomas and fibrosarcomas of the spleen (NCI, 1978f). Nitrosobenzene has been detected in the blood of dogs after injection of aniline in these animals (Kiese, 1959). Similarly, aniline has been shown to be N-hydroxylated with rat liver microsomes (Uehleke, 1963). However, both phenylhydroxylamine and nitrosobenzene, which are N-oxidation products of aniline, were found to be not carcinogenic when injected in rats (Belman et al., 1968; Miller et al., 1965, 1966). Similarly, N-ethyl-N-phenylhydroxylamine was also inactive as a carcinogen in the rat (Miller et al., 1966). Thus, it should be emphasized that not all N-hydroxy compounds of aromatic amines are carcinogenic.

On the basis of studies with AAF and several other carcinogenic aromatic amides, it was suggested that esterification of the N-hydroxyamides might be the second activation step in the carcinogenesis by aromatic amines and amides (Miller, 1970). Enzymatic sulfuric acid esterification of N-hydroxy-AAF appears to be the major ultimate carcinogenic metabolite of AAF for the liver (DeBaun et al., 1970; King and Phillips, 1969; Miller, 1970). Acyltransferase reaction, which transfers N-acetyl group from N-hydroxyacetamide to N-hydroxyarylamine, forming the very reactive N-acetoxyarylamine, appears to be one of the ultimate reactions for the nonhepatic tissues (Bartsch et al., 1972, 1973; King, 1974). Esterification may not be necessary for all compounds. In any event, the ultimate metabolite is unstable and is converted to an electrophile, which interacts with critical cellular macromolecules to initiate carcinogenesis.

In arylamine bladder carcinogenesis, esterification of N-oxidation products via sulfation or acetylation is not required. Thus, recent data by Kadlubar et al. (1977) support the concept that arylamine bladder carcinogens such as 1- and 2-naphthylamine and 4-biphenylamine are N-oxidized and N-glucuronidated in the liver and that the N-glucuronides are transported to the urinary bladder. The hydrolysis of these glucuronides to N-hydroxyarylamines and the conversion of the latter derivatives to highly reactive electrophilic arylnitrenium ions in the normally acidic urine of dogs and humans may be the critical reaction for tumor induction in the urinary bladder.

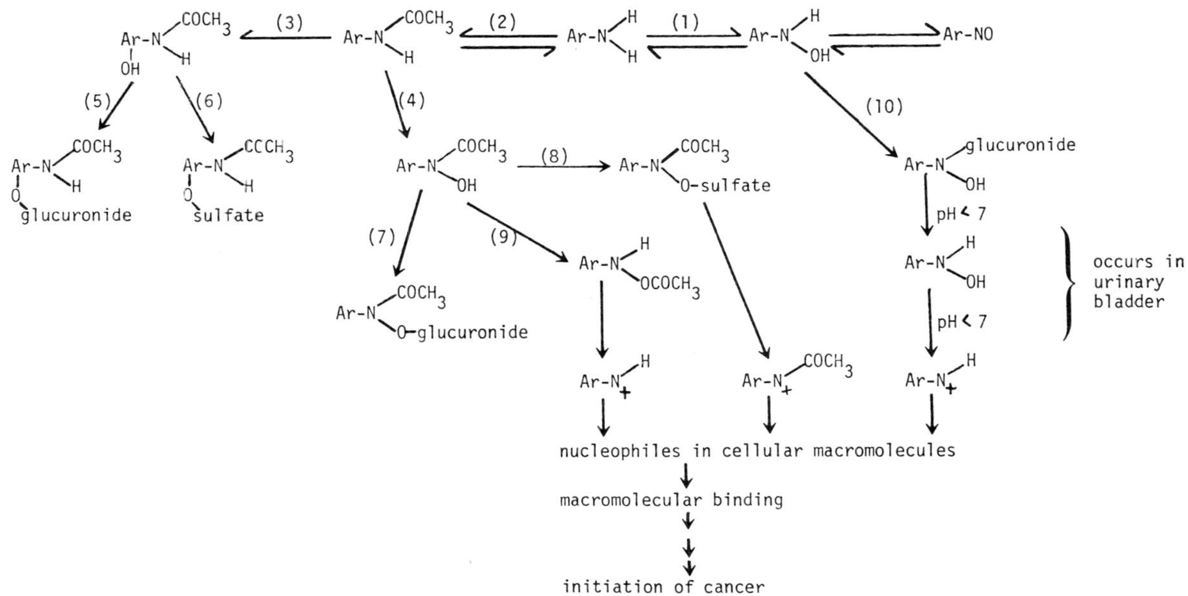

FIGURE 1 General metabolic pathways of aromatic amines. Various numbered enzyme catalyzed reactions represent as follows: (1), (3), and (4) are oxidation reactions catalyzed by tissue enzymes in the endoplasmic reticulum in the presence of NADPH and O_2; (2) is an acetylation reaction catalyzed by cytosolic enzyme in the presence of acetyl CoA; (5), (7), and (10) are glucuronidation reactions catalyzed by enzymes in the endoplasmic reticulum in the presence of uridine diphosphate glucuronic acid; (6) and (8) are sulfation reactions catalyzed by cytosolic enzymes in the presence of 3'-phosphoadenosine-5'-phosphosulfate; and (9) is an acetyltransfer reaction catalyzed by cytosolic enzyme. Ar = Aromatic.

Based on all the in vivo and in vitro evidence, the general metabolic pathways of aromatic amines are shown in Fig. 1.

Metabolic activation of aromatic amines has also been examined with the Ames bacterial mutation assay system using Salmonella bacteria with mammalian microsomes (McCann et al., 1975). In these studies mutagenic activity in the presence of mammalian liver microsomes is presumably due to the formation of N-oxidation products of aromatic amines during the test period. 2-Aminofluorene, 1- and 2-naphthylamine, benzidine, 4-biphenylamine, and 4,4-methylene-bis(2-chloroaniline) have been shown to be mutagenic in the Ames assay when tested on bacterial strain TA 1538, indicating the production of frameshift-type mutations (McCann et al., 1975). Some other aromatic amines, such as ortho-toluidine (Russfield et al., 1973a, b) and auramine (Williams and Bonser, 1962), which are hepatocarcinogens to rats and mice, were not mutagenic in the Ames assay. Aniline was also found to be inactive as a mutagen in this bacterial test system (McCann et al., 1975).

Among the various industrial aromatic amines discussed in this chapter, some are used in hair-dye formulations. Recently, several hair-dye formulations and several components of these hair dyes have been tested for mutagenicity in the Ames system (Ames et al., 1975). Among the three meta diamines, meta-phenylenediamine, 2,4-diaminotoluene, and 2,4-diaminoanisole—which were found to be mutagenic—2,4-diaminoanisole was about 30 times more reactive than the toluene derivative. Both 2,4-diaminoanisole (NCI, 1978o) and 2,4-diaminotoluene (Ito et al., 1969; Umeda, 1955) are carcinogenic to rats and mice; however, carcinogenicity of meta-phenlenediamine has not been tested adequately. Recent biochemical data by Dybing and Thorgeirsson (1977) strongly suggest that metabolic activation of 2,4-diaminoanisole to the hydroxylamine(s) may be the underlying reaction for the formation of mutagenic intermediates. para-Phenylenediamine was inactive, whereas 2,5-diaminotoluene was weakly active as a mutagen. However, both components became strongly mutagenic after oxidation by hydrogen peroxide (Ames et al., 1975). Based on these mutagenicity studies, it is very important to critically evaluate the carcinogenicity potencies of some of these active mutagens, which are being used in hair dyes and other consumer products.

III. AZO DYES

Azo dyes are used to color fabrics, paper, food, drugs, cosmetics, lubricants, and other products. Some of the azo dyes to be discussed in this chapter have either a free or substituted amino group on the molecule and hence are related to the aromatic amines. One azo dye derived from benzidine, direct brown 95, and all azo dyes derived from naphthylamine to be discussed in this chapter do not have a free amino group. However, amines may be generated from these dyes as a result of in vivo or in vitro reduction of azo linkage. All of the benzidine-derived dyes—direct blue 6, trypan blue, direct black 38, and direct brown 95—and three naphthylamine-derived dyes—Ponceau MX, Ponceau 3R, and amaranth—are sulfonic acid derivatives and hence are polar, whereas other dyes are nonpolar.

Excellent reviews on the carcinogenicity of aminoazo and related dyes are available (Clayson and Garner, 1976; Miller and Miller, 1953; Terrayama, 1967). Historically, the first conclusive evidence for the carcinogenicity of an azo dye was furnished by Yoshida (1932) and Sasaki (1935) who produced liver tumors in rats on feeding of ortho-aminoazotoluene (AAT). Early attempts to confirm these observations were unsuccessful in Germany because of the differences in animal diets in Germany and Japan. Thus, rats in Japan were fed a diet of polished white rice with virtually no additional nutrients, whereas rats in Germany were fed a nutritionally adequate regimen (see Miller and Miller, 1953). These experiments clearly emphasized the role of dietary factors in the induction of cancer by azo dyes. In later studies Kinosita (1936) demonstrated that para-dimethylaminoazobenzene was a more active hepatic carcinogen for the rat than AAT.

A. Aminoazobenzene and Related Dyes

para-Aminoazobenzene

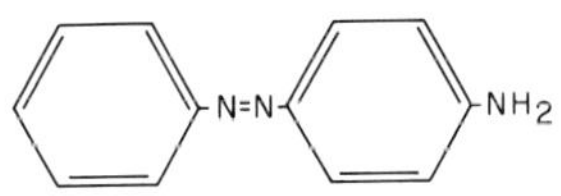

para-Aminoazobenzene, a brownish-yellow azo dye, was first produced on a commercial scale in the United States in 1924. According to the International Trade Commission, it is produced currently on a commercial scale in the United States (Chem. Eng. News, 1978). It is used as an intermediate in the manufacture of acid yellow, several diazo dyes and indulines, as a dye for lacquers, varnishes, wax products, and oil stains.

Experimental carcinogenesis

Oral administration of 0.2-1.0% para-aminoazobenzene in a restricted diet to male Wistar rats for a period of 2 years produced liver tumors in 7/16 rats. No liver tumors occurred in eight controls (Kirby and Peacock, 1947). In a skin-painting experiment that lasted for over 2 years, it was shown that p-aminoazobenzene induced skin tumors in all six albino male rats. No skin tumors were observed in six control animals. In this study no liver tumors were observed in either control or treated rats (Fare, 1966). Subcutaneous administration of this compound (2.3 mg) to male Charles River CD rats at twice weekly doses for 12 weeks did not produce any local or other tumors in 19 surviving rats 14 months after the initiation of the treatment. No local tumors but one skin tumor appeared in 20 controls (Poirier et al., 1967).

In stock mice on a restricted or normal diet several s.c. administrations of para-aminoazobenzene did not induce any local or liver tumors in any of these animals over a period of 18 months or more (Kirby, 1945).

Human data

No case reports or epidemiological data are yet available.

ortho-Aminoazotoluene

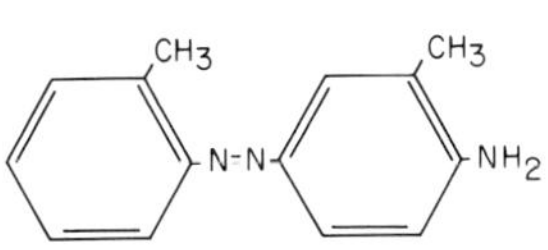

ortho-Aminoazotoluene is also known as 2-methyl-4[(2-methylphenyl)azo]benzenamine and AAT. It is a golden crystalline compound that melts at 101-102° C. ortho-Aminoazotoluene (AAT) was first produced on a commercial scale in the United States in 1914 (IARC, 1975). It is still being produced commercially in the United States (U.S. International Trade Commission, 1977). It is used to color oils, fats, and waxes (Society of Dyers and Colourists, 1971).

Experimental carcinogenesis

Oral administration of 0.1% AAT in the diet of male albino rats for about 1 year produced liver tumors in 4/6 surviving rats (Yoshida, 1932). Similar results have been obtained in later studies (Sasaki, 1935). Subcutaneous injection of this compound at weekly intervals for 1 year induced liver tumors in 12/21 albino rats surviving 1 year after the initiation of the treatment (Furukawa, 1939).

In mice oral feeding of 0.03% AAT in the diet for about 1 year produced liver tumors in 6/7 surviving animals (Nishiyama, 1935). This study has been confirmed in other laboratories (Baumann et al., 1939). Lung tumors have been induced in strain C mice of both sexes after oral feeding of AAT (Andervont et al., 1944). Such tumors were also obtained in strains A and C mice administered several doses of AAT s.c. (Andervont and Shimkin,

1940). Skin painting of mice on alternate days for 6 months induced liver tumors in 55% of animals. (Morosenskaya, 1938).

Liver and lung tumors were induced in 81 and 94% of surviving animals, respectively, when male Syrian golden hamsters were fed a diet containing 0.1% AAT for about 1 year (Tomatis et al., 1961).

Human data

Incidence of contact dermititis has been reported in people exposed to AAT (Meara and Martin-Scott, 1953). No epidemiological data are yet available.

para-Dimethylaminoazobenzene

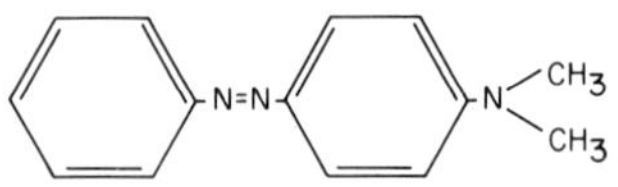

para-Dimethylaminoazobenzene is also known as butter yellow and DAB. It is a yellow crystalline compound that melts at 114-117°C. para-Dimethylaminoazobenzene (DAB) was first produced commercially in the United States in 1914 (IARC, 1975). According to the U.S. International Trade Commission, it is currently produced on a commercial scale in the United States (Chem. Eng. News, 1978). It is reportedly used for coloring polishes and other wax products, polystyrene, gasoline, and soap (Society of Dyers and Colourists, 1971).

Experimental carcinogenesis

Oral feeding of DAB in the diet was first shown to induce liver tumors in the rat (Kinosita, 1936). Since then oral feeding of 0.06% DAB in the diet has been shown to induce liver tumors equally well in Sherman, Wistar, and Evans strain rats (Sugiura and Rhoads, 1941). Liver tumors have also been induced in rats by administration of DAB by either s.c. (Maruya and Tanaka, 1936) or i.p. (Mori and Nakahara, 1940) route. In a skin-painting experiment all six male rats developed skin tumors after DAB application twice weekly for 90 weeks. No skin tumors were induced in six controls. In this study no liver tumors developed either in treated or control rats (Fare, 1966).

Oral administration of 0.015% DAB in the diet of stock albino mice for 4 months produced lung tumors in 27% of animals, whereas 15% of control mice developed lung tumors (Jaffe, 1947). In another study DAB was injected s.c. in newborn Swiss mice for 5 consecutive days. After 1 year liver tumors were observed in 26/28 treated males compared to 3/31 controls, and 4/25 treated females compared with 0/25 controls (Roe et al., 1971).

Oral feeding of DAB to hamsters and guinea pigs did not produce any tumors (Orr, 1940; Terracini and Della Porta, 1961). However, such a treatment produced bladder tumors in dogs (Nelson and Woodard, 1953).

Human data

Factory workers handling DAB were found to have contact dermatitis (National Research Council, 1971). No epidemiological data are yet available.

B. Benzidine-Derived Dyes

Direct Blue 6

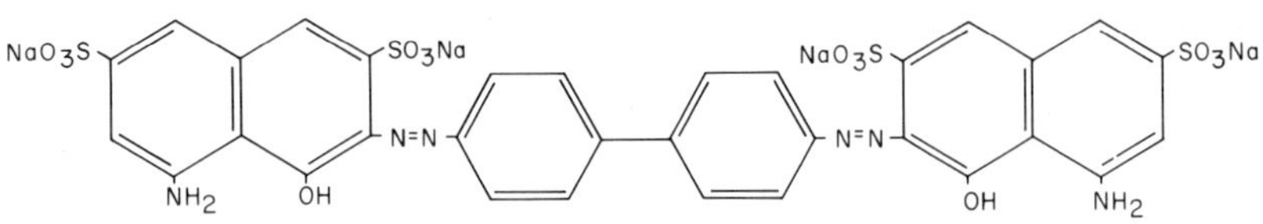

Exact data on its production are not available; however, it is believed that its production in the United States is greater than 5000 lb annually (U.S. International Trade Commission, 1977). Direct blue 6 is used for dyeing textiles such as cotton, silk, wool, nylon, and acetate, and also leather. It is also used in printing inks and paper (Society of Dyers and Colourists, 1971). Direct blue 6 has also been used in hair dyes (Comptroller General of the U.S., 1977).

Experimental carcinogenesis

Direct blue 6 was administered in the diet at 0.02, 0.04, 0.08, 0.15, and 0.30% levels to both male and female rats of Fischer 344 strain for a period of 13 weeks. Under these conditions direct blue 6 produced significant incidences of precancerous and cancerous changes in the liver of both male and female rats. Thus, direct blue 6 at 0.15% level produced liver tumors in 8/10 males and 0/10 females. At higher-dose level (0.3%), however, this dye produced liver tumors in 7/9 females. No liver tumors were produced in control males and females (NCI, 1978z; Thomas et al., 1978).

Oral administration of direct blue 6 in the diet of male and female B6C3F1 strain mice at various concentrations up to 1.25% of the diet for a 90-day period did not produce any tumors either in the liver or other organs (NCI, 1978z; Thomas et al., 1978).

Human data

Direct blue 6 is a benzidine-derived dye. The urine of workers at two benzidine-dye-manufacturing plants and two textile finishing companies contained benzidine or its metabolite monoacetylbenzidine. In one of the dye-manufacturing plants, workers exposed to the finished dyes had about 20 times more benzidine and up to 200 times more acetylated benzidine in their urine than if they had been exposed only to the residual benzidine content in the dyes. It is suggested that preventing the worker inhalation of the dye particles would greatly reduce benzidine absorption by the body (Thomas et al., 1978). No epidemiological studies are yet available implicating direct blue 6 in human cancer production.

Trypan Blue

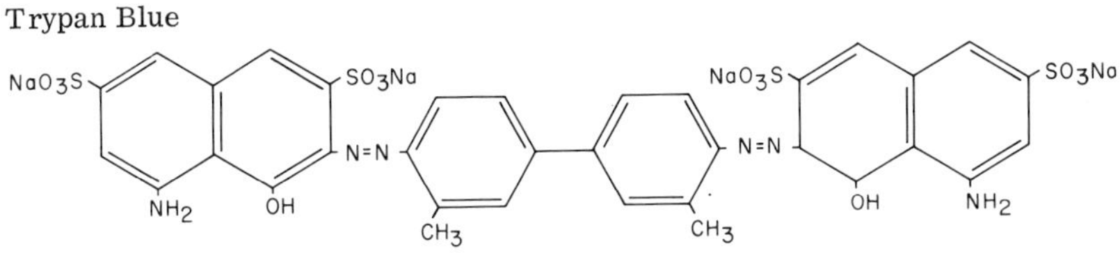

Trypan blue is a bluish gray powder which is soluble in water but almost insoluble in ethanol. Its first commercial production in the United States began in 1921 (IARC, 1975). According to the U.S. International Trade Commission, it is still produced on a commercial scale in the United States (Chem. Eng. News, 1978). It is used for dyeing textiles, leather, and paper (Society of Dyers and Colourists, 1971).

Experimental carcinogenesis

Trypan blue administered to both male and female rats by repeated s.c. injections induced tumors of the reticuloendothelial system, mainly of the liver in 56% of the surviving animals (Gillman et al., 1952). Several strains (Compton, Harwell Wistar, and Agricultural Research Council Wistar) of rats have recently been shown to be susceptible to the trypan blue carcinogenesis by this injection route (Gillman et al., 1973). In another study repeated s.c. injections of trypan blue to Wistar rats produced liver tumors and s.c. tumors at the injection site (Driessens et al., 1962). Sarcomas at the injection site were also induced in rats on i.p. administration of trypan blue (Papacharalampous, 1957).

Human data

No data are as yet available.

Direct Black 38

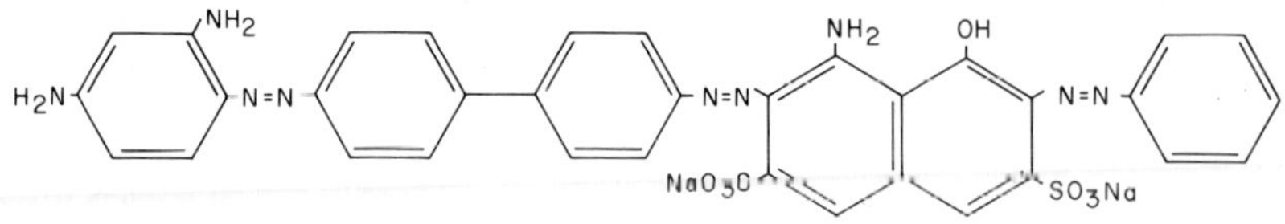

The commercial production of direct black 38 in the United States was about 3.8 million lb during the year 1976 (International Trade Commission, 1977). It is used for dyeing textiles such as cotton, wool, nylon, and acetate, and also leather. It is also used in printing inks, biological stains, in plastics, and wood stains (Society of Dyers and Colourists, 1971).

Experimental carcinogenesis

Oral administration of direct black 38 at 0.02-0.30% level in the diet of male and female Fischer 344 rats for 90 days produced liver tumors in 9/9 males and 5/9 females fed 0.15% dye in the diet. No liver tumors were observed in the control groups (NCI, 1978z; Thomas et al., 1978).

Subchronic toxicity studies of direct black 38 were also conducted in B6C3F1 mice of both sexes. No neoplastic lesions appeared in the liver or other tissues of animals fed the dye at 1.25% level of the diet for 90 days (NCI, 1978z; Thomas et al., 1978).

Human data

Large amounts of benzidine and its acetylated derivative are detected in the urines of workers at two benzidine-dye-manufacturing plants and two textile-finishing companies (Thomas et al., 1978). No epidemiological data are yet available.

Direct Brown 95

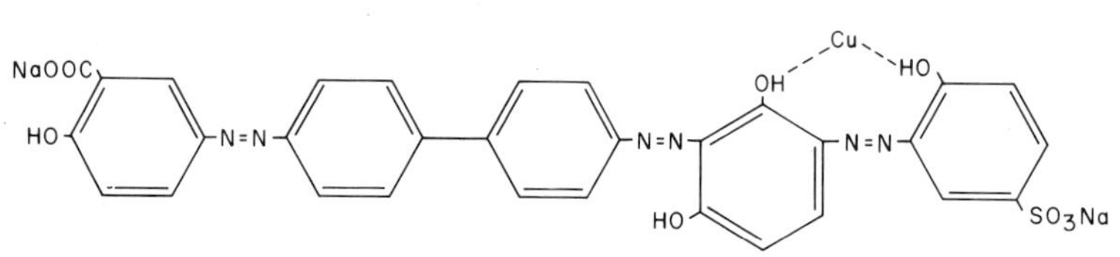

According to the U.S. International Trade Commission (1977), about 600,000 lb of direct brown 95 were produced commercially in the United States in 1976. This dye is used for dyeing textiles such as cotton, wool, silk, nylon, and acetate. In addition it is also used for dyeing leather, paper, and plastics (Society of Dyers and Colourists, 1971).

Experimental carcinogenesis

Fischer 344 rats of both sexes were given direct brown 95 in their diet at various dose levels from 0.02 to 0.30% levels for a 90-day period. Liver tumors did not develop in male rats fed this dye; however, preneoplastic lesions did develop in 7/8 male rats fed 0.15% level of this dye. This dose of the dye produced liver tumors in 5/8 females. No liver tumors or preneoplastic lesions occurred in control animals (NCI, 1978z; Thomas et al., 1978).

Oral feeding of this dye up to a dose of 1.25% of the diet to B6C3F1 mice of both sexes for a 90-day period did not produce any tumors either in the liver or any other organ (NCI, 1978z; Thomas et al., 1978).

Human data

Direct brown 95 is a benzidine-derived dye. Recently benzidine and its acetyl derivative have been detected in the urines of workers at two benzidine-dye-manufacturing plants and at two textile-finishing companies. Since benzidine is carcinogenic to experimental animals and humans, it is suggested that worker inhalation of the dye particles be kept minimum

(Thomas et al., 1978). No epidemiological data are yet available implicating direct brown 95 directly in cancer induction in humans.

C. Naphthylamine-Derived Dyes

Sudan I

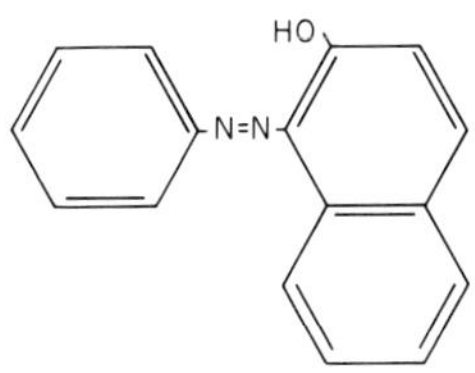

Sudan I, a red crystalline compound that melts at 134°C was first produced commercially in the United States in 1914. Its U.S. production was about 600,000 lb in 1972 (IARC, 1975). It is presumably still produced commercially in the United States. It is used for coloring oils, fats, waxes, shoe and floor polishes, varnishes, resins, gasoline, and soap (Society of Dyers and Colourists, 1971).

Experimental carcinogenesis

Addition of 0.1% Sudan I in the diet of rats and CBA strain mice for a 12-24-month period did not produce any tumors in these animals (Hackmann, 1951; Clayson et al., 1965). However, administration of Sudan I by s.c. route at 3-week intervals for 1 year produced liver tumors in 6/12 surviving male stock mice (Kirby and Peacock, 1949).

In another study Sudan I was implanted into the urinary bladder of (C57XIF)F_1 mice. After 40 weeks urinary bladder tumors were seen in 13/56 treated mice compared with 6/42 controls (Clayson et al., 1968).

Human data

No data are yet available.

Oil Orange SS

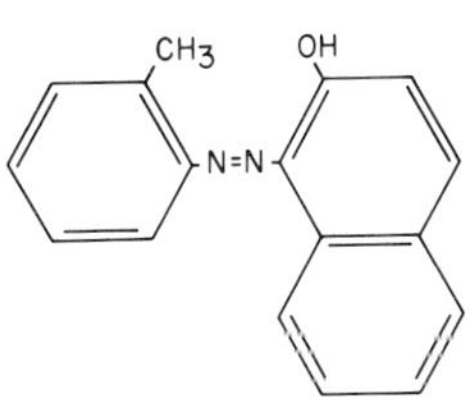

Oil orange SS, also known as FD&C Orange No. 2, was first produced on a commercial scale in the United States in 1940 (IARC, 1975). According to the U.S. International Trade Commission, it is currently produced commercially in the United States (Chem. Eng. News, 1978). It is reportedly used for coloring oils, fats, waxes, and varnishes (Society of Dyers and Colourists, 1971). This dye was used previously in the United States in foods, drugs, and cosmetics; however, because of its toxicity it has been removed from these uses (National Research Council, 1971).

Experimental carcinogenesis

Oil orange SS was administered to rats of both sexes at 0.03, 0.75, and 1.5% level in the diet. All animals on 0.75 and 1.5% levels died within 12-20 weeks. The animals on 0.03% level were sacrificed at 44 weeks. This time period was too short for induction of tumors. However, 2/20 females developed ovarian tumors. No tumors developed in 20 control animals (Allmark et al., 1956). Osborne-Mendel strain rats injected s.c. with oil orange SS once a week for 13 months did not develop tumors (Nelson and Davidow, 1957).

In contrast to rats, intestinal tumors developed in 9/12 surviving male mice when oil orange SS was administered in the diet of male and female stock albino mice at 0.1% level for 1 year. In the control group intestinal tumors appeared in 1/13 animals (Bonser et al., 1956a). In another study s.c. administration of oil orange SS induced sarcomas at the injection site in stock albino mice (Bonser et al., 1954). Bladder tumors were induced in mice on bladder implantation of oil orange SS (Clayson et al., 1958).

Human data

No data are yet available.

Sudan II

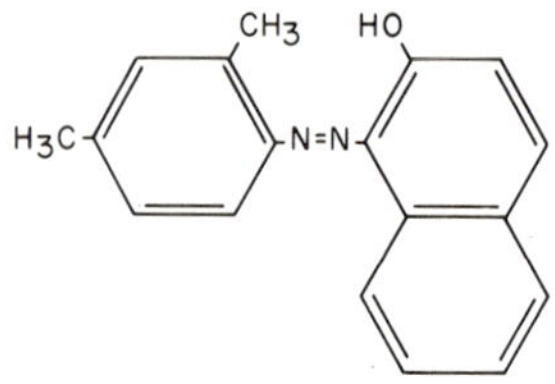

Sudan II, also known as FD&C Red No. 32, is a brownish-red crystalline compound that melts at 166°C. Its first U.S. commercial production was reported in 1921. Its production in the United States was about 76,000 lb in 1971 (IARC, 1975). It is probably still manufactured in the United States on a commercial scale. It is used for coloring oils, waxes, hydrocarbon solvents for polishes, and polystyrene resins (Society of Dyers and Colourists, 1971). It was previously used in foods, drugs, and cosmetics in the United States. However, because of its toxicological data, its use has been prohibited in food, drug, and cosmetic products since 1963 (National Research Council, 1971).

Experimental carcinogenesis

Oral and s.c. administrations of Sudan II to rats and mice did not induce tumors in these animals (Allmark et al., 1956; Bonser et al., 1956a). However, implantation of this compound in the urinary bladder of (C57XIF)F_1 mice produced bladder tumors in 43/44 of animals surviving 40 weeks after treatment. In control mice implanted with paraffin wax alone, only 6/142 mice developed bladder tumors (Clayson et al., 1968).

Human data

No data are yet available.

Scarlet Red

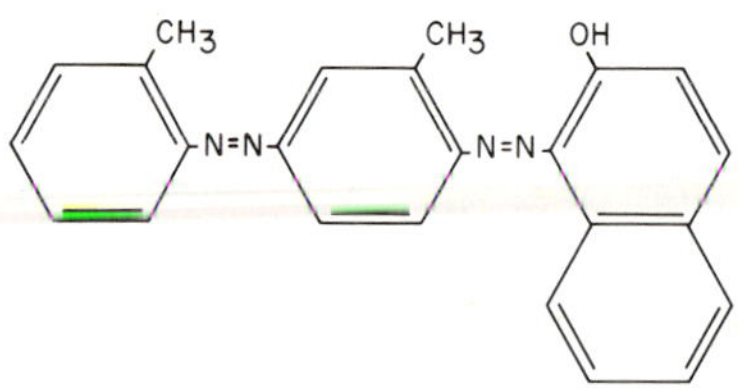

Scarlet red is a dark reddish brown crystalline compound that melts at 181-188°C. Commercial production of scarlet red was first reported in the United States in 1914 (IARC, 1975).

It is still produced commercially in the United States. It is used to color oils, fats, and waxes, shoe and floor polishes, and in petroleum oils and greases, wood stains, polystyrene, soap, cellulose acetate, and acrylic resins and varnishes (Society of Dyers and Colourists, 1971). Ointment containing scarlet red has been used as a wound-healing agent in humans.

Experimental carcinogenesis

Results of oral administration of scarlet red to rats and mice were not conclusive. However, toxicity to this compound was seen in these animals when scarlet red was administered by other routes. Scarlet red solution prepared in Tween 80 was injected s.c. at weekly intervals for about 56 weeks in male and female albino rats of Saitama strain. Of the eight rats that survived, four developed sarcomas at the site of injection. In this study no data of tumor incidence were given for controls, which received the injections of Tween 80 only (Umeda, 1957, 1958).

In a skin-painting experiment scarlet red was applied on the backs of mice thrice weekly for about 43 weeks. No tumors were observed in 64 mice which survived the treatment. However, 18/64 mice showed hyperplasia of the epithelial layer of the skin (Eckert et al., 1935).

Human data

Scarlet red has been used in medicine as a 4-8% ointment for stimulating wound healing. However, 8% ointment has been shown to cause skin irritation (Blacow, 1972). No other data are yet available.

Ponceau MX

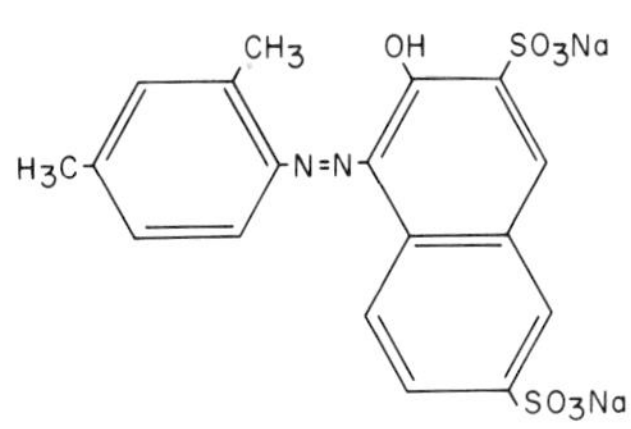

Commercial production of Ponceau MX in the United States was first reported in 1914, and is still produced commercially in the United States (Chem. Eng. News, 1978). Its primary use is as a dye for textile and leather industries. It is also used to color paper, pigment, wood stains, and inks (IARC, 1975).

Experimental carcinogenesis

A diet containing 0.2, 1.0, and 5.0% Ponceau MX was fed to a group of 20 male Wistar rats for a 15-month period. Under these conditions 4-6/15 surviving rats at these three dose levels developed liver tumors. No liver tumors were seen in any of 12 controls examined (Ikeda et al., 1966). High incidences of liver tumors were observed in male and female rats of CFE strain when they were fed similar concentrations of Ponceau MX for 2 years (Grasso et al., 1969).

A high incidence of liver tumors occurred in both male and female ddY strain mice when they were fed a diet containing 0.2, 1.0, and 5.0% Ponceau MX for 18 months (Ikeda et al., 1968).

Human data

No data are as yet available.

Ponceau 3R

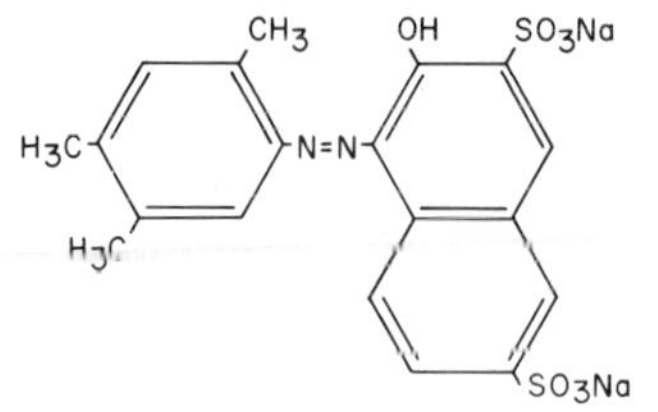

Ponceau 3R, also known as FD&C Red No. 1, is a dark-red crystalline compound that is very soluble in water. First commercial production of Ponceau 3R in the United States was reported in 1914 (IARC, 1975). According to the U.S. International Trade Commission, it is still manufactured commercially in the United States (Chem. Eng. News, 1978). It has been primarily used to dye wool. Since its initial production it was also used in foods, drugs, and cosmetics. However, because of its toxicity data in animals, its use in food, drugs, and cosmetics has been prohibited since 1966 (National Research Council, 1971).

Experimental carcinogenesis

Several chronic toxicity studies with Wistar and Osborne-Mendel strain rats of both sexes fed diets containing 0.3-3.0% Ponceau 3R for 16-24 months have shown that Ponceau 3R was carcinogenic in these animals, producing liver tumors (Grice et al., 1961; Hansen et al., 1963; Mannell, 1964).

Bladder implantation of Ponceau 3R in stock mice induced bladder tumors in 5/33 mice surviving 25 weeks compared to the appearance of bladder tumors in 1/82 controls (Bonser et al., 1963).

Human data

No data are available as yet.

Amaranth

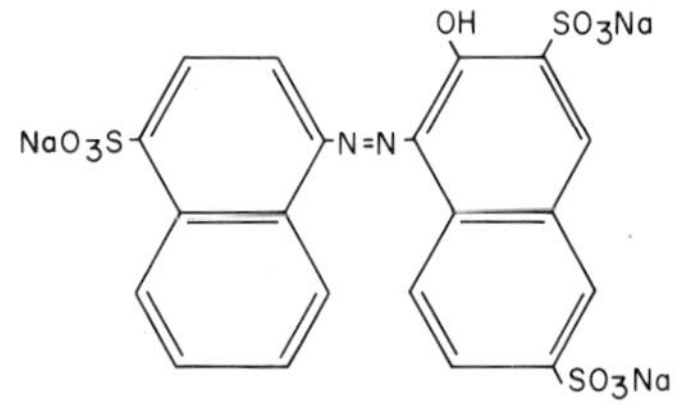

Amaranth is also known as 3-hydroxy-4-[(4-sulfo-1-naphthalenyl)azo]-2,7-naphthalenedisulfonic acid, trisodium salt, and FD&C Red No. 2. Amaranth, a dark reddish brown compound, was first produced on a commercial scale in the United States in 1914 (IARC, 1975). The latest U.S. International Trade Commission report indicates that it was produced commercially in the United States in 1975 (1977). Amaranth is used for dyeing textiles, paper, wood, leather, and phenol-formaldehyde resins (Society of Dyers and Colourists, 1971). It was also used extensively in various foods, cosmetics, and drugs. However, because of its carcinogenic activity, its use has been prohibited in food, cosmetics, and drugs in the United States (Burros, 1976).

Experimental carcinogenesis

In a recent study diet containing 2% amaranth was fed to a group of 50 noninbred rats for a period of 33 months. Under these conditions 13/48 surviving rats developed a total of 15 tumors of at least nine different tissues, including liver, mammary gland, ear duct gland, and intestine. Tumors were not observed in 50 surviving controls (Andrianova, 1970; IARC, 1975).

In another earlier study s.c. administration of amaranth to Osborne-Mendel rats of both sexes for a period of about 2 years did not induce any local or distant tumors in these animals (Nelson and Hagen, 1953).

Oral daily administration of 3-4 mg of amaranth to mice over a period of 15 months did not induce any tumors in 18 surviving mice (Cook et al., 1940).

Human data

No case reports or epidemiological data are yet available.

D. Metabolism of Azo Dyes

para-Dimethylaminoazobenzene (DAB) and related dyes have been used extensively as model compounds in studying structure-activity relationships and mechanism of activation of carcinogenesis by aminoazo dyes, in particular, and chemicals, in general. It was suggested that aminoazo dyes, like aromatic amines, must be metabolized in any animal for their carcinogenic activity, because several aminoazo dyes produced liver cancer in animals irrespective of the mode of administration of these compounds (Miller and Miller, 1953).

Earlier data on the metabolism of aminoazo and related dyes have been reviewed extensively by Miller and Miller (1953) and Terayama (1967). Recent metabolic studies of these compounds have also been reviewed (Clayson and Garner, 1976; Miller, 1970). Comprehensive metabolic studies on DAB and related dyes have been carried out in the laboratories of Drs. James and Elizabeth Miller at the University of Wisconsin. In earlier studies with aminoazo dyes it was suggested that it is not the parent dye (DAB) itself that initiates the carcinogenic process, but its azo reduction or split product, N,N-dimethyl-para-phenylenediamine (Kensler et al., 1942). However, N,N-dimethyl-para-phenylenediamine has not been found to be carcinogenic in the rat when fed at high levels for a long period of time (Miller and Miller, 1953). Mueller and Miller (1948, 1949, 1950) have shown that both N,N-dimethyl-para-phenylenediamine and aniline are formed in vitro by an enzymatic azo reduction of DAB with rat liver homogenate. In these studies it was shown that riboflavin is a component of a flavine adenine dinucleotide, which acts as an essential cofactor for the azoreductase enzyme (Mueller and Miller, 1950). Riboflavin in the diet was the factor responsible for protecting rat liver against DAB and ortho-aminoazotoluene carcinogenesis observed in earlier studies. Based on these and other studies, it has been suggested that azo reduction is an inactivation pathway in the carcinogenesis by aminoazo dyes (see Miller and Miller, 1953). Several other major metabolic reactions, such as N-demethylation, N-acetylation, and ring-hydroxylation have also been observed with DAB. The lack of carcinogenic activity with ring-hydroxylated metabolites of aminoazo dyes has indicated that ring-hydroxylation of aminoazo dyes, like aromatic amines, is also an inactivation pathway in the carcinogenesis by aminoazo dyes (Miller and Miller, 1953; Terayama, 1967).

N-Demethylation reactions are responsible for the conversion of DAB to N-methylaminoazobenzene (MAB) and aminoazobenzene (AB). MAB has been shown to be equipotent as DAB in liver tumor induction in rats, whereas AB was apparently not carcinogenic to rat liver when fed at equimolar dose levels. Thus, it appears that at least one methyl group on AB is essential for carcinogenicity to rat liver (Miller and Miller, 1953).

Sato et al. (1966) have demonstrated that, like aromatic amines, N-hydroxylation also occurs with the aminoazo dyes related to DAB. Thus, rats, mice, or hamsters administered AB, as well as rats given MAB or DAB, excrete N-hydroxy-N-acetyl-AB in the urine. Like AB, neither N-hydroxy-N-acetyl-AB nor N-hydroxy-AB was carcinogenic when administered to rats. The lack of carcinogenic activity of these compounds is apparently due to their lack of an N-methyl group, which has long been recognized as a structural feature essential for strong carcinogenic activity in this series (see Miller and Miller, 1953). These results suggested that N-hydroxy-MAB might be a proximate carcinogenic metabolite of MAB and DAB. Since N-hydroxy-MAB was labile and could not be readily synthesized, evidence for N-hydroxylation of MAB was obtained from the carcinogenic activity of a synthetic ester of N-hydroxy-MAB (Poirier et al., 1967) and its nonenzymatic interaction in vitro with constituents of proteins and nucleic acids (Lotlikar et al., 1966; Poirier et al., 1967). Lin et al. (1968, 1969, 1975) and Scribner et al. (1965) have shown the identity of several hydrolysis products of hepatic protein and nucleic acid-bound derivatives of MAB from rats given MAB with those obtained in vitro with ester of N-hydroxy-MAB. Recently Kadlubar et al. (1976a) have demonstrated that N-hydroxylation of MAB is not mediated via cytochrome P 450 enzyme system, but is mediated via microsomal amine oxidase system. Their current data indicate that enzymatic sulfuric acid esterification of N-hydroxy-MAB by rat liver cytosol may be the second and final activation step in the carcinogenesis by MAB and related aminoazo dyes (Kadlubar et al., 1976b). These data would support the enhancement of hepatocarcinogenesis by 3'-methyl-DAB in rats on supplementation of their diet with sodium sulfate (Blunck and Crowther, 1975).

In contrast to aminoazo dyes, few metabolic studies have been performed to understand the mechanism of action of azo dyes derived from either naphthylamine or benzidine. Radomski and Mellinger (1961) and Roxon et al. (1967) have shown that intestinal flora within animals and many animal hepatic enzyme systems are capable of splitting the azo bond in several azo dyes, releasing various types of aromatic amines.

Rinde and Troll (1975) demonstrated that rhesus monkeys fed benzidine-derived azo dyes with no residual benzidine excreted benzidine in their urine. The levels excreted were estimated as being almost as high as if an equal amount of pure benzidine as found in the dye moiety were fed to the monkeys. Recently benzidine and its acetyl derivative have been detected in the urine of workers at two benzidine-dye-manufacturing plants and at two textile-finishing companies (Thomas et al., 1978). It is estimated that about 20 times more benzidine and up to 200 times more monoacetylbenzidine were present in the urine of these dye workers than if they had been exposed only to the residual benzidine content in the dyes. These results in rhesus monkeys and humans definitely suggest that benzidine detected in the urine is produced by in vivo reduction of the azo bonds in benzidine-derived azo dyes. Such an azo reduction of trypan blue would generate 3,3'-dimethylbenzidine and its acetylated products.

Similarly, enzymatic azo reductions of several naphthylamine-derived dyes discussed in this chapter would also generate 1-amino-2-naphthol and several methylated anilines, such as 2-methylaniline (ortho-toluidine), 2,4-dimethylaniline (2,4-xylidine), and 2,4,5-trimethylaniline. ortho-Aminoazotoluene, a hepatocarcinogen, and 1-amino-2-naphthol would be generated by azo reduction of scarlet red.

Benzidine and its derivative 3,3'-dimethylbenzidine and ortho-toluidine have already been shown to be carcinogenic in several species. Carcinogenicity of 2,4-xylidine and 2,4,5-trimethylaniline has not been well established. The overall metabolism of these aromatic amines was discussed in Sec. II.E.

Azo reduction is considered to be an inactivation pathway in the carcinogenesis by aminoazo dyes, whereas azo reduction appears to be an activation pathway in carcinogenesis by benzidine-derived and naphthylamine-derived azo dyes.

IV. N-NITROSO COMPOUNDS

The N-nitroso compounds are substances that have a characteristic linkage of a secondary nitrogen atom to the nitroso group, -N=O. Several N-nitroso compounds have been used as industrial chemicals before their toxicities were discovered. There are now more than 100 N-nitroso compounds that are known to be carcinogenic in experimental animals largely because of the extensive studies by Dr. Druckrey and his colleagues in Heidelberg, Germany. Excellent reviews on the carcinogenicities of these compounds have been compiled by Druckrey et al. (1967a), Magee and Barnes (1967), and recently by Magee et al. (1976).

Historically, two laboratory workers accidentally exposed to dimethylnitrosamine (DMN) developed severe liver damage (Freund, 1937). Later, Barnes and Magee (1954) reported that DMN had produced acute or subacute poisoning in a few workers inadvertently exposed to this agent in industrial laboratories. Investigation of this condition in experimental animals revealed that DMN was not only a powerful hepatotoxin, but also a strong carcinogen in rats upon chronic intake (Magee and Barnes, 1956). It was later observed that small repeated doses of DMN to rats gave liver cancer, whereas a single large dose of this agent yielded kidney tumors in this species (Magee and Barnes, 1959). Other investigations indicate that different nitrosamines cause cancer in distinct main target organs although variations in dosage or the mode of administration yields diverse tumors in several organs (Druckrey et al., 1967a; Magee and Barnes, 1967; Magee et al., 1975, 1976).

N-Nitroso compounds discussed in this chapter are divided into two groups: (1) nitrosamines and (2) nitrosamides. The nitrosamines are the nitroso derivatives of secondary amines. In general, these compounds are relatively stable even in the presence of alkali and high temperatures if kept in the dark. However, they undergo rapid decomposition when exposed to ultraviolet light. Nitrosamides are the N-nitroso derivatives of monosubstituted acyl amides. In contrast to nitrosamines, nitrosamides are unstable under physiological conditions and decompose rapidly in alkali to yield diazoalkanes.

Since many N-nitroso compounds are carcinogenic in a wide range of experimental animals, it is believed that they are also carcinogenic in humans. Aspects of occurrence of nitrosamines in the environment and their possible hazards are discussed in Chapter 7. Many toxic and carcinogenic nitrosamines need not be consumed exogenously as such, but can be formed endogenously by the interaction of nitrite and secondary or tertiary amines. This aspect of nitrosamine formation is not reviewed here, but is discussed in Chapter 11.

A. Nitrosamines

N-Nitrosodimethylamine

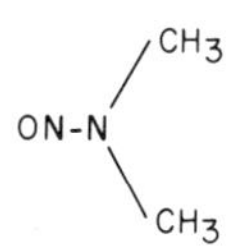

N-Nitrosodimethylamine, a yellow volatile liquid that boils at 151-153°C, is also known as dimethylnitrosamine and DMN. The International Trade Commission has identified N-nitrosodimethylamine (DMN) in commercial production in the United States (Chem. Eng. News, 1978). It has been used both as an industrial solvent and as an intermediate in the synthesis of the rocket fuel 1,1-dimethylhydrazine. Patents were issued for its use as a solvent in the fiber and plastics industry, as a softener for copolymers, as an additive for lubricants, and as an antioxidant. It has also been used as a nematocide (IARC, 1972).

Experimental carcinogenesis

It has been shown that oral administration of DMN is carcinogenic to rats, inducing liver and kidney tumors (Argus and Hoch-Ligeti, 1961; Magee and Barnes, 1956, 1962, 1967; Magee et al., 1976; Zak et al., 1960). Intraperitoneal or i.m. injection of DMN to rats has produced renal tumors (Murphy et al., 1966), whereas inhalation route of DMN has yielded tumors of the nasal cavity and kidney (Druckrey et al., 1967a, 1969). When pregnant rats were treated with DMN during the last week of pregnancy, their offspring developed renal tumors (Alexandrov, 1968).

Pulmonary and hepatic tumors are induced by DMN administered either orally or s.c. to several strains of mice (Toth et al., 1964; Takayama and Oota, 1965; Clapp et al., 1968; Otsuka and Kawahara, 1971). Administration of DMN to newborn mice produced both liver and lung tumors (Terracini et al., 1966; Toth and Shubik, 1967; Vesselinovitch, 1969). Single or repeated injections of DMN to pregnant mice during the last days of gestation produced lung and liver tumors in their offspring (Smetanin, 1971).

Oral administration of DMN has also produced liver tumors in hamsters (Tomatis et al., 1964), guinea pigs (LePage and Christie, 1969a), rabbits (LePage and Christie, 1969b), and even rainbow trout (Ashley and Halver, 1968).

Human data

Two cases of poisoning have been reported in laboratory workers involved in the production of DMN (Freund, 1937). According to this report, these two workers had repeatedly inhaled DMN in sufficient amounts to produce headache, backache, abdominal cramps, nausea, anorexia, weakness, and drowsiness. Toxicity of DMN in these workers produced liver cirrhosis.

No epidemiological data are as yet available to evaluate carcinogenic effect of DMN in humans.

N-Nitrosodiethylamine

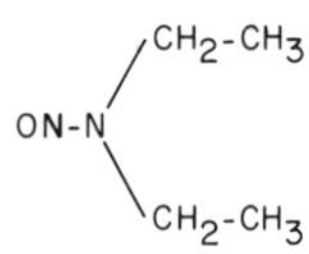

N-Nitrosodiethylamine, a slightly yellow volatile liquid that boils at 175-177° C, is also known as diethylnitrosomine and DEN. Patents were issued for the use of N-nitrosodiethylamine (DEN) as a solvent in the fiber industry, as an additive for lubricants, as a softener for copolymers, and as an intermediate in the synthesis of 1,1-diethylhydrazine (IARC, 1972). However, according to the International Trade Commission report, DEN is not produced commercially in the United States (Chem. Eng. News, 1978).

Experimental carcinogenesis

Schmahl et al. (1960) were the first to demonstrate carcinogenesis by DEN in the rat. These investigators showed that oral daily administration of DEN to rats produced liver tumors. This chemical in addition to inducing liver tumors has also produced esophageal and kidney tumors in this species (Druckrey et al., 1963a, 1964b). Other routes of administration, i.p. and i.m., have produced liver and kidney tumors, respectively (Svoboda and Higginson, 1968; Druckrey et al., 1963b, 1964b).

In several strains of mice studied oral administration of DEN has produced liver, lung, forestomach, and esophageal tumors (Schmahl et al., 1963; Takayama and Oota, 1965; Clapp and Craig, 1967; Clapp et al., 1970, 1971). Lung adenomas were obtained in this species when these animals were injected i.p. with DEN (Mirvish and Kaufman, 1970). However, s.c. administration of DEN produced both hepatomas and increased incidence of lung adenomas (Gargus et al., 1969). Even by transplacental route, DEN produced increased incidence of pulmonary tumors in the offspring when their mothers were given DEN from the 15th to 20th day of gestation (Mohr and Althoff, 1965).

Feeding DEN to Syrian golden hamsters resulted in tumors in the liver, lung, trachea, larynx, and nasal cavities (Dontenwill and Mohr, 1961; Dontenwill et al., 1962; Herrold and Dunham, 1963). However, either s.c. or intratracheal administration of this carcinogen gave high incidence of tumors in the respiratory tract but lower or no incidence of liver tumors (Dontenwill et al., 1962; Herrold and Dunham, 1963; Herrold, 1964). In transplacental studies, when pregnant hamsters were given DEN s.c. in the second half of the gestation period, tracheal tumors were produced both in the offspring and their treated mothers (Mohr et al., 1966).

Oral administration of DEN has produced predominantly liver tumors in several other species such as guinea pigs (Argus and Hoch-Ligeti, 1963), rabbits (Rapp et al., 1965), dogs (Schmahl et al., 1964), and monkeys (Kelly et al., 1966).

Human data

No epidemiological data are as yet available to evaluate the carcinogenic effect of DEN in humans.

N-Nitroso-Di-N-Butylamine

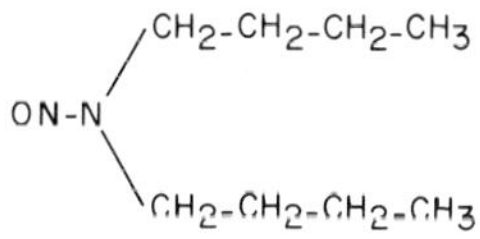

N-Nitroso-di-n-butylamine is also known as dibutylnitrosamine and DBN. It is a pale yellow liquid with a characteristic odor; it boils at about 234-237° C. N-Nitroso-di-n-butylamine (DBN) has been used in the synthesis of di-n-butylhydrazine. It is also used in the laboratories as a research chemical. However, there is no information available regarding its commercial production in the United States (IARC, 1974a).

Experimental carcinogenesis

Oral administration of DBN at various dose levels to both BD and Wistar strain rats induced bladder, esophageal, and liver tumors. It was shown in these studies that liver tumors occurred at high-dose levels only, whereas bladder and esophageal tumors were seen at both high- and low-dose levels (Druckrey et al., 1962b; 1967a; Okajima et al., 1971). Similar types of tumors arose in BD rats when they were given weekly s.c. injections of DBN; however, bladder tumor incidence by injection route was much higher than that with oral administration (Druckrey et al., 1967a).

In ICR strain mice it has been shown that feeding of DBN in the diet for 1 year induced forestomach tumors in all surviving animals. In addition, about 50% of surviving animals developed liver tumors; esophageal and lung tumors were also observed in some animals (Takayama and Imaizumi, 1969). In another study C57B1/6 mice of both sexes were given DBN in their drinking water at two dose levels. All animals of both sexes developed esophageal tumors at both dose levels. Tumors of the forestomach appeared in these animals only at the lower-dose level. Unlike ICR strain mice, no liver tumors developed in this strain. However, in this strain of mice bladder tumor was induced; males were more susceptible than females toward bladder tumor induction by DBN (Bertram and Craig, 1970). Bladder tumors were also induced in both sexes of IFxC57 mice when they were injected s.c. with DBN. However, liver tumors and not bladder tumors developed in both sexes in this strain when newborn animals were injected by the same route (Wood et al., 1970).

Differences in carcinogenic response on either oral or s.c. administration of DBN have also been observed with Syrian golden hamsters and Chinese hamsters. Thus, respiratory tract was very susceptible in the Syrian hamster, whereas it was resistant in the Chinese hamsters to tumor induction by DBN. Forestomach tumors developed to a larger extent in Chinese hamsters than in Syrian hamsters. Both strains also developed urinary bladder tumors on s.c. administration of DBN (Althoff et al., 1971).

Liver and bladder tumors were induced in guinea pigs on oral administration of DBN (Ivankovic and Bucholer, 1968).

Human data

No information is yet available on either exposure or toxicity of DBN in humans.

N-Methyl-N,4-Dinitrosoaniline

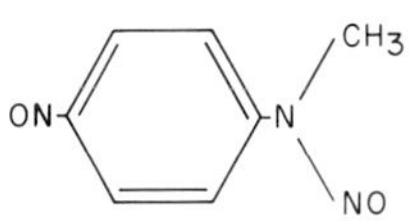

It is a crystalline green compound that melts at 101° C. It is very slightly soluble in water. Due to its antioxidant and anti-flex-cracking properties, it was used as a rubber additive. However, its present use as a rubber additive is not known (IARC, 1972).

Experimental carcinogenesis

Commercial preparations containing 33% of N-methyl-N,4-dinitrosoaniline were fed to rats at various dose levels from 0.1 mg to 30 mg/rat/day for 1 year. Under these conditions tumors developed in mammary glands, thyroid, pituitary, and testes. The percentage of tumor bearing animals at highest-dose levels was about 5 times higher than that in the control group (Weisburger et al., 1966; Hadidian et al., 1968). In another study this compound was administered i.p. at a dose level of 5 mg/animal/week for 6 months. Out of 24 rats undergoing such a treatment, only two local sarcomas, one hepatoma, one thymoma, one pancreatic, and one pituitary tumor were observed. In the control group only one hepatoma was seen (Boyland et al., 1968).

Human data

No information about exposure of workers to this chemical is yet available.

B. Nitrosamides

Nitrosomethylurea

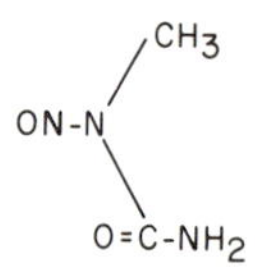

Nitrosomethylurea (NMU), a pale yellow crystalline compound that melts at 124°C with decomposition, is widely used in chemical laboratories for the generation of diazomethane. NMU and derivatives were also used in cancer chemotherapy. However, this compound is not produced commercially in the United States (Chem. Eng. News, 1978).

Experimental carcinogenesis

Oral administration of NMU at a level of 4-8 mg/kg body weight per day for life produced forestomach tumors in rats (Druckrey et al., 1961b, 1967a). Feeding of this compound at a slightly higher level intermittently over a period of 9 months induced malignant brain tumors, in addition to forestomach tumors, in rats (Schreiber and Janisch, 1967). In another study Leaver et al. (1969) have shown that a single intragastric dose of 90 mg NMU/kg body weight induced tumors in the kidney, forestomach, small and large intestine, skin, and the jaw in the rat.

Intravenous injection of a single dose of 70-100 mg NMU/kg body weight in rats produced tumors in various organs including the brain, kidney, stomach, and small and large intestine (Druckrey et al., 1963b, 1964b). In transplacental studies treatment of pregnant rats induced tumors of the kidney and the nervous system in the offspring and mammary tumors in the treated mothers (Alexandrov, 1969). In newborn mice topical application of NMU for 18 weeks induced malignant skin tumors (Graffi et al., 1967). Intraperitoneal injection of this chemical into newborn and 5-week-old mice produced lymphosarcomas and lung, liver, and forestomach tumors (Terracini and Testa, 1970). In these studies it was shown that newborn animals were more susceptible to the induction of all these tumors except those of the forestomach.

Oral administration of NMU in Syrian golden hamsters produced odontogenic tumors and epidermoid carcinomas of the oral cavity and intestinal tumors (Herrold, 1968, 1969). Intraperitoneal and intratracheal treatments induced intestinal and upper respiratory tract tumors, respectively (Herrold, 1969, 1970).

Human data

Epidemiological data are not yet available to evaluate the carcinogenic effect of NMU in humans.

Nitrosoethylurea

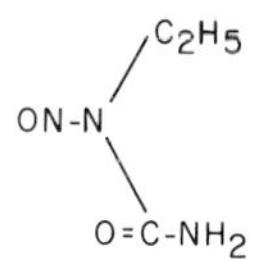

Nitrosoethylurea is also known as ethylnitrosourea and ENU. It is a yellowish-pink crystalline compound that melts at 103-104° C with decomposition. Industrial use of nitrosoethylurea (ENU) is not known. It is not produced commercially in the United States (Chem. Eng. News, 1978). It is, however, used in chemical laboratories for the generation of diazoethane.

Experimental carcinogenesis

Tumors in the central and peripheral nervous system developed in about 95% of the rats after oral administration of a single dose of ENU (Druckrey et al., 1970). Similar types of tumors appeared even by subcutaneous treatment. However, when rats were injected i.v. with ENU, in addition to the tumors of the nervous system, tumors of the kidney, ovary, and uterus also developed. More of such tumors were observed in the adult rats than in young or newborn animals (Druckrey et al., 1970). Neurogenic tumors also appeared in the offspring of BD rats when pregnant rats were injected with a single dose of ENU on the 14th day of gestation (Druckrey et al., 1966a).

Kidney and neurogenic tumors developed in mice when they were injected i.p. with ENU. The frequency and multiplicity of tumor types were shown to be dependent on age at the time of treatment (Vesselinovitch et al., 1973). In another study it has been demonstrated that when pregnant mice were injected i.p. with a single dose of ENU between the 12th and 19th day of gestation, pulmonary tumors appeared in the offspring at 12 weeks of age (Rice, 1969).

Human data

There is no information as yet available about exposure and toxicity of this chemical in humans.

N-Methyl-N'-Nitro-N-Nitrosoguanidine

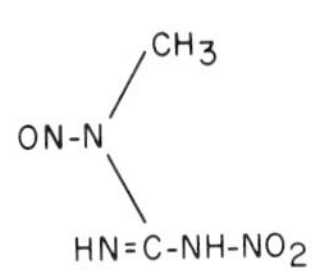

N-Methyl-N'-nitro-N-nitrosoguanidine (MNNG) is a pale yellow crystalline compound that melts at about 118-123° C with decomposition. MNNG was probably produced commercially during late 1940s and the 1950s when it was used extensively in the preparation of diazomethane solutions in the laboratories. At present it is not produced commercially in the United States (Chem. Eng. News, 1978). It is, however, produced on a small scale as a research chemical.

Experimental carcinogenesis

Glandular stomach tumors have been induced in male Wistar rats when they were given MNNG in their drinking water for a period of 6-12 months (Sugimura and Fujimura, 1967; Sugimura et al., 1969, 1970). Intragastric intubations of this chemical to rats produced, in addition, tumors of the forestomach (Schoental, 1966; Schoental and Bensted, 1969). In another study treatment of rats by s.c. injections induced sarcomas at the site of injections (Druckrey et al., 1966b; Sugimura et al., 1966). Gastrointestinal tumors, including tumors in the stomach, jejunum, and cecum developed in this species on i.p. treatment of MNNG (Schoental and Bensted, 1969).

In CH3 mice a single intragastric intubation of MNNG induced forestomach and intestinal tumors (Schoental and Bensted, 1969). In another study with C3H and CFW strain mice intestinal tumors developed on i.p. injection of this chemical (Schoental and Bensted, 1969). Topical application of MNNG to ICR strain mice induced skin tumors (Takayama et al., 1971).

Tumors of the glanudlar stomach developed in Syrian golden hamsters when they were given MNNG in their drinking water (Sugimura et al., 1969; Fujimura et al., 1970). On the other hand, no such tumors of the glandular stomach were induced in rabbits by such a treatment. Instead, this species developed lung tumors (Sugimura et al., 1969).

Human data

No epidemiological data are yet available to evaluate any carcinogenic effect of this chemical in humans.

N-Nitroso-N-Methylurethane

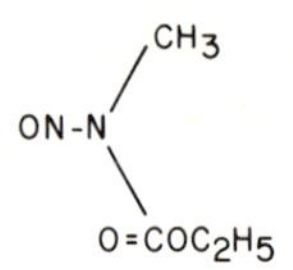

N-Nitroso-N-methylurethane is also known as N-methyl-N-nitrosourethane and MNUT. It is a yellowish to pink volatile oil that cannot be distilled at atmospheric pressure. N-Nitroso-N-methylurethane (MNUT) was used previously for the laboratory generation of diazomethane. There is no evidence that it is prepared on a commercial scale in the United States. However, it is used in the laboratories as a research chemical.

Experimental carcinogenesis

Oral administration of MNUT to rats produced forestomach and esophageal tumors (Druckrey et al., 1961b, 1967a; Schoental and Magee, 1962; Schoental, 1968). Lung and intestinal tumors developed on i.p. injection of this chemical in rats (Schoental and Bensted, 1968), whereas repeated i.v. treatment induced only lung tumors in this species (Druckrey et al., 1962a, 1967a).

Esophageal and forestomach tumors developed in mice on oral feeding of MNUT (Schoental, 1968). Lung tumors appeared in all mice on a single injection by i.p. route. Newborn mice appeared to be more susceptible to such a treatment than adult mice (Frei, 1970).

Syrian golden hamsters were susceptible to esophageal and forestomach tumor induction by MNUT on oral intubation (Herrold, 1966).

In another study guinea pigs developed stomach and pancreatic tumors on oral administration of MNUT in their drinking water (Druckrey et al., 1967a, 1968).

Human data

No data are available regarding exposure and toxicity of this chemical in humans.

Streptozotocin

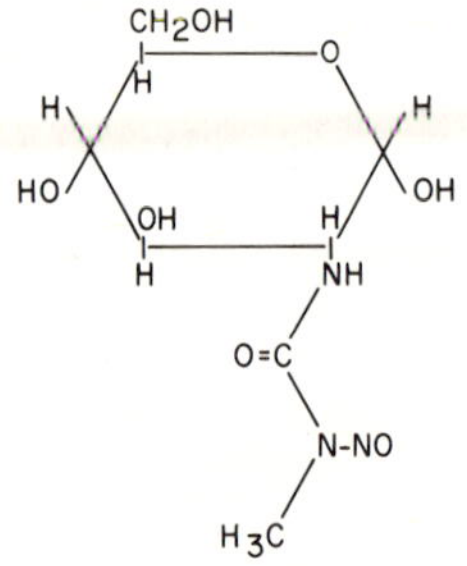

Streptozotocin, also known as N-D-glycosyl-(2)-N'-nitrosomethylurea, is a white to pale yellow crystalline compound. It was originally isolated as an antibiotic from Streptomyces achromogenes during fermentation. It has also been synthesized by various procedures. It is also produced commercially in the United States on a small scale (IARC, 1974a). Streptozotocin, though possessing antibacterial properties (Vavra et al., 1960), never found commercial use as an antimicrobial agent. It has a specific toxic effect on β-cells of the pancreas, producing hyperglycemia; therefore, it is being used in laboratories for research on diabetes (Rakieten et al., 1963). It can be used clinically in the treatment of pancreatic tumors of the β-cells (Rudas, 1972).

Experimental carcinogenesis

It has been demonstrated in two separate studies that a single dose of streptozotocin administered to rats by i.v. route induced kidney tumors (Arison and Feudale, 1967; Mauer et al., 1974).

In Chinese hamsters i.v. injection of streptozotocin produced liver tumors (Berman et al., 1973).

Human data

Streptozotocin has been used clinically for the treatment of pancreatic islet cell tumors. However, no epidemiological data are as yet available.

C. Metabolism of N-Nitroso Compounds

As indicated earlier, compared to nitrosamines, nitrosamides are very unstable compounds under physiological conditions. Both types of compounds when injected in laboratory animals are very rapidly and evenly distributed in all tissues of these animals. However, half-life of nitrosamides in various animal tissues is much shorter than that of nitrosamines, 5-10 min for nitrosamides compared to 5-10 hr for nitrosamines (see Druckrey et al., 1967a; Magee and Barnes, 1967; Magee et al., 1976).

In earlier studies Magee (1956) observed that metabolism of dimethylnitrosamine (DMN) occurs mainly in the liver. Heath (1962) later showed that following administration of ^{14}C-labeled DMN to rats, a large proportion of the injected radioactivity is expired as $^{14}CO_2$ within a few hours. In these studies very little of the unchanged nitrosamine was detected in the urine, feces, and exhaled air. Druckrey et al. (1964a) were the first to detect several nitroso metabolites in the urine of rats given di-n-butylnitrosamine (DBN). Since then Japanese investigators (Hashimoto et al., 1972; Okada, 1976; Okada et al., 1975) have shown several urinary nitroso metabolites of DBN to be carcinogenic to several tissues in rats. On the basis of detailed studies of the rates of metabolism of several dialkylnitrosamines, Heath (1962) concluded that the active molecular species involved in liver injury must be either the unstable monoalkylnitrosamine formed by the dealkylation of the dialkyl compound or an alkylating species derived from it. Since then there has been considerable evidence indicating that nitrosamines are inactive as such and that they must be metabolically activated for their carcinogenic effects. Good correlations have been obtained in in vitro studies between rat and hamster tissues in their capacity to metabolize radiolabeled DMN and diethylnitrosamine (DEN) and the response of these tissues to the carcinogenic effects by these chemicals (Bartsch et al., 1975; Montesano and Magee, 1974).

Oxidative metabolism of DMN and DEN has been shown to occur in the presence of endoplasmic reticulum of liver and other tissues from several species, NADPH, and molecular oxygen (Czygan et al., 1973; Lotlikar et al., 1975, 1976; Rao and Vesselinovitch, 1973; Venkatesan et al., 1968). Czygan et al. (1973), using mouse liver microsomes and Ames mutagenesis assay system, showed that both the oxidative demethylation and the activation of DMN to a mutagen were inhibited by carbon monoxide, and the inhibition was maximally reversed by monochromatic light at 450 nm. Their studies indicate that both microsomal metabolism and activation of DMN to a mutagen are cytochrome P-450 dependent. However, Lake et al. (1978), based on their studies with several other inhibitors, have suggested that DMN is not primarily metabolized by cytochrome P-450 mixed-function oxidase system but is metabolized by another noncytochrome P-450 enzyme system, that is, an amine oxidase system.

It is, however, generally accepted that oxidative dealkylation of dialkylnitrosamines is mediated via NADPH-dependent microsomal enzyme system. During such an enzyme reaction, a reactive species is generated which is responsible for mutation and carcinogenesis. Recently Montesano and Bartsch (1976) have reviewed the mutagenicity studies carried out with these and related compounds.

Unlike nitrosamines, nitrosamides do not require enzymatic activation. These compounds break down spontaneously in the body to yield alkylating intermediates that react covalently with tissue macromolecules. Sulfhydryl compounds enhance the breakdown of N-methylnitrosourethane and N-methyl-N'-nitro-N-nitrosoguanidine, but do not have any effect on the decomposition of N-nitrosomethylurea and N-nitrosoethylurea. Lee et al. (1977) have recently investigated the mutagenicity of several nitrosamides and related compounds using the Ames system without the presence of microsomal enzyme system.

Based on earlier studies in vivo and in vitro, it was believed that diazomethane was a reactive intermediate formed during oxidative dealkylation of DMN (Druckrey et al., 1967a; Magee and Barnes, 1967). However, in vivo studies by Lijinsky et al. (1968) have shown that the methyl group is transferred intact from the dimethylnitrosamine to nucleic acids and not via diazomethane intermediate. On the basis of available evidence, the metabolism of carcinogenic N-nitroso compounds can be shown with DMN and nitrosomethylurea (NMU) as representative compounds for nitrosamine and nitrosamide groups, respectively (Fig. 2). As indicated, DMN is first hydroxylated by a microsomal enzyme system to form an unstable metabolite which spontaneously decomposes to yield formaldehyde and an unstable intermediate, monomethylnitrosamine. The common unstable intermediate, obtained by the spontaneous breakdown of NMU, rearranges to yield a methyldiazonium hydroxide, which produces an alkylating species reacting covalently with tissue macromolecules such as RNA, DNA, and protein. Based on all the available evidence, it appears that DNA alkylation is responsible for mutagenicity and carcinogenicity by these compounds (Lawley, 1966, 1972; Magee et al., 1975, 1976).

Pegg has recently reviewed the extensive work on DNA alkylation by N-nitroso compounds (1977). It appears that even though there is extensive alkylation at N-7 position compared to 0^6-position of guanine, there is a much better correlation between 0^6-alkylguanine production in DNA and carcinogenesis. In addition, it is observed that 0^6-alkylguanine persists in the DNA of target tissues highly susceptible to carcinogenesis for much longer time than in tissues that are resistant. Thus, it is believed that the presence of 0^6-alkylguanine in DNA during cell division may be responsible for the initiation of the carcinogenic process.

V. HYDRAZINE AND RELATED COMPOUNDS

Hydrazine and some of its derivatives were originally used in rocket fuels. However, today many of these compounds are commercially used in herbicides, pesticides, blowing agents for plastics, and water treatment, and so on.

Historically, isonicotinic acid hydrazide, a hydrazine derivative used as an antitubercular agent, was shown to produce a very high incidence of pulmonary tumors in mice when administered orally (Mori et al., 1960). Hydrazine was known to be hepatotoxic, but it was not tested for carcinogenicity until Biancifiori and Ribbachi (1962) tested it to understand the mechanism of carcinogenicity of isonicotinic acid hydrazide. Their studies demonstrated that oral administration of hydrazine produced pulmonary tumors in 100% of female mice. Earlier investigations with rats (Argus and Hoch-Ligeti, 1961; Druckrey et al., 1961a) indicated that unsymmetrical 1,1-dimethylhydrazine was not carcinogenic in this species. This might have been due to administration of subeffective dose levels of this chemical. However, later studies with higher doses have shown that 1,1-dimethylhydrazine is carcinogenic to rats (Druckrey et al., 1967a) and mice (Roe et al., 1967; Toth, 1973). Among the hydrazine compounds investigated, symmetrical 1,2-dimethylhydrazine has been studied extensively in several laboratories because this compound produces tumors of the lower

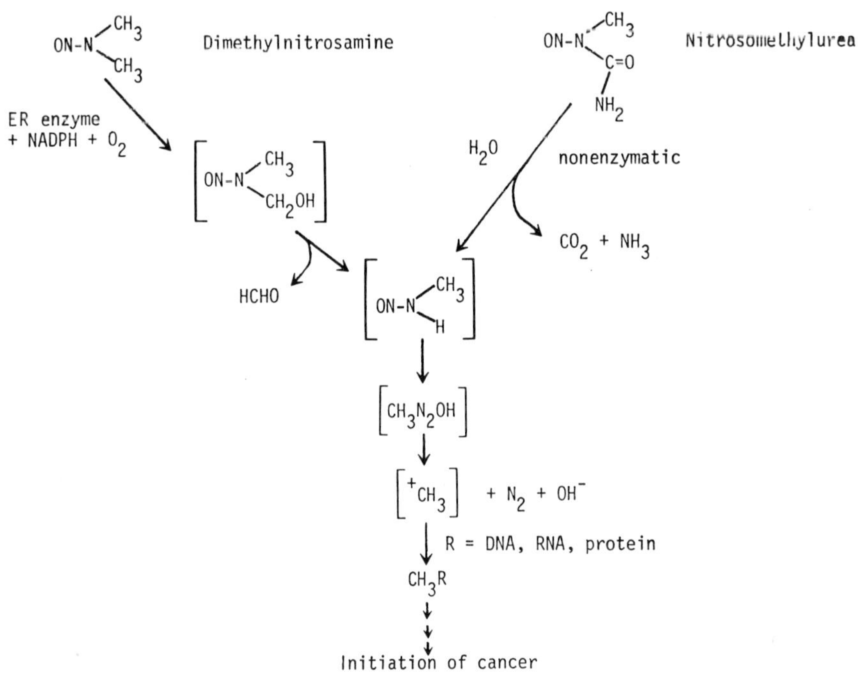

FIGURE 2 Probable metabolic pathways of dimethylnitrosamine and nitrosomethylurea.

intestinal tract, in addition to producing tumors at other sites in several rodent species (see Magee et al., 1976; Preussmann et al., 1969). Spontaneous tumors rarely develop in the colon or rectum of the laboratory animals (Grasso and Creasey, 1969). Therefore, 1,2-dimethylhydrazine has been used as one of the model compounds for studying colon cancers in experimental animals.

In this chapter only a few representative hydrazine compounds have been discussed. Carcinogenicity data on these and various other related compounds have been reviewed extensively by Druckrey et al. (1967a); Magee and Barnes (1967); Magee et al. (1976); and Preussmann et al. (1969).

Hydrazine

$H_2N\text{-}NH_2$

Hydrazine is a colorless oily liquid with ammonialike odor. Several million pounds of hydrazine are manufactured in the United States (IARC, 1974a). According to the recent International Trade Commission report, hydrazine is being manufactured in the United States on a commercial scale (Chem. Eng. News, 1978).

Originally used in rocket fuels, hydrazine is now used extensively in agricultural chemicals (maleic hydrazide and herbicide, 3-amino-1,2,4-triazole), antibacterial and antihypertension drugs, polymerization catalyst, blowing agents, antioxidant, scavenger for gases, explosives, photographic developers, and corrosion inhibitors (Hawley, 1977).

Experimental carcinogenesis

High incidences of lung and liver tumors have been produced in several strains of mice given oral administration of hydrazine as hydrazine sulfate (Biancifiori, 1970; Biancifiori and Ribacchi, 1962; Biancifiori and Severi, 1966; Roe et al., 1967; Toth, 1969).

Lung and liver tumors were also induced in both males and females in Cb/Se strain of rats administered hydrazine sulfate by stomach tube (Severi and Biancifiori, 1968). However, oral administration of this compound to hamsters did not produce any tumors in this species (Biancifiori, 1970; Biancifiori and Severi, 1966; Toth, 1972).

Human data

No epidemiological data implicating hydrazine in human cancer are yet available.

1, 1-Dimethylhydrazine

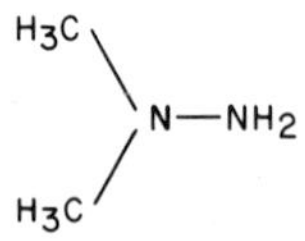

1, 1-Dimethylhydrazine, also known as unsymmetrical dimethylhydrazine and UDMH, is a hygroscopic flammable liquid with ammoniacal odor characteristic of aliphatic hydrazines. It fumes in air and gradually turns yellow. It is believed that the U.S. annual production of 1, 1-dimethylhydrazine (UDMH) is about 1 million lb (IARC, 1974a). It has been used as a component of jet and rocket fuels, chemical synthesis, stabilizer for organic peroxide fuel additives, and absorbent for acid gases. It has also been used in the manufacture of a plant growth regulator, N-dimethylamino-succinamic acid, and in photography (Hawley, 1977).

Experimental carcinogenesis

Lung tumors have been induced in female Swiss mice after oral administration of UDMH by gavage (Roe et al., 1967). In another study, when this compound was given in the drinking water (0.01% level), in addition to a high incidence of lung tumors, a high incidence of angiosarcomas located in various organs resulted in both male and female Swiss mice (Toth, 1973).

Large doses of this compound when administered via drinking water induced liver tumors in only 3/20 BD strain rats (Druckrey et al., 1967a).

Human data

No epidemiological data showing 1, 1-dimethylhydrazine as being responsible for induction of any human cancer are yet available. However, few cases of fatty livers (6/76) have been reported in personnel working with liquid rocket propellant for up to 5 years (Peterson et al., 1970).

1, 2-Dimethylhydrazine

$H_3C\text{-}NH—NH—CH_3$

1, 2-Dimethylhydrazine is also known as symmetrical dimethylhydrazine and SDMH. It is a flammable, hygroscopic liquid with characteristic ammoniacal odor of aliphatic hydrazines. It fumes in air and gradually turns yellow. There is no indication that this compound is produced in commercial quantities in the United States (IARC, 1974a). 1, 2-Dimethylhydrazine (SDMH) was used experimentally as a high-energy rocket fuel. Commercial uses for SDMH are not known.

Experimental carcinogenesis

High incidences of angiosarcomas mainly located in the muscle, liver, and pararenal tissues were observed in both male and female Swiss mice when they were administered SDMH in their drinking water. These animals also developed a higher incidence of lung tumors compared to their respective controls (Toth and Wilson, 1971).

Weekly oral doses (21 mg/kg body weight/week) of this compound to rats produced intestinal tumors in these animals (Druckrey et al., 1967b; Druckrey, 1970). However, a lower dose of this compound in their drinking water produced no intestinal tumors but a high incidence of hemangioendotheliomas of the liver (Druckrey, 1970).

Subcutaneous administration of SDMH to mice (Wiebecke et al., 1969; Thurnherr et al., 1973) and several strains of rats (Druckrey et al., 1967b; Druckrey, 1970; Preussmann et al., 1969) produced a high incidence of intestinal tumors in these two species.

In hamsters a very high incidence of angiosarcomas of the blood vessels, liver, lung, and muscle occurred in both males and females given SDMH in their drinking water (Toth, 1972).

Human data

No data suggesting the responsibility of 1,2-dimethylhydrazine for any cancer induction among industrial workers are available.

1,2-Diethylhydrazine

$H_3C-H_2C-NH-NH-CH_2-CH_3$

1,2-Diethylhydrazine is a colorless liquid that boils at 85-86° C. The compound was tested experimentally as a high-energy rocket fuel, but there are no known commercial uses for this compound. The compound is, however, used in chemical laboratories, that is, for the synthesis of symmetrical bases (IARC, 1974a).

Experimental carcinogenesis

Subcutaneous administration of this compound to several BD strains of rats produced tumors in the brain, mammary gland, and liver (Druckrey et al., 1966c).

A single i.v. injection of this compound to pregnant BD rats on the 15th day of gestation produced brain tumors in their offspring (Druckrey, 1973).

Human data

No epidemiological data are as yet available.

Hydrazobenzene

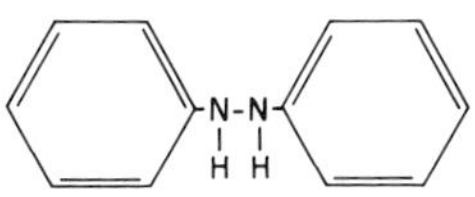

Hydrazobenzene is also known as 1,2-diphenylhydrazine. It is a powder that melts at 129-131° C. It is produced commercially in the United States, even though production data are not readily available (Stanford Research Institute, 1977). It is primarily used in the dye-manufacturing industry as a precursor of benzidine which is obtained by treatment of hydrazobenzene with hot mineral acid. Hydrazobenzene is also used in the preparation of phynylbutazone, a widely used agent against rheumatoid arthritis and related conditions (Wenner, 1967).

Experimental carcinogenesis

Hydrazobenzene was administered in the feed to male and female rats of Fischer 344 strain at two levels. The concentrations of hydrazobenzene were 0.008 and 0.03% for male and 0.004 and 0.01% for females. After 18 months of feeding of the compound in the diet, the animals were observed for an additional 6 months. Under these conditions hydrazobenzene was carcinogenic to both sexes, causing increased incidence of hepatocellular carcinoma and ear duct tumors in male rats and liver and mammary tumors in females. Thus, at the high-dose level hydrazobenzene induced liver and ear duct tumors in 31/49 and 5/49 male rats, respectively. In the control group only 1/48 males developed liver tumors, whereas 0/48 had ear duct tumors. Neoplastic nodules and mammary tumors developed in 6/50 females in the high-dose group, whereas none of the animals in the control group developed any of these tumors (NCI, 1978r). In a separate study s.c. injection of hydrazobenzene was found to be carcinogenic to rats producing tumors of the uterus, mammary gland, ear duct gland, and liver (Pliss, 1974).

Oral feeding of hydrazobenzene to B6C3F1 mice of both sexes at two levels for a period of 18 months induced hepatocellular carcinoma in 20/43 females given high dose of the compound. In the control group only 1/50 females developed liver tumor. The compound was found to be not carcinogenic to male mice at either of the two dose levels (NCI, 1978r). In another study in mice, s.c. treatment of this compound has produced liver tumors and sarcomas at the injection site in these animals (Pliss, 1974).

Human data

There is a great potential for exposure to hydrazobenzene among workers in the dye-manufacturing industry. It has been suggested that benzidine may be produced from hydrazobenzene, following ingestion, by acidity in the stomach (IARC, 1972). However, there is as yet no epidemiological data implicating hydrazobenzene in the induction of cancer in humans.

Isonicotinic Acid Hydrazine

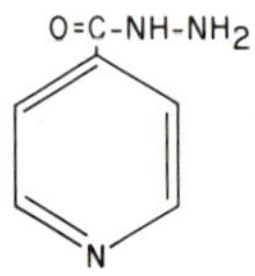

Isonicotinic acid hydrazide is also known as isoniazid or INH. It is a crystalline compound that melts at about 171-172°C. Isonicotinic acid hydrazide (INH) is produced commercially in the United States (Chem. Eng. News, 1978). It is also produced commercially in several countries, including India, Japan, Italy, and Germany (IARC, 1974a). Since 1952 INH has been used primarily as an antitubercular agent (Peters et al., 1965). It is taken either orally in the form of a syrup or a tablet (300 mg daily) or intramuscularly.

Experimental carcinogenesis

Prolonged oral administration of INH to several strains of rats did not induce any tumors in these animals (Biancifiori and Severi, 1966; Peacock and Peacock, 1966).

Like rats, hamsters have also been found to be resistant to the carcinogenic action of INH when given orally (Peacock and Peacock, 1966; Toth, 1972).

However, INH administered orally to several strains of mice produced a very high incidence of pulmonary tumors (Mori et al., 1960; Biancifiori and Severi, 1966).

A high incidence of pulmonary tumors was obtained in mice when INH was injected either s.c. (Mori et al., 1960) or i.p. (Juhasz et al., 1957).

Human data

Several studies have been reported regarding the effect of INH treatment on cancer incidence among tuberculosis patients (Hammond et al., 1967; Ferebee, 1970; Campbell and Guilfoyle, 1970). These studies do not demonstrate any significant increase of cancer among tuberculosis patients treated with INH.

Maleic Hydrazide

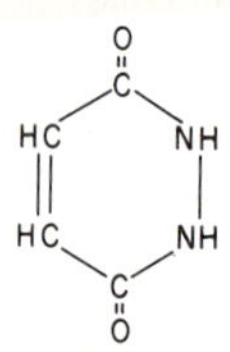

Several million pounds of maleic hydrazide, a crystalline compound, are produced commercially in the United States (IARC, 1974a). It is used exclusively as a plant growth inhibitor and herbicide. It is used mainly on tobacco in the control of sucker growth. It is used on potatoes and onions to control sprouting. In addition, it has been approved as a plant growth regulator on the following crops: beans, beets, citrus fruits, corn, lima beans, peas, strawberries, sugar beets, and tomatoes.

Experimental carcinogenesis

Oral administration of maleic hydrazide to rats (Barnes et al., 1957) and mice (Innes et al., 1969) did not show any significant increase in the incidence of tumors compared with their respective controls.

Subcutaneous administration of monosodium salt of maleic hydrazide to both rats and mice was also ineffective in demonstrating increase incidence of local and systemic tumors in these animals (Barnes et al., 1957). However, Epstein and Mantel (1968) reported the increased incidence of hepatomas in male Swiss mice injected s.c. with maleic hydrazide at birth. The significance of higher incidence of hepatoma cannot be assessed because of contamination of hydrazide (0.4%) in the maleic hydrazide preparations used in these studies (IARC, 1974a).

Human data

No epidemiological data are as yet available even though farmers and farm workers may have been exposed to maleic hydrazide during spraying of crops.

A. Metabolism of Hydrazine and Related Compounds

Some of the metabolic steps involved in the degradation of hydrazine and related compounds have been reviewed by Colvin (1960). Elevation of blood ammonia in dogs given hydrazine suggested that hydrazine is possibly degraded to ammonia in this species. The in vivo and in vitro metabolism of isonicotinic acid hydrazide (INH) in the rabbit and rat have yielded 1-acetyl-INH, isonicotinic acid, and ammonia, the latter being derived from a rapid breakdown of the hydrazine moiety. It has been reported that the major metabolite of INH excreted in the urine of humans and rhesus monkeys is 1-acetyl-INH (Hughes, 1953). Unlike rat, rabbit, and several other species, INH is metabolized in humans without the production of hydrazine (Vivien et al., 1972). The acetylated metabolite 1-acetyl-INH when given to mice in their drinking water for life has produced lung tumors in this species (Toth and Shimizu, 1973). Therefore, it appears that N-acetylation is not necessarily an inactivation pathway in the metabolism of INH. Recent studies with INH have indicated that the active metabolite of INH arises only from the acetylhydrazine moiety. The acetylhydrazine is now known to be oxidized by cytochrome P-450 enzymes in human and rat liver microsomes to a highly reacting acylating agent. These investigators have proposed that many monoacyl and monoalkyl hydrazines are oxidized by cytochrome P-450 enzyme system to N-hydroxyintermediates which then undergo dehydration to yield the reactive species (Nelson et al., 1976).

Since 1,2-dimethylhydrazine and 1,2-diethylhydrazine were inactive in inducing local tumors at the site of administration, Preussmann et al. (1969) indicated that these compounds were indirect carcinogens, that is, they require metabolic activation. They postulated that these hydrazoalkanes are easily oxidized to form the corresponding azoalkanes as a first step of activation. In their studies azoxymethane and azoxyethane were shown to be readily dealkylated by microsomal fraction from rat liver and other organs in the presence of NADPH and molecular oxygen. The same organotropic effects for all three compounds, hydrazo, azo, and azoxy alkanes, strongly suggested a common reactive intermediate. Fiala et al. (1976) have recently studied the in vivo metabolism of ^{14}C-labeled 1,2-dimethylhydrazine in rats and have detected labeled azomethane in the exhaled air as well as labeled azoxymethane and methylazoxymethanol (MAM) in the urine (Fiala, 1977; Fiala et al., 1976). Schoental (1973) proposed that further enzymatic activation of MAM to methylazoxyformaldehyde may be mediated via alcohol dehydrogenase. Evidence for this hypothesis has now been provided by the recent experiments of Grab and Zedeck (1977). Their studies indicate that alcohol de-

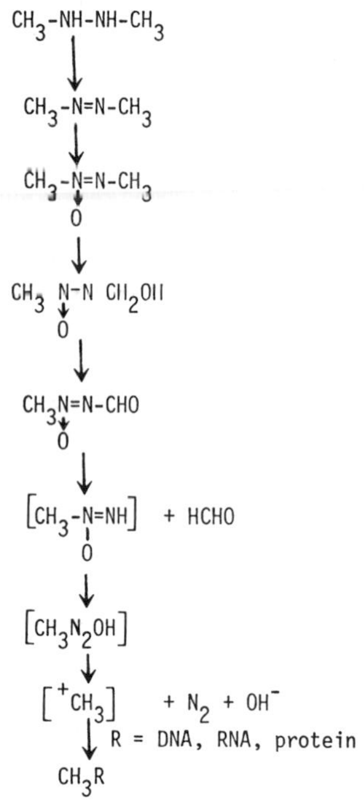

FIGURE 3 Probable metabolic pathway of 1,2-dimethylhydrazine and related compounds (Magee et al., 1975; Preussmann et al., 1969).

hydrogenase activity is not only involved in the metabolism of MAM but also plays a role in the organospecificity of MAM and therefore also of azoxymethane and 1,2-dimethylhydrazine.

It is generally believed that alkylation of DNA at 0^6-position of guanine and its persistence during DNA replication is possibly responsible for initiation of cancer by many alkylating agents (Magee et al., 1975, 1976; Pegg, 1977). Recent studies have shown the formation of 0^6-methylguanine by alkylation of rat liver, colon, and kidney DNA following administration of 1,2-dimethylhydrazine. Thus, persistence of 0^6-methylguanine in the colon DNA is suggested to be responsible for the initiation of carcinogenesis by this chemical in the colon (Rogers and Pegg, 1977). However, recent studies with DNA alkylation in mice with genetically different susceptibility to 1,2-dimethylhydrazine induced colon carcinogenesis indicate that the low carcinogenic response of C57BL/Ha mice compared to ICR/Ha strain is due to the smaller extent of initial alkylation of colon DNA, which probably reflects differences in the enzymatic metabolism of the carcinogen (Cooper et al., 1978).

Based on the earlier hypothesis (Preussmann et al., 1969) and recent experimental data (Fiala, 1977; Fiala et al., 1976; Grab and Zedeck, 1977), the overall metabolic pathway for 1,2-dimethylhydrazine is shown in Fig. 3.

VI. MISCELLANEOUS NITROGENOUS COMPOUNDS

Acetamide and urethane are two simple nitrogenous compounds that have been used extensively in several industries. In addition to these compounds, thioacetamide and several other thioamides, such as thiourea, ethylenethiourea, N,N-diethylthiourea, and trimethylthiourea are also discussed in this section because of their structural similarity to acetamide. All of these thioamides are also used extensively as industrial agents. Thiouracil, methylthiouracil, and propylthiouracil used as antithyroid agents are discussed briefly in this section. These antithyroid agents are discussed in detail in Chapter 12.

All the compounds discussed in this section have been shown to produce various types of tumors in experimental animals. However, there is as yet no epidemiological data implicating any of these compounds in induction of cancer in humans.

Acetamide

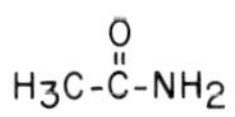

Acetamide is a crystalline compound that melts at 81°C. Molten acetamide is used as a solvent for many organic and inorganic compounds. It is also used as a plasticizer in leather, cloth, and coatings, as a wetting agent and penetration accelerator for dyes, as a component of urea molding compounds, as a humectant for paper, as an activator in bleach liquors, as a special food for molds, and as a chemical intermediate in the synthesis of methylamine, thioacetamide, hypnotics, insecticides, medicinals, and various plastics (IARC, 1974b). According to the International Trade Commission, acetamide is produced on a commercial scale in the United States (Chem. Eng. News, 1978).

Experimental carcinogenesis

Oral administration of acetamide in the drinking water at a dose level of 4 g/kg body weight/day for about 7 months produced liver tumors in 1/5 Rockland albino rats (Dessau and Jackson, 1955). In a later study these same investigators repeated this experiment using larger number of animals and feeding male Wistar rats 5% acetamide in the diet. Under these conditions liver tumors were observed after 14-40 weeks of acetamide treatment in 22/81 (27%) rats examined (Jackson and Dessau, 1961).

Simultaneous administration of arginine glutamate was shown to inhibit liver tumor induction in male Wistar rats. In this study one group of rats was fed 2.5% acetamide in the diet for 1 year and then a control diet for 3 more months. Another group of rats was fed a diet containing 2.5% acetamide and 5.6% arginine glutamate. In the acetamide-treated groups 7/16 (44%) rats developed liver tumors, whereas in the acetamide-arginine glutamate treated group only 1/11 (9%) rats developed liver tumors (Weisburger et al., 1969).

Human data

No information is as yet available regarding exposure and toxicity of acetamide in humans.

Thioacetamide

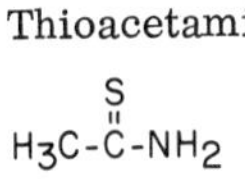

Thioacetamide is a crystalline compound with a slight odor of mercaptans. According to the International Trade Commission, thioacetamide is produced on a commercial scale in the United States (Chem. Eng. News, 1978). At present it is used as a substitute for hydrogen sulfide in the chemical laboratory. It has been reported that thioacetamide has also been used as an accelerator in rubber vulcanization, as a stabilizer of motor fuel containing tetraethyllead, and also as an organic solvent in the textile, leather, and paper industries (Hueper and Conway, 1964).

Experimental carcinogenesis

In one study with male albino rats thioacetamide in the diet at 0.025-0.05% level for a period of 18 months produced liver cell tumors (Fitzhugh and Nelson, 1948). In another study Wistar strain rats of both sexes fed 0.03% thioacetamide in the diet for 2-6 months developed bile duct tumors (Gupta, 1955).

Male and female Swiss mice fed 0.03% thioacetamide in their diet for a period of 17 months developed liver tumors in 6/6 males and 6/7 females (Gothoskar et al., 1970).

No carcinogenic effects were observed in Syrian golden hamsters on gastric intubation of thioacetamide (Terracini and Della Porta, 1961).

Human data

No information is available about exposure and toxicity of thioacetamide in humans.

Thiourea

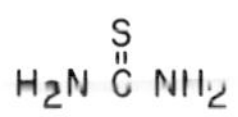

Thiourea is a crystalline compound that melts at 176–178°C. It was formerly used as an antithyroid agent; however, it is used in the United States as an intermediate in the production of other antithyroid agents, including thiouracil, propylthiouracil, and 5-iodo-2-thiouracil. It is also used as a photographic fixing agent and as a reagent to remove stains from negatives, in the manufacture of resins, as a vulcanization accelerator, and as a reagent for bismuth and selenite ions (IARC, 1974b). However, according to the International Trade Commission, it is not produced on a commercial scale in the United States (Chem. Eng. News, 1978).

Experimental carcinogenesis

Treatment of 0.25% thiourea in the drinking water for 16–24 months produced thyroid tumors both in Wistar and Norwegian strain rats of both sexes (Purves and Griesbach, 1946, 1947). In another study performed with Osborne-Mendel rats, oral feeding of 0.025–0.1% of thiourea in the diet for about 2 years induced liver tumors in 14/29 treated animals, compared with 0/18 in untreated controls (Fitzhugh and Nelson, 1948). Ear duct tumors appeared in albino rats of both sexes after either oral (Rosin and Ungar, 1957) or i.p. and oral administration of thiourea (Rosin and Rachmilewitz, 1954). No such tumors developed in untreated control animals.

Administration of 0.25–0.38% thiourea in the diet for 63 weeks did not produce any thyroid tumors in female C3H strain mice (Dalton et al., 1948).

Human data

Vanderlaan and Storrie (1955) have described the adverse effects of thiourea treatment in 525 patients. However, in this report no specific mention of cancer is made.

No other information is available.

Ethylenethiourea

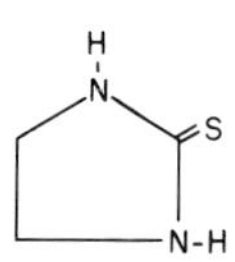

Ethylenethiourea (ETU) is a white crystalline compound that melts at 203–204°C. It is produced on a commercial scale in the United States. It has been used extensively as an accelerator for neoprene rubber, which is used in automotive products, industrial and mechanical goods, wire and cable production, and so on. It is also used as part of a curing system for polyacrylate rubber, which is used in automotive and aircraft industries for products such as seals, O-rings, and gaskets (IARC, 1974b).

Experimental carcinogenesis

Increased incidence of liver tumors was obtained in two strains of mice after oral feeding of ETU compared to their respective controls (Innes et al., 1969).

In another study oral administration of ETU to both sexes of Charles River CD rats produced thyroid tumors in 50–60% of animals (Ulland et al., 1972).

Human data

There is no information as yet available regarding exposure and toxicity of this chemical in humans.

N-N'-Diethylthiourea

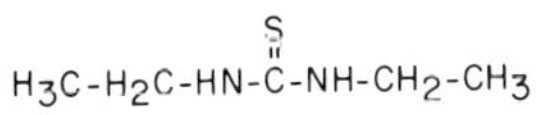

N, N'-Diethylthiourea is a buff solid that melts at 68-71°C (Hawley, 1977). Production data for N, N'-diethylthiourea are not readily available; however, it is known that this compound is produced commercially in the United States (Stanford Research Institute, 1977). N, N'-diethylthiourea is used as a corrosion inhibitor of iron and steel when it is used in solutions of HCl or H_2SO_4. It is also used for reducing the corrosion of ferrous metals and aluminum alloys in brine and as a vulcanization accelerator in the manufacture of elastomers (Hawley, 1977).

Experimental carcinogenesis

N, N'-Diethylthiourea was tested for possible carcinogenicity using Fischer 344 rats and B6C3F1 mice. The compound was administered in the diet at concentrations of 0.0125 and 0.025% for rats and 0.025 and 0.05% for mice for a period of 2 years. Under these conditions N, N'-diethylthiourea was found to be carcinogenic to rats. Thus, thyroid tumors developed in 15/48 males and 17/46 female rats on a high dose of the test compound. None of the control male or female rats developed thyroid tumors. There was no evidence for the carcinogenicity of this compound in mice (NCI, 1978p).

Human data

There is no epidemiological data implicating N, N'-diethylthiourea in cancer induction in humans.

Trimethylthiourea

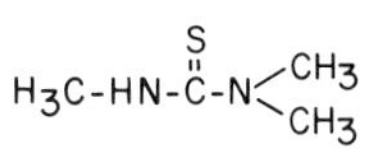

Trimethylthiourea is also known as 1, 1, 3-trimethyl-2-thiourea. This compound is produced commercially in the United States (Stanford Research Institute, 1977). It can be used to accelerate the vulcanization of various types of rubber (Langlade, 1976) and as a component of adhesives (Hauser and Malofsky, 1974). It is also used as an intermediate in the synthesis of pigments (Inuzuka et al., 1976) and substituted derivatives of penicillins (Rosati, 1973).

Experimental carcinogenesis

Trimethylthiourea was administered in the diet to Fischer 344 rats and B6C3F1 mice. The concentrations of the compound in the diet were 0.025 and 0.05% for rats and 0.05 and 0.10% for mice. After feeding of the test diet for about 18 months the animals were maintained for an additional 15-30 week period. Under these conditions trimethylthiourea was found to be carcinogenic to female rats, producing thyroid tumors in 14/47 surviving animals fed the high-dose diet. No thyroid tumors developed in the control group. There was not sufficient evidence for the carcinogenicity of this compound in male rats or mice of either sex. It should be pointed out that the trimethylthiourea preparations used in these studies contained about 20% contaminant as 1, 3-dimethylthiourea (NCI, 1978y).

Human data

No toxicity or epidemiological data are yet available.

Thiouracil

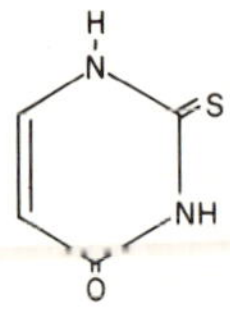

Thiouracil (TU) is a white crystalline compound without any definite melting point. It is produced on a commercial scale in the United States (Chem. Eng. News, 1978). Previously it was used as an antithyroid agent and in the treatment of angina pectoris and congestive heart failure. However, it is not known whether it is being used for these purposes any longer. Thiouracil is used as an intermediate in the synthesis of sodium salt of 5-iodo-2-thiouracil, which is being used as an antithyroid agent in the United States.

Experimental carcinogenesis

Thyroid tumors developed in 100% of the animals after Sprague-Dawley male rats were fed 0.1% TU in their drinking water for 14 weeks (Money et al., 1953). Similar results were obtained in another study with male Sprague-Dawley rats fed 0.2% TU in their drinking water for 24 months (Clausen, 1954). Several other strains of rats have also been found to be susceptible to thyroid tumor induction by oral feeding of TU (Laqueur, 1949; Wollman, 1961).

Administration of 0.3% TU in the diet of C3H strain male and female mice for a period of 17 months increased liver tumor incidence in both sexes. Thus, liver tumors developed in 12/13 males and 14/16 females, whereas in controls tumors appeared in only 2/32 males and 0/26 females. Liver tumors did not develop in either sex in TM strain mice on a similar treatment of TU (Casas, 1963).

Human data

No information is available regarding exposure and toxicity of thiouracil in humans.

Methylthiouracil

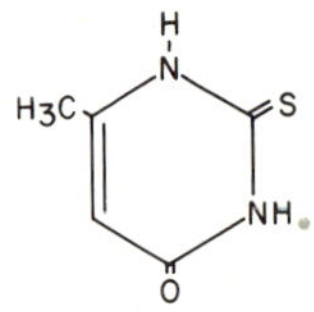

Methylthiouracil (MTU) is a white crystalline compound with a bitter taste. It has been used as an antithyroid agent. In this respect it is considered to be somewhat more effective than propylthiouracil. However, according to the International Trade Commission, MTU is not produced on a commercial scale in the United States (Chem. Eng. News, 1978).

At one time it was used for growing and fattening of swine and sheep. It is not known whether MTU is used presently for this purpose in the United States.

Experimental carcinogenesis

In Wistar strain female rats continuous administration of 0.01% MTU in their drinking water for 42-49 weeks produced thyroid tumors in several animals (Hall, 1948; Hall and Bielschowsky, 1949). In other studies thyroid tumors were induced in rats by oral feeding of MTU (Napalkov, 1959), whereas kidney tumors were observed in female rats fed this chemical orally (Akimova, 1962). Thyroid tumors and sarcomas at the site of implantation have been observed in this species on s.c. treatment (Napalkov and Saliamon, 1968).

Strain differences were observed in mice in tumor induction by MTU. Thus, oral feeding of MTU induced thyroid tumors in NZO/B_1 strain mice (Bielschowsky and Goodall, 1963), whereas such a treatment did not induce any thyroid tumors in C3H mice of both sexes (Israel and Ellis, 1960). Thyroid tumors were also induced in hamsters after oral treatment with MTU. The combined treatment with ^{131}I and MTU but not treatment with ^{131}I alone increased the incidence of thyroid tumors (Christov and Raichev, 1972).

Human data

Vanderlaan and Storrie (1955) have reviewed a large number of cases treated with MTU and have described the adverse effects of this treatment. However, no information is available regarding cancer incidence in these patients.

No other epidemiological data are yet available.

Propylthiouracil

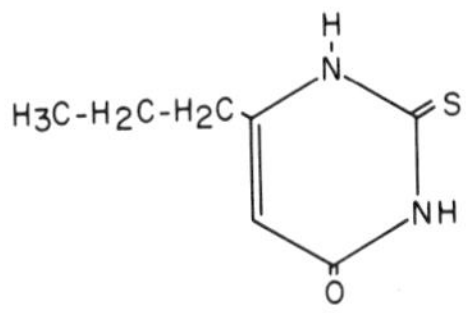

Propylthiouracil (PTU) is a white crystalline compound that is used as an antithyroid agent for the treatment of hyperthyroidism. Usually about 100-mg dose is recommended every 8 hr. At one time PTU was used as a metabolic depressant to promote fattening of swine and sheep. It is not known whether it is used presently for this purpose in the United States. According to the International Trade Commission, PTU is produced commercially in the United States (Chem. Eng. News, 1978).

Experimental carcinogenesis

Oral feeding of 0.2% PTU in the diet for 1 year produced thyroid tumors in female Wistar rats (Van Dyke, 1953). Incidence of thyroid tumor was increased considerably when rats were maintained on 0.1% PTU and 0.1% KF in their drinking water for 1 year. Thyroid tumors developed in 17/29 survivors in the PTU + KF groups, whereas only 4/15 survivors in the PTU group developed thyroid tumors (Zimmerman et al., 1954).

In two different strains of mice strains A and C57BL, PTU in the diet induced pituitary adenomas in addition to thyroid tumors (Moore et al., 1953; King et al., 1963).

Thyroid tumors also developed in Syrian golden hamsters (Sichuk et al., 1968) and guinea pigs (Hellwig and Welch, 1963) on oral administration of PTU.

Human data

A large number of cases treated with PTU have been reviewed (Vanderlaan and Storrie, 1955). Even though adverse effects of PTU treatment have been described, no information is available in this report regarding cancer incidence in these patients. No other epidemiological data are yet available.

Urethane

$$H_2N\text{-}\overset{O}{\overset{\|}{C}}\text{-}OC_2H_5$$

Urethane is also known as ethyl carbamate. It is a crystalline compound that melts at 48-50°C. According to the International Trade Commission report, urethane is produced on a commercial scale in the United States (Chem. Eng. News, 1978). It is used as an intermediate in the preparation and modification of amino resins, and as a solubilizer and cosolvent for pesticides, fumigants, and cosmetics. Urethane is believed to be primarily used as a chemical intermediate for reaction with formaldehyde to form N-hydroxymethyl derivatives, which are useful as cross-linking agents in textile treatments designed to impart wash-and-wear properties to fabrics. It was used formerly as an antineoplastic agent, as a hypnotic, as an adjunct to sulfonamide therapy, as a component with quinine of a sclerosing solution for varicose veins, and as a topical bactericide. In veterinary medicine it was infrequently used as a hypnotic and more often as an anesthetic in laboratory animals.

Experimental carcinogenesis

Some of the earlier carcinogenicity data on urethane have been reviewed by Mirvish (1968).

Oral administration of 0.1% urethane in the drinking water produced lymphomas and liver tumors in female Sprague-Dawley rats (Adenis et al., 1968). When August and Wistar strain newborn rats were given urethane s.c. over a period of 8 weeks, melanomas were induced only in the August strain rats of both sexes after a period of 9 months (Roe et al., 1963). When newborn Wistar strain rats were injected with urethane i.p. in addition to liver tumors, neurogenic, kidney, and ear duct tumors also developed (Vesselinovitch and Mihailovich, 1968a, b).

In several strains of mice (Swiss albino, CTM, C3H, and DBA) of both sexes administration of urethane in the drinking water induced lung tumors. Swiss albino and CTM strain mice in addition developed lymphomas (Toth et al., 1961; Tannenbaum and Maltoni, 1962; Della Porta et al., 1963).

Urethane has also been shown to be carcinogenic to mouse skin when it was given either orally or topically followed by croton oil treatment (Berenblum and Haran-Ghera, 1955, 1957).

The incidence of lung tumors was shown to be increased from 5% in untreated C3H female mice to 70% in mice treated with urethane i.p. (Nettleship et al., 1943). In C3H/HeA strain male mice such a treatment induced liver tumors in addition to lung tumors (Hollander and Bentvelzen, 1968). In newborn (C57BL X C3H)F_1 strain mice of both sexes injected with urethane i.p. at different times after birth, an increased incidence of lymphomas and lung, liver, ear duct, and ovarian tumors was observed. In these studies it appeared that only development of lung tumors was not modulated by age or sex of animals, whereas other tumors appeared at different frequencies according to the age at which treatment was started (Vesselinovitch and Mihailovich, 1967).

In transplacental studies it has been demonstrated that a single i.p. or i.v. injection of urethane to pregnant mice (Strain A or AXC) 1-5 days before parturition produced lung tumors in their respective offspring (Larsen, 1947; Klein, 1952). In another study with ICR/Jc1 strain mice it was shown that more pulmonary tumors appeared in sucklings when urethane was injected into lactating mothers soon after delivery (Nomura, 1973).

Continuous oral feeding of 0.2% urethane in the drinking water induced skin melanomas in the male Syrian golden hamsters (Pietra and Shubik, 1960). Injection of urethane by i.p. route in newborn hamsters of both sexes also induced skin melanomas in both sexes (Vesselinovitch et al., 1970).

Human data

No information is yet available about exposure and toxicity of urethane in humans.

Diazomethane

$$H_2C=\overset{+}{N}=\overset{-}{N}$$

Diazomethane is a very toxic yellow gas that is soluble in ethyl ether and dioxane. Because of its toxicity and explosive nature, diazomethane is not manufactured for distribution and sale. It is primarily used as a methylating agent in the laboratory. Previously diazomethane was generated from N-methyl-N'-nitro-N-nitrosoguanidine. However, in recent years it is believed to be generated from N-nitrosomethyl-para-toluenesulfonamide (Windholz, 1976).

Experimental carcinogenesis

Albino male rats of two strains (Porton and LAC 606p) were exposed to ethereal solutions of diazomethane twice weekly for 6 months. Control rats were exposed similarly to ether only. Lung tumors developed in 3/7 treated rats surviving longer than 10 months. No tumors developed in the four controls (Schoental and Magee, 1962).

Inhalation studies were carried out in A/2G strain mice, which were exposed to ethereal solutions of diazomethane twice weekly for 6 months. Multiple lung tumors were observed in 7/10 treated mice, compared with 2/8 in controls (Schoental and Magee, 1962). In another similar study with male Swiss mice lung tumors developed in 5/5 treated mice and 3/6 controls (Schoental, 1963). In skin carcinogenesis study male A/2G strain mice were used. Their shaved skin was painted with ethereal solution of diazomethane 5 times weekly for 5 months. All eight animals developed lung tumors. In this study no controls were used (Schoental and Magee, 1962).

Human data

Toxicity of diazomethane in humans has been recorded. Inhalation of diazomethane by humans, depending on the degree of exposure, caused chest pains, asthmatic symptoms, cough, fever, fulminating pneumonia, moderate cynosis, shock, and death (Sunderman et al., 1938; Sunderman, 1970).

No epidemiological data are as yet available to indicate that diazomethane is carcinogenic in humans.

A. Metabolism of Miscellaneous Nitrogenous Compounds

Among the miscellaneous nitrogenous compounds discussed in this section, urethane metabolism has been investigated most extensively. Earlier metabolic data on this compound have been reviewed by Mirvish (1968). Urethane is water soluble and is found to be rapidly and evenly distributed throughout the body when it is administered to rats and mice. It has been observed that about 90% of the administered dose in mice is excreted as CO_2 in the expired air within 24 hr, and about 5% of the dose is excreted in the urine. In addition to urethane, N-acetylated and N-glucuronide derivatives of N-hydroxy-urethane were also detected in the urine of several species including humans who were administered urethane (Boyland and Nery, 1965; Mirvish, 1966). It was therefore suggested that like aromatic amines (Miller et al., 1960) N-hydroxylation may be an activation step in the carcinogenesis by urethane (Boyland and Nery, 1965; Mirvish, 1968). Berenblum et al. (1959) have observed earlier that there is an absolute structural requirement for the biological activity of the urethane molecule. Thus, any chemical alteration of the molecular structure except by N-hydroxylation reduced the carcinogenic activity of urethane. However, it was later shown that N-hydroxy-urethane was not any more carcinogenic than the parent compound (see Mirvish, 1968). Recently another hypothesis has been proposed for metabolic activation of urethane. Thus, it is suggested that urethane (ethyl carbamate) is dehydrogenated in vivo to the proximate carcinogen vinyl carbamate, which then undergoes epoxidation to form a reactive electrophilic ultimate carcinogen (Dahl et al., 1978). In their studies vinyl carbamate was much more potent than ethyl carbamate in producing tumors in the skin or lungs of mice. Mutagenicity data obtained with Ames system support the hypothesis that vinyl carbamate is not carcinogenic per se, but requires cytochrome P-450 dependent oxidation to form an epoxide, an ultimate carcinogenic metabolite. It must be pointed out here that although Dahl et al. (1978) have not yet detected vinyl carbamate as a metabolite of ethyl carbamate in in vivo studies, their macromolecular binding data suggest the presence of desaturation in ethyl moiety.

Earlier studies by Weisburger et al. (1969) showing the inhibition of acetamide carcinogenicity to rat liver by arginine glutamate suggested involvement of ammonia in the toxicity and possibly carcinogenicity by acetamide. However, their direct studies with ammonium compounds ruled out this possibility. Like aromatic amines, N-hydroxylation hypothesis was also examined with acetamide (Poirier, 1965). However, no detectable level (<0.1 of administered dose) of N-hydroxy derivative of acetamide was detected in the urine of rats administered the parent compound. Moreover, the synthetic N-hydroxy-acetamide when tested for carcinogenicity was found to be inactive.

Thioacetamide is found to be 10-50 times more active than acetamide in inducing liver cancer in rats (Fitzhugh and Nelson, 1948; Gupta, 1955; Weisburger et al., 1969). Metabolic studies with thioacetamide indicate that almost all of thioacetamide is converted to acetate via acetamide within 24 hr. It is suggested that a metabolite produced by the liver is responsible for the carcinogenicity (Rees et al., 1966).

Some metabolic studies have been performed with antithyroid drugs. Thus, Maloof and Soodak (1957) demonstrated that drugs such as thiourea and thiouracil were not concentrated by the thyroid gland; they showed that thiourea was present in the thyroid gland mostly as sulfate, a metabolic oxidation product. Subsequent studies have indicated that compared to thiourea, other drugs such as thiouracil, methylthiouracil, and propylthiouracil are concentrated in the rat thyroid gland both as unmetabolized drugs and their metabolized oxidation products (Lees et al., 1973; Marchant et al., 1971; Sitar and Thornhill, 1972). Glucuronide of propylthiouracil has been identified as a major urinary metabolite of propylthiouracil in the rat (Sitar and Thornhill, 1972). However, in all of these studies no metabolic activation steps in the carcinogenesis by these compounds have been identified.

In earlier studies diazomethane was implicated as an intermediate both in the metabolic activation of dimethylnitrosamine and in the nonenzymatic breakdown of nitrosomethylurea (see Sec. IV.C on N-nitroso compounds in this chapter). Diazomethane is a potent direct-acting carcinogen. Its alkylating properties were first examined by its interaction with DNA (Kriek and Emmelot, 1964). In these studies several methylated bases in DNA were identified. Like dimethylnitrosamine and nitrosomethylurea, alkylation at 0^6-position of guanine in DNA by diazomethane may be involved in the initiation of cancer (see Pegg, 1977).

TABLE 1 Industrial Nitrogenous Chemicals Already Listed in OSHA's Category I[a]

1. Aromatic amines and related compounds
   o-Toluidine; 4-biphenylamine; 4-nitrobiphenyl; benzidine; 3,3'-dichlorobenzidine; 3,3'-dimethoxybenzidine; 4,4'-methylene-bis(2-methylaniline); 1-naphthylamine; 2-naphthylamine
2. Azo dyes
   p-Aminoazobenzene; p-dimethylaminoazobenzene; trypan blue; Ponceau 3R; Ponceau MX
3. N-nitroso compounds
   A. Nitrosamines
      N-Nitrosodimethylamine; N-nitrosodiethylamine; N-nitrosodibutylamine
   B. Nitrosamides
      Nitrosomethylurea; nitrosoethylurea; N-methyl-N'-nitro-N-nitrosoguanidine; N-nitroso-N-methylurethane
4. Hydrazine and related compounds
   Hydrazine; 1,1-dimethylhydrazine; 1,2-dimethylhydrazine; 1,2-diethylhydrazine; isonicotinic acid hydrazide
5. Miscellaneous compounds
   Acetamide; thioacetamide; thiourea; thiouracil; methylthiouracil; propylthiouracil; urethane

[a]OSHA's Category I includes chemicals that have been shown to be carcinogenic based on human data, or based on tests in two mammalian species, or one species if the tests have been replicated (Chem. Eng. News, 1978).

TABLE 2 Nitrogenous Chemicals Suggested for OSHA's Category I[a]

1. Aromatic amines and related compounds
   4-Chloro-m-phenylenediamine; 4-chloro-o-phenylenediamine; o-anisidine; 5-nitro-o-anisidine; 2,4-diaminoanisole; p-cresidine; N,N'-diacetylbenzidine; 3,3'-dimethylbenzidine; 4,4'-methylene-bis(2-chloroaniline); Michler's ketone; N,N'-bis(2-chloroethyl)-2-naphthylamine; auramine; 2-aminoanthraquinone; 1-amino-2-methylanthraquinone; 3-amino-9-ethylcarbazole; 5-nitroacenaphthene

2. Azo dyes
   o-aminoazotoluene

3. N-nitroso compounds
   A. Nitrosamines
      N-Methyl-N,4-dinitrosoaniline
   B. Nitrosamides
      Streptozotocin

4. Hydrazine and related compounds
   Hydrazobenzene

5. Miscellaneous compounds
   Ethylenethiourea; diazomethane

[a]All of these chemicals except N,N'-diacetylbenzidine and 3,3'-dimethylbenzidine have been shown to be carcinogenic in two or more mammalian species. Carcinogenicity data of benzidine derivatives in rats have been replicated.

VII. CONCLUSIONS

The Occupational Safety and Health Administration (OSHA) has issued a tentative carcinogen list which contains confirmed carcinogens into Category I (Chem. Eng. News, 1978). According to OSHA's guidelines, a chemical is included in Category I if it is shown to be carcinogenic based on human data, or based on tests in two mammalian species, or in one species if the tests have been replicated (Chem. Eng. News, 1978). Several of the chemicals discussed in this chapter have been shown to be carcinogenic in at least two mammalian species and therefore would fall into Category I of confirmed carcinogens. Actually, 33 out of 90 chemicals discussed in this chapter have already been listed in OSHA's Category I

TABLE 3 Industrial Nitrogenous Chemicals for OSHA's Category II[a]

1. Aromatic amines and related compounds
   Aniline; 5-nitro-o-toluidine; p-chloro-o-toluidine; 2,4-diaminotoluene; 1,4-diamino-2-nitrobenzene; 2,4-dinitrobenzene; 4-amino-2-nitrophenol; m-cresidine; 3-amino-4-ethoxyacetanilide; 4,4'-thiodianiline; N-phenyl-2-naphthylamine

2. Azo dyes
   Direct blue 6; direct black 38; direct brown 95; Sudan I; oil orange SS; amaranth

3. Miscellaneous compounds
   N,N'-Diethylthiourea; trimethylthiourea

[a]Carcinogenicity of these chemicals has been reported positively in only one species; these carcinogenicity data have not yet been replicated.

TABLE 4 Nitrogenous Chemicals Found to Be Not Carcinogenic[a]

Chemicals	References
2,5-Diaminotoluene	NCI, 1978x
3-Chloro-p-toluidine	NCI, 1978l
p-Anisidine	NCI, 1978h
Anthranilic acid	NCI, 1978i
Maleic hydrazide	Barnes et al., 1957; Innes et al., 1969

[a]Two mammalian species (rats and mice) used for carcinogenicity testing.

TABLE 5 Industrial Nitrogenous Chemicals Not Tested Adequately for Carcinogenicity

1. Aromatic amines and related compounds
   p-Phenylenediamine; m-phenylenediamine; 2,4-xylidine; 2,5-xylidine; 1,2-diamino-4-nitrobenzene; 2,4'-biphenyldiamine; 4,4'-diaminodiphenylether; 4,4'-methylenedianiline; magenta
2. Azo dyes
   Sudan II; scarlet red

(Table 1). In addition, 22 more chemicals are suggested to be included in Category I (Table 2). There is a group of chemicals including aniline whose positive carcinogenicity has been reported recently in only one species and whose data have not yet been replicated. According to OSHA's guidelines, such chemicals to be included in Category II are listed in Table 3. Thus, the majority of the industrial nitrogenous chemicals (74/90) listed in this chapter has been found to be carcinogenic to at least one or more mammalian species. The remaining compounds have been found to be either noncarcinogenic (Table 4) or inadequately tested (Table 5).

In general, these chemicals, with the exception of nitrosamides and diazomethane, are not carcinogenic per se, but they require metabolic activation via microsomal and/or cytosolic enzyme systems (Clayson and Garner, 1976; Druckrey et al., 1967a; Magee et al., 1975, 1976; Miller, 1970; Miller and Miller, 1967, 1976). It is believed that the ultimate metabolites are electrophiles which react covalently with critical cellular macromolecules. Based on the available evidence, it appears that covalent interaction of a chemical carcinogen with a specific site in a DNA molecule is one of the critical factors responsible for initiation of cancer.

ACKNOWLEDGMENTS

The author wishes to express his sincere thanks to Diana Smith for her great dedicated help in literature search and excellent typing, and to Sherry Battaglia and Dorothy Wyszynski for their excellent typing of this manuscript.

REFERENCES

Adenis, L., Demaille, A., and Driessens, J. (1968). Pouvoir cancerigene de l'urethane chez le rat Sprague. C. R. Soc. Biol. (Paris) 162:458-461.

Akimova, R. N. (1962). On the development of renal tumours in rats. Vrach. Delo 6:7-12.

Alexandrov, V. A. (1968). Blastogenic effect of dimethylnitrosamine on pregnant rats and their offspring. Nature 218:280-281.

Alexandrov, V. A. (1969). Transplacental blastogenic action of N-nitrosomethylurea in rat offspring. Vopr. Onkol. 15:55.

Allmark, M. G., Grice, H. C., and Mannell, W. A. (1956). Chronic toxicity studies on food colours. II. Observations on the toxicity of FD and C green No. 2 (light green SF yellowish), FD and C Orange No. 2 (orange SS) and FD and C Red No. 32 (oil red X0) in rats. J. Pharm. Pharmacol. 8:417-424.

Althoff, J., Kruger, F. W., Mohr, U., and Schmahl, D. (1971). Dibutylnitrosamine carcinogenesis in Syrian golden and Chinese hamsters. Proc. Soc. Exp. Biol. Med. 136:168-173.

Ames, B. N., Durston, W. E., Yamasaki, E., and Lee, F. D. (1973). Carcinogens are mutagens. A simple test system combining liver homogenates for activation and bacteria for detection. Proc. Natl. Acad. Sci. USA 70:2281-2285.

Ames, B. N., Kammen, H. O., and Yamasaki, E. (1975). Hair dyes are mutagenic: identification of a variety of mutagenic ingredients. Proc. Natl. Acad. Sci. USA 72: 2423-2427.

Andersen, R. A., Enomoto, M., Miller, E. C., and Miller, J. A. (1964). Carcinogenesis and inhibition of the Walker 256 tumor in the rat by trans-4-acetylaminostilbene, its N-hydroxy metabolite, and related compounds. Cancer Res. 24:128-143.

Andervont, H. B., and Shimkin, M. B. (1940). Biologic testing of carcinogens. II. Pulmonary-tumor-induction technique. J. Natl. Cancer Inst. 1:225-239.

Andervont, H. B., White, J. W., and Edwards, J. E. (1944). Effect of two azo compounds when added to the diet of mice. J. Natl. Cancer Inst. 4:583-586.

Andrianova, M. M. (1970). Carcinogenous properties of red food pigments—amaranth, SX purple, and 4R purple. Vopr. Pitan. 29:61-65.

Arcos, J. C., and Argus, M. F. (1974). Chemical Induction of Cancer, Vol. IIB. Academic Press, New York.

Argus, M. F., and Hoch-Ligeti, C. (1961). Comparative study of the carcinogenic activity of nitrosamines. J. Natl. Cancer Inst. 27:695-709.

Argus, M. F., and Hoch-Ligeti, C. (1963). Induction of malignant tumors in the guinea pig by oral administration of diethylnitrosamine. J. Natl. Cancer Inst. 30:533-551.

Arison, R. N., and Feudale, E. L. (1967). Induction of renal tumour by streptozotocin in rats. Nature 214:1254-1255.

Ashley, L. M., and Halver, J. E. (1968). Dimethylnitrosamine-induced hepatic cell carcinoma in rainbow trout. J. Natl. Cancer Inst. 41:531-552.

Baldwin, R. W., Smith, W. R., and Surtees, S. J. (1963). Carcinogenic action of N-hydroxy-4-acetylaminostilbene. Nature 199:613-614.

Barnes, J. M., and Magee, P. N. (1954). Some toxic properties of dimethylnitrosamine. Br. J. Ind. Med. 11:167-174.

Barnes, J. M., Magee, P. N., Boyland, E., Haddow, A., Passey, R. D., Bullough, W. S., Cruickshank, C. N., Salaman, M. H., and Williams, R. T. (1957). The nontoxicity of maleic hydrazide for mammalian tissues. Nature 180:62-64.

Bartsch, H., Dworkin, C., Miller, E. C., and Miller, J. A. (1973). Formation of electrophilic N-acetoxyarylamines in cytosols from rat mammary gland and other tissues by transacetylation from the carcinogen N-hydroxy-4-acetylaminobiphenyl. Biochim. Biophys. Acta 304:42-55.

Bartsch, H., Dworkin, C., Miller, J. A., and Miller, E. C. (1972). Electrophilic N-acetoxyaminoarenes derived from carcinogenic N-hydroxy-N-acetylaminoarenes by enzymatic deacetylation and transacetylation in liver. Biochim. Biophys. Acta 286:272-298.

Bartsch, H., Malaveille, C., and Montesano, R. (1975). In vitro metabolism and microsome-mediated mutagenicity of dialkylnitrosamines in rat, hamster, and mouse tissues. Cancer Res. 35:644-651.

Baumann, C. A., Jacobi, H. P., and Rusch, H. P. (1939). The effect of diet on experimental tumor production. Am. J. Hyg. 30:1-6.

Belman, S., Troll, W., Teebor, G., and Mukai, F. (1968). The carcinogenic and mutagenic properties of N-hydroxyaminonaphthalenes. Cancer Res. 28:535-542.

Berenblum, I., Ben-Ishai, D., Haran-Ghera, N., Lapidot, A., Simon, E., and Trainin, N. (1959). Skin initiating action and lung carcinogenesis by derivatives of urethane (ethyl carbamate) and related compounds. Biochem. Pharmacol. 2:168-176.

Berenblum, I., and Haran, N. (1955). The initiating action of ethyl carbamate (urethane) on mouse skin. Br. J. Cancer 9:453-456.

Berenblum, I., and Haran-Ghera, N. (1957). A quantitative study of the systemic initiating action of urethane (ethyl carbamate) in mouse skin carcinogenesis. Br. J. Cancer 11: 77-84.

Berman, L. D., Hayes, J. A., and Sibay, T. M. (1973). Effect of streptozotocin in the Chinese hamster (Cricetulus griseus). J. Natl. Cancer Inst. 51:1287-1294.

Bertram, J. S., and Craig, A. W. (1970). Induction of bladder tumors in mice with dibutylnitrosamine. Br. J. Cancer 24:352-359.

Biancifiori, C. (1970). Hepatomas in CBA/Cb/Se mice and liver lesions in golden hamsters induced by hydrazine sulfate. J. Natl. Cancer Inst. 44:943-949.

Biancifiori, C., and Ribacchi, R. (1962). Pulmonary tumours in mice induced by oral isoniazid and its metabolites. Nature 194:488-489.

Biancifiori, C., and Severi, L. (1966). The relation of isoniazid (INH) and allied compounds to carcinogenesis in some species of small laboratory animals: a review. Br. J. Cancer 20:528-538.

Bielschowsky, F., and Goodall, C. M. (1963). A reassessment of the thyroid tumors induced by goitrogens in mice. Proceedings of the University of Otago Medical School, Dunedin, New Zealand, 41:3-4.

Blacow, N. W. (Ed.) (1972). Martindale, the Extra Pharmacopoeia, 26th Ed. The Pharmaceutical Press, London.

Blunck, J. M., and Crowther, C. E. (1975). Enhancement of azo dye carcinogenesis by dietary sodium sulfate. Eur. J. Cancer 11:23-32.

Bonser, G. M. (1943). Epithelial tumors of the bladder in dogs induced by pure β-naphthylamine. J. Path. Bact. 55:1-6.

Bonser, G. M. (1962). Precancerous changes in the urinary bladder. In The Morphological Precursors of Cancer, L. Severi (Ed.), Perugia University, Perugia, p. 435.

Bonser, G. M., Boyland, E., Busby, E. R., Clayson, D. B., Grover, P. L., and Jull, J. W. (1963). A further study of bladder implantation in the mouse as a means of detecting carcinogenic activity: use of crushed paraffin wax or stearic acid as the vehicle. Br. J. Cancer 17:127-136.

Bonser, G. M., Clayson, D. B., and Jull, J. W. (1954). Induction of tumours with 1-(2-tolylazo)-2-naphthol (oil orange TX). Nature 174:879-880.

Bonser, G. M., Clayson, D. B., and Jull, J. W. (1956a). The induction of tumours of the subcutaneous tissues, liver and intestine in the mouse by certain dyestuffs and their intermediates. Br. J. Cancer 10:653-667.

Bonser, G. M., Clayson, D. B., and Jull, J. W. (1958). Some aspects of the experimental induction of tumours of the bladder. Br. Med. Bull. 14:146-152.

Bonser, G. M., Clayson, D. B., Jull, J. W., and Pyrah, L. N. (1952). The carcinogenic properties of 2-amino-1-naphthol hydrochloride and its parent amine 2-naphthylamine. Br. J. Cancer 6:412-424.

Bonser, G. M., Clayson, D. B., Jull, J. W., and Pyrah, L. N. (1956b). The carcinogenic activity of 2-naphthylamine. Br. J. Cancer 10:533-538.

Booth, J., and Boyland, E. (1964). The biochemistry of aromatic amines. 10. Enzymatic N-hydroxylation of arylamines and conversion of arylhydroxylamines into o-aminophenols. Biochem. J. 91:362-369.

Boutwell, R. K., and Bosch, D. K. (1959). The tumor-promoting action of phenol and related compounds for mouse skin. Cancer Res. 19:413-424.

Boyland, E. (1969). The correlation of experimental carcinogenesis and cancer in man. Prog. Exp. Tumor Res. 11: 222-234.

Boyland, E., Busby, E. R., Dukes, C. E., Grover, P. L., and Manson, D. (1964). Further experiments on implantation of materials into the urinary bladder of mice. Br. J. Cancer 18:575-581.

Boyland, E., Carter, R. L., Gorrod, J. W., and Roe, F. J. (1968). Carcinogenic properties of certain rubber additives. Eur. J. Cancer 4: 233-239.

Boyland, E., Dukes, C. E., and Grover, P. L. (1963). Carcinogenicity of 2-naphthylhydroxylamine and 2-naphthylamine. Br. J. Cancer 17: 79-84.

Boyland, E., Harris, J., and Horning, E. S. (1954). The induction of carcinoma of the bladder in rats with acetamidofluorene. Br. J. Cancer 8: 647-654.

Boyland, E., and Nery, R. (1965). The metabolism of urethane and related compounds. Biochem. J. 94: 198-208.

Boyland, E., and Williams, D. C. (1955). The estimation of tryptophan metabolites in the urine of patients with cancer of the bladder. Biochem. J. 60: v.

Bremner, D. A., and Tange, J. D. (1966). Renal and neoplastic lesions after injection of N,N'-diacetylbenzidine. Arch. Pathol. Lab. Med. 81: 146-151.

Brill, E., and Radomski, J. L. (1971). Comparison of the in vitro and in vivo N-oxidation of the carcinogenic aromatic amines. Xenobiotica 1: 347-348.

Brown, R. R., Friedell, G. H., and Leklem, J. E. (1972). Tryptophan metabolism in patients with bladder cancer of occupational etiology. Am. Ind. Hyg. Assoc. J. 33: 217-222.

Bryan, G. T. (1969). Role of tryptophan metabolites in urinary bladder cancer. Am. Ind. Assoc. J. 30: 27-34.

Burnett, C., Lanman, B., Giovacchini, R., Wolcott, G., Scala, R., and Keplinger, M. (1975). Long-term toxicity studies on oxidation hair dyes. Food Cosmet. Toxicol. 13: 353-357.

Burros, M. (1976). Popular red food dye banned as cancer agent (by FDA). Philadelphia Inquirer, Jan. 20, p. 1A.

Campbell, A. H., and Guilfoyle, P. (1970). Pulmonary tuberculosis, isoniazid and cancer. Br. J. Dis. Chest 64: 141-149.

Casas, C. B. (1963). Induction of hepatomas by thiouracil in inbred strains of mice. Proc. Soc. Exp. Biol. Med. 113:493-494.

Case, R. A., Hosker, M. E., McDonald, D. B., and Pearson, J. T. (1954). Tumours of the urinary bladder in workmen engaged in the manufacture and use of certain dyestuff intermediates in the British chemical industry. Part I. The role of aniline, benzidine, α-naphthylamine and β-naphthylamine. Br. J. Ind. Med. 11: 75-104.

Case, R. A., and Pearson, J. T. (1954). Tumours of the urinary bladder in workmen engaged in the manufacture and use of certain dyestuff intermediates in the British chemical industry. Part II. Further consideration of the role of aniline and of the manufacture of auramine and magenta (fuchsine) as possible causative agents. Br. J. Ind. Med. 11: 213-216.

Chem. Eng. News (1978). OSHA issues tentative carcinogen list, July 31, pp. 20-22.

Christov, K., and Raichev, R. (1972). Thyroid carcinogenesis in hamsters after treatment with 131-iodine and methylthiouracil. Z. Krebsforsch. 77: 171-179.

Clapp, N. K., and Craig, A. W. (1967). Carcinogenic effects of diethylnitrosamine in RF mice. J. Natl. Cancer Inst. 39: 903-916.

Clapp, N. K., Craig, A. W., and Toya, R. E., Sr. (1968). Pulmonary and hepatic oncogenesis during treatment of male RF mice with dimethylnitrosamine. J. Natl. Cancer Inst. 41: 1213-1228.

Clapp, N. K., Craig, A. W., and Toya, R. E., Sr. (1970). Diethylnitrosamine oncogenesis in RF mice as influenced by variations in cumulative dose. Int. J. Cancer 5: 119-123.

Clapp, N. K., Tyndall, R. A., and Otten, J. A. (1971). Differences in tumor types and organ susceptibility in BALB/c and RF mice following dimethylnitrosamine and diethylnitrosamine. Cancer Res. 31: 196-198.

Clausen, H. J. (1954). Experimental production of struma fibrosa. Arch Pathol. Lab. Med. 58: 222-226.

Clayson, D. B. (1962). Chemical Carcinogenesis. Little, Brown, Boston.

Clayson, D. B., and Ashton, M. J. (1963). The metabolism of 1-naphthylamine and its bearing on the mode of carcinogenesis of the aromatic amines. Acta Un. Int. Cancer 19: 539-542.

Clayson, D. B., and Cooper, E. H. (1970). Cancer of the urinary tract. Adv. Cancer Res. 13: 271-381.

Clayson, D. B., and Garner, R. C. (1976). Carcinogenic aromatic amines and related compounds. In Chemical Carcinogens, ACS Monograph 173, C. E. Searle (Ed.). American Chemical Society, Washington, D.C., pp. 366-461.

Clayson, D. B., Jull, J. W., and Bonser, G. M. (1958). The testing of ortho-hydroxy-amines and related compounds by bladder implantation and a discussion of their structural requirements for carcinogenic activity. Br. J. Cancer 12: 222-230.

Clayson, D. B., Lawson, T. A., and Pringle, J. A. (1967). The carcinogenic action of 2-aminodiphenylene oxide and 4-aminodiphenyl on the bladder and liver of C57 X 1F mouse. Br. J. Cancer 21: 755-762.

Clayton, D. B., Lawson, T. A., Santana, S., and Bonser, G. M. (1965). Correlation between the chemical induction of hyperplasia and of malignancy in the bladder epithelium. Br. J. Cancer 19: 297-310.

Clayson, D. B., Pringle, J. A., Bonser, G. M., and Wood, M. (1968). The technique of bladder implantation: further results and an assessment. Br. J. Cancer 22: 825-832.

Close, W. J. (1932). A case of poisoning from hair dye (paraphenylenediamine). Med. J. Aust. 1: 53-54.

Colvin, L. B. (1969). Metabolic fate of hydrazines and hydrazides. J. Pharm. Sci. 58: 1433-1443.

Comptroller General of the United States (1977). Cancer and coal tar hair dyes. An unregulated hazard to consumers. Report of the Comptroller General of the United States, HRD-78-22. General Accounting Office, Washington, D.C.

Conzelman, G. M., Jr., and Moulton, J. E. (1972). Dose-response relationships of the bladder tumorigen-2-naphthylamine: a study in beagle dogs. J. Natl. Cancer Inst. 49: 193-200.

Conzelman, G. M., Jr., Moulton, J. E., Flanders, L. E., III, Springer, K., and Crout, D. W. (1969). Induction of transitional cell carcinomas of the urinary bladder in monkeys fed 2-naphthylamine. J. Natl. Cancer Inst. 42: 825-831.

Cook, J. W., Hewett, C. L., Kennaway, E. L., and Kennaway, N. M. (1940). Effects produced in the livers of mice by azonaphthalenes and related compounds. Am. J. Cancer 40: 62-77.

Cooper, H. K., Buecheler, J., and Kleihues, P. (1978). DNA alkylation in mice with genetically different susceptibility to 1,2-dimethylhydrazine induced colon carcinogenesis. Cancer Res. 38: 3063-3065.

Corbett, J. F. (1973). The role of meta difunctional benzene derivatives in oxidative hair dyeing. I. Reaction with p-diamines. J. Soc. Cosmet. Chem. 24: 103-134.

Cramer, J. W., Miller, J. A., and Miller, E. C. (1960). N-hydroxylation: a new metabolic reaction observed in the rat with the carcinogen 2-acetylaminofluorene. J. Biol. Chem. 235: 885-888.

Czygan, P., Greim, H., Garro, A., Hutterer, F., Schaffner, F., Popper, H., Rosenthal, O., and Cooper, D. Y. (1973). Microsomal metabolism of dimethylnitrosamine and the cytochrome P-450 dependency of its activation to a mutagen. Cancer Res. 33: 2983-2986.

Dahl, G. A., Miller, J. A., and Miller, E. C. (1978). Vinyl carbamate as a promutagen and a more carcinogenic analog of ethyl carbamate. Cancer Res. 38: 3793-3804.

Dalton, A. J., Morris, H. P., and Dubnik, C. S. (1948). Morphologic changes in the organs of female C3H mice after long-term ingestion of thiourea and thiouracil. J. Natl. Cancer Inst. 9: 201-223.

Davison, C. (1943). para-Phenylenediamine poisoning with changes in the central nervous system. Arch. Neurol. Psych. 49: 254-265.

DeBaun, J. R., Miller, E. C., and Miller, J. A. (1970). N-Hydroxy-2-acetylaminofluorene sulfotransferase: its probable role in carcinogenesis and in protein-(methion-S-yl) binding in rat liver. Cancer Res. 30: 577-595.

Deichmann, W. B., MacDonald, W. M., Coplan, M. M., Woods, F. M., and Anderson, W. A. (1958a). para-Nitrobiphenyl, a new bladder carcinogen in the dog. Ind. Med. Surg. 27: 634-637.

Deichmann, W. B., Radomski, J. L., Anderson, W. A., Coplan, M. M., and Woods, F. M. (1958b). The carcinogenic action of p-aminobiphenyl in the dog. Ind. Med. Surg. 27: 25-26.

Deichmann, W. B., Radomski, J., Glass, E., Anderson, W. A., Coplan, M., and Woods, F. (1965). Synergism among oral carcinogens. III. Simultaneous feeding of four bladder carcinogens to dogs. Ind. Med. Surg. 34: 640-649

Della Porta, G., Capitano, J., Montipo, W., and Parmi, L. (1963). Studio sull' azione cancerogena dell' uretano nel topo. Tumori 49: 413-428.

Dessau, F. I., and Jackson, B. (1955). Acetamide-induced liver cell alterations in rats. Lab. Invest. 4: 387-397.

Dieteren, H. M. (1966). The biotransformation of o-tolidine. Arch. Environ. Health 12: 30-32.

Dontenwill, W., and Mohr, U. (1961). Carcinoma des Respirationstractus nach Behandlung von Goldhamstern met Diathylnitrosamin. Z. Krebsforsch. 64: 305-312.

Dontenwill, W., Mohr, U., and Zagel, M. (1962). Uber die unterschiedliche Lungen-carcinogene Wirkung des Diathylnitrosamins bei Hamster und Ratte. Z. Krebsforsch. 64: 499-502.

Driessens, J., Clay, A., Vanlerenberghe, J., and Adenis, L. (1962). Sarcomes au lieu d'injection sous-cutanee du bleu trypan chez le rat blanc. I. Etude histologique. C. R. Soc. Biol. (Paris) 156: 1099-1102.

Druckrey, H. (1950). Beitrageur Pharmakologie Cancerogener Substanzen. Versuche mit Anilin. Arch. Exp. Pathol. Pharmakol. 210: 137.

Druckrey, H. (1970). Production of colonic carcinomas by 1, 2-dialkylhydrazines and azoxyalkanes. In Carcinomas of the Colon and Antecedent Epithelium, W. J. Burdette (Ed.). Thomas, Springfield, Ill., pp. 267-279.

Druckrey, H. (1973). Chemical structure and action in transplacental carcinogenesis and teratogenesis. In Transplacental Carcinogenesis, L. Tomatis and U. Mohr (Eds.). IARC Scientific Publication No. 4, Lyon, France, pp. 45-58.

Druckrey, H., Ivankovic, S., Bucheler, J., Preussmann, R., and Thomas, C. (1968). Erzeugung von Magen-und Pankreas-Krebs beim Meersch-Weinchen durch Methylnitroso-harnstoff und-urethan. Z. Krebsforsch. 72: 167-182.

Druckrey, H., Ivankovic, S., and Preussmann, R. (1966a). Teratogenic and carcinogenic effects in the offspring after single injection of ethylnitrosourea to pregnant rats. Nature 210: 1378-1379.

Druckrey, H., Nieper, H. A., and Lo, H. W. (1956). Carcinogene Wirkung von Parafuchsin im Injektionsversuch an Ratten. Naturwissenschaften 13: 543.

Druckrey, H., Preussmann, R., Afkham, J., and Blum, G. (1962a). Erzeugung von Lungenkrebs durch Methylnitrosourethan bei intravenoser Gabe an Ratten. Naturwissenschaften 49: 451-452.

Druckrey, H., Preussmann, R., and Ivankovic, S. (1969). N-Nitroso compounds in organotropic and transplacental carcinogenesis. Ann. NY Acad. Sci. 163: 676-696.

Druckrey, H., Preussmann, R., Ivankovic, S., and Schmahl, D. (1967a). Organotrope Carcinogene Wirkungen bei 65 Verschiedenen N-Nitrosoverbindungen, an BD-Ratten. Z. Krebsforsch. 69: 103-201.

Druckrey, H., Preussmann, R., Ivankovic, S., Schmidt, C. H., Mennel, H. D., and Stahl, K. W. (1964a). Selektive Erzeugung von Blasenkrebs an Ratten durch Dibutyl-und N-Butyl-N-butanol-(4)-nitrosamin. Z. Krebsforsch. 66: 280-290.

Druckrey, H., Preussmann, R., Ivankovic, S., So, B. T., Schmidt, C. H., and Bucheler, J. (1966b). Zur Erzeugung subcutaner Sarkome an Ratten. Carcinogene Wirkung von Hydrazodicarbonsaure-bis(methyl-nitrosamid), N-Nitroso-N-n-butyl-harnstoff, N-Methyl-N-nitroso-nitroguanidin und N-Nitroso-imidazolidon. Z. Krebsforsch. 68:87-102.

Druckrey, H., Preussmann, R., Matzkies, F., and Ivankovic, S. (1966c). Carcinogene Wirkung von 1,2-Diathylhydrazin an Ratten. Naturwissenschaften 53:557-558.

Druckrey, H., Preussmann, R., Matzkies, F., and Ivankovic, S. (1967b). Selektive Erzeugung von Darm-Krebs bei Ratten durch 1,2-Dimethylhydrazin. Naturwissenschaften 54:285-286.

Druckrey, H., Preussmann, R., Schmahl, D., and Muller, M. (1961a). Chemische Konstitution und Carcinogene Wirkung bei Nitrosaminen. Naturwissenschaften 48: 134-135.

Druckrey, H., Preussmann, R., Schmahl, D., and Muller, M. (1961b). Erzeugung von Magenkrebs durch Nitrosamide an Ratten. Naturwissenschaften 48:165.

Druckrey, H., Preussmann, R., Schmahl, D., and Muller, M. (1962b). Erzeugung von Blasenkrebs an Ratten mit N,N-Dibutylnitrosamin. Naturwissenschaften 49:19.

Druckrey, H., Schagen, B., and Ivankovic, S. (1970). Erzeugung neurogener Malignome durch einmalige Gabe von Athylnitrosoharnstoff (ANH) an neugeborenen und junge BD IX-Ratten. Z. Krebsforsch. 74:141-161.

Druckrey, H., Schildbach, A., Schmahl, D., Preussmann, R., and Ivankovic, S. (1963a). Quantitative Analyse der Carcinogenen Wirkung von Diathylnitrosamin. Arznem. Forsch. 13:841-851.

Druckrey, H., Steinhoff, D., Preussmann, R., and Ivankovic, S. (1963b). Krebserzeugung durch einmaligne Dosis von Methylnitrosoharnstoff und verschiedenen Dialkylnitrosaminen. Naturwissenschaften 50:735.

Druckrey, H., Steinhoff, D., Preussmann, R., and Ivankovic, S. (1964b). Erzeugung von Krebs durch eine einmalige Dosis von Methylnitrosoharnstoff und verschiedenen Dialkylnitrosaminen an Ratten. Z. Krebsforsch. 66:1-10.

Dybing, E., and Thorgeirsson, S. (1977). Metabolic activation of 2,4-diaminoanisole, a hair dye component. I. Role of cytochrome P-450 metabolism in mutagenicity in vitro. Biochem. Pharmacol. 26:729-734.

Dzhioev, F. K. (1975). On carcinogenic activity of 4,4'-diaminodiphenyl ether. Vopr. Onkol. 21:69-73

Eckert, C. T., Cooper, Z. K., and Seelig, M. G. (1935). Scarlet red as a possible carcinogenic agent. Arch. Pathol. Lab. Med. 19:83-90.

Ehrilicher, H. von (1958). Benzidin in Arbeitsmedizinischer Sicht. Zentralbl. Arbeitsmed. Arbeitsschutz. Prophyl. 8:201-207.

Epstein, S. S. (1974). Environmental determinants of human cancer. Cancer Res. 34: 2425-2435.

Epstein, S. S., and Mantel, N. (1968). Hepatocarcinogenicity of the herbicide maleic hydrazide following parenteral administration to infant Swiss mice. Int. J. Cancer 3:325-335.

Fare, G. (1966). Rat skin carcinogenesis by topical applications of some azo dyes. Cancer Res. 26:2406-2408.

FDA (1977). File on Cosmetic Products. Ingredient Statements Registered in Accordance with 21 Code of Federal Regulations 720, Washington, D.C., Aug. 15.

Feinstein, R. N., and Lindahl, R. (1973). Detection of oxidases on polyacrylamide gels. Anal. Biochem. 56:353-360.

Ferebee, S. H. (1970). Controlled chemoprophylaxis trials in tuberculosis. A general review. Adv. Tuberc. Res. 17:28-106.

Fiala, E. S. (1977). Investigations into the metabolism and mode of action of the colon carcinogens 1,2-dimethylhydrazine and azoxymethane. Cancer 40:2436-2445.

Fiala, E. S., Kulakis, C., Bobotas, G., and Weisburger, J. H. (1976). Detection and estimation of azomethane in expired air of 1,2-dimethylhydrazine-treated rats. J. Natl. Cancer Inst. 56:1271-1273.

Fitzhugh, O. G., and Nelson, A. A. (1948). Liver tumors in rats fed thiourea or thioacetamide. Science 108:626-628.

Fox, A. J., and Collier, P. F. (1976). A survey of occupational cancer in the rubber and cablemaking industries: analysis of deaths occurring in 1972-74. Br. J. Ind. Med. 33: 249-264.

Frei, J. V. (1970). Toxicity, tissue changes and tumor induction in inbred Swiss mice by methylnitrosamine and -amide compounds. Cancer Res. 30:11-17.

Fruend, H. A. (1937). Clinical manifestations and studies in parenchymatous hepatitis. Ann. Intern. Med. 10:1144-1155.

Fujimura, S., Kogure, K., Oboshi, S., and Sugimura, T. (1970). Production of tumors in glandular stomach of hamsters by N-methyl-N'-nitro-N-nitrosoguanidine. Cancer Res. 30:1444-1448.

Furukawa, R. (1939). Experimentelle Entstehung des Leberkrebs durch subkutane Injektion von Olivenollosung des o-Amidoazotoluols. Nagasaki Igaku Zasshi 17:2370-2387.

Gargus, J. L., Paynter, O. E., and Reese, W. H., Jr. (1969). Utilization of newborn mice in the bioassay of chemical carcinogens. Toxicol. Appl. Pharmacol. 15:552-559.

Gehrmann, G. H., Foulger, J. H., and Fleming, A. J. (1949). Occupational tumours of the bladder. In Proc. 9th Int. Cong. Ind. Med., London, 1948, Bristol, Wright, pp. 472-475.

Gillman, J., Gillman, T., Gilbert, C., and Spence, I. (1952). The pathogenesis of experimentally produced lymphomata in rats (including Hodgkin's-like sarcoma). Cancer 5:792-846.

Gillman, T., Kinns, A. M., Hallowes, R. C., and Lloyd, J. B. (1973). Malignant lymphoreticular tumors induced by trypan blue and transplanted in inbred rats. J. Natl. Cancer Inst. 50:1179-1193.

Goldblatt, M. W. (1947). Occupational cancer of the bladder. Br. Med. Bull. 4:405-417.

Goldblatt, M. W. (1958). Occupational carcinogenesis. Br. Med. Bull. 14:136-140.

Goldwater, L. J., Rosso, A. J., and Kleinfeld, M. (1965). Bladder tumors in a coal tar dye plant. Arch. Environ. Health 11:814-817.

Gothoskar, S. V., Talwalkar, G. V., and Bhide, S. V. (1970). Tumorigenic effect of thioacetamide in Swiss strain mice. Br. J. Cancer 24:498-503.

Grab, D. J., and Zedeck, M. S. (1977). Organ-specific effects of the carcinogen methylazoxymethanol related to metabolism by nicotinamide adenine dinucleotide-dependent dehydrogenase. Cancer Res. 37:4182-4189.

Graffi, A., Hoffmann, F., and Schutt, M. (1967). N-methyl-N-nitrosourea as a strong topical carcinogen when painted on skin of rodents. Nature 214:611.

Grasso, P., and Creasey, M. (1969). Carcinoma of the colon in a rat. Eur. J. Cancer 5:415-419.

Grasso, P., Lansdown, A. B., Kiss, I. S., Gaunt, I. F., and Gangolli, S. D. (1969). Nodular hyperplasia in the rat liver following prolonged feeding of Ponceau MX. Food Cosmet. Toxicol. 7:425-442.

Grice, H. C., Mannell, W. A., and Allmark, M. G. (1961). Liver tumors in rats fed Ponceau 3R. Toxicol. Appl. Pharmacol. 3:509-520.

Griswold, D. P., Jr., Casey, A. E., Weisburger, E. K., and Weisburger, J. H. (1968). The carcinogenicity of multiple intragastric doses of aromatic and heterocyclic nitro or amino derivatives in young female Sprague Dawley rats. Cancer Res. 28:924-933.

Grundmann, E., and Steinhoff, D. (1970). Leber und Lungentumoren nach 3,3'-Dichlor-4,4'-diamino-diphenylmethan bei Ratten. Z. Krebsforsch. 74:28-39.

Gupta, D. N. (1955). Production of cancer of the bile ducts with thioacetamide. Nature 175:257.

Gutmann, H. R., and Bell, P. (1977). N-hydroxylation of arylamides by the rat and guinea pig: evidence for substrate specificity and participation of cytochrome P_1-450. Biochim. Biophys. Acta 498:229-243.

Hackmann, C. (1951). Untersuchungen uber die Cancerogene Wirkung einiger Fettloslicher Azofarbstuffe. Z. Krebsforsch. 57:530-541.

Hadidian, Z., Frederickson, T. N., Weisburger, E. K., Weisburger, J. H., Glass, R. M., and Mantel, N. (1968). Tests for chemical carcinogens. Report on the activity of derivatives of aromatic amines, nitrosamines, quinolines, nitroalkanes, amides, epoxides, aziridines and purine antimetabolites. J. Natl. Cancer Inst. 41: 985-1025.

Hall, W. H. (1948). The role of initiating and promoting factors in the pathogenesis of tumors of the thyroid. Br. J. Cancer 2: 273-280.

Hall, W. H., and Bielschowsky, F. (1949). The development of malignancy in experimentally-induced adenomata of the thyroid. Br. J. Cancer 3: 534-541.

Hamblin, D. O. (1967). Aromatic nitro and amino compounds. In _Industrial Hygiene and Toxicology_, 2nd Revised Ed., vol. II, _Toxicology_, F. A. Patty (Ed.), Interscience, New York, pp. 2105-2169.

Hamilton, S., and Sheridan, J. (1976). Aplastic anaemia and hair dye. Br. Med. J. 1: 834.

Hammond, E. C., Selikoff, I. J., and Robitzek, E. H. (1967). Isoniazid therapy in relation to later occurrence of cancer in adults and in infants. Br. Med. J. 2: 792-795.

Hansen, W. H., Davis, K. J., Fitzhugh, O. G., and Nelson, A. A. (1963). Chronic oral toxicity of Ponceau 3R. Toxicol. Appl. Pharmacol. 5: 105-118.

Hartwell, J. L., and Andervont, H. B. (1951). In: _Survey of Compounds Which Have Been Tested for Carcinogenic Activity_, P. Shubik and J. L. Hartwell (Eds.), Government Printing Office (U.S. Public Health Service Publication No. 149), Washington, D.C., p. 50.

Hashimoto, V., Suzuki, E., and Okada, M. (1972). Induction of urinary bladder tumors in ACI/N rats by butyl(3-carboxypropyl)nitrosamine, a major urinary metabolite of butyl(4-hydroxybutyl)nitrosamine. Gan. 63: 637-638.

Hauser, M., and Malofsky, B. M. (1974). Surface activator for anaerobic adhesives. Ger. Offen., 2,041,744 (Loctite Corp.), Chem. Abst. 82: 17949g.

Hawley, G. G. (Ed.) (1977). _The Condensed Chemical Dictionary_, 9th Ed. Van Nostrand Reinhold, New York.

Heath, D. F. (1962). The decomposition and toxicity of dialkylnitrosamines in rats. Biochem. J. 85: 72-91.

Hellwig, C. A., and Welch, J. W. (1963). Drug-induced tumors of the thyroid in guinea pigs with experimental thyroiditis. Growth 27: 305-315.

Herrold, K. M. (1964). Effect of route of administration on the carcinogenic action of diethylnitrosamine (N-nitrosodiethylamine). Br. J. Cancer 18: 763-767.

Herrold, K. M. (1966). Epidermoid carcinomas of esophagus and forestomach induced in Syrian hamsters by N-nitroso-N-methylurethan. J. Natl. Cancer Inst. 37: 389-394.

Herrold, K. M. (1968). Odontogenic tumors and epidermoid carcinomas of the oral cavity. An experimental study in Syrian hamsters. Oral Surg. 25: 262-272.

Herrold, K. M. (1969). Adenocarcinomas of the intestine induced in Syrian hamsters by N-methyl-N-nitrosourea. Pathol. Vet. 6: 403-412.

Herrold, K. M. (1970). Upper respiratory tract tumors induced in Syrian hamsters by N-methyl-N-nitrosourea. Int. J. Cancer 6: 217-222.

Herrold, K. M., and Dunham, L. J. (1963). Induction of tumors in the Syrian hamster with diethylnitrosamine (N-nitrosodiethylamine). Cancer Res. 23: 773-777.

Higginson, H. (1969). Present trends in cancer epidemiology. Can. Cancer Conf. 8: 40-75.

Hollander, C. F., and Bentvelzen, P. (1968). Enhancement of urethan induction of hepatomas in mice by prior partial hepatectomy. J. Natl. Cancer Inst. 41: 1303-1306.

Homburger, F., Friedell, G. H., Weisburger, E. K., and Weisburger, J. H. (1972). Carcinogenicity of simple aromatic amine derivatives in mice and rats. Toxicol. Appl. Pharmacol. 22: 280-281.

Hueper, W. C. (1942). _Occupational and Allied Diseases_. Thomas, Springfield, Ill.

Hueper, W. C. (1969). _Occupational and Environmental Cancers of the Urinary System_. Yale University Press, New Haven, Conn.

Hueper, W. C., and Conway, W. D. (Eds.) (1964). _Chemical Carcinogenesis and Cancers_. Thomas, Springfield, Ill.

Hueper, W. C., Wiley, F. H., and Wolfe, H. D. (1938). Experimental production of bladder tumors in dogs by administration of Beta-Naphthylaminc. J. Ind. Hyg. Toxicol. 20:46-84.

Hughes, H. B. (1953). On the metabolic fate of isoniazid. J. Pharmacol. Exp. Ther. 109: 444-452.

IARC (1972). Evaluation of Carcinogenic Risk of Chemicals to Man, IARC Monographs, Vol. 1. Lyon, France.

IARC (1974a). Some aromatic amines, hydrazine and related substances, N-nitroso compounds and miscellaneous alkylating agents. In Evaluation of Carcinogenic Risk of Chemicals to Man, IARC Monographs, Vol. 4. Lyon, France.

IARC (1974b). Some anti-thyroid and related substances, nitrofurans and industrial chemicals. In Evaluation of Carcinogenic Risk of Chemicals to Man, IARC Monographs, Vol. 7. Lyon, France.

IARC (1975). Some aromatic azo compounds. In Evaluation of Carcinogenic Risk of Chemicals to Man, IARC Monographs, Vol. 8. Lyon, France.

IARC (1978). Some aromatic amines and related nitro compounds—hair dyes, colouring agents and miscellaneous industrial chemicals. In Evaluation of Carcinogenic Risk of Chemicals to Man, IARC Monographs, Vol. 16. Lyon, France.

Ikeda, Y., Horiuchi, S., Furuya, T., and Omori, Y. (1966). Chronic toxicity of Ponceau MX in the rat. Food Cosmet. Toxicol. 4:485-492.

Ikeda, Y., Horiuchi, S., Kobayashi, K., Furuja, T., and Kohgo, K. (1968). Carcinogenicity of Ponceau MX in the mouse. Food Cosmet. Toxicol. 6:591-598.

Innes, J. R., Ulland, B. M., Valerio, M. G., Petrucelli, L., Fishbein, L., Hart, E. R., Pallotta, A. J., Bates, R. R., Falk, H. L., Gart, J. J., Klein, M., Mitchell, I., and Peters, J. (1969). Bioassay of pesticides and industrial chemicals for tumorigenicity in mice: a preliminary note. J. Natl. Cancer Inst. 42:1101-1114.

International Labour Office (1971). Encyclopedia of Occupational Health and Safety, Vol. 1. McGraw-Hill, New York, p. 96.

Inuzuka, Y., Kameyama, N., and Watanabe, K. (1976). Phthalocyanine pigments. Japan Kokai, 76 26, 933 (Toyo Ink Mfg. Co., Ltd.), Chem. Abst. 85:7367b.

Irving, C. C. (1964). Enzymatic N-hydroxylation of the carcinogen 2-acetylaminofluorene and the metabolism of N-hydroxy-2-acetylaminofluorene-9-^{14}C in vitro. J. Biol. Chem. 239:1589-1596.

Irving, C. C. (1970). Conjugates of N-hydroxy compounds. In Metabolic Conjugation and Metabolic Hydrolysis, Vol. 1, W. H. Fishman (Ed.). Academic Press, New York, pp. 53-119.

Irving, C. C. (1971). Metabolic activation of N-hydroxy compounds by conjugation. Xenobiotica 1:387-398.

Irving, C. C., Wiseman, R., Jr., and Young, J. M. (1967). Carcinogenicity of 2-acetylaminofluorene and N-hydroxy-2-acetylaminofluorene in the rabbit. Cancer Res. 27:838-848.

Israel, M. S., and Ellis, I. R. (1960). The neoplastic potentialities of mouse thyroid under extreme stimulation. Br. J. Cancer 14:206-211.

Israels, M. C., and Susman, W. (1934). Systemic poisoning by phenylenediamine with report of a fatal case. Lancet 1:508-510.

Ito, N., Hiasa, Y., Konishi, Y., and Marugami, M. (1969). The development of carcinoma in liver of rats treated with m-toluylenediamine and the synergistic and antagonistic effects with other chemicals. Cancer Res. 29:1137-1145.

Ivankovic, S., and Bucheler, J. (1968). Leber-und Blasen-Carcinome beim Meerschweinchen nach Di-n-butylnitrosamin. Z. Krebsforsch. 71:183-185.

Jackson, B., and Dessau, F. I. (1961). Liver tumors in rats fed acetamide. Lab. Invest. 10:909-923.

Jaffe, W. G. (1947). The response of mice to the simultaneous application of two different carcinogenic agents. Cancer Res. 1:529-530.

Jagow, R. V., Kiese, M., and Renner, G. (1966). Urinary excretion of N-hydroxylation derivatives of some aromatic amines by rabbits, guinea pigs, and dogs. Biochem. Pharmacol. 15:1899-1910.

Juhasz, J., Balo, J., and Kendrey, G. (1957). Uber die Geschwulsterzeugenden Wirkung des Isonicotinsaurehydrazid (INH). Z. Krebsforsch. 62:188-196.

Kadhim, A. M., and Peters, A. T. (1074). New intermediates and dyes for synthetic polymer fibers. Substituted benzimidazothioxanthenoisoquinolinones for polyester fibers. J. Soc. Dyers Colourists 90:199-202.

Kadlubar, F. F., Miller, J. A., and Miller, E. C. (1976a). Microsomal N-oxidation of the hepatocarcinogen N-methyl-4-aminoazobenzene and the reactivity of N-hydroxy-N-methyl-4-aminoazobenzene. Cancer Res. 36:1196-1206.

Kadlubar, F. F., Miller, J. A., and Miller, E. C. (1976b). Hepatic metabolism of N-hydroxy-N-methyl-4-aminoazobenzene and other N-hydroxyarylamines to reactive sulfuric acid esters. Cancer Res. 36:2350-2359.

Kadlubar, F. F., Miller, J. A., and Miller, E. C. (1977). Hepatic microsomal N-glucuronidation and nucleic acid binding of N-hydroxy-arylamines in relation to urinary bladder carcinogenesis. Cancer Res. 37:805-814.

Kaplow, L. S. (1975). Substitute for benzidine in myeloperoxidase stains. Am. J. Clin. Pathol. 63:451.

Kelly, M. G., O'Gara, R. W., Adamson, R. H., Gadekar, K., Botkin, C. C., Reese, W. H., and Kerber, W. T. (1966). Induction of hepatic cell carcinomas in monkeys with N-nitrosodiethylamine. J. Natl. Cancer Inst. 36:323-351.

Kensler, C. J., Dexter, S. O., and Rhoads, C. P. (1942). The inhibition of a diphosphopyridine nucleotide system by split products of dimethylaminoazobenzene. Cancer Res. 2:1-10.

Khlebnikova, M. I., Gladkova, E. V., Kurenko, L. T., Pshenitsyn, A. V., and Shalin, B. M. (1970). Problem of industrial hygiene and health status of workers engaged in the production of o-toluidine. Gig. Tr. Prof. Zabol. 14:7-10.

Kiese, M. (1959). Oxydation von Anilin zu Nitrosobenzol im Hunde. Naunyn Schmiedebergs Arch. Pharmacol. 235:354-359.

Kiese, M. (1966). The biochemical production of ferrihemoglobin-forming derivatives from aromatic amines and mechanisms of ferrihemoglobin formation. Pharmacol. Rev. 18:1091-1161.

Kiese, M., and Rauscher, E. (1968). The absorption of p-toluenediamine through human skin in hair dyeing. Toxicol. Appl. Pharmacol. 13:325-331.

Kiese, M., Renner, G., and Wiedemann, I. (1966). N-hydroxylation of 2-aminofluorene in the guinea pig and by guinea pig liver microsomes in vitro. Naunyn Schmiedebergs Arch. Pharmacol. 252:418-423.

Kilner, E., and Samuel, D. M. (1960). Applied Organic Chemistry. Interscience, New York, pp. 262, 266.

King, C. M. (1974). Mechanism of reaction, tissue distribution, and inhibition of arylhydroxamic acid acyltransferase. Cancer Res. 34:1503-1515.

King, C. M., and Phillips, B. (1969). N-Hydroxy-2-fluorenylacetamide. Reaction of the carcinogen with guanosine, ribonucleic acid, deoxyribonucleic acid, and protein following enzymatic deacetylation or esterification. J. Biol. Chem. 244:6209-6216.

King, D. W., Bock, F. G., and Moore, G. E. (1963). Dinitrophenol inhibition of pituitary adenoma formation in mice fed propylthiouracil. Proc. Soc. Exp. Biol. Med. 112: 365-366.

Kinkel, H. J., and Holzmann, S. (1973). Study of long-term percutaneous toxicity and carcinogenicity of hair dyes (oxidizing dyes) in rats. Food Cosmet. Toxicol. 11:641-648.

Kinosita, R. (1936). Researches on the cancerogenesis of the various chemical substances. Gan. 30:423-426.

Kirby, A. H. (1945). Studies in carcinogenesis with azo compounds. I. The action of four azo dyes in mixed and pure strain mice. Cancer Res. 5:673-682.

Kirby, A. H., and Peacock, P. R. (1947). The induction of liver tumours by 4-aminoazobenzene and its N,N-dimethyl derivative in rats on a restricted diet. J. Pathol. Bact. 59:1-7.

Kirby, A. H., and Peacock, P. R. (1949). Liver tumours in mice injected with commercial food dyes. Glasgow Med. J. 30:364-372.

Klein, M. (1952). The transplacental effect of urethan on lung tumorigenesis in mice. J. Natl. Cancer Inst. 12:1003-1010.

Koller, P. C. (1953). Dicentric chromosomes in a rat tumor induced by an aromatic nitrogen mustard. Heredity 6:181.

Kopelman, H., Robertson, M. H., Sanders, P. G., and Ash, I. (1966a). The Epping jaundice. Br. Med. J. 1:514-516.

Kopelman, H. Scheuer, P. J., and Williams, R. (1966b). The liver lesion of the Epping jaundice. Q. J. Med. 35:553-564.

Kriek, E. (1974). Carcinogenesis by aromatic amines. Biochim. Biophys. Acta 355:177-203.

Kriek, E., and Emmelot, P. (1964). Methylation of deoxyribonucleic acid by diazomethane. Biochim. Biophys. Acta 91:59-66.

Krisnan, R. M. (1975). 4-Chloro-1,3-benzenediamine. Ger. Offen., 2,428,141 (Goodyear Tire and Rubber Co.), Chem. Abst. 82:157140m.

Lake, B. G., Phillips, J. C., Cottrell, R. C., and Gangolli, S. C. (1978). The possible involvement of a microsomal amine oxidase enzyme in hepatic dimethylnitrosamine degradation in vitro. In Biological Oxidation of Nitrogen, J. W. Gorrod (Ed.). Elsevier-North Holland, Amsterdam, pp. 131-135.

Langlade, A. (1976). Extrusion and continuous vulcanization of polychloropropene rubbers. Hule Mex. Plast. 32 (364):18-20, 22-24. Chem. Abst. 85:161530t.

Laqueur, G. L. (1949). Nodular hyperplasiá of thyroid glands induced by thiouracil. Cancer Res. 9:247-255.

Larsen, C. D. (1947). Pulmonary-tumor induction by transplacental exposure to urethan. J. Natl. Cancer Inst. 8:63-70.

Laursen, B. (1970). Cancer of the bladder in patients treated with chlornaphazine. Br. Med. J. 3:684-685.

Lawley, P. D. (1966). Effects of some chemical mutagens and carcinogens on nucleic acids. Prog. Nucleic Acid Res. Mol. Biol. 5:89-131.

Lawley, P. D. (1972). The action of alkylating mutagens and carcinogens on nucleic acids: N-methyl-N-nitroso compounds as methylating agents. In Topics in Chemical Carcinogenesis, W. Nakahara, S. Takayama, T. Sugimura, and S. Odeshuma (Eds.). University of Tokyo Press, Tokyo, pp. 237-256.

Leaver, D. D., Swann, P. F., and Magee, P. N. (1969). The induction of tumours in the rat by a single oral dose of N-nitrosomethylurea. Br. J. Cancer 23:177-187.

Lee, K., Gold, B., and Mirvish, S. S. (1977). Mutagenicity of 22 N-nitrosamides and related compounds for Salmonella typhimurium TA1535. Mutat. Res. 48:131-138.

Lees, J., Alexander, W. D., and Marchant, B. (1973). Accumulation of S-thiouracil by the rat thyroid gland. Endocrinology 93:162-171.

LePage, R. N., and Christie, G. S. (1969a). Induction of liver tumors in the guinea pig by feeding dimethylnitrosamine. Pathology 1:49.

LePage, R. N., and Christie, G. S. (1969b). Induction of liver tumours in the rabbit by feeding dimethylnitrosamine. Br. J. Cancer 23:125-131.

Lijinsky, W., Loo, J., and Ross, A. E. (1968). Mechanism of alkylation of nucleic acids by nitrosodimethylamine. Nature 218:1174-1175.

Lin, J. K., Miller, J. A., and Miller, E. C. (1968). Studies on structures of polar dyes derived from the liver proteins of rats fed N-methyl-4-aminoazobenzene. II. Identity of synthetic 3-(homocystein-S-yl)-N-methyl-4-aminoazobenzene with the major polar dye P2b. Biochemistry 7:1889-1895.

Lin, J. K., Miller, J. A., and Miller, E. C. (1969). Studies on structures of polar dyes derived from the liver proteins of rats fed N-methyl-4-aminoazobenzene. III. Tyrosine and homocysteine sulfoxide polar dyes. Biochemistry 8:1573-1582.

Lin, J. K., Miller, J. A., and Miller, E. C. (1975). Structures of hepatic nucleic acid-bound dyes in rats given the carcinogen N-methyl-4-aminoazobenzene. Cancer Res. 35:844-850.

Linch, A. L., O'Connor, G. B., Barnes, J. R., Killian, A. S., Jr., and Neeld, W. E., Jr. (1971). Methylene-bis-ortho-chloroaniline (MOCA^R): evaluation of hazards and control. Am. Ind. Hyg. Assoc. J. 32:802-819.

Lotlikar, P. D., Baldy, W. J., Jr., and Dwyer, E. N. (1975). Dimethylnitrosamine demethylation by reconstituted liver microsomal cytochrome P-450 enzyme system. Biochem. J. 152:705-708.

Lotlikar, P. D., Baldy, W. J., Nyce, J. W., and Dwyer, E. N. (1976). Dealkylation of dimethyl- and diethyl-nitrosamine by tissue microsomal enzyme system. Proc. Am. Assoc. Cancer Res. 17:204.

Lotlikar, P. D., Enomoto, M., Miller, J. A., and Miller, E. C. (1967). Species variation in the N- and ring-hydroxylation of 2-acetylaminofluorene and effects of 3-methylcholanthrene pretreatment. Proc. Soc. Exp. Biol. Med. 125:341-346.

Lotlikar, P. D., Scribner, J. D., Miller, J. A., and Miller, E. C. (1966). Reactions of esters of aromatic N-hydroxy amines and amides with methionine in vitro: a model for in vivo binding of amine carcinogens to protein. Life Sci. 5:1263-1269.

Lotlikar, P. D., and Zaleski, K. (1974). Inhibitory effect of carbon monoxide on the N- and ring-hydroxylation of 2-acetamidofluorene by hamster hepatic microsomal preparations. Biochem. J. 144:427-430.

Magee, P. N. (1956). Toxic liver injury. The metabolism of dimethylnitrosamine. Biochem. J. 64:676-682.

Magee, P. N., and Barnes, J. M. (1956). The production of malignant primary hepatic tumours in the rat by feeding dimethylnitrosamine. Br. J. Cancer 10:114-122.

Magee, P. N., and Barnes, J. M. (1959). The experimental production of tumours in the rat by dimethylnitrosamine. Acta Un. Int. Cancer 15:187-190.

Magee, P. N., and Barnes, J. M. (1962). Induction of kidney tumours in the rat with dimethylnitrosamine (N-nitrosodimethylamine). J. Path. Bact. 84:19-31.

Magee, P. N., and Barnes, J. M. (1967). Carcinogenic nitroso compounds. Adv. Cancer Res. 10:163-246.

Magee, P. N., Montesano, R., and Preussmann, R. (1976). N-Nitroso compounds and related carcinogens. In <u>Chemical Carcinogens</u>, ACS Monograph 173, C. E. Searle (Ed.). American Chemical Society, Washington, D.C., pp. 491-625.

Magee, P. N., Pegg, A. E., and Swann, P. F. (1975). Molecular mechanisms in chemical carcinogenesis. In <u>Handbuch der Allgemeinen Pathologie</u>, E. Grundmann (Ed.), Springer-Verlag, Berlin, pp. 329-419.

Maloof, F., and Soodak, M. (1957). The uptake and metabolism of S^{35} thiourea and thiouracil by the thyroid and other tissues. Endocrinology 61:555-569.

Mancuso, T. F., and El-Attar, A. A. (1967). Cohort study of workers exposed to beta-naphthylamine and benzidine. J. Occup. Med. 9:277-285.

Mannell, W. A. (1964). Further investigations on the production of liver tumors in rats by Ponceau 3R. Food Cosmet. Toxicol. 2:169-174.

Manufacturing Chemists Association (1966). Properties and essential information for safe handling and use of dinitrotoluenes. Chemical Safety Data Sheet SD-93, London, England.

Marchant, B., Alexander, W. D., Robertson, J. W., and Lazarus, J. H. (1971). Concentration of ^{35}S-propylthiouracil by the thyroid gland and its relationship to anion trapping mechanism. Metabolism 20:989-999.

Marhold, J., Matrka, M., Hub, M., and Ruffer, F. (1968). The possible complicity of diphenyline in the origin of tumours in the manufacture of benzidine. Neoplasma 15: 3-10.

Maruya, H., and Tanaka, Y. (1936). Buttergelb. Osaka Igakkai Zasshi 35:2304.

Mattor, J. A., and Price, L. (1970). Color photographic materials. Ger. Offen., 1,937,230 (Scott Paper Co.), Chem. Abst. 73:50722q.

Mauer, S. M., Lee, C. S., Najarian, J. S., and Brown, D. M. (1974). Induction of malignant kidney tumors in rats with streptozotocin. Cancer Res. 34:158-160.

Mayer, R. L. (1954). Group-sensitization to compounds of quinone structure and its biochemical basis: role of these substances in cancer. Prog. Allergy 4:79-172.

McCann, J. E., Choi, E., Yamasaki, E. E., and Ames, B. N. (1975). Detection of carcinogens as mutagens in the Salmonella/microsome test: assay of 300 chemicals. Proc. Natl. Acad. Sci. USA 72:5135-5139.

Meara, R. H., and Martin-Scott, I. (1953). Contact dermatitis due to aminoazotoluene. Br. Med. J. 1:1142-1143.

Meigs, J. W., Brown, R. M., and Sciarini, L. J. (1951). A study of exposure to benzidine and substituted benzidines in a chemical plant. Arch. Ind. Hyg. Occup. Med. 4:533-540.

Meigs, J. W., Sciarini, L. J., and Van Sandt, W. A. (1954). Skin penetration by diamines of the benzidine group. Arch. Ind. Hyg. Occup. Med. 9:122-132.

Melick, W. F., Escue, H. M., Naryka, J. J., Mezera, R. A., and Wheeler, E. P. (1955). The first reported cases of human bladder tumors due to a new carcinogen—xenylamine. J. Urol. 74:760-766.

Melick, W. F., Naryka, J. J., and Kelly, R. E. (1971). Bladder cancer due to exposure to para-aminobiphenyl: 17 year follow-up. J. Urol. 106:220-226.

Miller, E. C., Lotlikar, P. D., Pitot, H. C., Fletcher, T. L., and Miller, J. A. (1966). N-Hydroxy-metabolites of 2-acetylaminophenanthrene and 7-fluoro-2-acetylaminofluorene as proximate carcinogens in the rat. Cancer Res. 26:2239-2247.

Miller, E. C., McKechnie, D., Poirier, M. M., and Miller, J. A. (1965). Inhibition of amino acid incorporation in vitro by metabolites of 2-acetylaminofluorene and by certain nitroso compounds. Proc. Soc. Exp. Biol. Med. 120:538-541.

Miller, E. C., and Miller, J. A. (1976). The metabolism of chemical carcinogens to reactive electrophiles and their possible mechanisms of action in carcinogenesis. In Chemical Carcinogens, ACS Monograph 173, C. E. Searle (Ed.). American Chemical Society, Washington, D.C., pp. 737-762.

Miller, E. C., Miller, J. A., and Enomoto, M. (1964). The comparative carcinogenicities of 2-acetylaminofluorene and its N-hydroxy metabolites in mice, hamsters, and guinea pigs. Cancer Res. 24:2018-2032.

Miller, E. C., Miller, J. A., and Hartmann, H. A. (1961a). N-Hydroxy-2-acetylaminofluorene: a metabolite of 2-acetylaminofluorene with increased carcinogenic activity in the rat. Cancer Res. 21:815-824.

Miller, E. C., Sandin, R., Miller, J. A., and Rusch, H. P. (1956). The carcinogenicity of compounds related to 2-acetylaminofluorene. III. Aminobiphenyl and benzidine derivatives. Cancer Res. 16:525-534.

Miller, J. A. (1970). Carcinogenesis by chemicals. An overview. Cancer Res. 30:559-576.

Miller, J. A., Cramer, J. W., and Miller, E. C. (1960). The N- and ring-hydroxylation of 2-acetylaminofluorene during carcinogenesis in the rat. Cancer Res. 20:950-962.

Miller, J. A., and Miller, E. C. (1953). The carcinogenic aminoazo dyes. Adv. Cancer Res. 1:339-396.

Miller, J. A., and Miller, E. C. (1967). Activation of carcinogenic aromatic amines and amides by N-hydroxylation in vivo. In Carcinogenesis: A Broad Critique. M. D. Anderson Tumor Institute, University of Texas. Williams and Wilkins, Baltimore, pp. 397-420.

Miller, J. A., and Miller, E. C. (1969). The metabolic activation of carcinogenic aromatic amines and amides. Prog. Exp. Tumor Res. 11:273-301.

Miller, J. A., Wyatt, C. S., Miller, E. C., and Hartmann, H. A. (1961b). The N-hydroxylation of 4-acetylaminobiphenyl by the rat and dog and strong carcinogenicity of N-hydroxy-4-acetylaminobiphenyl in the rat. Cancer Res. 21:1465-1473.

Mirvish, S. S. (1966). The metabolism of N-hydroxyurethane in relation to its carcinogenic action: conversion into urethane and an N-hydroxyurethane glucuronide. Biochim. Biophys. Acta 117:1-12.

Mirvish, S. S. (1968). The carcinogenic action and metabolism of urethan and N-hydroxyurethan. Adv. Cancer Res. 11:1-42.

Mirvish, S. S., and Kaufman, L. (1970). A study of nitrosamines and S-carboxyl derivatives of cysteine as lung carcinogens in adult SWR mice. Int. J. Cancer 6:69-73.

Mohr, U., and Althoff, J. (1965). Die diaplacentare Wirkung des Cancerogens Diäthylnitrosamin bei der Maus. Z. Krebsforsch. 67:152-155.

Mohr, U., Althoff, J., and Authaler, A. (1966). Diaplacental effect of the carcinogen diethylnitrosamine in the golden hamster. Cancer Res. 26:2349-2352.

Money, W. L., Fitzgerald, P. J., Godwin, J. T., and Rawson, R. W. (1953). The effect of thiouracil on the collection of radioactive iodine in experimentally induced thyroid tumors. Cancer 6:111-120.

Montesano, R., and Bartsch, H. (1976). Mutagenic and carcinogenic N-nitroso compounds: possible environmental hazards. Mutat. Res. 32:179-228.

Montesano, R., and Magee, P. N. (1974). Comparative metabolism in vitro of nitrosamines in various animal species including man. In Chemical Carcinogenesis Essays, R. Montesano and L. Tomatis (Eds.). IARC Scientific Publication No. 10, Lyon, France, pp. 39-56.

Moore, G. E., Brackney, E. L., and Bock, F. G. (1953). Production of pituitary tumors in mice by chronic administration of a thiouracil derivative. Proc. Soc. Exp. Biol. Med. 82:643-645.

Mori, K., and Nakahara, W. (1940). Effect of liver feeding on production of malignant tumors, based on injections of carcinogenic substances. Gan. 34:188-190.

Mori, K., Yasuno, A., and Matsumoto, K. (1960). Induction of pulmonary tumors in mice with isonicotinic acid hydrazid. Gan. 51:83-90.

Morosenskaya, L. S. (1938). ortho-Aminoazotoluene. Arch. Sci. Biol. (Moscow) 56:189-200.

Morris, H. P., Velat, C. A., Wagner, B. D., Dahlgard, M., and Ray, F. E. (1960). Studies of carcinogenicity in the rat of derivatives of aromatic amines related to N-2-fluorenylacetamide. J. Natl. Cancer Inst. 24:149-180.

Mueller, G. C., and Miller, J. A. (1948). The metabolism of 4-dimethylaminoazobenzene by rat liver homogenate. J. Biol. Chem. 176:535-544.

Mueller, G. C., and Miller, J. A. (1949). The reductive cleavage of 4-dimethylaminoazobenzene by rat liver: the intracellular distribution of the enzyme system and its requirement for triphosphopyridine nucleotide. J. Biol. Chem. 180:1125-1136.

Mueller, G. C., and Miller, J. A. (1950). The reductive cleavage of 4-dimethylaminoazobenzene by rat liver: reactivation of carbon dioxide treated homogenates by riboflavin-adenine dinucleotide. J. Biol. Chem. 185:145-154.

Mueller, P. (1976). Diazo pigment. Ger. Offen., 2,518,560 (Ciba-Geigy A.G.), Chem. Abst. 84:61181r.

Mull, R. L., and Giri, S. N. (1972). The role of renal aromatic N-deacetylase in selective toxicity of avicide 3-chloro-p-toluidine in birds. Biochim. Biophys. Acta 273:222-228.

Munn, A. (1967). Occupational bladder tumors and carcinogens: recent developments in Britain. In Bladder Cancer, A Symposium, K. F. Lampe (Ed.). Aesculapius, Birmingham, Ala., pp. 187-193.

Murphy, G. P., Mirand, E. A., Johnston, G. S., Schmidt, J. D., and Scott, W. W. (1966). Renal tumors induced by a single dose of dimethylnitrosamine: morphologic, functional, enzymatic and hormonal characterizations. Invest. Urol. 4:39-56.

Napalkov, N. P. (1959). Morphological characteristics of experimental thyroid tumours induced in rats with 6-methylthiouracil. Vopr. Onkol. 5:578-592.

Napalkov, N. P., and Saliamon, L. S. (1968). The incidence of sarcoma in rats during subcutaneous administration of 6-methylthiouracil. Vopr. Onkol. 14:41-42.

National Research Council (1971). Food colors. NAS, Washington, D.C.

NCI (1978a). Bioassay of 2-aminoanthraquinone for possible carcinogenicity. DHEW Publication No. (NIH)78-1399, U.S. Government Printing Office, Washington, D.C.

NCI (1978b). Bioassay of 3-amino-4-ethoxy-acetanilide for possible carcinogenicity. DHEW Publication No. (NIH)78-1367, U.S. Government Printing Office, Washington, D.C.

NCI (1978c). Bioassay of 3-amino-9-ethylcarbazole (hydrochloride) for possible carcinogenicity. DHEW Publication No. (NIH)78-1337, U.S. Government Printing Office, Washington, D.C.

NCI (1978d). Bioassay of 1-amino-2-methylanthraquinone for possible carcinogenicity. DHEW Publication No. (NIH)78-1366, U.S. Government Printing Office, Washington, D.C.

NCI (1978e). Bioassay of 4-amino-2-nitrophenol for possible carcinogenicity. DHEW Publication No. (NIH)78-1344, U.S. Government Printing Office, Washington, D.C.

NCI (1978f). Bioassay of aniline hydrochloride for possible carcinogenicity. DHEW Publication No. (NIH)78-1385, U.S. Government Printing Office, Washington, D.C.

NCI (1978g). Bioassay of o-anisidine hydrochloride for possible carcinogenicity. DHEW Publication No. (NIH)78-1339, U.S. Government Printing Office, Washington, D.C.

NCI (1978h). Bioassay of p-anisidine hydrochloride for possible carcinogenicity. DHEW Publication No. (NIH)78-1371, U.S. Government Printing Office, Washington, D.C.

NCI (1978i). Bioassay of anthranilic acid for possible carcinogenicity. DHEW Publication No. (NIH)78-836, U.S. Government Printing Office, Washington, D.C.

NCI (1978j). Bioassay of 4-chloro-m-phenylenediamine for possible carcinogenicity. DHEW Publication No. (NIH)78-1335, U.S. Government Printing Office, Washington, D.C.

NCI (1978k). Bioassay of 4-chloro-o-phenylenediamine for possible carcinogenicity. DHEW Publication No. (NIH)78-1313, U.S. Government Printing Office, Washington, D.C.

NCI (1978l). Bioassay of 3-chloro-p-toluidine for possible carcinogenicity. DHEW Publication No. (NIH)78-1701, U.S. Government Printing Office, Washington, D.C.

NCI (1978m). Bioassay of m-cresidine for possible carcinogenicity. DHEW Publication No. (NIH)78-1355, U.S. Government Printing Office, Washington, D.C.

NCI (1978n). Bioassay of p-cresidine for possible carcinogenicity. DHEW Publication No. (NIH)78-1397, U.S. Government Printing Office, Washington, D.C.

NCI (1978o). Bioassay of 2,4-diaminoanisole sulfate for possible carcinogenicity. DHEW Publication No. (NIH)78-1334, U.S. Government Printing Office, Washington, D.C.

NCI (1978p). Bioassay of N,N'-diethylthiourea for possible carcinogenicity. DHEW Publication No. (NIH)78-1705, U.S. Government Printing Office, Washington, D.C.

NCI (1978q). Bioassay of 2,4-dinitrotoluene for possible carcinogenicity. DHEW Publication No. (NIH)78-1360, U.S. Government Printing Office, Washington, D.C.

NCI (1978r). Bioassay of hydrazobenzene for possible carcinogenicity. DHEW Publication No. (NIH)78-1342, U.S. Government Printing Office, Washington, D.C.

NCI (1978s). Bioassay of Michler's ketone for possible carcinogenicity. DHEW Publication No. (NIH)79-1737, U.S. Government Printing Office, Washington, D.C.

NCI (1978t). Bioassay of 5-nitroacenaphthene for possible carcinogenicity. DHEW Publication No. (NIH)78-1373, U.S. Government Printing Office, Washington, D.C.

NCI (1978u). Bioassay of 5-nitro-o-anisidine for possible carcinogenicity. DHEW Publication No. (NIH)78-1382, U.S. Government Printing Office, Washington, D.C.

NCI (1978v). Bioassay of 2-nitro-p-phenylenediamine for possible carcinogenicity. DHEW Publication No. (NIH)78-1725, U.S. Government Printing Office, Washington, D.C.

NCI (1978w). Bioassay of 5-nitro-o-toluidine for possible carcinogenicity. DHEW Publication No. (NIH)78-1357, U.S. Government Printing Office, Washington, D.C.

NCI (1978x). Bioassay of 2,5-toluenediamine sulfate for possible carcinogenicity. DHEW Publication No. (NIH)78-1381, U.S. Government Printing Office, Washington, D.C.

NCI (1978y). Bioassay of trimethylthiourea for possible carcinogenicity. DHEW Publication No. (NIH)78-1384, U.S. Government Printing Office, Washington, D.C.

NCI (1978z). 13-week subchronic toxicity studies of direct blue 6, direct black 38 and direct brown 95 dyes. DHEW Publication No. (NIH)78-1358, U.S. Government Printing Office, Washington, D.C.

Nelson, A. A., and Davidow, B. (1957). Injection site fibrosarcoma production in rats by food colors. Fed. Proc. 16:367.

Nelson, A. A., and Hagan, E. C. (1953). Production of fibrosarcomas in rats at site of subcutaneous injection of various food dyes. Fed. Proc. 12:397-398.

Nelson, A. A., and Woodard, G. (1953). Tumors of the urinary bladder, gall bladder and liver in dogs fed o-aminoazotoluene or p-dimethylaminoazobenzene. J. Natl. Cancer Inst. 13:1497-1509.

Nelson, S. D., Mitchell, J. R., Timbrell, J. A., Snodgrass, W. R., and Cororan, G. B., III (1976). Isoniazid and iproniazid: activation of metabolites to toxic intermediates in man and rat. Science 193:901-903.

Nettleship, A., Henshaw, P. S., and Meyer, H. L. (1943). Induction of pulmonary tumors in mice with ethyl carbamate (urethane). J. Natl. Cancer Inst. 4:309-319.

NIOSH (1976). Current intelligence bulletin: metabolic precursors of a known human carcinogen, beta-naphthylamine. Rockville, Md., pp. 1-3.

Nishiyama, Y. (1935). Experimentelle Hepatombildung durch Futterung mit o-Amidoazotoluol bei dur Maus. Gan. 29:285-293.

Nomura, T. (1973). Carcinogenesis by urethan via mother's milk and its enhancement of transplacental carcinogenesis in mice. Cancer Res. 33:1677-1683.

NTIS (1968). Evaluation of Carcinogenic, Teratogenic and Mutagenic Activities of Selected Pesticides and Industrial Chemicals, Vol. 1, Carcinogenic Study. U.S. Department of Commerce, Washington, D.C.

Okada, M. (1976). Metabolic aspects in organotropic carcinogenesis by dialkylnitrosamines. In Proc. 6th Int. Symp. Princess Takamatsu, Cancer Research Fund, P. N. Magee, S. Takayama, T. Sugimura, and M. Matsushima (Eds.). Tokyo University Press, Tokyo, pp. 251-266.

Okada, M., Suzuki, E., Aoki, J., Iiyoshi, M., and Hashimoto, T. (1975). Metabolism and carcinogenicity of N-butyl-N-(4-hydroxybutyl)nitrosamine and related compounds, with special reference to induction of urinary bladder tumors. Gan. Monogr. Cancer Res. 17:161-176.

Okajima, E., Hiramatsu, T., Motomiya, Y., Iriya, K., Ijuin, M., and Ito, N. (1971). Effect of DL-tryptophan on tumorigenesis in the urinary bladder and liver of rats treated with N-nitrosodibutylamine. Gan. 62:163-169.

Orr, J. W. (1940). The histology of the rat's liver during the course of carcinogenesis by butter-yellow (p-dimethylaminoazobenzene). J. Path. Bact. 50:393-408.

Otsuka, H., and Kuwahara, A. (1971). Hemangiomatous lesions of mice treated with nitrosodimethylamine. Gan. 62:147-156.

Papacharalampous, N. X. (1957). Befunde an der Ratte nach Langfristigen Versuchen met Intraperitonealen Injecktionen von Trypanblau. Beitr. Pathol. 117:85-89.

Parkes, H. G. (1976). The epidemiology of the aromatic amine cancers. In Chemical Carcinogens, ACS Monograph 173, C. E. Searle (Ed.). American Chemical Society, Washington, D.C., pp. 462-480.

Peacock, A., and Peacock, P. R. (1966). The results of prolonged administration of isoniazid to mice, rats and hamsters. Br. J. Cancer 20:307-325.

Pegg, A. E. (1977). Formation and metabolism of alkylated purines: possible role in carcinogenesis by N-nitroso compounds and alkylating agents. Adv. Cancer Res. 25: 195-269.

Peters, J. H., Miller, K. S., and Brown, P. (1965). The determination of isoniazid and its metabolites in human urine. Anal. Biochem. 12:379-394.

Petersen, P., Bredahl, E., Lauritsen, O., and Laursen, T. (1970). Examination of the liver in personnel working with liquid rocket propellant. Br. J. Ind. Med. 27:141-146.

Pietra, G., and Shubik, P. (1960). Induction of melanotic tumors in the Syrian golden hamster after administration of ethyl carbamate. J. Natl. Cancer Inst. 25:627-630.

Pliss, G. B. (1959). The blastomogenic action of dichlorobenzidine. Vopr. Onkol. 5:524-533.

Pliss, G. B. (1962). Characteristics of the carcinogenic effect of N,N'-diacetylbenzidine. Vopr. Onkol. 8:11-15.

Pliss, G. B. (1963). On some regular relationships between carcinogenicity of aminodiphenyl derivatives and the structure of substance. Acta Un. Int. Cancer 19:499-501.

Pliss, G. B. (1965). Concerning carcinogenic properties of o-tolidine and dianisidine. Gig. Tr. Prof. Zabol. 9:18.

Pliss, G. B. (1974). Carcinogenic properties by hydrazobenzene. Vopr. Onkol. 20:53-57.

Pliss, G. B., and Zabezhinsky, M. A. (1970). Carcinogenic properties of ortho-tolidine (3,3'-dimethylbenzidine). J. Natl. Cancer Inst. 45:283-289.

Poirier, L. A. (1965). Carcinogenicity and metabolism of several aromatic amines and their N-oxidized derivatives. Ph.D. Thesis, University of Wisconsin, Madison, Wis., p. 194.

Poirier, L. A., Miller, J. A., Miller, E. C., and Sato, K. (1967). N-Benzoyloxy-N-methyl-4-aminoazobenzene: its carcinogenic activity in the rat and its reactions with proteins and nucleic acids and their constituents in vitro. Cancer Res. 27:1600-1613.

Preussmann, R., Druckrey, H., Ivankovic, S., and von Hodenberg, A. (1969). Chemical structure and carcinogenicity of aliphatic hydrazo, azo and azoxy compounds and of triazines, potential in vivo alkylating agents. Ann. NY Acad. Sci. 163:697-714.

Purves, H. D., and Griesbach, W. E. (1946). Studies on experimental goitre. VII: Thyroid carcinomata in rats treated with thiourea. Br. J. Exp. Pathol. 27:294-297.

Purves, H. D., and Griesbach, W. E. (1947). Studies on experimental goitre. VIII: Thyroid tumors in rats treated with thiourea. Br. J. Exp. Pathol. 28:46-53.

Radomski, J. L., and Brill, E. (1970). Bladder cancer induction by aromatic amines: Role of N-hydroxy metabolites. Science 167:992-993.

Radomski, J. L., and Brill, E. (1971). The role of N-oxidation products of aromatic amines in the induction of bladder cancer in the dog. Arch. Toxicol. 28:159-175.

Radomski, J. L., Brill, E., Deichmann, W. G., and Glass, E. M. (1971). Carcinogenicity testing of N-hydroxy and other oxidation and decomposition products of 1- and 2-naphthylamine. Cancer Res. 31:1461-1467.

Radomski, J. L., and Mellinger, T. J. (1961). The absorption, rate, and excretion in rats of the water soluble azo dyes, FD&C Red No. 2, FD&C Red No. 4, and FD&C Yellow No. 6. J. Pharmacol. Exp. Ther. 136:259-266.

Rakieten, N., Rakieten, M. L., and Nadkarni, M. V. (1963). Studies on the diabetogenic action of streptozotocin (NSC-37917). Cancer Chemother. Rep. 29:91-98.

Rao, K. V., and Vesselinovitch, S. D. (1973). Age- and sex-associated diethylnitrosamine dealkylation activity of the mouse liver and hepatocarcinogenesis. Cancer Res. 33:1625-1627.

Rapp, H. J., Carleton, J. H., Crisler, C., and Nadel, E. M. (1965). Induction of malignant tumors in the rabbit by oral administration of diethylnitrosamine. J. Natl. Cancer Inst. 34:453-458.

Rees, K. R., Rowland, G. F., and Varcoe, J. S. (1966). The metabolism of tritiated thioacetamide in the rat. Int. J. Cancer 1:197-206.

Rehn, L. (1895). Blasengeschwulste bei Fuchsin-Arbeitern. Arch. Klin. Chir. 50:588-600.

Rice, J. M. (1969). Transplacental carcinogenesis in mice by 1-ethyl-1-nitrosourea. Ann. NY Acad. Sci. 163:813-826.

Rinde, E., and Troll, W. (1975). Metabolic reduction of benzidine azo dyes to benzidine in rhesus monkey. J. Natl. Cancer Inst. 55:181-182.

Roe, F. J., Grant, G. A., and Millican, D. M. (1967). Carcinogenicity of hydrazine and 1,1-dimethylhydrazine for mouse lung. Nature 216:375-376.

Roe, F. J., Millican, D., and Mallett, J. M. (1963). Induction of melanotic lesions of the iris in rats by urethane given during the neonatal period. Nature 199:1201-1202.

Roe, F. J., Warwick, G. P., Carter, R. L., Peto, R., Ross, W. C., Mitchley, B. C., and Barron, N. A. (1971). Liver and lung tumors in mice exposed at birth to 4-dimethylaminoazobenzene or its 2-methyl or 3'-methyl derivatives. J. Natl. Cancer Inst. 47:593-601.

Rogers, K. J., and Pegg, A. E. (1977). Formation of O^6-methylguanine by alkylation of rat liver, colon and kidney DNA following administration of 1,2-dimethylhydrazine. Cancer Res. 37:4082-4087.

Rosati, R. L. (1973). Substituted acyl derivatives of α-aminopenicillins. Ger. Offen., 2,316,170 (Pfizer, Inc.), Chem. Abst. 80:82954c.

Rosin, A., and Rachmilewitz, M. (1954). The development of malignant tumors of the face in rats after prolonged treatment with thiourea. Cancer Res. 14:494-496.

Rosin, A., and Ungar, H. (1957). Malignant tumors in the eyelids and the auricular region of thiourea-treated rats. Cancer Res. 17:302-305

Roxon, J. J., Ryan, A. J., and Wright, S. E. (1967). Reduction of water soluble azo dyes by intestinal bacteria. Food Cosmet. Toxicol. 5:367-369.

Rudas, B. (1972). Streptozotocin. Arzneim. Forsch. 22:830-861.

Russfield, A. B., Boger, E., Homburger, F., Weisburger, E. K., and Weisburger, J. H. (1973a). Effect of structure of seven methyl anilines on toxicity and on incidence of subcutaneous and liver tumors in Charles River rats. Fed. Proc. 32:833.

Russfield, A. B., Homburger, F., Boger, E., Van Dongen, C. G., Weisburger, E. K., and Weisburger, J. H. (1975). The carcinogenic effect of 4,4'-methylene-bis(2-chloroaniline) in mice and rats. Toxicol. Appl. Pharmacol. 31:47-54.

Russfield, A. B., Homburger, F., Weisburger, E. K., and Weisburger, J. H. (1973b). Further studies on carcinogenicity of environmental chemicals including simple aromatic amines. Toxicol. Appl. Pharmacol. 25:446-447.

Saffiotti, U., Cefis, F., Montesano, R., and Sellakumar, A. R. (1967). Induction of bladder cancer in hamsters fed aromatic amines. In Bladder Cancer, a Symposium, K. F. Lampe (Ed.). Aesculapius, Birmingham, Ala., pp. 129-135.

Saruta, N., Yamaguchi, S., and Matsuoka, T. (1962). Sarcoma produced by subdermal administration of metaphenylenediamine and metaphenylenediamine hydrochloride. Kyushu J. Med. Sci. 13:175-179.

Saruta, N., Yamaguchi, S., and Nakatomi, Y. (1958). Sarcoma produced by subdermal administration of paraphenylenediamine. Kyushu J. Med. Sci. 9:94-101.

Sasaki, T. (1935). ortho-Aminoazotoluene. Gan. 29:52-64.

Sato, K., Poirier, L. A., Miller, J. A., and Miller, E. C. (1966). Studies on the N-hydroxylation and carcinogenicity of 4-aminoazobenzene and related compounds. Cancer Res. 26:1678-1687.

Sax, N. I. (1975). Dangerous Properties of Industrial Materials. Van Nostrand Reinhold, New York.

Schmahl, D., Preussmann, R., and Hamperl, H. (1960). Leberkrebs erzeugende Wirkung von Diathylnitrosamin nach oraler Gabe bei Ratten. Naturwissenschafter 47:89.

Schmahl, D., Thomas, C., and Koenig, K. (1963). Versuche zur Krebserzeugung mit Diathylnitrosamin bei Mausen. Naturwissenschaften 50:407.

Schmahl, D., Thomas, C., and Scheld, G. (1964). Carcerogene Wirkung von Diathylnitrosamin beim Hund. Naturwissenschaften 51:466-467.

Schoental, R. (1963). Experimental induction of squamous carcinoma of the lung, oesophagus and stomach. The mode of their induction. Acta Un. Int. Cancer 19:680-683.

Schoental, R. (1966). Carcinogenic activity of N-methyl-N-nitroso-N'-nitroguanidine. Nature 209:726-727.

Schoental, R. (1968). Experimental induction of gastro-intestinal tumors in rodents by N-alkyl-N-nitrosourethans and certain related compounds. Gan. Monogr. Cancer Res. 3:61.

Schoental, R. (1973). The mechanism of action of the carcinogenic nitroso and related compounds. Br. J. Cancer 28:436-439.

Schoental, R., and Bensted, J. P. (1968). Tumours of the intestines induced in rats by intraperitoneal injections of N-methyl- and N-ethyl-N-nitroso urethanes. Br. J. Cancer 22:316-323.

Schoental, R., and Bensted, J. P. (1969). Gastro-intestinal tumours in rats and mice following various routes of administration of N-methyl-N-nitroso-N'-nitroguanidine and N-ethyl-N-nitroso-N'-nitroguanidine. Br. J. Cancer 23:757-764.

Schoental, R., and Magee, P. N. (1962). Induction of squamous carcinoma of the lung and of the stomach and oesophagus by diazomethane and N-methyl-N-nitrosourethane, respectively. Br. J. Cancer 16:92-100.

Schreiber, D., and Janisch, W. (1967). Geschwulste bei Ratten nach wiederholter Applikation von N-Methyl-N-nitrosoharnstuff durch die Magensonde. Exp. Pathol. 1:331.

Scott, T. S. (1952). Incidence of bladder tumours in dyestuffs factory. Br. J. Ind. Med. 9:127-132.

Scott, T. S. (1962). Carcinogenic and Chronic Toxic Hazards of Aromatic Amines. Elsevier, Amsterdam.

Scribner, J. D., Miller, J. A., and Miller, E. C. (1965). 3-Methyl-mercapto-N-methyl-4-aminoazobenzene: an alkaline degradation product of a labile protein-bound dye in the livers of rats fed N,N-dimethyl-4-aminoazobenzene. Biochem. Biophys. Res. Commun. 20:560-565.

Searle, C. E., and Jones, E. L. (1977). Effects of repeated applications of two semi-permanent hair dyes to the skin of A and DBAf mice. Br. J. Cancer 36:467-478.

Sellakumar, A. R., Montesano, R., and Saffiotti, U. (1969). Aromatic amines carcinogenicity in hamsters. Proc. Am. Assoc. Cancer Res. 10:78.

Severi, L., and Biancifiori, C. (1968). Hepatic carcinogenesis in CBA/Cb/Se mice and Cb/Se rats by isonicotinic acid hydrazide and hydrazine sulfate. J. Natl. Cancer Inst. 41:331-340.

Shear, M. J., and Stewart, H. L. (1941). In: Survey of Compounds Which Have Been Tested for Carcinogenic Activity, P. Shubik and J. L. Hartwell (Eds.), Government Printing Office (U.S. Public Health Service Publication No. 149), Washington, D.C., p. 50.

Shimkin, M. B., Weisburger, J. H., Weisburger, E. K., Gubareff, N., and Suntzeff, V. (1966). Bioassay of 29 alkylating chemicals by the pulmonary-tumor response in strain A mice. J. Natl. Cancer Inst. 36:915-935.

Sichuk, G., Money, W. L., Der, B. K., and Fortner, J. G. (1968). Cancer of the thyroid, goitrogenesis and thyroid function in Syrian (golden) hamsters. Cancer 21:952-963.

Sielicka-Zuber, L. (1961). Skin changes due to N-phenyl-β-naphthylamine. Polski Tygod Lekar 16:1483-1486.

Sitar, D. S., and Thornhill, D. P. (1972). Propylthiouracil: absorption metabolism and excretion in the albino rat. J. Pharmacol. Exp. Ther. 183:440-448.

Smetanin, E. E. (1971). On transplacental blastogenic effect of dimethylnitrosamine and nitrosomethylurea. Vopr. Onkol. 17:75-81.

Society of Dyers and Colourists (1956). Colour Index, Vol. 3, 2nd Ed. Deanhouse, Picadilly, Yorkshire, England.

Society of Dyers and Colourists (1971). Colour Index, Vols. 1, 2, 3, & 4, 3rd Ed. Deanhouse, Picadilly, Yorkshire, England.

Spitz, S., Maguigan, W. H., and Dobriner, K. (1950). The carcinogenic action of benzidine. Cancer 3:789-804.

Stanford Research Institute (1976). 1976 Directory of Chemical Producers, USA, Menlo Park, California.

Stanford Research Institute (1977). 1977 Directory of Chemical Producers, USA, Menlo Park, California.

Stanley, L. N., and Farris, R. E. (1975). Azo dyes for polyester fibers. Ger. Offen., 2,364,476 (GAF Corp.), Chem. Abst. 82:5356y.

Steinhoff, D., and Grundmann, E. (1970). Zur Cancerogenen Wirkung von 4,4'-Diaminodiphenylmethan und 2,4'-Diaminodiphenylmethan. Naturwissenschaften 57: 247-248

Steinhoff, D., and Grundmann, E. (1971). Zur Cancerogenen Wirkung von 3,3'-Dichlor-4,4'-diaminodiphenylmethan bei Ratten. Naturwissenschaften 58:578.

Stula, E. F., Sherman, H., and Zapp, J. A., Jr. (1971). Experimental neoplasia in ChR-CD rats with the oral administration of 3,3'-dichlorobenzidine, 4,4'-methylene-bis(2-chloroaniline) and 4,4'-methylene-bis(2-methylaniline). Toxicol. Appl. Pharmacol. 19:380-381.

Stula, E. F., Sherman, H., Zapp, J. A., Jr., and Clayton, J. W., Jr. (1975). Experimental neoplasia in rats from oral administration of 3,3'-dichlorobenzidene, 4,4'-methylene-bis(2-chloroaniline) and 4,4'-methylene-bis(2-methylaniline). Toxicol. Appl. Pharmacol. 31:159-176.

Sugimura, T., and Fujimura, S. (1967). Tumor production in glandular stomach of rat by N-methyl-N'-nitro-N-nitroso guanidine. Nature 216:943-944.

Sugimura, T., Fujimura, S., and Baba, T. (1970). Tumor production in the glandular stomach and alimentary tract of the rat by N-methyl-N'-nitro-N-nitrosoguanidine. Cancer Res. 30:455-465.

Sugimura, T., Fujimura, S., Kogure, K., Baba, T., Saito, T., Nagao, M., Hosoi, H., Shimosato, Y., and Yokoshima, T. (1969). Production of adenocarcinomas in glandular stomach of experimental animals by N-methyl-N'-nitro-N-nitrosoguanidine. Gan. Monogr. Cancer Res. 8:157.

Sugimura, T., Nagao, M., and Okada, Y. (1966). Carcinogenic action of N-methyl-N'-nitro-N-nitrosoguanidine. Nature 210:962-963.

Sugiura, K., and Rhoads, C. P. (1941). Experimental liver cancer in rats and its inhibition by rice-bran extract, yeast and yeast extract. Cancer Res. 1:3-16.

Sunderman, F. W. (1970). Diazomethane poisoning. In _Laboratory Diagnosis of Diseases Caused by Toxic Agents_, F. W. Sunderman (Ed.). Ed. Proc. Appl. Semin., pp. 292-295.

Sunderman, F. W., Connor, R., and Fields, H. (1938). Diazomethane poisoning. First clinical case report. Am. J. Med. Sci. 195:469-473.

Svoboda, D., and Higginson, J. (1968). A comparison of ultrastructural changes in rat liver due to chemical carcinogens. Cancer Res. 28:1703-1733.

Synalloy Corporation (1977). Material safety data sheet on fast scarlet G base. Blackman Uhler Chemical Division, Spartanburg, S.C.

Takayama, S., and Imaizumi, T. (1969). Carcinogenic action of N-nitrosodibutylamine in mice. Gan. 60:353.

Takayama, S., Kuwabara, N., Azama, Y., and Sugimura, T. (1971). Skin tumors in mice painted with N-methyl-N'-nitro-N-nitrosoguanidine and N-ethyl-N'-nitro-N-nitrosoguanidine. J. Natl. Cancer Inst. 46:973-980.

Takayama, S., and Oota, K. (1965). Induction of malignant tumors in various strains of mice by oral administration of N-nitrosodimethylamine and N-nitrosodiethylamine. Gan. 56:189-199.

Takemura, N. (1970). Carcinogenic action of the intermediates of fluorescent whitening agents, 5-nitroacenaphthene and 5-aminoacenaphthene. Tenth Int. Cancer Cong., Houston, Texas, p. 79.

Takemura, N., Hashida, C., and Terasawa, M. (1974). Carcinogenic action of 5-nitroacenaphthene. Br. J. Cancer 30:481-483.

Tannenbaum, A., and Maltoni, C. (1962). Neoplastic response of various tissues to the administration of urethan. Cancer Res. 22:1105-1112.

Terayama, H. (1967). Aminoazo carcinogenesis—methods and biochemical problems. In _Methods in Cancer Research_, Vol. 1, H. Busch (Ed.). Academic Press, New York, pp. 399-449.

Terracini, B., and Della Porta, G. (1961). Feeding with aminoazo dyes, thioacetamide and ethionine. Arch. Pathol. Lab. Med. 71:566-575.

Terracini, B., Palestro, G., Ramella Gigliardi, M., and Montesano, R. (1966). Carcinogenicity of dimethylnitrosamine in Swiss mice. Br. J. Cancer 20:871-876.

Terracini, B., Palcotro, G., Ramella Gigliardi, M., and Montesano, R. (1966). Carcinogenicity of dimethylnitrosamine in Swiss mice. Br. J. Cancer 20:871-876.

Terracini, B., and Testa, M. C. (1970). Carcinogenicity of a single administration of N-nitrosomethylurea: a comparison between newborn and five-week old mice and rats. Br. J. Cancer 24:588-598.

Thiede, T., Chievitz, E., and Christensen, B. C. (1964). Chlornaphazin as a bladder carcinogen. Acta Med. Scand. 175:721-725.

Thiede, T., and Christensen, B. C. (1969). Bladder tumours induced by chlornaphazine: a five-year follow-up study of chlornaphazine-treated patients with polycynthaemia. Acta Med. Scand. 185:133-137.

Thomas, A. W., Boeniger, M. F., Weber, M. G., Stein, H. P., Upton, A. C., and Millar, J. D. (1978). Direct black 38, Direct blue 6, Direct brown 95, benzidine derived dyes. Am. Ind. Hyg. Assoc. J. 39:A18-A24.

Thorgeirsson, S. S., Jollow, D. J., Sasame, H., Green, I., and Mitchell, J. R. (1973). The role of cytochrome P-450 in N-hydroxylation of 2-acetylaminofluorene. Mol. Pharmacol. 9:398-404.

Thurnherr, N., Deschner, E. E., Stonehill, E. H., and Lipkin, M. (1973). Induction of adenocarcinomas of the colon in mice by weekly injections of 1,2-dimethylhydrazine. Cancer Res. 33:940-945.

Toghill, P. J., and Wilcox, R. G. (1976). Aplastic anaemia and hair dye. Br. Med. J. 1:502-503.

Tomatis, L., Della Porta, G., and Shubik, P. (1961). Urinary bladder and liver cell tumors induced in hamster with o-aminoazotoluene. Cancer Res. 21:1513-1517.

Tomatis, L., Magee, P. N., and Shubik, P. (1964). Induction of liver tumors in the Syrian golden hamster by feeding dimethylnitrosamine. J. Natl. Cancer Inst. 33:341-345.

Toth, B. (1969). Lung tumor induction and inhibition of breast adenocarcinomas by hydrazine sulfate in mice. J. Natl. Cancer Inst. 42:469-475.

Toth, B. (1972). Tumorigenesis studies with 1,2-dimethylhydrazine dihydrochloride, hydrazine sulfate and isonicotinic acid in golden hamsters. Cancer Res. 32:804-807.

Toth, B. (1973). 1,1-Dimethylhydrazine (unsymmetrical) carcinogenesis in mice. Light microscopic and ultrastructural studies on neoplastic blood vessels. J. Natl. Cancer Inst. 50:181-187.

Toth, B., Della Porta, G., and Shubik, P. (1961). The occurrence of malignant lymphomas in urethan-treated Swiss mice. Br. J. Cancer 15:322-326.

Toth, B., Magee, P. N., and Shubik, P. (1964). Carcinogenesis study with dimethylnitrosamine administered orally to adult and subcutaneously to newborn BALB/c mice. Cancer Res. 24:1712-1721.

Toth, B., and Shimizu, H. (1973). Lung carcinogenesis with 1-acetyl-2-isonicotinoylhydrazine, the major metabolite of isoniazid. Eur. J. Cancer 9:285-289.

Toth, B., and Shubik, P. (1967). Carcinogenesis in AKR mice injected at birth with benzo(a)pyrene and dimethylnitrosamine. Cancer Res. 27:43-51.

Toth, B., and Wilson, R. B. (1971). Blood vessel tumorigenesis by 1,2-dimethylhydrazine dihydrochloride (symmetrical). Gross, light and electron microscopic descriptions. I. Am. J. Pathol. 64:585-600.

Troll, W., and Nelson, N. (1961). N-Hydroxy-2-naphthylamine, a urinary metabolite of 2-naphthylamine in man and dog. Fed. Proc. 20:41.

Troll, W., Tessler, A. N., and Nelson, N. (1963). Bis(2-amino-1-naphthyl) phosphate, a metabolite of beta-naphthylamine in human urine. J. Urol. 89:626-627.

Ubelin, F., and Pletscher, A. (1954). Atiologie und Prophylaxe gewerblicher Tumoren in der Farbstuffindustrie. Schweiz. Med. Wochenschr. 84:917-920.

Uehleke, H. (1963). N-Hydroxylation of carcinogenic amines in vivo and in vitro with liver microsomes. Biochem. Pharmacol. 12:219-221

Ulland, B. M., Weisburger, J. H., Weisburger, E. K., Rice, J. M., and Cypher, R. (1972). Thyroid cancer in rats from ethylene thiourea intake. J. Natl. Cancer Inst. 49:583-584.

Umeda, M. (1955). Production of rat sarcoma by injections of propylene glycol solution of m-toluylenediamine. Gan. 46:597-604.

Umeda, M. (1957). Production of rat sarcoma by injections of Tween 80 solution of scarlet red. Gan. 48:579-580.

Umeda, M. (1958). Production of rat sarcoma by injections of Tween 80 solution of scarlet red. Gan. 49:27-31.

U.S. International Trade Commission (1977). Synthetic organic chemicals. U.S. production and sales, 1975. USITC Publication 804, U.S. Government Printing Office, Washington, D.C.

U.S. Tariff Commission (1973). Synthetic organic chemicals, U.S. Production and Sales, 1971. USTC Publication 614, U.S. Government Printing Office, Washington, D.C.

U.S. Tariff Commission (1974). Synthetic organic chemicals, U.S. Production and Sales, 1972. USTC Publication 681, U.S. Government Printing Office, Washington, D.C.

Vanderlaan, W. P., and Storrie, V. M. (1955). A survey of the factors controlling thyroid function with especial reference to newer views on antithyroid substances. Pharmacol. Rev. 7:301-334.

Van Dyke, J. H. (1953). Experimental thyroid tumorigenesis in rats: predominance of neoplasm type and influence of age. Arch. Pathol. Lab. Med. 56:613-628.

Vavra, J. J., DeBoer, C., Dietz, A., Hanka, L. J., and Sokolski, W. T. (1960). Streptozotocin, a new antibacterial antibiotic. Antibiot. Ann. 7:230-235.

Venkatesan, N., Arcos, J. C., and Argus, M. G. (1968). Differential effect of polycyclic hydrocarbons on the demethylation of the carcinogen dimethylnitrosamine by rat tissues. Life Sci. 7:1111-1119.

Vesselinovitch, S. D. (1969). The sex-dependent differences in the development of liver tumors in mice administered dimethylnitrosamine. Cancer Res. 29:1024-1027.

Vesselinovitch, S. D., Itze, L., Mihailovich, N., Rao, K. V., and Manojlovski, B. (1973). Role of hormonal environment, partial hepatectomy, and dose of ethylnitrosourea in renal carcinogenesis. Cancer Res. 33:339-341.

Vesselinovitch, S. D., and Mihailovich, N. (1967). The neonatal and infant age periods as biologic factors which modify multicarcinogenesis by urethan. Cancer Res. 27:1422-1429.

Vesselinovitch, S. D., and Mihailovich, N. (1968a). The induction of benign and malignant liver tumors by urethan in newborn rats. Cancer Res. 28:881-887.

Vesselinovitch, S. D., and Mihailovich, N. (1968b). The development of neurogenic neoplasms, embryonal kidney tumors, harderian gland adenomas, anitschkow cell sarcomas of the heart and other neoplasms in urethan-treated newborn rats. Cancer Res. 28:888-897.

Vesselinovitch, S. D., Mihailovich, N., and Richter, W. R. (1970). The induction of malignant melanomas in Syrian white hamster by neonatal exposure to urethan. Cancer Res. 30:2543-2547.

Veys, C. A. (1969). Two epidemiological inquiries into the incidence of bladder tumors in industrial workers. J. Natl. Cancer Inst. 43:219-226.

Videbaek, A. (1964). Chlornaphazin (Erysan^{R}) may induce cancer of the urinary bladder. Acta Med. Scand. 176:45-50.

Vivien, J. N., Thibier, R., and Lepeuple, A. (1972). Recent studies on isoniazid. Adv. Tuberc. Res. 18:148.

Wall, F. E. (1972). Bleaches, hair colorings and dye removers. In Cosmetics Science and Technology, Vol. 2, Balsam, M.S. and E. Sagarm (Eds.). Wiley-Interscience, New York, pp. 306-308.

Walpole, A. L. (1963). On substances inducing cancer of the bladder. Acta Un. Int. Cancer 19:483.

Walpole, A. L., Williams, M. H., and Roberts, D. C. (1952). Carcinogenic action of 4-aminodiphenyl and 3,2'-dimethyl-4-aminobiphenyl. Br. J. Ind. Med. 9:255-263.

Walpole, A. L., Williams, M. H., and Roberts, D. C. (1954). Tumours of urinary bladder in dogs after ingestion of 4-aminodiphenyl. Br. J. Ind. Med. 11:105-109.

Weast, R. C. (Ed.) (1977-1978). CRC Handbook of Chemistry and Physics. CRC, Cleveland, Ohio.

Weisburger, J. H., and Weisburger, E. K. (1973). Biochemical formation and pharmacological, toxicological and pathological properties of hydroxylamine and hydroxamic acids. Pharmacol. Rev. 25:1-66.

Weisburger, J. H., Weisburger, E. K., Mantel, N., Hadidian, Z., and Frederickson, T. (1966). New carcinogenic nitrosamines in rats. Naturwissenschaften 53:508.

Weisburger, J. H., Yamamoto, R. S., Glass, R. M., and Frankel, H. H. (1969). Prevention by arginine glutamate of the carcinogenicity of acetamide in rats. Toxicol. Appl. Pharmacol. 14:163-175.

Wenner, W. (1967). Malonic acid derivatives. In Kirk-Othmer Encyclopedia of Chemical Technology, 2nd Ed., Vol. 12, Wiley Interscience, New York, p. 857.

Wiebecke, B., Lohrs, U., Gimmy, J., and Eder, M. (1969). Erzeugung von Darmtumoren bei Mausen durch 1,2-Dimethylhydrazin. Z. Gesamte Inn. Med. 149:277-278.

Wignall, T. H. (1929). Incidence of disease of the bladder in workers in certain chemicals. Br. Med. J. ii:291-293.

Williams, M. H., and Bonser, G. M. (1962). Induction of hepatomas in rats and mice following the administration of auramine. Br. J. Cancer 16:87-91.

Windholz, M. (Ed.) (1976). The Merck Index, 9th Ed. Merck & Co., Rahway, N.J.

Wollman, S. H. (1961). Effects of feeding thiouracil on thyroid glands of rats. J. Natl. Cancer Inst. 26:473-487.

Wood, M., Flaks, A., and Clayson, D. B. (1970). The carcinogenic activity of dibutylnitrosamine in IFXC57 mice. Eur. J. Cancer 6:433-440.

Yoshida, T. (1932). Uber die Experimentelle Erzeugung von Hepatom durch die Futterung mit o-Amidoazotoluol. Proc. Imp. Acad. Jap. 8:464-467.

Zak, F. G., Holzner, J. H., Singer, E. J., and Popper, H. (1960). Renal and pulmonary tumors in rats fed dimethylnitrosamine. Cancer Res. 20:96-99.

Zavon, M. R., Hoegg, U., and Bingham, E. (1973). Benzidine exposure as a cause of bladder tumors. Arch. Environ. Health 27:1-7.

Zimmerman, L. M., Shubik, P., Baserga, R., Ritchie, A. C., and Jacques, L. (1954). Experimental production of thyroid tumors by alternating hyperplasia and involution. J. Clin. Endocrinol. Metab. 14:1367-1373.

10

Carcinogens in Foods

HAROLD C. GRICE,* DAVID J. CLEGG, D. EARLE COFFIN, MEI-TEIN LO, EDWARD J. MIDDLETON, EMIL SANDI, PETER M. SCOTT, NRISINHA P. SEN, BARRY L. SMITH, and JAMES R. WITHEY / Bureau of Chemical Safety, Ottawa, Ontario, Canada

I. REGULATORY CONTROL OF CHEMICAL CARCINOGENS IN FOODS—AN INTERNATIONAL OVERVIEW

A. Introduction

For simplicity carcinogenic substances in foods may be classified as to source—those of intentional origin and those of unintentional or environmental origin.

1. Substances of Intentional Origin

The term "intentional origin" is somewhat misleading in that such substances are generally permitted to be present under regulatory control as food additives or flavoring agents until

*Present affiliation: F.D.C. Consultants, Inc., Nepean, Ontario, Canada

new toxicological data becomes available indicating carcinogenic potential to be associated with these compounds. Of course, once the toxic potential becomes known, most countries take action to revoke provision for the use of the subject agent from a positive listing of food additives and/or alternately enacting or adding the substance to a list of adulterating substances that shall not be present in food. Examples of substances that may be controlled in this manner are synthetic food colors, nonnutritive sweeteners, and flavoring agents.

2. Substances of Unintentional or Environmental Origin—Mycotoxins

It has long been recognized that the feeding of mouldy grain or hay to animals may cause serious illness or death. Investigations that started in the 1960s have demonstrated that some molds can produce powerful carcinogens called "aflatoxins," capable of producing fatal liver cancers in poultry, fish, some animals, and possibly humans. Improper control over temperature and moisture during storage can favor the production of mold toxins in products such as peanuts, Brazil nuts, copra, cottonseed meal, filberts, pistachio nuts, and cereals.

3. Agricultural and Environmental Contaminants with Carcinogenic Potential

Use of pesticides, fungicides, and herbicides has grown rapidly since World War II. The population explosion and the movement of people from rural to metropolitan areas have put tremendous pressure on the agricultural sector to grow more food. To meet these needs, farmers have resorted to using more and more insecticides, fungicides, and herbicides. Unfortunately, some of these agricultural agents are highly toxic. Consequently, many countries have elaborated positive listings providing for maximum residue levels of agricultural chemicals that may occur in a food before that food is considered to be adulterated.

In addition to contamination from the agricultural use of chemicals, toxic and potentially carcinogenic industrial wastes may enter the food supply from contaminated soil, air, or water.

4. Basic Concepts Used for the Regulatory Control of Carcinogens in Foods

The basic food control legislation of many countries contains a general provision that prohibits the sale of any food that contains a poisonous or harmful substance or is adulterated. This particular provision then permits the enactment of specific regulations in the form of positive lists to control the use of intentional food additives and to prescribe maximum residue levels for agricultural chemicals and maximum permitted tolerances for certain unintentional contaminants. Thus, if a substance defined as a food additive is not listed in an appropriate table of food additives, then that substance may not be used in or on any foodstuff. Similarly, if the residue for an agricultural chemical or a tolerance for a particular contaminant exceeds the established level, then the food is considered to be adulterated. This provides an effective regulatory control mechanism on which to base enforcement action without having to resort to the general safety provision, which would require proving the existence of a hazard based on expert toxicological testimony.

Finally, a number of countries utilize the concept of a negative list, which specifies substances, frequently carcinogenic, that may not be added to foods. The addition or presence of these substances is usually defined as an act of adulteration, which again offers an effective mechanism for enforcement and control.

5. International Overview of Regulatory Control of Carcinogens in Foods

The following are examples of how 13 countries exercise regulatory control over the occurrences of carcinogenic substances in foodstuffs through the use of some or all of the basic concepts previously described.

a. Belgium

Belgium does not have any specific regulations concerning carcinogenic agents in foodstuffs. However, the legal framework in that country permits the king to regulate the method of manufacture of food products. In particular, certain processes utilizing high processing temperatures that have the potential to produce carcinogenic agents may be regulated in this manner. Furthermore, an ordinance exists stipulating that liquid smokes (dextrose and salt in an infusion of wood smoke) and products manufactured using such flavoring agents contain no carcinogenic substances that could develop in the wood smoke (i.e., benzopyrenes, benzophenanthrene). The other part of the same ordinance stipulates that the king may regulate, by prohibiting or limiting, the sale of foods containing contaminants. This applies in particular to certain heavy metals suspected of having carcinogenic potential.

Finally, a royal decree of January 3, 1975 relative to foodstuffs considers, inter alia, foods containing toxic levels of pathogenic microorganisms or toxins of microbial origin (i.e., mycotoxins) which are considered to be carcinogenic (Belgium Ministry of Public Health and the Environment).

b. Canada

The basic Canadian food law is embodied in the Food and Drugs Act and Regulations (Canadian Department of National Health and Welfare). Section 4(a) and 4(d) of this act states that:

> No person shall sell an article of food that
> (a) has in or upon it any poisonous or harmful substance
> (b) is adulterated

The authority to enact specific regulations declaring certain substances as adulterating agents is derived from the aforementioned Section 4. In particular, Section B.01.046 specifies that a food is adulterated if any of the following substances are present therein or have been added thereto:

(a) mineral oil or paraffin wax or any preparation thereof;
(b) coumarin, an extract of tonka beans, the seed of _Dipleryx odorata_ Willd. or _Dipleryx oppositifolia_ Willd.;
(c) non-nutritive sweetening agents;
(d) cottonseed flour that contains more than four hundred and fifty parts per million of free gossypol;
(e) fatty acids and their salts containing chickedema factor or other toxic factors;
(f) dihydrosafrole;
(g) isosafrole;
(h) oil of American sassafras from _Sassafras albidum_ (Nutt). Nees;
(i) oil of Brazilian sassafras from _Ocolea cymbarum_ H.B.K.;
(j) oil of camphor sassafrassy from _Cinnamomum Camphorum_ Sieb.;
(k) oil of micranthum from _Cinnamomum micranthum_ Hayata;
(l) safrole, or
(m) oil, extract or root of calamus from _Acorus calamus_ L.;
(n) nut and nut products that contain more than fifteen parts per billion of aflatoxin; or
(o) ethylene thiourea.

Notwithstanding the prohibitions in B.01.046, Section B.01.047 permits the use of mineral oil, paraffin wax, and petrolatum under the following carefully defined conditions:

(a) a food, other than collagen sausage casing, is not adulterated by reason only that it contains 0.3 percent or less mineral oil, if good manufacturing practice requires the use of mineral oil;
(b) chewing gum is not adulterated by reason only that it contains a paraffin wax base;

(c) fresh fruits and vegetables, except turnips, are not adulterated by reason only that they are coated with not more than 0.3 percent paraffin wax and petrolatum, if good manufacturing practices require the use of such coating;
(d) turnips and cheese are not adulterated by reason only that they are coated with paraffin wax in accordance with food manufacturing practice; and
(e) edible collagen sausage casing is not adulterated by reason only that it contains 5 percent or less mineral oil by weight, if good manufacturing practice requires the use of mineral oil.

Canada utilizes the concept of positively listing food additives, maximum residue limits for pesticides, and maximum permissible levels for the presence of certain inorganic contaminants in specified food products.

c. Denmark

Section 12 of the Danish Food Act (Danish Food Act, 1973) of June 6, 1973 contains the following general provision which prevents the sale of food containing poisonous or toxic substance:

> No food shall be sold if it is assumed that, when used in the normal manner, it may transmit or cause disease or result in poisoning, or if, on account of morbid alteration, putrefaction, pollution, faulty manufacturing or for some other reason, the food must be deemed to be unfit for human consumption.

The positive listing concept is used for the purpose of regulating both food additives and other food constituents. Recently Denmark issued a decree on vinyl chloride monomer in polyvinyl chloride with reference to cancer risk. A draft decree on flavoring agents has also been prepared to ban a number of suspected carcinogens (Danish Ministry of Environmental Protection).

d. Federal Republic of Germany

The Federal Republic of Germany feels the problem of chemical carcinogens in foods cannot be viewed in isolation from the total exposure of man to chemical substances. The following extensive legislative measures incorporating the total environmental concept have been implemented to deal with food contamination (Focke, 1976):

(a) Law or overall reform of food legislation of August 15, 1974
(b) Statutory Ordinance on Drinking Water and on Industrial Waste for Food Plants of January 31, 1975
(c) Fourth Ordinance amending the Ordinance on Foods for Special Dietary Uses of April 14, 1975
(d) Law amending the Law on Drugs of June 5, 1974
(e) Law on Fodder of July 2, 1975
(f) Second Ordinance amending the Ordinance on the Enforcement of the Law on Fodder of April 19, 1975
(g) 6th, 7th and 9th Ordinance on the Enforcement of the Law on the Modification of Foodstuff Regulations of July 17, 1973, March 28, 1974 and December 12, 1974
(h) Ordinance amending the enforcement regulations concerning the examination and sanitary treatment of slaughter animals of January 20, 1975
(i) Maximum quantities ordinance (DDT and other Pesticides) in foods of animal origin of November 15, 1973 amended May 16, 1975
(j) Ordinance on maximum quantities of mercury in fish, crustaceae, shellfish and molluscs of February 6, 1972
(k) Ordinance amending the maximum quantities ordinance—Plant protection of December 14, 1972
(l) Second law amending the plant protection law of August 15, 1975
(m) Law on the trade in DDT of August 7, 1972

(n) Ordinance on the revision of the ordinance on the prohibitions and restrictions of the use of plant protection agents of May 31, 1974

e. Hungary

Section 13 (7) of the Hungarian food law states that only those substances may be added to foods for the purpose of coloring, flavoring, clarification, enrichment, or preserving, or for other purposes that are harmless to human health at the prescribed level of use (Hungarian Food Law).

f. Ireland

The presence of dangerous or toxic substances in food is controlled by the Sale of Food and Drugs Act of 1875, which makes it an offense to sell food which has been mixed with any substance likely to render that food injurious to the consumers' health.

In addition, the Minister of Health has the power to prescribe specific regulations to prevent danger to the public health arising from the manufacture, preparation, importation, storage, distribution, and sale of food intended for human consumption. The following regulations govern the use of additives and the presence of contaminants in foods (Irish Department of Health):

(1) Health (Cyclamate in Food) Regulations, 1970
(2) Health (Arsenic and Lead in Food) Regulations, 1972
(3) Health (Mineral Hydrocarbons in Food) Regulations, 1972
(4) Health (Solvents in Food) Regulations, 1972
(5) Health (Preservatives in Food) Regulations, 1973
(6) Health (Colouring Agents in Food) Regulations, 1973
(7) Health (Antioxidants in Food) Regulations, 1973

g. Israel

Specific legislation governing the presence or addition of chemical carcinogens is not included in the Israeli legal code. Problems in this area are handled administratively or in regulations based on the powers granted to the Minister of Health "to take measure to prevent dangers arising to public health" and to make rules "to define, where necessary, what additions of extraneous matter—shall constitute proof—that it is injurious to health" (Israeli Ministry of Health).

h. Netherlands

In the Netherlands a general regulation exists that makes it an offense to sell or offer for sale a food or drink that is or could be a health hazard when normally used for human consumption (Netherlands Committee for the Codex Alimentarius).

The only specific legislation operative with respect to a carcinogenic substance deals with aflatoxin. This regulation decrees that aflatoxin shall not be detectable in peanuts (Arachis hypogaea) nor in parts of peanuts, nor in foods and drinks prepared from or manufactured with peanuts and intended for human consumption.

The Dutch legal system uses the concept of positive lists to regulate intentional food additives and maximum residue levels for pesticides. Finally, the carry-over possibility of carcinogens from animal feed to food products of animal origin destined for human consumption is restricted by domestic regulations harmonized with an European Economic Community (EEC) directive. Maximum levels of aflatoxin in cattle feed are set at 0.05 mg/kg for non-milking cows and at 0.02 mg/kg for milking cows.

i. Norway

Norwegian food legislation states that food must not contain substances that are hazardous to human health. Special reference to carcinogenic agents has not been made (Royal Norwegian Ministry of Social Affairs).

j. Switzerland

The Swiss food legislation contains a general section that stipulates that food must be free of all substances that may represent a hazard to health (Swiss Federal Office of Public Health, Foodstuffs Control). On September 1, 1976, a specific regulation was introduced with reference to the presence of aflatoxin in almonds. This substance is tolerated at the level of 5 ppb for the B_1 fraction and 10 ppb for total aflatoxin. Commencing January 1, 1978, the Swiss food legislation will be amended to introduce a zero tolerance for aflatoxin. This will apply to nuts, kernels, seed, grain, and so on.

k. Sweden

The Swedish Food Regulations prohibit the sale of food containing foreign substances that are defined as a "substance which, if present in or on food, can constitute a risk to health or change the normal composition of the food or its quality in other respects" (Swedish National Food Administration, 1977). However, the Swedish National Food Administration has laid down certain exceptions to the foregoing rules in the form of maximum acceptable levels for pesticide residues and maximum permitted levels for other contaminants, namely, aflatoxin, lead, and vinyl chloride. The permitted levels of aflatoxin, lead, and vinyl chloride are as follows:

Substance	Food	Maximum permitted level (PPM)
Aflatoxin (as sum of aflatoxins B_1, B_2, G_1, G_2)	All	0.005
Lead	All	3 (Under review with a view to reducing permitted level)
Vinyl chloride	All	0.01

The Swedish National Food Administration has set an actionable level of 5 mg/kg for the presence of PCB in the edible portion of fish. Sweden also uses the concept of positive listing for food additives (Swedish National Food Administration, 1977).

l. New Zealand

New Zealand regards aflatoxins, polycyclic aromatic hydrocarbons, nitrosamines, and asbestos (filters for beverages) as carcinogens or possible carcinogens. Specific regulations have not been promulgated to control these substances (New Zealand Department of Health). When necessary the general provisions of the 1969 Food and Drug Act are invoked. Section 6(4) states the following (New Zealand Department of Health, 1969):

> No person shall sell
> (a) any food which is unsound or unfit for human consumption
> (b) any food or drug containing or having attached to it or enclosed with it any extraneous thing which is harmful or dangerous, or which is offensive.

m. United States

The Food, Drug, and Cosmetic Act is the basic legislation instrument used to insure food safety in the United States. In addition to general food safety provisions, the Delaney amendment of 1958 sets out certain rigorous provisions concerning the safety of food additives. These provisions that are found in Section 409[348](c) of the Food, Drug, and Cosmetic Act states the following (Code of Federal Regulations):

> No such regulation shall issue if a fair evaluation of the data before the Secretary
> (A) fails to establish that the proposed use of the food additive, under the conditions of use to be specified in the regulations, will be safe: Provided, that no additive shall be deemed to be safe if it is found to induce cancer when ingested by man or animal, or if it is found, after tests which are appropriate for the evaluation of the safety of food additives, to induce cancer in man or animal, except that

> this proviso shall not apply with respect to the use of a substance as an ingredient of feed for animals which are raised for food production, if the Secretary finds (i) that, under the conditions of use and feeding specified in proposed labeling and reasonably certain to be followed in practice, such additive will not adversely affect the animals for which such feed is intended, and (ii) that no residue of the additive will be found (by methods of examination prescribed or approved by the Secretary by regulations, which regulations shall not be subject to subsections (f) and (g)) in any edible portion of such animal after slaughter or in any food yielded by or derived from the living animal.

The United States also uses the concept of positive listing of food additives, and flavors as well as maximum residue limits for pesticides. In addition, Section 121.106 lists the following substances that are prohibited from use in human food and thus adulterate any food to which they have been added (Code of Federal Regulations).

(a) Calamus oil, oil of calamus, extract of calamus
(b) Dulcin (4-ethoxyphenylurea)
(c) P-4000 (5-nitro-2-n-propoxyaniline)
(d) Coumarin
(e) Cyclamate; calcium, sodium, magnesium, potassium
(f) Safrole
(g) Monochloroacetic acid
(h) Thiourea
(i) Cobaltous salts; acetate, chloride and sulfate
(j) NDGA (nor dihydroguaiaretic acid)
(k) DEPC (diethylpyrocarbonate)

5. Role of the Joint FAO/WHO Food Standards Program in Harmonizing Food Legislation on an International Scale

In 1962 the Joint FAO/WHO Food Standards Program was conceived to elaborate international food standards aimed at protecting the health of the consumer and ensuring fair practices in the food trade. In addition to some 100 commodity standards that have been issued for acceptance, the Codex Alimentarius Commission has issued recommended international maximum limits for residues associated with 45 pesticides (Recommended International Maximum Limits for Pesticide Residues), a list of food additives that have been evaluated for their safety-in-use in food (List of Additives Evaluated for Safety-in-Use in Foods), and a list of maximum levels recommended for contaminants (List of Maximum Levels Recommended for Contaminants).

The Codex Alimentarius Commission in collaboration with the United Nations Environment Programme have prepared a model food law suitable for adoption by countries wishing to strengthen or implement basic national food control legislation. It is interesting to note that this model law contains a basic provision which prohibits the sale of poisonous, unwholesome, or adulterated food. It also recommends that positive lists to control food additives should be the goal of legislators (Guidelines for Developing an Effective National Food Control System, 1976).

II. INTENTIONAL FOOD ADDITIVES

A. Artificial Sweeteners

1. Origin and Use in Foods

Interest in the adverse effects of artificial sweeteners such as dulcin, cyclamates, and saccharin has centered largely on their potential to produce cancer in laboratory animals, with particular emphasis on the development of urinary bladder neoplasms.

2. Dulcin (4-Ethoxyphenylurea)

Dulcin does not occur in nature. It was first prepared in 1883 by Berlinerblau by reacting p-phenetidine with phosgene and ammonia. Since that time various methods of preparation, as well as numerous methods for its determination by paper, thin-layer, and gas chromatography, have been reported (IARC, 1976).

Dulcin, when administered per os to rats was rapidly absorbed (Akagi et al., 1965; Kojima et al., 1966). Although tissue distribution was widespread, the liver, kidneys, brain, and lungs showed the highest concentration. Studies on the excretion of dulcin in the rabbit indicated that this compound was eliminated primarily in the urine as p-hydroxyphenylurea and its o-sulfate and o-glucuronide (40%), as the n-glucuronide (27%), and unchanged dulcin (3%), as well as small amounts of p-aminophenol (Akagi et al., 1966).

a. Carcinogenicity

This sweetener was demonstrated to induce hepatomas when fed in the diet of rats at 0.1, 0.25, 0.5, or 1.0% for 2 years. No tumors occurred in rats fed 0.01% dulcin or in the control group (Fitzhugh et al., 1951). In other studies (Lettré and Wrba, 1955; Bekemeier et al., 1958; Ikeda et al., 1960) rats were fed dulcin at graded levels from 0 to 1% for 18 to 22 months without noticeable effect on the incidence of malignant tumors. However, in further investigations (Bär and Griepentrog, 1958; Griepentrog, 1959) rats fed dulcin at the 1% level for 22-24 months developed papillomas of the pelvis and of the bladder. Stones were associated with the papillomas, but the papillomas did not always occur in the area of the urinary tract where the stones were located.

Although this substance has been used by humans without apparent adverse effects, it has been deemed unacceptable for use as a food additive because of its tumorigenic potential.

3. Cyclamates (Salts of Cyclohexylsulfamic Acid)

In 1937 Audrieth and Sveda (1944) were the first to discover and report on the sweetness of the salts of cyclohexylsulfamic acid. Cyclohexylsulfamic acid was derived from the sulfonation of cyclohexylamine, and the process was patented in the United States in 1942. Commercial production of the sodium and calcium salts was begun in 1950. Methods for the determination of the cyclamates and their impurities have been published in the National Formulary (13th Edition, 1970).

a. Metabolism

The metabolism of cyclamate has been studied extensively in the rat, rabbit, guinea pig, dog, and monkey, as well as the human. Studies using ^{14}C- or ^{35}S-labeled cyclamate showed a wide species variation in the ability to absorb this chemical. However, the rate of elimination from the body appeared to be comparable in the various species tested, with 96-98% being excreted within 96 hours (Audrieth and Sveda, 1944; Taylor et al., 1951; Richards et al., 1951; Schoenberger et al., 1953; Hwang, 1966; Kojima et al., 1966; Miller et al., 1966; Sonders et al., 1968; Parekh et al., 1970; Wallace et al., 1970; Renwick and Williams, 1972). Cyclamate, once regarded as metabolically inert, is now known to be partially metabolized; the primary metabolite is cyclohexylamine. The partial conversion of cyclamate to cyclohexylamine has been demonstrated in the rat (Oser et al., 1968; Renwick and Williams, 1969), dog (Golberg et al., 1969; Kojima and Ichibagase, 1966), rabbit and guinea pig (Renwick and Williams, 1970), rhesus monkey (Parekh et al., 1970), and in the human (Leahy et al., 1967; Davis et al., 1969). Conversion has been shown to take place in the gastrointestinal tract involving the bacteria flora (Renwick and Williams, 1969; Golberg et al., 1969). Other urinary metabolites detected in small amounts include cyclohexanol and cyclohexanone (Kojima and Ichibagase, 1966; Golberg et al., 1969; Parekh et al., 1970; Ichibagase et al., 1972). The metabolic conversion of cyclamate to cyclohexylamine has been extensively reviewed by the Temporary Committee for the Review of Data on Carcinogenicity of Cyclamate (1976). The urinary excretion levels of cyclohexylamine have been reported to be extremely variable not only from species to species and individual to individual, but also from day to day in the same individual. The incidence of human subjects who convert cyclamate to cyclohexylamine appears to be roughly 10-30%. Of those individuals who are converters, the majority convert from less than 0.1% to approximately 8%, a relatively few individuals converting up to approximately 60%.

b. Carcinogenicity

The first chronic study of sodium cyclamate was conducted by Fitzhugh et al. (1951), who fed groups of Osborne-Mendel rats 1 and 5% sodium cyclamate in the diet for 2 years and found no increase in tumor incidence over the controls. Since that time hundreds of research investigations have been carried out dealing with the toxicity of cyclamate. Up to the 1965-1967 period the vast collection of medical and scientific evidence available strongly suggested that cyclamate was safe under normal conditions of use (Berryman et al., 1968).

In 1969 a study was conducted by Price et al. (1970) in which a mixture of cyclamate/saccharin (10:1) was fed in the diet of rats at 0, 500, 1120, or 2500 mg/kg body weight/day for 2 years. Since a significant number of animals were shown to convert cyclamate to cyclohexylamine, especially at the upper dosage level, cyclohexylamine was also added to the diet of half the animals of each treated group from the 79th week of this study. Urinary bladder carcinoma was demonstrated at the level of 2500 mg/kg body weight.

At that time the evidence indicating the carcinogenic potential of cyclamate or its breakdown product, cyclohexylamine, was sufficient to result in the banning or severe restriction in the use of this nonnutritive sweetener in over 30 countries. Since that time, however, further long-term studies have been conducted on both cyclamate and cyclohexylamine. Friedman et al. (1972) reported on two studies in which rats were fed sodium and calcium cyclamate at various dose levels in a semisynthetic diet and a chow diet. This study was not designed specifically as a test for carcinogenicity but to study the conversion of cyclamate to cyclohexylamine. Three non-dose-related bladder carcinomas were detected in male rats, two at the level of 0.4% calcium cyclamate in a chow diet. In a further study from this laboratory (Taylor and Friedman, 1974) no bladder tumors were observed in rats that were exposed in utero and were continued on the parental diet containing 5% calcium cyclamate for their lifetime. In other studies in which rats (Schmähl, 1973; Furuya et al., 1975; Gaunt et al., 1976) were fed diets containing either sodium cyclamate, a mixture of cyclamate: saccharin, or cyclohexylamine, no apparent increase in bladder carcinoma was observed. Mice have also been exposed to diets containing sodium cyclamate (Roe et al., 1970; Brantom et al., 1973), cyclohexylamine (Hardy et al., 1976), and a mixture of cyclamate: saccharin in which the animals were exposed in utero; and a parental group and two progeny generations were maintained on treatment for 21 months (Kroes et al., 1975). No carcinogenic or tumor-promoting activity was demonstrated. Similar results were observed in the hamster when exposed to either sodium or calcium cyclamate at several dose levels in their drinking water (Althoff et al., 1975). Thus it would appear from the available toxicological data that neither cyclamate or its metabolites are tumorigenic.

4. Saccharin (Salts of 2,3-Dihydro-3-Oxobenziososulfonazole)

Saccharin is synthesized by using such starting materials as toluene (Remsen and Fahlberg, 1879), phthalic anhydride, or phthalic acid (Maumee, 1951), and o-chlorotoluene (Bungard, 1967). Each procedure results in a final product with different impurities. The most widely used methods for the manufacture of saccharin are the Remsen-Fahlberg and the Maumee processes (Munro et al., 1975b).

a. Analysis

No universal analytical method for the identification of impurities present in saccharin, regardless of the production method, is presently available. However, a method for isolating and identifying the organic (Stavric et al., 1976) and water-soluble (Stavric et al., 1974a, 1974b) impurities present in Remsen-Fahlberg-produced saccharin has been reported, while Nelson (1976) has only examined the water-soluble impurities.

b. Metabolism

Metabolic studies have been conducted with the mouse, rat, hamster, guinea pig, dog, monkey, and human. Rates of saccharin elimination appear to be similar in the various species studied. Orally administered saccharin is almost completely eliminated from the body within 96 hr, 70-90% being excreted by way of the urine (Pitkin et al., 1971; Kennedy et al., 1972; Minegishi et al., 1972; Byard and Golberg, 1973; Byard et al., 1974). Kennedy et al. (1972) reported the presence of two hydrolytic products of saccharin, o-sulfamoylbenzoic acid and ammonium o-carboxylbenzenesulfonate, in the urine of rats, while Lethco and Wallace (1975) detected only o-sulfamoylbenzoic acid. In both instances the hydrolytic products accounted for less than 1% of the orally administered dose. The presence of these hydrolytic products was observed in the urine of female monkeys after the oral administration of saccharin (Pitkin et al., 1971). In a similar study with male monkeys Byard and Golberg (1973) reported that saccharin was excreted unchanged in the urine and that the two hydrolytic products were artifactual metabolites produced during the extraction procedure. No changes in the excretion pattern or the metabolism of saccharin was observed during 79 months of the later study (McChesney et al., 1977). Other investigators (Byard, 1972; Minegishi et al., 1972; Matthews et al., 1973; Ball et al., 1974; Ball et al., 1977) did not detect metabolites of saccharin in the urine of animals receiving either single or multiple oral doses of saccharin. In humans more than 90% of orally ingested saccharin is excreted unchanged in the urine and up to 6% may be excreted in the feces within 48 hr of dosing (Herter and Folin, 1911; Staub and Staehelin, 1936; McChesney and Golberg, 1973; Byard et al., 1974; Ball et al., 1977).

c. Carcinogenicity

An assessment of the chronic toxicity of saccharin was first undertaken by Fitzhugh et al. (1951), who fed groups of rats of 1 or 5% saccharin in the diet for 2 years and found no increase in tumor incidence over controls apart from an increased incidence of lymphosarcomas in animals given the highest dose. The importance of this finding was discounted by the authors. The urinary bladders were apparently not examined. Lessel (1970) noted that rats fed a diet containing 5% saccharin for 2 years had an increased incidence of urinary bladder calculi compared to controls. He presumed that the bladder-stone formation was causally related to the high intake of saccharin. Increased tumor incidence was not noted in the treated rats, although epithelial proliferative lesions of the bladder and the presence of one papilloma were noted in the 5% dose group. The author concluded that the benign proliferative lesions may have been related to the irritant effects of bladder stones. In another study, Roe et al. (1970) fed mice 5% saccharin in the diet for 18 months and found no evidence of carcinogenesis, although the urinary bladders were not examined histologically.

The anticipated increase in saccharin usage following the cyclamate ban in 1969-1970, coupled with previous findings, led to a worldwide effort to determine the carcinogenic potential of saccharin. Studies were undertaken in several countries, including Canada, Germany, Great Britain, Japan, The Netherlands, and the United States. Some of these studies have not appeared in the literature to date; however, they were included in the report by the National Research Council (NRC) of the United States (1974). At the National Institute of Health in The Netherlands diets containing up to 0.5% sodium saccharin were fed to mice during a six-generation study in which the animals from the F_0, F_{3b}, and F_{6a} generation remained on test for 20 months. No significant treatment-related effects were noted. In studies performed at Bio-Research in Canada saccharin was fed at dietary levels of 0, 1, or 5% to mice and rats for 24 months, with no significant difference in the incidence of bladder tumors between the various groups. Miyagi of the Institute of Pathology in Japan fed mice and rats diets containing 0, 0.2, 1.0, or 5% saccharin for 21 and 28 months, respectively. No treatment effects were noted. Furuya et al. (1975) found no bladder abnormalities when rats received 2.5 g/kg/day sodium saccharin for 28 months. In 1973, Schmähl reported spontaneous tumors in rats consuming diets containing 0, 100, or 250 mg/kg/day saccharin. The only significant finding was reticulum cell sarcoma in five animals at the highest-dose level. No increase in tumor incidence was observed in a study conducted by the Health Protection Branch in Canada (Munro et al., 1975a) in which sodium saccharin was fed in the diet to rats at levels of 0, 90, 270, 810, or 2430 mg/kg/day for 26 months. Five bladder tumors were noted; however, they were not considered to be compound or dose related.

In studies conducted at the Wisconsin Alumni Research Foundation (WARF) and the FDA (NRC, 1974) rats were fed diets containing graded levels of sodium saccharin for 3 months prior to mating. The F_1 progeny were weaned to the diet of their parents, which was consumed ad libitum until the studies were terminated at 24 and 28 months, respectively. An increase in bladder tumors was noted in both the WARF and FDA studies, especially in the male at levels of 5 and 7.5% sodium saccharin, respectively.

In the WARF and FDA studies the animals were exposed in utero to saccharin that contained levels of orthotoluene sulfonamide (OTS) up to 4660 ppm (Stavric et al., 1974b). It was suggested (NRC, 1974) that OTS might be the chemical responsible for the observed bladder tumors. This in turn led to a study by Arnold et al. (1977), who fed rats OTS at 0, 2.5, and 250 mg/kg, as well as a group receiving 250 mg/kg of OTS with drinking water containing 1% NH_4Cl. A further group received 5% sodium saccharin containing no detectable amounts of OTS in the diet. Animals were bred after being on test for 3 months, and F_1 pups weaned on the diet of parental groups and both generations remained on respective diets for a lifetime (30-32 months). OTS did not produce bladder tumors; however, in the 5% saccharin group free of OTS there was an increase in the incidence of malignant bladder tumors in males of both generations. This was the first study in which an increase in bladder tumors was observed in the F_0 generation.

5. Model Systems Used to Study the Carcinogenicity of Nonnutritive Sweeteners Other than by Dietary Exposure

Studies by Allen et al. (1957), Bryan et al. (1970), and Bryan and Yoshida (1971) in which paraffin or cholesterol pellets containing saccharin were implanted into the urinary bladders of mice and rats, demonstrated that the saccharin-containing pellets produced an increased incidence of bladder neoplasms when compared with controls implanted with the vehicle alone. The significance of the results of such tests has been questioned. Hicks et al. (1973a, 1973b, 1975) reported a rat model system for testing bladder carcinogens. Each rat was subjected to pretreatment with a single instillation into the bladder of 2 mg methyl-n-nitrosourea (MNU). Rats were then given sodium saccharin or sodium cyclamate added either to the diet or drinking water at dosage levels of up to 4 g/kg/day. Significantly higher incidences of bladder tumors were produced with a dramatically reduced latent period in the animals treated with MNU plus saccharin or cyclamate, compared to the untreated control or animals receiving a single instillation of MNU or animals receiving saccharin or cyclamate without MNU pretreatment. This has been shown to be a controversial procedure, and more research is needed to confirm and evaluate the biological significance of this model system.

6. Epidemiology of Nonnutritive Sweeteners

There have been very few epidemiological studies dealing specifically with nonnutritive sweetener effects in humans. Mortality rates from bladder cancer were examined in Britain (Armstrong and Doll, 1974) and the United States (Burbank and Fraumeni, 1970), and no increase was revealed that might be attributable to saccharin consumption. Extensive studies of cancer in relation to diabetus mellitus (Armstrong and Doll, 1975; Armstrong et al., 1976; Kessler, 1970) showed no excessive mortality from bladder cancer although saccharin consumption was greater than average. Kessler (1976) and Morgan and Jain (1974) conducted studies in which bladder cancer patients were matched against appropriate controls and questioned as to their intake of nonnutritive sweeteners. Use of these sweeteners was not associated with an increased risk of bladder cancer.

Recently Howe et al. (1977) have produced the first positive association between the use of nonnutritive sweeteners, particularly saccharin, and risk of bladder cancer in males.

In a case control study of 480 men and 152 women in three provinces in Canada the risk ratio for ever versus never used was 1.6 for males and a significant dose-response relationship was obtained for both duration and frequency of use. The population attributable risk for males was estimated at 7% and for diabetics, who have a similar risk factor, the attributable risk is 33%. However, this is in direct contradiction to another recent study by Wynder and Goldsmith (1977). They analyzed nonnutritive sweetener use in 146 cases and 132 matched controls and found no apparent increase in the incidence of bladder cancer.

B. Food Colors

1. Origin and Use in Foods

Of the colors available for use in food, "coal-tar colors," synthetic organic cyes, or azo dyes are employed in the largest quantities principally because they are stable under varied conditions of processing and storage. The number of synthetic colors permitted for use varies from a high of 33 in Denmark to none in Greece. The countries of the European Economic Community permit 22, Canada 9, the United States 8, and the Soviet Union 3.

A synthetic food color may contain (1) subsidiary dyes that are colored compounds of various molecular weights resembling one another in chemical structure, or isomers of the same molecular weight but with functional groups at different molecular positions, and (2) unreacted noncolored compounds known as intermediates. Concentrations of volatile matter, subsidiary dyes, intermediates, water-insoluble matter, and ether extracts may vary from one color to another; their total may be as high as 15%. A color having less than 85% of the principal dye (98% for citrus red) and more than 2 ppm of arsenic, 10 ppm of lead, and a total of 100 ppm of iron and copper is generally not permitted for use in food.

The safety of azo dyes was first questioned in 1936 following demonstration of the carcinogenic potential of o-aminoazotoluene and p-dimethylaminoazobenzene (butter yellow). The latter was then used in concentrations of 0.5-1 g/100 kg of butter fat (Meuron, 1955). Food colors manufactured from β-naphthylamine by interaction with aniline (yellow AB or FD&C Yellow No. 3), with o-toluidine (yellow OB or FD&C Yellow No. 4), and with m-xylidine (oil red XO or FD&C Red No. 32) were disallowed for use in food of many countries, although no evidence of carcinogenicity was established. In most instances food colors that were found to have carcinogenic potential or other adverse effects were removed from permitted lists.

It is not the intent of the authors to discuss in detail each of the food colors permitted in various countries nor their carcinogenic potential since excellent reviews are available (Radomski, 1974; Drake, 1975). This section of the chapter on food additive carcinogens is devoted to a brief review of those food colors that were shown to be carcinogenic and those whose carcinogenicity is suspect or controversial. Amaranth, Ponceau SX, citrus red no. 2, and other food colors, such as Brilliant Blue FCF, that have been shown to be carcinogenic when injected subcutaneously, fall into one or the other of these categories and are considered in some detail.

2. Brilliant Blue FCF

a. Carcinogenicity on parenteral injection

Brilliant Blue FCF, indigotine, and Blue VRS produced sarcomas at the site of subcutaneous or intramuscular injections in rodents (Hansen et al., 1966; Grice and Mannell, 1966). A shorter series of injections given twice weekly induced histologic changes such as macrophagic accumulation, macrophagic necrosis, and fibroblastic proliferation (Gangolli et al., 1967) and were consistent with the type of lesions that would initiate sarcoma formation (Grasso and Golberg, 1966a). The oncogenic effect following dye injections was, reportedly, related to physiochemical characteristics, protein-binding ability, and pH of the dye solutions, and was not considered as a true measure for evaluating carcinogenic hazard of substances intended for oral ingestion (Grasso and Golberg, 1966b; Gangolli et al., 1972).

3. Ponceau 3R

a. Uses

Ponceau 3R was used as a food color in many countries until bioassay studies showed it to be carcinogenic.

b. Metabolism

Ponceau 3R undergoes azo reduction to give several aromatic amines as well as trimethylanilines and xylidines (Lindstrom, 1961). Of these, mesidine (2, 4, 6-trimethylaniline) and pseudocumidine (2, 4, 5-trimethylaniline or 4-cumidine) were highly toxic, perhaps because of their greater resistance to oxidative metabolism and their conversion into metabolites of high toxicity (Lindstrom et al., 1969). 2,4, 6-Trimethylaniline has been reported to produce transplantable hepatic carcinomas in rats when fed in the diet at a level of 150 mg/kg of diet for 18 months (Mannell, 1964). The xylidine isomers, 2,4-, 2,5-, and 2, 6-xylidine, were hepatotoxic in rats and dogs (Lindstrom et al., 1963).

c. Carcinogenicity

Ponceau 3R, also known as FD&C Red No. 1, produced liver tumors in rats (Grice et al., 1961; Mannell, 1964) and pathologic changes in the liver of dogs (Hansen et al., 1963).

4. Amaranth

a. Uses

Amaranth until recently was one of the most widely used food colors. Whether amaranth (FD&C Red No. 2)—a color permitted in food in 63 countries—is or is not carcinogenic became an important issue recently. The issue focused attention on the growing concern for current methods of toxicity testing and resulted in the imposition of more stringent criteria for safety evaluation of food additives in general and food colors in particular, with emphasis on purity, metabolism, and testing procedures.

b. Metabolism

One important reason for the confusion that surrounded amaranth has been the lack of data on human metabolism that could provide the much needed basis for selecting a metabolically analogous animal species for carcinogenicity testing. Metabolic studies conducted in the rat have revealed that amaranth underwent azo reduction in the gut to produce 1-amino-4-naphthalene sulfonic acid (naphthionic acid), 1-amino-2-naphthol-3, 6-disulfonic acid (amino R-acid), and 1, 2-naphthoquinone-3, 6-disulfonic acid (Radomski and Mellinger, 1962; Honohan et al., 1976). These metabolites crossed the intestinal wall, migrated into major body tissues, and were excreted within 24 hr of ingestion of amaranth (Report of the Comptroller General of United States, Food and Drug Administration, 1975). Only 2.8% of the intact molecule of amaranth was absorbed (Pritchard et al., 1976).

c. Carcinogenicity

Amaranth was universally accepted as safe for use in food until 1968, when its safety was challenged on the basis of the development of sarcomas in male rats fed 1 g/kg body weight for 25 months (Baigusheva, 1968). The study is inconclusive since the sample of amaranth tested in this study was of undefined purity. In another study amaranth at a dietary concentration of 2% was considered to be associated with malignant tumors in 13 of the 50 rats (Andrianova, 1970). This study is questioned on the basis that none of the 50 control rats developed tumors. A zero incidence in the control rats is highly unusual, particularly if the control animals live sufficiently long to serve as effective controls.

In an FDA study amaranth fed at dietary concentrations of 0, 0.003, 0.03, 0.3, and 3% produced no significant difference in total number of tumors, both benign and malignant, in the high-dose and lowest-dose groups, but there was a significant increase in the number of malignant tumors found in female rats maintained at the 3% dose. The experiment formed the basis for delisting amaranth in the United States. The experimental conditions and evaluation of the data have been questioned (Boffey, 1976). Tumors did not appear to have toxicologic significance since they were neither organ specific nor unusual for the strain of rats tested. Further, the increased tumor incidence was confined to female rats, and, except for mammary tumors, the tumors were not sex related.

5. Ponceau SX

a. Uses

Ponceau SX has been disallowed in several countries including the United States. Its use in Canada is restricted to coloring of fruit peel, glacé fruits, and maraschino cherries with a maximum level of 150 ppm.

b. Purity

The commercial samples may contain isomeric xylidines, dimethylanilines, and their intermediates, and, therefore, may give subsidiary colors (Graichen and Heine, 1954; Wenninger et al., 1960). In the rat the dye is metabolized to 2-amino-1-hydroxy-4-naphthalene sulfonic acid, 1-amino-2,4-dimethyl-5-benzene sulfonic acid, and 2 acetamino-1-hydroxy-4-naphthalene sulfonic acid (Radomski and Mellinger, 1962).

c. Carcinogenicity

Suspicion regarding carcinogenicity was raised by the occurrence of one mesenteric lymphosarcoma in 7 rats fed Ponceau SX at 4% concentration in the diet for 18 months (Willheim and Ivy, 1953). This suspicion was removed by definitive studies in rats and mice fed as high as 5% concentration in the diet for 2 years with no untoward effects (Davis et al., 1966). In dogs dietary feeding at 1% level for 7 years resulted in chronic follicular cystitis and atrophy in the adrenal, hematomatous projections into the urinary bladder, and hemosiderotic foci in the liver (Davis et al., 1966). Adrenal changes following long-term feeding were not observed in the rat, pointing out an important species difference in toxicity to Ponceau SX.

6. Citrus Red No. 2

a. Uses

Citrus red no. 2 is approved for coloring the skin of mature oranges with levels not exceeding 2 ppm in the whole orange.

b. Purity

There are two major subsidiary colors found in citrus red, dimethoxy color and benzidine color (Stein, 1970).

c. Metabolism

Several metabolites resulting from reductive fission of the azo group by the intestinal flora and in vivo metabolism were found in the rat's urine, of which the O-glucuronide conjugate of the unmodified dye (in the highest quantity), and 1-amino-2-naphthyl, 1-amino-2-naphthyl glucuronide, and 1-amino-2-naphthyl sulfate were identified. There was no evidence of the production of N-hydroxy metabolites or metabolites considered to be actively carcinogenic (Radomski, 1974).

d. Carcinogenicity

Evidence of carcinogenic potential of citrus red was obtained upon finding hyperplasia and tumors of the urinary bladder wall in rats and mice maintained for 2 years on diets containing 0, 0.05, and 0.25% of citrus red (Dacre, 1965). This hyperplasia was similar to that found in the bladder of mice fed on a diet of 0.01% of 4-ethyl-sulfonylnaphthalene-1-sulfonamide, a well-known bladder carcinogen (Bonser and Clayson, 1964). In another study mice were fed diets containing various levels of citrus red for periods of up to 80 weeks; diets containing 0.3, 1.0, and 3.0% of the dye were toxic, but the other of the dietary levels (0.01, 0.03, and 0.1%) were well tolerated and produced no significant effect on tumor induction in either sex (Sharratt et al., 1966).

Fifty subcutaneous injections of a 10% suspension of citrus red no. 2 in 0.1 ml of tricaprylin, given over a period of 80 weeks, caused an increased incidence of malignant tumors (adenocinomas of lung and lymphosarcomas) in female mice (Sharratt et al., 1966).

C. Food Packaging Materials and Associated Carcinogens

1. Origin in Foods

A wide range of materials varying from metallic cans and foils to waxed paper and plastics is used in the food-packaging industry. Only recently (Fed. Reg., 1975) has the association of cancer with a material leached from a container to the food contents caused concern. This arose as a consequence of the discovery that the then newly introduced beverage containers, fabricated from a rigid polyvinyl chloride formulation, retained sufficient vinyl chloride monomer so that up to 20 ppm of the monomer was leached into the contents.

The migration of polymeric materials, additives, and residual reactants from plastics to food has been discussed at some length (Briston and Katan, 1974). The principles of safety evaluation, test procedures, the fundamental principles of the diffusion processes involved, and some examples of the leaching of undesirable materials are discussed in this publication, but no mention of the presence of carcinogenic materials in plastics is included. A review of a range of potential mutagens, teratogens, and carcinogens used as additives in the fabrication of plastics has been published recently (Withey, 1977).

2. Vinyl Chloride Monomer

The presence of vinyl chloride monomer in alcoholic beverages had been discovered in May of 1973 when complaints were received by the U.S. Bureau of Tobacco, Firearms, and Alcohol of the Department of Justice that alcoholic beverages packaged in rigid polyvinyl chloride bottles for use on airlines had a "tainted taste." Subsequent analyses by the U.S. Food and Drug Administration failed to reveal the unequivocal identity of the substance responsible for the unpalatable taste of the beverages (although it was thought to have been probably a mercapto ester stabilizer), but the presence of a substance of high volatility, which was later confirmed as vinyl chloride monomer, was discovered. In its initial action to withdraw the prior sanctioned use of rigid polyvinyl chloride for food packaging (Fed. Reg., 1973) the FDA had pointed out that "vinyl chloride monomer is a poisonous and deleterious substance" and that "it knew of no studies which had established a safe level of consumption for this chemical."

a. Analysis in foods

Since vinyl chloride monomer is a gas at room temperature (boiling point, b.p. -13°C), the technique of headspace analysis (Curry et al., 1962) has been used with high sensitivity and reproducibility for this and other monomers in foods (Williams and Miles, 1975).

b. Occurrence and concentration

Vinyl chloride monomer has been found, usually at concentrations of about 1-5 ppm, but as high as 10-20 ppm in a very wide variety of foodstuffs packaged in rigid polyvinyl chloride containers (van Esch and van Logten, 1975; Williams and Miles, 1975; Fed. Reg., 1975).

c. Metabolism

Vinyl chloride monomer is known to be metabolized both by mixed function oxidases and by the alcohol dehydrogenase pathways. The principal metabolites are trichloroacetic acid and its glucuronide derivative (Hefner et al., 1975). Metabolic intermediates are known to be chlorethanol, chloracetaldehyde, and vinylchloroepoxide, all of which have been demonstrated to be mutagens. The most labile of these intermediates and a powerful alkylating agent, is vinyl chloroepoxide which is believed to be the ultimate carcinogen.

d. Carcinogenicity

In January of 1974 a press release on the findings of Dr. John L. Creech of the B. F. Goodrich chemical plant in Louisville, Kentucky, stated that there appeared to be an association of industrial exposure to vinyl chloride monomer and the induction of a rare liver tumor, hemangiosarcoma, which were later confirmed by further epidemiological studies (IARC, 1975) and bioassay cancer studies with animals (Maltoni and Lefemine, 1974). In addition to hemangiosarcoma, animal studies also revealed zymbal gland carcinoma, nephroblastomas, osteochondromas, and squamous cell papillomas of the skin. This topic has been the subject of a number of excellent reviews (Haley, 1975; Holmberg and Molina, 1974; van Esch and van Logten, 1975). Regulatory agencies throughout the world have now moved to prohibit the use of rigid polyvinyl chloride for food-packaging use or have required the demonstration by food packagers or manufacturers that no detectable vinyl chloride monomer, using official analytical methods, is leached to the foodstuff.

Largely as a consequence of the concern generated by the problem of vinyl chloride monomer in foods, numerous carcinogenic bioassay studies as well as an examination of the toxicology, metabolism, and pharmacokinetics, have been initiated on a number of monomers that are used in the manufacture of plastics. Some of these are used either for packaging materials or as food contact surfaces (e.g., disposable cutlery, drinking cups, and tableware).

3. Vinylidene Chloride

Vinylidene chloride, used as a copolymer with vinyl chloride to produce a thin film wrap for foods and as an adjunct for other food-use plastics, has been shown to cause tumors in animals (Food Chem. News, 1977a) and must now be considered as a suspect carcinogen. Mice exposed to 25 ppm of vinylidene chloride by the inhalation route were reported to develop kidney tumors and bacterial test systems have shown this compound to be mutagenic (Bartsch et al., 1975). No reports of analytical methodology or of the presence of this compound in foods have yet been published, although one report claims that the levels in thin film food wrap were only on the order of 10 ppm and that methods that were sensitive to 40 ppb failed to detect any in food simulating solvents (Food Chem. News, 1977a).

4. Acrylonitrile

Acrylonitrile, used as a copolymer with butadiene and styrene to form rigid containers for fats and as a "barrier resin" for the lining of carbonated beverage bottles, has recently been implicated as a mutagen, teratogen, tumorogen, and possibly as a carcinogen in recent animal bioassay and epidemiological studies (Food Chem. News, 1977b). Acrylonitrile has proven to be an extremely valuable material for the production of plastic food containers in view of their low permeability to gases such as oxygen, which prevents fatty foods from going rancid, and to carbon dioxide, which allows the storage of carbonated beverages. No evidence of its presence in foods has been reported and no analytical methodology for its determination in foods has yet been published, although the determination of acrylonitrile with a sensitivity of 1 ppm in plastics and in food simulants to 13 ppb using a nitrogen-phosphorus-specific detector was recently reported (Brown et al., 1977).

5. Styrene Monomer

The volume use of polystyrene formulations probably ranks second only to those of polyethylene in the plastics food packaging industry. Both in the crystalline and amorphous forms, as well as in the copolymerized form with butadiene and acrylonitrile, polystyrene is used to package a very wide variety of foods (Withey and Collins, 1977).

a. Analysis in foods

Analytical methods, similar to those that were developed for vinyl chloride monomer, have been reported with a sensitivity of less than 1 ppb for many foods (Withey and Collins, 1977).

b. Occurrence and concentration

Residual styrene monomer has been found in food packaging in concentrations greater than 3000 ppm, although the amount leached to the food contents was less than 0.5 ppm by weight (Withey and Collins, 1977; Withey, 1976).

c. Metabolism

Since the metabolism of styrene monomer proceeds via the formation of styrene epoxide (El Masri et al., 1958; Ohtsuji and Ikeda, 1971) and the epoxide formed from vinyl chloride, rather than vinyl chloride per se, has been suggested as an ultimate carcinogen (Hefner et al., 1975), a number of cancer bioassays with styrene monomer and styrene epoxide are now underway (Tox-Tips, 1977). Styrene epoxide has been demonstrated to be a mutagen (Parkki et al., 1976; Stoltz and Withey, 1977) and to produce tumors in skin-painting tests on mice (Van Duuren, 1969).

d. Carcinogenicity

No information is yet available on the mutagenic or carcinogenic activity of styrene, although a number of cancer studies in which animals have been dosed with styrene monomer by the inhalation and oral routes are now nearing completion (Tox-Tips, 1977).

6. Other Concerns

A number of other polymeric materials that are used in the food-packaging industry, for example, polyethylene, polycarbonates, cellulose acetate, cellulose propionate, and so on, have not yet given cause for concern in terms of their carcinogenic potential. A recent review (Withey, 1977), however, pointed out that a wide variety of substances, which are necessarily used as plastics additives in order to confer desirable physical and mechanical properties to a polymer, have been demonstrated to have a carcinogenic potential.

III. PRODUCTS OF CHEMICAL REACTIONS

A. N-Nitrosamines

N-Nitrosamines are simple organic compounds formed by the interaction of nitrous acid and secondary or tertiary amines. While investigating a case report of cirrhosis of liver in three men working in a large industrial research laboratory, Barnes and Magee (1954) observed an association of the liver disease with the use of N-nitrosodimethylamine (NDMA) as a chemical solvent. The suspicion that NDMA was the causative agent was later confirmed by feeding studies in laboratory animals. Subsequent work by Magee and Barnes (1956) showed that in addition to being a hepatotoxic agent, NDMA is also a potent carcinogen in rats, causing malignant liver and kidney tumors within 26-40 weeks of oral feeding. Soon it became apparent that this carcinogenic property was not restricted to NDMA alone, but to many other N-nitrosamines and, in general, to most N-nitroso compounds, such as nitrosamino acids, nitrosoureas, nitrosoguanidines, and so on (Schoental, 1960; Druckrey et al., 1961; Druckrey et al., 1969; Magee et al., 1976). Thus far about 130 N-nitroso compounds have been tested, and approximately 80% of them have been found to be carcinogenic (Preussmann et al., 1976).

Since many foods contain naturally occurring amines and some contain nitrates and nitrites (which could occur naturally or be added as food additives), traces of nitrosamines may be formed in these foods. In addition, there is the potential for formation of nitrosamines in the acidic environment of the human stomach from ingested nitrite and amines in foods (Lijinsky and Epstein, 1970; Sen, 1974). Extensive research during the last 10 years has resulted in many positive findings of nitrosamines in food and the demonstration of their formation in the stomach of experimental animals and humans. A brief account of these findings is considered in this section. A detailed review of the subject has recently been published by Magee et al. (1976).

1. Chemical Structure

The N-nitrosamines can be simply described by the general formula $R_1R_2N\text{-}N{=}O$, where R_1 and R_2 can be either an aliphatic or aromatic group, or they can be replaced by a cyclic ring as in N-nitrosopiperidine (NPIP) or N-nitrosomorpholine (NMOR). In some cases the compound may contain functional groups (as in nitrosoproline) or it may be the N-nitroso derivative of an amide such as nitrosomethylurea. Chemical formulae of some common nitrosamines and nitrosamides are shown in Fig. 1.

2. Physical and Chemical Properties

Some of the important physical properties of N-nitroso compounds are given in Table 1. In general, the low molecular weight nitrosamines are pale brown liquid and steam volatile. They all show the characteristic UV absorption maxima due to the >N-N=O group. All N-nitroso compounds are sensitive to light, especially UV radiation. For this reason they should be stored in the dark, preferably in brown bottles. Further details can be obtained in the published literature quoted in Table 1.

Nitrosamines are generally stable in aqueous solution, but they slowly decompose in the presence of strong acids (Fieser and Fieser, 1968). They can be reduced to unsymmetrical hydrazines (Hatt, 1943; Serfontein and Hurter, 1966) or oxidized to nitramines (Emmons, 1954). Nitrosamides are very unstable in aqueous solution, especially under alkaline conditions; they break down spontaneously to diazoalkanes (Fieser and Fieser, 1968).

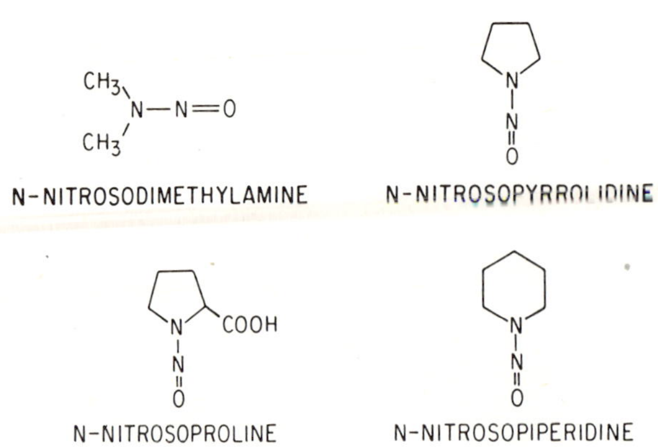

FIGURE 1 Chemical formulae of some N-nitroso compounds.

TABLE 1 Physical and Chemical Properties of Some N-Nitroso Compounds

Name	Mol wt	b.p. or m.p.	Density D_4^{20}	Refractive index n_D^{20}	UV absorption[a] characteristics λ_{max}(nm)	log ε	Stability
N-Nitrosodimethylamine (NDMA) (yellow liquid)	74.1	150°C (760 mm) b.p.	1.0048	1.4368	230 332	3.86 1.98	Stable, sensitive to light
N-Nitrosodiethylamine (NDEA) (pale yellow liquid)	102.1	177°C (760 mm) b.p.	0.9422	1.4386	230 332	3.86 1.98	Stable, sensitive to light
N-Nitrosodi-n-butylamine (NDBA) (pale yellow liquid)	158.2	234–237°C (760 mm) b.p. 104–105°C (8 mm) b.p.	0.9009		233 347	3.85 1.95	Stable, sensitive to light
N-Nitroso-n-butyl(4-hydroxybutyl)amine (NBHBA)	174.2	115–116°C (0.01 mm) b.p.			232 346	3.95 2.26	Stable, sensitive to light
N-Nitrosopyrrolidine (NPYR) (pale yellow liquid)	100.2	98°C (12 mm) b.p.	1.085	1.4896	230 333	3.91 2.03	Stable, sensitive to light
N-Nitrosopiperidine (NPIP) (pale yellow liquid)	114.2	100°C (14 mm) b.p.	1.0631[b]	1.4933[b]	235 337	3.98 1.92	Stable, sensitive to light
N-Nitrosoproline (NPRO) (white to pale yellow crystals)	144	100–101°C m.p. (decomp.)			238 343	3.81 1.96	Unstable in aqueous solution, sensitive to light
N-Nitrososarcosine (NSAR) (white to pale yellow crystals)	118.1	66–67°C m.p.			234 337	3.96 1.89	Unstable in aqueous solution, sensitive to light
N-Nitroso-N-methylurea (NMU) (pale yellow crystals)	103.1	124°C (decomp.) m.p.			231	3.77	Unstable in aqueous solution at pH > 7, sensitive to light
N-D-Glucosyl-(2)-N'-nitrosomethylurea (streptozotocin) (white to pale yellow crystals)	265	115°C (decomp.) m.p.			228	6360	Unstable in aqueous solution especially under acidic and alkaline conditions, sensitive to light

[a]In most cases in aqueous solvents.

[b]At 18°C.

Sources: For reference see Druckrey et al., 1967; IARC, 1972, 1974; Chemical Rubber Company, 1973; Lijinsky et al., 1970.

3. Precursors and Formation

Secondary and tertiary amines are the major amine precursors of nitrosamines. Recent studies, however, indicate that tertiary amine oxides and quaternary amines such as neurine, choline, and carnitine can also be precursors of nitrosamines (Ender et al., 1967; Fiddler et al., 1972). Besides these naturally occurring amines there are other N-nitrosatable organic compounds, which, under suitable conditions, can yield nitrosamines. For example, nitrogen-containing pesticides such as Carbaryl, Atrazine, Thiram, Ziram, and Alar, and drugs such as piperazine and tetracyclines, have been shown to undergo nitrosation and form nitrosamines (Lijinsky et al., 1972; Sen et al., 1974a; Eisenbrand et al., 1974). Naturally occurring ureas and guanidines can also form nitroso derivatives, many of which are potent carcinogens and mutagens (Mirvish, 1975). These compounds can be of either natural origin or present in foods as undesirable contaminants (e.g., pesticide and drug residues).

Secondary, tertiary, and quaternary amines, and trimethylamine oxide occur ubiquitously in nature and have been reported to occur in various foods such as fish (especially marine fish), seafoods, meat, eggs, cheese, vegetables, spices, wine, spirits, beer, and many other foods (Rea and Shewan, 1951; Sander, 1971; Neurath et al., 1976; Castell et al., 1971; Ishidate et al., 1971; Singer and Lijinsky, 1976). Many ureas and guanidines also occur in foods that can be potential precursors of N-nitroso compounds (Mirvish, 1972a).

The major portion of nitrate in our diet comes from vegetables, but some is also obtained from cured meats, and nitrate- or nitrite-treated fish or cheese (White, 1975). Nearly all vegetables (e.g., spinach, cauliflower, radish, celery, lettuce, cabbage, turnip, beets) contain fairly high levels of nitrate, sometimes over 1000 ppm (Siciliano et al., 1975; White, 1975). The concentration of nitrite in vegetables is normally negligible, although fairly high levels have been reported to occur in storage-abused spinach and beets (Heisler et al., 1974). Nitrates and nitrites are used as food additives in many countries for the preservation of meats, fish, and cheese (Canadian Food and Drugs Act and Regulations, 1965; U.S. Food Additive Regulations, Code of Federal Regulations 121.1063, 121.1064, 1972; Meester, 1973). Nitrite is used mainly to control the growth of *Clostridium botulinum* spores or other unwanted bacteria (Ingram, 1973), but it also plays an important role in the development of the typical color and flavor of cured meat products. Nitrate per se is inactive, but it can be converted to nitrite by microorganisms present in the meat products, and thus serve as a reservoir of nitrite.

Recent studies have shown that traces of nitrite are being constantly excreted in human saliva, and in some cases, especially after a high-vegetable diet, the salivary nitrite concentration may reach as high as 300-400 ppm (Tannenbaum et al., 1976; Harada et al., 1975). This finding suggests that the nitrite in saliva could play a major role in the in vivo formation of nitrosamines in the stomach.

The rate of nitrosation of secondary amines depends on many factors, such as the concentration of the reactants, basicity of the amine, pH, and temperature. It is directly proportional to the concentration of the amine and square of the nitrite concentration (Mirvish, 1972a). In the absence of thiocycanate ions, the optimum pH of nitrosation of most secondary amines lies between 3-3.4, but in the human gastric juice, which contains thiocyanate ions, the pH optima would be much lower, probably in the range of pH 1-2 (Boyland and Walker, 1974; Fan and Tannenbaum, 1973). Thiocyanate and a few other ions (e.g., Cl^-, Br^-, I^-) have been shown to have a catalytic effect on the formation of nitrosamines (Boyland, 1972). The ease of nitrosation greatly depends on the basicity of the amine; the higher the basicity, the lower the reaction rate (Sander et al., 1968; Mirvish, 1972a, b). Thus, morpholine, having a pK_a value of 8.7, nitrosates about 148 times faster than dimethylamine, whose pK_a value is 10.72. For a detailed review of the kinetics of nitrosamines formation see Mirvish (1975).

Formaldehyde, which is a constituent of many foodstuffs, can catalyze the formation of nitrosamines even under unfavorable conditions, that is, under alkaline pHs (Keefer and Roller, 1973). Conversely, ascorbate and other antioxidants such as ascorbyl palmitate, propyl gallate, α-tocopherol, and so on, can markedly inhibit the nitrosamine formation (Mirvish et al., 1972; Fiddler et al., 1973; Herring, 1973; Sen et al., 1976a; Walters et al.,

1976). Since many of these compounds are naturally present in foods or added as additives, their presence or absence will greatly influence the formation of nitrosamines. In fact, the incorporation of ascorbate, ascorbyl palmitate, or α-tocopherol to frankfurters and bacon has been shown to markedly reduce the concentration of nitrosamines in these foods (Herring, 1973; Mergens et al., 1977).

Considerable amounts of data are available to suggest that traces of nitrosamines can be formed in the human stomach, but it is difficult to estimate the extent of this formation. Early studies by Sander et al. (1968) and Sen et al. (1969) clearly demonstrated the formation of nitrosamines in human gastric juice from the added secondary amines and nitrite. The latter group of workers showed that the formation of NDEA was more rapid in the gastric juice of human and rabbit (pH 1-2) than in the gastric juice of rat (pH 4-5). Similar results were obtained by others (Asahina et al., 1971; Alam et al., 1971). The weakly basic amines such as morpholine, methylbenzylamine, and piperazine produced the higher yields of nitrosamines than the strongly basic amines (e.g., piperidine, diethylamine, dimethylamine) (Sander et al., 1968). Montesano and Magee (1971) and Epstein (1972) observed the expected biochemical changes (incorporation of $^{14}CH_3$ groups into nucleic acids) after feeding ^{14}C-dimethylamine or ^{14}C-N-methylurea, and sodium nitrite to rats or mice, thus confirming the in vivo formation of N-nitroso compounds. Administration of ^{14}C-dimethylamine or ^{14}C-N-methylurea alone gave negative results.

Numerous studies carried out over the past few years have pointed out that simultaneous feeding of weakly basic secondary amines and nitrite can induce cancer in experimental animals (Sander and Buerkle, 1969; Greenblatt et al., 1971; Shank and Newberne, 1976). Similar studies with the strongly basic secondary amines (e.g., dimethylamine, diethylamine, pyrrolidine, and piperidine) and nitrite, however, have given negative results (Druckrey et al., 1963; Greenblatt et al., 1971; Garcia and Lijinsky, 1973; Sen et al., 1976c).

4. Occurrence in Foods

There have been many reports of the occurrence of both low and high levels of nitrosamines in various foodstuffs such as cured meat products, fresh, smoked, or salted fish, cheese, vegetables, a solanaceous fruit, and some alcoholic drinks. Since the likelihood of formation of nitrosamines is greater in nitrate-treated foods most of the positive findings came from the analysis of cured meats and nitrate or nitrite treated fish and fish meal (animal feed). In fact, the discovery of high levels of NDMA in nitrite preserved fish meal in the early sixties (Ender et al., 1964) sparked the worldwide interest in nitrosamine research in human foods.

Since it is beyond the scope of this presentation to list or discuss all the reported occurrences of nitrosamines in foods, the main findings have been summarized in Table 2. It should be pointed out, however, that the validity of some of the earlier results is in doubt, for the specificity of the analytical method used in those studies was inadequate. Only more recently, with the introduction of the highly sophisticated and specific gas-chromatographic-high-resolution mass-spectrometric (GC-MS) techniques, has unequivocal proof of the presence of nitrosamines in foods been obtained.

It is clear from the data in Table 2 that all cured meat products, cured fish, beer, and Chinese salted fish are the main sources of nitrosamines in our diet. Bacon represents a unique case; uncooked bacon is usually free of nitrosamines, but fairly high levels of nitrosamines are formed during cooking. The concentration of nitrosamines, mainly NPYR and NDMA, in the cooked bacon is dependent on many factors, including cooking temperature, mode of cooking, age of bacon, and the level of nitrite used in preparing the bacon (Gray, 1977). The cooked-out fat usually contains more nitrosamines than the cooked lean. There are some reports that the concentration of nitrosamines in a few other cured meat products such as country-style ham, spiced ham and salami also increases upon cooking (Greenberg, 1976; Eisenbrand et al., 1976). Recent surveys in Canada, the United Kingdom, the United States, and West Germany, however, indicate that nitrosamine levels in various meat products have been decreasing steadily over the past few years, and except in bacon, the levels normally

TABLE 2 Reported Occurrences of Nitrosamines in Foods

Item	Nitrosamines[a]	Level, ppb	
		Highest level reported	Typical average[c]
Cooked bacon	NDMA	6	3
	NDEA	43	Traces
	NPYR	108	10
	NPIP	8	Traces
Cooked-out bacon fat	NDMA	28	6
	NDEA	—[b]	—
	NPYR	207	22
	NPIP	—	—
Frankfurters	NDMA	84	Traces
	NDEA	7	—
	NPYR	8	—
	NPIP	15	—
Spiced sausages, salami, and ham	NDMA	54	Traces
	NDEA	25	Traces
	NPYR	105	Traces
	NPIP	250	Traces
Miscellaneous meat products (meat loaf, corned beef, bologna, etc.)	NDMA	48	Traces
	NDEA	91	Traces
	NPYR	19	Traces
	NPIP	50	Traces
Fish (untreated)	NDMA	18	2
	NDEA	13	—
Fish (treated with nitrate or nitrite)	NDMA	26	12
Chinese salted and dried fish and other seafoods	NDMA	300	4
	NPYR	37	Traces
Cheese	NDMA	19	1
	NDEA	2	—
	NPYR	4	—
Beer	NDMA	68	2.7

[a]NDMA = N-nitrosodimethylamine, NDEA = N-nitrosodiethylamine, NPYR = N-nitrosopyrrolidine, NPIP = N-nitrosopiperidine.

[b]Either negative or not enough data available.

[c]Based on most recent data (Sen, unpublished data). Older (when nitrite-spice premixes were used) average values would be much higher.

Sources: For references see Sen, 1974; Crosby, 1976; Sen et al., 1976b, 1977; Panalaks et al., 1974; Eisenbrand et al., 1976, 1977; Gorenen et al., 1976; Stephany et al., 1976; Gough and Walters, 1976; Iyengar et al., 1976; Magee et al., 1976; Spiegelhalder et al., 1979.

found are extremely low—usually in the low ppb range, and even those are detected only sporadically (Gough et al., 1977; Eisenbrand et al., 1977; Havery et al., 1977; Sen et al., 1976b; Sen et al., 1977).

The discovery of high levels (up to 25,000 ppb) of nitrosamines in spice-nitrite premixes (which were until recently used for the commercial preparation of a wide variety of cured meat products) and discontinuation of this practice have been major factors in reducing the concentration of nitrosamines in these products (Sen et al., 1973; Sen et al., 1974b; Sen et al., 1976b; Sen and McKinley, 1974; Rubin, 1977; Gough and Goodhead, 1975). The decline in the concentration of NPYR in cooked bacon may be attributed to a variety of factors, such as elimination of nitrate combined with a reduction of the permissible level of nitrite used for preparation of the bacon, greater control of the input of these additives by meat industries, or the addition of ascorbate, and so on, to inhibit the formation of nitrosamines (Sen et al., 1977; Havery et al., 1977). Similarly, the studies by Fong and Chan (1976) indicate that the use of pure sodium chloride instead of crude salt (which contains nitrate as an impurity) and the addition of benzoic acid preservative (to control the bacterial population) in the manufacture of Chinese dried salted fish can significantly reduce the formation of nitrosamines in these foods.

5. Analysis

The detection and quantitative estimation of trace levels of nitrosamines in a complex system such as food extracts may pose many problems because of the presence of interfering materials, which are invariably present at much higher concentration than the nitrosamines. Because of the carcinogenic nature of these compounds the method used for their detection must be highly reliable. To be applicable for trace analysis, the detection techniques must be highly specific (selective) and moderately accurate and precise. Various methods, including polarographic, spectrophotometric, thin-layer chromatographic, high pressure liquid chromatographic (HPLC), and gas-liquid chromatographic (GLC) techniques have been proposed for the detection of nitrosamines, but only a few are suitable for food analysis (Sen, 1974; Foreman and Goodhead, 1975). Prior to the actual determinative step the food sample is taken through various isolation and clean-up procedures in an effort to increase the relative (to impurities) concentration of the nitrosamines in the final extract. The procedures are usually lengthy and tedious and may take up to 2 days for the complete analysis of a sample (Crosby, 1976; Sen, 1974).

The most widely used screening methods are usually based on GLC analysis using either a thermionic detector or a nitrogen-specific Coulson or Hall detector. Each has its advantages and disadvantages. Nitrosamines can be oxidized to nitramines which are highly sensitive to electron capture detector. As little as 16 picograms of NDMA can be detected by this technique. Alternatively, nitrosamines can be reduced or cleaved to secondary amines which can be analyzed by GLC-electron capture technique after suitable derivatization (Crosby, 1976; Sen, 1974).

The most reliable method for the determination of nitrosamines is believed to be that involving the use of a combined GLC-MS technique (Foreman and Goodhead, 1975; Telling et al., 1971). The analysis can be carried out either in the low- or high-resolution mode. For trace analysis in the presence of interfering materials, it is preferable to use the latter. In this mode, the MS is set up to monitor a specific ion (either the NO^+ or molecular ion) at a resolution of 5000-10,000. The interference is minimal provided the sample has been carried through some extraction and cleanup procedures. Even then, one may occasionally encounter false-positive results. For this reason, the analyst must be very careful in interpreting the results. High-resolution specific-ion monitoring for more than one fragment ion can provide additional confidence in the results (Sen et al., 1976b). Figure 2 gives a typical example of GLC-MS tracings obtained from the analysis of two cured meat products.

More recently Fine and Rufeh (1974) and Fine et al. (1976b) have developed a chemiluminescent detector which is extremely sensitive and highly specific to N-nitroso compounds. The instrument is called the "Thermal Energy Analyzer" or simply TEA, and it can be inter-

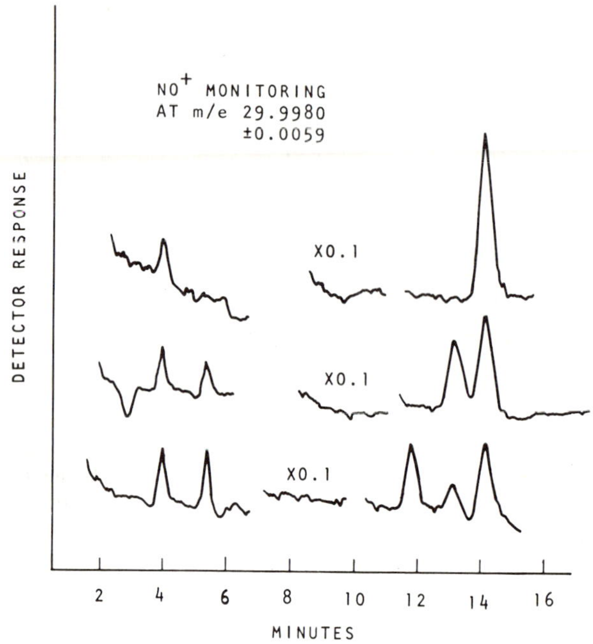

FIGURE 2 GLC-MS tracings for the NO^+ peak at a resolution of 5000. Bottom line: 2-3 ng each of NDMA, NDEA, NDBA, NPIP, and NPYR (left to right); middle line: 2 μl of final extract of a Chinese sausage. The gaps in the chromatograms represent areas where the recorder pen was lifted for accurate peak matching. Attenuation, 0.1

GLC conditions: 6 ft × 1/8 in. OD stainless-steel column packed with 25% 20 M Carbowax and 2% sodium hydroxide on 60-80 mesh Chromosorb P. Helium flow, 30 ml/min; column temperature, 140°C for 4 min, then programmed at 10°C/min to 180°C.

Source: Sen et al. (1976c).

faced with a GLC or HPLC apparatus. The available data obtained thus far (Fine et al., 1976a; Castegnaro and Walker, 1977) indicate that the instrument is highly reliable and useful for rapid screening of foodstuffs for nitrosamines.

6. Metabolism and Mechanism of Action

The dialkylnitrosamines are fairly stable chemically and they need enzymic activity for decomposition (Magee et al., 1976). Various studies have clearly shown that the simple N-nitrosamines are metabolized very rapidly in vivo in experimental animals. NDMA, for example, is broken down completely within 6 hr of parenteral injection to rats. By tracer studies with ^{14}C-labeled NDMA it has been found that about 65% of the injected radioactivity is expired as CO_2 within the first 12 hr (Dutton and Health, 1956). NDEA is metabolized by rats at an approximate rate of 4% of the dose per hr (Magee et al. 1976).

The available evidence indicates that NDMA and other N-nitrosamines are probably nontoxic and noncarcinogenic by themselves, and only after enzymic breakdown in the liver or other organs do they become transformed into the active carcinogens (Magee, 1971; Magee et al., 1976). The isolation of 7-methylguanine and other alkylated products from the liver and kidney of rats treated with N-nitrosocompounds gave support to the theory that some form of alkylating agent is formed as a result of the metabolic breakdown (Craddock and Magee, 1963, 1965; Loveless, 1969). In vitro studies with human liver slices suggest that

NDMA is metabolized by human liver in a similar fashion (Montesano and Magee, 1970). It was concluded that humans are probably as sensitive as rats to the carcinogenic action of NDMA.

The first step in the enzymic activation process of dialkylnitrosamines is believed to be hydroxylation at the α-carbon atom in one of the side-chains, followed by heterolysis to monoalkylnitrosamines and finally to diazoalkanes or carbonium ions (Druckrey et al., 1969). The diazoalkanes or the carbonium ions are probably responsible for alkylating nucleic acids and other cellular components and for initiating the changes in the normal cell growth process. Although this α-C hydroxylation and alkylation theory fits well with some compounds, data obtained with others are dissonant with this theoretical concept (Magee et al., 1976).

The requirement for enzymic activation to promote α-C hydroxylation explains the organotropic (organospecific) properties of various N-nitrosamines. A particular nitrosamine can be hydroxylated only if the necessary enzyme is present in that specific organ (Druckrey et al., 1969). It also explains the lack of carcinogenicity of some nitrosamines (e.g., N-nitrosodiphenylamine, tertiarybutylethylnitrosamine, etc.). On chemical grounds these compounds cannot form either an α-hydroxy intermediate or a diazoalkane.

The nitrosamides, on the other hand, are very unstable, and they can undergo spontaneous hydrolysis even at neutral pH (Magee et al., 1976). For this reason these compounds do not need metabolic activation in order to manifest their biological action. N-Nitrosomethylurea, for example, induces cancer of the forestomach after oral feeding to rats and produces skin neoplasms after topical application. After repeated intravenous injection some nitrosamides induce tumors in a distant organ, thus indicating some organotropism (Magee, 1973). The nitrosamides are also strong mutagens, but the chemically stable nitrosamines need some form of enzymic activation before they are able to exert their mutagenic properties.

Research on the metabolism of long-chain dialkylnitrosamines has produced some interesting results. Druckrey et al. (1964) have reported that metabolism of NDBA proceeds mainly through terminal hydroxylation of one of the side-chains, forming NBHBA which is a strong bladder carcinogen. This hydroxylation is probably carried out by the enzymes present in the bladder mucosa. More recently a few other metabolites, namely, N-nitrosobutyl-3-carboxypropylamine, N-nitrosobutyl-3-carboxy-2-hydroxypropylamine, and the glucuronide of NBHBA, have been detected in rat urine (Magee et al., 1976). Kruger (1972) has provided evidence for the β-oxidation of dialkylnitrosamines.

7. Carcinogenicity

Since the discovery of carcinogenicity of NDMA by Magee and Barnes (1954) various N-nitrosamines and N-nitrosamides have been tested for carcinogenicity and in a majority of the cases results have been positive (Druckrey et al., 1967; Magee et al., 1976). The carcinogenic potency, however, varies widely among various compounds, ranging from the highly potent NDMA and NDEA to weakly carcinogenic NSAR and N-nitrosodiethanolamine. Archer and Wishnok (1977) have calculated the relative potency of three N-nitrosamines commonly found in foods. Their data indicate that at equivalent daily doses NDMA and NDEA are about 6 to 7 times more potent than NPYR. NDMA has been shown to be carcinogenic in more than six species and NDEA in about 20 species including subhuman primates (Preussmann et al., 1976). No animal species tested has been found to be resistant to the carcinogenic action of this compound. It is, therefore, highly likely that humans are also susceptible to the carcinogenic action of nitrosamines, although direct evidence of their carcinogenicity in humans has not been reported.

The dose required for tumor induction depends somewhat on the species and ages of the animals. In the first study of Magee and Barnes (1956) 19 out of 20 rats fed NDMA in diet at a level of 50 ppm developed liver tumors. Later studies by Druckrey et al. (1963) and Terracini et al. (1967) demonstrated that even a much lower daily dose of NDEA (0.075 mg/kg body weight) or NDMA (2 ppm in the diet), if continued for a prolonged period, could be carcinogenic. One of the remarkable features of the N-nitroso compounds is that some of them can

TABLE 3 Carcinogenic Properties of Some Common N-Nitroso Compounds

Compound[a]	Species	Organs affected
NDMA	Mouse, hamsters, rat, rabbit, guinea pig, mink, rainbow trout	Liver, lung, kidney, nasal cavities
NDEA	Rat, mouse, hamsters, guinea pig, rabbit, dog, pig, trout, parakeet, monkey	Liver, kidney, esophagus, lung, forestomach, nasal cavities, trachea, bronchi, larynx
NDBA	Rat, mouse, hamsters, guinea pig	Bladder, esophagus, liver, forestomach, tongue, lung, trachea
N-Nitrosodiphenylamine	Rat	Negative
N-Nitrosomethyl-n-pentylamine	Rat	Esophagus
N-Nitroso-N-methylaniline	Rat, mouse	Esophagus, pharynx, forestomach, lung
NBHBA	Rat, mouse	Bladder, pelvis
NPRO	Mouse	Negative
NPYR	Rat, mouse, hamster	Forestomach, liver, esophagus, lung, nasal cavities, larynx, trachea
NMU	Rat, mouse, hamster, guinea pig, rabbit, dog	Central and peripheral nervous system, intestine, kidney, forestomach, jaw, bronchi, esophagus, trachea, bladder, vagina, skin, pancreas, ear ducts

[a]For abbreviations see Table 1.

Source: Adapted from Magee et al., 1976.

cause tumors after only a single dose. Thus, a single oral dose of 30 mg NDMA/kg body weight to adult rats or a single subcutaneous injection of 1 mg NDMA/kg body weight to newborn mice has been shown to be carcinogenic (Magee and Barnes, 1954; Toth et al., 1964). Many N-nitroso compounds can also cross the placental barrier and cause cancer in the offsprings (Magee et al., 1976).

The site of action varies from compound to compound, and many of the N-nitroso compounds exhibit striking structure-activity relationship. The site of action is also dependent on the dose level, mode of application, age, and nutritional status of the animals. A single dose of NDMA, for example, produces kidney tumors in adult rats, but a similar treatment induces mainly liver tumors in the newborn animals (Magee et al., 1976). In general, the symmetrical dialkylnitrosamines induce liver and occasionally kidney tumors, whereas the cyclic nitrosamines induce cancer at various sites such as liver, lung, stomach, esophagus, and so on. Among the symmetrical dialkylnitrosamines NDBA and N-nitrosodipentylamine are selective inducers of bladder tumors and lung tumors, respectively. The carcinogenic properties of some of the common N-nitroso compounds are described in Table 3.

Several dose-response studies carried out in rats suggest that the carcinogenic no-effect level of NDMA, NDEA and NPYR probably lies in the range of 1-5 ppm in the diet—NDMA and NDEA being more potent than NPYR (Preussmann et al., 1976).

B. Polycyclic Aromatic Hydrocarbons

1. Formation and Origin in Foods

Polycyclic aromatic hydrocarbons (PAHs), also known as polynuclear aromatic hydrocarbons, represent a group of hydrocarbons consisting of two or more benzenic ring structures, which may or may not have attached substituted groups. PAHs are formed in nature normally as a result of incomplete combustion or pyrolysis of organic matter (Badger, 1962), although endogenous biosynthesis in some higher plants, algae, and other organisms has been demonstrated (Borneff et al., 1968; Knorr and Schenk, 1968; Mallet and Tissier, 1969; Niaussat et al., 1970).

To date over 100 different PAHs have been identified in the environment and in foods, and about 22 of them are recognized carcinogens (Tilgner and Daun, 1969; Andelman and Suess, 1970; Gunther et al., 1967; NAS, 1972; EPA, 1975). Twelve of the 22 had been detected in foods (Table 4).

TABLE 4 Carcinogenic PAHs Identified in the Environment and in Foods

Abbreviation	Compound	Carcinogenic activity	Occurrence
B(a)A; BA	Benz(a)anthracene*	+	E, F, S
B(a)P; BP; 1,2-BP	Benzo(a)pyrene; 1,2-benzpyrene*	+++	E, F, S
B(e)P; 4,5-BP	Benzo(e)pyrene; 4,5-benzpyrene*	+	E, F, S
B(b)FL	Benzo(b)fluoranthene*	++	E, F
B(c)PA	Benzo(c)phenanthrene	+++	E
B(j)AC	Benz(j)aceanthrylene; cholanthrene	++	E, S
B(j)FL	Benzo(j)fluoranthene*	++	E, F
3,4-BFL	3,4-Benzofluoranthene	++	E
10,11-BFL	10,11-Benzofluoranthene	++	E
CH	Chrysene*	++	E, F, S
DB(ac)A	Dibenz(a,c)anthracene	+	F
DB(ah)A; DBA	Dibenz(a,h)anthracene*	+++	E, F
DB(ag)F	Dibenzo(a,g)fluorene	+	E
DB(ah)P	Dibenzo(a,h)pyrene*	+++	E, F, S
DB(aj)A	Dibenz(a,j)anthracene	+	E, F, S
DB(ai)P	Dibenzo(a,i)pyrene	+++	E, S
DB(el)P	Dibenzo(e,l)pyrene	+	E
DMB(a)A; DMBA	7,12-Dimethylbenz(a)anthracene	+++	E, F, S
IP	Indeno(1,2,3-cd)pyrene*	+	E, F
MCA; 3-MCA	Methylcholanthrene; 3-methylcholanthrene*	+++	E, F
2-MFL	2-Methylfluoranthene	+	E
TBP	Tribenzo(a,e,i)pyrene	+	E

+ Carcinogenic; ++, +++ Strongly carcinogenic.

* Considered as carcinogens by US PHS (EPA, 1975) and IARC, 1973.

E = Water, air, tobacco smoke, and gasoline or diesel exhaust.

F = Foods.

S = Curing smoke.

Source: Derived from Lo and Sandi, 1978.

The origin of PAHs in foods can be ascribed to a number of sources. The most significant ones are the pyrolysis products of fats resulting from roasting, toasting, barbecuing, or grilling of meats (Lijinsky and Shubik, 1964; Lijinsky and Ross, 1967) and the curing smoke of "liquid smoke" (Tilgner and Daun, 1969; Lijinsky and Shubik, 1965a; White et al., 1971). Although washing and filtration can reduce considerably the PAH concentration in curing smoke (Toth and Blass, 1972a, 1972b, 1972c; Toth 1969, 1971; Filipovic and Toth, 1971), at least some 6 to 11 different PAHs may not be removed completely by such processes. Commercial wax ("dairy wax"), hexane, and food grade carbon blacks have also been reported to contribute PAHs to foods, in various degrees (Howard and Haenni, 1963; Lijinsky and Raha, 1961; Panalaks, personal communication, 1976).

Natural forest and prairie fires and combustion of fossil fuels by humans also generate PAHs, which may then migrate into the food chain (Blumer and Youngblood, 1975; Dorr, 1965; Andelman and Suess, 1970; Hites et al., 1977; Laflamme and Hites, 1978). Another source of some importance is human-made pollution. Grimmer (1966) noticed a significant increase in a number of PAHs in samples of lettuce, kale, spinach, leeks, and tomatoes grown in regions with polluted atmosphere. Guerrero et al. (1976) reported that clams collected from petroleum-polluted surroundings contained up to 16 ppb benzopyrene (B(a)P), whereas those from nonpolluted areas contained only 1.5 ppb. Dunn and Stich (1976) found that the B(a)P concentration in mussels from Vancouver Harbor ranged from 2 to 30 ppb as compared to 54-215 ppb in those grown in the immediate vicinity of the wharf and of the creosoted barricade. When a similar study was conducted in southern California only 0.1 ppb B(a)P was found in mussels taken 1 km from pier or wharfs, and up to 0.4-8.2 ppb in those grown on piers or creosoted pilings (Dunn and Young, 1976).

2. Analysis

The procedure of PAH analysis in foods usually involves several steps—organic solvent extraction, chromatographic separation, and identification and quantitation. Various modifications of extracting techniques are often necessary prior to chromatographic separation. Liquid-liquid partition is frequently used to isolate PAHs from liquid smoke (White et al., 1971), and saponification following the initial extraction is required to remove fats from the extract in the case of meats with high fat content (Bailey and Dungal, 1958).

Thus methods of analyzing PAHs depend very much on the characteristics of the samples. Using isooctane extraction, washing with alkali solution, water, phosphoric acid, dimethylsulfoxide, followed by column or thin-layer chromatography separation, White et al. (1971) were able to determine B(a)P content in liquid smoke flavors, with the aid of ultraviolet (UV) and fluorometric procedure (Haenni, 1968; Tilgner and Daun, 1969); similar methods were also reported suitable for B(a)P, benz(a)anthracene (B(a)A), and dibenz(a,h)anthracene (DB(ah)A) determination in vegetable oils and in solvents used for the extraction of edible oils (Howard et al., 1966b; Howard et al., 1968a).

In a study of controlling PAH contamination in petroleum waxes Lijinsky et al. (1963) described a method involving chromatography separations on silica gel, partition between cyclohexane and nitromethane, and UV spectral analysis for dibenz(a,h)pyrene (DB(ah)P) and DB(ah)A determination. Employing dimethyl sulfoxide-phosphoric acid mixture as extracting solvents, and chromatography on magnesia-celite column, Haenni et al. (1962a, b) and Howard et al. (1965) extended the detection limit to include B(a)P, benzo(c)pyrene (B(c)P), B(a)A, DB(ah)P, DB(ah)A, and 7,12-dimethylbenz(a)anthracene (DMBA) in mineral oils and waxes.

For smoked foods an early method of Bailey and Dungal (1958) was available specifically for B(a)P. With some modifications it was established that B(a)P, B(a)A, and DB(ah)A can be determined in smoked food products, as well as in "total diet" composite samples at the level of 2 ppb (Howard et al., 1966a, 1968b). These methods consist of extraction with ethanol, saponification with potassium hydroxide, further extraction with isooctane and partition on paper or thin-layer chromatography, and finally measurement by UV and spectrophotofluorometry. Lijinsky and Shubik (1965a, b), on the other hand, reported that benzene or acetone extraction, partition with dimethylsulfoxide and cyclohexane or isooctane, and chromatography on paper or on silica gel column are effective for cooked, broiled, or grilled meats.

Others reported that methanol extraction followed by methanol-cyclohexane or methanol-benzene-hexane partition is effective for separating PAHs from oysters (Cahnmann and Kuratsune, 1957), and ether-hexane extraction plus similar partition for clams (Warner, 1974). Procedures developed by Grimmer and Hildebrandt (1965a, b, 1966) are used for determining B(a)A and DB(ah)A in vegetables, grains, coffee, and tea.

More recently methods of liquid-liquid partition, with methanol-water-cyclohexane and dimethylformamide-water-cyclohexane systems, combined with high-pressure liquid chromatographic separation, using UV and fluorescence detectors, were introduced. With these techniques a total of 10 carcinogens, including B(a)P, chrysene (CH), B(a)A, benzo(b)fluoranthene (B(b)FL), benzo(j)fluoranthene (B(j)FL), B(e)P, dibenz(a, i)anthracene (DB(ai)A), DB(ah)A, indeno (1, 2, 3-cd)pyrene (IP), and DMBA, can be extracted, separated, and determined in smoked foods, vegetables, fats, and broiled meats (Grimmer and Bohnke, 1975; Panalaks, 1976).

3. Occurrence and Concentration

The review of Howard and Fazio (1969) indicated that B(a)P, B(e)P, B(a)A, and CH had been detected in edible vegetable oils by European workers from 1962-1965. Later Howard et al. (1966b) in the United States found up to 1.6 ppb B(a)P or B(e)P and 8.6 ppb B(a)A in some soybean, cottonseed, corn, olive, and peanut oils, but not in safflower oil, and Fritz in Europe reported about 0.4 ppb B(a)P and 2.2 ppb B(a)A to be present in margarine or mayonnaise (Grasso and O'Hare, 1976). In re-used cooking oil, the B(a)P content is apparently higher; a level of 0.9-1.9 ppb has been reported (Malanoski et al., 1968).

Raw meats and raw fish from unpolluted waters normally are free of PAHs (Howard et al., 1966a, c), but may contain varying amounts after being smoked or cooked. Data published over a decade ago from Europe revealed that the concentration of B(a)P alone in smoked fish, mutton, and sausage ranged from 0.1 to 60 ppb (Howard and Fazio, 1969), depending on the condition of smoke generation and of smoking process (Draudt, 1963). Since then, investigation has been expanded to include other carcinogenic PAHs and conducted also in other parts of the world. Accumulated information up to 1970 are summarized in Table 5. As indicated, the most common carcinogenic PAHs present in commercially smoked fish and meats were B(a)A, B(a)P, B(e)P, and CH, and their concentrations were well below 10 ppb; similar concentrations were also noted for commercially broiled or barbecued meats. However, home-smoked and laboratory-broiled meats generally contain much more PAH.

Recently, with the aid of modern techniques for analysis, more data of carcinogenic PAH in foods have been generated (Table 6). These data seem to confirm the observation referred to earlier that the smoked meats and fish produced in North America in general contain relatively low levels of B(a)A, B(a)P, B(e)P, and CH; however, other carcinogenic PAHs such as 3-methylcholanthrene (MCA), IP, DMBA, DB(ah)P, dibenz(aj)anthracene (DB(aj)A), and DB(ah)A are readily detectable. One other noticeable finding is that some carcinogenic PAH levels in both smoked and nonsmoked oysters are rather high. The B(a)P levels in the smoked meats reported in Table 6 also appear to be significantly lower than recent data reviewed by Walker (1977), in which up to 4, 14, 11, and 33 ppb were being found in smoked bacon, ham, meats, and sausages, respectively. Most recent analyses by Lintas et al. (1979) of commercially available Italian foods, however, revealed that the levels in smoked, cooked, or toasted food products (not including fish or shellfish) are rather low (0.05-1.28 ppb) but relatively high in toasted tea leaves (9.51 ppb), olive oil (2.36-3.59 ppb), and butter (0.47-0.91 ppb).

Various workers in Japan and in Europe have reported the presence of carcinogenic PAHs in fruits, vegetables, and related products as well. The amounts detected are represented in Table 7. The higher concentration in kale was probably due to environmental contamination (IARC, 1973). Recently Walker (1977) further reported that

TABLE 5 Carcinogenic PAHs Found in Foods, Published Prior to 1970

Food	ppb							Reference
	B(a)A	B(a)P	B(e)P	CH	B(b)FL	B(j)FL	DB(aj)A	
Commercially smoked								
Eel, lumpfish, trout	Trace	0–1.0	Trace	ND	ND	ND	ND	Thorsteinsson, 1969
Herring, salmon, sturgeon, whitefish	0.5–1.7	0.8–1.0	0.4–1.2	ND	ND	ND	—	Howard et al., 1966a
Salmon, haddock	0–0.2	0.3–1.0	—	0.3–0.6	ND	ND	ND	Lijinsky and Shubik, 1965b
Chubs, salmon, whitefish, kippers, cod	—	1.3–6.6	—	1.4	ND	ND	ND	Malanoski et al., 1968
Horse mackerel	0.6–2.9	0.3–0.9	0.2–1.2	0.4–2.1	0.1–1.2	Trace–0.5	ND	Masuda et al., 1966
Beef, pork, sausages, frankfurters, ham	0.4–2.8	3.2	1.2	ND	ND	ND	—	Howard et al., 1966a
Sausages, ham	0.5–9.6	0.4–0.7	0	0.5–2.6	ND	ND	ND	Malanoski et al., 1968
Mutton, sausages	0.5–2.0	Trace	Trace–5.0	ND	ND	ND	ND	Thorsteinsson, 1969
Barbecued beef	13.2	3.2	1.7	9.6	ND	ND	ND	Malanoski et al., 1968
Commercially broiled or barbecued								
Steaks, ribs	1.4–3.6	5.8–10.5	5.5–7.5	0.6–2.2	ND	ND	ND	Lijinsky and Shubik, 1964, 1965b
Home smoked:[a] mutton, lamb	3–115	3–107	2–27	ND	ND	ND	ND	Thorsteinsson, 1969
Laboratory broiled								
Steak, hamburger, pork, chicken (charcoal)	2.7–31	2.6–50	3.4–17	0.3–25	ND	ND	ND	Lijinsky and Ross, 1967
T-bone steak (flame)	3.9	4.4	5.7	2.0	ND	ND	ND	

[a]At various conditions such as close to or far from heat source, or with casings.

ND = Not determined or not detectable by the method used.

TABLE 6 Carcinogenic PAHs Found in Foods, Published After 1970

Food	ppb B(a)A	B(a)P	B(e)P	B(b)FL	B(j)FL	CH	DB(ah)A	DB(aj)A	DB(ah)P	DMBA	IP	MCA	Reference
Commercially smoked													
Bacon, ham, others[a]	0.5–8.0	1.0–2.0	0.2–5.0	—	ND	ND	ND	0.6	0.5–8.0	—	0.5–1.0	ND	Panalaks 1976
Sausages	0.4–0.55	0.05–0.08	ND	ND	ND	ND	0.04–1.10	ND	ND	0.05–2.15	ND	0.04–0.15	Frethein, 1976
Ham, sausages, mortadella, salami	0.5–9.0	0.2–4.4	0.5–2.9	0.7–3.5	ND	0–9.2	ND	ND	ND	ND	ND	ND	Filipovic and Toth, 1971; Toth and Blass, 1972a
Heavy smoked ham and bacon	6–33	5–26	3.6–55	3.6–33	ND	2.6–66	ND	ND	ND	ND	ND	ND	
Mussels	10.0	—	—	—	ND	ND	ND	—	—	—	—	ND	Panalaks 1976
Fish[b]	1–20	0.5–15	1.0–2.0	—	ND	ND	ND	—	5.0	—	—	ND	
Oysters	30.0	2.0	16.0	25.0	ND	ND	ND	1.0	—	38.0	5.0	ND	
Nonsmoked oysters	15–30	—	1.0	—	ND	ND	ND	—	—	25.0	2.0	ND	
Fish[c]	6–59	2–37	3–29	4–37	2–30	10–173	ND	ND	ND	ND	ND	ND	Masuda and Kuratsune, 1971
Laboratory broiled													
Meats[d]	1–50	3–25	1–20	2–30	ND	ND	ND	8.0	ND	—	2–10	ND	Panalaks, 1976

[a]Bologna, frankfurters, salami, pepperoni, sausages, beef, pork, and gouda cheese.

[b]Herring and other unspecified fish including canned fish.

[c]Katsuwonus vagans, Scomber japonicus, or Saronnia melanosticta.

[d]Steak, chicken, hamburger, frankfurters, and Chinese sausages.

TABLE 7 Carcinogenic PAHs Found in Fruits and Plant Products

Food	ppb					
	B(a)A	B(a)P	B(e)P	B(b)FL	CH	DB(ah)A
Kale	43-230	12.6-48	1.1-67.2		58-395	0.1-2.6
Other vegetables[a]	4.6-16	2.8-7.4	3.7-14.7		5.7-28	0.3-1.0
Fruits[b]	0-0.3	0.2-8.0	0-0.2		0-0.5	0-0.04
Cereals	0.4-6.8	0.2-4.1	0.3-4.9		0.8-14	0.1-0.6
Tea[c]		3.9-21.0	1.9-22		4.6-6.0	
Dry yeast	2.5-93.5	1.8-40.4	3.1-55.0		42-203	0.9
Roast peanuts	0.9		0.4		0.01-0.7	
Roast coffee (powder)	0.5-14	0.1-4.0	0.3-7.0	1.2-2.1	0.6-19.1	
Heavy roast coffee (powder)	43	15	20.5	1.2-3.0		

[a]Includes spinach, salad, soybean.

[b]Apples, tomatoes, and unspecified fruits.

[c]Includes tea extracts.

Source: Based on data from IARC, 1973.

while most of the alcoholic beverages consumed in northwest France contained no detectable amounts of PAH, 15 farm-produced apple brandies were found to contain 5-10 ppb B(a)P, with one of the samples also containing 4.5 ppb B(a)A, 5.3 ppb CH, 3.5 ppb B(b)FL, 2.0 ppb B(e)P, 0.3 ppb DB(aj)A, and 0.6 ppb IP.

4. Metabolism

In a rat study with isotope-labeled PAH, Daniel et al. (1967) showed that intragastrically administered DB(ah)A, MCA, DMB(a)A, and dibenz(ac)anthracene (DB(ac)A) were mostly rapidly absorbed, held for a short period in the liver and kidneys, and then excreted, via bile, in the feces and the urine. Some of the absorbed PAHs are retained in the tissues for several days. While the chemical form of the excreted PAH in this study was not determined, it was reported that when mice were injected with DB(ah)A, a large quantity of acidic and phenolic compounds, along with small amounts of unchanged DB(ah)A, was present in the excreta and in the tissues (Heidelberger et al., 1948). Follow-up studies, however, identified three quinones in the liver of mice which had received intravenous injection of DB(ah)A (Heidelberger et al., 1953).

When radioactive B(a)P was injected into rats, the metabolic products collected from biliary fistulae were mostly of four different oxidation products in conjugated form with sulfuric and glucuronic acids (Falk et al., 1962). Further investigation by Boyland and Sims (1964) found four phenols and four dihydrodiols, also as sulfuric or glucuronic acid conjugates, in the urine, bile, and feces of B(a)A-treated rats.

In vitro systems of liver preparations have also been studied extensively. The metabolites that have been identified in these two systems are listed and compared in Table 8 (Lo and Sandi, 1978). It seems that most of the carcinogenic PAHs are similarly metabolized both in intact animals and in liver preparations, and give rise to phenols, quinones, and dihydrodiols. Although in vivo studies with DMB(a)A and MCA appear to be lacking in the literature, in tissue cultures, these two, B(a)P, and DBA were shown to be metabolized comparably to those in liver preparations (Huberman et al., 1971c).

In recent years metabolism of B(a)P has also been examined in liver and lung microsome preparations from monkey (Leber et al., 1976) and from humans (Selkirk et al., 1976; Freudenthal et al., 1978). Results of the chromatographic profiles again reveal the presence of

TABLE 8 Metabolites of Carcinogenic PAHs Found in Rat or Mouse Studies

PAH	Group	In vitro	In vivo
B(a)A	Dihydrodiols	5,6-diH-5,6-diOH-BA[a]	3,4-diH-3,4-diOH-BA
		7,8-diH-7,8-diOH-BA	5,6-diH-5,6-diOH-BA
		8,9-diH-8,9-diOH-BA	8,9-diH-8,9-diOH-BA
		—	10,11-diH-10,11-diOH-BA
	Phenols	2-OH-BA	—
		3-OH-BA	3-OH-BA
		4-OH-BA	4-OH-BA
		—	8-OH-BA
		—	9-OH-BA
	Quinones	BA-7,12-dione	BA-7,12-dione
DB(ah)A	Dihydrodiols	1,2-diH-1,2-diOH-DBA	—
		3,4-diH-3,4-diOH-DBA[a]	—
		5,6-diH-5,6-diOH-DBA[a]	—
	Phenols	3-OH-DBA	—
		4-OH-DBA	—
	Quinones	—	DBA-9,10-dione
		—	DBA-3,4-dione
		—	4,8-diOH-DBA-9,10-dione
DMBA[b]	Dihydrodiols	8,9-diH-8,9-diOH-DMBA	
		5,6-diH-5,6-diOH-DMBA[a]	
	Derivatives	Hydroxymethyl derivatives	
MCA[b]	Dihydrodiols	11,12-diH-11,12-diOH-MCA[a]	
	Phenols	1-OH-MCA	
		2-OH-MCA	
		1,2-diOH-MCA	
	Derivatives	3-Hydroxymethyl derivatives	
B(a)P	Dihydrodiols	1,2-diH-1,2-diOH-BP	—
		4,5-diH-4,5-diOH-BP[a]	—
		7,8-diH-7,8-diOH-BP	—
		9,10-diH-9,10-diOH-BP	—
		—	1,6-diH-1,6-diOH-BP
		—	3,6-diH-3,6-diOH-BP
	Phenols	1-OH-BP	1-OH-BP
		3-OH-BP	3-OH-BP
		7-OH-BP	—
		9-OH-BP	—
		—	6-OH-BP
		—	1,6-diOH-BP
		—	3,6-diOH-BP
	Quinones	BP-1,6-dione	—
		BP-3,6-dione	BP-3,6-dione
		BP-6,12-dione	—
B(e)P	Dihydrodiols	4,5-diH-4,5-diOH-BeP	—
CH	Dihydrodiols	1,2-diH-1,2-diOH-CH	—
		3,4-diH-3,4-diOH-CH	—
		—	3-OH-CH

[a]K-region epoxide.

[b]In vivo studies with these two compounds have not been conducted.

Abbreviations: OH = hydroxy; diH = dihydro; diOH = dihydroxy.

a number of dihydrodiols and quinones, including 9,10-dihydro-9,10-dihydroxy-benzo(a)pyrene (BP-9,10-diol), benzo(a)pyrene-6,12-dione (BP-6,12-quinone), 4,5-dihydro-4,5-dihydroxy-benzo(a)pyrene (BP-4,5-diol), 7,8-dihydro-7,8-dihydroxy-benzo(a)pyrene (BP-7,8-diol), benzo(a)pyrene-1,6-dione (BP-1,6-quinone), benzo(a)pyrene-3,6-dione (BP-3,6-quinone), 9-hydroxy-benzo(a)pyrene (9-OH-BP), and 3-hydroxy-benzo(a)pyrene (3-OH-BP).

The latter six compounds have also been detected (15% of the dose) by Hecht et al. (1979) in the feces of rats, along with another 6-13% of unchanged B(a)P, at 48 hr after oral administration of B(a)P at 36 μmol/rat. In this study B(a)P provided in the form of charcoal-broiled hamburger (containing 52 ppb B(a)P) was investigated as well. When rats and humans were fed this hamburger at the B(a)P levels, respectively, 0.06 μg/rat and 24 μg/kg body weight to humans, it was shown that the excretion of unmetabolized B(a)P in the feces was 11% of the dose in rats, whereas nil in humans at 48-72 hr after the ingestion.

The primary enzyme system responsible for the metabolism of PAHs is the microsomal cytochrome mixed function oxygenase, also known as aryl hydrocarbon hydroxylase (Gelboin et al., 1972). This enzyme system is known to be present in various tissues of rodents (Aitio, 1973) and in human liver (Kuntzman et al., 1966), skin (Levin et al., 1972), and placenta (Nebert et al., 1969). Recent experiments further demonstrated that the enzymes present in human placentas, and in fetal livers, lungs, kidneys, and adrenal glands were able to convert B(a)P and DMBA to their mutagenic metabolites (Juchau et al., 1978).

In the course of metabolism the most important group of intermediate metabolites is epoxides (arene oxides). The type most commonly believed to be responsible for the biological effects of their parent compounds is so-called K-region epoxides (Grover et al., 1972; Selkirk et al., 1975). B(a)A, B(a)P, DB(ah)A, DMB(a)A, MCA, and B(e)P all can form such K-region epoxides (Grover et al., 1971; Keysell et al., 1973; Burki et al., 1972; Sims, 1966; Grover et al., 1972; Sims, 1970). For example, the K-region epoxide of B(a)A forms at 5- and 6-position, and for B(a)P at 4- and 5- position.

Although under biological conditions these K-region epoxides are converted to their respective phenols, dihydrodiols, or conjugated glutathione, some K-region epoxides were known to react covalently with DNA and exhibit higher levels of biological activity leading to malignant transformation (Grover et al., 1971; Huberman et al., 1971b, 1972; Marquardt et al., 1972), and higher mutagenic activity than their parent compounds (Ames et al., 1972; Huberman et al., 1971a).

However, in whole animal studies, either with topical or parenteral route of administration, the K-region epoxides of B(a)P, CH, B(a)A, DB(ah)A, DM(a)A, and MCA were found to exhibit less carcinogenic activity than their parent compounds (Boyland and Sims, 1967; Miller and Miller, 1967; Sims, 1967; Grover et al., 1975). Moreover, in studies with B(a)P and B(a)A evidence seems to indicate that BP-7,8-diol and BA-3,4-diol and bay-region epoxides, such as BP-7,8-diol-9, 10-epoxides, and BA-3,4-diol-1,2-epoxides, are in fact more mutagenic and carcinogenic than their parent compounds or K-region epoxides (Levin et al., 1976; Kapitulnik et al., 1977; Wood et al., 1976, 1977a, b; Mager et al., 1977). Most recent investigations further suggested that B(a)P-7β, 8α-diol, 9α-, 10α-epoxide, produced from BP(-)trans-7,8-diol, is the most potent carcinogen among several epoxides or diols of B(a)P tested (Huberman et al., 1976, 1977; Slaga et al., 1978).

Apart from the aforementioned possibility of activation by formation of epoxide, some workers think that carbonium ions on methyl groups and radical cations generated by one-electron oxidation are the ultimate carcinogens (Dipple et al., 1968; Hulbert, 1975; Fried and Schumm, 1967; Umans et al., 1969; Cavalieri et al., 1975, 1976). Others are even of the opinion that carcinogenic PAHs are active per se and need no activation (Farber, 1968; Burki and Bresnick, 1975).

5. Carcinogenicity

After the early observation of high incidence of scrotum cancer in chimney sweeps (Pott, 1775), Yamagiwa and Ichikawa (1915) developed skin cancer in the ear of rabbits by repeated application with coal tar, and Kennaway (1925) succeeded in producing carcinogenic tars from

TABLE 9 Tumorigenic Effects of Carcinogenic PAH via Oral Routes

Compound	Animal	Levels causing no effects	Levels causing effects	Tumorigenic effects	Reference
B(a)A	Mice	Single dose of 0.5 mg	8 × 0.5 mg in 24 days	Forestomach papilloma, 16 months	Bock and King, 1959
	Infant mice	—	15 × 1.5 mg in 15 weeks	Lung adenoma, hepatoma, and stomach papilloma, within 500 days	Klein, 1963
B(a)P	Mice	30 ppm in diet for 100 days	Over 50 ppm in diet for 100 days or 25 ppm over 100 days, or 250 ppm for 90 days	Gastric tumors, papilloma and squamous cell carcinoma (stomach), leukemia, and pulmonary adenoma	Neal and Rigdon, 1967; Rigdon and Neal, 1966, 1969; Rigdon et al., 1969
	Rats	—	Single dose of 100 mg or daily dose of 2.5 mg	Papilloma (esophagus and forestomach) and mammary tumors	Gibel 1964; Huggins and Yang, 1962
DB(ah)A	Mice	—	0.4 mg daily in drinking water for 166 days	Forestomach papilloma	Lorenz and Stewart, 1948
		—	0.2 mg/ml drinking water for 200 days	Pulmonary adenoma, alveologenic carcinoma, and mammary carcinoma	Snell and Stewart 1962, 1963
DMB(a)A	Mice	—	Single dose of 0.5 mg	Gastric papilloma, 8–10 months	Bock and King, 1959
		—	8 × 0.5 mg in 24 days	Gastric papilloma and carcinoma, 8–10 months	Bock and King, 1959
	Mice	—	1.0 mg weekly for 8 weeks	Carcinoma, mammary glands, 5 weeks after treatment	Biancifiori et al., 1961
	Mice	—	6 × 1.0 mg in 6 weeks	Lymphoma, latent period, 26 weeks	Chen, 1970
	Rats	Single dose of 5.0 mg	Single dose of 5–10 mg	Mammary tumors, latent period, 40 days	Eskin et al., 1968; Flesher and Sydnor, 1970

(Table 9 continued)

Compound	Animal	Levels causing no effects	Levels causing effects	Tumorigenic effects	Reference
	Rats	Single dose of 350 mg/kg body weight	8 × 40 mg/kg body weight in 16 weeks	Mammary carcinoma and leukemia, in 100 days	Yoshida and Fukunishi, 1977; Huggins et al., 1974
MCA	Mice	—	Single dose of 0.5 mg	Gastric papilloma, 8–10 months	Bock and King, 1959
		—	8 × 0.5 mg in 24 days	Gastric papilloma and carcinoma, 8–10 months	Bock and King, 1959
	Infant mice	—	15 × 1.5 mg in 15 weeks	Stomach papilloma, hepatoma, and pulmonary adenoma	Klein, 1963
	Rats	—	10 × 5 mg	Leukemia	Moloney et al. 1971

petroleum, coal, and organic matter. Since then hydrocarbons have been investigated extensively and many proved to have carcinogenic activity both in whole animals and in cultures.

Following B(a)P or MCA treatment in beef serum based culture, Berwald and Sachs (1963) observed morphologic alterations and piled-up colonies of hamster embryonic fibroblasts. Further studies revealed that B(a)A, B(e)P, B(a)P, DB(ac)A, DB(ah)A, MCA, and DMB(a)A can all induce in vitro transformation of normal cells to tumor cells (Berwald and Sachs, 1965; Dipaolo et al., 1969a, b); several cell lines derived from B(a)P-treated colonies were also capable of producing fibrosarcomas on injection to hamsters.

When organ cultures of mouse ventral prostate were treated with MCA, Lasnitzki (1963) noticed hyerplastic and preneoplastic changes in prostate cells. In another similar culture it was found that not only MCA but also DB(ah)A and DMB(a)A could induce similar changes; however, none of them can produce tumors when injected into isologous mice (Roller and Heidelberger, 1967). With additional treatment of pronase, Heidelberger and Iype (1967) succeeded in producing transplantable tumors in C3H mice with DMB(a)A and MCA. Several B_1 prostate cell lines developed by Chen and Heidelberger (1969a) were also shown to induce fibrosarcomas in mice by pretreatment of B(a)P, MCA, DMB(a)A, or DB(ah)A (Chen and Heidelberger, 1969b, c).

There is vast literature on whole animal studies which is briefly outlined. Data published during 1947 to 1969 were documented in the U.S. PHS survey (Hartwell 1951; Shubik and Hartwell, 1957, 1969). These data had been reviewed by EPA (1975), NAS (1972), and IARC (1973). According to these and more recent surveys by the U.S. PHS (Tracor/Jitco, 1973), and by Lo and Sandi (1978), apparently only five known carcinogenic PAH have actually been tested and demonstrated to induce tumor formation by the oral route of administration; these are B(a)A, B(a)P, DB(ah)A, DMB(a)A, and MCA. Some published data which have demonstrated tumorigenic effects at relatively low levels are summarized in Table 9. These data showed that the most common encountered effects were leukemia, forestomach tumors, hepatoma, pulmonary adenoma, and mammary tumors, and that the levels required to induce these effects, although some may not be regarded as minimum toxic effect levels, were extremely high as compared to the concentrations that may normally be expected in foods.

Despite the fact that some PAHs are well known carcinogens in humans and can produce serious adverse effects in animals like those noted here, cases of human cancer directly attributed to PAH contamination in foods have not been reported. Neither is there adequate epidemiological evidence to link foodborne PAHs to any specific cancer or diseases in the literature, although the high incidence of stomach cancer in Iceland was suggested to be associated with the high consumption of smoked fish and meats (Dungal, 1961).

IV. UNINTENTIONAL FOOD ADDITIVES

A. Mycotoxins

Toxic metabolites (mycotoxins) produced by filamentous fungi in improperly stored agricultural products, or, as is becoming increasingly evident, in crops before harvest, may result in mycotoxicoses of farm animals or be carried through in trace amounts into the human food supply. Only a very small percentage of the known mycotoxins are demonstrated carcinogens by the oral route. They are aflatoxins B_1, G_1, B_2, and M_1, sterigmatocystin, cyclochlorotine, (-)-luteoskyrin, and (+)-rugulosin; to these may be added griseofulvin, a fungal metabolite not usually considered a mycotoxin, and from recent reports, ochratoxin A, and T-2 toxin. Local tumors have been produced by subcutaneous injection of penicillin G and the mycotoxins patulin and penicillic acid. Extracts of whole cultures of certain fungi, *Candida parapsilosis* and other pathogens for humans, *Penicillium viridicatum*, and *P. camemberti* are also reported to have carcinogenic properties. Methods of analysis and natural occurrence in agricultural commodities and foods have been published for the aflatoxins, sterigmatocystin, patulin, penicillic acid, penicillins, ochratoxin A, and T-2 toxin. Of these only the aflatoxins have been epidemiologically associated with cancer in humans.

1. Aflatoxins

The aflatoxins were discovered during investigations into the deaths of over 100,000 turkey poults in England in 1960 (Goldblatt, 1969). The cause was traced to Brazilian groundnut meal in the feeds, which contained several ppm of aflatoxins formed by *Aspergillus flavus*. Aflatoxins B_1, B_2, G_1, G_2, and M_1 are produced by this species and by *A. parasiticus*, and are of particular concern to regulatory authorities because of their carcinogenicity.

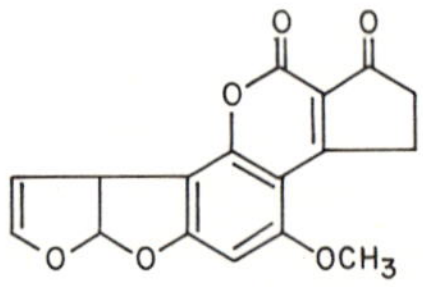

B_1

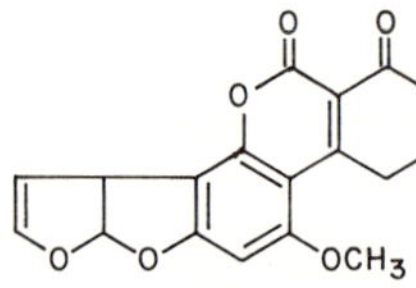

G_1

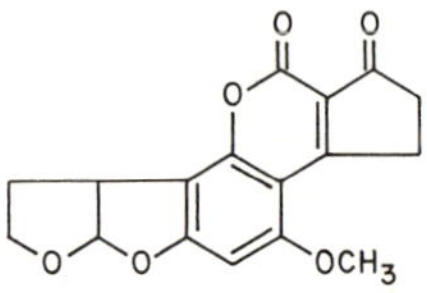

B_2

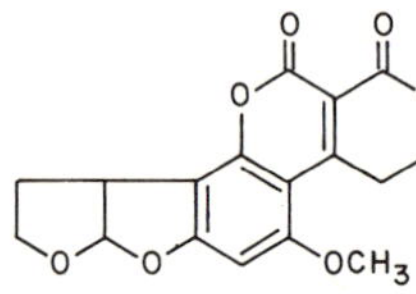

G_2

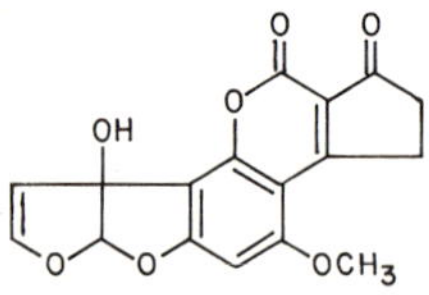

M_1

AFLATOXINS

a. Carcinogenicity

Aflatoxin B_1 has induced liver carcinoma in male Fischer rats at concentrations in the diet as low as 1 ppb (Wogan et al., 1974). Aflatoxin G_1 and (by injection) aflatoxin B_2 are also carcinogenic to the rat liver, but there is no evidence that aflatoxin G_2 is a carcinogen (Wogan et al., 1971). High doses of aflatoxin B_1 or G_1 have also caused renal neoplasms when fed to rats (Butler et al., 1969; Epstein et al., 1969).

b. Metabolism

Aflatoxin M_1, which may accompany the other aflatoxins in minor amounts in fungal cultures, is formed by metabolism of aflatoxin B_1 in many animal species and has been detected in commercial milk and cheese samples, in concentrations generally below 1 ppb (Kiermeier et al., 1977; Polzhofer, 1977; Purchase, 1972). Aflatoxin M_1 has been shown to cause hepatocarcinoma in the rainbow trout, and there is some evidence that the synthetic racemic mixture is a hepatocarcinogen in the rat (Butler, 1974; Wogan and Paglialunga, 1974). In addition to aflatoxin M_1, aflatoxin B_1 is metabolized in the liver to a variety of demethylated, reduced, hydrated, and/or hydroxylated products—aflatoxin P_1, aflatoxin B_{2a}, aflatoxicol, aflatoxin Q_1, and aflatoxicol H_1—whose formation may depend on the animal or avian species concerned (Büchi et al., 1974; Patterson, 1973; Salhab and Hsieh, 1975). Strong indirect evidence has indicated that aflatoxin B_1-2,3-oxide, in itself unstable, is the major activated metabolite responsible for macromolecular binding of aflatoxin B_1 (Swenson et al., 1977). The identification of a major DNA adduct as 2,3-dihydro-2(N^7-guanyl)-3-hydroxyaflatoxin B_1, released by formic acid from aflatoxin B_1 bound to calf thymus DNA, lends support to this hypothesis (Essigmann et al., 1977).

c. Occurrence

Aflatoxins B_1, B_2, G_1, and G_2 have been shown to occur naturally in many agricultural commodities, with serious contamination possible in corn, cottonseed, copra, and nuts, particularly peanuts (Stoloff, 1976b). A relatively high temperature (25–45°C) and a water activity (a_W) of 0.84–0.86 favor the molds responsible for aflatoxin production. Hence tropical and subtropical products are particularly susceptible to contamination, a fact illustrated by the generally higher incidences and levels of aflatoxins found in corn from the southeast United States compared to those from the corn belt (Shotwell, 1977; Stoloff, 1976a). Fortunately, aflatoxins do not survive the refining operations used in the manufacture of vegetable oils (Parker and Melnick, 1966), and the main sources of aflatoxin in the human diet in North America are nuts and nut products such as peanut butter. Maximum levels of total aflatoxins permitted in these foods in Canada are 15 ppb (proposed also as a tolerance in the United States). In the underdeveloped world exposure of the human population to aflatoxins is sufficiently high in several countries (The Philippines, Thailand, Kenya, Uganda, Swaziland, and Mozambique) to have enabled epidemiological correlations (not necessarily causative) to be made between aflatoxin contamination and incidences of primary hepatoma (Bulato-Jayme et al., 1976; Campbell and Stoloff, 1974; van Rensburg et al., 1974; Shank, 1976). Reports of the presence of aflatoxin B_1 in human liver provide additional evidence of human exposure to aflatoxin, which may be associated with acute encephalopathy and fatty degeneration of the viscera (EFDV) in Thai children (Phillips et al., 1976; Richir et al., 1976; Shank et al., 1971).

d. Analysis

Analysis of foodstuffs for aflatoxins is facilitated by their intense fluorescence when irradiated by long-wave UV light. Less than 1 ng of each aflatoxin can be detected by thin-layer chromatography (TLC), and detection limits for peanut butter, for example, are on the order of 2 ppb. High-pressure liquid chromatography (HPLC) offers even greater sensitivity (Panalaks and Scott, 1977). The Association of Official Analytical Chemists (AOAC) has published TLC methods for the determination of aflatoxins in peanuts and peanut products, cocoa beans, coconut products, corn, cottonseed products, green coffee, pistachio nuts, eggs and soybeans, and for alfatoxin M_1 in dairy products, together with chemical and biological (chick embryo) confirmatory procedures (AOAC, 1980). Sampling of lots of whole peanuts, corn, and so on, is the greatest source of error in aflatoxin analysis because of the great variability in aflatoxin content of individual kernels, which can be as high as 1,100,000 ppb aflatoxin B_1 (Cucullu et al., 1966; Whitaker and Dickens, 1974). Electronic sorting following by careful handpicking can reduce the aflatoxin concentration in a lot of shelled peanuts by up to 79% (Dickens and Whitaker, 1975). The only chemical detoxification processes currently in commercial use are the destruction of aflatoxin in cottonseed meal by ammoniation in the southwest United States (Stoloff, 1976a) and treatment of groundnut protein for human food with hydrogen peroxide in India (Parpia and Sreenivasamurthy, 1971).

2. Sterigmatocystin

Sterigmatocystin, first isolated from _Aspergillus versicolor_ (van der Watt, 1974), is structurally related to the aflatoxins. It is in fact also a metabolite of _A. flavus_ and _A. parasiticus_, among other fungal species (Schroeder and Kelton, 1975), and a biogenetic precursor of aflatoxin B_1 (Singh and Hsieh, 1976). Although acute oral toxicity in rats and mice is not high—LD_{50} values (male) are, respectively, 166 mg/kg and 800 mg/kg (van der Watt, 1974)—long-term feeding of 5 ppm sterigmatocystin to mice induced pulmonary neoplasms (Zwicker et al., 1974) and 10–15 ppm in the diet of male Wistar rats caused hepatocellular carcinoma

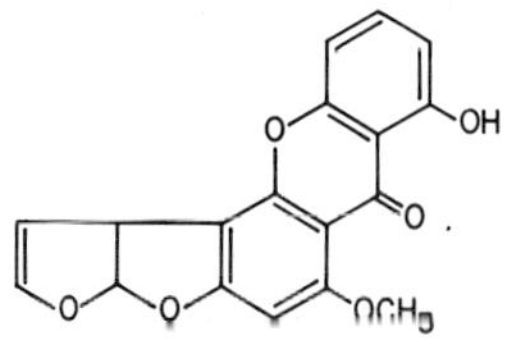

STERIGMATOCYSTIN

(Purchase and van der Watt, 1970). The major metabolite of sterigmatocystin in the urine of vervet monkeys has been identified as the glucuronide (Thiel and Steyn, 1973).

a. Occurrence

Although sterigmatocystin is generally considered dangerous because of the high yields (5-12 g/kg) that can be obtained in laboratory cultures on maize (Steyn and Rabie, 1975), it should be noted that yields of aflatoxin B_1 on grain substrates may also be high (2.9 g/kg) (Hesseltine, 1976) and that natural contamination of grains by sterigmatocystin appears to be extremely limited. Isolated cases of occurrence in rice (Manabe and Tsuruta, 1975), feed grain (Scott et al., 1972; Shreeve et al., 1975), coffee beans (Purchase and Pretorius, 1973), and pecans (Schroeder and Hein, 1977) have been reported, but a 2-year survey of 457 small grains in the United States was negative (Stoloff, 1976c).

b. Analysis

Sensitivity of the AOAC method for analysis of grains (AOAC, 1975) is only about 30 ppb (Stack and Rodricks, 1971); sterigmatocystin is detected by TLC as a bright yellow fluorescent spot in short-wave UV light after spraying and heating with aluminum chloride. High-pressure liquid chromatography (Stack et al., 1976) and gas-liquid chromatography (GLC) (Manabe et al., 1973) have also been used in methods for the determination of sterigmatocystin in grains.

3. Penicillium Islandicum Toxins

Long-term feeding to rats and mice of rice inoculated with P. islandicum has been shown to cause liver cirrhosis and hepatoma (Uraguchi et al., 1972). (-)-Luteoskyrin, one of numerous pigments isolated from this fungus (Enomoto and Ueno, 1974), produced hepatoma when fed to mice in amounts as low as 50 μg/day (Uraguchi et al., 1972). (+)-Rugulosin, a metabolite of P. rugulosum, is the optical antipode of (-)-rugulosin, which has been isolated from P. islandicum (Takeda et al., 1973). The former is stated to produce liver tumors in mice (Ueno and Nakajima, 1974). Isolated together with (-)-luteoskyrin in low yield was a highly toxic (oral LD_{50} in mice, 6.55 mg/kg) water-soluble chlorine-containing peptide, cyclochlorotine, which produced hepatoma in mice given daily oral doses of 40 μg (Uraguchi et al., 1972; Yoshioka et al., 1973). There is a lack of adequate methodology for luteoskyrin and cyclochlorotine, and their natural occurrence in foods has not been reported (Enomoto and Ueno, 1974).

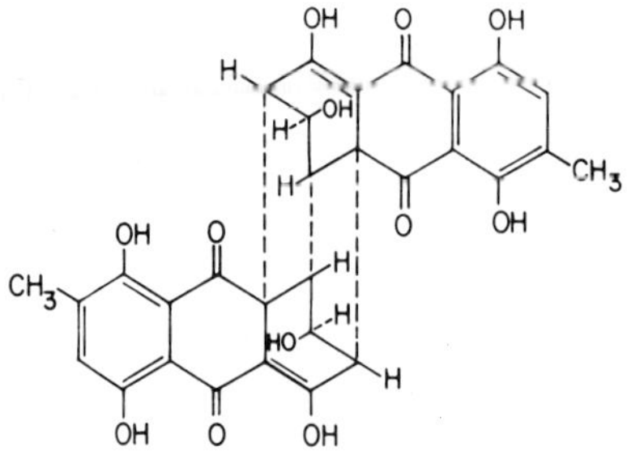

(-)-LUTEOSKYRIN

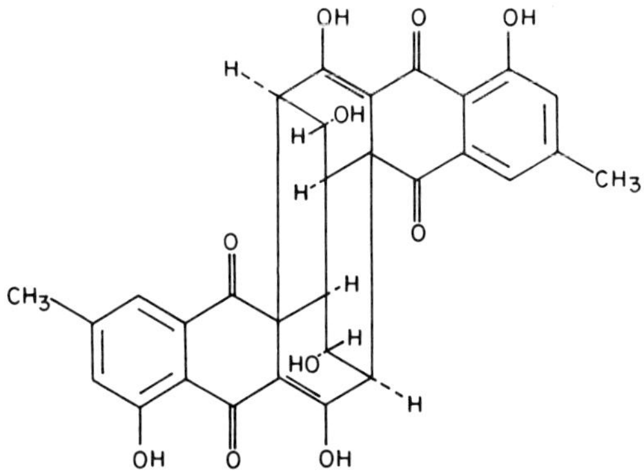

(+) - RUGULOSIN

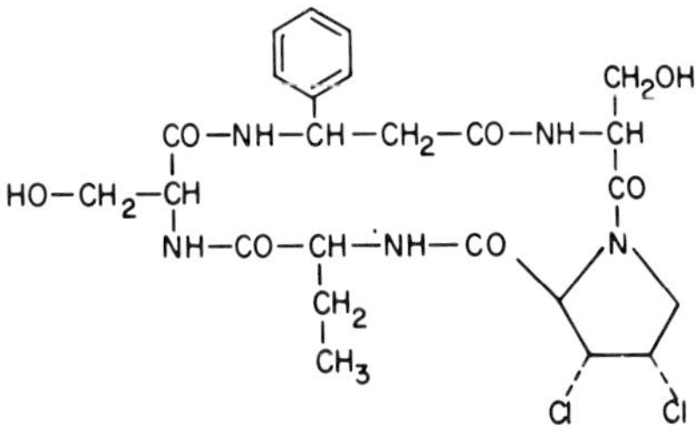

CYCLOCHLOROTINE

4. Griseofulvin

A therapeutic agent for cutaneous fungal infections, griseofulvin has produced hepatoma when fed to mice in large doses (up to 2.5% of the diet) (Wilson, 1971; DeMatteis et al., 1966). It is a metabolite of several Penicillium spp., but no attempt has been made to search for it in foodstuffs and it is still available as a prescription drug.

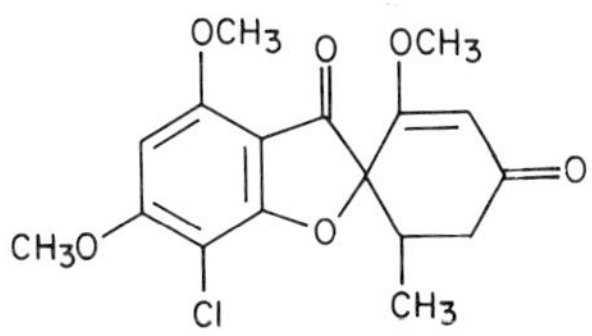

GRISEOFULVIN

5. Patulin and Penicillic Acid

Patulin and penicillic acid are antibiotic metabolites of several Aspergillus and Penicillium species; in addition patulin is produced by two Byssochlamys species (Escoula, 1975; Scott, 1974; Wilson, 1971). Both compounds are carcinogenic to rodents on repeated subcutaneous injection of 0.2-mg doses (Dickens and Jones, 1961, 1963, 1965), observations that have stimulated searches for their natural occurrence in foods and chronic feeding trials in laboratory animals that are currently underway in the United States (Dailey et al., 1977). Since one of the fungi that produce patulin, P. expansum, is a common storage rot of apples, patulin may occur frequently in apple juice; a survey in the United States in 1973 revealed 37% incidence of patulin at an average contamination level of 69 µg/liter (Stoloff, 1976b). The detection limit of the AOAC method for apple juice is 20 µg/liter; patulin forms a yellow-brown fluorescent spot on the TLC plate with 3-methyl-2-benzothiazolinone hydrazone

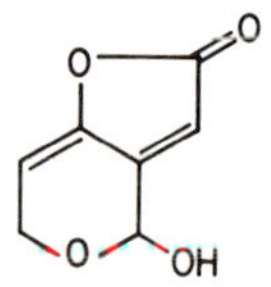

PATULIN

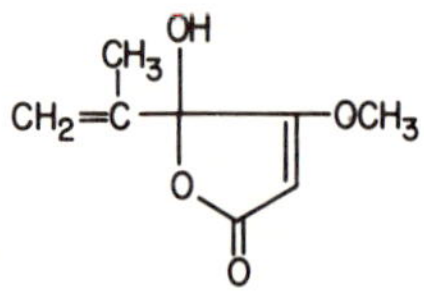

PENICILLIC ACID

hydrochloride solution at 130°C (AOAC, 1980; Scott and Kennedy, 1973). Patulin has also been detected in samples of moldy silage (Escoula, 1974), moldy baked goods, and wheat straw residues (Scott, 1974). Natural occurrence of penicillic acid has been demonstrated by GLC in samples of corn, beans, and tobacco (Snow et al., 1972; Stoloff, 1976b; Thorpe and Johnson, 1974).

6. Miscellaneous

Penicillin G, commercially produced by mutants of Penicillium chrysogenum (Turner, 1971). produced fibrosarcomas in rats on continued twice weekly subcutaneous injection of 2 mg of sodium salt (Dickens and Jones, 1961, 1963). Assay methods are available for penicillin

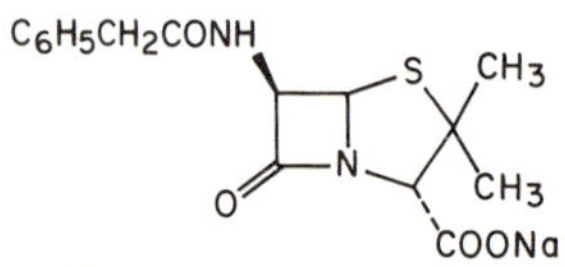

PENICILLIN G (Na SALT)

residues (Kramer et al., 1968). Extracts of Candida parapsilosis and Microsporum quinckeanum, two fungi often found associated with cutaneous disorders in humans, produced a high incidence of sarcomas in mice at the site of repeated subcutaneous injection (Blank et al., 1968). Frequency of lymphomas increased significantly in mice receiving extracts of several other pathogenic fungi, notably Candida albicans and Trichophyton spp., and there were cases of increased numbers of primary pulmonary tumors, particularly with extracts of Microsporum spp. and Scopulariopsis brevicaulis (Blank et al., 1968). Zwicker and coworkers (1974) found that inclusion of 7.5% of a rice culture of Penicillium viridicatum in the diet of mice also caused an increase in pulmonary neoplasms. Carcinogenic effects have been shown in rats after long-term oral administration and subcutaneous injection with a culture of Penicillium camemberti var. candidum, a fungus used in the manufacture of certain soft ripened cheeses (Gibel et al., 1971). The compounds responsible for the carcinogenic effects of all the aforementioned fungi have not been isolated.

7. Some Recent Developments

Kanisawa and Suzuki (1978) have reported that ochratoxin A was carcinogenic to the liver and kidneys of mice when fed at a level of 40 ppm in the diet. Ochratoxin A is a nephrotoxic metabolite of several species of Aspergillus and Penicillium, notably A. ochraceus and P. viridicatum, and many cases of its natural occurrence in grains and feeds have been documented (Scott, 1978). A causal association between ochratoxin A and mycotoxic porcine nephropathy was observed in Denmark (Krogh and Elling, 1977). There is also some evidence

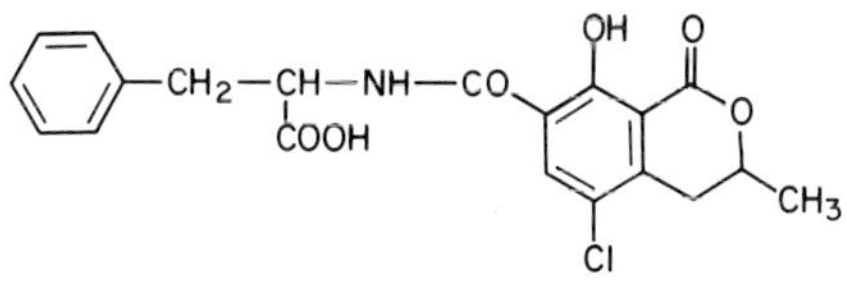

OCHRATOXIN A

for a hypothesis that ochratoxin A is a disease determinant in a human nephropathy endemic in the Balkans (Pavlović et al., 1979).

T-2 toxin is one of over 40 trichothecene mycotoxins produced by certain Fusarium species and other fungal genera (Ueno, 1977). Recently Schoental et al. (1979) showed that T-2 toxin given to rats by stomach tube contributed significantly to development of benign and malignant tumors in several organs, including the gastrointestinal tract. Occasional

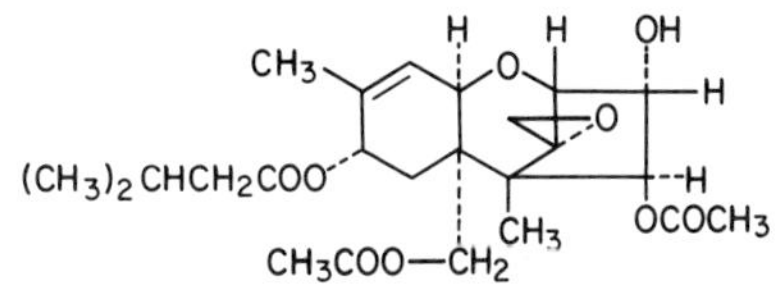

T-2 TOXIN

contamination of grains by T-2 toxin has been reported (Scott, 1978), and the difficult problem of analysis for trichothecenes in foods and feeds has been reviewed by Eppley (1979).

No carcinogenic action attributable to orally administered patulin was observed in a 64-week study with rats and a transplacental study with pregnant mice (Osswald et al., 1978). Nevertheless, regulatory limits of 50 ng/ml of patulin in apple juice have been set by Sweden, Switzerland, and Norway (Stoloff, 1979; Stray, 1978).

B. Agricultural Chemicals

The use of naturally occurring organic insecticides and rodenticides has been known to humans for several hundred years, and inorganic pesticides have been in use for over 100 years (DHEW, 1969). However, the widespread use of pesticides in agriculture is a relatively recent phenomenon, arising from the development and use of synthetic organic pesticides during World War II. During the period from 1945 to 1969, in the United States alone, production of synthetic organic pesticides increased from negligible amounts to over 1×10^9 lb/year (Matsumura, 1972).

Public concern about possible ill effects of pesticides on nontarget organisms remained minimal for many years. However, the publication of Silent Spring by Rachel Carson in 1962 crystallized public concern. Even so, it was not until the late 1960s that the first accepted evidence of possible carcinogenic activity of pesticides was recognized.

To attempt to review the carcinogenic potential of the several hundred pesticides presently in use throughout the world would require several volumes. It is proposed, therefore, to consider the major groups of synthetic organic pesticides and briefly discuss the carcinogenic potential of compounds within each group.

1. Occurrence

Some organochlorine pesticide residues and metabolites are very persistent and occur in many parts of the environment. These compounds are lipid soluble and are concentrated in both plant and animal lipids. Their levels tend to be magnified in each succeeding step of the food chain, and high levels are found in the larger carnivorous fish and marine mammals, in certain fish-eating birds, and in humans. These compounds are very persistent in soils from which they are taken up to varying degrees by growing plants. Residues of DDT and its metabolites are still found in practically all samples of animal fat, even several years after drastic reduction or elimination of the use of DDT in many areas. Some fish from waters containing only a few parts per trillion of DDT may contain as much as a few parts per million of DDT and its metabolites. Certain plants such as carrots are capable of concentrating considerable quantities of DDT and other organochlorine pesticides from soil. Canadian studies conducted between 1972 and 1975 involving more than 2000 samples of 15 food commodities serve to illustrate the levels of organochlorine pesticide residues in the food supply. The average levels of total DDT (DDT + DDE + TDE) were 13 μg/kg in beef fat and 35-60 μg/kg in the fat of milk, pork, poultry, and eggs. Carrots contained an average of 39 μg/kg, potatoes 4 μg/kg, while a variety of other vegetables and fruit all averaged not more than 1 μg/kg. The average dieldrin levels in the fat of animal products ranged from 6 μg/kg in beef to 15 μg/kg in milk. The only plant commodity containing more than 1 μg/kg of dieldrin was carrots at an average level of 4 μg/kg. Average BHC levels of 15-20 μg/kg were found in milk and beef fats, 7 μg/kg in flour, and 6 μg/kg in vegetable oils. Lower levels were found in all of the other commodities examined. Essentially all of the BHC residues in flour were present as lindane, whereas the residues in all other commodities consisted of a mixture of several isomers of BHC. Levels averaging up to 2 μg/kg of heptachlor epoxide, endrin, and chlordane were found in animal fats. These compounds were detected only occasionally at very low levels in plant products. Endosulfan residues were detected in some vegetables, the highest average level of which was 7 μg/kg in tomatoes, and dicofol residues averaging 5 μg/kg and 52 μg/kg were found in apples and oranges, respectively. Canadian total diet studies from 1969 to 1974 indicate a major decrease in the dietary intake of organochlorine pesticides. The total DDT intake decreased from 19 to 2 μg/person/day, while the total organochlorine pesticide intake decreased from 30 to 5 μg/person/day (Smith, 1971; Smith et al., 1972, 1973, 1975).

Organophosphate residues occur only occasionally in foods, usually at low levels and almost exclusively in plant products. In the earlier mentioned Canadian survey of over 2000 food samples, 14 different organophosphate pesticides were detected. Of these, the only ones occurring in more than a few isolated samples were diazinon in carrots and oranges, ethion and parathion in oranges, imidan and phosalone in apples, and malathion in flour and vegetable oils. Canadian total diet studies have indicated that the dietary intake of organophosphate pesticide residues from 1970 to 1974 was in the range of 2-5 μg/person/day.

There is very little information on the occurrence of carbamate residues in foods. The use patterns and rapid degradation of most of these compounds indicate that there would be little likelihood of significant residues in foods. Residues of the ethylene-bis-dithiocarbamates have been shown to persist for some time on food crops (Newsome et al., 1975; Newsome, 1976; Yip et al., 1971). The presence of ethylenethiourea and ehtylenethiuram monosulfide on crops treated with ethylene-bis-dithiocarbamates has been demonstrated (Engst et al., 1968; Newsome et al., 1975; Newsome, 1976) and the conversion of ethylene-bis-dithiocarbamate residues in foods to ethylenethiourea by heating has been demonstrated (Newsome and Laver, 1973).

2. Analysis

The analysis of the minute quantities of agricultural chemical residues present in foods is a complex procedure involving extraction to separate the chemicals from the bulk of the sample, cleanup to further isolate the residues from extraneous sample material, and separation, detection, and measurement of the individual chemical residues. Complete analysis of any pesticide residue in foods also requires confirmation of the identity and quantity of the residue by a completely independent method or, at least, by a different detection and measurement procedure. Solvent extraction, solvent partitioning, adsorption chromatography, and gas chromatography are probably the most commonly applied techniques for the analysis of pesticide residues, but many other approaches have been employed for the isolation and measurement of these residues. Gas chromatography using a variety of specific detectors has been the major tool for the detection, identification, and measurement of pesticide residues. High-performance liquid chromatography shows particular promise for the analysis of the more polar pesticide residues and metabolites, which are difficult to analyze by gas chromatography. A variety of chromatographic and spectrometric techniques has been used for confirmation of residue analysis results.

While there have been many analytical methods developed for the determination of specific agricultural chemical residues, the more practical approach, for regulatory purposes, has been to develop methods capable of simultaneously isolating, identifying, and measuring all of a group of similar chemicals (e.g., the organochlorine pesticides).

There are several compilations of methods for the analysis of pesticide residues in foods (AOAC, 1975; Health Protection Branch, 1973; DHEW, 1977) which outline the methodology for the analysis of pesticide residues in foods.

3. Metabolism

Many agricultural chemicals are readily metabolized in biological systems to produce both toxic and relatively nontoxic metabolites.

Dechlorination, dehydrochlorination, and epoxidation are the major processes involved in the formation of toxic metabolites of the organochlorine pesticides. DDT is readily metabolized in biological systems by dechlorination to form TDE [1,1-dichloro-2,2-di(chlorophenyl)ethane] and by dehydrochlorination to form DDE [1,1-dichloro-2,2-di(chlorophenyl)ethylene]. This metabolism occurs to the extent that p,p'-DDE, is commonly the major residue in foods, with smaller amounts of p,p'-DDT and p,p'-TDE. Residues of o,p'-DDT are sometimes detected in foods but o,p'-DDE and o,p'-TDE are only rarely detected as residues. Mirex has been shown to be dechlorinated to form photomirex (Hallett et al., 1976). Epoxidation is also a significant metabolic process in the case of certain organochlorine pesticides. Aldrin is converted to dieldrin and heptachlor to heptachlor epoxide so readily that residues of aldrin and heptachlor are rarely detected in foods. Chlordane is converted to oxychlordane to such an extent that oxychlordane is detected in essentially all samples of human milk and human adipose tissue (Mes et al., 1977; Mes and Davies, 1978). Most of these organochlorine pesticides and the metabolites formed by the processes of dechlorination, dehydrochlorination, and epoxidation are only very slowly metabolized to relatively nontoxic compounds by hydroxylation and other reactions. This very slow detoxification combined with the lipid solubility of compounds such as DDT, dieldrin, and chlordane accounts for their prolonged persistence in the environment.

The metabolic conversion of organophosphates to form toxic metabolites is primarily a reaction involving sulfur in the organophosphate ester molecule. Many of these pesticides are thionophosphates that require activation by conversion to the phosphate form. This conversion occurs readily in both plants and animals. Some of these compounds (e.g., phorate, carbophenothion, demeton) also contain thioether groups that readily form sulfoxides and sulfones. It has been shown that many of these thioether organophosphate compounds rapidly disappear from plants, to be replaced by as many as five metabolites, which are the thionophosphate and phosphate sulfoxides and sulfones and the phosphate oxon (Coffin, 1964).

Organophosphate pesticides and their metabolites are rapidly metabolized in plants and animals to relatively nontoxic compounds by deesterification or by specific reactions involving one or more of the ester groups.

The carbamate pesticides are in general rapidly metabolized in soils, plants, and animals with the production of a large number of metabolites. The predominant metabolic process affecting the herbicidal carbamates in soils is cleavage of the carbamate bond to yield an alcohol and an amine, which may be further metabolized by the soil-plant system. The predominant mode of metabolism of these compounds in animals is by hydrolysis or aryl hydroxylation followed by the conjugation and elimination in the feces and urine (Still and Herrett, 1976). The methyl carbamate insecticides are metabolized in plants and animals by hydrolysis to the alcohol and amine, but the major metabolic pathways appear to involve oxidation or hydroxylation followed by conjugation to glycosides in plants and sulfates or glucuronides in animals (Casida, 1972; Miyamoto, 1972; Slade, 1972). Thiocarbamate herbicides also do not persist as plant residues for any appreciable length of time. Relatively little work has been done to investigate their possible metabolic products. It is generally believed that upon hydrolysis, thiocarbamates yield a molecule of mercaptan, carbon dioxide, and dialkylamine (Fang, 1975; Slade, 1972). Several conjugates of thiocarbamates have been demonstrated in rat urine, indicating that hydroxylation of aliphatic side-chains or N-alkyl groups must take place (Fang et al., 1964). Ethylenebisdithiocarbamate fungicides are metabolized by plant and animal systems to yield ethylenethiourea, ethylenethiuram monosulfide, 2-imidazoline, and ethylene urea, as well as ethylenediamine, carbon disulfide, hydrogen sulfide, and sulfur (Vonk, 1975; Lyman, 1971; Iverson et al., 1977; Newsome et al., 1975). The parent fungicides are also degraded to form ethylenethiourea during the cooking of foods (Newsome and Laver, 1973).

4. Organochlorine Pesticides

The most extensively studied pesticide to date is the organochlorine compound, 1,1,1-trichloro-2,2,di(chlorophenyl)ethane, more commonly known as DDT.

Prior to 1966, long-term feeding studies in rats and monkeys had been reported for DDT. Of the three rat studies, one did not report any tumor incidence (Treon and Cleveland, 1955), one reported an increase in leukemia, attributed to the use of a purified diet (Kimbrough et al., 1964), and the third concluded that DDT was not carcinogenic, despite the observations of "hepatic cell tumors," and "nodular adenomatoid hyperplasia" (Fitzhugh and Nelson, 1947). The single monkey study did not result in the detection of any tumors using biopsy techniques after $7\frac{1}{2}$ years exposure to DDT (Durham et al., 1963). On the basis of these studies, all performed at dose levels considerably in excess of human exposure levels, DDT was considered to be noncarcinogenic.

In 1966 Kemeny and Tarjan published a preliminary note (later amplified) (Tarjan and Kemeny, 1969) indicating that in a mouse multigeneration study a significant increase in the incidence of leukemia was detectable in the F_3 generation, and a similar increase in the incidence of malignant tumors was detectable in the F_2 generation, following exposure to levels of 3 ppm DDT in the diet. The significance of the effects, as compared to controls, increased with successive generations.

During the subsequent decade several papers have reported the results of carcinogenicity studies on DDT. In the mouse increased incidence of hepatomas have been reported in single generation studies at 140 ppm (Innes et al., 1969), and at 50 and 100 ppm (Walker et al., 1973; Thorpe and Walker, 1973), while in another study an increased incidence of lung adenomas has been reported by Shabad et al. (1973) at the 50-ppm dose level. Fitzhugh (1969) reported that in BALB/cJ mice fed 100 ppm DDT for 2 years no increase in tumor incidence was noted, although survival in all groups was low. In contrast, female C_3HeB/FeJ mice showed a significant increase in hepatoma incidence. However, incidence of other tumors was reduced so that overall tumor incidence was comparable between control and DDT-treated groups. Laws (1971) using C57B1 mice exposed to 5.5 mg/kg/day failed to induce any tumors in the livers of 14 mice, which survived for 16 months on the experimental diet. Saline suspensions of the Zimmerman ependymoma resulted in a 100% "take" in control mice compared with a 92.1% "take" in DDT-treated mice. Rate of tumor development was reduced in DDT-treated mice.

In mouse multigeneration studies at dose levels ranging from 2 to 250 ppm in CF1 mice and BALB/c mice incidence of liver tumors increased with dose and with generation (Tomatis et al., 1972; Terracini et al., 1973; Turosov et al., 1973).

In the Fischer rat a single-generation study by Weisburger and Weisburger (1968) did not yield any significant increase in hepatomas following 10 mg/rat DDT for one year succeeded by 6 months observation period prior to slaughter. In two further single-generation studies with Osborne-Mendel rats fed 80 or 200 ppm DDT for 2 years no dose-related changes in tumor incidence was shown (Deichmann et al., 1967; Radomski et al., 1965).

A single-generation study in the hamster at 500 and 1000 ppm DDT in the diet did not indicate any increase in either specific or general tumor incidence (Agthe et al., 1970).

The data on DDT carcinogenesis indicates that tumorigenic induction occurs in the mouse (possibly only in certain strains of mice), and that the main site of action in this species is the liver. In the rat, data do not provide convincing evidence of tumorigenicity. Negative data exist regarding the potential for tumor induction in the hamster and the monkey.

Considering next aldrin and its metabolite dieldrin, data are available following long-term oral exposure in only two species, the rat and the mouse. The mouse studies on both compounds (Davies and Fitzhugh, 1962; Walker et al., 1969; Thorpe and Walker, 1973) indicate that liver cell tumors were induced in all studies, even at dose levels as low as 0.1 ppm dieldrin in the diet. In contrast, in the rat studies on both aldrin and dieldrin separately (Treon and Cleveland, 1955; Fitzhugh et al., 1964; Deichmann et al., 1970), one study on aldrin (Deichmann et al., 1967), and one study on dieldrin (Walker et al., 1969), no evidence of tumorigenicity has occurred even at dose levels of up to 50 ppm in the diet. Thus, as with DDT, both aldrin and dieldrin appear to be species specific, exerting tumorigenic activity in mouse, but not in rat.

In the case of lindane and the other benzene hexachloride (BHC) isomers, a similar pattern emerges. Again mouse studies on technical BHC, containing a mixture of isomers resulted in hepatic tumors at high-dose levels (660 ppm) after 24 weeks, at which point the mice were killed. Lower doses (6.6 and 66 ppm) did not cause tumors over this short time span (Nagasaki et al., 1971). In a subsequent experiment the α-, β-, γ-, or δ-isomers were fed separately at 100, 250, or 500 ppm in the diet, over a 24-week period. Doses of 250 and 500 ppm α-BHC caused mouse liver tumors but over the short time period of the study, all other isomers failed to result in tumor induction (Nagasaki et al., 1972). However, longer-term studies (110 weeks) showed β-BHC (200 ppm) and γ-BHC (400 ppm) induced liver tumors in CF1 mice with lung metastases in males receiving β- or γ-BHC, and in females receiving γ-BHC (Thorpe and Walker, 1973). These results confirmed those of Goto et al. (1972) who showed tumor induction in mouse livers following 6 months dietary administration of 600 ppm α-, β-, γ-, δ-, and ε-BHC. Similarly, Hanada et al. (1973), feeding 0, 100, 300, or 600 ppm technical BHC to dd mice induced liver tumors in 100% of the animals at the two higher doses following 32 weeks administration, followed by 5-6 weeks on basal diet prior to killing. Further studies by Nagasaki et al. (1975) on the α-BHC also resulted in tumor induction in mice. The paper also indicated a strain difference in susceptibility to tumor induction.

In contrast to these studies, a study with NMRI mice at 12.5, 25, and 50 ppm γ-BHC for 80 weeks failed to induce tumors (Herbst et al., 1975). Neither is there clear evidence of tumor induction in the recent NCI Carcinogenic Bioassay of Lindane in the mouse.

In the rat Fitzhugh et al. (1950) fed 0, 5, 10, 50, 100, 400, 800, or 1600 ppm in 10% oil solution of γ-BHC, 10, 100, or 800 ppm of technical BHC, 10, 50, 100, or 800 ppm α-BHC, or 10, 100 or 800 ppm of β-BHC. Doses of 800 ppm or more of all compounds decreased life span. Tumor incidence in all groups was comparable to that in control groups. Similarly, the NCI Carcinogenesis Bioassay on lindane at maximum tolerated dose levels does not indicate any carcinogenic effect. The 1965 FAO/WHO Monograph of the Joint Meeting on Pesticide Residues summarizes three additional rat studies by Truhaut (1954), Ortega et al. (1957), and Klimmer (1955). The study by Truhaut, utilizing 10 male and 10 female rats per group, fed 25, 50, or 100 ppm lindane for their life span does not show any compound related effect on tumor incidence. The Ortega et al. study (six male and six female rats fed 50 or 100 ppm) is also negative, as is the Klimmer study (25 rats dosed at 10 μg/kg body weight, by stomach tube for 17 months). The only positive rat study, by Ito et al. (1975) reports that 3/13 rats fed 1500 ppm α-BHC, and 1/16 rats fed 1000 ppm α-BHC for 72 weeks developed liver carcinomas. Hyperplastic nodules were noted in other animals of these groups, and also after 48 weeks exposure to 1000 ppm α-BHC. β- and δ-BHC given for 24 or 48 weeks at doses up to 1000 ppm did not induce tumors or hyperplastic nodules.

Once again, the pattern of positive carcinogenic activity with regard to induction of mouse liver tumors is apparent. The majority of available data on the rat tends to indicate that lindane has little tumorigenic effect in this species. The study by Ito et al. (1975) has not been evaluated and hence its significance is uncertain.

The general pattern established by the foregoing data on carcinogenic studies on DDT, aldrin, dieldrin, and lindane continues to be found when considering other organochlorine insecticides. Reference to the IARC monograph on organochlorine pesticides (IARC, 1974) shows the following evaluations:

a. Compound

Chlorobenzilate Two strains of mice show increased hepatoma incidence (Innes et al., 1969). Two rat studies (inadequate for evaluation according to IARC) did not show any compound related changes in tumor incidence (Horn et al., 1955; Bartsch et al., 1971).

Endrin Mouse data are not available. In two rat studies (Treon and Cleveland, 1955; Deichmann et al., 1970) no compound-induced tumors were reported. (IARC indicates that in one of these studies, details of pathology are not provided.)

Heptachlor In the mouse details of a DHEW study (1969) were not available. The study was considered to be positive for tumor induction. In the rat five unpublished studies (cited by the FAO/WHO Joint Meeting on Pesticide Residues, 1967) were considered. In four of these studies (at doses of 12.5 ppm (three studies) and 10 and 20 ppm) no tumorigenic effects were observed. In the fifth study tumor incidence, when combined for all groups (i.e., 0.5, 2.5, 5, 7.5, and 10 ppm) showed an increase in the incidence of tumor-bearing rats. No dose response relationship was observed for hepatic tumors.

Methoxychlor No mouse data are available. Four studies in rat (Nelson and Fitzhugh, unpublished, quoted by Deichmann et al., 1967; Hodge et al., 1952; Radomski et al., 1965) did not provide any evidence of carcinogenic activity.

Mirex In a mouse-screening study (Innes et al., 1969) increased hepatoma incidence was observed in both sexes of two strains of mice.

Quintozene In mouse a screening study (Innes et al., 1969) indicated increased hepatic tumor incidence in males in one of two mouse strains tested. In a rat study (Finnegan et al., 1958) tumor incidence is not given.

Strobane Increased hepatoma incidence was observed in males only, in one of two mouse strains (Innes et al., 1969). No rat data are available.

Thus, as a generalization, it seems probable that organochlorine pesticides result in the induction of liver tumors in the mouse, but rarely in other species. In light of the concern regarding the suitability of the mouse hepatoma as a predictive parameter indicating potential human carcinogenicity (as exemplified by Butler and Newberne, 1975), considerable caution should be exercised in basing regulatory decisions on organochlorine insecticides on mouse carcinogenicity studies alone.

5. Organophosphates

Published data on carcinogenicity studies on organophosphate pesticides are extremely limited. The following data are therefore mainly based on abstract reports from FAO/WHO Monographs of the Joint Meetings on Pesticide Residues.

No increase in tumor incidence is specifically mentioned with reference to 2-year rat studies for the following compounds:

Compound	Maximum dose	Reference
Azinphos methyl	20 ppm	Huntingdon Research Center, 1966
Bromophos	350 mg/kg body weight	Kinkel and Sann, 1965
Bromophos ethyl	7.2 mg/kg body weight	Leuschner et al., 1971
Carbophenothion	80 ppm	Johnston, 1967
Chlorfenvinphos	300 ppm (95 weeks)	Ambrose et al., 1970
Chlorpyrifos methyl	1 mg/kg body weight	Hunter et al., 1974
Coumaphos[a]	100 ppm	Doull et al., 1960
Cyanofenphos[a]	100 ppm	Kadota et al., 1974
Dichlorvos	500 ppm	Witherup et al., 1967

Compound	Maximum dose	Reference
Fenamiphos	30 ppm	Loser, 1972; Cherry and Newman, 1973
Fenchlorphos[b]	50 mg/kg body weight	McCollister et al., 1959
Fenitrothion	100 ppm	Rutter and Nelson, 1974
Fensulfothion[a]	20 ppm	Doull et al., 1966
Formothion[a]	320 ppm	Klotzsche and Carpy, 1970
Leptophos[a]	30 ppm	Smith et al., 1973
Malathion[a]	5000 ppm	Hazelton and Holland, 1953
Methidathion	64 ppm	Johnston, 1967
Monocrotophos[a]	100 ppm	Johnston et al., 1967
Parathion	100 ppm	Lehman, 1952
Phosalone[a]	250 ppm	Woodard et al., 1967

[a]Tumors not specifically mentioned. Stated no compound related histologic lesions found.

[b]No direct reference to tumors, but histology reported on various organs.

In the only mouse studies noted on organophosphate pesticides, fenamiphos at 50 ppm in the diet (Smith et al., 1972) or leptophos at 100 ppm in the diet (Smith et al., 1973) for 18 months, did not affect tumor incidence. Thus, for the majority of organophosphate pesticides, oral administration over 2 years, in the rat at least, does not indicate any carcinogenic potential. The single exception identified is trichlorfon. For this compound conflicting data have been reported. Gibel et al. (1971) report that in Wistar rats, intubated thrice weekly for their life span with 30 mg/kg, exophytic papillomas of the forestomach occurred in three rats. In a second study (Gibel et al., 1973) twice weekly intubation with 15 mg/kg induced benign tumors in 19/28 rats (cf., 3/36 in controls) and malignant tumors in 7/28 rats (cf., 0/36 in controls). Doull and co-workers (1962) fed groups of 25 male and 25 female rats 50, 250, 500, or 1000 ppm trichlorfon in the diet for 2 years. Life span was reduced at 1000 ppm. Gross mammary tumor incidence was 14%, 8%, 20%, 21%, and 25% at 0, 50, 250, 500, and 1000 ppm, respectively. Appearance of the first tumor was 1.7, 1.6, 1.8, 1.5, and 1.1 years after commencement of dosing at 0, 50, 250, 500, and 1000 ppm. In a second study (Doull et al., 1965) at 0, 100, 200, or 400 ppm (terminated at 70 weeks because of high mortality in all groups) mammary tumor incidence was 8, 11, and 15% at 0, 200, and 400 ppm, respectively. Latent period was unaffected by dose. A dose-related increase in cystic granular ovaries (8, 14, 33, and 40% at 0, 100, 200, and 400 ppm, respectively) and an increase in nonneoplastic ovarian cyst incidence at 400 ppm were also reported. In a fifth study, however, 2-year feeding of diets containing 0, 50, 250, 500, or 1000 ppm trichlorfon did not result in any change in the incidence of rat mammary tumors (9, 18, 12, 10, and 8% at 0, 50, 250, 500, and 1000 ppm). A total of 35 malignant tumors were identified, of which 15 occurred in controls, and five at 1000 ppm trichlorfon. Thus in the case of trichlorfon, data are conflicting. Tumorigenic activity of this compound has not been satisfactory resolved (Lorke and Loser, 1966; Grundmann and Hobik, 1966).

The limited data, usually on a single species, available on organophosphate pesticides do not appear to indicate that these compounds possess carcinogenic potential. It is interesting to speculate, however, that with these highly toxic materials acting as cholinesterase inhibitors, the possibility of lethality occurring prior to tumor induction at high-dose levels may be occurring (i.e., in cancer studies in rodents, negative data may be more likely with highly toxic compounds).

6. Carbamates

In 1976, IARC examined the available published data on some carbamates, and ethylene bisdithiocarbamates for which a carcinogenic effect or a suspicion of carcinogenicity has been reported. Of the 10 pesticides reviewed, an assessment was deemed impossible in nine cases, while in the 10th case (Monuron), the data suggest Monuron to be a carcinogen (IARC, 1976).

In the cases in which either an assessment was stated to be considered impossible, or in which no assessment is given, the following data were cited:

Compound	Species	Maximum dose	Comment and result	Reference
Carbaryl	Mouse	MTD[a]	Negative	Innes et al., 1969
	Rat	16 mg/kg	Negative	Carpenter et al., 1961
	Rat	30 mg/kg	Poor survival, sarcoma incidence increased	Adrianova and Alekseev, 1970
Chlorpropham	Mouse	MTD[a]	Negative	Innes et al., 1969
	Mouse	1000 ppm	Negative	van Esch and Kroes, 1972
	Rat	20,000 ppm	Negative	Larson et al., 1960
	Hamster	2000 ppm	Negative	van Esch and Kroes, 1972
Diallate	Mouse	MTD[a]	Liver cell tumor increase	Innes et al., 1969
	Rat	MTD[a]	Incidence of tumor-bearing animals increased, not site specific	Ulland et al., 1973
Ferbam	Mouse	MTD[a]	Negative	Innes et al., 1969
	Rat	2500 ppm	Negative (low survival)	Hodge et al., 1956
Maneb	Mouse	MTD[a]	Negative	Innes et al., 1969
	Mouse	500 mg/kg	9-month study showing increased lung adenomas in A strain, but no effect in C 57 RL strain	Balin, 1970
	Rat	335 mg/kg	Poor survival, no result	Adrianova and Alekseev, 1970
Propham	Mouse	MTD[a]	Negative	Innes et al., 1969
	Mouse	0.1%	Negative	Heuper, 1952
	Rat	2.0%	No tumors, but survival very low	Heuper, 1952
	Hamster	2000 ppm	Negative	van Esch and Kroes, 1972
Thiram	Mouse	MTD[a]	Negative	Innes et al., 1969
Zectran	Mouse	MTD[a]	Increased lung adenomas in one of two strains	Innes et al., 1969
Zincb	Mouse	MTD[a]	Negative	Innes et al., 1969
	Rat	285 mg/kg	Poor survival, 2/10 tumors cf. 1/46 in controls	Adrianova and Alekseev, 1970
	Rat	10,000 ppm	Group sizes inadequate	Blackwell-Smith et al., 1953

[a]MTD Maximum tolerated dose.

From the limited information frequently involving inadequate studies, it is not possible to determine whether a pattern exists in the "carbamate" type pesticides, with regard to potential carcinogenic activity.

It is not possible to discuss the carcinogenicity of the carbamate pesticides without reference to two major points; first, the reaction of these compounds with nitrite, and second, the consideration of the carcinogenicity of the metabolite, ethylenethiourea, formed by the breakdown of ethylene-bis-dithiocarbamates.

Sen et al. (1974) showed that dimethyl nitrosamine could be formed by the reaction of nitrite with ziram, or thiram or ferbam, both in vitro and in vivo, while NO-derivatives of carbaryl and propoxur were identified by Eisenbrand et al. (1974) in vitro when 1mM pesticide: 5mM nitrite were reacted under acid conditions at 37° C for 15 min. Nitrosodimethyl amine is a known carcinogen (Magee and Barnes, 1956; Schmahl and Osswald, 1967), while N-nitrosocarbaryl known to be a potent mutagen (Elespuru et al., 1974), induces local sarcomas at the injection site after a single subcutaneous (s.c.) injection of 1000 mg/kg in rats (Eisenbrand et al., 1975) and is carcinogenic in rats after oral administration (Eisenbrand et al., 1976; Lijinsky and Taylor, 1976). Thus, the nitroso products resulting from nitrite reaction with carbamate pesticides are known to be, or are highly suspected of being, carcinogens. The extent of N-nitroso derivative formation in vivo is not presently known, and hence further work is required to delineate this potential problem.

Ethylenethiourea is a known degradation product of ethylene-bis-dithiocarbamates, which has been shown to occur at very low levels on some food crops (Newsome et al., 1975). Degradation of residues of parent compound also occur during cooking of foods bearing residues (Newsome and Laver, 1973).

Carcinogenesis studies on ethylenethiourea in C57B1/6 × C_3H/Anf and C57BL/6 × ARK cross bred mice have resulted in increased hepatoma incidence in both strains, and a slightly increased lymphoma incidence in the C57BL/6 × ARK F_1 mice (Innes et al., 1969). In the rat Ulland et al. (1972) fed 175 or 350 ppm ETU to rats for 18 months, when five rats/sex at 350 ppm were sacrificed. Hyperplastic goitre was observed in all males and in 4/5 females. Three rats of each sex showed follicular thyroid carcinoma. The remaining rats were fed control diet from 18-24 months when they were killed. At 350 ppm, 17/26 males and 8/26 females showed thyroid carcinomas. In two of the males lung metastases were observed. At 175 ppm, three per sex showed thyroid carcinomas, and nine males and six females showed hyperplastic goitre. Liver hyperplastic nodules occurred in one male at 350 ppm and two males and one female at 175 ppm. In a subsequent 12-month study (Graham et al., 1973) nodular hyperplasia at 125 ppm and carcinomas at 250 ppm in males, and carcinomas at 500 ppm in females were observed. Extension of this study to 2 years (Graham et al., 1975) showed thyroid hyperplasia (minimal) at 5 ppm, and an increase in thyroid benign and malignant tumors at 125 ppm and above. These data indicate that ETU is a rat thyroid carcinogen. ETU may, at high doses, induce tumors in mice. The latter fact remains to be confirmed.

It would appear that the thyroid carcinogenesis in rats is preceded by a thyroid hyperplasia (which is now known to be reversible (Arnold, personal communication, 1977). Since the levels of ETU in the diet are insufficient to induce such hyperplasia, the potential for human thyroid carcinoma induction by ETU is believed to be negligible.

REFERENCES

Section I

Actionable level guideline for the presence of PCBs in fishery products. Provided by the Legal Division, Swedish National Food Administration in a letter to the author, August 6, 1977.

Belgium Ministry of Public Health and the Environment. Regulatory information provided in a letter to the author, August 9, 1977.

Department of National Health and Welfare, Ottawa, Canada. Office Consolidation of the Food and Drugs Act and of the Food and Drug Regulations.

21 Code of Federal Regulations, Parts 1-119, 120-129 (Food and Drugs). Superintendent of Documents, U.S. Government Printing Office, Washington, D.C.

Danish Food Act No. 310 (1973). Danish Ministry of Environmental Protection, Dep. 1972, File No. 600-1.

Danish Ministry of Environmental Protection. Regulatory information provided in a letter to the author, August 14, 1977.

Department of Health, Dublin, Ireland. Regulatory information provided in a letter to the author, August 24, 1977.

Focke, K. (1976). Environmental chemicals, problems - situation - measures in the Federal Republic of Germany. Report of a German interdepartmental project group, "Environmental Chemicals," under the chairmanship of the Federal Ministry of Youth, Family Affairs and Health, Bon-Bad Godesberg (9-14), March 20.

Guidelines for Developing an Effective National Food Control System (1976). FAO Food Control Series No. 1, WHO Food Control No. 1. Food and Agriculture Organization, World Health Organization in collaboration with the United Nations Environment Program.

Hungarian Food Law. Provided by the Hungarian Office for Standardization, Budapest, Hungary, in a letter to the author, September 9, 1977 (English translation).

List of Additives Evaluated for their Safety-in-Use in Foods, First Series and Suppl. 1. Joint FAO/WHO Food Standards Program, Publication Nos. CAC/FAL 1-1973, CAC/FAL 1-1973 (Supp. 1).

List of Maximum Levels Recommended for Contaminants by the Joint FAO/WHO Codex Alimentarius Commission, First Series. Joint FAO/WHO Food Standards Program, Publication No. CAC/FAL 2-1973.

List of Maximum Levels Recommended for Contaminants by the Joint FAO/WHO Codex Alimentarius Commission, Second Series. Joint FAO/WHO Food Standards Program, Publication No. CAC/FAL 3-1969.

Ministry of Health, State of Israel. Regulatory information provided in a letter to the author, September 7, 1977.

New Zealand Department of Health. Food and Drugs Act (1969).

Recommended International Maximum Limits for Pesticide Residues, Fourth Series. Joint FAO/WHO Food Standards Program, Publication No. CAC/RS 65-1974.

Recommended International Maximum Limits for Pesticide Residues, Fifth Series. Joint FAO/WHO Food Standards Program, Publication No. CAC/RS 71-1976.

Royal Norwegian Ministry of Social Affairs. Regulatory information provided in a letter to the author, August 9, 1977.

Secretary, Netherlands Committee for the Codex Alimentarius. Regulatory information provided in a letter to the author, July 26, 1977.

Swedish National Food Administration. Foreign Substance in Food (SLVFS 1977:7) (English translation).

Swiss Federal Office of Public Health, Foodstuffs Control. Regulatory information provided in a letter to the author, August 31, 1977.

Section II.A

Akagi, M., Aoki, I., and Uematsu, T. (1966). Studies on food additives. X. The metabolism of p-ethoxyphenylurea in the rabbit. Chem. Phar. Bull. (Tokyo) 14:1.

Akagi, M., Oketani, Y., and Uematsu, T. (1965). Studies on food additives. IX. Estimation of p-ethoxyphenylurea in biological materials and physiological disposition in animals. Chem. Pharm. Bull. (Tokyo) 13:1200.

Allen, M. J., Boyland, E., Dukes, C. E., Horning, E. S., and Watson, J. G. (1957). Cancer of the urinary bladder induced in mice with metabolites of aromatic amines and tryptophan. Br. J. Cancer 11:212.

Althoff, J., Cardesa, A., Pour, P., and Shubik, P. (1975). A chronic study of artificial sweeteners in Syrian golden hamsters. In Report of the Temporary Committee for the Review of Data on the Carcinogenicity of Cyclamate. Natl. Cancer Inst., Feb. 1976.

Armstrong, B., and Doll, R. (1974). Bladder cancer mortality in England and Wales in relation to cigarette smoking and saccharin consumption. Br. J. Prev. Soc. Med. 28: 233.

Armstrong, B., and Doll, R. (1975). Bladder cancer mortality in diabetics in relation to saccharin consumption and smoking habits. Br. J. Prev. Soc. Med. 29: 73.

Armstrong, B., Lea, A. J., Adelstein, A. M., Donovan, J. W., White, G. C., and Ruttle, S. (1976). Cancer mortality and saccharin consumption in diabetics. Br. J. Prev. Soc. Med. 30: 151.

Arnold, D. L., Carbonneau, S. M., Moodie, C. A., and Munro, I. C. (1977). Long term toxicity study with o-toluene sulphonamide and saccharin. 16th Annual meeting, Society of Toxicology, Toronto, Canada.

Audrieth, L. F., and Sveda, J. (1944). Preparation and properties of some N-substitute sulfamic acids. J. Org. Chem. 9: 89.

Ball, L. M., Renwick, A. G., and Williams, R. T. (1974). The fate of ^{14}C-saccharin in rats chronically fed on saccharin. Biochem. Soc. Trans. 2: 1084.

Ball, L. M., Renwick, A. G., and Williams, R. T. (1977). The fate of ^{14}C-saccharin in man, rat and rabbit and of 2-sulphamoyl-^{14}C-benzoic acid in the rat. Xenobiotica 7: 189.

Bär, F., and Griepentrog, F. (1958). Zur chronischen Toxizität von Dulcin (p-Äthoxy-phenylharnstoff). Naturwissenschaften 45: 390.

Bekemeier, H., Hannig, E., and Pfennigsdorf, G. (1958). Zur kennthnis von Vertröglichkeit und Cancerogenität des p-Athoxy-phenylharnstoffes. Arzneim. Forsch. 8: 150.

Berryman, G. H., Hazel, G. R., Taylor, J. D., Sanders, P. G., and Weinberg, M. S. (1968). A case of safety of cyclamate and cyclamate-saccharin combinations. Am. J. Clin. Nutr. 21: 673.

Brantom, P. G., Gaunt, I. F., and Grasso, P. (1973). Long-term toxicity of sodium cyclamate in mice. Food Cosmet. Toxicol. 11: 735.

Bryan, G. T., Erturk, E., and Yoshica, O. (1970). Production of urinary bladder carcinomas in mice by sodium saccharin. Science 168: 1238.

Bryan, G. T., and Yoshida, O. (1971). Artificial sweeteners as urinary bladder carcinogens. Arch. Environ. Health 23: 6.

Bungard, G. (1967). Die substoffe. Dor. Deut. Apoth. 19: 150.

Burbank, F., and Fraumeni, J. F. (1970). Synthetic sweeteners consumption and bladder cancer trends in the United States. Nature 227: 296.

Byard, J. L. (1972). Observations on the metabolism of saccharin. Toxicol. Appl. Pharmacol. 22: 291 (Abst. No. 46).

Byard, J. L., and Golberg, L. (1973). The metabolism of saccharin in laboratory animals. Food Cosmet. Toxicol. 11: 391.

Byard, J. L., McChesney, E. W., Golberg, L., and Coulston, F. (1974). Excretion and metabolism of saccharin in man. II. Studies with ^{14}C-labelled and unlabelled saccharin. Food Cosmet. Toxicol. 12: 175.

Davis, T. R., Adler, N., and Opsahl, J. C. (1969). Excretion of cyclohexylamine in subjects ingesting sodium cyclamate. Toxicol. Appl. Pharmacol. 15: 106.

Fitzhugh, O. G., Nelson, A. A., and Frawley, J. P. (1951). A comparison of the chronic toxicities of synthetic sweetening agents. J. Am. Pharm. Assoc. 40: 583.

Friedman, L., Richardson, H. L., Richardson, M. E., Lethco, E. J., Wallace, W. C., and Sauro, F. M. (1972). Toxic response of rats to cyclamates in chow and semi-synthetic diets. J. Natl. Cancer Inst. 49: 751.

Furuya, T., Kawamata, K., Kanebo, T., Uchida, O., Horiuchi, S., and Ikeda, Y. (1975). Long-term toxicity study of sodium cyclamate and sodium saccharin in rats. Jpn. J. Pharmacol. 25 (Suppl. 55) (Abst.).

Gaunt, I. F., Hardy, J., Grasso, P., Gangolli, S. D., and Butterworth, K. R. (1976). Long-term toxicity of cyclohexylamine hydrochloride in the rat. Food Cosmet. Toxicol. 14:255.

Golberg, L., Parekh, C., Patti, A., and Soike, K. (1969). Cyclamate degradation in mammals and in vitro. Toxicol. Appl. Pharmacol. 14:654.

Griepentrog, F. (1959). Tumoren der Harnwege und Harnsteine in chronischen Versuchen mit Süsstoff p-phenetylcarbamid. Arzneim. Forsch. 9:123.

Hardy, J., Gaunt, I. F., Hooson, J., Hendy, R. J., and Butterworth, K. R. (1976). Long-term toxicity of cyclohexylamine hydrochloride in mice. Food Cosmet. Toxicol. 14:269.

Herter, C. A., and Folin, O. (1911). Influence of saccharin on the nutrition and health of man. Report No. 94, U.S. Department of Agriculture, Washington, D.C.

Hicks, R. M., Wakefield, J. S., and Chowaniec, J. (1973a). Carcinogenic action of saccharin in the chemical induction of bladder cancer. Nature 243:347.

Hicks, R. M., Wakefield, J. S., and Chowaniec, J. (1973b). Impurities in saccharin and bladder cancer. Nature 243:424.

Hicks, R. M., Wakefield, J. S., and Chowaniec, J. (1975). Evaluation of a new model to detect bladder carcinogens or cocarcinogens. Results obtained from saccharin, cyclamate and cyclophosphamide. Chem. Biol. Interact. 11:225.

Howe, G. R., Burch, J. D., Miller, A. B., Morrison, B., Gordon, P., Weldon, L., Chambers, L. W., Fodor, G., and Winsor, G. M. (1977). Artificial sweeteners and human bladder cancer. Lancet 578: Sept. 17.

Hwang, K. (1966). Mechanism of the laxative effect of sodium sulfate, sodium cyclamate and calcium cyclamate. Arch. Int. Pharmacodyn. Ther. 163:302.

IARC (1976). Dulcin. In Evaluation of Carcinogenic Risk of Chemicals to Man, IARC Monographs, Vol. 12, p. 97.

Ichibagase, H., Kojima, S., Suenaga, A., and Inoue, K. (1972). Studies on synthetic sweetening agents. XVI. Metabolism of sodium cyclamate (5). The metabolism of sodium cyclamate in rabbits and rats after prolonged administration of sodium cyclamate. Chem. Pharm. Bull. (Tokyo) 20:1093.

Ikeda, Y., Omori, Y., Oka, S., Shinoda, M., and Tsuzi, K. (1960). Studies on chronic toxicity of dulcin. J. Food Hyg. Soc. Jap. 1:62.

Kennedy, G. L., Jr., Faucher, O. E., Calandra, J. C., and Keller, R. E. (1972). Metabolic fate of saccharin in the albino rat. Food Cosmet. Toxicol. 10:143.

Kessler, I. I. (1970). Cancer mortality among diabetics. J. Natl. Cancer Inst. 44:673.

Kessler, I. I. (1976). Non-nutritive sweeteners and human bladder cancer: Preliminary findings. J. Urol. 115:143.

Kojima, S., and Ichibagase, H. (1966). Studies on synthetic sweeteners. VIII. Cyclohexylamine, a metabolite of sodium cyclamate. Chem. Pharm. Bull. (Tokyo) 14:971.

Kojima, S., Ichibagase, H., and Iguchi, S. (1966). Studies on synthetic sweetening agents. VII. Absorption and excretion of sodium cyclamate. Chem. Pharm. Bull. (Tokyo) 14: 965.

Kroes, R., Berkvens, J. M., Peters, P. W., Verschuusen, H. G., Helleman, P. W., deVries, T., and van Esch, G. J. (1975). Long-term toxicity and reproduction study with cyclamate, saccharin and cyclohexylamine. In Report of the Temporary Committee for the Review of Data on Carcinogenicity of Cyclamate. Feb. 1976, Natl. Cancer Inst., Washington, D.C.

Leahy, J. S., Wakefield, N., and Taylor, T. (1967). Urinary excretion of cyclohexylamine following oral administration of sodium cyclamate to man. Food Cosmet. Toxicol. 5: 447.

Lessel, B. (1970). Carcinogenic and teratogenic aspects of saccharin. Proc. 3rd Int. Cong. Food Sci. Technol. 764.

Lethco, E. J., and Wallace, W. C. (1975). The metabolism of saccharin in animals. Toxicology 3:287.

Lettré, H., and Wrba, H. (1955). Die Wirkung des Susstoffes Dulcin bei langdauernder Futterung. Naturwissenschaften 42:217.

Matthews, H. B., Fields, M., and Fishbein, L. (1973). Saccharin: distribution and excretion of a limited dose in the rat. J. Agric. Food Chem. 21:916.

Maumee (1951). American Patent Number 2667503. Che. Eng. News (1963) 41:76.

McChesney, E. W., Coulston, F., and Benitz, K. F. (1977). Six year study of saccharin in rhesus monkeys. 16th Annual meeting, Society of Toxicology, March 27-30, 1977. Toronto, Canada (Abst. 70).

McChesney, E. W., and Golberg, L. (1973). The excretion and metabolism of saccharin in man. I. Methods of investigation and preliminary results. Food Cosmet. Toxicol. 11:403.

Miller, J. P., Crawford, L. E., Sonders, R. C., and Cardinal, E. V. (1966). Distribution and excretion of ^{14}C-cyclamate sodium in animals. Biochem. Biophys. Res. Commun. 25:153.

Minegishi, K. I., Asahina, M., and Yamaha, T. (1972). The metabolism of saccharin and the related compound in rats and guinea pigs. Chem. Pharm. Bull. (Tokyo) 20:1351.

Morgan, R. W., and Jain, M. G. (1974). Bladder cancer: smoking, beverages and artificial sweeteners. Can. Med. Assoc. J. 111:1067.

Munro, I. C., Moodie, C. A., Krewski, D., and Grice, H. C. (1975a). A carcinogenicity study of commercial saccharin in the rat. Toxicol. Appl. Pharmacol. 32:513.

Munro, I. C., Stavric, B., and Lacombe, R. (1975b). The current status of saccharin. In Toxicology Annual, 1974, C. L. Winek (Ed.). p. 71.

National Formulary (1970). 13th Ed. 642.

National Research Council (1974). Safety of saccharin and sodium cyclamate in the human diet. Prepared for the U.S. Food and Drug Administration, Washington, D.C.

Nelson, J. J. (1976). Quantitation of o and p-sulfamoylbenzoic acids in commercial saccharin by high performance liquid chromatography. J. Assoc. Off. Anal. Chem. 59:243.

Oser, B. L., Carson, S., Vogin, E. E., and Sonders, R. C. (1968). Conversion of cyclamate to cyclohexylamine in rats. Nature 220:178.

Parekh, C., Goldberg, E. K., and Golberg, L. (1970). Fate of sodium cyclamate -C^{14} in the rhesus monkey (M. mulatta). Toxicol. Appl. Pharmacol. 17:282.

Pitkin, R. M., Anderson, D. W., Reynolds, W. A., and Filer, L. J., Jr. (1971). Saccharin metabolism in Macaca mulatta. Proc. Soc. Exp. Biol. Med. 137:803.

Price, J. M., Biava, C. G., Oser, B. L., Vogin, E. E., Steinfield, J., and Ley, H. L. (1970). Bladder tumors in rats fed cyclohexylamine or high doses of a mixture of cyclamate and saccharin. Science 167:1131.

Remsen, I., and Fahlberg, C. (1879). On the oxidation of substitution products of aromatic hydrocarbons. IV. On the oxidation of orthotoluenesulphonamide. Am. Chem. J. 1: 426.

Renwick, A. G., and Williams, R. T. (1969). Gut bacteria and the metabolism of cyclamate in the rat. Biochem. J. 114:78 pages.

Renwick, A. G., and Williams, R. T. (1970). The metabolism of cyclamate. In Proc. 1st Int. Sugar Research Conf., Brussels, p. 3.

Roe, F. J., Levy, L. S., and Carter, R. L. (1970). Feeding studies on sodium cyclamate, saccharin and surcrose for carcinogenic and tumor-promoting activity. Food Cosmet. Toxicol. 8:135.

Richards, R. K., Taylor, J. D., O'Brien, J. L., and Duescher, H. O. (1951). Studies on cyclamate sodium (Sucaryl Sodium), a new caloric sweetening agent. J. Am. Pharm. Assoc. E (40):1.

Schmähl, D. (1973). Absence of carcinogenic activity of cyclamate, cyclohexylamine and saccharin in rats. Arzneim. Forsch. 23:1466.

Schoenberger, J. A., Rix, D. M., Sakamoto, A., Taylor, J. D., and Kark, R. M. (1953). Metabolic effects, toxicity and excretion of calcium n-cyclohexylsulfamate (Sucaryl) in man. Am. J. Med. Sci. 225:551.

Sonders, R. C., Wiegand, R. G., and Netwal, . (1968). Excretion of cyclamate in the rat. J. Assoc. Off. Anal. Chem. 51:136.

Staub, H., and Staehelin, R. (1936). Med. Press Circ. 193:2.

Stavric, B., Klassen, R., and By, A. W. (1976). I. Impurities soluble in inorganic solvents. J. Assoc. Off. Anal. Chem. 59:1051.

Stavric, B., Lacombe, R., Munro, I. C., By, A. W., Klassen, R., and Ethier, J. (1974a). Studies on water soluble impurities in commercial saccharins. 107th AOC Natl. Meeting, Los Angeles, 31 March-5 April, 1974, ANAL. 171.

Stavric, B., Lacombe, R., Watson, J. R., and Munro, I. C. (1974b). Isolation and quantitation of o-toluenesulphonamide, a major impurity in commercial saccharins. J. Assoc. Off. Anal. Chem. 57:678.

Taylor, J., and Friedman, L. (1974). Combined chronic feeding and three generation reproduction study of sodium saccharin in the rat. Toxicol. Appl. Pharmacol. 29: 154.

Taylor, J. D., Richards, R. K., and Davin, J. C. (1951). Excretion and distribution of radioactive ^{35}S-cyclamate sodium (Sucaryl Sodium) in animals. Proc. Soc. Exp. Biol. Med. 78:530.

Temporary Committee for the Review of Data on Carcinogenicity of Cyclamate (1976). Report by the Division of Cancer Cause and Prevention. National Cancer Institute, Washington, D.C.

Wallace, W. C., Lethco, E. J., and Brouwer, E. A. (1970). The metabolism of cyclamates in rats. J. Pharmacol. Exp. Ther. 175:325.

Wynder, F., and Goldsmith, R. (1977). Unpublished referred to in the Lancet, 592: September 17.

Section II.B

Andrianova, M. M. (1970). Carcinogenic properties of the red food dyes—amaranth, SX purple, and 4R purple. Vopr. Pitan. 29:61-65.

Baigusheva, M. M. (1968). Carcinogenic properties of amaranth paste. Vopr. Pitan. 27: 46-50.

Boffey, P. M. (1976). Color additives: botched experiment leads to banning of red dye No. 2. Science 191:450-451.

Bonser, G. M., and D. B. Clayson (1964). A sulphonamide derivative which induces urinary tract epithelial hyperplasia and carcinomas of the bladder epithelium in the mouse. Br. J. Urol. 36:26-34.

Dacre, J. C. (1965). Chronic toxicity and carcinogenicity studies on citrus red no. 2. Proc. Univ. Otago Med. Sch. 43:31-33.

Davis, K. J., Nelson, A. A., Zwickey, R. E., Hansen, W. H., and Fitzhugh, O. G. (1966). Chronic toxicity of Ponceau SX in rats, mice, and dogs. Toxicol. Appl. Pharmacol. 8:306-317.

Drake, J. J. (1975). Food colors—harmless aesthetics or epicurean luxuries. Toxicology 5:3-42.

Gangolli, S. D., Grasso, P., and Golberg, L. (1967). Physical factors determining the early local tissue reactions produced by food colourings and other compounds injected subcutaneously. Food Cosmet. Toxicol. 5:601-621.

Gangolli, S. D., Grasso, P., Golberg, L., and Hooson, J. (1972). Protein binding by food colourings in relation to the production of subcutaneous sarcoma. Food Cosmet. Toxicol. 10:449-462.

Graichen, C., and Heine, K. S. (1964). Studies on coal-tar colors in foods. XVI FD&C Red No. 4. J. Assoc. Off. Anal. Chem. 37:905-912.

Grasso, P., and Golberg, L. (1966a). Early changes at the site of repeated subcutaneous injection of food colourings. Food Cosmet. Toxicol. 4:269-282.

Grasso, P., and Golberg, L. (1966b). Subcutaneous sarcomas as an index of carcinogenic potency. Food Cosmet. Toxicol. 4:297-320.

Grice, H. C., and Mannell, W. A. (1966). Rhabdomyosarcomas induced in rats by intramuscular injections of Blue VRS. J. Natl. Cancer Inst. 37:845-857.

Grice, H. C., Mannell, W. A., and Allmark, M. G. (1961). Liver tumors in rats fed Ponceau 3R. Toxicol. Appl. Pharmacol. 3:509-520.

Hansen, W. H., Davis, K. J., Fitzhugh, O. G., and Nelson, A. A. (1963). Chronic oral toxicity of Ponceau 3R. Toxicol. Appl. Pharmacol. 5:105-118.

Hansen, W. H., Fitzhugh, O. G., Nelson, A. A., and Davis, K. J. (1966). Chronic toxicity of two food colors, Brilliant Blue FCF and indigotine. Toxicol. Appl. Pharmacol. 8: 29-36.

Honohon, T., Enderlin, F. E., and Ryerson, B. A. (1976). Absorption, metabolism and excretion of the azo food dyes, amaranth, sunset yellow and tartrazine after oral administration to rats. Fed. Proc. Fed. Am. Soc. Exp. Biol. 35:328 (Abst.).

Lindstrom, H. V. (1961). The metabolism of FD&C Red No. 1. I. The fate of 2,4-metaxylidine in rats. J. Pharmacol. Exp. Ther. 132:306-310.

Lindstrom, H. V., Bowie, W. C., Wallace, W. C., Nelson, A. A., and Fitzhugh, O. G. (1969). Toxicity and metabolism of mesidine and pseudocumidine in rats. J. Pharmacol. Exp. Ther. 167:223-234.

Lindstrom, H. V., Hansen, W. H., Nelson, A. A., and Fitzhugh, O. G. (1963). The metabolism of FD&C Red No. 1. II. The fate of 2,5-para-xylidine and 2,6-meta-xylidine in rats and observations on the toxicity of xylidine isomers. J. Pharmacol. 142:457-264.

Mannell, W. A. (1964). Further investigations on production of liver tumors in rats by Ponceau 3R. Food Cosmet. Toxicol. 2:169-174.

Meuron, G. (1955). L'état actuel de la question des colorants pour denrées alimentaires. Mitt. Lebensm. Hyg. 46:97-120.

Pritchard, A. B., Holmes, P. A., and Kirschman, J. C. (1976). The fate of FD&C Red No. 2 and its metabolite, naphthionic acid, after different routes of administration in the rat. Toxicol. Appl. Pharmacol. 35:1-10.

Radomski, J. L. (1974). Toxicology of food colors. J. Annu. Rev. Pharmacol. 14:127-137.

Radomski, J. L., and Mellinger, T. J. (1962). Absorption, fate, and excretion in rats of the water-soluble azo dyes, FD&C Red No. 2, FD&C Red No. 4, and FD&C Yellow No. 6. J. Pharmacol. Exp. Ther. 136:259-266.

Sharratt, M., Farzer, A. C., and Paranjoti, I. S. (1966). Biological effects of citrus red #2 in the mouse. Food Cosmet. Toxicol. 4:493-502.

Stein, C. (1970). TLC and spectrophotometric determination of 1[4-(2,5-dimethoxyphenylazo)-2,5-dimethoxyphenylazo]-2-naphthol and 1,1'-(2,2',5,5'-tetramethoxy-4,4'-biphenylenebisazo)-di-2-naphthol in citrus red no. 2. J. Assoc. Off. Anal. Chem. 53: 26-28.

Wenninger, J. A., Jones, J. H., and Dolinsky, M. (1960). Studies on coal-tar colors. XXIV. FD&C Red No. 4. J. Assoc. Off. Anal. Chem. 43:805-809.

Willheim, R., and Ivy, A. C. (1953). A preliminary study concerning the possibility of dietary carcinogenesis. Gastroenterology 23:1-19.

Section II.C

Bartsch, H., Malaveille, C., and Montesano, R. (1975). Human, rat and mouse liver-mediated mutagenicity of vinyl chloride in Salmonella tryphimurium strains. Int. J. Cancer 15:429-437.

Briston, J. H., and Katan, L. L. (1974). Plastics in Contact with Food. Food Trade Press, London.

Brown, M. E., Breder, C. B., and McNeal, T. P. (1977). Gas-solid chromatographic procedures for the determination of acrylonitrile monomer in acrylonitrile containing polymers and food simulating solvents. Assoc. Off. Anal. Chem. Meeting, Oct. 17-20, Washington, D.C.

Curry, A. S., Hurst, G., Kent, N. R., and Powell, H. (1962). Rapid screening of blood samples for volatile poisons by gas chromatography. Nature 195:603-604.

El Masri, A. M., Smith, J. N., and Williams, R. T. (1958). The metabolism of alkylbenzenes: phenyl acetylene and phenylethylene (styrene). Biochem. J. 68:199-204.

Fed. Reg. (1975). Prior sanctioned polyvinyl chloride resin, termination of notice of proposed rule making. 40(171):40529.

Food Chem. News (1977a). 18(50):43-46.

Food Chem. News (1977b). 19(21):29-31.

Haley, T. J. (1975). Vinyl chloride: how many unknown problems? Environ. Health Perspect. 1:47-64.

Hefner, R. E., Watanabe, P. G., and Gehring, P. J. (1975). Preliminary studies on the fate of vinyl chloride monomer (VCM) in rats. Environ. Health Perspect. 11:85-95.

Holmberg, B., and Molina, G. (1974). The industrial toxicology of vinyl chloride. A review. Work Environ. Health 11:138-144.

IARC (1975). Report of working group on epidemiological studies on vinyl chloride exposed people. Internal Technical Report, No. 75/001, Lyon, France.

Maltoni, C., and Lefemine, G. (1974). Carcinogenicity bioassays of vinyl chloride. Environ. Res. 7:387-405.

Ohtsuji, H., and Ikeda, M. (1971). The metabolism of styrene in the rat and the stimulatory effect of phenobarbital. Toxicol. Appl. Pharmacol. 18:321-328.

Parkki, M. G., Marieni, J., and Vanio, H. (1976). Action of Styrene and its metabolites, styrene oxide and styrene glycol, on activities of xenobiotic biotransformation enzymes in rat liver in vivo. Toxicol. Appl. Pharmacol. 38:59-70.

Stoltz, D. R., and Withey, J. R. (1977). Mutagenicity of styrene and styrene epoxide. Bull. Environ. Contam. Toxicol. 18:739-742.

Tox-Tips (1977). January, pp. 41, 43, 45, 47.

Van Duuren, B. L. (1969). Carcinogenic epoxides, lactones and haloethers and their mode of action. Ann. NY Acad. Sci. 163:633.

van Esch, G. J., and van Logten, M. J. (1975). Vinyl chloride: a report of a European assessment. Food Cosmet. Toxicol. 13:121-139.

Williams, D. T., and Miles, W. F. (1975). Gas-liquid chromatographic determination of vinyl chloride monomer in alcoholic beverages, vegetable oils and vinegars. J. Assoc. Off. Anal. Chem. 58:272-275.

Withey, J. R. (1976). Quantitative analysis of styrene monomer in polystyrene and foods including some preliminary studies of the uptake and pharmacodynamics of the monomer in rats. Environ. Health Perspect. 17:125-133.

Withey, J. R. (1977). Mutagenic, carcinogenic and teratogenic hazards arising from exposure to plastics additives. In Origins of Human Cancer, H. H. Hiatt, J. D. Watson, and J. A. Winston (Eds.). Cold Spring Harbor Conferences of Cell Proliferation, IV, Cold Spring Harbor, N.Y.

Withey, J. R., and Collins, P. G. (1977). Styrene monomer in foods: a limited Canadian survey. Bull. Environ. Contam. Toxicol. 19:1.

Section III. A

Alam, B. S., Saporoschetz, I. B., and Epstein, S. S. (1971). Formation of N-nitrosopiperidine from piperidine and sodium nitrite in the stomach and the isolated intestinal loop of the rat. Nature 232:116-118.

Archer, M. C., and Wishnok, J. S. (1977). Quantitative aspects of human exposure to nitrosamines. Food Cosmet. Toxicol. 15:233-235.

Asahina, S., Friedman, M. A., Arnold, E., Millar, G. N., Mishkin, M., Bishop, Y., and Epstein, S.S. (1971). Acute synergistic toxicity and hepatic necrosis following oral administration of sodium nitrite and secondary amines to mice. Cancer Res. 31:1201-1205.

Barnes, J. M., and Magee, P. N. (1954). Some toxic properties of dimethylnitrosamine. Br. J. Ind. Med. 11:167-174.

Boyland, E. (1972). The effect of some ions of physiological interest on nitrosamine synthesis. In N-Nitroso Compounds: Analysis and Formation. P. Bogovski, R. Preussmann, and E. A. Walker (Eds.). IARC Scientific Publication No. 3, Lyon, France, 124-126.

Boyland, E., and Walker, S. A. (1974). Thiocyanate catalysis of nitrosamine formation and some dietary implications. In N-Nitroso Compounds in the Environment, P. Bogovski and E. A. Walker (Eds.). IARC Scientific Publication No. 9, Lyon, France, pp. 132-136.

Canadian Food and Drug Act and Regulations (1965). Table XI. Queen's Printer and Controller of Stationery, Ottawa.

Castegnaro, M., and Walker, E. A. (1977). New data on collaborative studies on analysis of nitrosamines. Presented at the 5th IARC Meeting on Analysis and Formation of N-Nitroso Compounds, Aug. 21-24, University of New Hampshire, Durham, N.H.

Castell, C. H., Smith, B., and Neal, W. (1971). Production of dimethylamine in muscle of several species of gadoid fish during frozen storage, especially in relation to presence of dark muscle. J. Fish Res. Board Can. 28:1-5.

Chemical Rubber Company (CRC) (1973). Handbook of Chemistry and Physics, 54th Ed., R. C. Weast (Ed.). Cleveland, Ohio.

Craddock, W. M., and Magee, P. N. (1963). Reaction of the carcinogen dimethylnitrosoamine with nucleic acids in vivo. Biochem. J. 89:32-37.

Craddock, V. M., and Magee, P. N. (1965). Methylation of liver DNA in the intact animal by the carcinogen dimethylnitrosamine during carcinogenesis. Biochim. Biophys. Acta 95:677-678.

Crosby, N. T. (1976). Nitrosamines in foodstuffs. Res. Rev. 64:77-135.

Druckrey, H., Preussmann, R., and Ivankovic, S. (1969). N-nitroso compounds in organotropic and transplacental carcinogenesis. Ann. NY Acad. Sci. 163:676-696.

Druckrey, H., Preussmann, R., Ivankovic, S., and Schmaehl, D. (1967). Organotrope carcinogene Wirkungen bei 65 verschiedenen N-Nitroso-Verbindungen an BD-Ratten. Z. Krebsforsch. 69:103-201.

Druckrey, H., Preussmann, R., Ivankovic, S., Schmidt, C. H., Mennel, H. D., and Stahl, K. W. (1964). Selektive Erzeugung von Blasenkrebs an Ratten durch Dibutyl- und N-Butyl-N-butanol(4)-nitrosamin. Z. Krebsforsch. 66:280-290.

Druckrey, H., Preussmann, R., Schmaehl, D., and Mueller, M. (1961). Chemische Konstitution und carcinogene Wirkung bei Nitrosaminen. Naturwissenschaften 48: 134-135.

Druckrey, H., Steinhoff, D., Beuthner, H., Schneider, H., and Klaerner, P. (1963). Pruefung von Nitrit auf toxische Wirkung an Ratten. Arzneim. Forsch. 13:320-323.

Dutton, A. H., and Heath, D. F. (1956). Demethylation of dimethylnitrosamine in rats and mice. Nature 178:644.

Eisenbrand, G., Janzowski, C., and Preussmann, R. (1976). Analysis, formation, and occurrence of volatile and non-volatile N-nitroso compounds: recent results. Proc. 2nd Int. Symp. Nitrite Meat Prod., B. J. Tinbergen and B. Krol (Eds.). Zeist, Pudoc, Wagenigen, pp. 155-169.

Eisenbrand, G., Spiegelhalder, B., Janzowski, C., Kann, J., and Preussmann, R. (1977). Volatile and non-volatile N-nitroso compounds in foods and other environmental media. Presented at the 5th IARC Meeting on Analysis and Formation of N-Nitroso Compounds, Aug. 21-24, University of New Hampshire, Durham, N.H.

Eisenbrand, G., Ungerer, O., and Preussmann, R. (1974). Formation of N-nitroso compounds from agricultural chemicals and nitrite. In N-Nitroso Compounds in the Environment, P. Bogovski and E. A. Walker (Eds.). IARC Scientific Publication No. 9, Lyon, France, pp. 71-74.

Emmons, W. D. (1954). Peroxytrifluoroacetic acid. I. The oxidation of nitrosamines to nitramines. J. Am. Chem. Soc. 76:3468-3470.

Ender, F., Havre, G., Helgebostad, A., Koppang, N., Madsen, R., and Cěh, L. (1964). Isolation and identification of a hepatotoxic factor in herring meal produced from sodium nitrite preserved herring. Naturwissenschaften 51:637-638.

Ender, F., Havre, G., Madsen, R., Cěh, L., and Helgebostad, A. (1967). Studies on conditions under which N-nitrosodimethylamine is formed in herring meal produced from nitrite-preserved herring. Z. Tierphysiol. 22:181-189.

Epstein, S. S. (1972). In vivo studies on interactions between secondary amines and nitrite or nitrates. In N-Nitroso Compounds: Analysis and Formation, P. Bogovski, R. Preussmann, and E. A. Walker (Eds.). IARC Scientific Publication No. 3, Lyon, France, pp. 109-115.

Fan, T.-Y., and Tannenbaum, S. R. (1973). Factors influencing the rate of formation of nitrosomorpholine from morpholine and nitrite: acceleration by thiocyanate and other ions. J. Agric. Food Chem. 21:237-240.

Fiddler, W., Pensabene, J. W., Doerr, R. C., and Wassermann, A. E. (1972). Formation of N-nitrosodimethylamine from naturally occurring quaternary ammonium compounds and tertiary amines. Nature 236:307.

Fiddler, W., Pensabene, J. W., Piotrowski, E. G., Doerr, R. C., and Wassermann, A. E. (1973). Use of sodium ascorbate or erythorbate to inhibit formation of N-nitrosodimethylamine in frankfurters. J. Food Sci. 38:1084.

Fieser, L. F., and Fieser, M. (1968). In Advanced Organic Chemistry. Reinhold, New York, pp. 377, 508, 717-718.

Fine, D. H., Rounbehler, D. P., and Sen, N. P. (1976a). A comparison of some chromatographic detectors for the analysis of volatile N-nitrosamines. J. Agric. Food. Chem. 24:980-984.

Fine, D. H., Rounbehler, D. P., Silvergleid, A., and Ross, R. (1976b). Trace analysis of polar and apolar N-nitroso compounds by combined high-performance liquid chromatography and thermal energy analysis. Proc. 2nd Int. Symp. Nitrite Meat Prod., Zeist, Pudoc, Wagenigen, pp. 191-199.

Fine, D. H., and Rufeh, F. (1974). Description of the thermal energy analyser for N-nitroso compounds. In N-Nitroso Compounds in the Environment, P. Bogovski and E. A. Walker (Eds.). IARC Scientific Publication No. 9, Lyon, France, pp. 40-44.

Fong, Y. Y., and Chan, W. C. (1976). Methods for limiting the content of dimethylnitrosamine in Chinese marine salt fish. Food Cosmet. Toxicol. 14:95-98.

Foreman, J. K., and Goodhead, K. (1975). The formation and analysis of N-nitrosamines. J. Sci. Food Agric. 26:1771-1783.

Garcia, H., and Lijinsky, W. (1973). Studies of the tumorigenic effect of feeding of nitrosamino acids and low doses of amines and nitrite to rats. Z. Krebsforsch. 79: 141-144.

Gorenen, P. J., de Cock-Bethbeder, M. W., Jonk, R. J., and van Ingen, C. (1976). Further studies on the occurrence of volatile N-nitrosamines in meat products by combined gas chromatography and mass spectrometry. Proc. 2nd Int. Symp. Nitrite Meat Prod., Zeist, Pudoc, Wageningen, pp. 227-237.

Gough, T. A., and Goodhead, K. (1975). Occurrence of volatile nitrosamines in spice premixes. J. Sci. Food Agric. 26:1473-1478.

Gough, T. A., McPhail, M. F., Webb, K. S., Wood, B. J., and Coleman, R. F. (1977). An examination of some foodstuffs for the presence of volatile nitrosamines. J. Sci. Food Agric. 28:345-351.

Gough, T. A., and Walters, C. L. (1976). Volatile nitrosamines in fried bacon. In Environmental N-Nitroso Compounds: Analysis and Formation, E. A. Walker, P. Bogovski, and L. Griciute (Eds.). IARC Scientific Publication No. 14, Lyon, France, pp. 195-203.

Gray, J. I. (1977). Nitrosamine precursors in bacon. Can. Inst. Food Sci. Technol. 10: A15-A17.

Greenberg, R. A. (1976). Nitrosopyrrolidine in United States cured meat products. Proc. 2nd Int. Symp. Nitrite Meat Prod., Zeist, Pudoc, Wageningen, pp. 203-210.

Greenblatt, M., Mirvish, S., and So, D. T. (1971). Nitrosamine studies: induction of lung adenomas by concurrent administration of sodium nitrite and secondary amines in Swiss mice. J. Natl. Cancer Inst. 46:1029-1034.

Harada, M., Ishiwata, H., Nakamura, Y., Tanimura, A., and Ishidate, M. (1975). J. Food Hyg. Soc. 16:11-18.

Hatt, H. H. (1943). In Organic Synthesis, Collective Volume II, A. H. Blatt (Ed.). Wiley, New York, pp. 211-213.

Havery, D. C., Fazio, T., and Howard, J. W. (1977). Survey of cured meat products for volatile N-nitrosamines: comparison of two analytical methods. Presented at the 5th IARC Meeting on Analysis and Formation of N-Nitroso Compounds, Aug. 21-24, University of New Hampshire, Durham, N.H.

Heisler, E. G., Siciliano, J., Krulick, S., Feinberg, J., and Schwarts, J. H. (1974). Changes in nitrate and nitrite content and search for nitrosamines in storage-abused spinach and beets. J. Agric. Food Chem. 22:1029-1032.

Herring, H. K. (1973). Effect of nitrite and other factors on the physico-chemical characteristics and nitrosamine formation in bacon. In Proc. Meat Industry Research Conf., Univ. of Chicago, pp. 47-60.

IARC (1972). Evaluation of Carcinogenic Risk of Chemicals to Man. IARC Monographs, Vol. 1. Lyon, France, pp. 95-140.

IARC (1974). Evaluation of Carcinogenic Risk of Chemicals to Man. IARC Monographs, Vol. 4. Lyon, France, pp. 183-227.

Ingram, M. (1973). The microbiological effects of nitrite. In Proc. of the Int. Symp. Nitrite Meat Prod., B. Krol and B. J. Tinbergen (Eds.). Zeist, The Netherlands, pp. 63-75.

Ishidate, M., Tanimura, A., Ito, Y., Sakai, A., Sakuta, H., Kawamura, T., Sakai, K., Miyazawa, F., and Wade, H. (1971). Secondary amine, nitrite and nitrosamines in Japanese foods. Nippon Yakuza. Zasshi 23:47-51.

Iyengar, J. R., Panalaks, T., Miles, W. F., and Sen, N. P. (1976). A survey of fish products for volatile N-nitrosamines. J. Sci. Food Agric. 27:527-530.

Keefer, L. K., and Roller, P. P. (1973). N-Nitrosation by nitrite ion in neutral and basic medium. Science 181:1245-1247.

Kruger, F. W. (1972). New aspects in metabolism of carcinogenic nitrosamines. In Topics in Chemical Carcinogenesis (Proc. 2nd Int. Symp. Princes Takamatsu Cancer Res. Found.), W. Nakahara, S. Takayama, T. Sugimura, and S. Odashima (Eds.). University Park Press, Baltimore, pp. 213-232.

Lijinsky, W., Conrad, E., and van de Bogart, R. (1972). Formation of carcinogenic nitrosamines by interactions of drugs with nitrite. In N-Nitroso Compounds: Analysis and Formation, P. Bogovski, R. Preussmann, and E. A. Walker (Eds.). IARC Scientific Publication No. 3, Lyon, France, pp. 130-133.

Lijinsky, W., Keefer, L., and Loo, J. (1970). The preparation and properties of some nitrosamino acids. Tetrahedron 26:5137-5135.

Loveless, A. (1969). Possible relevance of O-6 alkylation of deoxyguanosine to the mutagenicity and carcinogenicity of nitrosamines and nitrosamides. Nature 233:206-207.

Magee, P. N. (1971). Toxicity of nitrosamines: their possible human health hazards. Food Cosmet. Toxicol. 9:207-218.

Magee, P. N. (1973). Nitrosamines: Ubiquitous carcinogens? New Scientist 59:432-434.

Magee, P. N., and Barnes, J. M. (1956). The production of malignant primary hepatic tumours in the rat by feeding dimethylnitrosamine. Br. J. Cancer 10:114-122.

Magee, P. N., Montesano, R., and Preussmann, R. (1976). N-Nitroso compounds and related carcinogens. In Chemical Carcinogens, ACS Monograph 173, C. E. Searle (Ed.). American Chemical Society, Washington, D.C., pp. 491-625.

Meester, J. (1973). Nitrate and nitrite allowances in meat products. In Proc. Int. Symp. Nitrite Meat Prod., B. Krol and B. J. Tinbergen (Eds.). Zeist, The Netherlands, pp. 265-268.

Mergens, W. J., Kamm, J. J., Newmark, H. L., Fiddler, W., and Pensabene, J. (1977). Alpha-tocopherol: uses in preventing nitrosamine formation. Presented at the 5th IARC Meeting on Analysis and Formation of N-Nitroso Compounds, Aug. 21-24, University of New Hampshire, Durham, N.H.

Mirvish, S. S. (1972a). Kinetics of N-nitrosation reactions in relation to tumorigenesis experiments with nitrite plus amines or ureas. In N-Nitroso Compounds: Analysis and Formation, P. Bogovski, R. Preussmann, and E. A. Walker (Eds.). IARC Scientific Publication No. 3, Lyon, France, pp. 104-108.

Mirvish, S. S. (1972b). Studies on N-nitrosation reactions: kinetics of nitrosation, correlation with mouse feeding experiments, and natural occurrence of nitrosatable compounds (ureides and guanidines). In Topics in Chemical Carcinogenesis, W. Nakahara, S. Takayama, S. Sugimura, and S. Odashima (Eds.). University of Tokyo Press, Tokyo, pp. 279-295.

Mirvish, S. S. (1975). Formation of N-nitroso compounds: chemistry, kinetics, and in vivo occurrence. Toxicol. Appl. Pharmacol. 31:325-351.

Mirvish, S. S., Wallcave, L., Eagen, M., and Shubik, P. (1972). Ascorbate-nitrite reaction: possible means of blocking the formation of carcinogenic N-nitroso compounds. Science 177:65-68.

Montesano, R., and Magee, P. N. (1970). Metabolism of dimethylnitrosamine by human liver slices in vitro. Nature 228:173-174.

Montesano, R., and Magee, P. N. (1971). Evidence of formation of N-methyl-N-nitrosourea in rats given N-methylurea and sodium nitrite. Int. J. Cancer 7:249-255.

Neurath, G. B., Duenger, M., Pein, F. G., Ambrosius, D., and Schreiber, O. (1976). Primary and secondary amines in the human environment. Food Cosmet. Toxicol. 15: 275-282.

Panalaks, T., Iyengar, J. R., Donaldson, B., Miles, W. F., and Sen, N. P. (1974). Further survey of cured meat products for volatile N-nitrosamines. J. Assoc. Off. Anal. Chem. 57:806-812.

Preussmann, R., Schmaehl, D., Eisenbrand, G., and Port, R. (1976). Dose-response study with N-nitrosopyrrolidine and some comments on risk evaluation of environmental N-nitroso compounds. In Proc. 2nd Int. Symp. Nitrite Meat Prod., B. J. Tinbergen and B. Krol (Eds.). Zeist, The Netherlands, pp. 261-268.

Rea, G. A., and Shewan, J. M. (1951). The spoilage of fish and its preservation by chilling. Adv. Food Res. 2:343-398.

Rubin, L. J. (1977). Nitrites and nitrosamines in perspective. Can. Inst. Food Sci. Technol. 10:A11-A13.

Sander, J. (1971). Untersuchungen ueber die Entstehung cancerogener Nitrosoverbindungen im Magen von Versuchstieren und ihre Bedeutung fuer den Menschen. Arzneim. Forsch. 21:1572-1580, 1707-1713, 2034-2039.

Sander, J., and Buerkle, G. (1969). Induktion maligner Tumoren bei Ratten durch gleichzeitige Verguetterung von Nitrit und sekundaeren Aminen. Z. Krebsforsch. 73:54-66.

Sander, J. Schweinsberg, F., and Menz, H. P. (1968). Untersuchungen ueber die Entstehung cancerogener Nitrosamine im Magen. Hoppe Seylers Z. Physiol. Chem. 349:1691-1697.

Schoental, R. (1960). Carcinogenic action of diazomethane and of nitroso-N-methyl urethan. Nature 188:420-421.

Sen, N. P. (1974). Nitrosamines. In Toxic Constituents of Animal Foodstuffs, I. E. Liener (Ed.). Academic Press, New York, pp. 131-194.

Sen, N. P., Donaldson, B., and Charbonneau, C. (1974a). Formation of nitrosodimethylamine from the interaction of certain pesticides and nitrite. In N-Nitroso compounds in the Environment, P. Bogovski and E. A. Walker (Eds.). IARC Scientific Publication No. 9, Lyon, France, pp. 75-79.

Sen, N. P., Donaldson, B., Charbonneau, C., and Miles, W. F. (1974b). Effect of additives on the formation of nitrosamines in meat curing mixtures containing spices and nitrite. J. Agric. Food Chem. 22:1125-1130.

Sen, N. P., Donaldson, B., Seaman, S., Collins, B., and Iyengar, J. R. (1977). Recent nitrosamine analysis in cooked bacon. Can. Inst. Food Sci. Technol. 10:A13-A15.

Sen, N. P., Donaldson, B., Seaman, S., Iyengar, J. R., and Miles, W. F. (1976a). Inhibition of nitrosamine formation in fried bacon by propyl gallate and L-ascorbyl palmitate. J. Agric. Food Chem. 24:397-401.

Sen, N. P., Iyengar, J. R., Miles, W. F., and Panalaks, T. (1976b). Nitrosamines in in cured meat products. In Environmental N-Nitroso Compounds Analysis and Formation, E. A. Walker, P. Bogovski, and I. Griciute (Eds.). IARC Scientific Publication No. 14, Lyon, France, pp. 333-342.

Sen, N. P., and McKinley, W. P. (1974). Meat curing agents as one source of nitrosamines. In Proc. 4th Int. Cong. Food Sci. and Technol. Vol. III, pp. 476-482.

Sen, N. P., Miles, W. F., Donaldson, B., Panalaks, T., and Iyengar, J. R. (1973). Formation of nitrosamines in a meat curing mixture. Nature 245:104-105.

Sen, N. P., Smith, D. C., Moodie, C. A., and Grice, H. C. (1976c). Failure to induce tumours in guinea pigs after concurrent administration of nitrite and diethylamine. Food Cosmet. Toxicol. 13:423-425.

Sen, N. P., Smith, D. C., and Schwinghamer, L. (1969). Formation of N-nitrosamines from secondary amines and nitrite in human and animal gastric juice. Food Cosmet. Toxicol. 7:301-307.

Serfontein, W. J., and Hurter, P. (1966). Nitrosamines as environmental carcinogens. II. Evidence for the presence of nitrosamines in tobacco smoke condensate. Cancer Res. 26:575-579.

Shank, R. C., and Newberne, P. M. (1976). Dose-response study of the carcinogenicity of dietary sodium nitrite and morpholine in rats and hamsters. Food Cosmet. Toxicol. 14:1-8.

Siciliano, J., Krulick, S., Heisler, E. G., Schwartz, J. H., and White, J. W. (1975). Nitrate and nitrite content of some fresh and processed market vegetables. J. Agric. Food Chem. 23:461-464.

Singer, G. M., and Lijinsky, W. (1976). Naturally occurring nitrosatable compounds. I. Secondary amines in foodstuffs. J. Agric. Food Chem. 24:550-553.

Spiegelhalder, B., Eisenbrand, G., and Preussmann, R. (1979). Contamination of beer with trace quantities of N-nitroso-dimethylamine. Food Cosmet. Toxicol. 17:29-31.

Stephany, R. W., Fruedenthal, J., and Schuller, P. L. (1976). Quantitative and qualitative determination of some volatile nitrosamines in various meat products. In Environmental N-Nitroso Compounds Analysis and Formation, E. A. Walker, P. Bogovski, and L. Griciute (Eds.). IARC Scientific Publication No. 14, Lyon, France, pp. 343-354.

Tannenbaum, S. R., Weisman, M., and Fett, D. (1976). The effect of nitrate intake on nitrite formation in human saliva. Food Cosmet. Toxicol. 14:549-552.

Telling, G. M., Bryce, T. A., and Althorpe, J. (1971). Use of vacuum distillation and gas chromatography-mass spectrometry for determining low levels of volatile nitrosamines in meat products. J. Agric. Food Chem. 19:937-940.

Terracini, B., Magee, P. N., and Barnes, J. M. (1967). Hepatic pathology in rats on low dietary levels of diemthylnitrosamine. Br. J. Cancer 21:559-565.

Toth, B., Magee, P. N., and Shubik, P. (1964). Carcinogenesis study with dimethylnitrosamine administered orally to adult and subcutaneously to newborn BALB/c mice. Cancer Res. 24:1712-1721.

U.S. Food Additive Regulations (1972). Code of Federal Regulations, Office of the Federal Register, Washington, D.C.

Walters, C. L., Edwards, M. W., Elsey, T. S., and Martin, M. (1976). The effect of antioxidants on the production of volatile nitrosamines during the frying of bacon. Z. Lebensm. Unters. Forsch. 162:377-385.

White, J. W. (1975). Relative significance of dietary sources of nitrate and nitrite. J. Agric. Food Chem. 23:886-891.

Section III.B

Aitio, A. (1973). Extrahepatic microsomal drug metabolism with special reference to glucuronide synthesis. Academic dissertation, Monistepalvelu, Turkey. Cited by O. Pelkonen in Polynuclear Aromatic Hydrocarbons: Chemistry, Metabolism and Carcinogenicity, R. I. Freudenthal and P. Jones (Eds.). Raven Press, New York (1976), pp. 9-21.

Ames, B. N., Sims, P., Grover, P. L. (1972). Epoxides of carcinogenic polycyclic hydrocarbons are frameshift mutagens. Science 176:47-49.

Andelman, J. B., and Suess, M. J. (1970). Polynuclear aromatic hydrocarbons in the water environment. Bull. WHO 43:479-508.

Badger, G. M. (1962). Mode of formation of carcinogens in human environment. Natl. Cancer Inst. Monogr. 9:1-16.

Bailey, E. J., and Dungal, N. (1958). Polycyclic hydrocarbons in Icelandic smoked food. Br. J. Cancer 12:348-350.

Berwald, Y., and Sachs, L. (1963). In vitro cell transformation with chemical carcinogens. Nature 200:1182-1184.

Berwald, Y., and Sachs, L. (1965). In vitro transformation of normal cells to tumor cells by carcinogenic hydrocarbons. J. Natl. Cancer Inst. 35:641-661.

Biancifiori, C., Bonser, G. M., and Caschera, F. (1961). Ovarian and mammary tumors in intact C_3Hb virgin mice following a limited dose of four carcinogenic chemicals. Br. J. Cancer 15:270-283.

Blumer, M., and Youngblood, W. W. (1975). Polycyclic aromatic hydrocarbons in soils and recent sediments. Science 188:53-55.

Bock, F. G., and King, D. W. (1959). A study of the sensitivity of the mouse forestomach toward certain polycyclic hydrocarbons. J. Natl. Cancer Inst. 23:833-839.

Borneff, J., Selenka, F., Kunte, H., and Maximos, A. (1968). Experimental studies on the formation of polycyclic aromatic hydrocarbons in plants. Environ. Res. 2:22-29.

Boyland, E., and Sims, P. (1964). Metabolism of polycyclic compounds. 24. The metabolism of benz(a)anthracene. Biochem. J. 91:493-506.

Boyland, E., and Sims, P. (1967). The carcinogenic activities in mice of compounds related to benz(a)anthracene. Int. J. Cancer 2:500-504.

Burki, K., and Bresnick, E. (1975). Early morphologic alterations in mouse skin after topical application of 3-methylcholanthrene and its metabolites. J. Natl. Cancer Inst. 55:171-175.

Burki, K., Seibert, R. A., and Bresnick, E. (1972). Induction of benzpyrene hydroxylase activity in fetal rat liver explants. I. Metabolism of 3-methylcholanthrene and differential effects of its derivatives of benzpyrene hydroxylase activity. Biochem. Biophys. Acta 260:98-109.

Cahnmann, J. J., and Kuratsune, M. (1957). Determination of polycyclic aromatic hydrocarbons in oysters collected in polluted water. Anal. Chem. 29:1312-1317.

Cavalieri, E., Garcia, H., Mailander, P., and Patil, K. (1975). Isotope effect on the carcinogenicity of 3-methylcholanthrene in mouse skin by selective deuteration of the 1-methylene group: biological evidence for a mechanism of tumor initiation. Chem. Biol. Interact. 11:179-189.

Cavalieri, E., Roth, R., and Rogan, E. G. (1976). Metabolic activation of aromatic hydrocarbons by one-electron oxidation in relation to the mechanism of tumor initiation. In Polynuclear Aromatic Hydrocarbons: Chemistry, Metabolism and Carcinogenicity, R. I. Freudenthal and P. Jones (Eds.). Raven Press, New York, 1:181-190.

Chen, L. (1970). Further studies of the effect of bone marrow cells on chemically induced lymphoma in C_{57}BL/6 mice. Br. J. Cancer 24:554-560.

Chen, T. T., and Heidelberger, C. (1969a). Cultivation in vitro of cells derived from adult C3H mouse ventral prostrate. J. Natl. Cancer Inst. 42:903-914.

Chen, T. T., and Heidelberger, C. (1969b). In vitro malignant transformation of cells derived from mouse prostrate in the presence of 3-MCA. J. Natl. Cancer Inst. 42: 915-925.

Chen, T. T., and Heidelberger, C. (1969c). Quantitative studies on the malignant transformations of mouse prostrate cells by carcinogenic hydrocarbons in vitro. Int. J. Cancer 4:166-178.

Daniel, P. M., Pratt, O. E., and Prichard, M. M. (1967). Metabolism of labelled carcinogenic hydrocarbons in rats. Nature 215:1142-1146.

Dipaolo, J. A., Donovan, P., and Nelson, R. (1969a). Quantitative studies of in vitro transformation by chemical carcinogens. J. Natl. Cancer Inst. 42:867-874.

Dipaolo, J. A., Nelson, R. L., and Donovan, P. J. (1969b). Sarcoma-producing cell lines derived from clones transformed in vitro by benzo(a)pyrene. Science 165:917-918.

Dipple, A., Lawley, P. D., and Brookes, P. (1968). Theory of tumor initiation by chemical carcinogens: dependence of activity on structure of ultimate carcinogen. Eur. J. Cancer 4:493-506.

Dorr, R. (1965). Die Aufnahme von Alkaloiden und Benzpyren durch intakte Pflanzenwurzeln. Naturwissenschaften 52:166.

Draudt, H. N. (1963). The meat smoking process: a review. Food Technol. 17:85-90.

Dungal, N. (1961). The special problem of stomach cancer in Iceland with particular reference to dietary factor. JAMA 178:789-798.

Dunn, B. P., and Stich, H. F. (1976). Monitoring procedures for chemical carcinogens in coastal waters. J. Fish Res. Board Can. 33:2040-2046.

Dunn, B. P., and Young, D. R. (1976). Baseline levels of benzo(a)pyrene in southern California mussels. Marine Poll. Bull. 7:231-234.

EPA (1975). Scientific and technical assessment report on particulate polycyclic organic matter. U.S. Environmental Protection Agency, Washington, D.C.

Eskin, B. A., Murphey, S. A., and Dunn, M. R. (1968). Induction of breast cancer in altered thyroid states. Nature 218:1162.

Falk, H. L., Kotin, P., Lee, S. K., and Nathan, A. J. (1962). Intermediary metabolism of benzo(a)pyrene in the rat. J. Natl. Cancer Inst. 28:699-724.

Farber, E. (1968). Biochemistry of carcinogenesis. Cancer Res. 28:1859-1869.

Filipovic, J., and Toth, L. (1971). Polycyclische Kohlenwasserstoffe in geraeucherten jugoslawischen Fleischwaren. Fleischwirtschaft 51:1323-1325.

Flesher, J. W., and Sydnor, K. L. (1970). Comparative studies on distribution of DMBA-^{3}H and 7-hydroxy-DMBA-^{3}H and their carcinogenic activity. Int. J. Cancer 5:253-259.

Frethein, K. (1976). Carcinogenic polycyclic aromatic hydrocarbons in Norwegian smoked meat. J. Agric. Food Chem. 24:976-979.

Fried, J., and Schumm, D. E. (1967). One electron transfer oxidation of 7,12-dimethylbenz(a)anthracene, a model for the metabolic activation of carcinogenic hydrocarbons. J. Am. Chem. Soc. 89:5508-5509.

Freudenthal, R. I., Hundley, S. G., and Cattaneo, S. M. (1978). A comparison of the metabolites of benzopyrene by lung mixed function oxidase from rat, rhesus, and humans. In Polynuclear Aromatic Hydrocarbons: 2nd Int. Symp. Analysis, Chemistry and Biology, R. I. Freudenthal and P. Jones (Eds.). Raven Press, New York, 3:313-323.

Gelboin, H. V., Kinoshita, N., and Wiebel, F. J. (1972). Microsomal hydroxylase: induction and role in polycyclic hydrocarbon carcinogenesis and toxicity. Fed. Proc. 31:1298-1309.

Gibel, W. von (1964). Experimenteller Beitrag zur Synkarzinogense bein Speiserohrenkarzainom. Krebsarzt 19: 268. In Evaluation of Carcinogenic Risk of Chemicals to Man, IARC Monographs, Vol. 3. Lyon, France, p. 103.

Grasso, P., and O'Hare, C. (1976). Carcinogens in foods. In Chemical Carcinogens, C. E. Searle (Ed.). ACS Monograph 173, American Chemical Society, Washington, D.C., pp. 701-728.

Grimmer, G. (1966). Cancerogeme Kohlenwasserstoffe in der Umgebung des Menschen. Erdoel Kohle 19:578-583.

Grimmer, G., and Bohnke, H. (1975). Polycyclic aromatic hydrocarbon profile analysis of high-protein foods, oils, and fats by gas chromatography. J. Assoc. Off. Anal. Chem. 58:725-733.

Grimmer, G., and Hildebrandt, A. (1965a). Content of polycyclic hydrocarbon in different vegetables. III. Hydrocarbons in the human surroundings. Deut. Lebensm. Rundschau. 61:237-239. Reported in Chem. Abst. (1965), 63:16769g.

Grimmer, G., and Hildebrandt, A. (1965b). Hydrocarbons in the human environment. II. Content of polycyclic hydrocarbons in bread grains from various localities. Z. Krebsforsch. 67:272-277. Reported in Chem. Abst. (1966), 64:7272g.

Grimmer, G., and Hildebrandt, A. (1966). Hydrocarbons in the human environment. IV. Polycyclic hydrocarbons in coffee and tea. Deut. Lebensm. Rundschau. 62:19-21. Reported in Anal. Abst. (1966), 14:3591.

Grover, P. L., Hewer, A., and Sims, P. (1971). Epoxides as microsomal metabolites of polycyclic hydrocarbons. Fed. Eur. Biochem. Soc. Lett. 18:76-80.

Grover, P. L., Hewer, A., and Sims, P. (1972). Formation of K-region epoxides as microsomal metabolites of pyrene and benzopyrene. Biochem. Pharmacol. 21:2713-2726.

Grover, P. L., Sims, P., Huberman, E., Marquardt, H., Kuroki, T., and Heidelberger, C. (1971). In vitro transformation of rodent cells by K-region derivatives of polycyclic hydrocarbon. Proc. Natl. Acad. Sci. USA 68:1098-1101.

Grover, P. L., Sims, P., Mitchley, B. C., and Roe, F. J. (1975). The carcinogenicity of polycyclic hydrocarbon epoxides in new born mice. Br. J. Cancer 31:182-188.

Guerrero, H., Biehl, E. R., and Kenner, C. T. (1976). High-pressure liquid chromatography of benzo(a)pyrene and benzo(ghi)perylene in oil-contaminated shellfish. J. Assoc. Off. Anal. Chem. 59:989-992.

Gunther, F. A., Buzzetti, F., and Westlake, W. E. (1967). Residue behavior of polynuclear hydrocarbons on and in oranges. Residue Rev. 17:81-104.

Haenni, E. O. (1968). Analytical control of polycyclic aromatic hydrocarbons in food and food additives. Residue Rev. 24:41-78.

Haenni, E. O., Howard, J. W., and Joe, F. L., Jr. (1962a). Dimethyl sulfoxide: a superior analytical extraction solvent for polynuclear hydrocarbons and for some highly chlorinated hydrocarbons. J. Assoc. Off. Anal. Chem. 45:67-70.

Haenni, E. O., Joe, F. L., Jr., Howard, J. W., and Leibel, R. L. (1962b). A more sensitive and selective ultraviolet absorption criterion for mineral oil. J. Assoc. Off. Anal. Chem. 45:59-66.

Hartwell, J. (1951). Survey of compound which have been tested for carcinogenic activity. Public Health Service, Publication No. 149, U.S. Government Printing Office, Washington, D.C.

Hecht, S. S., Grabowski, W., and Groth, K. (1979). Analysis of faeces for benzo(a)pyrene after consumption of charcoal-broiled beef by rats and humans. Food Cosmet. Toxicol. 17:223-227.

Heidelberger, C., Hadler, H. I., and Wolf, G. (1953). The metabolic degradation in the mouse of 1,2,5,6-dibenzanthracene-9,10-C^{14}. IV. Some quinone metabolites retaining the intact ring system. J. Am. Chem. Soc. 75:1303-1308.

Heidelberger, C., and Iype, P. T. (1967). Malignant transformation in vitro by carcinogenic hydrocarbons. Science 155:214-217.

Heidelberger, C., Kirk, M. R., and Perkins, M. S. (1948). The metabolic degradation in the mouse of dibenzanthracene labelled in the 9 and 10 positions with carbon 14. Cancer 1:261-275.

Hites, R. A., Laflamme, R. E., and Farrington, J. W. (1977). Sedimentary polycyclic aromatic hydrocarbons: the historical record. Science 198:829-831.

Howard, J. W., and Fazio, T. (1969). A review of polycyclic aromatic hydrocarbons in foods. J. Agric. Food Chem. 17:527-531.

Howard, J. W., Fazio, T., and White, R. H. (1968a). Polycyclic aromatic hydrocarbons in solvents used in extraction of edible oils. J. Agric. Food Chem. 16:72-76.

Howard, J. W., Fazio, T., White, R. H., and Klimeck, B. A. (1968b). Extraction and estimation of polycyclic aromatic hydrocarbons in total diet composites. J. Assoc. Off. Anal. Chem. 51:122-129.

Howard, J. W., and Haenni, E. O. (1963). The extraction and determination of polynuclear hydrocarbons in paraffin waxes. J. Assoc. Off. Anal. Chem. 46:933-941.

Howard, J. W., Haenni, E. O., and Joe, F. L., Jr. (1965). An ultraviolet absorption criterion for total polynuclear aromatic hydrocarbon content of petroleum waxes in food additive use. J. Assoc. Off. Anal. Chem. 48:304-315.

Howard, J. W., Teague, R. T., White, R. H., and Fry, B. E., Jr. (1966a). Extraction and estimation of polycyclic aromatic hydrocarbons in smoked foods. I. General method. J. Assoc. Off. Anal. Chem. 49:595-611.

Howard, J. W., Turicchi, E. W., White, R. H., and Fazio, T. (1966b). Extraction and estimation of polycyclic hydrocarbons in vegetable oils. J. Assoc. Off. Anal. Chem. 49:1236-1244.

Howard, J. W., White, R. H., Fry, B. E., Jr., and Turicchi, E. W. (1966c). Extraction and estimation of polycyclic aromatic hydrocarbons in smoked foods. II. Benzo(a)pyrene. J. Assoc. Off. Anal. Chem. 49:611-617.

Huberman, E., Aspiras, L., Heidelberger, C., Grover, P. L., and Sims, P. (1971a). Mutagenicity to mammalian cells of epoxides and other derivatives of polycyclic hydrocarbons. Proc. Natl. Acad. Sci. USA 68:3195-3199.

Huberman, E., Grover, P. L., Kuroki, T., Sims, P., and Heidelberger, C. (1971b). K-region epoxides are more active than hydrocarbons in producing transformation in vitro. Proc. Am. Assoc. Cancer Res. 12:79

Huberman, E., Kuroki, T., Marquardt, H., Selkirk, J. K., Heidelberger, C., Grover, P. L., and Sims, P. (1972). Transformation of hamster embryo cells by epoxides and other derivatives of polycyclic hydrocarbons. Cancer Res. 32:1391-1396.

Huberman, E., Sachs, L., Yang, S. K., and Gelboin, H. V. (1976). Identification of mutagenic metabolites of benzo(a)pyrene in mammalian cells. Proc. Natl. Ada. Sci. USA 73:607-611.

Huberman, E., Selkirk, J. K., and Heidelberger, C. (1971c). Metabolism of polycyclic aromatic hydrocarbons in cell cultures. Cancer Res. 31:2161-2167.

Huberman, E., Yang, S. K., McCourt, D. W., and Gelboin, H. V. (1977). Mutagenicity to mammalian cells in culture by (+) and (-) trans-7,8-dihydroxy-7,8-dihydrobenzo(a)pyrenes and the hydrolysis and reduction products of two stereoisomeric benzo(a)pyrene 7,8-diol-9,10-epoxides. Cancer Lett. 4:35-43.

Huggins, C., and Yang, N. C. (1962). Induction and extinction of mammary cancer. Science 137:257-262.

Huggins, C. B., Yoshida, H., and Bird, C. C. (1974). Hormone-dependent stem-cell rat leukemia evoked by a series of feeding of 7,12-dimethylbenz(a)anthracene. J. Natl. Cancer Inst. 52:1301-1306.

Hulbert, P. B. (1975). Carbonium ion as ultimate carcinogen of polycyclic aromatic hydrocarbons. Nature 256:146-148.

IARC (1973). Evaluation of Carcinogenic Risk of Chemicals to Man, IARC Monographs, Vol. 3, Lyon, France.

Juchau, M. R., Jones, A. H., Namkung, M. J., and DiGiovanni, J. (1978). Extrahepatic bioactivation of 7,12-dimethylbenz(a)anthracene and benzo(a)pyrene in human fetal tissues. In Polynuclear Aromatic Hydrocarbons: 2nd Int. Symp. Analysis, Chemistry and Biology, R. I. Freudenthal and P. Jones (Eds.). Raven Press, New York, 3:361-370.

Kapitulnik, J., Levin, W., Conney, A. H., Yagi, H., and Jerina, D. M. (1977). Benzo(a)pyrene 7,8-dihydrodiol is more carcinogenic than benzo(a)pyrene in newborn mice. Nature 266:378-380.

Kennaway, E. L. (1925). Experiments on cancer-producing substances. Br. Med. J. 2: 1-4.

Keysell, G. R., Booth, J., Grover, P. L., Hewer, A., and Sims, P. (1973). The formation of "K-region" epoxides as hepatic microsomal metabolites of 7-methylbenz(a)anthracene and 7,12-dimethylbenz(a)anthracene and their 7-hydroxymethyl derivatives. Biochem. Pharmacol. 22:2853-2867.

Klein, M. (1963). Susceptibility of strain BbAF1/J hybrid infant mice to tumorigenesis with 1,2-benzanthracene, deoxycholic acid and 3-methylcholanthrene. Cancer Res. 23: 1701-1707.

Knorr, M., and Schenk, D. (1968). Synthesis of polycyclic aromatic compounds by bacteria. Arch. Hyg. Bakteriol. 152:282-285. Reported in Chem. Abst. (1968), 69:74645.

Kuntzman, R., Mark, L. C., Brand, L., Jacobson, M., Levin, W., and Conney, A. H. (1966). Metabolism of drugs and carcinogens by human liver enzymes. J. Pharmacol. Exp. Ther. 152:151-156.

Laflamme, R. E., and Hites, R. A. (1978). The global distribution of polycyclic aromatic hydrocarbons in recent sediments. Geochim. Cosmochim. Acta 42:289-303.

Lasnitzki, I. (1963). Growth pattern of the mouse prostate gland in organ culture and its response to sex hormones, vitamin A and 3-methylcholanthrene. Natl. Cancer Inst. Monogr. 12:381-403.

Leber, P., Kerchner, G., and Freudenthal, R. I. (1976). A comparison of benzo(a)pyrene metabolism by primates, rats, and miniature swine. In Polynuclear Aromatic Hydrocarbons: Chemistry, Metabolism and Carcinogenesis, R. I. Freudenthal and P. Jones (Eds.). Raven Press, New York, pp. 35-43.

Levin, W., Conney, A. H., and Alvares, A. P. (1972). Induction of benzo(a)pyrene hydroxylase in human skin. Science 176:419-420.

Levin, W., Wood, A. W., Yagi, H., Dansette, P. M., Jerina, D. M., and Conney, A. H. (1976). Carcinogenicity of benzo(a)pyrene 4,5-, 7,8- and 9,10-oxides on mouse skin. Proc. Natl. Acad. Sci. USA 73:243-247.

Lijinsky, W., Domsky, I., and Raha, C. R. (1963). A short method of testing petroleum waxes for the presence of polycyclic aromatic hydrocarbons. J. Assoc. Off. Anal. Chem. 49:725-731.

Lijinsky, W., and Raha, C. R. (1961). Polycyclic aromatic hydrocarbons in commercial solvents. Toxicol. Appl. Pharmacol. 3:469-473.

Lijinsky, W., and Ross, A. E. (1967). Production of carcinogenic polynuclear hydrocarbons in the cooking of food. Food Cosmet. Toxicol. 5:343-347.

Lijinsky, W., and Shubik, P. (1964). Benzo(a)pyrene and other polynuclear hydrocarbons in charcoal-broiled meat. Science 145:53-55.

Lijinsky, W., and Shubik, P. (1965a). The detection of polycyclic aromatic hydrocarbons in liquid smoke and some foods. Toxicol. Appl. Pharmacol. 7:337-343.

Lijinsky, W., and Shubik, P. (1965b). Polynuclear hydrocarbon carcinogens in cooked meat and smoked food. Ind. Med. Surg. 34:152-154.

Lintas, C., and DeMatthaeis, M. C, and Merbi, F. (1979). Determination of benzo(a)pyrene in smoked, cooked and toasted food products. Food Cosmet. Toxicol. 17:325-328.

Lo, M.-T., and Sandi, E. (1978). Polycyclic aromatic hydrocarbons (polynuclears) in foods. Residue Rev. 69:35-86.

Lorenz, E., and Stewart, H. L. (1948). Tumors of alimentary tract in mice fed carcinogenic hydrocarbons in mineral oil emulsions. J. Natl. Cancer Inst. 9:173-180.

Mager, R., Huberman, E., Yang, S. K., Gelboin, H. V., and Sachs, L. (1977). Transformation of normal hamster cells by benzo(a)pyrene diol-epoxide. Int. J. Cancer 19: 814-817.

Malanoski, A. J., Greenfield, E. L., Barnes, C. J., Worthington, J. M., and Joe, F. L., Jr. (1968). Survey of polycyclic aromatic hydrocarbons in smoked foods. J. Assoc. Off. Anal. Chem. 51:114-121.

Mallet, L., and Tissier, M. (1969). Biosynthesis expérimentale des hydrocarbures polybenzniques du type benzo3-4pyréne aux dépens des terres de forêts. C. R. Soc. Biol. (Paris) 163:63-65. Reported in Chem. Abst. (1970), 73:44301k.

Marquardt, H., Kuroki, T., Huberman, E., Selkirk, J. K., Heidelberger, C., Grover, P. L., and Sims, P. (1972). Malignant transformation of cells derived from mouse prostate by epoxides and other derivatives of polycyclic hydrocarbons. Cancer Res. 32:716-720.

Masuda, Y., and Kuratsune, M. (1971). Polycyclic aromatic hydrocarbons in smoked fish, "Katsuobushi." Gan. 62:27-30.

Masuda, Y., Mori, K., and Kuratsune, M. (1966). Polycyclic aromatic hydrocarbons in common Japanese foods. I. Broiled fish, roasted barley, shoyu and caramel. Gan. 57:133-142.

Miller, E. C., and Miller, J. A. (1967). Low carcinogenicity of the K-region epoxides and 7-methylbenz(a)anthracene and benz(a)anthracene in mouse and rat. Proc. Soc. Exp. Biol. Med. 124:915-919.

Moloney, W. C., Batata, M., and King, V. (1971). Leukomogenesis in the rat: further observations. J. Natl. Cancer Inst. 46:1139-1144.

NAS (1972). Particulate polycyclic organic matter. U.S. National Academy of Science, Washington, D.C.

Neal, J., and Rigdon, R. H. (1967). Gastric tumors in mice fed benzo(a)pyrene: a quantitative study. Tex. Rep. Biol. Med. 25:553-557.

Nebert, D. W., Winker, J., and Gelboin, H. V. (1969). Aryl hydrocarbon hydroxylase activity in human placenta from cigarette smoking and nonsmoking women. Cancer Res. 29:1763-1769.

Niaussat, P., Auger, C., and Mallet, L. (1970). Apparition relative de quantités d'hydrocarbures cancérigenes dans des cultures pures de Bacillus badius, en fonction de la présence, dans le milieu, de certains composés chimiques. C. R. Acad. Sci. (Paris) 270:1042-1045. Reported in Chem. Abst. (1970), 72:129595.

Panalaks, T. (1976). Determination and identification of polycyclic aromatic hydrocarbons in smoked and charcoal-broiled food products by high pressure liquid chromatography and GAS chromatography. J. Environ. Sci. Health 4:299-315.

Pott, P. (1775). Chirurgical observations relative to the cataract, the polypus of the nose, the cancer of the scrotum, the different kinds of ruptures, and the mortification of the toes and feet. London, L. Hawes, W. Clarke, and R. Collins p. 208.

Rigdon, R. H., Benge, M. C., Kirschoff, H., Mack, J., and Neal, J. (1969). Leukemia in mice fed benzo(a)pyrene: a clinical, pathologic and hematologic study. Tex. Rep. Biol. Med. 27:803-820.

Rigdon, R. H., and Neal, J. (1966). Gastric carcinomas and pulmonary adenomas in mice fed benzo(a)pyrene. Tex. Rep. Biol. Med. 24:195-207.

Rigdon, R. H., and Neal, J. (1969). Relationship of leukemia to lung and stomach tumors in mice fed benzo(a)pyrene. Proc. Soc. Exp. Biol. Med. 130:146-148.

Roller, M. R., and Heidelberger, C. (1967). Attempts to produce carcinogenesis in organ cultures of mouse prostate with polycyclic hydrocarbons. Int. J. Cancer 2:509-520.

Selkirk, J. K., Croy, R. G., and Gelboin, H. V. (1975). Isolation by high pressure liquid chromatography and characterization of benzo(a)pyrene-4,5-epoxide as a metabolite of benzo(a)pyrene. Arch. Biochem. Biophys. 168:322-326.

Selkirk, J. K., Yang, S. K., and Gelboin, H. V. (1976). Analysis of benzo(a)pyrene metabolism in human liver and lymphocytes and kinetic analysis of benzo(a)pyrene in rat liver microsomes. In Polynuclear Aromatic Hydrocarbons: Chemistry, Metabolism and Carcinogenesis, R. I. Freudenthal and P. Jones (Eds.). Raven Press, New York, 1:153-169.

Shubik, P., and Hartwell, J. (1957). Survey of compounds which have been tested for carcinogenic activity. Public Health Service, Publication No. 149 (Suppl.), U.S. Government Printing Office, Washington, D.C.

Shubik, P., and Hartwell, J. (1969). Survey of compounds which have been tested for carcinogenic activity. Public Health Service, Publication No. 149 (Suppl. 2), U.S. Government Printing Office, Washington, D.C.

Sims, P. (1966). The metabolism of 3-methylcholanthrene and some related compounds by rat-liver homogenates. Biochem. J. 98:215-228.

Sims, P. (1967). The carcinogen activities in mice of compounds related to 3-methylcholanthrene. Int. J. Cancer 2:505-508.

Sims, P. (1970). The metabolism of some aromatic hydrocarbons by mouse embryo cell cultures. Biochem. Pharmacol. 19:285-297.

Slaga, T. J., Bracken, W. M., Viaje, A., Berry, D. L., Fisher, S. M., Miller, D. M., Levin, W., Conney, A. H., Yagi, H., and Jerina, D. M. (1978). Tumor initiating and promoting activities of various benzo(a)pyrene metabolites in mouse skin. In Polynuclear Aromatic Hydrocarbons 2nd Int. Symp. Analysis, Chemistry and Biology, R. I. Freudenthal and P. Jones (Eds.). Raven Press, New York, 3:371-382.

Snell, K. C., and Stewart, H. L. (1962). Pulmonary adenomatosis induced in DBA/2 mice by oral administration of dibenz(a,h)anthracene. J. Natl. Cancer Inst. 28:1043-1051.

Snell, K. C., and Stewart, H. L. (1963). Induction of pulmonary adenomatosis in DBA/2 mice by the oral administration of dibenz(a,h)anthracene. Acta Un. Int. Cancer 19: 692-694.

Thorsteinsson, T. (1969). Polycyclic hydrocarbons in commercially and home smoked food in Iceland. Cancer 23:455-457.

Tilgner, D. J., and Daun, H. (1969). Polycyclic aromatic hydrocarbons (polynuclears) in smoked foods. Residue Rev. 27:19-41.

Toth, L. (1969). Cancerogene Stoffe in geraeucherten Fleischwaren. Fleischwirtschaft 49: 1611-1614.

Toth, L. (1971). Polycyclische Kohlenwasserstoffe in geraeucherten Schinken und Bauchspeck. Fleischwirtschaft 51:1069-1970.

Toth, L., and Blass, W. (1972a). Einfluss der Raeuchertechnologie auf den Gehalt von geraeucherten Fleischwaren an cancerogenen Kohlenwasserstoffen. Fleischwirtschaft 52:1121-1124.

Toth, L., and Blass, W. (1972b). 4-Benspyren-Gehalt verschiedener Raeucherpraeparate. Fleischwirtschaft 52:1171.

Toth, L., and Blass, W. (1972c). Einfluss der Raeuchertechnologie auf den Gehalt von geraeucherten Fleischwaren an cancerogenen Kohlenwasserstoffen. Fleischwirtschaft 52:1419-1422.

Tracor/Jitco, Inc. (1973). Survey of compounds which have been tested for carcinogenic activity. Public Health Service, Publication No. 149, U.S. Government Printing Office, Washington, D.C.

Umans, R. S., Lesko, S. A., and Ts'o, P. O. (1969). Chemical linkage of carcinogenic 3,4-benzpyrene to DNA in aqueous solution induced by peroxide and iodine. Nature 221:763-764.

Walker, E. A. (1977). Some facts and legislation concerning polycyclic aromatic hydrocarbons in smoked foods. Pure Appl. Chem. 49:1673-1686.

Warner, J. S. (1974). Quantitative determination of hydrocarbons in marine organisms. Natl. Bur. Stand. USA (Spec. Publ.) 409:195-196.

White, R. H., Howard, J. W., and Barnes, C. J. (1971). Determination of polycyclic aromatic hydrocarbons in liquid smoke flavors. J. Agric. Food Chem. 19:143-146.

Wood, A. W., Chang, R. L., Levin, W., Lehr, R. E., Schaeffer-Ridder, M., Karle, J. M., Jerina, D. M., and Conney, A. H. (1977a). Mutagenicity and cytotoxicity of benzo(a)anthracene diol epoxides and tetrahydro epoxides: Exceptional activity of the bay region 1,2-epoxides. Proc. Natl. Acad. Sci. USA 74:2746-2750.

Wood, A. W., Levin, W., Chang, R. L., Lehr, R. E., Schaeffer-Ridder, M., Karle, J. M., Jerina, D. M., and Conney, A. H. (1977b). Tumorigenicity of five dihydrodiols of benz(a)anthracene on mouse skin: exceptional activity of benz(a)anthracene 3,4-dihydrodiol. Proc. Natl. Acad. Sci. USA 74:3176-3179.

Wood, A. W., Levin, W., Lu, A. Y., Ryan, D., West, S. B., Lehr, R. E., Schaefer-Ridder, M., Jerina, D. M., and Conney, A. H. (1976). Mutagenicity of metabolically activated benzo(a)anthracene 3,4-dihydrodiol: evidence for bay region activation of carcinogenic polycyclic hydrocarbons. Biochem. Biophys. Res. Commun. 72:680-686.

Yamagiwa, K., and Ichikawa, K. (1915). Experimentelle Studie über die Pathogenese der Epithelialgeschwulste. Mitt. Med. Fak. Univ. Tokyo 15:295-334.

Yoshida, H., and Fukunishi, R. (1977). Mammary tumor and leukemia in male Sprague-Dawley rats evoked by a series of intragastric administration of 7,12-dimethylbenz(a)anthracene. Gan. 68:237-239.

Section IV.A

AOAC (1980). Natural poisons. In Official Methods of Analysis. Association of Official Analytical Chemists, Washington, D.C., 22 pages.

Blank, F., Chin, O., Just, G., Meranze, D. R., Shimkin, M. B., and Wieder, R. (1968). Carcinogens from fungi pathogenic for man. Cancer Res. 28:2276-2281.

Büchi, G. H., Müller, P. M., Roebuck, B. D., and Wogan, G. N. (1974). Aflatoxin Q_1: a major metabolite of aflatoxin B_1 produced by the human liver. Res. Commun. Chem. Pathol. Pharmacol. 8:585-592.

Bulatao-Jayme, J., Almero, E. M., and Salamat, L. (1976). Epidemiology of primary liver cancer in the Philippines with special consideration of a possible aflatoxin factor. J. Philippine Med. Assoc. 52:129-150.

Butler, W. H. (1974). Aflatoxin. In Mycotoxins, I. F. Purchase (Ed.). Elsevier, Amsterdam, pp. 1-28.

Butler, W. H., Greenblatt, M., and Lijinsky, W. (1969). Carcinogenesis in rats by aflatoxins B_1, G_1, and B_2. Cancer Res. 29:2206-2211.

Campbell, T. C., and Stoloff, L. (1974). Implications of mycotoxins for human health. J. Agric. Food Chem. 22:1006-1015.

Cucullu, A. F., Lee, L. S., Mayne, R. Y., and Goldblatt, L. A. (1966). Determination of aflatoxins in individual peanuts and peanut sections. J. Am. Oil Chem. Soc. 43:89-92.

Dailey, R. E., Brouwer, E., Blaschka, A. M., Reynaldo, E. F., Green, S., Monlux, W. S., and Ruggles, D. I. (1977). Intermediate-duration toxicity study of patulin in rats. J. Toxicol. Environ. Health 2:713-725.

DeMatteis, F., Donnelly, A. J., and Runge, W. J. (1966). The effect of prolonged administration of griseofulvin in mice with reference to sex differences. Cancer Res. 26 (Part 1):721-726.

Dickens, F., and Jones, H. E. (1961). Carcinogenic activity of a series of reactive lactones and related substances. Br. J. Cancer 15:85-100.

Dickens, F., and Jones, H. E. (1963). Further studies on the carcinogenic and growth-inhibitory activity of lactones and related substances. Br. J. Cancer 17:100-108.

Dickens, F., and Jones, H. E. (1965). Further studies on the carcinogenic action of certain lactones and related substances in the rat and mouse. Br. J. Cancer 19:392-403.

Dickens, J. W., and Whitaker, T. B. (1975). Efficacy of electronic color sorting and handpicking to remove aflatoxin contaminated kernels from commercial lots of shelled peanuts. Peanut Sci. 2:45-50.

Enomoto, M., and Ueno, I. (1974). Penicillium islandicum (toxic yellowed rice)-luteoskyrin-islanditoxin-cyclochlorotine. In Mycotoxins, I. F. Purchase (Ed.). Elsevier, Amsterdam, pp. 303-326.

Eppley, R. M. (1979). Trichothecenes and their analysis. J. Am. Oil Chem. Soc. 56: 824-829.

Epstein, S. M., Bartus, B., and Farber, E. (1969). Renal epithelial neoplasms induced in male Wistar rats by oral aflatoxin B_1. Cancer Res. 29:1045-1050.

Escoula, L. (1974). Moisissures toxinogènes de fourrages ensilés. I. Présence de patuline dans les fronts de coupe d'ensilages. Ann. Rech. Vet. 5:423-432.

Escoula, L. (1975). Moisissures toxinogènes de fourrages ensilés. IV. Production de patuline en milieu liquide par des espèces fongiques isolées des ensilages. Ann. Rech. Vet. 6:303-310.

Essigmann, J. M., Croy, R. G., Nadzan, A. M., Busby, W. F., Jr., Reinhold, V. N., Büchi, G., and Wogan, G. N. (1977). Structural identification of the major DNA adduct formed by aflatoxin B_1 in vitro. Proc. Natl. Acad. Sci. USA 74:1870-1874.

Gibel, W., Wegner, K., and Wildner, G. P. (1971). Experimentelle Untersuchungen zur Frage einer kanzerogenen Wirkung von _Penicillium camemberti_ var. _candidum_. Arch. Geschwulstforsch. 38:1-6.

Goldblatt, L. A. (Ed.) (1969). _Aflatoxin_. _Scientific Background, Control and Implications_. Academic Press, New York, 472 pages.

Hesseltine, C. W. (1976). Conditions leading to mycotoxin contamination of foods and feeds. In _Mycotoxins and Other Fungal-Related Food Problems, Advances in Chemistry Series_, Number 149, J. V. Rodricks (Ed.). American Chemical Society, Washington, D.C., pp. 1-22.

Kanisawa, M., and Suzuki, S. (1978). Induction of renal and hepatic tumors in mice by ochratoxin A, a mycotoxin. Gan. 69:599-600.

Kiermeier, F., Weiss, G., Behringer, G., Miller, M., and Ranfft, K. (1977). Vorkommen und Gehalt an Aflatoxin M_1 in Molkerei-Anlieferungsmilch. Z. Lebensm. Unters. Forsch. 163:171-174.

Kramer, J., Carter, G. G., Arret, B., Wilner, J., Wright, W. W., and Kirschbaum, A. (1968). Assay methods for antibiotics in milk, dairy products, and animal tissues. In _Antibiotic Residues in Milk, Dairy Products, and Animal Tissues: Methods, Reports, and Protocols_, Food and Drug Administration, Washington, D.C., pp. 1-41.

Krogh, P., and Elling, F. (1977). Mycotoxic nephropathy. Vet. Sci. Commun. 1:51-63.

Manabe, M., Minamisawa, M., and Matsuura, S. (1973). Extraction and clean-up method for the sterigmatocystin analysis of rice (gas-liquid chromatographic assay of sterigmatocystin Part II). J. Agric. Chem. Soc. Jap. 47:209-215.

Manabe, M., and Tsuruta, O. (1975). Mycological damage of domestic brown rice during storage in warehouse under natural condition. (Part 2) Natural occurrence of sterigmatocystin on rice during a long time storage. Trans. Mycol. Soc. Jap. 16: 399-405.

Osswald, H., Frank, H. K., Komitowski, D., and Winter, H. (1978). Long-term testing of patulin administered orally to Sprague Dawley rats and Swiss mice. Food Cosmet. Toxicol. 16:243-247.

Parpia, H. A., and Sreenivasamurthy, V. (1971). Importance of aflatoxin in foods with reference to India. Proc. 3rd Int. Cong. Food Sci. Technol (SOS/70), Washington, D.C. (1970):701-704.

Panalaks, T., and Scott, P. M. (1977). Sensitive silica gel-packed flowcell for fluorometric detection of aflatoxins by high pressure liquid chromatography. J. Assoc. Off. Anal. Chem. 60:583-589.

Parker, W. A., and Melnick, D. (1966). Absence of aflatoxin from refined vegetable oils. J. Am. Oil Chem. Soc. 43:635-638.

Patterson, D. S. (1973). Metabolism as a factor in determining the toxic action of the aflatoxins in different animal species. Food Cosmet. Toxicol. 11:287-294.

Pavlović, M., Pleština, R., and Krogh, P. (1979). Ochratoxin A contamination of foodstuffs in an area with Balkan (endemic) nephropathy. Acta Pathol. Microbiol. Scand. [B] 87:243-246.

Phillips, D. L., Yourtee, D. M., and Searles, S. (1976). Presence of aflatoxin B_1 in human liver in the United States. Toxicol. Appl. Pharmacol. 36:403-406.

Polzhofer, K. (1977). Aflatoxinbestimmung in Milch und Milchprodukten. Z. Lebensm. Unters. Forsch. 163:175-177.

Purchase, I. F. (1972). Aflatoxin residues in food of animal origin. Food Cosmet. Toxicol. 10:531-544.

Purchase, I. F., and Pretorius, M. E. (1973). Sterigmatocystin in coffee beans. J. Assoc. Off. Anal. Chem. 56:225-226.

Purchase, I. F., and Watt, J. J., van der (1970). Carcinogenicity of sterigmatocystin. Food Cosmet. Toxicol. 8:289-295.

Richir, C., Paccalin, J., Larcebeau, S., Faugeres, J., Morard, J.-L., and Lamant, M. (1976). Présence d'aflatoxine B_1 dans le foie humain. Cah. Nutr. Diét. 11:223-226.

Salhab, A. S., and Hsieh, D. P. (1975). Aflatoxicol H_1: a major metabolite of aflatoxin B_1 produced by human and rhesus monkey livers in vitro. Res. Commun. Chem. Pathol. Pharmacol. 10:419-431.

Schoental, R., Joffe, A. Z., and Yagen, B. (1979). Cardiovascular lesions and various tumors found in rats given T-2 toxin, a trichothecene metabolite of Fusarium. Cancer Res. 39:2179-2189.

Schroeder, H. W., and Hein, H., Jr. (1977). Natural occurrence of sterigmatocystin in in-shell pecans. Can. J. Microbiol. 23:639-641.

Schroeder, H. W., and Kelton, W. H. (1975). Production of sterigmatocystin by some species of the genus Aspergillus and its toxicity to chicken embryos. Appl. Microbiol. 30:589-591.

Scott, P. M. (1974). Patulin. In Mycotoxins. I. F. Purchase (Ed.). Elsevier, Amsterdam, pp. 383-403.

Scott, P. M. (1978). Mycotoxins in feeds and ingredients and their origin. J. Food Prot. 41:385-398.

Scott, P. M., and Kennedy, B. P. (1973). Improved method for the thin layer chromatographic determination of patulin in apple juice. J. Assoc. Off. Anal. Chem. 56:813-816.

Scott, P. M., Walbeek, W., van, Kennedy, B., and Anyeti, D. (1972). Mycotoxins (ochratoxin A, citrinin and sterigmatocystin) and toxigenic fungi in grains and other agricultural products. J. Agric. Food Chem. 20:1103-1109.

Shank, R. C. (1976). The role of aflatoxin in human disease. In Mycotoxins and Other Fungal Related Food Problems, Advances in Chemistry Series, Number 149, J. V. Rodricks (Ed.). American Chemical Society, Washington, D.C., pp. 51-57.

Shank, R. C., Bourgeois, C. H., Keschamras, N., and Chandavimol, P. (1971). Aflatoxins in autopsy specimens from Thai children with an acute disease of unknown etiology. Food Cosmet. Toxicol. 9:501-507.

Shotwell, O. L. (1977). Aflatoxin in corn. J. Am. Oil Chem. Soc. 54:216A-224A.

Shreeve, B. J., Patterson, D. S., and Roberts, B. A. (1975). Investigation of suspected cases of mycotoxicosis in farm animals in Britain. Vet. Rec. 97:275-278

Singh, R., and Hsieh, D. P. (1976). Enzymatic conversion of sterigmatocystin into aflatoxin B_1 by cell-free extracts of Aspergillus parasiticus. Appl. Environ. Microbiol. 31:743-745.

Snow, J. P., Lucas, G. B., Harvan, D., Pero, R. W., and Owens, R. G. (1972). Analysis of tobacco smoke condensate for penicillic acid. Appl. Microbiol. 24:34-36.

Stack, M. E.. Nesheim, S., Brown, N. L., and Pohland, A. E. (1976). Determination of sterigmatocystin in corn and oats by gel permeation and high-pressure liquid chromatography. J. Assoc. Off. Anal. Chem. 59:966-970.

Stack, M., and Rodricks, J. V. (1971). Method for analysis and chemical confirmation of sterigmatocystin. J. Assoc. Off. Chem. 54:86-90.

Steyn, M., and Rabie, C. J. (1975). Production of sterigmatocystin. J. Assoc. Off. Anal. Chem. 58:622-623.

Stoloff, L. (1976a). Incidence, distribution, and disposition of products containing aflatoxins. Proc. Am. Phytopathol. Soc. 3:156-172.

Stoloff, L. (1976b). Occurrence of mycotoxins in foods and feeds. In Mycotoxins and Other Fungal Related Food Problems, Advances in Chemistry Series, Number 149, J. V. Rodricks (Ed.). American Chemical Society, Washington, D.C., pp. 23-50.

Stoloff, L. (1976c). Report on mycotoxins. J. Assoc. Off. Anal. Chem. 59:317-323.

Stoloff, L. (1979). Report on mycotoxins. J. Assoc. Off. Anal. Chem. 62:356-362.

Stray, H. (1978). High pressure liquid chromatographic determination of patulin in apple juice. J. Assoc. Off. Anal. Chem. 61:1359-1362.

Swenson, D. H., Lin, J.-K., Miller, E. C., and Miller, J. A. (1977). Aflatoxin B_1-2,3-oxide as a probable intermediate in the covalent binding of aflatoxins B_1 and B_2 to rat liver DNA and ribosomal RNA in vivo. Cancer Res. 37:172-181.

Takeda, N., Seo, S., Ogihara, Y., Sankawa, U., Iitaka, I., Kitigawa, I., and Shibata, S. (1973). Studies on fungal metabolites. XXXI. Anthraquinonoid colouring matters of Penicillium islandicum Sopp and some other fungi. (-) Luteoskyrin, (-)rubroskyrin, (+)rugulosin and their related compounds. Tetrahedron 29:3703-3719.

Thiel, P. G., and Steyn, M. (1973). Urinary excretion of the mycotoxin, sterigmatocystin by vervet monkeys. Biochem. Pharmacol. 22:3267-3273.

Thorpe, C. W., and Johnson, R. L. (1974). Analysis of penicillic acid by gas-liquid chromatography. J. Assoc. Off. Anal. Chem. 57:861-865.

Turner, W. B. (1971). Fungal Metabolites. Academic Press, London, 446 pages.

Ueno, Y. (1977). Trichothecenes: overview address. In Mycotoxins in Human and Animal Health, J. V. Rodricks, C. W. Hesseltine, and M. A. Mehlman (Eds.). Pathotox Publishers, Park Forest South, Ill., pp. 189-207.

Ueno, Y., and Nakajima, M. (1974). Production of respiratory-deficient mutants of Saccharomyces cerevisiae by (-)luteoskyrin and (+)rugulosin. Chem. Pharm. Bull. (Tokyo) 22:2258-2262.

Uraguchi, K., Saito, M., Noguchi, Y., Takahashi, K., Enomoto, M., and Tatsuno, T. (1972). Chronic toxicity and carcinogenicity in mice of the purified mycotoxins, luteoskyrin and cyclochlorotine. Food Cosmet. Toxicol. 10:193-207.

van Rensburg, S. J., Watt, J. J., van der, Purchase, I. F., Coutinho, L. P., and Markham, R. (1974). Primary liver cancer rate and aflatoxin intake in a high cancer area. S. Afr. Med. J. 48:2508a-2508d.

Watt, J. J., van der (1974). Sterigmatocystin. In Mycotoxins, I. F. Purchase (Ed.). Elsevier, Amsterdam, pp. 369-382.

Whitaker, T. B., and Dickens, J. W. (1974). Variability of aflatoxin test results. J. Am. Oil Chem. Soc. 51:214-218.

Wilson, B. J. (1971). Miscellaneous Penicillium toxins. In Microbial Toxins. Vol. VI, A. Ciegler, S. Kadis, and S. J. Ajl (Eds.). Academic Press, New York, pp. 459-521.

Wilson, D. M. (1976). Patulin and penicillic acid. In Mycotoxins and Other Fungal Related Food Problems, Advances in Chemistry Series, Number 149, J. V. Rodricks (Ed.). American Chemical Society, Washington, D.C., pp. 90-109.

Wogan, G. N., Edwards, G. S., and Newberne, P. M. (1971). Structure-activity relationships in toxicity and carcinogenicity of aflatoxins and analogs. Cancer Res. 31:1936-1942.

Wogan, G. N., and Paglialunga, S. (1974). Carcinogenicity of synthetic aflatoxin M_1 in rats. Food Cosmet. Toxicol. 12:381-384.

Wogan, G. N., Paglialunga, S., and Newberne, P. M. (1974). Carcinogenic effects of low dietary levels of aflatoxin B_1 in rats. Food Cosmet. Toxicol. 12:681-685.

Yoshioka, H., Nakatsu, K., Sato, M., and Tatsuno, T. (1973). The molecular structure of cyclochlorotine, a toxic chlorine-containing cyclic pentapeptide. Chem. Lett. 1319-1322.

Zwicker, G. M., Carlton, W. W., and Tuite, J. (1974). Long-term administration of sterigmatocystin and Penicillium viridicatum to mice. Food Cosmet. Toxicol. 12: 491-497.

Section IV.B

Adrianova, M. M., and Alekseev, I. V. (1970). On the carcinogenic properties of the pesticides, sevin, maneb, ciram and cineb. Vopr. Pitan 29:71.

Agthe, C., Garcia, H., Shubik, P., Tomatis, L., and Wenyon, E. (1970). Studies of the potential carcinogenicity of DDT in the Syrian golden hamster. Proc. Soc. Exp. Biol. Med. 134:113.

Ambrose, A. M., Larson, P. S., Borzellica, J. F., and Hennigar, G. R., Jr. (1970). Toxicologic studies on diethyl-1-(2,4-dichlorophenyl)-2-chlorovinyl phosphate. Toxicol. Appl. Pharmacol. 17:323.

AOAC (1975). Official Methods of Analysis, W. Horwitz (Ed.). Association of Official Analytical Chemists, Washington, D.C.

Balin, P. N. (1970). Experimental data on the blastomogenic activity of the fungicide, maneb. Vrach. Delo 4:21.

Bartsch, E., Eberle, D., Ramsreiner, K., Tomann, A., and Spindler, M. (1971). The carbinole acaricides: chlorobenzilate and chloropropylate. Residue Rev. 39:1.

Blackwell-Smith, R., Jr., Finnegan, J. K., Larson, P. S., Sahyoun, P. F., Dreyfuss, M. L., and Haag, H. B. (1953). Toxicologic studies on zinc and disodium ethylenebis-dithiocarbamates. J. Pharmacol. Exp. Ther. 109:159.

Butler, W. H., and Newberne, P. M. (Eds.) (1975). Mouse Hepatic Neoplasia. Elsevier, Amsterdam.

Carpenter, C. P., Weil, C. S., Palm, P. E., Woodside, M. W., Nair, J. H., III, and Smyth, H. F., Jr. (1961). Mammalian toxicity of 1-naphthyl-N-methyl carbamate (Sevin). J. Agric. Food Chem. 9:30.

Carson, R. (1962). Silent Spring. Houghton-Mifflin, Boston.

Casida, J. E. (1972). Chemistry and metabolism of terminal residues of organophosphorus compounds and carbamates. In Pesticide Chemicals, Vol. 6, Fate of Pesticides in the Environment, A. S. Tahori (Ed.). Gordon and Breach, New York.

Cherry, C., and Newman, A. (1973). Huntingdon Research Centre unpublished report cited by FAO/WHO, JMPR, 1975.

Coffin, D. E. (1964). The metabolism and persistence of Systox, Diazinon and Phosdrin on field-sprayed lettuce. J. Assoc. Off. Anal. Chem. 47:632.

Davies, K. J., and Fitzhugh, O. G. (1962). Tumorigenic potential of aldrin and dieldrin for mice. Toxicol. Appl. Pharmacol. 4:187.

Deichmann, W. B., Keplinger, M., Sala, F., and Glass, F. (1967). "Synergism" among oral carcinogens. IV. Simultaneous feeding of four tumorigens to rats. Toxicol. Appl. Pharmacol. 11:88.

Deichmann, W. B., MacDonald, W. E., Blum, E., Bevilacqua, M., Radomski, J. L., Keplinger, M., and Balkus, M. (1970). Tumorigenicity of aldrin, dieldrin, and endrin in the rat. Ind. Med. Surg. 39:426.

Doull, J., DiGiacomo, R., Root, M., and Meskauskas, J. (1966). University of Chicago, unpublished report cited by FAO/WHO, JMPR, 1972.

Doull, J., Root, M., Vesselinovitch, D., Meskauskas, J., and Fitch, F. (1962). University of Chicago, unpublished report cited by FAO/WHO, JMPR, 1972.

Doull, J., Vesselinovitch, D., Fitch, F., Root, M., and Meskauskas, J. (1960). University of Chicago, unpublished report cited by FAO/WHO, Joint Meeting on Pesticide Residues (JMPR), 1968.

Doull, J., Vesselinovitch, D., Root, M., Cowen, J., Meskauskas, J., and Fitch, F. (1965). University of Chicago, unpublished report cited by FAO/WHO, JMPR, 1972.

Durham, W. F., Ortega, P., and Hayes, W. J., Jr. (1963). The effect of various dietary levels of DDT on liver function cell morphology and DDT storage in the rhesus monkey. Arch. Int. Pharmacodyn. Ther. 141:111.

Eisenbrand, G., Schmähl, D., and Preussmann, R. (1976). Carcinogenicity in rats of high doses of N-nitrosocarbaryl, a nitrosated pesticide. Cancer Lett. 1:281.

Eisenbrand, G., Ungerer, O., and Preussmann, R. (1974). Formation of N-nitroso compounds from agricultural chemicals and nitrite. In N-Nitroso Compounds in the Environment, P. Bogovski, R. Preussmann, and E. A. Walker (Eds.). IARC Scientific Publication No. 9, Lyon, France.

Eisenbrand, G., Ungerer, O., and Preussmann, R. (1975). The reaction of nitrite with pesticides. II. Formation, chemical properties and carcinogenic activity of the N-nitroso-derivative of N-methyl-1-naphthyl carbamate (carbaryl). Food Cosmet. Toxicol. 13:365.

Elespuru, R., Lijinsky, W., and Setlow, J. K. (1974). Nitrosocarbaryl as a potent mutagen of environmental significance. Nature 247:386.

Engst, R., Schnaak, W., and Rattba, H. (1968). Fungicidal effect and residue formation of decomposition products of Maneb and Zineb in tomatoes. Nachrechtenbl. Deut. Pflanzenschutzdienstes (Braunschweig) 22:26.

Fang, S. C. (1976). Thiocarbamates. In Herbicides, Vol. I, P. C. Kearney and D. D. Kaufman (Eds.). Marcel Dekker, New York.

Fang, S. C., George, M., and Freed, V. H. (1964). Metabolism of S-propyl-1-^{14}C-butylethylthiocarbamate. J. Agric. Food Chem. 12:37.

Finnegan, J. K., Larson, P. S., Smith, R. B., Jr., Haag, H. B., and Hennigar, G. R. (1958). Acute and chronic studies on pentachloronitrobenzene. Arch. Int. Pharmacodyn. Ther. 114:38.

Fitzhugh, O. G. (1969). Quoted in the monographs of FAO/WHO, JMPR (DDT), p. 61.

Fitzhugh, O. G., and Nelson, A. A. (1947). The chronic toxicity of DDT. J. Pharmacol. Exp. Ther. 89:18.

Fitzhugh, O. G., Nelson, A. A., and Frawley, J. P. (1950). The chronic toxicities of technical benzene hexachloride and its α, β and γ isomers. J. Pharmacol. Exp. Ther. 100:5.

Fitzhugh, O. G., Nelson, A. A., and Quaife, M. L. (1964). Chronic oral toxicity of aldrin and dieldrin in rats and dogs. Food Cosmet. Toxicol. 2:551.

Gibel, von W., Lohs, Kh., Wildner, G. P., and Ziebarth, D. (1971). Tier experimentelle untersuchungen uber die hepatotoxische und Kanzerogene Wirkung phosphororganischer Verbind ungen. I. Mitteilung: Trichlorphon. Arch. Geschwulstforsch. 37:303.

Gibel, von W., Lohs, Kh., Wildner, G. P., Ziebarth, D., and Steiglitz, R. (1973). Uber die Kanzerogene, haematotoxische und hepatotoxische Wirkung pesticider organischer Phosphorverbindungen. Arch. Geschwulstforsch. 41:311.

Goto, M., Hattori, M., Miyagawa, T., and Enomoto, M. (1972). Hepatoma-Bildung in Mausen nach Verabreichung von HCH-isomerin in hohen Dosen. Chemosphere 6:279.

Graham, S. L., Davis, K. J., Hansen, W. H., and Graham, C. H. (1975). Effects of prolonged ethylenethiourea ingestion on the thyroid of the rat. Food Cosmet. Toxicol. 13:493.

Graham, S. L., Hansen, W. H., Davis, K. J., and Perry, C. H. (1973). Effects of one-year administration of ethylenethiourea upon the thyroid of the rat. J. Agric. Food Chem. 21:324.

Grundmann, E., and Hobik, H. P. (1966). Farbenfabriken Bayer A. G., unpublished report cited by FAO/WHO, JMPR, 1972.

Hallett, D. J., Norstrom, R. J., Onuska, F. I., Comba, M. C., and Sampson, R. (1976). Mass spectral confirmation and analysis by the hall detector of mirex and photomirex in herring gulls from Lake Ontario. J. Agric. Food Chem. 24:1189.

Hanada, M., Gutani, C., and Miyaji, T. (1973). Induction of hepatomas in mice by benzene hexachloride. Gan. 65: 511. Reported in Fed. Reg., Oct. 19, 1976, p. 46025.

Hazelton, L. W., and Holland, E. G. (1953). Arch. Ind. Hyg. 8:399. Cited by FAO/WHO, JMPR, 1963.

Herbst, M., Weisse, I., and Koellmer, H. (1975). A contribution to the question of the possible hepatocarcinogenic effects of lindane. Toxicology 4:91.

Hodge, H. C., Maynard, E. A., and Blanchard, H. J., Jr. (1956). Chronic oral toxicity tests of methoxychlor (2,2-di-(p-methoxyphenyl)-1,1,1-trichloroethane) in rats and dogs. J. Pharmacol. Exp. Ther. 104:60.

Hodge, H. C., Maynard, E. A., Downs, W. L., Coye, R. D., Jr., and Steadman, L. T. (1952b). Chronic oral toxicity of ferric dimethyl dithiocarbamate (Ferbam) and zinc dimethyldithiocarbamate (Ziram). J. Pharmacol. Exp. Ther. 118:174.

Horn, H. J., Bruce, R. B., and Paynter, O. E. (1955). Toxicology of chlorobenzilate. J. Agric. Food Chem. 3:752.

Hueper, W. C. (1952). Carcinogenic studies on isopropyl-N-phenyl carbamate. Ind. Med. Surg. 21:71.

Hunter, B., Graham, C., and Brooks, P. N. (1974). Huntingdon Research Centre, unpublished report cited by FAO/WHO, JMPR, 1976.

Huntingdon Research Centre (1966). Unpublished study, cited by FAO/WHO, JMPR, 1968

IARC (1974). Some organochlorine pesticides. In Evaluation of Carcinogenic Risk of Chemicals to Man, IARC Monographs, Vol. 5. Lyon, France.

IARC (1976). Some carbamates, thiocarbamates and carbazides. In Evaluation of Carcinogenic Risk of Chemicals to Man, IARC Monographs, Vol. 12. Lyon, France.

Innes, J. R., Ulland, B. M., Valerio, M. G., Petrucelli, L., Fishbein, L., Hart, E. R., Pallotta, A. J., Bates, R. R., Falk, H. L., Gart, J. J., Klein, M., Mitchell, I., and Peters, J. (1969). Bioassay of pesticides and industrial chemicals for tumorigenicity in mice: a preliminary note. J. Natl. Cancer Inst. 42:1101.

Ito, N., Nagasaki, H., Ade, H., Sugihara, S., Miyata, Y., Asai, M., and Shirai, T. (1975). Development of hepatocellular carcinomas in rats treated with benzene hexachloride. J. Natl. Cancer Inst. 54:801. Reported in Fed. Reg., Oct. 19, 1976, p. 46028.

Iverson, F., Newsome, W. H., and Hierlihy, S. L. (1977). Tissue distribution of ethylenethiuram monosulfide (ETM) in the rat. Bull. Environ. Contam. Toxicol. 18:541.

Johnston, C. D. (1967). Woodard Research Corp. unpublished report cited by FAO/WHO, JMPR, 1972.

Johnston, C. D., Thompson, W. M., and Donoso, J. (1967). Woodard Research Corp., unpublished report cited by FAO/WHO, JMPR, 1972.

Kadota, T., Hosokawa, T., Kohda, H., Miyamoto, J., and Itoh, N. (1974). Research Department Sumitomo, unpublished report cited by FAO/WHO, JMPR, 1976.

Kemeny, T., and Tarjan, R. (1966). Investigations on the effect of chronically administered small amounts of DDT in mice. Experientia 22:748.

Kimbrough, R., Gaines, T. B., and Sherman, J. D. (1964). Nutritional factors, long term DDT intake and chloroleukemia in rats. J. Natl. Cancer Inst. 33:215.

Kinkel, H. J., and Sann, E. (1965). Batelle Institute, unpublished report, cited by FAO/WHO, JMPR, 1972.

Klimmer, O. R. (1955). Arch. Exp. Pathol. Pharmakol. 227:183. Quoted in the monographs of FAO/WHO, JMPR, 1965.

Klotzsche, C., and Carpy, S. (1973). Sandoz Chemical, unpublished report cited by FAO/WHO, JMPR, 1973.

Larson, P. S., Crawford, E. M., Blackwell-Smith, R., Jr., Hennigar, G. R., Haag, H. B., and Finnegan, J. K. (1960). Chronic toxicologic studies on isopropyl N-(3-chlorophenyl) carbamate (CIPC). Toxicol. Appl. Pharmacol. 2:659.

Laws, E. R. (1971). Evidence of antitumorigenic effects of DDT. Arch. Environ. Health 23:181.

Lehman, A. J. (1952). Q. Bull. Assoc. Food Drug Off. 16:47, cited by FAO/WHO, JMPR, 1963.

Leuschner, F., Leuschner, A., Schwerdtfeger, W., Pliess, G., and Dontenwiller, W. (1971). C. H. Boehringer Sohn, unpublished report, cited by FAO/WHO, JMPR, 1972.

Lijinsky, W., and Taylor, H. W (1976). Carcinogenesis in Sprague-Dawley rats by N-nitroso-N-alkyl-carbamate esters. Cancer Lett. 1:275.

Lorke, D., and Loser, E. (1966). Farbenfabriken Bayer A. G., unpublished report cited by FAO/WHO, JMPR, 1972.

Loser, E. (1972). Institute for toxicology, bayer, unpublished report cited by FAO/WHO, JMPR, 1975.

Lyman, W. R. (1971). Pesticide Terminal Residues. Butterworths, London.

Magee, P. N., and Barnes, J. M. (1956). The production of malignant primary hepatic tumors in the rat by feeding dimethylnitrosamine. Br. J. Cancer 10:114.

Matsumura, F. (1972). Current pesticide situation in the United States: environmental toxicology of pesticides. F. Matsumura, G. M. Bousch, and T. Misato (Eds.). Academic Press, New York.

McLeod, H. A., and Ritcey, W. R. (Eds.) (1973). Analytical Methods for Pesticide Residues in Foods. Ottawa, Canada. Department of National Health and Welfare.

McCollister, D. D., Oyen, F., and Rowe, V. K. (1959). Toxicological studies of o,o-dimethyl-o-(2,4,5-tri-chlorophenyl) phosphorothioate (Ronnel) in laboratory animals. J. Agric. Food Chem. 7:689, cited by FAO/WHO, JMPR, 1968.

McMahon, B. M., and Sawyer, L. D. (Eds.) (1977). Pesticide Analytical Manual. U.S. FDA, Washington, D.C.

Mes, J., Campbell, D. S., Robinson, R. N., and Davies, D. J. (1977). Polychlorinated biphenyl and organochlorine pesticide residues in adipose tissue of Canadians. Bull. Environ. Contam. Toxicol. 17:196.

Mes, J., and Davies, D. J. (1978). The presence of polychlorinated biphenyl and organochlorine pesticide residues and the absence of polychlorinated terphenyls in Canadian human milk. Bull. Environ. Contam. Toxicol. In Press.

Miyamoto, J. (1972). Metabolism of organophosphorus compounds and carbamate insecticides. In Pesticide Chemicals, Vol. VI, Fate of Pesticides in the Environment, A. S. Tahori (Ed.). Gordon and Breach, New York.

Nagasaki, H., Kawabata, H., Miyata, Y., Inoue, K., Hirao, K., and Aoe, H. (1975). Various factors on induction of liver tumours in animals by alpha isomers of benzene hexachloride. Gann. 2: 185.

Nagasaki, H., Tomii, S., Mega, T., Marugami, M., and Ito, N. (1971). Development of hepatomas in mice treated with benzene hexachloride. Gan. 62:431.

Nagasaki, H., Tomii, S., Mega, T., Marugami, M., and Ito, N. (1972). Hepatocarcinogenic effect of α-, β-, γ- and δ-isomers of benzene hexachloride in mice. Gan. 63:393.

Nagasaki, H., Kawabata, H., Miyata, Y., Indue, K., Hirao, K., Aoe, H. (1975). Various factors on induction of liver tumours in animals by alpha isomer of benzene hexachloride. Gan. 2:185.

Newsome, W. H. (1976). Residues of four ethylenebis(dithiocarbamates) and their decomposition products on field sprayed tomatoes. J. Agric. Food Chem. 24:999.

Newsome, W. H., and Laver, G. W. (1973). Effect of boiling on the formation of ethylenethiourea in Zineb-treated foods. Bull. Environ. Contam. Toxicol. 10:151.

Newsome, W. H., Shields, J. B., and Villeneuve, D. C. (1975). Residues of Maneb, ethylenethiuram monosulphide ethylenethiourea and ethylenediamine on beans and tomatoes field treated with Maneb. J. Agric. Food Chem. 23:756.

Ortega, P., Hayes, W. J., and Durham, W. F. (1957). Arch. Pathol. Lab. Med. 64:614. Quoted in the monographs of FAO/WHO, JMPR, 1965.

Radomski, J. L., Deichmann, W. B., MacDonald, W. E., and Glass, E. M. (1965). Synergism among oral carcinogens. I. Results of simultaneous feeding of four tumorigens to rats. Toxicol. Appl. Pharmacol. 7:652.

Rutter, H. A., and Nelson, L. W. (1974). Hazelton Laboratories, unpublished report, cited by FAO/WHO, JMPR, 1975.

Schmähl, D., and Osswald, H. (1967). Carcinogenesis in different animal species by dimethylnitrosamine. Experientia 23:497.

Sen, N. P., Donaldson, B., and Charbonneau, S. (1974). Formation of nitrosodimethylamine from the interaction of certain pesticides and nitrite. In N-Nitroso Compounds in the Environment. P. Bogovski and E. A. Walker (Eds.). IARC Scientific Publication No. 9 (1975), Lyon, France.

Shabad, L. M., Kolesnichenko, T. S., and Nikonova, T. V. (1973). Transplacental and combined long-term effects of DDT in five generations of A strain mice. Int. J. Cancer 11:688.

Slade, P. (1972). Metabolism of carbamate and thiocarbamate herbicides. In Pesticide Chemistry, Vol. VI, Fate of Pesticides in the Environment, A. S. Tahori (Ed.). Gordon and Breach, New York.

Smith, D. C. (1971). Pesticide residues in the total diet in Canada. Pestic. Sci. 2:92.

Smith, D. C., Leduc, R., and Charbonneau, C. (1973). Pesticide residues in the total diet in Canada. III. 1971. Pestic. Sci. 4:211.

Smith, D. C., Leduc, R., and Tremblay, L. (1975). Pesticide residues in the total diet in Canada. IV. 1972 and 1973. Pestic. Sci. 6:75.

Smith, D. C., Sandi, E., and Leduc, R. (1972). Pesticide residues in the total diet in Canada. II. 1970. Pestic. Sci. 3:207.

Smith, P., Wright, P., and Keplinger, M. (1972). Industrial Biotest Laboratories, unpublished report, cited by FAO/WHO, JMPR, 1975.

Smith, P. S., Plank, J. B., Wright, P. L., and Keplinger, M. (1973). Industrial Biotest Laboratories, unpublished report cited by FAO/WHO, JMPR, 1976.

Still, G. G., and Herrett, R. A. (1976). Methylcarbamates, carbanilates and acylanilides. In Herbicides, Vol. II, P. C. Kearney and D. D. Kaufman (Eds.). Marcel Dekker, New York.

Tarjan, R., and Kemeny, T. (1969). Multigeneration studies on DDT in mice. Food Cosmet. Toxicol. 7:215.

Terracini, B., Carbal, R. J., and Testa, M. C. (1973). A multigeneration study on the effects of continuous administration of DDT to BALB/C mice. In Proc. 8th Inter-American Conf. on Toxicology, W. B. Deichmann (Ed.). London Intercontinental Medical Book Co., New York, p. 77.

Thorpe, E., and Walker, A. I. (1973). The toxicology of dieldrin (HEOD). II. Comparative long-term oral toxicity studies in mice with dieldrin, DDT, phenobarbitone, β-HCH and γ-BHC. Food Cosmet. Toxicol. 11:433.

Tomatis, L., Turosov, V. S., Day, N. E., and Charles, R. T. (1972). The effect of long-term exposure to DDT of CF1 mice. Int. J. Cancer 10:489.

Treon, J. F., and Cleveland, F. P. (1955). Toxicity of certain chlorinated hydrocarbon insecticides for laboratory animals with special reference to aldrin and dieldrin. J. Agric. Food Chem. 3:402.

Truhaut, R. (1954). Communication au symposium intern. de la prévention du cancer, Sao Paulo. Reported in FAO/WHO JMPR, 1965.

Turosov, V. S., Day, N. E., Tomatis, L., Gati, E., and Charles, R. T. (1973). Tumors in CF1 mice exposed for six consecutive generations to DDT. J. Natl. Cancer Inst. 51:983.

Ulland, B., Weisburger, E. K., and Weisburger, J. H. (1973). Chronic toxicity and carcinogenicity of industrial chemicals and pesticides. Toxicol. Appl. Pharmacol. 25:446.

Ulland, B. M., Weisburger, J. H., Weisburger, E. K., Rice, J. M., and Cypher, R. (1972). Thyroid cancer in rats from ethylenethiourea intake. J. Natl. Cancer Inst. 49:1972.

U.S. Department of Health, Education, and Welfare (1969). Report of the Secretary's Commission on Pesticides and Their Relationship to Environmental Health. Washington, D.C., p. 44.

van Esch, G. J., and Keroes, R. (1972). Long term toxicity studies of chlorpropham and propham in mice and hamsters. Food Cosmet. Toxicol. 10:373.

Vonk, J. W. (1975). Chemical decomposition of bisdithiocarbamate fungicides and their metabolism by plants and microorganisms. Ph.D. Thesis, Elinkwijk Bv., Utrecht, The Netherlands.

Walker, A. I., Stevenson, D. E., Robinson, J., Thorpe, E., and Roberts, M. (1969). The toxicology and pharmacology of dieldrin (HEOD); two-year oral exposure of rats and dogs. Toxicol. Appl. Pharmacol. 15:345.

Walker, A. I. T., Thorpe, E., and Stevenson, D. E. (1973). The toxicology of dieldrin (HEOD). 1. Long term oral toxicity studies in mice. Food and Cosmetics Toxicology, 11:415-432.

Weisburger, J. H., and Weisburger, E. K. (1968). Food additives and chemical carcinogens: on the concept of zero tolerance. Food Cosmet. Toxicol. 6:235.

Witherup, S., Stemmer, K. L., and Pfitzer, E. A. (1967). Shell International, unpublished report cited by FAO/WHO, JMPR, 1967.

Woodard, M. W., Imming, R. J., Thompson, W., and Woodard, G. (1967). Woodard Research Corp., unpublished report cited by FAO/WHO, JMPR, 1972.

Yip, G., Onley, J. H., and Howard, S. F. (1971). Residues of Maneb and ethylenethiourea on field-sprayed lettuce and kale. J. Assoc. Off. Anal. Chem. 54:1373.

11

Naturally Occurring Carcinogens in Higher Plants

ADRIANNE E. ROGERS / Massachusetts Institute of Technology, Cambridge, Massachusetts

I. INTRODUCTION

Chemical induction of cancer in experimental animals and wide geographic variations in human cancer incidence have led to the idea that many, perhaps most, cancers are the result of exposure to chemical carcinogens present in the natural environment, or added to it accidentally or intentionally by human activities. Many environmental carcinogens or their sources have been identified; they include tobacco smoke, the major etiologic agent for lung cancer, which is responsible for the greatest number of cancer deaths in the United States, and aflatoxins, mold metabolites that may be etiologic agents for liver cancer, which is responsible for the greatest number of cancer deaths in parts of Africa. There are no substances in the external environment that are at present strong candidates for consideration as etiologic agents for two other major cancers in the United States, colon and breast cancer, but dietary components are possible causative or conditioning factors.

As epidemiologic studies improve and expand and as methods for environmental monitoring improve, the contribution of naturally occurring environmental carcinogens to human cancer incidence will be more readily assessed. Identification of toxins or carcinogens of plant or microbial origin often has been made from observation of their effects in domestic animals. The aflatoxins were discovered following outbreaks of toxic hepatic damage in poultry given contaminated feed and then related to earlier episodes of toxicity in other domestic animals. Subsequently their possible role in toxic hepatitis and hepatocarcinoma in people was recognized. Several other mycotoxins that are known or suspected carcinogens have caused serious illness in domestic animals and, in some cases, in people (Chapter 10.IV).

The pyrrolizidine alkaloid-bearing plants and bracken fern, both environmental sources of carcinogens discussed in this chapter, were investigated first in connection with toxicity in domestic animals. Cycasin, a carcinogen present in seeds from which flour is made for human consumption, was found as a result of a search for a human neurotoxin in the same food source.

These are the major groups of chemical carcinogens to which significant exposure may occur in the natural environment. Other carcinogens such as metals and their compounds, polycyclic aromatic hydrocarbons (PAHs), and nitrosamines (Chapter 7) are normally present in air, water, or food in minute quantities that do not constitute a significant hazard. They may be added to the environment by industrial processes or other human activities and become hazardous.

Some of the carcinogens contained in plants which may be important in human disease are discussed in this chapter. Four recent reviews of the chemistry, biochemistry, toxicity, and carcinogenicity of these and other plant products are available (Culvenor and Jago, 1978; Farnsworth et al., 1976; Mattocks, 1978; Schoental, 1976).

II. PYRROLIZIDINE ALKALOIDS

The pyrrolizidine alkaloids are compounds toxic to liver, lung, vasculature, and other tissues and are in some cases carcinogenic for liver, mesenchymal tissues, and possibly other sites. They are produced by many plants in the genera *Senecio* and *Petasites*, in species of *Crotolaria*, *Heliotroprium*, *Amsinckia*, *Echium*, and *Trichodesma*, and less commonly other plants (Bull et al., 1968). Common names for some of the pyrrolizidine alkaloid-producing plants in the United States are fiddleneck, tarweed, fireweed, rattlebox, viper's bugloss, potato weed, stinking Willie (tansy ragwort), other ragworts, and groundsels (McLean, 1970). One or more of the alkaloids can be isolated from roots, leaves, seeds, and flowers in concentrations that vary with species and conditions of growth. Many are not toxic, but those that are have caused considerable economic loss, particularly in North America, Australia, New Zealand, and South Africa through poisoning of domestic animals. Consumption of the alkaloids by people has been associated with acute and chronic liver disease.

Human poisoning by ingestion of grain contaminated with alkaloid-bearing seeds or other plant parts and ingestion of alkaloids in medicinal herb teas have been reported in the West Indies, South Africa, and Central Asia (Bras and Hill, 1956; McLean, 1970; Selzer and Parker, 1951).

Human pyrrolizidine poisoning has been reported recently in the United States, Afghanistan, and India (Lyford et al., 1976; Mohabbat et al., 1976; Stillman et al., 1977; Tandon et al., 1976). Two American cases were infants from Mexican-American families treated with herbal teas that contained toxic pyrrolizidine alkaloids; one child died with acute hepatic necrosis, and the other survived but developed cirrhosis (Huxtable et al., 1977; Stillman et al., 1977). A third case was a patient from Ecuador who had ingested teas made from herbs which included *Crotolaria* species. She had hepatic veno-occlusive disease which resolved following portocaval shunt and cessation of ingestion of the tea (Lyford et al., 1976). In Afghanistan approximately 23% of people examined in an area that had suffered severe drought and famine 3-5 years earlier had liver disease, and there was a history of many deaths, apparently from liver disease, over the preceding year. Evidence of contamination of wheat flour by heliotrine and possibly lasiocarpine from seeds of *Heliotropium* plants growing in the wheat fields was found. Autopsy or liver biopsy showed hepatic veno-occlusive disease. It was concluded that the population had been exposed to toxic alkaloids, particularly during the drought period (Mohabbat et al., 1976). The Indian cases, again, were reported from an area of recurrent drought and famine in which cereal grains probably were contaminated by

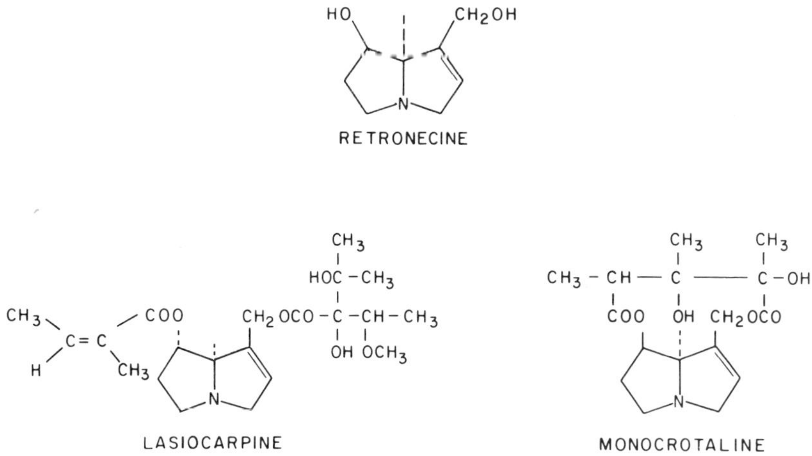

FIGURE 1

Crotolaria seeds, although the contamination was not clearly demonstrated (Tandon et al., 1976).

In patients who died from acute poisoning hemorrhagic hepatic necrosis, occlusion of central and small hepatic veins, and development of ascites and other signs of portal hypertension were described (Bras and Hill, 1956; Selzer and Parker, 1951). Patients who survived recovered or developed progressive liver disease culminating in portal hypertension and hepatic failure (Stuart and Bras, 1957). Reference to medicinal uses of pyrrolizidine alkaloid-bearing plants was made in western pharmacopiae, as well as in developing countries (Schoental, 1968).

Toxic alkaloids or metabolites are secreted into milk by rats and cows, and damage to suckling young has been reported in rats (Dickinson et al., 1976; Schoental, 1976). This may pose a health hazard, but none has been recognized.

The alkaloids have a role in the life cycle of several butterfly and moth species. Males feed on pyrrolizidine-containing plants, metabolize the alkaloids, and secrete metabolites that facilitate mating and repel other males. Some species use the plants as larval hosts (Edgar et al., 1976; Culvenor, 1978). Honey from bees which have fed on the plants may contain the alkaloids (Deinzer et al., 1977).

The alkaloids are primarily branched chain esters of retronecine, and the toxic compounds are esters of basic aminoalcohols with branched chain, unsaturated, epoxide, or hydroxyl C_4-C_6 acids (Fig. 1). A 1,2-double bond in the pyrrolizidine nucleus is required for hepatotoxicity (Schoental, 1976).

Toxicity to grazing animals was recognized in cattle in Canada in the late nineteenth and early twentieth centuries. The plants and alkaloids responsible have been identified by studies in domestic and experimental animals (Bull et al., 1968; McLean, 1970). Sensitivity of animals to poisoning varies with species, age, sex, and the toxin tested. Structure-activity relationships have been defined (Schoental, 1976). Sheep, cattle, horses, pigs, dogs, turkeys, and chickens are susceptible to toxicity of one or more alkaloids. Experimental studies have demonstrated toxicity of many alkaloids to rats and of several of the compounds to monkeys, mice, and hamsters. Guinea pigs are resistant to the alkaloids which have been tested in them, probably because of their inability to form the toxic metabolites (Chesney and Allen, 1973b).

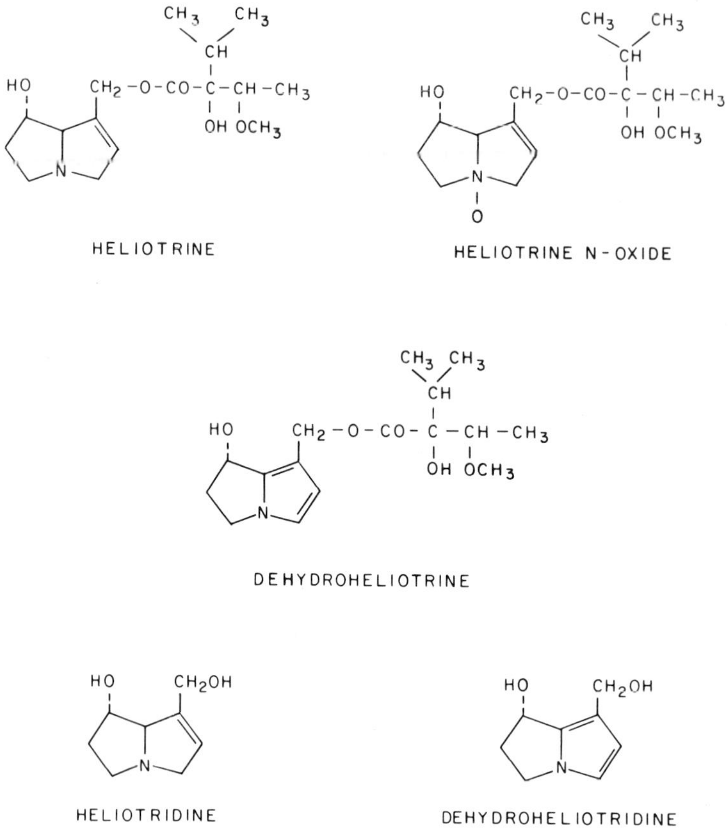

FIGURE 2

The dependence of toxicity and carcinogenicity of many chemicals on metabolism to reactive forms is discussed in Chapter 14. Experiments with pyrrolizidine alkaloids have contributed to knowledge in this area and help explain certain experimental observations. Hydrolysis of the alkaloids to aminoalcohols, for example, heliotridine (Fig. 2), or metabolism to N-oxides and pyrrolic derivatives have been demonstrated. The N-oxides, for example, heliotrine N-oxide (Fig. 2), may occur in plants along with the parent alkaloid and are less toxic than or equally toxic to the parent alkaloid. The pyrrole derivatives appear to be responsible for toxicity of the compounds. These derivatives are dehydroalkaloids, for example, dehydroheliotrine (Fig. 2), and dehydroaminoalcohols, for example, dehydroheliotridine (Fig. 2). They are formed by liver in vivo and in vitro, are more toxic than the parent alkaloids, and their concentration in liver and lung is correlated with manifestations of toxicity (Culvenor and Jago, 1978; Mattocks, 1968, 1972, 1978). Unchanged alkaloids, their N-oxides, and pyrrolic metabolites are excreted in the urine, and pyrrolic metabolites may be identified bound to tissue constituents. Presence of "metabolic pyrroles" in tissues or urine can be demonstrated by reaction with the Ehrlich pyrrole reagent 4-dimethylaminobenzaldehyde (Mattocks, 1968).

The dehydroaminoalcohols that have been tested are not hepatotoxic but are toxic to other tissues, probably because of their antimitotic activity; the N-oxides, which can be converted to the parent alkaloids in the gut, are toxic when given by the gastrointestinal tract but less toxic or nontoxic when given parenterally. The dehydroalkaloids are more toxic and reactive than the dehydroaminoalcohols; both are alkylating agents in vitro. The 1,2-double bond in the hepatotoxic alkaloids apparently enhances aromatization of the ring in which it occurs; alkaloids with a saturated ring are not hepatotoxic and are metabolized to pyrrolic derivatives in which the other ring is unsaturated (Culvenor and Jago, 1978). The dehydroalkaloids have not been isolated from tissues but have been synthesized and shown to be toxic to lung and liver (Butler et al., 1970). The dehydroalkaloid of monocrotaline was tested for carcinogenicity and gave a small increase in incidence of injection site sarcomas, but the results were not significant and require further study (Hooson and Grasso, 1976). The dehydroaminoalcohol of monocrotaline, dehydroretronecine, inhibited mitosis and induced rhabdomyosarcomas at the injection site in rats and malignant skin tumors in mice (Allen et al., 1975; Johnson et al., 1978; Shumaker et al., 1976). Dehydroheliotridine given intraperitoneally to rats induced benign or malignant tumors of liver, lungs, pancreas, gut, or subcutis (Culvenor and Jago, 1978).

Dietary, chemical, and species effects on pyrrolizidine alkaloid toxicity can be explained in part by measurement of tissue pyrrole concentration (Table 1). Hepatic pyrrole content after LD_{50} doses of different toxic alkaloids are similar (Mattocks, 1972). Allen et al. (1972) studied the effect of microsomal oxidase induction by phenobarbital or inhibition by chloramphenicol on monocrotaline toxicity and found, as had Mattocks, that phenobarbital pretreatment increased toxicity of monocrotaline and hepatic pyrrole content. Enzyme inhibition decreased monocrotaline toxicity and the amount of pyrrole in the liver. However, the results of oxidase manipulations are not consistent for all alkaloids. Lasiocarpine toxicity was decreased by phenobarbital or other inducing treatment despite increased production of pyrrole metabolites; heliotrine toxicity was increased by the same treatment, again with increased pyrrole production (Jago, 1971; Tuchweber et al., 1974). Changes induced in retrosine

TABLE 1 Dietary and Other Treatment Effects on Toxicity of Pyrrolizidine Alkaloids and Hepatic Pyrrole Content in Male Rats

Alkaloid	Route of administration	Pretreatment	LD_{50} (mg/kg)	Hepatic pyrroles per 100 mg/kg alkaloid
Retrorsine (Mattocks, 1972)	i.p.	None	34	1.88 ± 0.07
		Phenobarbital	67	1.67 ± 0.12
		SKF 525 A	53	~1.21
		Sucrose diet	120	1.32 ± 0.08
Monocrotaline (Mattocks, 1972)	i.p.	None	109	0.64 ± 0.03
		Phenobarbital	98	0.96 ± 0.03
Monocrotaline (Hayashi and Lalich, 1968)	s.c.	None	<30	a
		Mercaptoethylamine	>30	
		Cysteine	>30	
Monocrotaline (Newberne et al., 1971)	i.g.	None	71	2-3+
		Lipotrope-deficient diet	104	0-1+
Lasiocarpine (Rogers and Newberne, 1971)	i.g.	None	~110	a
		Lipotrope-deficient diet	~150	
		Mercaptoethylamine	>110, <150	

[a]Not measured.

toxicity by phenobarbital treatment in mice and guinea pigs did not correlate consistently with pyrrole production (White et al., 1973). Dietary treatment in rats, which reduced hepatic pyrrole production from monocrotaline reduced its toxicity and also toxicity of lasiocarpine (Newberne et al., 1971; Rogers and Newberne, 1971).

Studies in guinea pigs, which are resistant to pyrrolizidine toxicity, support the role of the metabolic pyrroles in toxicity of the alkaloids. Hepatic microsomes from rats and guinea pigs formed N-oxides in vitro, but guinea pig microsomes formed little if any pyrrole metabolites, while rat microsomes formed readily detectable amounts. In vivo conversion by guinea pigs could not be detected, again in contrast to extensive conversion by rats. Administration of the pyrrolic compound dehydromonocrotaline to guinea pigs caused severe hepatic damage comparable to the damage induced in rats (Chesney and Allen, 1973b).

Mattocks (1972) reviewed the data on metabolism and toxicity of the alkaloids and concluded that the effects of enzyme inducers or inhibitors were not the result of production of different metabolites, but rather the result of changes in rate of further metabolism of the active compounds. However, apparent separation of hepatotoxicity from carcinogenicity in the two classes of pyrrole metabolites, the dehydroalkaloids and the dehydroaminoalcohols, and the retention of alkylating and antimitotic activity by both classes suggests that examination of specific metabolite production may elucidate the variable effects of hepatic microsomal enzyme induction or inhibition on alkaloid toxicity and carcinogenicity (Table 1).

Antimitotic effects of the alkaloids and their pyrrole metabolites have been demonstrated in liver, bone marrow, gut mucosa, lymphopoetic organs, testis, and hair follicles (Allen and Hsu, 1974; Hsu et al., 1973; Jago, 1969; Peterson, 1965; Peterson et al., 1972; Rogers and Newberne, 1971).

Sheep can detoxify the alkaloids in the rumen (Bull et al., 1968). The microorganism and reactions responsible have been defined and trials made of methods to increase rumen detoxification, but significant protection has not been achieved (Culvenor, 1977; Lanigan, 1976). Another approach to protection has been to immunize animals against the alkaloids. Initial studies in immunized rats showed increased rather than decreased toxicity and higher and more persistent blood content of alkaloid, probably because reversible binding of alkaloid to antibody prevented excretion in the urine (Culvenor, 1977).

Toxicity of the alkaloids is directed against vascular endothelium, hepatic parenchymal cells, red cells and the central nervous system (McLean, 1970). Endothelial proliferation, vasculitis, and perivascular fibrosis lead to occlusion of alveolar capillaries, pulmonary arterioles and venules, and hepatic central veins. Pulmonary damage varies in severity with the alkaloid used, occurs following treatment with N-oxides as well as parent compounds and appears to be secondary to vascular toxicity rather than to a primary effect on pulmonary epithelium. Most studies have used either monocrotaline or intravenous injection of the pyrrole metabolites of several different alkaloids. Fibrin thrombi in alveolar capillaries, vasculitis involving small vessels, particularly pulmonary arterioles, perivascular fibrosis, endothelial swelling, and muscular spasm or hypertrophy are prominent in lungs of poisoned animals and result in pulmonary hypertension and edema. Disruption of vessels may occur, followed by death from hemorrhage. Enlarged alveolar macrophages may be seen, but the respiratory epithelium does not appear to be a primary site of damage (Chesney and Allen, 1973a; Fishman, 1974; Kay et al., 1967; Lalich and Merkow, 1961; McLean, 1970). Vascular damage may be prominent in the liver and has been described in humans and cattle poisoned accidentally and in experimental studies.

Hepatocyte lesions range from acute necrosis to megalocytosis and include persistent inhibition of mitosis which probably is the cause of the megalocytosis (Jago, 1969; Peterson, 1965; Rogers and Newberne, 1971). The enlarged parenchymal cells do not appear degenerated but show proliferation of endoplasmic reticulum and, in some cases, abnormalities of nucleus and nucleolus. Liver function deteriorates in chronic pyrrolizidine poisoning as cirrhosis develops, although as in other types of cirrhosis, the degree of dysfunction cannot be correlated with the histologic appearance of the liver (McLean, 1970). Tissue changes may progress long after exposure to toxins ceases. Hepatic necrosis and gradual development of chronic liver lesions follow injection of pyrrole metabolites into the portal venous system, which provides further evidence that the metabolites are the active toxic agents (Butler et al., 1970).

The question of carcinogenicity of the alkaloids was debated until recently, but several laboratories have demonstrated induction of hepatocarcinoma and other tumors by parenteral or oral administration of monocrotaline or lasiocarpine (Shumaker et al., 1976; Svoboda and Reddy, 1972, Newberne and Rogers, 1973; Rao and Reddy, 1978).

Monocrotaline given subcutaneously to rats induced injection site sarcomas (rhabdomyosarcoma, primarily) and a low incidence of hepatocarcinomas and pulmonary adenocarcinomas. A metabolite, dehydroretronecine, induced injection site sarcomas and was postulated to be the ultimate carcinogen (Shumaker et al., 1976). The same compound induced basal and squamous cell carcinomas in mice exposed by topical application or subcutaneous (s.c.) injection (Johnson et al., 1978). Monocrotaline induced hepatocarcinomas when given by gavage (Newberne and Rogers, 1973). Intraperitoneal lasiocarpine induced hepatocarcinoma and cutaneous squamous cell carcinomas in rats (Svoboda and Reddy, 1973), and lasiocarpine fed in the diet induced parenchymal and vascular liver tumors (Rao and Reddy, 1978). Petasitene or the plant from which it was isolated induced hepatocarcinomas and hepatic hemangioendothelial sarcomas (Hirono et al., 1977). In the same laboratory two additional alkaloids present in plants used medicinally in Japan have been studied. Senkirkine, extracted from <u>Tussilago farfara</u> L. or colts foot, induced hepatic adenoma but no malignant tumors in rats. Symphytine, extracted from <u>Symphytum officinale</u> L. or Russian comfrey, induced hepatic adenoma or hemangioendothelial sarcoma in rats (Hirono et al., 1979).

Another alkaloid, heliotrine, was associated with development of pancreatic adenomas in rats protected against toxicity of the compound by nicotinamide (Schoental, 1977). There are reports of tumor induction by other alkaloids, but the malignancy of the tumors induced has not been conclusively demonstrated. Retrorsine and its N-oxide, isatidine, administered orally or intragastrically induced tumors in a few animals (Schoental, 1976) and were considered carcinogenic in the IARC review (IARC, 1976), but the evidence is not strong and more extensive studies are needed. Problems in interpretation of early studies have been discussed, and the importance of dosage schedules and other aspects of methodology has been pointed out (Schoental, 1976).

Extracts from several plants induced vascular hepatic tumors and hepatocarcinomas when fed or given in drinking water to rats but the agent(s) responsible was (were) not identified (IARC, 1976).

Induction of chromosome abnormalities and mutations in <u>Drosophila</u>, bacteria and plants and of teratogenesis in rats by the alkaloids have been reported (Schoental, 1976). Alkylation of cellular macromolecules by pyrrole metabolites and formation of adducts with DNA have been demonstrated (Culvenor and Jago, 1978; White and Mattocks, 1972). Dehydroretronecine binds covalently to proteins and the thiol compounds cysteine and glutathione (Robertson et al., 1977), which may explain the ability of thiol compounds to block monocrotaline toxicity (Table 1) and raises the possibility that the same compounds may block pyrrolizidine carcinogenicity. Certain thiol compounds block tumor induction by PAH or 1,2-dimethylhydrazine (Wattenberg et al., 1977). Sulfhydryl administration increased hepatocyte glutathione concentration and decreased pyrrolic metabolites detectable in the liver (White, 1976).

Attempts to exploit the antimitotic activity of pyrrolizidine alkaloids for tumor therapy have been unsuccessful until recently because of the toxicity of the compounds. However, indicine N-oxide, a compound of low toxicity which differs from heliotrine N-oxide (Fig. 2) only by replacement of the methoxy group on the penultimate carbon atom of the side-chain by a hydroxyl group, has significant antitumor activity in experimental systems and is undergoing clinical trial (Powis et al., 1979). The compound is reduced to indicine in rabbits and humans; studies in rabbits demonstrated that the reduction took place in hepatic microsomes and in the gut through the activity of the microbial flora (Powis et al., 1979). Small amounts of retronecine were detected after metabolism of indicine by rabbit liver homogenates, and the authors pointed out that this compound would be expected to produce the (carcinogenic) metabolite dehydroretronecine already discussed.

Despite known exposure of humans and domestic animals to the pyrrolizidine alkaloids in foods and herbal medicines, there is no evidence that relates such exposure to the incidence of liver or other tumors. Exposure of people to compounds of unquestioned carcinogenicity for animals must always be a source of concern, even in the absence of positive epidemiologic data, and should be considered in investigations of geographic or other variations in cancer incidence. An example is the marked geographic variation in esophageal cancer, which is increased in incidence in the West Indies and parts of South Africa and central Asia, all areas in which human pyrrolizidine poisoning has occurred. This has led to the suggestion that the alkaloids should be investigated for a possible role in the etiology of esophageal cancer (Schoental, 1976). Studies in an area of high incidence in Iran have demonstrated an association with consumption of wheat rather than rice and with poverty and malnutrition, particularly with respect to vitamins A and C and riboflavin (Joint Iran-IARC Study Group, 1977). Contamination of wheat flour by pyrrolizidine alkaloids has been a major source of human poisoning and is a possibility in Iran although not found in the recent studies. The investigators have not identified other recognized carcinogenic food contaminants (PAHs, aflatoxins, nitrosamines) in higher concentration in high- than in low-incidence regions and have not shown an association with medicinal or other use of plants except opium.

The association of esophageal cancer with poverty and malnutrition is worldwide, although partially obscured in the West by the effects of cigarette smoking and alcohol consumption (Day, 1975; Rothman, 1975). The search for its environmental cause(s) emphasizes the importance of including nutritional evaluations. Many nutritional influences on chemical carcinogenesis have been demonstrated in experimental animals and are thought to operate in people (Cancer Research, 1975; Newberne and Rogers, 1976). The particular deficiencies identified in Iran have not been tested experimentally for their effect on esophageal carcinogenesis, but vitamin A and riboflavin influence tumor induction in other target organs in rats, and vitamin C might have an influence if tested in animals that require it.

III. BRACKEN FERN CARCINOGEN

Bracken fern (Polypodiacea, pteridium aquilinium) grows in many areas in the northern hemisphere and has caused severe toxicity in grazing animals. It contains several toxins and the enzyme thiaminase, which can induce nervous system lesions of thiamin deficiency. Other toxic effects of bracken ingestion include intestinal ulceration, bone marrow suppression with anemia, leukopenia, thrombocytopenia, and the expected sequelae, that is, hemorrhage and marked abnormalities of immunologic responses (Evans, 1968, 1976a, b).

Carcinogenicity of bracken fern was suspected because of association of tumors in grazing animals with its ingestion (Evan, 1976a, b; Pirie, 1973; Price and Pamukcu, 1968). The first and most frequent association reported from several areas was with benign and malignant bladder tumors in cattle, but esophageal and rumenal squamous carcinomas were reported in association with bladder tumors and bracken ingestion in Brazil (Dobereiner et al., 1967) and were recognized in Kenya in cattle with and without bladder tumors (Plowright et al., 1971). In Kenya wild grazing animals (giant forest hogs) also had esophageal and gastric squamous carcinomas. Subsequently, oral and esophageal carcinomas and papillomas, sometimes multifocal, were reported from western Scotland where cattle grazed on bracken fern (Evans, 1976a, b).

Experimental induction of bladder tumors in cattle and guinea pigs and of intestinal tumors in rats, Japanese quail, and guinea pigs by feeding bracken fern supported the epidemiologic observations (Evans, 1968; Evans and Mason, 1965; Price and Pamukcu, 1968). Tumors induced in the urinary bladder were hemangiomas, hemangioendotheliomas, transitional cell papillomas, papillary adenocarcinomas, and mucinous adenocarcinomas. Intestinal tumors were adenocarcinomas. In pilot experiments, sheep and hamsters developed intestinal adenocarcinomas following ingestion of bracken fern (Evans, 1968). In all species tested the intestinal tumors occurred primarily in small intestine and cecum. Gastric and other tumors have been induced in mice by a single dose of bracken extract (Evans, 1976a).

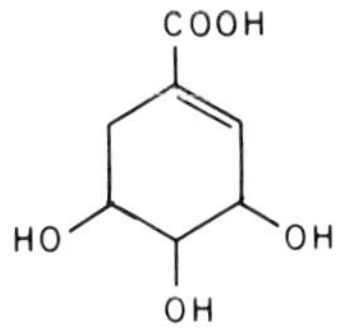

SHIKIMIC ACID FIGURE 3

In rats the toxicology and carcinogenesis of bracken fern for the intestine were related to the geographical area in which the bracken grew and the part of the plant fed, being greatest in the rhizome (Evans et al., 1961; Hirono et al., 1973). Activity was reduced by treatment of bracken with boiling water, alkali, and sodium chloride, methods used in Japan to prepare it for human consumption. Unprocessed material occasionally induced bladder tumors as well as intestinal tumors in rats (Hirono et al., 1972). Heating or drying did not influence tumor induction (Mori et al., 1977). Thiamin administration increased tumor induction in the bladder but did not alter the incidence of intestinal tumors (Pamukcu et al., 1970). Significant reduction of bracken tumor induction in rat intestine by butylated hydroxyanisole (BHA), disulfiram, or calcium chloride ($CaCl_2$) and in rat urinary bladder by $CaCl_2$ or polyvinyl pyrrolidone was reported, but no protective mechanism was defined. Bicarbonate feeding decreased induction of intestinal tumors but increased induction of bladder tumors (Pamukcu et al., 1977).

Milk from cows fed bracken fern induced intestinal, renal, and bladder tumors when fed to rats, but no conclusive correlation of human tumor incidence with consumption of bracken fern or milk from cattle consuming the plant has been demonstrated. Data suggesting a link with increased risk of esophageal carcinoma have been reported (Pamukcu et al., 1978).

Many chemicals have been isolated from bracken fern, but the carcinogenic principles have not been fully defined. There has been considerable interest in the tannins present because of their possible association with esophageal carcinoma in humans, but their carcinogenicity in rats or other laboratory animals has not been adequately demonstrated (Farnsworth et al., 1976; Pamukcu et al., 1978).

Shikimic acid (Fig. 3), a common plant constituent (Yoshida et al., 1975), was isolated from carcinogenic bracken and induced tumors in mice. Carcinogenicity in rats has not been demonstrated. Bracken preparations free of shikimic acid also are carcinogenic (Evans, 1976, 1979*).

IV. CYCASIN

Cycasin and other β-glycosides of methylazoxymethanol (MAM) are present in seeds, roots, and leaves of species of Gymnospermae in the family Cycadaceae and owe their toxicity and carcinogenicity to the aglycone methylazoxylmethanol (MAM) (Fig. 4). A description and photographs of the plants are given by Binsey (1972). Flour made from the seeds provides human food in tropical and subtropical areas, but no epidemiologic evidence exists for its carcinogenicity in humans, probably because the glycosides are removed from the flour by soaking and washing with water (Magee et al., 1976; Laquer and Spatz, 1968; Whiting, 1964).

---

*Two extracts have been separated and partially characterized. One, as mentioned, contains shikimic acid, which is toxic, teratogenic, and carcinogenic in mice and mutagenic in fungi and bacteria. Carcinogenicity in rats has not been demonstrated. The second is toxic to mice and calves and carcinogenic in mice, and contains a 1-indanone derivative, which is toxic but not carcinogenic, and other compounds which are not yet identified.

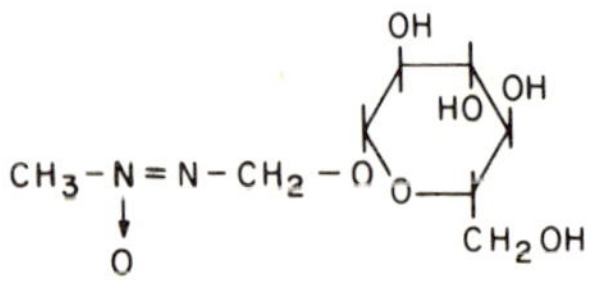

CYCASIN FIGURE 4

Carcinogenicity of cycad flour, cycasin, and MAM have been demonstrated in rats by induction of hepatic and renal parenchymal or vascular tumors and of intestinal adenocarcinomas; tumors can be induced by a single dose. Occasionally tumors of lung, CNS, or mammary gland have been reported (Hirono, 1972; Laquer and Spatz, 1968; Magee et al., 1976). The compounds are carcinogenic also in mice, hamsters, and other laboratory animals (Hirono, 1972). Characteristics of cycasin and MAM carcinogenicity that vary with respect to age, sex, and species of experimental animals and metabolism of the compounds were reviewed at a symposium in 1972 (Hirono, 1972). Neurotoxicity of the compounds, which was the original reason for studying them, also was reviewed at that time (Fed. Proc., 1972).

Studies in germ-free rats demonstrated the requirement for hydrolysis of the glycoside for carcinogenicity and toxicity, a reaction carried out by intestinal bacteria which contain β-glucosidase (Spatz et al., 1967). MAM and its acetate are alkylating agents and are directly carcinogenic in rat colon. MAM is directly mutagenic to bacteria and *Drosophila*. Its chemical and biological activities are similar to N-nitrosodimethylamine (DMN) (Magee et al., 1976).

V. SAFROLE, ESTRAGOLE

Allyl and propenyl benzene derivatives, safrole (Fig. 5), and chemically related compounds that occur in oils and spices derived from several different plants are carcinogenic in rats and mice (Culvenor and Jago, 1978; IARC, 1976). Safrole is found in oils of sassafras, camphor and nutmeg, cinnamon, mace, star anise, ginger, and black pepper, and has been used in perfume and soaps as well as in foods (IARC, 1976). The parent compound or its metabolites induced hepatic and esophageal tumors in rats and hepatic tumors in mice (Borchert et al., 1973; Hagan et al., 1965). Carcinogenicity, mutagenicity, covalent binding to macromolecules, and alkylation of nucleotide bases of several safrole derivatives have been demonstrated (Culvenor and Jago, 1978; Wislocki et al., 1977). A related compound, estragole (Fig. 5), present in tarragon, basil, and fennel, and its hydroxylated derivative are hepatocarcinogenic by s.c. injection in newborn mice (Drinkwater et al., 1976).

Detailed analysis of urinary and biliary metabolites in rats showed that o-demethylation to the phenol and alteration of the allylic side-chain were the major pathways of metabolism (Solheim and Scheline, 1973). The compounds are hepatoxic in rats (Taylor et al., 1964). There are no epidemiologic data in people that indicate a relationship between ingestion of the compounds and incidence of carcinoma.

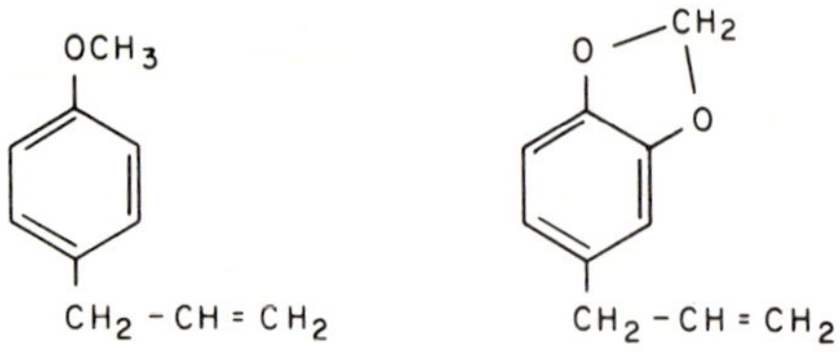

ESTRAGOLE SAFROLE FIGURE 5

VI. OTHER CARCINOGENS PRESENT IN PLANTS

There are other chemicals such as shikimic acid and tannins which are present in plants and which may be carcinogenic but require more extensive study (Farnsworth et al., 1976; Mattocks, 1978). Plant products that are chewed for their pharmacological effects and are or may be carcinogenic include tobacco, betel, nass, and coca. The alkaloid content and possible carcinogenicity of the latter three have been reviewed (Farnsworth et al., 1976; IARC, 1976; Mattocks, 1978). Farnsworth et al., published an extensive list of plants containing proven or potentially carcinogenic compounds and discussed evidence for carcinogenicity of crude extracts or other mixtures of compounds from plants. There is not sufficient evidence to include them as carcinogens at present. Kapadia et al. (1976, 1978) induced malignant mesenchymal tumors in rats at the site of injection of aqueous extracts from plants used medicinally. Further studies to identify the compound(s) responsible and to determine carcinogenicity by other routes of administration are needed to evaluate the significance of the results.

Yeast or mold products that may contribute to development of tumors either directly or indirectly, in addition to the compounds of major importance discussed in Chapter 10.IV, include ethanol and substances such as zearalenone, which are produced by *Fusarium* species and other microorganisms and have estrogenic activity (Schoental, 1977). Carcinogenicity by the naturally occurring estrogenic substances has not been demonstrated but is of interest because of the implication of several estrogenic compounds in causation of experimental and human tumors (Lemon, 1977; Chapter 12). Ethanol is not known to be carcinogenic, but, again, it is of interest because intake of alcoholic beverages is associated with increased risk of tumors of the upper gastrointestinal and respiratory tracts and tumors of the liver (Rothman, 1975; Chapter 12).

Finally, mention should be made of plant products that are cocarcinogens or promoters of tumor development when applied with or after a carcinogen, but not inducers of tumors by themselves, at least under most experimental conditions. Croton oil, derived from seeds of *Croton tiglium*, was described as a promoter of skin-tumor induction by PAHs, and its active principles have been identified as phorbol esters. Related compounds have been isolated from other plants of the family *Euphorbia* to which *Croton tiglium* belongs (Boutwell, 1977; Farnsworth et al., 1976; Weinstein et al., 1977). Cyclopropenoid fatty acids present in cottonseed and other plant oils promoted aflatoxin B_1 tumor induction in rainbow trout (Sinnhuber et al., 1968).

In summary, there are several compounds or groups of compounds produced by higher plants that are carcinogenic in experimental animals and therefore pose a threat to humans exposed to them in foods, medicines, or elsewhere. The compounds that are known carcinogens include the pyrrolizidine alkaloids, the bracken fern carcinogen(s), cycasin and safrole, and related compounds. Many other chemicals or mixtures in plant extracts are toxic and probably or possibly carcinogenic, but require further study.

The magnitude of the human risk from the known or suspected plant carcinogens cannot be accurately assessed at present. Esophageal and gastric cancer in the high-incidence areas may be related to ingestion of bracken, pyrrolizidine, or other plant carcinogens, but epidemiologic data are not yet sufficient to permit conclusions. Nutritional status may be a significant factor in determining cancer induction and development at these two or other sites by plant or other environmental carcinogens.

REFERENCES

Allen, J. R., Chesney, C. F., and Frazee, W. J. (1972). Modifications of pyrrolizidine alkaloid intoxication resulting from altered hepatic microsomal enzymes. Toxicol. Appl. Pharmacol. 23:470-479.

Allen, J. R., Hsu, I. C., and Carstens, L. A. (1975). Dehydroretronecine induced rhabdomyosarcomas in rats. Cancer Res. 35:997-1002.

Allen, J. R., and Hsu, I. C. (1974). Antimitotic effects of dehydroretronecine pyrrole. Proc. Soc. Exp. Biol. Med. 147:546.

Binsey, M. R. (1972). A brief description of the cycads. Fed. Proc. 31:1467-1469.

Borchert, P., Miller, J. A., and Miller, E. C., and Shires, T. K. (1973). 1-Hydroxyl safrole, a proximate carcinogenic metabolite of safrole in the rat. Cancer Res. 33: 590-600.

Boutwell, R. K. (1977). The role of the induction of ornithine decarboxylase in tumor promotion. In Origins of Human Cancer, H. H. Hiatt, J. D. Watson, and J. A. Winsten (Eds.). Cold Spring Harbor Laboratory, Cold Spring Harbor, N.Y., pp. 773-783.

Bras, G., and Hill, K. R. (1956). Veno-occlusive disease of the liver, essential pathology. Lancet ii:161-163.

Bull, L. B., Culvenor, C. C., and Dick, A. T. (1968). The Pyrrolizidine Alkaloids. Their Chemistry, Pathogenicity and other Biological Properties. North Holland, Amsterdam.

Butler, W. H., Mattocks, A. R., and Barnes, J. M. (1970). Lesions in the liver and lungs of rats given pyrrole derivatives of pyrrolizidine alkaloids. J. Pathol. 100: 169-175.

Cancer Res. Symp. (1975). Nutrition in the causation of cancer. 35:3235-3550.

Chesney, C. F., and Allen, J. R. (1973a). Endocardial fibrosis associated with monocrotaline-induced pulmonary hypertension in non-human primates (Macaca arcotoides). Am. J. Vet. Res. 34:1577-1581.

Chesney, C. F., and Allen, J. R. (1973b). Resistance of the guinea pig to pyrrolizidine alkaloid intoxication. Toxicol. Appl. Pharmacol. 26:385-392.

Culvenor, C. C. (1978). Prevention of pyrrolizidine alkaloid poisoning. Animal adaptation or plant control. In Effects of Poisonous Plants on Livestock, K. R. Van Campen and L. F. James (Eds.). Academic Press, New York, pp. 189-200.

Culvenor, C. C., and Jago, M. V. (1978). Carcinogenic plant products and DNA. In Chemical Carcinogens and DNA. Cleveland, Ohio.

Day, N. E. (1975). Some aspects of the epidemiology of esophageal cancer. Cancer Res. 35:3304-3307.

Deinzer, M. L., Thomson, P. A., Burgett, D. M., and Isaacson, D. L. (1977). Pyrrolizidine alkaloids: their occurrence in honey from tansy ragwort (Senecio Jacobaca L.). Science 195:497-499.

Dickinson, J. O., Cooke, M. P., King, R. R., and Mohamed, P. A. (1976). Milk transfer or pyrrolizidine alkaloids in cattle. J. Am. Vet. Med. Assoc. 169:1192-1196.

Dobereiner, J. C., Tokarnia, C. A., and Canella, F. C. (1967). Occurrence of enzootic hematuria and epidermoid carcinoma of the upper digestive tract of cattle in Brazil. Pesq. Agropec. Brasil 2:489-504.

Drinkwater, N. R., Miller, E. C., Miller, J. A., and Pitot, H. C. (1976). Hepatocarcinogenicity of estragole (1-allyl-4 methoxybenzene) and 1'-hydroxy estragole in the mouse and mutagenicity of 1'-acetoxy-estragole in bacteria. J. Natl. Cancer Inst. 57:1323-1331.

Edgar, J. A., Cockrum, P. A., and Frahn, J. L. (1976). Pyrrolizidine alkaloids in Danaus plexippus L. and Danaus chryssippus L. Experientia 32:1535-1537.

Evans, I. A. (1968). The radio mimetic nature of bracken toxin. Cancer Res. 28:2252-2261.

Evans, I. A. (1976a). Relationship between bracken and cancer. Bot. J. Linnean Soc. 73:105-112.

Evans, I. A. (1976b). The bracken carcinogen. In Chemical Carcinogens, ACS Monograph 13, C. E. Searle (Eds.). American Chemical Society, Washington, D.C., pp. 691-700.

Evans, I. A. (1979). Bracken carcinogenicity. Res. Vet. Sci. 26:339-348.

Evans, I. A., and Mason, J. (1965). Carcinogenic activity of bracken. Nature 208:913-914.

Evans, W. C., Evans, I. A., Axford, R. F. E., Threlfall, G., Humphreys, D. A., and Thomas, A. J. (1961). Studies in bracken poisoning in cattle. VII. The toxicity of bracken rhizomes. Vet. Rec. 73:852-853.

Farnsworth, N. R., Bingel, A. S., Fong, H. H. S., Harry, H. S., Saleh, A. A., Christenson, G. M., and Saufferer, S. M. (1976). Oncogenic and tumor-promoting spermatophytes and pteridophytes and their active principles. Cancer Treat. Rep. 60:1171-1214.

Fed. Proc. (1972). Neurotoxicity of cycad derivatives and related compounds. 31:1503-1542.

Fishman, A. P. (1974). Dietary pulmonary hypertension. Circ. Res. 35:657-660.

Hagan, E. C., Jenner, P. M., Jones, W. I., Fitzhugh, O. G., Long, E. L., Bronwer, J. G., and Webb, W. K. (1965). Toxic properties of compounds related to safrole. Toxicol. Appl. Pharmacol. 7:18-24.

Hayashi, Y., and Lalich, J. J. (1968). Protective effect of mercapto-ethylamine and cysteine against monocrotaline intoxication in rats. Toxicol. Appl. Pharmacol. 12:36-43.

Hirono, I. (1972). Carcinogenicity and neurotoxicity of cycasin with special reference to species differences. Fed. Proc. 31:1493-1497.

Hirono, I., Haga, M., Fujii, M., Matsuura, S., Matsubara, N., Nakayama, M., Furiya, T., Hikichi, M., Takanashi, H., Uchida, E., Hosaka, S., and Ueno, I. (1979). Induction of hepatic tumors in rats by senkirkine and symphytine. J. Natl. Cancer Inst. 63: 469-472.

Hirono, I., Mori, H., Yamada, K., Hirata, Y., Haga, M., Tatematsu, H., and Kame, S. (1977). Carcinogenic activity of petasitenine, a new pyrrolizidine alkaloid isolated from petasites Japonicus maxim. J. Natl. Cancer Inst. 58:1155-1157.

Hirono, I., Shibuya, C., Mori, H., Miwa, T., and Haga, M. (1973). Comparative study of carcinogenic activity of each part of bracken, J. Natl. Cancer Inst. 50:1367-1371.

Hirono, I., Shibuya, C., Shimizu, M., and Fushimi, K. (1972). Carcinogenic activity of processed bracken used as human food. J. Natl Cancer Inst. 48:1248-1250.

Hooson, J., and Grasso, P. (1976). Cytotoxic and carcinogenic response to monocrotaline pyrrole. J. Pathol. 118:121-128.

Hsu, I. C., Allen, J. R., and Chesney, C. F. (1973). Identification and toxicological effects of dehydroretronecine, a metabolite of monocrotaline. Proc. Soc. Exp. Biol. Med. 144:834-838.

Huxtable, R., Stillman, A., and Ciaramitaro, D. (1977). Characterization of alkaloids involved in human Senecio (pyrrolizidine) poisoning. Proc. West. Pharmacol. Soc. 20:455-459.

IARC (1976). Evaluation of Carcinogenic Risk of Chemicals to Man. Some Naturally Occurring Substances. IARC Monographs, Vol. 10. Lyon, France.

Jago, M. V. (1969). The development of the hepatic megalocytosis of chronic pyrrolizidine alkaloid poisoning. Am. J. Pathol. 56:405-422.

Jago, M. V. (1971). Factors affecting the chronic hepatotoxicity of pyrrolizidine alkaloids. J. Pathol. 105:1-11.

Johnson, W. D., Robertson, K. A., Pounds, J. G., and Allen, J. R. (1978). Dehydrorchronecine induced skin tumors in mice. J. Natl. Cancer Inst. 61:85-89.

Joint Iran and IARC Study Group (1977). Esophageal cancer studies in the Caspian littoral of Iran: Results of population studies—a prodrome. J. Natl. Cancer Inst. 59:1127-1138.

Kapadia, G. J., Chung, E. B., Ghosh, B., Shukla, Y. N., Basak, S. P., Morton, J. F., and Pradhan, S. N. (1978). Carcinogenicity of some folk medicinal herbs in rats. J. Natl. Cancer Inst. 60:683-686.

Kapadia, G. J., Paul, B. D., Chung, E. B., Ghosh, B., and Pradhan, S. N. (1976). Carcinogenicity of Camellia sinensis (tea) and some tannin-containing folk medicinal herbs administered subcutaneously in rats. J. Natl. Cancer Inst. 207-209.

Kay, J. M., Harris, P., and Heath, D. (1967). Pulmonary hypertension produced in rats by ingestion of Crotolaria spectabilis seeds. Thorax 22:176-179.

Lalich, J. J., and Merkow, M. S. (1961). Pulmonary arteritis produced in rats by feeding Crotolaria spectabilis. Lab. Invest. 10:744-750.

Lanigan, G. W. (1976). Peptococcus heliotrinreducans Sp. Nov., a cytochrome-producing anaerobe which metabolizes pyrrolizidine alkaloids. J. Gen. Microbiol. 94:1-10.

Laquer, G. L., and Spatz, M. (1968). Toxicology of cycasin. Cancer Res. 28:2262-2267.

Lemon, H. M. (1977). Experimental basis for multiple primary carcinogenesis by sex hormones. Cancer 40:1825-1832.

Lyford, C. L., Vergara, G. G., and Moeller, D. D. (1976). Hepatic veno-occlusive disease originating in Ecuador. Gastroenterology 70:105-108.

Magee, P. N., Montesano, R., and Preussmann, O. (1976). N-nitroso compounds and related carcinogens. In Chemical Carcinogens, ACS Monograph 173, C. E. Searle (Ed.). American Chemical Society, Washington, D.C., pp. 491-625.

Mattocks, A. R. (1968). Toxicity of pyrrolizidine alkaloids. Nature 217:723-728.

Mattocks, A. R. (1972). Acute hepatotoxicity and pyrrolic metabolites in rats dosed with pyrrolizidine alkaloids. Chem. Biol. Interact. 5:227-242.

Mattocks, A. R. (1978). Plant toxins. In Trace Substances and Health, A Handbook. Part II, P. M. Newberne (Ed.). Marcel Dekker, New York, NY.

McLean, E. K. (1970). The toxic actions of pyrrolizidine (Senecio) alkaloids. Pharmacol. Rev. 22:429-483.

Mohabbat, O., Younos, M. S., Merzad, A. A., Srivastava, R. N., Sedig, G. G., and Aram, G. N. (1976). An outbreak of hepatic veno-occlusive disease in north-western Afghanistan. Lancet 2:269-271.

Mori, H., Kato, K., Ushimaru, Y., Kato, T., and Hirono, I. (1977). Effect of drying with hot forced fraft and of mincing bracken fern on its carcinogenic activity. Gan. 68: 517-520.

Newberne, P. M., and Rogers, A. E. (1973). Nutrition, monocrotaline and aflatoxin B_1 in liver carcinogenesis. Plant Foods Man. 1:23-31.

Newberne, P. M., and Rogers, A. E. (1976). Nutritional modulation of carcinogenesis. In Fundamentals in Cancer Prevention, P. N. Magee, S. Takayama, T. Sugimura, and T. Matsushima (Eds.). University of Tokyo Press, Tokyo/University Press, Baltimore, pp. 15-40.

Newberne, P. M., Wilson, R., and Rogers, A. E. (1971). Effects of a low-lipotrope diet on the response of young male rats to the pyrrolizidine alkaloid, monocrotaline. Toxicol. Appl. Pharmacol. 18:387-397.

Pamukcu, A. M., Erdogan, E., Yalciner, S., Milli, U., and Bryan, G. T. (1978). Carcinogenic and mutagenic activities of milk from cows fed bracken fern (Pteridium aguclinim). Cancer Res. 38:1556-1560.

Pamukcu, A. M., Yalciner, S., and Bryan, G. T. (1977). Inhibition of carcinogenic effect of bracken fern (Pteridium aguilinum) by various chemicals. Cancer 40:2450-2454.

Pamukcu, A. M., Yalciner, S., Price, J. M., and Bryan, G. T. (1970). Effects of the administration of thiamine on the incidence of urinary bladder carcinomas in rats fed bracken fern. Cancer Res. 30:2671-2674.

Peterson, J. E. (1965). Effects of the pyrrolizidine alkaloid, lasiocarpine N-oxide on nuclear and cell division in the liver of rats. J. Path. Bact. 89:153-171.

Peterson, J. E., Samuel, A., and Jago, M. V. (1972). Pathological effects of dehydroheliotridine, a metabolite of heliotridine-based pyrrolizidine alkaloids, in the young rat. J. Pathol. 107:175-189.

Pirie, H. M. (1973). Unusual occurrence of squamous carcinoma of the upper alimentary tract in cattle in bracken. Res. Vet. Sci. 15:135-138.

Plowright, W., Linsell, C. A., and Peers, F. O. (1971). A focus of rumenal cancer in Kenyan cattle. Br. J. Cancer 25:72-80.

Powis, G., Ames, M. M., and Kovach, J. S. (1979). Metabolic conversion of indicine N-oxide to indicine in rabbits and humans. Cancer Res. 39:3564-3570.

Price, J. M., and Pamukcu, A. M. (1968). The induction of neoplasms of the urinary bladder of the cow and the small intestine of the rat by feeding bracken fern. Cancer Res. 28:2247-2251.

Rao, M. S., and Reddy, J. K. (1978). Malignant neoplasms in rats fed lasiocarpine. Br. J. Cancer 37:289-293.

Robertson, K. A., Seymour, J. L., Hsia, M.-T., and Allen, J. R. (1977). Covalent interaction of dehydroretronecine, a carcinogenic metabolite of the pyrrolizidine alkaloid, monocrotaline, with cysteine and glutathione. Cancer Res. 37:3141-3144.

Rogers, A. E., and Newberne, P. M. (1971). Lasiocarpine: factors influencing its toxicity and effects on liver cell division. Toxicol. Appl. Pharmacol. 18:356-366.

Rothman, K. J. (1975). Alcohol. In Persons at High Risk of Cancer. An Approach to Cancer Etiology and Control, J. F. Fraumeni, Jr. (Ed.). Academic Press, New York, pp. 139-150.

Schoental, R. (1968). Toxicology and carcinogenic action of pyrrolizidine alkaloids. Cancer Res. 28:2237-2246.

Schoental, R. (1976). Carcinogens in plants and micro-organisms. In Chemical Carcinogens, ACS Monograph 13, C. E. Searle (Ed.). American Chemical Society, Washington, D.C., pp. 626-689.

Schoental, R. (1977). The role of nicotinamide and certain other modifying factors in diethylnitrosamine carcinogenesis. Cancer 40:1833-1840.

Selzer, G., and Parker, R. G. (1951). Senecio poisoning exhibiting as Chiari's syndrome. Amer. J. Pathol. 27:885-907.

Shumaker, R. C., Robertson, K. A., Hsu, I. C., and Allen, J. R. (1976). Neoplastic transformation in tissues of rats exposed to monocrotaline or dehydroretronecine. J. Natl. Cancer Inst. 56:787-790.

Sinnhuber, R. O., Lee, D. J., Wales, J. H., and Ayres, J. L. (1968). Dietary factors and hepatoma in rainbow trout (Salmo gairdneri). II. Cocarcinogenesis by cyclopropenoid fatty acids and the effect of gossypol and altered lipids on aflatoxin-induced cancer. J. Cancer Inst. 41:1293-1301.

Solheim, E., and Scheline, R. R. (1973). Metabolism of alkenebenzene derivatives in the rat. I. p-Methoxyallylbenzene (estragole) and p-methoxypropenylbenzene (anethole). Xenobiotica 3:493-510.

Spatz, M., McDaniel, E. G., and Laquer, G. L. (1967). Role of intestinal micro-organisms in determining cycasin toxicity. Proc. Soc. Exp. Biol. Med. 124:691-697.

Stillman, A. E., Huxtable, R. J., Fox, D., Hart, M., and Bergeson, P. (1977). Pyrrolizidine (Senecio) poisoning in Arizona: severe liver damage due to herbal teas. Ariz. Med. 34:545-546.

Stuart, K. L., and Bras, G. (1957). Veno-occlusive disease of the liver. Q. J. Med. 26: 291-315.

Svoboda, D. J., and Reddy, J. K. (1972). Malignant tumors in rats given lasiocarpine. Cancer Res. 32:908-912.

Tandon, B. N., Tandon, H. D., Tandon, R. K., Narndranathan, M., and Joshi, Y. K. (1976). An epidemic of veno-occlusive disease of the liver in Central India. Lancet 2:271-272.

Taylor, J. M., Jenner, P. M., and Jones, W. I. (1964). A comparison of the toxicity of some allyl, propenyl and propyl compounds in the rat. Toxicol. Appl. Pharmacol. 6: 378-387.

Tuchweber, D., Kovacs, K., Jago, M. V., et al. (1974). Effect of steroidal and non-steroidal microsomal enzyme inducers on the hepatotoxicity of pyrrolizidine alkaloids in rats. Res. Commun. Chem. Pathol. and Pharmacol. 7:459-480.

Wattenberg, L. W., Lam, L. K., Fladmoe, A. V., and Borchert, P. (1977). Inhibitors of colon carcinogenesis. Cancer 40:2432-2435.

Weinstein, I. B., Wigler, M., and Pietropaolo, C. (1977). The action of tumor-promoting agents in cell culture. In Origins of Human Cancer, H. H. Hiatt, J. D. Watson, and J. A. Winsten (Eds.). Cold Spring Harbor Laboratory, Cold Spring Harbor, N.Y., pp. 751-772.

White, I. N. (1976). The role of liver glutathione in the acute toxicity of retrorsine to rats. Chem. Biol. Interact. 13:333-342.

White, I. N., Mattocks, A. R., and Butler, W. H. (1973). The conversion of the pyrrolizidine alkaloid retrorsine to pyrrolic derivatives in vivo and in vitro and its acute toxicity to various animal species. Chem. Biol. Interact. 6: 207-218.

White, I. N., and Mattocks, A. R. (1972). Reaction of dehydropyrrolizines with deoxyribonucleic acids in vitro. Biochem. J. 128: 291-297.

Whiting, M. G. (1964). Food practices in ALS foci in Japan, the Marianas and New Guinea. Fed. Proc. 23: 1343-1344.

Wislocki, P. G., Miller, E. C., Miller, J. A., McCoy, E. C., and Rosenkranz, H. S. (1977). Carcinogenic and mutagenic activities of safrole, 1'-hydroxysafrole and some known or possible metabolites. Cancer Res. 37: 1883-1891.

Yoshida, S., Tazaki, K., and Minimikawa, T. (1975). Occurrence of shikimic and quinic acids in angiosperms. Phytochemistry 14: 195-197.

12

Therapeutic Agents and Procedures in Cancer Induction

DAVID BARRINGER CLAYSON / University of Nebraska Medical Center, Omaha, Nebraska

I. INTRODUCTION

Carcinogenic drugs are of great concern and fascination to those interested in environmentally mediated carcinogenesis. Extensive but definable human populations are exposed often to high levels of these agents to aid in the clinical management of real, or sometimes imagined,

---

The author wishes to acknowledge Public Health Service Contract NO1 CP33278 from the National Cancer Institute, which provided financial support during the writing of this chapter.

disease. Drugs differ from other carcinogens insofar as the benefits of using them are often more apparent than the benefits of many environmental agents. In consequence, risk-benefit evaluations are accepted with far less question than with carcinogenic food contaminants, such as pesticides or agricultural chemicals.

In the treatment of chronic disease, particular drugs may be used in large amounts. Thus, a patient receiving only 100 mg drug (1.4 mg/kg) daily will, in the course of less than 3 years, have been exposed to 100 g of the agent. This may help to explain the relatively short latency of some drug-associated tumors. Other biologic properties of the drug may also contribute to the rapidity of tumor development.

Ideally, medical records should help to define those exposed to specific drugs and the level at which they have been given. Unfortunately, access to medical records is often difficult, due to the entirely proper desire to maintain confidentiality between physician and patient, and, when they are reached, records are found to contain woefully incomplete information. The degree of accuracy in records of drug use decreases from those drugs that are usually administered only in hospitals, to those prescribed and subsequently consumed at home. The lack of accuracy is due to the fact that there can be little certainty that drugs consumed at home are used completely, if at all. Drugs sold over the counter without prescription present quite a different problem, and their consumption, in both qualitative and quantitative aspects, must depend on each individual patient's ability to recall past use.

Pharmaceutic agents should be one of the major areas in which human carcinogens are sought. At the time of the great advances in drug therapy of a wide range of infectious and other diseases, 1935-1960, and the concurrent expansion of the pharmaceutical industry, there were many fewer premarketing tests for adverse reactions than are required today. As a consequence, we should expect that many drugs with carcinogenic properties came unnoticed into clinical use. The need before and after World War II to treat many diseases, such as tuberculosis—"the captain of the kings of death"—was rightly seen as the first priority. Even now, the adverse effects of drugs must always be subject to an unbiased risk-benefit evaluation before their use is discarded. For example, with cancer chemotherapeutic agents, the idea of not using a life-prolonging drug, because it might give the patient another cancer many years later must be carefully balanced against the probable prognosis of the primary tumor in the absence of the drug. As cancer therapy becomes increasingly successful, the balance between risk and benefit will slowly alter.

A further hazard of drug use is the possible contamination of those attending the patient. This possibility has not been much investigated in the cancer area, but there are disquieting reports that female anesthetists and operating room nurses have, as a consequence of exposure to volatile anesthetics (Corbett et al., 1974), given birth to a greater number of deformed babies than would have been predicted. In a similar vein, there are slight data to support the conclusion that nurses and technicians who formerly used the human bladder carcinogen benzidine to test for occult blood in feces have developed more bladder tumors than would have been expected (Anthony and Thomas, 1970). At the beginning of this century radiologists were exposed to a considerable hazard in the use of improperly screened machines and developed leukemia (March, 1944, 1950; Brown and Doll, 1958).

This chapter is concerned with the evidence that certain pharmaceutic agents are carcinogenic in humans and/or laboratory animals. The data on humans are considered in greater depth than those in animals because: (1) they are most relevant to the human condition, and (2) much of the data on the possible carcinogenicity of new drugs are buried in the files of the drug manufacturer or regulatory agency and cannot readily be obtained.

The carcinogenic effects of drugs are not a consequence only of the use of new, powerfully effective agents developed in the past 40 years. Some of the relatively ineffective remedies in medieval herbals were based on treatments with plant materials which we now know to be potently toxic and carcinogenic. Culpepper (1950), for example, recommended groundsel (Senecio vulgaris) for a variety of conditions: animal tests have clearly demonstrated that the pyrrolizidine alkaloids present in this, and other species, are very toxic and carcinogenic to the liver of rodents (Cook et al., 1950). The more recent use of prescriptions of radium-containing medicaments for the palliation of rheumatic complaints and other conditions has similarly led to cancers in the patient (Aub et al., 1952).

II. DRUGS AND PROCEDURES INVESTIGATED AS HUMAN CARCINOGENS

The first three drugs (Fig. 1) to be considered in this section were chosen not because of their clinical usefulness or widespread prescription, but because they illustrate: (1) how much information may be obtained in the case of a drug used exclusively under strict medical control, (2) how much information may be obtained in the case of a popular nonprescription medicament, and (3) how a specific drug may lead to difficulties in interpreting epidemiologic results.

A. Chlornaphazin, β-Naphthylamine Mustard Bis(2-Chloroethyl)2-Naphthylamine

Chlornaphazin was originally devised by Sir Alexander Haddow and his colleagues in London for treatment of leukemia and lymphoma, both of which in the late 1940s had a pitifully poor prognosis of only a few months. Clearly the need for carcinogenicity testing under these conditions was minimal. Chlornaphazin, however, found favor in Denmark for the treatment of the blood disorder polycythemia vera, which had a much better prognosis. It was most effective when used in combination with ^{32}P-phosphate.

The first indication of an impending disaster was contained in reports that polycythemia was associated with bladder cancer (Videbaek, 1950, 1964; Chievitz and Thiede, 1962). Chlornaphazin was soon recognized as the likely cause. Thiede and his colleagues (Thiede

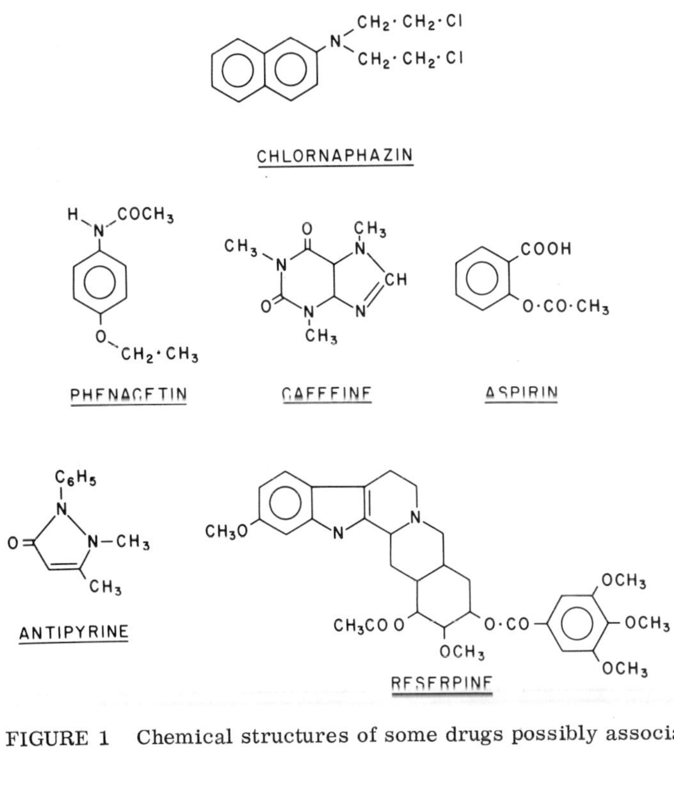

FIGURE 1 Chemical structures of some drugs possibly associated with cancer in humans.

et al., 1964; Thiede and Christensen, 1969, 1975) assembled a population of 61 polycythemia patients treated with this drug, which has now been followed for over 10 years. Other groups of polycythemia patients, with equivalent survival, were investigated to show that neither the disease itself nor treatment with ^{32}P-phosphate was responsible for the bladder tumors. These groups consisted of 40 and 46 patients, respectively. Thirteen of the 61 patients receiving chlornaphazin had developed bladder cancer at the time of the 10 year follow-up. Eight others had abnormal urinary cytology, indicative of an impending bladder tumor (Clayson, 1975a). That is to say, with 17 of the original patients still surviving, 34% of those treated had neoplastic or potentially neoplastic bladder lesions. The doses administered varied from 2 to 360 g/patient and tumor latency from 2.5 to 11 years, a much shorter time than has been observed for occupationally induced bladder tumors (Clayson, 1976). There was, even in this small series, evidence of dose dependency (Table 1). Four of five patients receiving more than 200 g of chlornaphazin developed bladder cancer, whereas only three of the 31 patients receiving less than 50 g of the drug did so. The latency period also was shown to be reduced by increasing dosages of the drug.

Chlornaphazin has been relatively little investigated in animals other than to show it induced lung adenomas in sensitive mice. Further animal experiments are clearly unneeded insofar as human risk assessment is concerned. The induction of bladder tumors is almost certainly due to the metabolism of chlornaphazin to the same active constituents as the potent human carcinogen 2-naphthylamine (Boyland and Manson, 1963), but the possibility that this drug is also immunosuppressive may help to explain the very short latency of these tumors. Immunosuppression has led to bladder cancer formation in rats treated parenterally with methylnitrosourea (Denlinger et al., 1973).

The extent of use of chlornaphazin on a worldwide scale is unknown. However, medical journals in Italy and South America have in the past advertised this drug.

B. Analgesics

Analgesics containing phenacetin, caffeine, and aspirin or antipyrene were commonly used in many places. The overconsumption of these analgesics, which was particularly prevalent in parts of northern Sweden, is associated primarily with renal papillary necrosis and sometimes with renal pelvic cancer. Rathert et al. (1975), in a survey of the world literature, reported 118 cases of renal pelvic cancer associated with this drug combination.

Bengtsson and her colleagues (1968) investigated the epidemiology of these conditions, and identified 242 cases of renal papillary necrosis, of which 142 had each previously consumed more than 1 kg analgesic. Of the 142 drug-exposed patients, nine developed renal pelvic cancer, whereas no such tumors were present in the 100 not exposed to high levels of these analgesics. Similar findings have been reported from other countries. For example, Mahoney et al. (1977) discussed the connection between habituation to these analgesics and renal pelvic cancer in Australia.

TABLE 1 Chlornaphazin and the Induction of Bladder Cancer in Polycythemia Patients

Dose of chlornaphazin (g)	Number of patients	Bladder carcinomas No.	Bladder carcinomas %	Abnormal cytology No.	Abnormal cytology %	Bladder carcinoma latency (years)
200+	5	4	80	0	0	4.0
50-200	25	6	24	2	8	7.2
50	31	3	9	6	19	8.7
All doses	61	13	13	8	13	—

Source: Thiede and Christensen, 1975.

Nephropathy and renal pelvic cancer are endemic in certain parts of southeastern Europe (Chernozemsky et al., 1977). It appears less likely that this Balkan nephropathy is due to analgesic abuse. Recent reports have associated the condition with a product of the mold Penicillin verrucosum var cyclopium in model systems (Barnes et al., 1977). In such an area it would therefore be more difficult to associate particular cases of renal pelvic cancer with analgesic use.

The components of the analgesic responsible for tumor induction are not definitely known. Phenacetin seems most likely, as it is an aromatic amine; that is, it is structurally analogous to the known human urinary tract carcinogens (Clayson, 1975a). Furthermore, it is metabolized to N-hydroxyphenacetin (Hinson and Mitchell, 1976) analogously to the metabolic activation of other carcinogenic aromatic amines, and N-hydroxyphenacetin has been demonstrated to be carcinogenic to rat liver (Calder et al., 1976). More direct information that phenacetin itself is carcinogenic derives from a report (Johansson and Angervall, 1976) that feeding 0.535% phenacetin to female rats led to four of 17 developing ear duct carcinomas and five of 17 developing mammary adenocarcinomas, compared to one mammary carcinoma in 18 controls. Among noncancerous changes, severe urothelial hyperplasia and severe vascular changes associated with the renal papillae were frequent. Nevertheless, antipyrene is a hydrazine derivative (Toth, 1975), which implies the possibility of carcinogenicity, while neither caffeine nor aspirin has yet been adequately tested in animals.

C. Reserpine (Rauwolfia Alkaloids)

Rauwolfia alkaloids are used extensively in the management of hypertension. Three separate epidemiologic surveys published in 1974 indicated that this medication might be associated with mammary cancer in women (Boston Collaborative Drug Surveillance Program, 1974; Heinonen et al., 1974; Armstrong et al., 1974). In the succeeding year, three further epidemiologic studies failed to confirm the association (Laska et al., 1975; O'Fallon et al., 1975; Mack et al., 1975). The increase in risk due to treatment was relatively small, but with a disease as common as mammary cancer any increase in risk can involve a substantial number of individual cases. The explanation of these contradictory observations may lie in the fact that mammary cancer is more prevalent in women of affluent social status than in those who are less well off, possibly because of a more adequate diet and less exercise. The effect of changes in caloric intake in animals on the incidence of naturally occurring and induced tumors is well-documented (Clayson, 1975b). The more affluent woman is also more able to seek medical advice and is thus more likely to have been prescribed a specific drug, such as reserpine. The examination of the correlation between mammary cancer and reserpine use, carried out completely within a retirement community, which housed only well-to-do, failed to show any association, thus supporting the contention that rauwolfia does not lead to mammary carcinoma in women (Mack et al., 1975).

D. Estrogens

Estrogens (Fig. 2) are the greatest cause for concern of all currently used drugs. They have been shown to be tumorigenic to humans when administered during pregnancy to prevent spontaneous abortion. They have been used to suppress the adverse effects of the menopause, and again cancer has resulted. Recently it has become clear that in combination with progestogens in oral contraceptives, they present a small, but disturbing, risk of inducing benign liver tumors and endometrial cancer in those women who use this medication for long periods without intermission. Animal experiments have likewise indicated that abnormally high levels of estrogen administration may lead to the induction of a wide variety of tumors, ranging from mammary carcinoma in mice carrying the mammary tumor virus (Bittner, 1939) to renal tumors in Syrian golden hamsters (Kirkman and Bacon, 1952). Despite the vast volume of evidence that estrogens induce cancer, doubt still remains whether the tumors are induced by a direct carcinogenic mechanism or as a result of modification of the action of other, unknown, carcinogens.

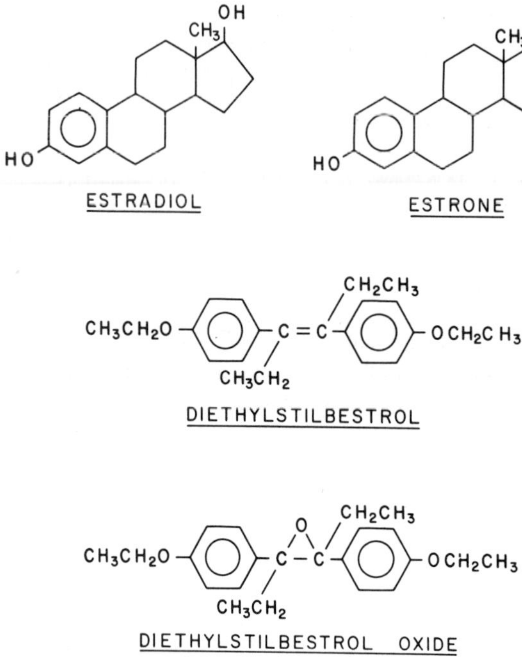

FIGURE 2 Chemical structures of estrogens.

1. Diethylstilbestrol in Pregnancy

Diethylstilbestrol (DES) was advocated in 1949 for the maintenance of pregnancy in women with a history of spontaneous abortion (Smith and Smith, 1949). The treatment schedule varied considerably; for example, in some women the initial treatment was 5 mg/day, increasing progressively to 125 mg/day at term. This therapy was enthusiastically used so that there is now an estimated population of 0.5 to 2.0 million young women and an equal number of young men whose mothers were exposed to this drug during pregnancy (Herbst, personal communication to Dr. M. Rustia, 1975).

The discovery in 1971 (Herbst et al., 1971) of seven young women whose mothers had received DES during pregnancy, and who had a very rare tumor, clear cell adenocarcinoma of the vagina, suggested the need for great caution in the use of this medication. The suspicion raised by those case reports was rapidly followed by a confirmatory epidemiological survey (Greenwald et al., 1971). The present position has been summarized by Poskanzer and Herbst (1977), who have indicated that the frequency of adenocarcinoma of the vagina and cervix in the exposed population between the ages of 15 and 27 years is low. On the other hand, proliferative lesions of the reproductive tract, such as adenosis of the vagina and cervix, after in utero exposure to DES, is relatively frequent and affects from 30% (Poskanzer and Herbst, 1977) to 90% of the exposed population. The appearance of fibrous ridges in the vagina and a failure of the cervix and vagina to stain with iodine on colposcopic examination were also noted. The male population exposed to DES in utero has also been studied. Failure of the testes to attain their normal size, and cystic lesions of the testes and tissues ancillary to the spermatogenic system were the principal lesions (Bibbo et al., 1977).

The use of DES in the first trimester of pregnancy appears to be most closely associated with tumorigenesis (Poskanzer and Herbst, 1977). Similarly, adenosis occurred in 75% of young women whose mothers were treated with DES before the eighth week of pregnancy, but in none of a group of 19 whose treatment commenced after the 18th week (Poskanzer and Herbst, 1977). This timing suggests a teratogenic rather than a direct carcinogenic effect. Adenocarcinoma was found to be associated with a wide range of daily doses of DES (1.5-225 mg); total doses during pregnancy ranged from 300-18,200 mg (Poskanzer and Herbst, 1977).

Transplacental DES in high doses leads to similar, but not identical, proliferative changes in hamsters (Rustia and Shubik, 1976). This system could be used to determine more accurately the dose requirements for the observed changes and whether estrogens other than DES and its analogs are effective, a possibility that the evidence in human cases does not make clear. The hamster model has also been used to show that in utero exposure to DES has a profound effect on the response to other chemical carcinogens administered after birth. The potent carcinogen 7,12-dimethylbenz(a)anthracene (DMBA), when administered at a high dose to female hamsters, yields mainly benign mammary tumors. Transplacental DES, followed after birth by DMBA, leads to a high yield of malignant mammary tumors (Rustia and Shubik, 1978). This experiment suggests that those exposed in utero to DES may be more sensitive to the tumorigenic effects of environmental carcinogens on tissues other than the reproductive tract and that they may require special surveillance for a variety of tumors.

DES provides the first example of a transplacental carcinogen in humans. Studies in animals have provided many examples of the effects of in utero exposure to carcinogens (Rice, 1979). Tumors induced in this way are no less dangerous than those induced later in life, as evidenced by the 16% mortality rate from adenocarcinoma of the vagina and cervix (Poskanzer and Herbst, 1977).

2. Postmenopausal Estrogens

Cancer of the endometrium appears to be increasing in frequency in the United States. In certain areas this increase has amounted to as much as 10% per year during the last decade (Weiss et al., 1976; Shanklin, 1974; Kistner et al., 1973), a truly frightening increase even of a comparatively rare tumor.

It appears that the use of estrogens to alleviate the distressing side effects of the menopause may be a major contributing factor in the genesis of endometrial cancer. Smith and his associates (1975) compared the histories of 243 patients with endometrial cancer with 317 matched controls; Ziel and Finkle (1975) reviewed 94 cancer patients with two equal-sized groups of matched controls. It was estimated that the risk of developing endometrial cancer was 4.5 to 7.6 times greater among estrogen users than among controls. Both studies carefully excluded the effects of use of other drugs, such as valium, reserpine, or thyroid-active substances.

Nevertheless, because post-menopausal estrogen therapy is so valuable in combating the adverse symptoms of the menopause, and also in delaying effects such as aging of the skin, many clinicians have been unwilling to accept this evidence. Apart from criticisms of the employed epidemiologic techniques, the major argument is that in the United States the more affluent women seek medical advice more frequently and are therefore more likely to be prescribed estrogen. These women, because of their affluence, have a different life style, which is established as enhancing the incidence of certain endocrine-related tumors, for example, of the breast. Therefore, it is possible that the endometrial tumors are a consequence of some factor other than estrogen. These criticisms were met by Mack et al. (1976), who investigated cases of endometrial cancer and controls drawn from the residents of a single California retirement community of a fairly uniform, high level of affluence. A further advantage of the use of this population was that a common pharmacy was used by most residents, thus making the accurate assessment of histories of drug prescription more possible. A total of 63 endometrial cancer cases were compared with 396 controls. Estrogen use presented a risk ratio of 8.0, while users of conjugated estrogens (Premarin), which is the treatment of choice for postmenopausal symptoms, demonstrated a risk ratio of 5.6.

This survey, combined with several that have appeared recently (Schindler, 1976; McDonald et al., 1977; Gray et al., 1977), all of which led to similar results, must be taken as establishing that the use of estrogens to counteract postmenopausal symptoms carried a significant risk from endometrial cancer.

This conclusion places a substantial burden on the busy clinician wishing to prescribe this therapy, who must be assured that the symptoms he or she is attempting to relieve are, in fact, sufficiently intense to justify this added risk. Furthermore, the desirability of advising the patient of this risk and of the need for periodic examination for endometrial cancer should be considered, so that if the condition develops, it may be detected and treated at an early stage.

3. Oral Contraceptives: Benign Liver Tumors and Endometrial Cancer

Oral contraceptives generally consist of mixtures of synthetic estrogens and progestogens; the level of estrogen has in recent years been progressively lowered. Such chronic animal bioassays of oral contraceptives as have been conducted have officially been accepted as negative, but have not been completely satisfactory. For example, in a review by the United Kingdom Committee on the Safety of Medicines (1972), the oral contraceptives were accepted as safe, despite a dose-related incidence of rodent hepatomas in certain instances (Barnes, 1972; British Medical Journal, 1972). The reason the Committee failed to attach any significance to these tumors is not clear, but at that time, the relevance of rodent hepatomas to human disease was being seriously questioned.

The first report of tumors associated with the use of these drugs by women was by Baum et al. (1973), who described seven oral contraceptive-associated cases of benign liver tumors. Several hundred instances of this previously very uncommon condition in young women have subsequently been reported. Despite the benign nature of the lesion, generally reported as adenoma, focal nodular hyperplasia, or hamartoma, the condition is life threatening, as patients may present with hemoperitoneum due to ruptured liver. This means that cases are treated as surgical emergencies rather than being referred to specialists in liver disease, and, therefore, they do not readily attract attention because no one surgeon sees many of them. This, combined with the former absence of a registry for reporting benign liver tumors, has made adequate epidemiology difficult. Mahboubi and Shubik (1977), as a result of repeated questioning of surgeons in the State of Nebraska, found 20 cases of benign liver tumors in women between 19 and 44 years of age, all of whom had used oral contraceptives. These cases occurred between 1966 and 1975, in a total population (males and females of all ages) of 1.4 million. It may, therefore, be deduced that the frequency of this condition is currently low.

Many small (Edmondson et al., 1976) and a few large (Christopherson and Mays, 1977) series have been reported. Christopherson and Mays (1977) discussed their experience with the first 100 cases reported to their Louisville, Ky. registry. In three cases, aged 14, 15, and 15 years, oral contraceptives had not been used; a fourth patient with streak ovaries who had not used oral contraceptives presented with a malignant rather than a benign liver tumor. Three cases had used conjugated estrogens (Premarin), one had an ovarian thecoma, and six others who were pregnant or immediately postpartum also had elevated estrogen levels during pregnancy. The remaining 86 were all contraceptive users (in 19, the type used could not be identified). It was also noted that the occurrence of liver lesions was often associated with long-term exposure to oral contraceptives. In a few cases, resection of the lesion, followed by continued oral contraceptive use, led to recurrence, while in others, discontinuation of drug administration resulted in the disappearance of the lesions without surgery. That is to say, these benign lesions depended on the presence of estrogen for their maintenance. Christopherson and Mays (1977) concluded from their observations that benign, but probably not the normally more common malignant, liver tumors were associated with the use of this medication and that in view of the large number of oral contraceptive users, the risk of developing these tumors is probably small. Whether the use of these drugs with their great social benefits is justified, in view of the low, but real, probability of developing a life-threatening disease, may be debated.

There have been two attempts to develop a national overview of the seriousness of the benign liver tumor problem. The American College of Surgeons (Vana et al., 1976) forwarded questionnaires to its members concerning the number of patients with this condition and their oral contraceptive use. The association between drug use and the condition was held to be established, but was far less definite than in the earlier and smaller surveys. This is probably due to the weakness in the questionnaire approach, which depends entirely on the conscientiousness of the answerer in providing the required information. Recently the U.S. Center for Disease Control carried out another survey through the Armed Forces Institute of Pathology (Morbid. Mortal. Weekly Rep., 1977). They concluded that continuous drug use for 7 or more years in women aged 27 or more presented the greatest risk. Their survey of 79 living cases and 237 matched neighborhood controls involved formal interviews and is not, therefore, subject to the same criticisms as the American College of Surgeons' Report.

There are also grounds to suspect that oral contraceptive use may be associated with endometrial cancer. This is based on a series of case reports in which drug use was prolonged (Lyon and Frisch, 1976; Kaufman et al., 1976; Cohen and Deppe, 1977). It must be regarded seriously in view of the association between replacement estrogen therapy after the menopause and this form of cancer.

Tumor development may be regarded as a relatively minor hazard of oral contraceptive use. A recent survey by the Royal College of General Practitioners of the United Kingdom (1977) retrospectively studied approximately 46,000 women of child-bearing age. It was concluded that the risk of mortality among regular oral contraceptive users was 40% higher than among nonusers. The most impressive finding was that the risk of dying of disease of the circulatory system increased seven-fold.

4. Other Evidence Relating to Estrogen Use

Attempts have been made to associate oral contraceptive and other estrogen use with tumors other than those already described. The current evidence for such associations is not particularly convincing, but the proportion of women of child-bearing age who have used oral contraceptives for most of their reproductive life is still probably relatively small. There will be a special need to investigate these women who continuously use oral contraceptives and are subsequently prescribed estrogens to mitigate the adverse effects of the menopause. Such studies will go far to elucidate the cancer burden associated with human estrogen use.

There are presently disquieting reports that mammary cancer and carcinoma of the uterine cervix may be associated with estrogen use. Hoover et al. (1976) reported a doubling in mammary cancer in women using conjugated estrogens, especially for prolonged periods. Fasal and Paffenbarger (1975) found a similar increase in this form of cancer, limited to those women who had taken oral contraceptives for more than 2, but fewer than 4, years. They suggested that the synthetic steroids might accelerate development of preexisting tumors. The level of suspicion of excess cervical cancer associated with estrogen use is less convincing (Choi et al., 1976; Sandmire et al., 1976). The difficulties which make a clear appreciation of the effects of oral contraceptive use on this tissue have been summarized (Lancet, 1977b).

The effective treatment for prostatic cancer over the past 30 years has involved administration of the synthetic estrogen DES. There have been reports that this therapy led to mammary cancer in some patients (Bulow et al., 1973). Such reports cannot be accepted, unless in each case there is a full comparative pathological study to differentiate between secondary deposits of prostatic carcinoma and primary mammary carcinoma.

E. Other Hormones

1. Thyroxine

The longest known cancer-associated hormone-induced aberration is the result of iodide deficiency in the drinking water and diet. This leads first to overstimulation of the thyroid, thus to goiter, and subsequently to an excess incidence of benign and malignant thyroid neoplasms in the affected population (Walmer et al., 1966). These are follicular in nature (Hedinger, 1969). Excess iodide, however, is equally undesirable, as it has been shown in both Hawaii and Iceland to lead to papillary thyroid cancer (Hedinger, 1969).

The mechanism of thyroid tumor formation associated with iodide deficiency rests on the fact that the major function of the thyroid is to convert iodide into thyroxine and other related thyroid hormones. An iodide deficiency leads to a deficiency in these hormones which exist in homeostatic balance with the pituitary-produced thyroid stimulating hormone (TSH). Thus, deficiency in thyroid hormone levels leads to unblocking of TSH synthesis by the pituitary and overstimulation of the thyroid occurs. In experimental animals a number of treatments lead to thyroid neoplasms, including iodide deficiency, an excessive dietary ratio of chloride compared to iodide ions, goitrogens (i.e., chemicals that specifically block thyroid hormone synthesis), and surgical or radiological partial thyroidectomy. Doniach (1958) showed that in rats partial radiological thyroidectomy using ^{131}I, combined with chronic exposure to goitrogens, led to thyroid malignancies, whereas either ^{131}I administration or goitrogen treatment alone led only to benign tumors. He cautioned against the use of the combined therapy in clinical practice.

2. Androgens

A limited number of case reports have indicated that chronic administration of androgens may be associated with the development of hepatocellular carcinoma. This has been found particularly in patients with Fanconi's anemia, and usually concerns the use of oxymetholone or methyltestosterone derivatives (Recant and Lacy, 1965; Johnson et al., 1972; Guy and Alexander, 1973; Meadows et al., 1974; Farrell et al., 1975; Sweeney and Evans, 1975; Bernstein et al., 1971). Epidemiologic study is required to determine whether the reported effect of androgens is significant, and whether it exerts its effects only in patients with Fanconi's anemia, or has a more generalized effect.

3. Animal Studies on Hormones

It is undoubtedly true that hormones induce tumors in humans, but at this time it is not completely certain whether they act in the same manner as other chemical carcinogens or in some other way. Most direct-acting chemical carcinogens decompose spontaneously or are converted enzymically to reactive positively charged entities (electrophiles), which covalently combine with DNA, RNA, protein, and other cellular macromolecules (Miller, 1970). Hormones appear to exert their effects by interaction with a specific cytoplasmic receptor protein, which after modification, passes into the nucleus and localizes on the DNA to modify its expression (Jensen, 1975). The suggestion by Metzler (1976; 1978) that DES metabolism could best be explained by the formation of an epoxide, which might also be a reactive electrophile, requires further investigation to establish first that the postulated intermediate is actually formed, and second, if it is formed, that it has strong electrophilic properties. The lack of activity of diethylstilbestrol and natural steroid hormones in the various microbial mutagenesis screening tests now proposed for the detection of chemical carcinogens suggests that it acts through a different mechanism.

In the 6 years following Lacassagne's (1932) observation that a crude estrogen preparation substantially increased the incidence of mammary cancer in male mice, Bittner (1939) was able to demonstrate the multifactorial nature of this disease. He found that mammary cancer depended on the presence of murine mammary tumor virus which was transmitted from mother to offspring in the milk, on the presence of the correct hormonal regimen, and

TABLE 2 Examples of the Minimum Hormonal Requirements for the Development of the Breast and the Induction of Mammary Cancer in C3H/He/Crgl Mice Which Had Been Hypophysectomized, Ovariectomized, and Adrenalectomized

State of development of breast	Hormonal requirements						
	Estrogen	Progesterone	Cortisol acetate	Deoxycorticol acetate	Corticosterone	GH	MH
Duct branching stimulated	+ +			+ +		+	 +
Ductal and alveolar development highly stimulated	+	+		+		+	
Breast as in early pregnancy	+ +	+ +				+	 +
Lactogenesis initiated in developed breast			+ +			+	 +
Growth and neoplastic development of nodules				+	+	+	

on the use of a mouse of the right genetic constitution. The validity of this classic series of experiments has recently been massively confirmed at the U.S. National Center for Toxicological Research (National Center for Toxicological Research, 1977). The virus rather than the hormone appears to be the carcinogenic factor, since in virus-free mice administration of a chemical carcinogen was necessary for mammary tumor induction, even in the presence of high levels of estrogen (Strong and Smith, 1939; Bonser and Orr, 1939). The virus or a limited treatment with a chemical carcinogen were both effective in combination with estrogen.

Nandi and his colleagues (Nandi, 1958, 1959, 1961; Nandi et al., 1960), using mice from which the pituitary, gonads, and adrenals had been surgically resected and replaced by various combinations of protein and steroid hormones, demonstrated that the mouse mammary gland was dependent for its development and maintenance on a range of hormones (Table 2). Estrogen and prolactin (or growth hormone) appeared to be of particular importance. Whereas most pituitary hormones exist in homeostatic equilibrium, through a feedback mechanism with their corresponding steroid hormone the secretion of prolactin is stimulated by estrogen. That is to say, estrogen administration results in an increase in circulating levels of both estrogen and prolactin. The question should therefore be asked whether estrogen or prolactin, or both, play a part in the carcinogenic process. A partial answer to this may be gained from a consideration of the induction of hamster renal tumors by diethylstilbestrol and certain other estrogens. Co-administration of bromocryptine led to the nearly complete abolition of estrogen-induced renal tumors (Hamilton et al., 1975). Bromocryptine was formerly thought to inhibit the secretion of prolactin by the pituitary. The position now is less precise, as further interference with secretion of pituitary hormones has been demonstrated (Hamilton et al., 1977).

It seems most probable that hormones are mainly effective in tumor formation through their natural role of maintaining endocrine and endocrine-responsive tissues in a developed state and through their ability to induce proliferation in these tissues. This, however, does not rule out the possibility that individual synthetic hormones, because of vagaries in their chemical structure, may be transformed to a reactive electrophile. Such considerations are of major importance in view of the widespread use of hormones as human and animal drugs. The use of diethylstilbestrol as an animal drug (growth promoter) is presently contraindicated, because residues of 1-3 ppb are found in the liver of treated cattle. The hazard due to such levels of this agriculturally useful drug depends on whether diethylstilbestrol is a true carcinogen or merely exerts its effect as an estrogen.

In summary, estrogens are undoubtedly capable of inducing cancer in humans and animals under appropriate conditions. The major questions that arise concern the mechanism by which they exert their effect and whether the benefits of their use outweigh the hazards they present.

F. Radiation, Radioisotopes, and Cancer Chemotherapeutic Agents

The discovery that combinations of chemotherapeutic drugs and radiation are more effective in the treatment of cancer than are single therapeutic regimes makes it logical to consider these agents together. The knowledge that both radiation and the alkylating chemotherapeutic agents are genotoxic reinforces this conclusion. In humans and animals these agents are well known as cancer inducers, either separately or together, but their continued use may be justified, because at this time their beneficial effects in improving the prognosis of otherwise fatal diseases outweigh their harmful effects. The use of these agents for less essential purposes has, however, been disastrous.

1. Radiation

Several forms of radiation are associated with cancer induction in humans or animals, including ionizing radiation (roentgen or gamma radiation), alpha and beta particles, protons, neutrons, and ultraviolet light (Upton, 1977). In humans this information has been gained from studies of occupational exposure to radiation and radioisotopes, from the effects of the socially desirable habit of sunbathing, from the populations exposed to atomic bombs, as well as from radiation used for medical purposes.

The medical use of ionizing radiation in the treatment of ankylosing spondylitis (Brown and Doll, 1965) led to a 10-fold increase in leukemia incidence. In this survey 5.48 cases of leukemia were expected and 52 cases were found, the rate of induction being 6 cases/1000 over an average of 13 years. Each case was diagnosed clinically and cytologically. Aplastic anemia was increased by 29-fold from an expected 0.51 to an observed 15 cases. Cancers of the heavily irradiated areas around the spine were increased only 1.6-fold, from 127 expected to 200 observed cases. The authors were concerned at the time of their study that they could not exclude the possibility that the observed tumors were a consequence of the disease rather than the irradiation. This possibility was excluded by a recent survey (Radford et al., 1977).

Head and neck irradiation of children has been carried out for a variety of reasons, such as for treatment of thymic enlargement—a condition which would have righted itself without treatment—destruction of tonsilar or adenoid tissue, and even the eradication of tinea capitis. The consequences of these therapeutic uses of radiation have been the induction of cancer, particularly of the thyroid.

A group of 2872 children who were irradiated, mainly for thymic enlargement, have been surveyed at intervals for adverse effects. Hemplemann et al. (1975) used as a control 5005 nonirradiated brothers and sisters of children in the study group. They concluded that the dose of radiation reaching the thyroid was essentially linearly related to the excess risk of thyroid cancer, and that females were more at risk than males. It appeared from their investigations that the excess risk was approximately 2.5 cases/10^6 population/rad/year. Of particular interest is the presence of a subgroup of 261 patients in this population who were mainly of Jewish extraction. They had been treated by a single radiotherapist who used high doses of radiation with less than the usual degree of beam focusing. This subgroup had a relative risk of thyroid cancer of 3.4, compared to that of controls. The Jewish females within the group were shown to be at a relative risk 17 times greater than the controls. DeGroot and Paloyan (1973) commented on the high frequency of thyroid carcinoma in the Chicago area. The thyroid cancer cases who had had childhood irradiation developed their tumors some 20 years later at a mean age of 28 years. Patients who had not been irradiated developed their tumors at an average age of 42.4 years. Refetoff et al. (1975) discussed 100 irradiated patients and commented that the thyroid carcinoma incidence showed no evidence of declining with time after irradiation. When it is considered that many of these irradiated children still have a major part of their lifespan left, it should also be remembered that present findings in this population may represent little more than the tip of the iceberg.

Children immigrating into Israel, if found to have tinea capitis, were irradiated to prevent them from carrying the infection into their new homeland. The consequence of this cavalier and injudicious use of irradiation has been to increase the incidence of parotid, thyroid, and possibly brain tumors. Modan et al. (1974) studied some 11,000 irradiated children treated in this fashion for ringworm of the scalp some 12-13 years previously. Tumor incidences were compared with those of the general population and of nonirradiated siblings. Head and neck tumors occurred in 2.5/1000 of the irradiated group, compared to 0.6 and 0.4/1000 in the two control groups, respectively. These authors claimed that brain tumors were also increased, but there were only six definitely diagnosed tumors in the irradiated group, compared to two and zero in the control groups, and these are too few cases to be fully convincing.

Radiation has been used to treat other benign conditions. Radiological sterilization has been used to treat metropathia hemorrhagica, excessive and often continuous uterine bleeding induced by ovarian dysfunction. Smith and Doll (1976) reported on 2068 women who were irradiated, and of whom only 103 had been lost to follow-up for various reasons. These women were treated between 1940 and 1960 and showed a 2.6-fold increase in leukemia, compared to the general population (seven cases observed, 2.69 expected) and a 1.29-fold increase in tumors of heavily irradiated sites, including the intestines, rectum and uterus. Mammary cancer, as might be expected in women who had had their ovarian function suppressed radiologically, was reduced to 0.52 times the expected level.

Other nonmalignant conditions for which radiation has been used include postpartum mastitis (Shore et al., 1977) and fluoroscopic chest examination in tuberculosis patients (Boice and Monson, 1977). Both treatments are reported to increase the incidence of breast cancer. Among the women treated for postpartum mastitis, the relative risk was estimated to be 2.2-fold if all women 10-34 years after irradiation were considered and 3.6-fold in those between 20 and 34 years postirradiation. It should be realized that although the increase may seem small, breast cancer is very prevalent among women, and such an increase, induced by a total of 247 rads administered to both breasts, represents a considerable number of individual cases of this disease.

These observations on the induction of breast cancer by radiation are of the utmost importance to the use of mammography in population-based screening studies for early detection of breast malignancy. Mammography involves low level (diagnostic) irradiation of the breast tissue, involving under the best modern conditions a fraction of a rad of exposure. It, therefore, must be considered to carry some risk for breast cancer induction. The problems are whether the benefits of mammography outweigh the potential risks, and whether we presently have people sufficiently skilled to interpret the results. Clearly, if the routine use of this screening technique enables a considerable proportion of breast cancers to be detected at a successfully treatable stage, an appreciable level of risk might be justified. This argument would be enhanced if those at highest risk of breast cancer development were shown to gain the greatest benefit. As long as this technique remains relatively unexploited and highly controversial (Wolfe, 1977), it should be used only in women who have been informed of the possible risks and subsequently voluntarily accept them. Key questions that can only be answered by practical experience include: (1) are the lesions detected by routine mammography at a "curable" stage? (2) how frequently must mammography be carried out to ensure that most detected lesions are "curable," and (3) is the integrated risk of repeated irradiation acceptable?

A U.S. National Cancer Institute Panel has examined these questions (Perry, 1978). It drew attention to the difference between the use of mammography to diagnose preexisting lesions and its use in healthy women for screening purposes. The level of risk to the mammary tissue was estimated to be less than 1%/rad, that is to say, the national incidence of breast cancer in women through this exposure would be increased from 7 to 7.07%. The panel indicated that mammography combined with self-examination was presently the optimal approach and recommended that radiological screening be restricted to women over 50, unless the patient had a previous history of breast cancer or her mother or sister had developed the disease.

Diagnostic radiation has previously been considered as at too low a level to be a major factor in cancer induction, except in the example of pelvic irradiation of pregnant women, when the sensitive fetus is exposed. Questions may, however, be raised about the adverse effects of repeated diagnostic radiation, as, for example, sequential chest X rays in patients with tuberculosis or other lung diseases.

MacMahon (1962) reported a survey of 734,243 children for the effects of in utero radiation. A 1% sample was contacted. It was established that pelvic irradiation had been used in 770 of 7242 pregnancies (10.6%). In the total population, 584 childhood cancers were identified and the medical records of 569 were available for study. Eighty-five of these (15.3%) had histories of pelvic irradiation in utero, which after corrections were made for the effects of birth order, etc., suggested that perhaps there was a 40% excess of childhood cancer in the study population associated with in utero irradiation. This excess was mainly leukemia and central nervous system tumors. The relative risk in children between 5 and 7 years of age was 2.0. There was an inexplicable excess of leukemia in first-born children.

Similarly, in England Stewart and her colleagues have analyzed large populations of children to determine whether in utero exposure to diagnostic radiation influenced the incidence of childhood tumors of several types (Stewart and Kneale, 1970). She found that childhood tumors were more frequent in those who had been irradiated in utero than in those who had not been irradiated. Her work has, however, been criticized on the grounds that no allowance was made for maternal age, which is recognized to influence the incidence of childhood leukemia. The importance of radiation as a factor in the genesis of these tumors was, however, emphasized by the observations that higher tumor incidences (mainly of leukemia) were observed after irradiation in the first trimester, and that the greater the number of films taken, the greater the leukemia risk.

Stewart (1973) speculated on the increase in childhood leukemia following World War II. This, it was suggested, resulted from the innovative use of antibiotics to control pneumonia at this time. As pneumonia frequently precedes childhood leukemia, it is possible that children formerly reported as dying from pneumonia were, in fact, victims of leukemia (Kneale, 1971). Stewart (1973) also commented on a report (Schneiderman and Peters, 1972) that data from California and Connecticut cancer registries demonstrated that leukemia notifications in the 0 to 4-year old age range had recently fallen by half. This, she suggested, might be because of more prudent use of diagnostic radiation during pregnancy. She presented a comparison of stillbirths in single and twin pregnancies. The latter group was more frequently subjected to in utero irradiation and had a greater frequency of difficult parturitions involving some degree of anoxia to the baby. It is, therefore, possible that as the leukemic is more sensitive than the normal child to anoxia, these stillbirths might conceal cases of leukemia. As pelvic irradiation is usually carried out late in pregnancy, it would seem that either leukemias leading to these stillbirths have an extremely short latency or they are dependent on other factors.

The number of tumors known to be induced as a result of medically mandated radiation is relatively small and demands that large populations be studied in epidemiologic surveys of tumor morbidity. The reality of these effects cannot, however, be denied, as they fit closely with data from occupational and other exposures (Upton, 1977), and with a great mass of experimental animal studies. Childhood cancers are now one of the more frequent causes of death in the first decade, and the consequent mortality at the beginning of life represents an even more tragic loss than do cancers in the elderly. While it is necessary to agree with Mole's (1975) dictum that great care must be taken to ensure that random variation in mortality statistics are not mistakenly confused with radiation effects, the after effects of radiation exposure must continue to be vigorously explored.

2. Radioisotopes

Radioisotopes are especially hazardous to health, if localized at specific body sites. For example, the use of radium-containing solutions at the beginning of the century to treat rheumatic disease led to deposition of the radioisotope in bone and the consequent low level irradiation of bone and bone marrow. These patients, like the population of young women who, during World War I ingested quantities of mesothorium-based luminous paint, developed radiation sickness, leukemia, and osteosarcoma (Aub et al., 1952).

Thorotrast, colloidal thorium dioxide, has been used extensively as a radiological contrast medium. Two particular types of adverse reaction followed. When injected into a sinus or hollow organ to enable the radiologist to outline its surface, traces of thorotrast were sometimes left behind with the consequence that the surrounding tissue was cumulatively exposed to heavy doses of radiation. If, on the other hand, thorotrast was administered intravenously, it was drained by the reticuloendothelial cells of the liver and the surrounding tissue exposed to radiation. Dahlgren (1961) found more than 60 cancers in the world literature in which a long-standing local thorotrast deposit indicated a possible causal relationship. More recent epidemiological studies demonstrate thorotrast to be clearly associated with human carcinogenesis. Boyd et al. (1968) studied all cases to whom thorotrast had been administered between 1926 and 1955 in the University of Edinburgh's Department of Neurological Surgery. Cancer in this group of 168 patients was three times as common as in the general population. Moreover, there were four cases of primary liver cancer, which is very rare in Western Europeans. A similar survey in Japan using 147 thorotrast-treated war veterans reached similar conclusions (Mori et al., 1967).

The most convincing study on the carcinogenic effect of thorotrast (Da Silva Horta et al., 1972) used all 2468 patients who had received the drug between 1930 and 1955 in Portugal. At the time of the report 49.5% of this population had been traced, compared to 36.6% of 1867 control patients treated with a nonradioactive contrast medium. Thorotrast treatment was followed by a high risk of leukemia, primary liver cancer and two or three cases of bone cancer. Lung cancer was also increased, but as cigarette smoking histories were not available, the significance of these tumors is in doubt. Recent reports on this and other studies have further consolidated these conclusions (Farber, 1979; Cayolla da Motta et al., 1979; Mole, 1979).

Selbie (1938) showed that thorotrast gave subcutaneous sarcomas on injection into rats and mice. The potential significance of this observation to exposed humans was not, however, apparent at this time, and thorotrast continued to be used. Subsequently, the carcinogenicity of other natural and human-made radioisotopes has been investigated in animals (Clayson, 1962).

3. Chemicals Used in Cancer Therapy

There are three major classes. From the viewpoint of cancer induction, the most important class is the biological alkylating agents (Fig. 3), such as nitrogen or sulfur mustards, nitrosamides, and so on. Metabolic inhibitors have not been incriminated as carcinogens in humans or animals (Schmähl and Osswald, 1970; Schmähl, 1977), but the possibility cannot be excluded that specific examples of this class may be metabolically activated to a carcinogenic form. Hormones are used in cancer therapy and have been discussed (Secs. II.D and II.E).

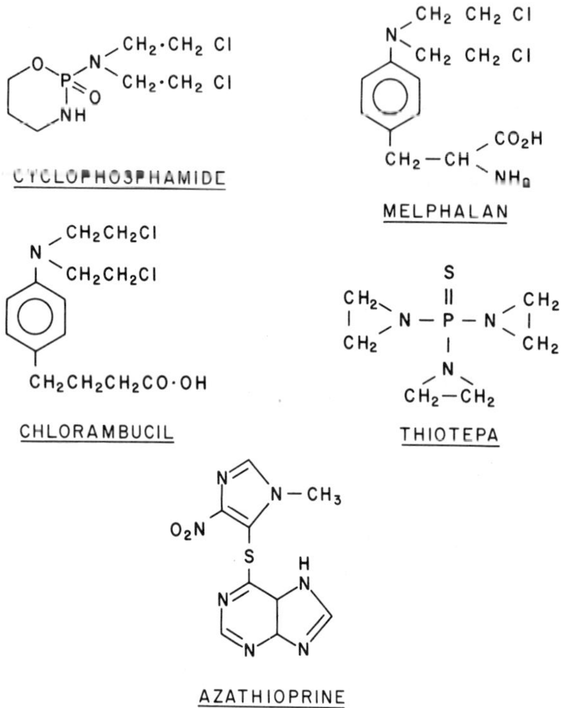

FIGURE 3 Chemical structures of cancer chemotherapeutic agents.

Biological alkylating agents are useful in cancer therapy and as immunosuppressants because of their toxic effects on lymphocytes. Thus, the present interest in immune disease has led to their use for conditions other than cancer. In general, the relatively short survival of many cancer patients has prevented full manifestation of the oncogenic potential of these agents. The experience with chlornaphazin (p. 537) in treatment of polycythemia serves as a warning of the possible consequences of the use of such drugs for conditions with a longer prognosis. These agents are established as carcinogenic in animals (Lawley, 1976), and their potential in humans is being revealed in epidemiologic surveys and numerous case reports.

Ovarian cancer is stated to be best treated with alkylating agents. Reimer et al. (1977) surveyed the results of therapy in 70 separate centers that had treated a total of 5455 cases. A historical control population not treated with alkylating agents contained 13,309 cases and served for comparison. Thirteen of the 5455 cases developed nonlymphoid leukemia, whereas only 0.62 were expected. When patients surviving for 2 or more years were considered, the relative risk rose 171.4-fold. Nine of the 13 leukemia patients were also exposed to radiation, but as in the historical control group radiation did not affect the incidence of nonlymphocytic leukemia, this was discounted as a major factor. The alkylating agents used in the treatment were phenylalanine mustard (five patients), chlorambucil (three), cyclophosphamide (two), thiotepa (one), and uracil mustard (one). A similar report from Sweden (Einhorn, 1978) considered 474 ovarian cancer patients treated with melphalan. Forty-eight survived for 3 or more years, and of these, four developed leukemia (two blast cell type, one myeloic, and one erythro). These tumors arose 36, 40, 58, and 77 months after the start of treatment with more than 800 mg melphalan. Radiotherapy was again a complicating factor.

There are many literature references to single patients developing a second tumor after cancer chemotherapy (Sieber and Adamson, 1975). Only a few are mentioned here. Cyclophosphamide has been reported to be associated with cancer induction in humans on 34 occasions leading to a total of 64 individual cases (Puri and Campbell, 1977). Of these tumors, 27 were leukemia, 10 lymphomas, 13 cancers of the urinary bladder, and 16 of other tissues. The tumors were approximately evenly distributed between patients who had received only cyclophosphamide and those receiving this agent and other therapy. Wall and Clausen (1975) reported on five patients given cyclophosphamide in high doses for long periods (Total dose, mean 200 g, range 114-295 g); all of these patients developed bladder cancer. The population from which these patients were drawn and their smoking and occupational histories were not given. This observation was predictable, however, since cyclophosphamide has a markedly cytotoxic effect on the urinary bladder epithelium, leading to stripping and regeneration of the normally quiescent transitional epithelium in humans and in many experimental animals (Philips et al., 1961). Among others, Roberts (1976) refers to the use of massive amounts of cyclophosphamide to treat renal disease, leading to three cases of acute myeloid leukemia. This is of special interest as radiotherapy was not a confusing factor. Fairchild et al. (1979) reported a ninefold increase in the development of bladder tumor in patients treated for a first neoplasm with cyclophosphamide. In no case was the first tumor in the genitourinary tract.

Some investigators are of the opinion that the cancer risk involved in the use of these agents is small (Symington et al., 1977). The fact that Reimer and his associates (1977) found that only 13 of 5455 women at risk developed nonlymphoid leukemia superficially tends to support that view. When, however, the high mortality of these women from the primary ovarian cancer and the extremely short latencies of 5 years or less are considered, the cancer risk in the survivors is seen to be exceptionally high. This will merit most serious consideration as cancer therapy is improved and more patients survive for longer periods.

Too much confidence should not be put into individual case reports, unless they are mutually supporting (e.g., Puri and Campbell, 1977). Special care must be taken to exclude other known causes of tumors, as illustrated in a report by Thorpe et al. (1976) who described the trial of chlorambucil for treatment of rheumatoid arthritis. Three cancers were found in 22 subjects; one was a bronchial carcinoma in a heavy smoker of 20 years' duration; one was a renal pelvic tumor in an analgesic abuser (p. 358), and the third was a basal cell carcinoma, the commonest tumor in Australia from whence the report emanated. Direct causation by chlorambucil seems unlikely in these cases.

4. Combination Therapy

This procedure is increasingly used in tumor management. With Hodgkin's disease in particular, the hazards to patients are much better understood than with other forms of cancer therapy. A population of 452 patients treated for Hodgkin's disease was compared with an equivalent section of the general population for cancer incidence (Arseneau et al., 1972; Canellos et al., 1975). The entire group showed three to four times the expected cancer incidence. Patients receiving either intensive chemotherapy or intensive radiotherapy had relative risks of developing cancer of 4.0 and 3.8, respectively, while the 62 patients who had received both intensive radiotherapy and chemotherapy developed six tumors, the relative risk being 14.5. Nevertheless, as the authors emphasize, without treatment, Hodgkin's disease has a most dismal prognosis.

Arseneau et al. (1977) explored the uncertainties in this type of analysis. The major difficulty lies in the fact that it is not possible to assemble an untreated group of Hodgkin's disease patients because of their poor survival. Therefore, one cannot exclude the objection that the increase in second tumors is a consequence of the disease rather than of treatment. Attention was drawn to the association of treatment with acute nonlymphocytic leukemia, which may be the sequel of cytotoxic drug therapy (Lancet, 1977a; Chabner, 1977). The number of such cases appears to have markedly increased since the introduction of modern modes of cytotoxic drug therapy.

It should not be imagined that cancer is the only adverse reaction to afflict patients in remission from Hodgkin's disease or after other forms of cancer therapy. Effects on general condition, pulmonary and cardiac functions, hematology, thyroid function, neurological performance, and epithelial tissue have been summarized (Slanina et al., 1977). Nevertheless, despite the fact that these other adverse effects may considerably diminish the quality of life for the individual patient, second malignancies attract much attention. The similarity of response to radiation and cytotoxic agents, whether encountered environmentally, occupationally, or therapeutically, helps to confirm the general validity of the overall hazards of these agents (Hodgin and Webster, 1976).

G. Renal Transplantation

Renal transplantation requires immunosuppression to prevent rejection of the grafted kidney. Immunosuppression is achieved by a variety of agents and procedures, including splenectomy, azathioprine, prednisone, cytotoxic drugs, radiation and antilymphocyte serum or globulin. The first reported tumors were reticulum cell sarcomas (Penn and Starzl, 1972). Other authors reported tumors of other tissues. For example, Starzl et al. (1970) described 10 tumors in 149 renal transplant recipients who survived for 4 or more postoperative months. These were six tumors of the skin and lip, three reticulum cell sarcomas, and one carcinoma of the cervix. There was no evidence that these existed before the operation. Marshall (1973) referred to the skin cancer incidence in renal transplant recipients in Australia.

The facts were established in a survey of all renal transplant patients reported to an internationally based Human Renal Transplant Registry. There were 6297 individual patients from 200 hospitals in 30 countries who survived at least 1 month after operation. Six cases were excluded because it was possible that tumors had been introduced with the graft. The risk ratio was 30-40-fold for lymphoma. This was almost entirely reticulum cell sarcoma, which had a 350-fold relative risk. Comparison of the incidence of other tumors and especially of skin tumors, with the expected incidence in the areas from which the cases were drawn, suggested that these other tumors were not greatly in excess (Hoover and Fraumeni, 1973). The induction of reticulum cell sarcomas at a high rate with a relatively short latency (5 months or more) raises a series of questions about the etiology of the disease. The specific site has not been reported to the same extent following cytotoxic agent administration and deserves further study.

Immunosuppression in animals leads to an enhancement in tumor yield, particularly if viruses are the inciting agent. Thus, Law (1970) showed that adult BALB/C mice, which are resistant to Moloney leukemia virus, were highly susceptible if immunosuppressed, and developed leukemia about 45 days after inoculation. Chemically induced tumors, on the other hand, do not appear as susceptible to the effects of immunosuppression (Jeejeebhoy, 1970; Woods, 1969; Wagner and Haughton, 1971), except in specific instances (Denlinger et al., 1973). The differences in site between cytotoxic drug-induced tumors and those seen in immunosuppressed renal graft recipients, combined with the short latency of these tumors and results in animal experiments, suggests these reticulum cell sarcomas in immunosuppressed patients may have a viral factor in their etiology.

H. Other Drugs

1. Arsenic

Neubauer (1947) in his survey of the relationship between exposure to inorganic arsenic and cancer, described a number of patients who had been treated with Fowler's solution (potassium arsenite) and subsequently developed cancer. Conditions treated included psoriasis, syphilis, asthma, anxiety, and epilepsy. Inorganic arsenic was also used as a general tonic. In only 16 of 143 patients was the total arsenic dose recorded and ranged from 0.19 g to about 121 g. In view of the paucity of this evidence, the present inability of scientists to induce cancer in animals with inorganic arsenicals, and the rather diffuse nature of the evidence relating arsenical exposure to cancer in environmental and occupational settings (Hernberg, 1977), this author has difficulty in regarding inorganic arsenic as a carcinogen in the normally accepted sense. The use of inorganic arsenicals in medicine has largely been discarded, either because new and better drugs are available, or because of the possible risk of cancer as an adverse reaction.

2. Laxatives

Boyd and Doll (1954), in a retrospective analysis of 614 gastrointestinal cancer patients and 1313 patients with diseases other than gastrointestinal, found no correlation between cancer and laxative consumption. However, there was an appreciable excess of patients using liquid paraffin among those with gastrointestinal cancer. Attempts to confirm this observation have failed. Thus, it may be a chance observation or be due to the fact that the liquid paraffin used by the patients in Boyd and Doll's study contained carcinogenic impurities.

3. Leukemia-Associated Drugs

A number of drugs, including phenylbutazone, chloramphenicol, certain sulfonamides, aminopyrine, and amphetamine sulfate are associated in some patients with bone marrow depression (Fraumeni, 1967). Leukemia induction is a further suspected complication. The relevant literature has been surveyed by McCarthy and Chalmers (1964), who found seven cases of aplastic anemia associated with phenylbutazone use, although other blood dycrasias were more common. The Australian position was summarized by Bean (1960) and by Woodliff and Dougan (1964). The number of cases involved was small. Fraumeni (1967) was unable to demonstrate an association between drug use and blood dycrasias or leukemia, but further work is needed, especially in view of the poor response obtained to the questionnaires used.

III. DRUGS DEMONSTRATED TO BE CARCINOGENIC IN LABORATORY ANIMALS

The drugs considered in the first part of this chapter have been directly demonstrated to lead to cancer in humans. Some, such as the biological alkylating agents, require only a brief latent period to induce their effects; others, like the analgesics, take much longer. Clearly, such results have been obtained only because these agents were used in humans and have had time to induce their effects. Control of an effective therapeutic agent subsequent to an epidemiologic survey may be difficult, as clinicians often dispute the validity of epidemiologic evidence which could deprive them of useful drugs.

Drugs may, however, be tested for carcinogenicity before introduction into general clinical practice using standardized protocols in animals (Sontag et al., 1976). Such safety evaluations were not part of normal procedures between 1935 and 1960 at the time of the great expansion in the number of clinically valuable drugs, but are now used more frequently. It cannot be assumed that all drugs proved carcinogenic in animals will necessarily have the same effect in humans, but prudence indicates that such a position be taken unless there are strong reasons to the contrary. In the drug area the results of animal tests are best assessed in terms of the potential clinical usefulness of the agent for a specific condition and the carcinogenic potency demonstrated in the animal tests. For example, does the agent show promise of controlling an otherwise incurable disease, such as cancer? Carcinogenic drugs should never knowingly be considered in the management of conditions that do not seriously affect the quality of life of the patient and that have a good prognosis.

Unfortunately, carcinogenicity tests in animals take at least 3 to 4 years to complete, during which time much effort may be expended on the experimental and clinical development of a new drug. Therefore, the demonstration that a new drug is carcinogenic results in a considerable financial loss to the developer and ultimately, to the community. The introduction of a series of short-term tests as predictors of carcinogenicity promises, if they can be standardized and validated, the opportunity to discard potentially carcinogenic drugs at an early stage of their development. These short-term prescreening tests include the induction of microbial and mammalian cell mutagenesis, cell transformation in vitro, DNA repair, and techniques such as sister chromatid exchange. The major advance by Ames and his group (Ames et al., 1973a, b) was to incubate bacteria with a microsomal activating system capable of metabolizing procarcinogens to their ultimate form. Ames claims an 80-90% correlation between carcinogenicity in animal studies and mutagenicity in his microbial systems (McCann and Ames, 1977).

The following pages discuss some of the evidence from laboratory studies demonstrating the carcinogenicity of clinically useful drugs. Clearly, this cannot be complete, because, first, many of the test results have not been published, but are hidden in the records of regulatory agencies and drug manufacturers, and second, positive results in animal tests may prevent potentially useful drugs from clinical investigation and use.

A. Isoniazid and Other Hydrazine-Based Drugs

Isoniazid, with streptomycin and para-aminosalicyclic acid, has proved highly effective in the control of tuberculosis. Together with improved sanitation, these drugs have reduced tuberculosis mortality, especially in children and young adults, from a high to a low level in less than one generation.

The discovery, first by Juhasz and his associates (1957), that isoniazid markedly increases the incidence of lung tumors in susceptible mice, has been confirmed by many other investigators (e.g., Schwan, 1961, 1962; Biancifiori and Ribacchi, 1962; Toth and Shubik, 1966). Biancifiori and Ribacchi (1962) demonstrated that hydrazine administered as the sulfate also induced these tumors leading to the study of a range of hydrazine derivatives for carcinogenicity (Toth, 1975). Toth and Shubik (1966) observed that, in mice, naturally occurring lymphoma and mammary tumor induction were inhibited by isoniazid, although pulmonary tumors were induced by this drug.

The implication that isoniazid is a carcinogen in mice, although not in any other tested species, raises serious questions about its potential carcinogenicity in humans. Treated tuberculosis patients are not a suitable study population because the disease itself may possibly predispose to cancer, and other therapeutic or diagnostic measures might themselves be cancer inducing, as, for example, repeated diagnostic radiation to assess the progress of the disease. Ferebee (1970), therefore, assembled a population that, although in good health, had been administered isoniazid as a prophylactic to prevent transmission of the disease from tuberculosis-infected contacts. The most recent reports on such continuing studies (Glassroth et al., 1977; Goldman et al., 1977) indicate that isoniazid is not carcinogenic in humans. For example, no excess of tumors due to isoniazid has been observed over a period of 15 years in populations of 12,400 given isoniazid, compared to 12,600 given placebo. It is to be hoped that this study will be actively pursued, because in humans some carcinogens have latency periods in excess of 30 years.

Other hydrazine-based drugs (Fig. 4) have been shown to be carcinogenic (Toth, 1975). The most carcinogenic of these is procarbazine (Natulan) or N-4-isopropylcarbamoylbenzyl-N'-methylhydrazine, which induced tumors of lung, lymphoreticular tissue, and kidneys in mice, and breast, lung, and blood vessel tumors in rats (Kelly et al., 1964, 1968). Hydrazine itself has been useful as an antineoplastic agent. Toth and his co-workers have shown that 1-acetyl-2-isonicotinic acid hydrazide, a metabolite of isoniazid (Toth and Shimizu, 1973), and phenylethylhydrazine or phenelzine, an antidepressant, are carcinogenic (Toth, 1976). In light of Toth's (1975) observation that 19 of 19 hydrazine derivatives that had been tested in animals were tumorigenic, it is probable that other hydrazine-containing drugs such, for example, as clinically used monoamineoxidase inhibitors, will, when tested, also be carcinogenic. Unfortunately, short-term prescreening tests for carcinogenicity have not yet been successful with these chemicals (Eppley Institute, unpublished results).

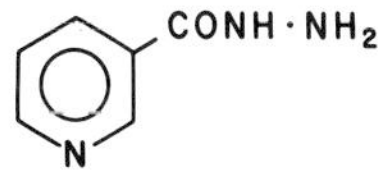

ISONIAZID

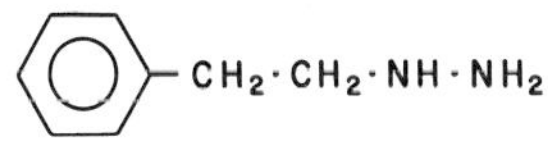

PHENYLETHYLHYDRAZINE

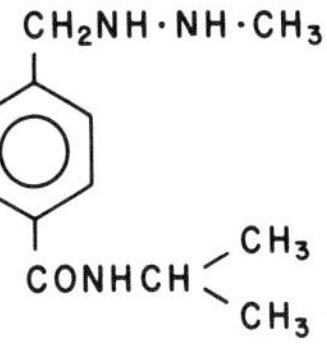

PROCARBAZINE
(NATULAN)

$NH_2 \cdot NH_2$

HYDRAZINE

FIGURE 4 Chemical structures of hydrazines.

B. Schistosomacides

Bilharzia is a consequence of infestation by schistosomes, digenetic parasites that, to complete their life cycle, require two hosts, a mammal, such as a human, and a specific snail. Bilharzia is thus common in situations that favor the survival of the particular species of snail; that is to say, tropical or subtropical areas where irrigation projects to support agriculture are widespread. It is estimated that there are about 200,000,000 cases of this type of debilitating disease among the world's population. In the Nile Valley and Delta region of Egypt, there are perhaps 26,000,000 cases.

Attempts to contain bilharzia by eradicating the snail vector have not proved successful. The antimonial drugs formerly used to treat this disease are toxic and only marginally effective. Neither tartar emetic, which is highly toxic, nor stibophen, which is an organic antimonial, have been adequately investigated for carcinogenicity. This may be a cause for concern since there is evidence linking urinary tract bilharzia induced by *Schistosomum haematobium* with the prevalence of bladder tumors, especially in Egypt (Clayson, 1975a). The hepatic form of bilharzia, induced by *S. mansoni* and *S. japonica*, is not as clearly related to cancer.

Recently introduced treatments for *S. mansoni*- and *S. haematobium*-related disease include the organophosphate metrifonate, niridazole, hycanthone, and oxamiquine (Fig. 5). Niridazole is both a potent bacterial mutagen and an animal carcinogen, while hycanthone is a potent mutagen, but has given relatively equivocal evidence of animal carcinogenicity. The suspicion engendered against hycanthone is particularly unfortunate because it is effective in only a single dose of 1.5-2.0 mg/kg in more than 75% of *S. mansoni* and *S. haematobium* cases, and in those whom it fails to cure, it reduces the worm count by more than 75% (WHO Reports, 1971).

Feeding niridazole in the diet to mice led to induction of papillomas and carcinomas of the forestomach and lungs, to ovarian and mammary tumors, and in a few mice, to bladder tumors (Urman et al., 1975). In hamsters forestomach and bladder papillomas were induced (Bulay et al., 1977), while in rats kidney carcinomas were the principal neoplastic response (Bulay, 1979b). In mouse and hamster experiments niridazole was given to animals carrying a mild *S. mansoni* infection to determine whether it enhanced tumor induction. No difference could be detected in the response of infected and uninfected animals. Niridazole appears to be of like potency to the standard experimental carcinogen, N-2-fluorenylacetamide.

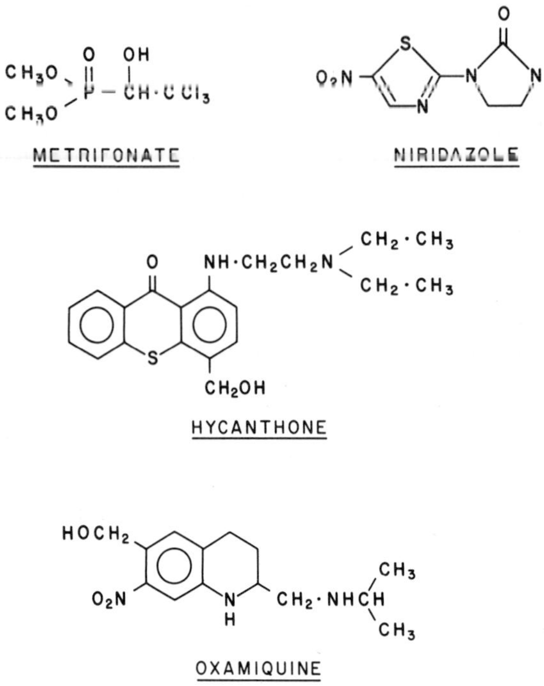

FIGURE 5 Chemical structures of antischistosomal drugs.

Hycanthone was stated by Haese and his associates (1973) to be carcinogenic in S. mansoni-infected mice on the grounds that a single intraperitoneal dose of 3 or 60 mg/kg body weight led to a 6% incidence of hepatomas. Twenty-five percent of the treated animals had hyperplastic nodules, and only these latter lesions were found in untreated control mice. In a second experiment the same dose of hycanthone given on three occasions led to incidences of 20% hyperplastic nodules and 12% hepatomas in mice surviving for 60 weeks or more (Haese and Bueding, 1976). Yarinsky et al. (1974) failed to confirm the first result in a repeat experiment. Our own results failed to show any carcinogenic activity attributable to hycanthone in hamsters (Bulay, 1979b). In mice there was an increase in hepatoma incidence from control levels of 1-4% to, on the average, 9-10%. Statistical analysis, using the age-based prevalence of these tumors, showed that in contradistinction to Haese's observations, S. mansoni infection had a relatively small effect on tumor yield. In fact, infection only slightly increased the incidence of hepatomas in control mice. Male mice did not develop a statistically significant response to hycanthone, while noninfected females developed an increased incidence of hepatomas after intraperitoneal or intramuscular injection of hycanthone significant only at the 95 and 92% levels of confidence. The major experimental difference in approach between these experiments and those of Haese and his colleagues was that near maximum tolerated and repeated doses of hycanthone were given by Bulay and his associates (1978b). In view of these observations, hycanthone in mice is at most a weak carcinogen. It may lead to the slightly increased tumor incidence by an indirect mechanism.

Despite these relatively unconvincing carcinogenicity studies, hycanthone is a potent mutagen in several systems (Bueding and Batzinger, 1977). This could, at least in part, be due to its ability to intercalate between the bases in the DNA helix. The possibility that hycanthone is carcinogenic, combined with its potency as a microbial mutagen, makes its use in population-based bilharzia eradication campaigns a difficult clinical decision.

C. Nitro- and Amino-Heterocyclic Compounds

Doubly unsaturated, five-membered heterocyclic ring systems, such as furans, thiophenes, pyrazoles, or thiazoles, have aromatic characteristics (Fig. 6). The aromatic sextet of electrons is contributed by two electrons from each double bond and a "lone pair" of electrons from the heteroatom. We might, therefore, expect the nitro and amino derivatives of these substances to share a number of properties, including carcinogenicity, with carbocyclic aromatic amines and nitro compounds. The relevant literature was summarized by Clayson and Garner (1976).

There are many five-membered, doubly unsaturated heterocyclic compounds with amino and nitro substituents among potentially useful pharmaceutic products in the areas of both clinical and veterinary medicine (Merck Index, 1976). Attention was drawn to the potential carcinogenicity of these compounds by the work of Price and Bryan and their colleagues (Price et al., 1966; Stein et al., 1966). Certain of these chemicals are very potent carcinogens; N-[4-(5-nitro-2-furyl)-2-thiazolyl]formamide, for example, is now a standard experimental bladder carcinogen (Ertürk et al., 1970a, b). A closely related chemical, N-[4-(5-nitro-2-furyl)-2-thiazolyl]acetamide, has been used against human infectious disease in parts of Europe. In female rats it led to mammary gland adenocarcinomas, renal pelvic tumors, lung adenocarcinomas, and salivary gland adenocarcinomas. In dogs and hamsters both the formamide and acetamide induced tumors of bladder, while in mice treated with the acetamide, leukemia and stomach tumors were observed (Ertürk et al., 1970a; Croft and Bryan, 1973; Cohen et al., 1970; Ertürk et al., 1970b). These results show a carcinogenic potency similar to that of niridazole, [1-(5-nitro-2-thiazolyl)-1-imidazolidinone], which was discussed in the previous section. Clearly, this aspect of carcinogenicity in the pharmaceutical area needs urgent attention; a point of view that is reinforced by the many positive microbial mutagenesis assays on these substances.

Nevertheless, there are some drugs of this chemical type which have given less convincing evidence of carcinogenicity, but are still disturbing because of their widespread clinical use. Metronidazole (Flagyl), for example, on chronic administration to Swiss mice markedly increased the incidence of lymphoma and lung tumors (Rustia and Shubik, 1972). Such results are to some extent warnings that the drug may be a human carcinogen, although Beard et al. (1979), as a result of a survey of tumor frequency in 771 women developing vaginitis from 1960-1969 and treated with metronidazole at some subsequent time, found no evidence of human carcinogenicity. The relatively short latency period, combined with possibly short periods of exposure to the drug, indicates that this evidence is not adequate

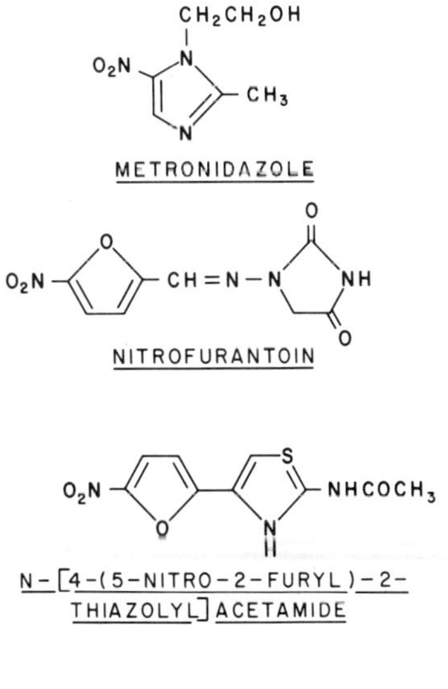

FIGURE 6 Chemical structures of nitroheterocyclic drugs.

to demonstrate metronidazole is not a human carcinogen. Other rodent studies (e.g., Rustia and Shubik, 1978) have shown consistently increased incidences of relatively common tumors in rats and mice. It is a matter of debate whether the potential risk is sufficient to justify discontinuation of the use of a drug which is exceptionally valuable in the treatment of infective vaginitis, a painful disease.

Attention must also be drawn to those drugs used as urinary tract antibacterial agents, such as nitrofurantoin [N-(5-nitro-2-furfurylidene)-1-aminohydantoin], which in a single test in rats gave relatively benign mammary tumors. The need for further critical work to define the carcinogenicity of these chemicals should be apparent.

D. Antibiotics

Mold-produced antimicrobial agents, or antibiotics (Fig. 7), have proven effective in combating morbidity and mortality from bacterial infection. Perhaps because of their effectiveness against infectious disease, there appears to have been a marked reluctance to examine their carcinogenic potency.

It is difficult to assess earlier investigations in which relatively large quantities of a number of natural products with strained lactone or lactam rings were injected into the subcutaneous tissues of rats, because of the small number of animals employed and the difficulty in interpreting the significance of rodent sarcomas following local injection of large amounts of chemical (Dickens and Jones, 1961). In these studies penicillin induced two sarcomas in eight rats. In view of the large-scale use of penicillins, terramycins, and erythromycins, test results in this area are urgently required.

Highly toxic antibiotics have found use in the treatment of more serious diseases, as in attempts at cancer chemotherapy. Actinomycin D following multiple intraperitoneal injections

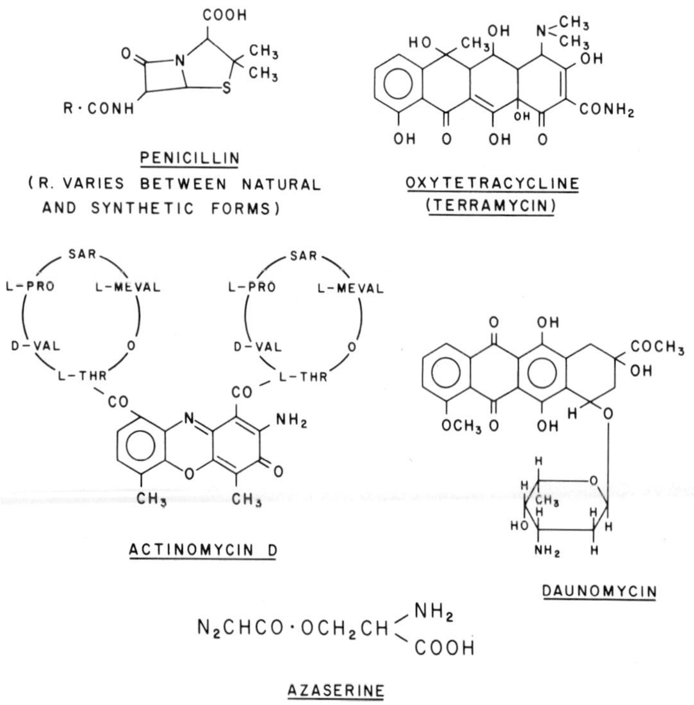

FIGURE 7 Chemical structures of antibiotics.

into Fischer 344 rats in a total dose of 0.050-0.005 mg/kg reduced survival in general to less than 50 weeks and led to induction of invasive tumors in the peritoneal lining and mesentery (Svoboda et al., 1970). Daunomycin has been examined on two occasions. Bertazzoli and his colleagues (1971) showed that a single intravenous instillation of 12.5 mg/kg into female Sprague-Dawley rats led to 11 of 25 developing mammary adenocarcinomas and three of 25 fibroadenomas. Adriamycin, on the other hand, gave only one mammary adenocarcinoma and six fibroadenomas, whereas untreated rats in this study had no breast tumors. Sternberg and his associates (1972) gave daunomycin intravenously to female Sprague-Dawley rats at the toxic level of 20 mg/kg and at 10 or 5 mg/kg. Sixteen of 27 surviving rats developed kidney tumors and seven tumors of the genital tract.

Ikegami et al. (1967) reported that mitomycin C, a direct alkylating agent, gave sarcomas on injection in mice. Intraperitoneal injection of this drug into rats led to peritoneal tumors (Weisburger et al., 1975), while intravenous injection led to a miscellany of malignancies in 34% of the rats (Schmähl and Osswald, 1970).

Griseofulvin is widely used in the treatment of tinea pedis and other ringworm infections. Individual daily doses may be as high as 0.5-1.0 g by ingestion in adults. Hepatomas were induced when griseofulvin was fed in the diet to mice (Hurst and Paget, 1963; De Matteis et al., 1966; Rustia and Shubik, 1978). In rats feeding griseofulvin for 2-2.5 years led to a dose-related increase in the incidence of thyroid tumors (Rustia and Shubik, 1978). These observations stress the need for caution to prevent misuse of this valuable drug.

Finally, mention must be made of azaserine, another cancer chemotherapeutic agent. This led to pancreatic adenocarcinomas in nine of 23 rats injected intraperitoneally with 5 mg/kg drug twice weekly for 6 months. Five of 18 rats given once weekly injections developed this tumor (Longnecker and Curphey, 1975).

E. Other Drugs (Fig. 8)

1. Phenobarbital

Phenobarbital, a sedative and hypnotic that is used to control epilepsy, and more commonly, as a sleep inducer, leads to liver tumors in rats and mice. Thus, feeding 0.05% phenobarbital in the diet to CF1 mice led, after 109 weeks, to liver tumors in 24 of 30 males and 21 of 28 females, compared to incidences in untreated mice of 11 of 45 and 10 of 44, respectively (Thorpe and Walker, 1973). Similar results have been obtained in C3H mice (Peraino et al., 1973) and further CF1 mice (Ponomarkov et al., 1976), while in male Wistar rats only benign tumors were observed (Rossi et al., 1976).

These animal studies suggest that phenobarbital is carcinogenic (IARC, 1977a), but there is no evidence for this effect of the agent in humans, although possibly phenobarbital during pregnancy increases the level of birth defects (IARC, 1977a). Clemmesen and his colleagues (1974) reported on the cancer incidence in 9136 epileptic patients admitted to the neuropsychiatric hospital of Filadelfia in Denmark between 1933 and 1962. These patients were treated with phenobarbital and phenytoin or primidone. Cancer incidence at all sites, except the liver, was the same as or lower than in the general population. In cases treated for more than 10 years, there were three cases of liver cancer in males (1.1 expected) and 1 case (0.7 expected) in females. In males treated for less than 10 years there was one case (0.4 expected). The significance of these tumors has been hotly debated (Schneiderman, 1974), but seems most unlikely to be related to phenobarbital in view of Clemmesen's (1975) observation that three of the four male cases of liver cancer arose in patients who had previously received the radio-opaque medium thorotrast (p. 549).

It thus appears that phenobarbital is hepatocarcinogenic in rodents, but in the one study reported it is nontumorigenic in humans. The concept that liver cancer is a multistage disease and that phenobarbital acts by a modifying or promotional mechanism, rather than as an initiating carcinogen, may offer some explanation of the discrepancy. Peraino and his associates (1971, 1973, 1975) demonstrated that while in rats phenobarbital was a weak tumor inducer, when preceded by a relatively nontumorigenic dose of N-2-fluorenylacetamide, it

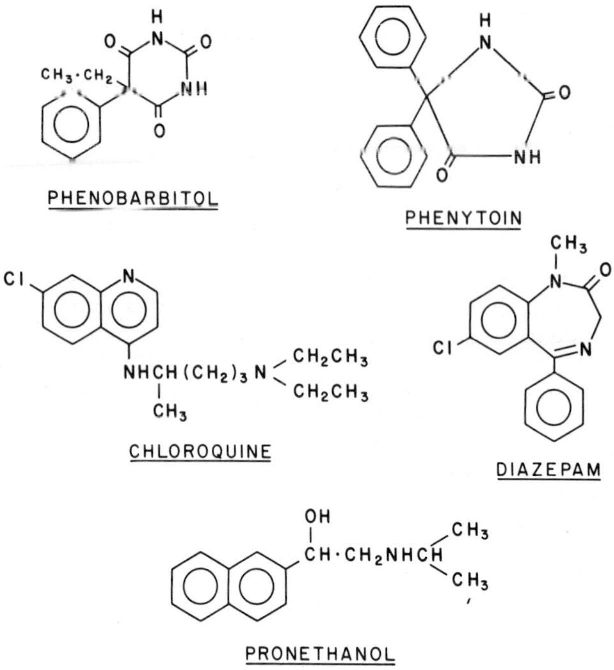

FIGURE 8 Chemical structures of other drugs.

became markedly more effective. The pesticide DDT resembled phenobarbital in its effect in this system, but two other drugs, amobarbital and diphenylhydantoin, did not. These observations suggest that in rats, at least, phenobarbital is deficient in the power to induce liver tumors, but is able to enhance their development once they are initiated. They clearly demonstrate that our present state of knowledge of how to interpret the significance of animal tumors to the human situation is rudimentary. This is especially true with regard to the rodent liver tumor.

2. Phenytoin or Phenytoin Sodium

These are used often in conjunction with phenobarbital in the management of epilepsy. Maintenance doses range from 300 mg to 600 mg/day. Oral administration or intraperitoneal injection of phenytoin in mice led to a relatively low incidence of lymphomas, whereas none was seen in controls (Krüger et al., 1972; Juhasz et al., 1968). Phenytoin, like phenobarbital, is associated with case reports of birth deformities (IARC, 1977b). The negative report of Clemmesen et al. (1974), which concerned patients treated with phenytoin, as well as phenobarbital, is relevant, but in the case of phenytoin there are a number of other case reports and a small series of patients indicating the drug may induce lymphoma or leukemia (Anthony, 1970; Charlton and Lunsford, 1971; Li et al., 1975). Further investigations of phenytoin are needed.

3. Antimalarial Drugs

These play a major role in current efforts to combat the debilitating effects of endemic malaria. This disease is prevalent in many tropical and subtropical areas. The World Health Organization is making strenuous efforts to control it, both by pesticide spraying on the breeding grounds of the mosquito vector and by drug treatment of the affected populations. It is, therefore, surprising how little published information there is on the carcinogenic potency of these drugs. The suggestion that malarial infection or one of the antimalarial drugs is a contributing factor to the etiology of Burkitt's lymphoma emphasizes our lack of knowledge in this area.

Chloroquine was originally developed as an antimalarial agent. The evidence for its carcinogenicity was reviewed by IARC (1977c), who noted only one negative study (Fitzhugh et al., 1948; Nelson and Fitzhugh, 1948). Rustia and Shubik (1978) have also obtained negative results with this drug and with primaquine.

4. Diazepam

This drug is mainly used at a dose of 5-20 mg/day for treatment of anxiety. Its major metabolite, oxazepam, led to liver cell adenomas in mice, but none were seen in controls (Fox and Lakcen, 1974).

5. Pronetalol Hydrochloride

This is a potent β-adrenergic blocking agent, but was withdrawn from use when it was shown to induce thymic tumors in mice (Howe, 1965). Other members of this class may come under suspicion of animal carcinogenicity.

The possible carcinogenicity of a number of other pharmaceutic systems in animals is discussed in Vol. 13 and other volumes of the IARC monographs on the Evaluation of Carcinogenic Risk of Chemicals to Man (IARC, 1977a, b, c). This chapter does not pretend to have considered all pharmaceutic agents for which tests for potential carcinogenicity have been published. An attempt is made to describe agents of major concern as human cancer risks and those that illustrate the difficulties of interpreting and using available data.

IV. CONCLUSIONS

There can be no reasonable doubt that drugs and therapeutic procedures, such as radiation, contribute to the human cancer burden. Two major questions remain to be answered. What is the overall extent of iatrogenic cancer in the population, and taking into account political sensitivity to agents which induce malignancies, can the excess risk be justified in terms of the reduction in morbidity and mortality from cancer itself or from other diseases? Both these questions are at this time difficult to answer.

If one or more epidemiologic surveys have quantitatively demonstrated a specific increase in cancer risk associated with a certain therapeutic regimen, it should be possible to calculate the number of tumors to be expected in the total population, provided the number of patients under treatment can be determined. Unfortunately, this is seldom the case. Alternative approaches are suggested by the observation that endometrial cancer among white U.S. women may be increasing by 10% each year and that this increase is mainly associated with the use of postmenopausal estrogen (p. 541). A 10% per year increase is equivalent to a doubling of incidence in about 9 years. If present therapy for the effects of postmenopausal symptoms continues unabated, an extra mortality of about 5000 endometrial cancer cases per year might be expected every 9 years. Epidemiologic estimates suggesting an increase in a more common form of cancer, for example of the mammary gland, if associated with a commonly used drug, may indicate a really considerable increase in cancer cases. However, even this relatively crude approach is difficult in view of our relative lack of knowledge of the drugs prescribed to individual patients. This generally unsatisfactory state of affairs is likely to remain until properly financed record linkage surveillance of large populations can be established. The recording of drug prescription history, occupation, diet, and other personal habits, although extremely costly and an intrusion into personal privacy, would go far to resolve questions of how much cancer is associated with drug use, occupation, and other suspected factors. At this stage it is only possible to conclude in very general terms that drug treatment is probably as, or more, important than occupation in the genesis of human cancer, but certainly far less important than cigarette smoking.

The justification for the continued use of a drug indicted as a human carcinogen is difficult to assess in quantitative terms. One approach would be to assess mortality, or life-spoiling morbidity, from the disease being treated using the best alternate treatment available, and to compare this with the mortality and morbidity using the carcinogenic drug. A treatment that does not improve prognosis is clearly unjustified. If, at this time, a carcinogenic drug substantially improves survival and/or the quality of life of the patient, its use is commendable. However, if in the future a further treatment is developed that is not carcinogenic, but is at least as good as that involving a risk of inducing cancer, the carcinogenic regimen should be immediately discarded. We know enough at this time to avoid using agents, such as thorotrast (p. 549), when equally effective and safer treatments exist. This approach, however, will require an enlightened approach and considerable self-discipline on the part of therapy-prescribing physicians.

REFERENCES

Ames, B. N., Durston, W. E., Yamasaki, F., and Lee, F. D. (1973a). Carcinogens are mutagens—a simple test system combining liver homogenates for activation and bacteria for detection. Proc. Natl. Acad. Sci. USA 70:2281-2285.

Ames, B. N., Lee, F. D., and Durston, W. E. (1973b). An improved bacterial test system for the detection and classification of mutagens and carcinogens. Proc. Natl. Acad. Sci. USA 70:782-786.

Anthony, H. M., and Thomas, G. M. (1970). Tumors of the urinary bladder: an analysis of the occupations of 1,030 patients in Leeds, England. J. Natl. Cancer Inst. 45:879-895.

Anthony, J. J. (1970). Malignant lymphoma associated with hydantoin drugs. Arch. Neurol. 22:450-454.

Armstrong, B., Stevens, N., and Doll, R. (1974). Retrospective study of the association between use of rauwolfia derivatives and breast cancer in English women. Lancet 2: 672-675.

Arseneau, J. C., Canellos, G. P., Johnson, R., and DeVita, V. T. (1977). Risk of new cancers in patients with Hodgkin's disease. Cancer 40:1912-1916.

Arseneau, J. C., Sponzo, R. W., Levin, D. L., Schnipper, L. E., Bonner, H., Young, R. C., Canellos, G. P., Johnson, R. E., and DeVita, V. T. (1972). Non-lymphomatous malignant tumors complicating Hodgkin's disease: possible association with intensive therapy. N. Engl. J. Med. 287:1119-1122.

Aub, J. C., Evans, R. D., Hemplemann, L. H., and Martland, H. S. (1952). The late effects of internally-deposited radioactive materials in man. Medicine 31:221-329.

Barnes, J. M. (1972). Tests on the pill for carcinogenicity. Br. Med. J. 4:359.

Barnes, J. M., Austwick, P. K., Carter, R. L., Flynn, F. V., Peristianis, G. C., and Aldridge, W. N. (1977). Balkan (endemic) nephropathy and a toxin-producing strain of _Penicillin verrucosum var cyclopium_: an experimental model in rats. Lancet 1: 671-675.

Baum, J. K., Holtz, F., Bookstein, J. J., and Klein, E. W. (1973). Possible association between benign hepatomas and oral contraceptives. Lancet 2:926-929.

Bean, R. H. (1960). Phenylbutazone and leukaemia: a possible association. Br. Med. J. ii:1552-1555.

Beard, C. M., Nollar, K. L., O'Fallon, W., Kurland, L. T., and Dockerty, M. B. (1979). Lack of evidence for cancer due to use of metronidazole. N. Engl. J. Med. 301:519-522.

Bengtsson, U., Angervall, L., Ekman, H., and Lehmann, L. (1968). Transitional cell tumours of the renal pelvis in analgesic abusers. Scand. J. Urol. Nephrol. 2:145-150.

Bernstein, M. S., Hunter, R. L., and Yachnin, S. (1971). Hepatoma and peliosis hepatitis developing in a patient with Fanconi's anemia. N. Engl. J. Med. 284:1135-1136.

Bertazzoli, C., Chieli, T., and Solcia, E. (1971). Different incidence of breast carcinoma or fibroadenomas in daunomycin or adriamycin-treated rats. Experientia 27:1209-1210.

Bibbo, M., Gill, W. B., Azizi, F., Blough, R., Fang, V. S., Rosenfield, R. I., Schumacher, R. I., Sleeper, K., Sonek, M. G., and Weid, G. L. (1977). Follow-up study of male and female offspring of DES-exposed mothers. J. Obstet. Gynecol. 49:1-8.

Biancifiori, C., and Ribacchi, R. (1962). Pulmonary tumours in mice induced by oral isoniazid and its metabolites. Nature 194:488-489.

Bittner, J. J. (1939). "Influences" of breast cancer development in mice. Public Health Rep. 54:1590-1597.

Bolce, J. D., and Monson, R. R. (1977). Breast cancer in women after repeated fluoroscopic examinations of the chest. J. Natl. Cancer Inst. 59:823-835.

Bonser, G. M., and Orr, J. W. (1939). The morphology of 160 tumours induced by carcinogenic hydrocarbons in the subcutaneous tissues of mice. J. Path. Bact. 49:171-183.

Boston Collaborative Drug Surveillance Program, Boston University Med. Ctr. (1974). Reserpine and breast cancer. Lancet 2:669-671.

Boyd, J. T., and Doll, R. (1954). Gastro-intestinal cancer and the use of liquid paraffin. Br. J. Cancer 8:231-237.

Boyd, J. T., Langlands, A. O., and MacCabe, J. J. (1968). Long-term hazards of thorotrast. Br. Med. J. 2:517-521.

Boyland, E., and Manson, D. (1963). Ann. Rep. Porit, Emp. Cancer Camp. 41:691.

Br. Med. J. (1972). Tests on the pill for carcinogenicity. Br. Med. J. 4:190

Brown, W. M., and Doll, R. (1958). Expectation of life and mortality from cancer among British radiologists. Br. Med. J. 2:181-187.

Brown, W. M., and Doll, R. (1965). Mortality from cancer and other causes after radiotherapy for ankylosing spondylitis. Br. Med. J. 2:1327-1332.

Bueding, E., and Batzinger, R. P. (1977). Hycanthone and other antischistosomal drugs: lack of obligatory association between chemotherapeutic effects and mutagenic activity. In Origins of Human Cancer, H. H. Hiatt, J. D. Watson, and J. A. Winsten (Eds.). Cold Spring Harbor Conference on Cell Proliferation, Vol. 4, Cold Spring Harbor, New York, pp. 445-463.

Bulay, O., Patil, K., Wilson, R., and Shubik, P. (1979a). Kidney tumors induced in rats by the antischistosomal drug niridazole. Cancer Res. 39:4996-5002.

Bulay, O., Urman, H., Patil, K., Clayson, D. B., and Shubik, P. (1979b). Carcinogenic potential of hycanthone in mice and hamsters. Int. J. Cancer, 23:97-104.

Bulay, O., Urman, H., Clayson, D. B., and Shubik, P. (1977). Carcinogenic effects of niridazole on rodents infected with Schistosoma mansoni. J. Natl. Cancer Inst. 59:1625-1629.

Bulow, H., Wullstein, H. K., Bottiger, G., and Schroder, F. H. (1973). Carcinoma of the breast under estrogen treatment for prostatic carcinoma. Urologe [A] 12:249-253.

Calder, I. C., Goss, D. E., Williams, P. J., Funder, C. C., Green, C. R., Ham, K. N., and Tange, J. D. (1976). Neoplasia in the rat induced by N-hydroxyphenacetin, a metabolite of phenacetin. Pathology 8:1-6.

Cannelos, G. P., De Vita, V. T., Arseneau, J. C., Whang-Peng, J., and Johnson, R. E. (1975). Second malignancies complicating Hodgkin's disease in remission. Lancet 1:947-949.

Cayolla da Motta, L., Da Silva Horta, J., and Tavereses, M. H. (1979). Prospective epidemiological study of Thorotrast—exposed patients in Portugal. Environ. Res. 18:152-179.

Chabner, B. A. (1977). Second neoplasia—a complication of cancer chemotherapy (editorial). N. Engl. J. Med. 297:213-215.

Charlton, M. H., and Lunsford, D. (1971). Le sostanze di idantoina come possibili cause del linfoma maligns. Minerva Med. 62:2185-2190.

Chernozemsky, I. N., Stoyanov, I. S., Petkova-Bocharova, T. K., Nicolov, I. G., Dragonov, I. V., Stoichev, I. I., Tanchev, Y., Naidenov, D., and Kalcheva, N. D. (1977). Geographic correlation between the occurrence of endemic nephropathy and urinary tract tumors in Vratza district, Poland. Int. J. Cancer 19:1-11.

Choi, N. W., Nelson, N. A., and Abu-Zeid, H. A. (1976). Cervical cancer and contraceptive pill use. Am. J. Epidemiol. 104:317-318.

Chievitz, E., and Thiede, T. (1962). Complications and causes of death in polycythaemia vera. Acta Med. Scand. 172:513-523.

Christopherson, W. M., and Mays, E. T. (1977). Guest editorial—liver tumors and contraceptive steroids: experience with the first 100 registry patients. J. Natl. Cancer Inst. 58:167-171.

Clayson, D. B. (1962). *Chemical Carcinogenesis*. Churchill, London.

Clayson, D. B. (1975a). Epidemiology of bladder cancer. In *The Biology and Clinical Management of Bladder Cancer*, E. H. Cooper and R. E. Williams (Eds.). Blackwell, Oxford, England, pp. 65-86.

Clayson, D. B. (1975b). Nutrition and experimental carcinogenesis: a review. Cancer Res. 35:3292-3300.

Clayson, D. B. (1976). Occupational bladder cancer. Prev. Med. 5:228-244.

Clayson, D. B., and Garner, R. C. (1976). Carcinogenic aromatic amines and related compounds. In *Chemical Carcinogens*, ACS Monograph 173, C. E. Searle (Ed.). American Chemical Society, Washington, D.C., pp. 366-461.

Clemmesen, J. (1975). Phenobarbitone, liver tumors, and thorotrast. Lancet i:37-38.

Clemmesen, J., Fuglsang-Frederiksen, V., and Plum, C. M. (1974). Are anti-convulsants oncogenic? Lancet i:705-707.

Cohen, C. J., and Deppe, G. (1977). Endometrial carcinoma and oral contraceptive agents. J. Obstet. Gynecol. 49:390-392.

Cohen, S. M., Ertürk, E., and Bryan, G. T. (1970). Carcinogenicity of N-[4-(5-nitro-2-furyl)-2-thiazolyl]acetamide in female Swiss mice. Cancer Res. 30:906-912.

Committee on Safety of Medicines (1972). Carcinogenicity tests of oral contraceptives. A report of the Committee on Safety of Medicines, H. M. Stationery Office, London.

Cook, J. W., Duffy, E., and Schoental, R. (1950). Primary liver tumors in rats following feeding with alkaloids of *Senecio jacobeac*. Br. J. Cancer 4:405-410.

Corbett, T. H., Cornell, R. G., Linde, H. W., and Endres, J. L. (1974). Birth defects of children among nurse-anesthetists. A 20-year survey. Anesthesiology 41:341-344.

Croft, W. A., and Bryan, G. T. (1973). Production of urinary bladder carcinomas in male hamsters by N[4-(5-nitro-2-furyl)-2-thiazolyl]formamide, N[4-(5-nitro-2-furyl)-2-thiazolyl]acetamide or formic acid 2-[4-(5-nitro-2-furyl)-2-thiazolyl]hydrazide. J. Natl. Cancer Inst. 51:941-949.

Culpepper, N. (ca. 1750). *The British Herbal and Family Physician to Which Is Added a Dispensatory for the Use of Private Families*. Garlick, Halifax.

Dahlgren, S. (1961). Thorotrast tumours. Acta Pathol. Microbiol. Scand. 53:147-161.

Da Silva Horta, J., Abbott, J. O., Da Motta, L. C., and Tavares, M. H. (1972). Leukaemia, malignancies and other late effects following administration of thorotrast. Z. Krebsforsch. 77:202-216.

DeGroot, L., and Paloyan, E. (1973). Thyroid carcinomas and radiation. A Chicago epidemic. JAMA 225:487-491.

DeMatteis, F., Donnelly, A. J., and Runge, W. J. (1966). The effect of prolonged administration of griseofulvin in mice with reference to sex differences. Cancer Res. 26:721-726.

Denlinger, R. H., Swenberg, J. A., Koestner, A., and Wechsler, W. (1973). Differential effects of immunosuppression on the induction of nervous system and bladder tumors by N-methyl-N-nitrosourea. J. Natl. Cancer Inst. 50:87-93.

Dickens, F., and Jones, H. E. (1961). Carcinogenic activity of a series of reactive lactones and related substances. Br. J. Cancer 15:85-100.

Doniach, I. (1958). Experimental induction of tumours of the thyroid by radiation. Br. Med. Bull. 14:181-183.

Edmondson, H. A., Henderson, B., and Benton, B. (1976). Liver cell adenomas associated with use of oral contraceptives. N. Engl. J. Med. 294:470-472.

Einhorn, N. (1978). Acute leukemia after chemotherapy (Melphalan). Cancer 41:444-447.

Ertürk, E., Atassi, S. A., Yoshida, O., Cohen, S. M., Price, J. M., and Bryan, G. T. (1970a). Comparative gall bladder and urinary carcinogenicity of N-[4-(5-nitro-furyl)-2-thiazolyl]formamide and N-[4-(5-nitro-2-furyl)-2-thiazolyl]acetamide in the dog. J. Natl. Cancer Inst. 45:535-542.

Ertürk, E., Cohen, S. M., and Bryan, G. T. (1970b). Urinary bladder carcinogenicity of N-[4-(5-nitro-2-furyl)-2-thiazolyl]formamide in female Swiss mice. Cancer Res. 30:936-941.

Fairchild, W. V., Spence, C. R., Solomon, H. D., and Gangai, M. P. (1979). The incidence of bladder cancer after cyclophosphamide therapy. J. Urol. 122:163-164.

Farber, M. (1979). Twenty-eight years of continuous follow-up of patients injected with thorotrast for cerebral angiography. Environ. Res. 18:37-43.

Farrell, G. C., Joshua, D. E., Uren, R. F., Baird, P. U., Perkins, K. W., and Kronenberg, H. (1975). Androgen-induced hepatoma. Lancet 1:430-432.

Fasal, E., and Paffenbarger, R. S., Jr. (1975). Oral contraceptives as related to cancer and benign lesions of the breast. J. Natl. Cancer Inst. 55:767-773.

Ferebee, S. H. (1970). Controlled chemoprophylaxis trials in tuberculosis. Adv. Tuberc. Res. 17:28-106.

Fitzhugh, O. G., Nelson, A. A., and Holland, O. L. (1948). The chronic oral toxicity of chloroquine. J. Pharmacol. Exp. Ther. 93:147-152.

Fox, K. A., and Lakcen, R. B. (1974). Liver-cell adenomas and peliosis hepatitis in mice associated with oxazepam. Res. Commun. Chem. Pathol. Pharmacol. 8:481-488.

Fraumeni, J. F. (1967). Bone marrow depression induced by chloramphenicol or phenylbutazone. Leukemia and other sequelae. JAMA 201:828-834.

Glassroth, J. L., White, M. C., and Snider, D. E. (1977). An assessment of the possible association of isoniazid with human cancer deaths. Am. Rev. Respir. Dis. 116:1065-1074.

Goldman, P., Ingelfinger, J. A., and Friedman, P. A. (1977). Metronidazole, isoniazid, and the threat of human cancer. In Origins of Human Cancer, H. H. Hiatt, J. D. Watson, and J. A. Winsten (Eds.). Cold Spring Harbor Symposium on Cell Proliferation. Vol. 4, Cold Spring Harbor, New York, pp. 465-474.

Gray, L. A., Christopherson, W. M., and Hoover, R. N. (1977). Estrogens and endometrial carcinoma. J. Obstet. Gynecol. 49:385-389.

Greenwald, P., Barlow, J. J., and Masca, P. C. (1971). Vaginal cancer after maternal treatment with synthetic estrogens. N. Engl. J. Med. 285:390-392.

Guy, J. T., and Auslander, M. O. (1973). Androgenic steroids and hepatocellular carcinoma. Lancet 1:148.

Haese, W. H., and Bueding, E. (1976). Long-term hepatocellular effects of hycanthone and of two other antischistosomal drugs in mice infected with Schistosomum mansoni. J. Pharmacol. Exp. Ther. 197:703-713.

Haese, W. H., Smith, D. L., and Bueding, E. (1973). Hycanthone-induced hepatic changes in mice infected with Schistosomum mansoni. J. Pharmacol. Exp. Ther. 186:430-440.

Hamilton, J. M., Flaks, A., Saluja, P. G., and Maquire, S. (1975). Hormonally induced renal neoplasia in the male Syrian hamster and the inhibitory effect of 2-bromo- -ergocryptine methanesulfonate. J. Natl. Cancer Inst. 54:1385-1400.

Hamilton, J. M., Saluja, P. G., Thody, A. J., and Flaks, A. (1977). The pars intermedia and renal carcinogenesis in hamsters. Eur. J. Cancer 13:29-32.

Hedinger, C. E. (1969). Articles and discussion in section 2. Epidemiology of thyroid cancers. UICC Monograph 12. Springer-Verlag, Berlin, 1969.

Heinonen, O. P., Shapiro, S., Tuominen, L., and Turunen, M. I. (1974). Reserpine use in relation to breast cancer. Lancet 2:675-677.

Hemplemann, L. H., Hall, W. J., Phillips, M., Cooper, R. A., and Ames, W. R. (1975). Neoplasms in persons treated with x-rays in infancy: 4th survey in 20 years. J. Natl. Cancer Inst. 55:519-530.

Herbst, A. L., Ulfelder, H., and Poskanzer, D. C. (1971). Adenocarcinoma of the vagina. Association of maternal stilbestrol therapy with tumor appearance in young women. N. Engl. J. Med. 284:878-881.

Hernberg, S. (1977). Incidence of cancer in population with exceptional exposure to metals. In Origins of Human Cancer, H. H. Hiatt, J. D. Watson, and J. A. Winsten (Eds.). Cold Spring Harbor Conferences on Cell Proliferation, Vol. 4, Cold Spring Harbor, New York, pp. 147-157.

Hinson, J. A., and Mitchell, J. R. (1976). N-Hydroxylation of phenacetin by hamster liver microsomes. Drug Metab. Dispos. 4:430-435.

Hodgin, J. D., and Webster, P. D. (1976). Malignancies in blood-forming organs following diagnostic and therapeutic procedures: a review. South. Med. J. 69:1363-1366.

Hoover, R., and Fraumeni, J. F., Jr. (1973). Risk of cancer in renal transplant recipients. Lancet 2:55-57.

Hoover, R., Fraumeni, J. F., and Everson, R. (1976). Cancer of the uterine corpus after hormonal treatment for breast cancer. Lancet 1:885-887.

Howe, R. (1965). Carcinogenicity of "Alderlin" (pronethalol) in mice. Nature 207:594-595.

Hurst, E. W., and Paget, G. E. (1963). Protoporphyrin, cirrhosis and hepatomata in the livers of mice given griseofulvin. Br. J. Dermatol. 75:105-112.

IARC (1977a). Phenobarbital and phenobarbital sodium. In Evaluation of Carcinogenic Risk of Chemicals to Man, IARC Monographs, Vol. 13. Lyon, France, pp. 157-181.

IARC (1977b). Phenytoin and phenytoin sodium. In Evaluation of Carcinogenic Risk of Chemicals to Man, IARC Monographs, Vol. 13. Lyon, France, pp. 201-225.

IARC (1977c). Chloroquine. In Evaluation of Carcinogenic Risk of Chemicals to Man, IARC Monographs, Vol. 13. Lyon, France, pp. 47-55.

Ikegami, R., Akamatsu, Y., and Haruta, M. (1967). Subcutaneous sarcomas induced by mitomycin C in mice. Acta Pathol. Jpn. 17:495.

Jeejeebhoy (1970). Discussion of Law, L. W. (See below.)

Jensen, E. V. (1975). Estrogen receptors in hormone-dependent breast cancers. Cancer Res. 35:3362-3364.

Johansson, S., and Angervall, L. (1976). Urothelial hyperplasia of the renal papillae in female Sprague-Dawley rats induced by long term feeding of phenacetin. Acta Pathol. Microbiol. Scand. 84:353-354.

Johnson, F. L., Feagler, J. R., Lerner, K. G., Majerus, P. W., Siegle, M., Hartmann, J. R., and Thomas, E. D. (1972). Association of androgenic-anabolic steroid therapy with development of hepatocellular carcinoma. Lancet 2:1273-1278.

Juhasz, J., Balo, J., and Szende, B. (1968). Experimental tumors developing upon the effect of diphenylhydantoin treatment. Magy. Onkol. 12:39-44.

Juhasz, J., Balo, J., and Kendrey, G. (1957). Uber die geschwulster-zeugende Wirkung des Isonicotinsaurehydrazid (INH). Z. Krebsforsch. 62:188-196

Kaufman, R. H., Reeves, K. O., and Dougherty, C. M. (1976). Severe atypical endometrial changes and sequential contraceptive use. JAMA 236:923-926.

Kelly, M. G., O'Gara, R., Gadekar, K., Yancey, S. T., and Oliverio, V. T. (1964). Carcinogenicity activity of a new anti-tumor agent, n-isopropyl-α-(2-methylhydrazine)p-toluamide hydrochloride (NSC 77213). Cancer Chemother. Rep. 39:77-80.

Kelly, M. G., O'Gara, R., Yancey, S. T., and Botkin, C. (1968). Tumors in rats with procarbazine hydrochloride. J. Natl. Cancer Inst. 40:1027-1051.

Kirkman, H., and Bacon, R. L. (1952). Estrogen-induced tumors of the kidney. I. Incidence of renal tumors in intact and gonadectomized male golden hamsters treated with diethylstilbestrol. J. Natl. Cancer Inst. 13:745-756.

Kistner, R. W., Krantz, K. E., Lebherz, T. B., Lewis, G. L., Reagan, J. W., Smith, J., Tobin, J. J., and Weid, G. L. (1973). Endometrial cancer: rising incidence, detection and treatment. J. Reprod. Med. 10:53-74.

Kneale, G. W. (1971). Excess sensitivity of pre-leukaemics to pneumonia. A model situation for studying the interaction of an infectious disease with cancer. Br. J. Prev. Soc. Med. 25:152-159.

Krüger, G., Harris, D., and Sussman, P. (1972). Effect of dilantin in mice. II. Lymphoreticular tissue atypia and neoplasia after chronic exposure. Z. Krebsforsch. 78:290-302.

Lacassagne, A. (1932). Apparition de cancers de la mamelle chez la souris male, soumise a des injections de folliculine. C. R. Acad. Sci. [D] (Paris) 195:630.

Lancet (1977a). Therapy-linked leukaemia (editorial). 1:519-520.

Lancet (1977b). Cervical neoplasia and the pill. 2:644.

Laska, E. M., Siegle, C., Meisner, M., Fischer, S., and Wanderling, J. (1975). Matched-pairs study of reserpine use and breast cancer. Lancet 2:296-300.

Law, L. W. (1970). Effect of antilymphocyte serum on the induction of neoplasms of lymphoreticular tissues. Fed. Proc. 29:171-174.

Lawley, P. D. (1976). Carcinogenesis by alkylating agents. In *Chemical Carcinogens*, ACS Monograph 173, C. E. Searle (Ed.). American Chemical Society, Washington, D.C., pp. 83-244.

Li, F. P., Willard, D. R., Goodman, R., and Vawter, G. (1975). Malignant lymphoma after diphenylhydantoin (dilantin) therapy. Cancer 36:1359-1362.

Longnecker, D. S., and Curphey, T. J. (1975). Adenocarcinomas of the pancreas in azaserine-treated rats. Cancer Res. 35:2249-2258.

Lyon, F. A., and Frisch, M. J. (1976). Endometrial abnormalities occurring in young women on long term sequential oral contraception. J. Obstet. Gynecol. 47:639-643.

Mack, T. M., Henderson, B. E., Gerkins, V. R., Baptista, J., and Pike, M. C. (1975). Reserpine and breast cancer in a retirement community. N. Engl. J. Med. 292:1366-1371.

Mack, T. M., Pike, M. C., Henderson, B. E., Pfeffer, R. I., Gerkins, V. R., Arthur, M., and Brown, S. E. (1976). Estrogens and endometrial cancer in a retirement community. N. Engl. J. Med. 294:1262-1267.

MacMahon, B. (1962). Prenatal x-ray exposure and childhood cancer. J. Natl. Cancer Inst. 28:1173-1191.

Mahboubi, E., and Shubik, P. (1977). Epidemiological relationship between steroid hormones and liver lesions. J. Toxicol. Environ. Health 3:207-218.

Mahoney, J. F., Storey, B. G., Ibanez, R. C., and Stewart, J. H. (1977). Analgesic abuse, renal parenchymal disease, and carcinoma of the kidney or ureter. Aust.-NZ J. Med. 7:463-469.

March, H. C. (1944). Leukemia in radiologists. Radiology 43:275-278.

March, H. C. (1950). Leukemia in radiologists in a 20-year period. Am. J. Med. Sci. 220:282-285.

Marshall, V. C. (1973). Skin tumours in immunosuppressed patients. Aust.-NZ J. Surg. 43:214-222.

McCann, J., and Ames, B. N. (1977). The *Salmonella* microsome mutagenicity test: predictive value for animal carcinogenicity. In *Origins of Human Cancer*, H. H. Hiatt, J. D. Watson, and J. A. Winsten (Eds.). Cold Spring Harbor Symposia on Cell Proliferation, Vol. 4, Cold Spring Harbor, New York, pp. 1431-1450.

McCarthy, D. D., and Chalmers, T. M. (1964). Hematological complications of phenylbutazone therapy. Review of the literature and report of two cases. Can. Med. Assoc. J. 90:1061-1067.

McDonald, T. W., Annegers, J. F., O'Fallon, W. M., Dockerty, M. B., Malkasian, G. D., and Kurland, L. T. (1977). Exogenous estrogen and endometrial carcinoma: case-control and incidence study. Gynecology 127:572-580.

Meadows, A. T., Nailman, J. L., and Valdes-Sapena, M. (1974). Hepatoma associated with androgen therapy for aplastic anemia. J. Pediatr. 84:109-113.

Merck Index (1976). 9th Ed., Merck & Co., Rahway, N.J.

Metzler, M. (1976). Metabolic activation of carcinogenic diethylstilbestrol in rodents and humans. J. Toxicol. Environ. Health (Supp.) 1:21-35.

Metzler, M. (1978). Physiological mechanisms of diethylstilbestrol organotropic carcinogenesis. Abstracts of Eur. Soc. Toxicol. Meeting, June.

Miller, J. A. (1970). Carcinogenesis by chemicals: an overview. G.H.A. Clowes Memorial Lecture. Cancer Res. 30:559-576.

Modan, B., Baidatz, D., Mark, H., Steinitz, R., and Levin, S. G. (1974). Radiation-induced head and neck tumors. Lancet i:277-279.

Mole, R. H. (1975). Ionizing radiation as a carcinogen: practical questions and academic pursuits. Br. J. Radiol. 48:157-169.

Mole, R. H. (1979). Carcinogenesis by thorotrast and other sources of irradiation, especially alpha-emitters. Environ. Res. 18:192-215.

Morbid. Mortal. Weekly Rep. (1977). Increased risk of hepatocellular adenoma in women with long term use of oral contraceptives (editorial). 26:293.

Mori, T., Sakai, T., Nozue, Y., Okamoto, T., Wada, T., Tanaka, T., and Tsuya, A. (1967). Malignancy and other injuries following thorotrast administration: follow-up study of 147 cases in Japan. Strahlentherapie 134:229-254.

Nandi, S. (1958). Endocrine control of mammary-gland development and function in the C3H/He Crgl mouse. J. Natl. Cancer Inst. 21:1039-1064.

Nandi, S. (1959). Hormonal control of mammogenesis and lactogenesis in the C3H/He Crgl mouse. Univ. Calif. Pub. Zool. 65:1-128.

Nandi, S. (1961). Effect of hormones on maintenance of hyperplastic alveolar nodules in mammary glands of various strains of mice. J. Natl. Cancer Inst. 27:187-201.

Nandi, S., Bern, H. A., and Deome, K. B. (1960). Effect of hormones on growth and neoplastic development of transplanted hyperplastic alveolar nodules in hypophysectomized-ovariectomized-adrenalectomized C3H/Crgl mice. J. Natl. Cancer Inst. 27:173-185.

National Cancer for Toxicological Research (1977). Annual Report.

Nelson, A. A., and Fitzhugh, O. G. (1948). Chloroquine (SN-7618). Pathologic changes observed in rats which for 2 years had been fed various proportions. Arch. Pathol. 45:454-462.

Neubauer, O. (1947). Arsenical cancer: a review. Br. J. Cancer 1:192-251.

O'Fallon, W. M., Labarthe, D. R., and Kurland, L. T. (1975). Rauwolfia derivatives and breast cancer: a case/control study in Olmsted County, Minnesota. Lancet 2:292-296.

Penn, I., and Starzl, T. E. (1972). Malignant tumours arising de novo in immunosuppressed organ transplant recipients. Transplant 14:407-417.

Peraino, C., Fry, R. J., and Staffeldt, E. (1971). Reduction and enhancement by phenobarbital of hepatocarcinogenesis induced in the rat by 2-acetylaminofluorene. Cancer Res. 31:1506-1512.

Peraino, C., Fry, R. J., Staffeldt, E., and Christopher, J. P. (1975). Comparative enhancing effects of phenobarbital, amobarbital, diphenylhydantoin, and dichlorodiphenyltrichloromethane on 2-acetylaminofluorene-induced hepatic tumorigenesis in the rat. Cancer Res. 35:2884-2890.

Peraino, C., Fry, R. J., Staffeldt, E., and Kisieleski, W. E. (1973). Effects of varying the exposure to phenobarbital in its enhancement of 2-acetylaminofluorene-induced hepatic tumorigenesis in the rat. Cancer Res. 33:2701-2705.

Perry, S. (1978). Recommendations of the consensus development panel on breast cancer screening. Cancer Res. 38:476-477.

Philips, F. S., Sternberg, S. S., Cronin, A. P., and Vidal, P. M. (1961). Cyclophosphamide and urinary bladder toxicity. Cancer Res. 21:1577-1589.

Ponomarkov, V., Tomatis, L., and Turusov, V. (1976). The effect of long term administration of phenobarbitone in CF-1 mice. Cancer Lett. 1:165-172.

Poskanzer, D. C., and Herbst, A. L. (1977). Epidemiology of vaginal adenosis and adenocarcinoma associated with exposure to stilbestrol in utero. Cancer 39:1892-1895.

Price, J. M., Morris, J. E., and Lalich, J. J. (1966). Evaluation of the carcinogenic activity of 5-nitrofuran derivatives in the rat. Fed. Proc. 25:410.

Puri, H. C., and Campbell, R. A. (1977). Cyclophosphamide and malignancy. Lancet 1: 1306.

Radford, E. P., Doll, R., and Smith, P. G. (1977). Mortality among patients with ankylosing spondylitis not given x-ray therapy. N. Engl. J. Med. 297:572-576.

Rathert, P., Melchoir, H., and Lutzeyer, W. (1975). Phenacetin, a carcinogen for the urinary tract. J. Urol. 113:653-657.

Recant, L., and Lacy, L. (1965). Fanconi's anemia and hepatic cirrhosis. Am. J. Med. 39:464-475.

Refetoff, S., Harrison, J., and Karanfilski, B. T., Kaplan, E. L., De Groot, L. J., and Beberman, C. (1975). Continuing occurrence of thyroid carcinoma after irradiation to the neck in infancy and children. N. Engl. J. Med. 292:171-175.

Reimer, R. R., Hoover, P., Fraumeni, J. F., and Young, R. C. (1977). Acute leukemia after alkylating agents therapy of ovarian cancer. N. Engl. J. Med. 297:177-181.

Rice, J. (1979). Editor - Perinatal Carcinogenesis, NCI Monographs No. 51, pp. i-ix, 1-282.

Roberts, M. M. (1976). Acute leukaemia after immunosuppressive therapy. Lancet 2: 768-770.

Rossi, L., Ravera, M., Repetti, G., and Santi, L. (1976). Long term administration of DDT or phenobarbital-Na in Wistar rats. Int. J. Cancer 19:179-185.

Royal College of General Practitioners' Oral Contraceptive Study (1977). Mortality among oral contraceptive users. Lancet 2:727-731.

Rustia, M., and Shubik, P. (1972). Induction of lung tumors and malignant lymphoma in mice by metronidazole. J. Natl. Cancer Inst. 48:721-729.

Rustia, M., and Shubik, P. (1976). Transplacental effects of diethylstilbestrol on the genital tract of hamster offspring. Cancer Lett. 1:139-146.

Rustia, M., and Shubik, P. (1978). Thyroid tumors in rats and hepatomas in mice after griseofulvin treatment. Br. J. Cancer 38:237-249.

Sandmire, H. F., Austin, S. D., and Bechtell, R. C. (1976). Carcinoma of the cervix in oral contraceptive users and IUD users and non-users. Am. J. Obstet. Gynecol. 125: 339-345.

Schindler, A. E. (1976). Estrogens and endometrial cancer: aspects of etiology and survival rate. Arch. Geschwulstforsch. 46:345-349.

Schmähl, D. (1977). Carcinogenic action of anticancer drugs with special reference to immunosuppression. Cancer 40 (Supp.):1927-1929.

Schmähl, D., and Osswald, H. (1970). Experimentelle Untersuchungen uber carcinogene Wirkungen von Krebs-Chemotherapeutica and Immunosuppressiva. Arzneim. Forsch. 20:1461-1467.

Schneiderman, M. A. (1974). Phenobarbitone and liver tumors. Lancet 2:1085.

Schneiderman, M. A., and Peters, J. A. (1972). Cancer prevention. Science 178:697-698.

Schwan, S. (1961). Isonicotinic acid hydrazide (INH) as a "carcinogenic" factor in mice. I. Patol. Pol. 12:53-56.

Schwan, S. (1962). Isonicotinic acid hydrazide as a carcinogenic agent in mice. II. Patol. Pol. 13:42.

Selbie, F. R. (1938). Tumours in rats and mice following the injection of thorotrast. Br. J. Exp. Pathol. 19:100-107.

Shanklin, D. R. (1974). Endometrial cancer: a worsening problem. Consultant 14:94-99.

Shore, R. E., Hemplemann, L. H., Kowaluk, E., Mansur, P. S., Pasternack, B. S., Albert, R. E., and Haughie, G. E. (1977). Breast neoplasms in women treated with x-rays for acute post-partum mastitis. J. Natl. Cancer Inst. 59:813-822.

Sieber, S. M., and Adamson, R. H. (1975). Toxicity of antineoplastic agents in man, chromosomal aberrations, antifertility effects, congenital malformations and carcinogenic potential. Adv. Cancer Res. 22:57-155.

Slanina, J., Musshoff, K., Rahner, T., and Stasny, R. (1977). Long-term side effects in irradiated patients with Hodgkin's disease. Int. J. Radiat. Oncol. Biol. Phys. 2: 1-19.

Smith, D. C., Prentice, R., Thompson, D. J., and Herrmann, W. L. (1975). Association of exogenous estrogen and endometrial carcinoma. N. Engl. J. Med. 293:1164-1167.

Smith, P. G., and Doll, R. (1976). Late effects of x-irradiation in patients treated for metropathia haemorrhagica. Br. J. Radiol. 49:224-232.

Smith, O. W., and Smith, G. V. (1949). Use of diethylstilbestrol to prevent fetal loss from complications of late pregnancy. N. Engl. J. Med. 241:562-568.

Sontag, J. M., Page, N. P., and Saffiotti, U. (1976). Guidelines for carcinogen bioassay in small rodents, NCI-CG-TR-1. Carcinogenesis Technical Report Series 1, NCI, U.S. Dept. of Health, Education, and Welfare, Washington, D.C.

Starzl, T. E., Porter, K. A., Andres, G., Halgrimson, C. C., Hurwitz, R., Giles, C., Terasaki, P. I., Penn, I., Schroter, G. T., Lilly, J., Starkie, S. J., and Putnam, C. W. (1970). Long-term survival after renal transplantation in humans: with special reference to histocompatibility matching, thymectomy, homography, glomerulonephritis, heterologous ALG and recipient malignancy. Ann. Surg. 172:437-472.

Stein, R. J., Yost, D., Petroilunas, F., and Von Esch, A. (1966). Carcinogenic activity of nitrofurans: a histological evaluation. Fed. Proc. 25:291.

Sternberg, S. S., Philips, F. S., and Cronin, A. P. (1972). Renal tumors and other lesions in rats following a single intravenous injection of daunomycin. Cancer Res. 32:1029-1036.

Stewart, A. M. (1973). Cancer as a cause of abortions and stillbirths: the effects of these early deaths on the recognition of radiogenic leukaemias. Br. J. Cancer 27:465-472.

Stewart, A., and Kneale, G. W. (1970). Radiation dose effects in relation to obstetric x-rays and childhood cancers. Lancet 1:1185-1188.

Strong, L. C., and Smith, G. M. (1939). The local induction of carcinoma of the mammary gland by methylcholanthrene. Yale J. Biol. Med. 11:589-592.

Svoboda, D., Reddy, J., and Harris, C. (1970). Invasive tumors induced in rats with actinomycin D. Cancer Res. 30:2271-2279.

Sweeney, E. C., and Evans, D. J. (1975). Liver lesions and androgenic steroid therapy. Lancet 2:1042.

Symington, G. R., Mackay, I. R., and Lambert, R. P. (1977). Cancer and teratogenesis: infrequent occurrence after medical use of immunosuppressive drugs Aust.-NZ J. Med. 7:368-372.

Thiede, T., Chievitz, E., and Christensen, B. C. (1964). Chlornaphazine as a bladder carcinogen. Acta Med. Scand. 175:721-725.

Thiede, T., and Christensen, B. C. (1969). Bladder tumours induced by chlornaphazine: a 5-year follow-up study of chlornaphazine-treated patients with polycythaemia. Acta Med. Scand. 185:133-137.

Thiede, T., and Christensen, B. C. (1975). Blaeretumoret inducerede af Klornafazinbehandling. Ugeskrift for Laeger 137:661-666.

Thorpe, P., Hassall, J. E., and York, J. R. (1976). Rheumatoid arthritis treated with chlorambucil: a 5-year follow-up. Med. J. Aust. 2:197-199.

Thorpe, E., and Walker, A. I. (1973). The toxicology of dieldrin (HEOD). II. Comparative long term oral toxicity studies in mice with dieldrin, DDT, phenobarbitone, β-BHC and γ-BHC. Food Cosmet. Toxicol. 11:433-442.

Toth, B. (1975). Synthetic and naturally-occurring hydrazines as possible cancer causative agents. Cancer Res. 35:3693-3697.

Toth, B. (1976). Tumorigenicity of β-phenylethylhydrazine sulfate in mice. Cancer Res. 36:917-921.

Toth, B., and Shimizu, H. (1973). Lung carcinogenesis with 1-acetyl-2-isonicotinoylhydrazine, the major metabolite of isoniazid. Eur. J. Cancer 9:285-289.

Toth, B., and Shubik, P. (1966). Carcinogenesis in Swiss mice by isonicotinic acid hydrazide. Cancer Res. 26:1473-1475.

Upton, A. C. (1977). Radiation effects. In Origins of Human Cancer, H. H. Hiatt, J. D. Watson, and J. A. Winsten (Eds.). Cold Spring Harbor Conference on Cell Proliferation, Vol. 4, Cold Spring Harbor, New York, pp. 477-500.

Urman, H. K., Bulay, O., Clayson, D. B., and Shubik, P. (1975). Carcinogenic effects of niridazole. Cancer Lett. 1:69-74.

Vana, J., Murphy, G. P., Arnoff, B. L., and Baker, H. W. (1976). Study of association between liver tumors and oral contraceptive use. Interim Report, November 15, 1976, Commission on Cancer, American College of Surgeons, pp. 1-18.

Videbaek, A. (1950). Polycythaemia vera, course and prognosis. Acta Med. Scand. 138: 179-187.

Videbaek, A. (1964). Blaercancer opstaet under behandling med klornafazin (Erysan). Ugeskr. Laeg. 126:62-66.

Wagner, J. L., and Haughton, G. (1971). Immunosuppression by antilymphocyte serum and its effect on tumors induced by 3-methylcholanthrene in mice. J. Natl. Cancer Inst. 46:1-10.

Wahner, H. W., Cuello, C., and Correa, P. (1966). Thyroid cancer in an endemic goiter area—Cali. Colombia. Am. J. Med. 40:58-66.

Wall, R. L., and Clausen, K. P. (1975). Carcinomas of the urinary bladder in patients receiving cyclophosphamide. N. Engl. J. Med. 293:271-273.

Weisburger, J. H., Griswold, D. P., Prejean, J. D., Casey, A. E., Wood, H. B., and Weisburger, E. K. (1975). The carcinogenic properties of some of the principal drugs used in cancer chemotherapy. Recent Results Cancer Res. 52:1-17.

Weiss, N. S., Szekely, D. R., and Austin, D. F. (1976). Increasing incidence of endometrial cancer in the United States. N. Engl. J. Med. 294:1259-1262.

Wolfe, J. N. (1977). Mammography: a radiologist's view. JAMA 237:2223-2224.

Woodliff, H. J., and Dougan, I. (1964). Acute leukaemia associated with phenylbutazone treatment. Br. Med. J. 5385:744-746.

Woods, D. A. (1969). Influence of antilymphocyte serum on DMBA induction of oral carcinomas. Nature 224:276-277.

World Health Organization (1971). WHO reports on schistosomicidal drugs. Bull. Offic. Sanit. Pan. Amer. (English Ed.) 6:82.

Yarinsky, A., Drobeck, H. P., Freele, S., Wiland, J., and Gumaer, K. I. (1974). An 18-month study of the parasitological and tumorigenic effects of hycanthone in Schistosoma mansoni infected and non-infected mice. Toxicol. Appl. Pharmacol. 27: 169-182.

Ziel, H. K., and Finkle, W. D. (1975). Increased risk of endometrial carcinoma among users of conjugated estrogens. N. Engl. J. Med. 293:1167-1170.

13

Cosmetics

FRANCIS N. MARZULLI* / Food and Drug Administration, Washington, D.C.
ELIZABETH K. WEISBURGER / National Cancer Institute, Bethesda, Maryland

I. INTRODUCTION

The Federal Food, Drug, and Cosmetic Act, enforced by the U.S. Food and Drug Administration, requires that food additives and drugs be shown to be safe prior to marketing. Cosmetics, on the other hand, require no premarketing safety testing. They may be removed from the market only if the FDA can show that they may be harmful to consumers under conditions of customary cosmetic use.

Cosmetics are used to cleanse or adorn the body (soaps are not classed as cosmetics) and are generally thought to be without significant physiologic or pharmacologic impact when used according to directions. Legally, some cosmetics are also drugs because an ingredient is claimed to have a pharmacologic effect. Sun-screening agents and antiperspirant chemicals, such as aluminum chlorohydrate, are recent examples.

*Present affiliation: National Academy of Sciences, Washington, D.C.

In view of the thousands of ingredients which go into the formation of cosmetics, many of which may be used over the greater part of a lifetime, it was reasonable to expect that some substances would emerge the safety of which during chronic use would be questioned by toxicologists. Some of those recently identified substances have been removed from the market; others are under further investigation because tests for mutagenesis or carcinogenesis suggest a hazard in human use.

This paper reports some of the findings of a review of cosmetic ingredients the safety of which is now, or has been, questioned.

II. COSMETICS CATEGORIES AND COMPONENTS

A. Hair-Coloring Preparations

The possibility that some ingredients used in coloring hair may be both carcinogenic and capable of penetrating scalp skin has been explored by scientists of the FDA from time to time. A wide variety of chemical substances are used in "temporary," "semipermanent," and "permanent" coloring systems,* few of which have been specifically tested for their carcinogenic potential. These include acid dyes, basic dyes, benzidine-derived dyes, anthraquinone types, azo dyes, nitro dyes, metabolized dyes, and the many aromatic amines, diamines, aminophenols, and others that are either direct dyes or intermediates forming dyes on oxidation.

The carcinogenic potential of 2,4-toluenediamine (2,4-TDA), a component of some permanent (oxidation) hair-dye systems, came to light when Japanese workers reported that it caused hepatocellular tumors when fed to rats (Ito et al., 1969). Its skin penetration potential was demonstrated somewhat later (Marzulli et al., 1978, in press); however, most manufacturers of hair-dye products voluntarily eliminated it soon after its carcinogenicity was brought to their attention. The carcinogenic potential of this substance was later confirmed under the National Cancer Institute Bioassay program (cited in Marzulli et al., 1978, in press).

As stated in the Federal Register of January 6, 1978, another oxidation hair-dye ingredient reported to be carcinogenic when fed to rats and mice is 2,4-diaminoanisole (2,4-DAA), also called 4-methoxy-m-phenylenediamine. It is related structurally to 2,4-TDA and is also absorbed through skin following topical application. On this basis, the FDA concluded that it may pose a hazard to users of products containing it and proposed that this hazard be made known to consumers through an appropriate label warning (Fed. Reg., 1978). Exemptions in the FD&C Act do not now permit the FDA to prohibit the use of cancer-causing coal-tar hair dyes such as 2,4-DAA if they bear a statutory warning regarding their potential for producing local skin reactions. Congress may change the law to eliminate this deficiency and to require that the safety of hair dyes be demonstrated as for other color additives.

Lead Acetate, a "progressive" hair dye recommended for darkening gray hair, produces renal tumors (Van Esch et al., 1962) when administered chronically to rats at 1% of the diet. When used daily (applied to hair) at a 2% concentration in certain marketed formulations, absorption and systemic retention of some lead may occur, as has been reported in human experiments (Marzulli et al., 1977).† The question of whether lead acetate may be safely used as a hair-dye ingredient is under review by FDA, in view of certain reported negative findings.

---

*"Temporary" dyes are defined as easily removable by shampooing; "semipermanent" are those which require several shampoos for removal; "permanent" are those which are not removed by shampooing.

†Lead acetate hair dye was applied to scalp hair and the systemic uptake of lead was measured by its increase in hair growing in other sites (underarm and pubic areas).

B. Make-Up Preparations

Talc is a naturally occurring hydrated magnesium silicate compound which is used in baby powders, aftershave powders, dusting powders, and many cosmetic make-up products. To be acceptable for cosmetic use, talc must generally be free of asbestos, a chemically related silicate mineral. Asbestos fibers are known to pose an inhalation hazard to asbestos miners and other workers, causing asbestosis, a fibrotic disease. Asbestos may also lead to mesothelioma and lung cancer (Baris et al., 1978; Haley, 1975; Selikoff, 1975). The carcinogenic potential of asbestos is thought to be related to physical characteristics such as fineness (0.25 μm diameter) and length (>8 μm) of fibers.

The problem of distinguishing asbestos fibers in talc is complicated, requiring a determination of refractive indices, other optical crystallographic properties, and morphology, using a polarizing or electron microscope (Fed. Reg., 1973a).

C. Skin-Care Preparations

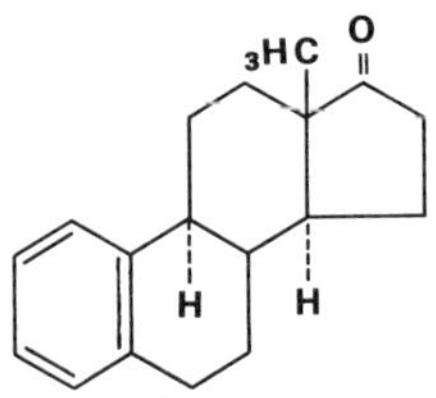

Estrone

Skin preparations (usually creams and lotions) containing estrogens (steroid-type female hormones) have been marketed for approximately 4 or more decades. These preparations are mainly promoted for reversing the effects of age on skin. Some hormone preparations are advertised as stimulating the growth of hair. Because estrogens are potent pharmacodynamic substances* which affect functions of the human body, preparations containing them, although considered cosmetics by users, are legally drugs, as well as cosmetics. As topical application results in skin penetration the labels of these products are required to reveal the quantity or proportion of hormone (not to exceed 10,000 I.U. of estrogen/ounce) and limit the amount of product applied to not more than 20,000 I.U. of estrogen/month (FDA Trade Correspondence, Administration Information Letter No. 265, 1953). Among the estrogenic substances used in topical preparations are estrone, pregnenolone, estradiol, estriol, equiline, and progesterone.

Beneficial effects of some of these products on skin have been claimed by Goldzieher (1946) and Eller and Eller (1949). Adverse systemic physiological effects have been reported by Goldberg and Harris (1952) and by Ramos and Bower (1969). The FDA drug bulletin (1976) reports epidemiologic studies showing an increased risk of cancer of the endometrium from prolonged therapeutic use of estrogens by postmenopausal women (Ziel and Finkle, 1975; Smith et al., 1975). As approximately 1/10 to 1/7 of topically applied estrogen may be absorbed systemically (Goldzieher, 1946), the use of estrogen-containing preparations is not without some risk. There are numerous animal studies suggesting that estrogens have a carcinogenic potential when administered in certain amounts.

D. Preservatives

Dimethoxane (2,6-dimethyl-1,3-dioxan-4-ol acetate, mol wt 174.2, $C_8H_{14}O_4$) is a light amber liquid, which is miscible with water and organic solvents. It has been marketed for some

*Marked proliferative effects occur with primary and secondary sex tissues, with a wide array of complex physiologic effects on sex and other organ systems. Breast enlargement and endometrial hyperplasia have been reported.

time for use as a preservative in cosmetics under the trade name "Giv Gard DXN" (Am. Perfum. Cosmet., 1962). It is claimed that its broad spectrum antimicrobial activity makes it suitable for this purpose.

Dioxanes, of which dimethoxane is a member, represent a relatively new class of compounds with oncogenic potential. Dioxane itself is a strong promoter of 7,12 dimethylbenz(a)anthracene-induced skin tumors in mice, similar in potency to croton oil (Hoch-Ligeti et al., 1974). When administered orally to rats dimethoxane produced hepatomas, leukemia, and tumors of kidney, skin, subcutaneous, and lymphoid tissue. At this time it is speculated that oncogenic effects of this compound are due to metabolic transformation (Hoch-Ligeti et al., 1974).

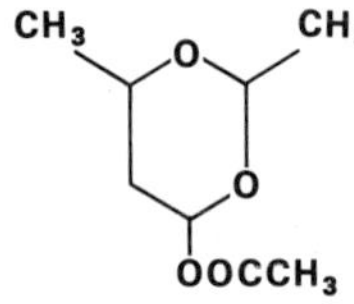

Dimethoxane

Captan ($C_9H_8Cl_3NO_2S$, mol wt 300.57) is used in shampoos, eye shadows, face powders, skin-care products, and hair conditioners. It is employed as a preservative or bactericide/fungicide. In predictive skin sensitization tests in humans it sensitized 9/205 subjects, demonstrating a capacity to penetrate human skin when topically applied (Marzulli and Maibach, 1974). It was recently found to produce carcinoma of the duodenum when fed to mice (NCI, 1977).

E. Fragrances

Cosmetics are now required to display the name of each ingredient on product labels; nevertheless, fragrances or flavors are exempted from this requirement (Code of Federal Regulations, 1977). Currently, perfumery materials are thought to be present at only low levels in finished cosmetics. Although little is known about the systemic effects of fragrance materials, a few of the many compounds used in perfumes have shown some carcinogenic activity when fed to animals at relatively high levels. One of these, safrole, accounts for up to 93% of sassafras oil; it is present to a much lower extent in oils from nutmeg, mace, ginger, cinnamon, black pepper, and star anise. The isomer isosafrole also occurs in low quantities in spice oils. Both safrole and isosafrole caused liver tumors in mice and rats (IARC, 1976b). Dihydrosafrole, a synthetic material, is also used in fragrances. It is an animal carcinogen (IARC, 1976b).

Compounds with certain structural similarities to safrole are β-asarone, a constituent of oil of calamus, and estragole, present in oil of estragen or oil of tarragon. β-asarone led to intestinal tumors upon feeding to rats (Taylor et al., 1967), while estragole caused hepatomas in infant mice (Drinkwater et al., 1976).

Coumarin (1,2-benzopyrone) is an organic lactone (mol wt 146.14, $C_9H_6O_2$) found in various oils, tonka bean, cassia, and plant extracts, and said to be a component of peru balsam. It is readily soluble in alcohol, ether, and oils, but relatively insoluble in water. Its pleasant, vanillalike odor is responsible for its incorporation in perfumery and flavoring formulations. Coumarin induced bile duct tumors in rats upon oral administration at high dose levels (Bär and Griepentrog, 1967; Griepentrog, 1973; IARC Monograph, 1976a). The hazard of these substances to consumers under conditions of cosmetic use is under review.

F. Propellants and Solvents

Certain chlorinated hydrocarbons that have been used in cosmetics are thought to pose a carcinogenic potential based on animal test data. These include vinyl chloride (C_2H_3Cl), trichloroethylene (C_2HCl_3), and chloroform ($CHCl_3$). Methylene chloride (CH_2Cl_2), an alternative to low-pressure chlorofluorocarbons in aerosol products, is currently under investigation for possible carcinogenicity by toxicologists at Dow Chemical Company. It has been reported to be strongly mutagenic to Salmonella typhimurium.

Vinyl chloride, (C_2H_3Cl), a colorless gas (b.p. 14°C), has been used as an aerosol propellant for marketed cosmetics. It is also the precursor of polyvinyl chloride, the ubiquitous solid plastic found in containers for mouthwash, shampoo, and baby oil preparations. As vinyl chloride monomer is carcinogenic to animals and humans when inhaled or ingested (Viola et al., 1971; Maltoni and Lefemine, 1974a, b), its presence in cosmetics is unacceptable and its use as an ingredient of hair sprays is no longer permitted (Fed. Reg., 1974b). The regulation prohibiting the use of vinyl chloride as a propellant in cosmetic aerosols and requiring an approved new drug application for the marketing of aerosol drugs containing vinyl chloride as a propellant was published in the Federal Register of August 26, 1974.

Hepatic angiosarcoma, a rare liver cancer has been associated with exposure of workers to vinyl chloride in vinyl chloride polymerization plants (Falk et al., 1974; Makk et al., 1974). Toxic effects may include degeneration of bone in fingers and hands. Acute inhalation toxicity from high concentrations is manifested by dizziness, headache, disorientation, and unconsciousness (Fed. Reg., 1974a).

As little as 50 ppm vinyl chloride in the atmosphere has induced tumors in chronically exposed rats (Maltoni and Lefemine, 1975).

A review of the British experience with environmental, clinical, epidemiological, and pathological effects of exposure to vinyl chloride is contained in a symposium report (Gauvain, 1976).

After the finding that alcoholic liquors packaged in polyvinyl chloride bottles were contaminated with vinyl chloride extracted from the plastic, mouthwashes became suspect and were investigated (Fed. Reg., 1973b). At first, quantities up to 8 ppm of vinyl chloride were found in some mouthwashes. Later with improved technology contamination was reduced by one or two orders of magnitude. The contamination of cosmetics with vinyl chloride from residues that might be present in polyvinyl chloride containers would be undesirable.

Findings with vinyl chloride have prompted a closer look at chlorinated analogues such as vinylidene chloride and trichloroethylene. Vinylidene chloride is now undergoing tests (Dow Co.) for its potential as a carcinogen.

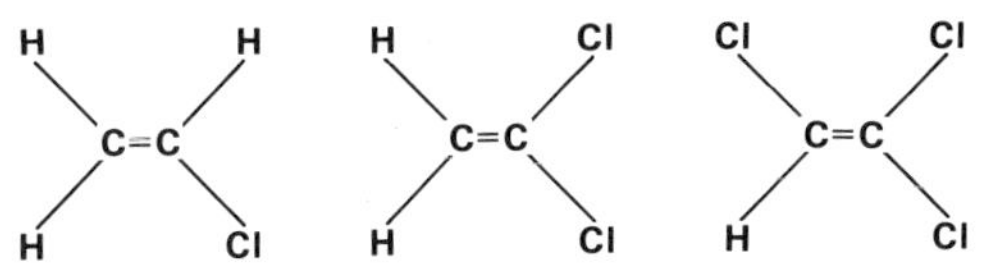

Vinyl chloride **Vinylidine chloride** **Trichloroethylene**

Trichloroethylene (TCE) (C_2HCl_3) is a volatile, nonflammable solvent which has been used in cosmetics as an adhesive remover and as a solvent ingredient in lash cleaners and other cosmetics. It has also been used in food preparation, particularly for the purpose of decaffeination of coffee. Trichloroethylene has been found to produce hepatocellular carcinomas in mice (NCI, 1976a). Because of its carcinogenic activity, the FDA proposed that its use as an ingredient of cosmetics be prohibited (Fed. Reg., 1977).

Chloroform ($CHCl_3$), a well known volatile solvent, has been used for many years as a flavoring agent in dentrifrices and mouthwashes. DeSalva et al. (1975) reported that chloroform is safe, based on liver function tests that showed no change in monitored humans who used chloroform-containing dentrifrices and mouthwashes over a period of 5 years. Following disclosure under an NCI bioassay program that it produces hepatocellular carcinomas (NCI, 1976a; Weisburger, 1977) when orally administered to mice and renal tumors when administered to male rats, the FDA considered it a deleterious substance which may be injurious to consumers under conditions of customary cosmetic use and prohibited its further use as a cosmetic ingredient by regulation (Fed. Reg., 1976a, b). Some industry cosmetic scientists have objected to the characterization of chloroform as a carcinogen on the basis that this effect is produced by high nonphysiologic (liver damaging) doses.

G. Amine-Reaction Products

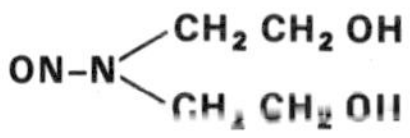

N-Nitrosodiethanolamine

Pioneer work by Magee and Barnes (1956) disclosed that nitrosamines have a significant potential for producing cancer. In subsequent studies on 65 nitrosamines conducted by Druckrey et al. (1967) it was reported that following chronic oral administration, N-nitrosodiethanolamine (NDELA) produces carcinoma of the liver in rats, often with metastases to lung and kidney. A study by Hilfrich et al. (1977) showed that NDELA was carcinogenic when administered to Syrian golden hamsters at 1/10th the total amount used by Druckrey (15 versus 150 g/kg). Neoplasms of the nasal cavity and tracheal tumors, as well as some hepatocellular adenomas and sarcomas at the injection site, were observed. The possibility that NDELA can be formed in vitro and in vivo by chemical reaction between nitrites or oxides of nitrogen and secondary and tertiary amines was investigated by Zingmark and Rappe (1976) and others. This led ultimately to the finding that many currently marketed cosmetics (and other products*) which contain appropriate precursors (triethanolamine, sodium nitrite, or other nitrosating agents), including some cosmetics that do not appear to have traceable precursor chemicals, have amounts of NDELA ranging from less than 1 ppb to 130 ppm (Fan et al., 1977a, b).

NDELA has been found in shampoos, sun-screening preparations, skin-care products for face, hands, and body, and make-up (Fan et al., 1977a, b). The skin penetration capacity of NDELA in cosmetics is expected to be variable, as the vehicles include aqueous or oily solutions, water-in-oil and oil-in-water emulsions. The fact that NDELA is both water- and fat-soluble, however, suggests that it is capable of skin penetration. Diethylnitrosamine (DEN), a related compound, has been reported to produce carcinoma of the nasal cavity when applied to the skins of mice (Hoffmann and Graffi, 1964). These findings have stimulated additional research by the FDA and other involved agencies to define more accurately the carcinogenic potential of NDELA in cosmetics and other products.

III. CARCINOGENIC BURDEN

A. Promotion and Inhibition

A few compounds used in cosmetics have the capacity to either promote (enhance) or inhibit the action of chemical carcinogens in model experiments. Among those that have promoting or cocarcinogenic activity are various surface active agents or fatty acid esters, such as linalyl acetate and synthetic esters, the Tweens and Spans (Van Duuren, 1969; Van Duuren et al., 1971). These materials probably enhance the transfer of the carcinogen into the skin cells by damaging the integrity of the skin barriers.

Still other representative perfumery materials have the ability to inhibit the effects of chemical carcinogens. Terpenes and flavones of varying types fall into this category and have lessened the tumor incidence from certain potent carcinogens such as benzo(a)pyrene (Benko et al., 1963; Wattenberg and Leong, 1970) and benzo(rst) pentaphene (Homburger et al., 1971).

In view of the possible tumor-promoting action of some substances, the cumulative toxicological impact of ingredients must be given careful consideration in the formulation of cosmetics. Furthermore, obvious promoting agents such as dodecane (Bingham and Falk, 1969) have no place in cosmetic formulations.

*Cutting oils (Thermo Electron Corporation, 83 First Avenue, Waltham, Mass. 02154) and pesticides.

Recently, it was reported that ethoxylated emulsifiers used in many cosmetics (such as polysorbate 60 and polysorbate 80) may contain small amounts of p-dioxane (up to 665 ppm), a carcinogen, as a contaminant (Birkel et al., 1979; IARC, 1976c; FDA, 1979). Some suppliers of these ingredients have already resolved the problem. In any case, the small penetration capacity of p-dioxane under use conditions suggests a negligible hazard.

IV. CONCLUSIONS

The current list of chemical cosmetic ingredients that may pose a human carcinogenic hazard is not long. On the other hand, the carcinogenic potential of most chemicals has only come to light in recent years as a result of an increase in investigative efforts. This explains the need for specific testing to disclose the carcinogenic potential of cosmetic ingredients and products, rather than arriving at safety substantiation by guess work, no matter how educated it appears.

Limitations in the usefulness of so-called "white lists" of safe cosmetic ingredients must also share our attention. For years cosmetic toxicologists have adhered to an empirical tenet that a formulation made up of safe ingredients might not in fact be safe after compounding, if reaction between components produced a new compound. We now have an example of this in the reaction of nitrosating agents with di- or triethanolamine (much used cosmetic ingredients) to form nitrosodiethanolamine, a carcinogen.

The lesson to be learned is that it behooves the toxicologist to remain ever alert not only to the inherent toxicity of an ingredient, but also to hazards resulting from cumulative action; that is, cocarcinogenesis and formation of a carcinogen by chemical interaction. In the meantime, it appears that the FDA is now and will continue for some time to be confronted with an increasing number of decisions regarding the hazards of marketed cosmetics, based on tests showing the cancer potential of specific ingredients in animals.

ACKNOWLEDGMENTS

We acknowledge helpful suggestions made in preparation of this manuscript by Mr. Heinz Eiermann, Director, Division of Cosmetics Technology and Program Manager for Cosmetics, FDA, and Mr. Martin Greif, Acting Chief, Registration and Product Experience Branch, Division of Cosmetics Technology, FDA.

The views expressed in this chapter do not necessarily reflect the official position of the FDA.

REFERENCES

Am. Perfum. Cosmet. (1962). Dimethoxane, a new preservative effective with non ionic agents. 77:32-32.

Bär, von F., and Griepentrog, F. (1967). Die Situation in der gesundheitlichen Beurteilung der Aromatishierungsmittel für Lebensmittel. Med. Ernähr. 8:244-251.

Baris, Y. I., Sahin, A. A., Ozesmi, M., Kerse, I., Ozen, E., Kolacan, B., Altinörs, M., Göktepeli, A. (1978). An outbreak of pleural mesothelioma and chronic fibrosing pleurisy in the village of Karain/Urgüp in Anatolia. Thorax 33(2):181-92.

Benko, A., Tiboldi, T., and Bardos, J. (1963). The effect of painting with cyclical terpenes on the skin of white mice and on the skin carcinoma developed by benzpyrene painting. Acta Intern. Contra Cancrum 19:786-788.

Bingham, E., and Falk, H. (1969). Environmental carcinogens. The modifying effect of cocarcinogens on the threshold response. Arch. Environ. Health 19:779-783.

Birkel, T. J., Warner, C. R., and Fazio, T. (1979). Gas chromatographic determination of 1,4-dioxane in polysorbate 60 and polysorbate 80. J. Assoc. Off. Anal. Chem. 62(4): 931-936.

21 Code of Federal Regulations (Sept. 16, 1977). Subchapter: G-cosmetics, designation of ingredients, par. 701.3.

DeSalva, S., Volpe, A., Leigh, G., and Regan, T. (1975). Long-term safety studies of a chloroform-containing dentrifrice and mouth-rinse in man. Food Cosmet. Toxicol. 13: 529-532.

Drinkwater, N. R., Miller, E. C., Miller, J. A., and Pitot, H. C. (1976). Hepatocarcinogenicity of estragole (1-allyl-4-methoxybenzene) and 1'-hydroxyestragole in the mouse and mutagenicity of 1'-acetoxyestragole in bacteria. J. Natl. Cancer Inst. 57: 1313-1331.

Druckrey, H., Preussmann, R., Ivankovic, S., and Schmähl, D. (1967). Organotrope carcinogene Wirkung bei 65 verschiedenen N-Nitroso-verbindungen an BD-Ratten. Z. Krebsforsch. 69: 103-201.

Eller, J. J., and Eller, W. D. (1949). Estrogenic ointments, cutaneous effects of topical application of natural estrogens, with report of 321 biopsies. Arch. Dermatol. Syphilol. 59: 449-464.

Falk, H., Creech, J. L., Heath, C. W., Johnson, M., and Key, M. (1974). Hepatic disease among workers at a vinyl chloride polymerization plant. JAMA 230: 56-63.

Fan, T. Y., Goff, U., Song, L., and Fine, D. H. (1977a). N-Nitrosodiethanolamine in consumer cosmetics, lotions and shampoos. Presented to American Chemical Society, March 23, New Orleans.

Fan, T. Y., Goff, U., Song, L., Fine, D. H., Arsenault, G. P., and Biemann, K. (1977b). N-Nitrosodiethanolamine in cosmetics, lotions and shampoos. Food Cosmet. Toxicol. 15: 423-430.

FDA Drug Bull. (1976). Estrogens and endometrial cancer. 6(1): 18-20.

FDA Trade Correspondence, Administration Information Letter No. 265 (Mar. 30, 1953). Labeling for estrogenic skin cream. 526.1-.10 (581.8).

FDA (1979). Summary of FDA 1,4-dioxane analyses of ethoxylated cosmetic raw materials, samples analyzed by Division of Cosmetics Technology.

Fed. Reg. (1973a). Asbestos particles in foods and drugs. 38: 27076-27081 (Sept. 28).

Fed. Reg. (1973b). 38: 12931 (May 17).

Fed. Reg. (1974a). 39: 14215-14216 (Apr. 22).

Fed. Reg. (1974b). 39: 30830 (Aug. 26).

Fed. Reg. (1976a). 41: 23449 (June 10).

Fed. Reg. (1976b). 41: 26842-26846 (Jan. 29).

Fed. Reg. (1977). 42: 4967-4968 (Sept. 27).

Fed. Reg. (1978). 43: 1101-1106 (Jan. 6).

Gauvain, S. (1976). Vinyl chloride. Proc. R. Soc. Med. 69: 275-310.

Goldberg, M. B., and Harris, F. I. (1952). Severe hemorrhage in a 40 year old after 3 years of estrogens at 10,000 I.U./week. JAMA 150: 790-791.

Goldzieher, M. A. (1946). The effects of estrogen on senile skin. J. Gerontol. 1: 196-200.

Griepentrog, F. (1973). Pathologisch-anatomische Befunde zur karzinogenen Wirkung von Coumarin im Tierversuch. Toxicology 1: 93-102.

Haley, T. J. (1975). Asbestosis: A reassessment of the overall problem. J. Pharm. Sci. 64: 1435-1449.

Hilfrich, J., Schmeltz, I., and Hoffmann, D. (1977). Effects of N-nitrosodiethanolamine and 1,1-diethanol-hydrazine in Syrian golden hamsters. Cancer Lett. 4: 56-60.

Hoch-Ligeti, C., Argus, M. F., and Arcos, J. C. (1974). Oncogenic activity of an m-dioxane derivative: 2,6-Dimethyl-m-dioxan-4-ol acetate (dimethoxane). J. Natl. Cancer Inst. 53: 791-793.

Hoffmann, F., and Graffi, A. (1964). Nasenhohlentumoren bei Mausen nach percutaner Diäthylnitrosamin-applikation. Arch. Geschwulstforsch. 23: 274-288.

Homburger, F., Treger, A., and Boger, E. (1971). Inhibition of murine subcutaneous and intravenous benzo [rst] pentaphene carcinogenesis by sweet orange oils and d-limonene. Oncology 25: 1-10.

IARC (1976a). Evaluation of Carcinogenic Risk of Chemicals to Man—Some Naturally Occurring Substances. Coumarin, IARC Monographs, Vol. 10. Lyon, France, pp. 113-119.

IARC (1976b). Evaluation of Carcinogenic Risk of Chemicals to Man—Some Naturally Occurring Substances. Safrole, isosafrole and dihydrosafrole. IARC Monographs, Vol. 10. Lyon, France, pp. 231-244.

IARC (1976c). Evaluation of Carcinogenic Risk of Chemicals to Man. IARC Monographs, Vol. 112. Lyon, France, p. 247.

Ito, N., Hiasa, Y., Konishi, Y., and Marugami, M. (1969). The development of carcinoma in liver of rats treated with m-toluylenediamine and the synergistic and antagonistic effects with other chemicals. Cancer Res. 29:1137-1145.

Magee, P. N., and Barnes, J. M. (1956). The production of malignant hepatic tumours in the rat by feeding dimethylnitrosamine. Br. J. Cancer 10:114-122.

Makk, L., Creech, J., Whelan, J., and Johnson, M. (1974). Angiosarcoma in vinyl chloride workers. JAMA 230:64-68.

Maltoni, C., and Lefemine, G. (1974a). Carcinogenicity bioassays of vinyl chloride. Environ. Res. 7:387-405.

Maltoni, C., and Lefemine, G. (1974b). Le Potenzialità dei Saggi sperimentali nella predizione dei rischi oncogeni ambienti. Un essempio il choruro di vinile. Accad. Nazionale Linzei 56:1-11.

Maltoni, C., and Lefemine, G. (1975). Carcinogenicity bioassays of vinyl chloride: current results. Ann. NY Acad. Sci. 246:195-218.

Marzulli, F., and Maibach, H. (1974). The use of graded concentrations in studying skin sensitizers: experimental contact sensitizers in man. Food Cosmet. Toxicol. 12:219-227.

Marzulli, F., Watlington, P., and Maibach, H. (1977). Exploratory skin penetration findings relating to the use of lead acetate hair dyes: hair as a test tissue for monitoring uptake of systemic lead. Presented at 22nd OHOLO Conference on Skin, Israel Institute for Biological Research, Ness Ziona, P. O. Box 19, Israel.

Marzulli, F., Green, S., and Maibach, H. (1978). Hair dye toxicity—A review. J. Environ. Pathol. Toxicol. 1:509-530.

NCI (1976a). Carcinogenesis Technical Report Series 2. Bioassay of trichloroethylene. DHEW Publication No. (NIH) 76-802, U.S. Government Printing Office, Washington, D.C.

NCI (1976b). Report on the carcinogenesis bioassay of chloroform. Bethesda, Md.

NCI (1977). Carcinogenesis Technical Report Series 15. DHEW Publication (NIH) 77-815, U.S. Government Printing Office, Washington, D.C.

Ramos, A. S., and Bower, B. F. (1969). Pseudoisosexual precocity due to cosmetic ingestion. JAMA 207:369.

Selikoff, I. J. (1975). Recent perspectives in occupational cancer. Ambio 4:14-17.

Smith, D. C., Prentice, R., Thompson, D. J., and Herrman, W. L. (1975). Association of exogenous estrogen and endometrial carcinoma. N. Engl. J. Med. 293:1164-1167.

Taylor, J. M., Jones, W. I., Hagen, E. C., Gross, M. A., Davis, D. A., and Cook, E. L. (1967). Toxicity of oil of calamus (Jammu variety). Toxicol. Appl. Pharmacol. 10:405.

Van Duuren, B. L. (1969). Tumor promoting agents in two-stage carcinogenesis. Prog. Exp. Tumor Res. 11:31-68.

Van Duuren, B. L., Blazej, T., Goldschmidt, B. M., Katz, C., Melchionne, S., and Sivak, A. (1971). Cocarcinogenesis studies on mouse skin and inhibition of tumor induction. J. Natl. Cancer Inst. 46:1039-1044.

Van Esch, G., Van Gendern, H., and Vink, H. (1962). The induction of renal tumors by feeding basic lead acetate to rats. Br. J. Cancer 16:289-207.

Viola, P. L., Bigotti, A., and Caputo, A. (1971). Oncogenic response of rat skin, lungs and bones to vinyl chloride. Cancer Res. 31:516-522.

Wattenberg, L. W., and Leong, J. L. (1970). Inhibition of the carcinogenic action of benzo[a]pyrene by flavones. Cancer Res. 30:1922-1925.

Weisburger, E. K. (1977). Carcinogenicity studies on halogenated hydrocarbons. Environ. Health Perspect. 21:7-16.

Ziel, H. K., and Finkle, W. D. (1975). Increased risk of endometrial carcinoma among users of conjugated estrogens. N. Engl. J. Med. 293:1167-1170.

Zingmark, P. A., and Rappe, C. (1976). On the formation of N-nitrosodiethanolamine from a grinding fluid under simulated gastric conditions. <u>Ambio</u> 5:80-81.

14

N-2-Fluorenylacetamide and Derivatives

ELIZABETH K. WEISBURGER / National Cancer Institute, Bethesda, Maryland

I. INTRODUCTION

In this chapter the emphasis is on a chemical that is used as a model for research purposes. For this reason, polycyclic aromatic hydrocarbons, nitrosamines, halogenated compounds, urethane, and others are not mentioned, since they occur environmentally. Of all model compounds employed in research on chemical carcinogenesis, N-2-fluorenylacetamide (FAA) (2-acetylaminofluorene) and its derivatives continue to hold a prominent position. The studies with these compounds encompass a wide range of disciplines in physical, chemical, and biological sciences. The last comprehensive review on fluorenylacetamide appeared over 20 years ago. Therefore it seems a propitious time to update and summarize the research efforts on the fluorenamine derivatives.

II. CHEMICAL ASPECTS

A. Synthetic

1. Ring Substituted Compounds

Of particular interest for a time in the study of FAA was the preparation of various ring-substituted fluoro derivatives. The purpose was to determine what effect blocking the different ring positions with fluorine, a substituent not readily removed metabolically, had on the carcinogenicity of FAA. Thus 1-, 3-, 4-, 5-, 6-, 7-, and 8-fluoro-FAA were all synthesized (Fletcher et al., 1959, 1960a, b; Suzuki et al., 1959, 1961a, b). For the same reason various difluoro analogues were prepared in which the more important detoxication positions were occupied by the halogen substituents (Namkung and Fletcher, 1961, 1967; Namkung et al., 1965). Although the monofluoro derivatives were all tested for carcinogenicity in animals (Miller et al., 1962), the difluoro compounds apparently were not. In the course of these studies various interesting techniques that could be applied for the synthesis of 2-fluorenamine (2-FA) derivatives were developed. These included the use of dimethyl sulfoxide as a solvent and/or reactant to facilitate various reactions (Fletcher and Pan, 1959; Fletcher, 1968; Namkung and Fletcher, 1968a; Pan and Fletcher, 1968), the use of tetrahydrofuran to improve yields when fluorofluorenes were prepared through a diazonium fluoborate from the amine (Schiemann reaction) (Fletcher and Namkung, 1961), and the discovery that lithium bromide with trialkylphosphates, -phosphites, or -phosphonates afforded good yields of alkylamino-fluorenes (Pan and Fletcher, 1962).

Synthetic methods for various ring hydroxylated derivatives of FAA except for the 4- and 6-hydroxy compounds were reviewed previously (Weisburger and Weisburger, 1958b). The 6-hydroxy-FAA (6-OH-FAA) (Weisburger and Weisburger, 1958a) proved to be a minor metabolite of FAA (Weisburger et al., 1959a). Although 4-hydroxy-FAA apparently was not an initial metabolite of FAA (Pan and Fletcher, 1960), it was formed by conversion of the activated carcinogen N-acetoxy-FAA, presumably through a nitrenium ion (Scribner, 1977).

The N-OH-FAA and N-acetoxy-FAA share a common end product, 3-chloro-FAA, when heated with HCl or NH_4Cl (Weisburger and Weisburger, 1973; Scribner, 1977). The reaction is reminiscent of the Bamberger reaction in which aryl hydroxylamines rearrange to o- and p-substituted phenols. Thermal rearrangement of N-acetoxy-FAA in nitrobenzene afforded an o-acetoxy-2-FAA; the half time of the reaction was approximately 52 hr at 60° (Calder and Williams, 1975).

The various ortho-aminofluorenols and N-OH-FAA all formed 2:1 chelates with various bivalent metal ions (Weisburger et al., 1963). Some of the insoluble chelates of N-OH-FAA were carcinogenic, probably because of their immobilization at the injection site (Poirier et al., 1965).

A 3-methylthio-2-FAA was synthesized from the reaction of N-acetoxy-FAA with methionine (Lotlikar et al., 1966), while 3-methylthio- and 1-methylthio-4-FAA were formed from N-acetoxy-4-FAA (Yost et al., 1975). Additional methylthio derivatives of FAA and 2-FA were synthesized by more conventional methods, starting from substituted fluorenamines (Fletcher et al., 1967; Namkung and Fletcher, 1968b; Pan et al., 1968). Other 2,3-disubstituted fluorenes and related compounds (Ishikawa and Okazaki, 1958) included 3-methoxy-2-FA and various chloro derivatives from 2-FAA (Sieglitz, 1964). Pan and Fletcher (1964) reported the synthesis of many polyhalogenated derivatives of 2-FAA.

Despite the carcinogenic effect of FAA and the corresponding amine 2-FA, derivatives of these compounds have been synthesized for various experimental purposes. Thus quaternary ammonium salts derived from 2-FA or the 2,5- and 2,7-fluorenediamines all had curare-like activity (Dobrescu et al., 1966). Interferon-inducing activity in mice, comparable to that of the drug Tilorone was noted for 2,7-bis[(diethylamino)acetylamino]fluoren-9-one (Meindl et al., 1976). Nitrogen mustards derived from 2-FA have been synthesized for testing as chemotherapeutic agents (Fletcher and Wetzel, 1960; Fletcher et al., 1966), as well as other nitro and amino derivatives of 2-FA (Namkung and Fletcher, 1960).

2-FA has also been employed as a starting material for heterocyclic compounds (Buu-Hoi et al., 1970). Schiff bases (Dobrescu et al., 1971) and other derivatives have been prepared, many as reference materials for metabolic studies. These include 2,2'-hydrazofluorene and derivatives (Namkung and Fletcher, 1969; Fletcher and Namkung, 1970), azoxyfluorene (Yost, 1969), and fluorene-1,2-quinone 2-acetimide (Burtle and Morath, 1965). Spin-labeled 2-FA was made to investigate carcinogen-DNA intercalation mechanisms (Hong and Piette, 1976).

Several studies on use of electron spin resonance to study possible free radicals arising in rat liver after feeding 2-FAA have been reported (Abdurasulov et al., 1967; Duchesne et al., 1969; Commoner et al., 1970; Dardas and Carraz, 1974). The utility of this approach was perhaps negated when the complex giving the signal could also be observed in yeast cultured with nitrate; it was identified as an iron-NO complex with a thiol-containing protein (Woolum and Commoner, 1970).

The 2,5- and 2,7-fluorenediamine have been employed to some extent as reagents for cytochemical localization of peroxidase (Ohkawa et al., 1976) or as peroxidase reagents for blood smears (Inagaki et al., 1976). Although the chief reason was to replace benzidine, the fluorenediamines also were better reagents for these purposes.

Oxidation of 2-FA by peracetic acid yielded not only 2-nitrofluorene, but other products such as 2,2'-azoxybisfluorene and the azofluorene (Gutmann, 1964; Gorrod, 1968; Yost, 1969). On the other hand, reduction by hydrazine and Raney nickel afforded aminofluoren-9-ols from nitrofluorenone (Pan and Fletcher, 1972). Some of these oxidation-reduction methods were employed in the synthesis of tritiated 2-FAA or analogues (Neumann, 1967; Gutmann and Bell, 1974). In addition, acid-catalyzed exchange of 2-nitrosofluorene, followed by catalytic reduction afforded nonspecifically labeled ^{3}H-2-FA (Breeman et al., 1978).

Extensive studies of many variously substituted fluorenamines did not show any apparent relationship between the ionization constants and possible carcinogenicity (Grantham et al., 1961; Davey et al., 1967). Likewise, magnetic susceptibility showed no relationship to carcinogenicity (French and Pritchard, 1961).

2. N-Hydroxy Derivatives

The N-hydroxy derivative of FAA (N-OH-FAA) was first synthesized as a reference material for identification of a metabolic product (Cramer et al., 1960b). The method involved controlled reduction of 2-nitrofluorene in the presence of triethylamine and acetic anhydride, followed by hydrolysis of the diacetyl derivative to N-OH-FAA. Various improvements in technique have increased yields and reduced the possiblity of rearrangement to unwanted byproducts (Kadlubar et al., 1977). In addition, synthetic methods have afforded the probable metabolic intermediates, 2-nitrosofluorene, 2-fluorenylhydroxylamine, and the sulfate and acetate esters of N-OH-FAA.

N-OH-FAA and N-OH-FA can be oxidized to 2-nitrosofluorene (Baumgarten et al., 1965). In turn 2-nitrosofluorene can be diazotized and coupled with N-(1-naphthyl)ethylenediamine to form a chromophore. This system was used to determine the amount of N-OH-FA excreted in the urine of guinea pigs given large doses of 2-FA (Kiese and Wiedemann, 1968). Some of the reactions of N-OH-FAA and analytical methods for this compound have been reviewed (Weisburger and Weisburger, 1973).

B. Analytical

In this area recent emphasis has been on chromatographic methods suitable for determining 2-FAA and its ring- or N-hydroxylated derivatives. Thus chromatography on alumina has been applied to separate the free compounds, glucuronic acid conjugates, and sulfuric acid conjugates formed during metabolism of FAA (Weisburger et al., 1961a). Ion-exchange chromatography was also adapted for the same purpose (Grantham, 1967). Thin-layer chromatography has afforded a rapid means to examine metabolic profiles (Irving, 1964; Ikan et al., 1965). Gas-liquid chromatographic separation of FAA and its ring-hydroxylated derivatives was feasible; however, N-OH-FAA was dehydroxylated unless a derivative was first made (Irving, 1970; Lhoest et al., 1976). A recent paper proposed that N-OH-FAA formed from in vitro metabolism of FAA be treated with HCl to form N-chloro-2-FA; trifluoroacetic anhydride then afforded N-chloro-2-trifluoroacetamidofluorene which was determined by an electron capture detector (Razzouk et al., 1977). The method actually was a measure of N-hydroxylase activity; there was no mention of possible rearrangement products that might also be present.

Combinations of extraction procedures along with chromatography have led to finding traces of fluorenamines and many other aromatic amines in tobacco smoke, probably formed through pyrolytic reactions (Schmeltz and Hoffmann, 1977).

Much emphasis has been placed on developing high-pressure liquid chromatographic (HPLC) systems for separation of metabolites and analogues of FAA (Gutmann, 1974; Gutmann et al., 1975; Fullerton and Jackson, 1976; Young and McNair, 1976; Thorgeirsson and Nelson, 1976; Weisburger et al., 1978). With some of the systems not all the FAA metabolite could be separated cleanly with one solvent program and a second run was often necessary. Preparative HPLC was essential for obtaining pure samples of FAA or 7-OH-FAA for a comparative mutagenicity test in Salmonella strains (Donahue et al., 1978). Some recent papers have reported determinations of FAA or FAA metabolites in animal diets or cell culture media with good recovery or separation from interfering materials (Bowman and King, 1974; West and Oller, 1978; Raineri et al., 1978).

Proper application of HPLC facilitated the separation of the various products from reaction of deoxyguanosine with N-acetoxy-FAA, thus enabling better characterization of these adducts (Goodman, 1976). RNA- and DNA-adducts of FAA could be separated on hydroxyapatite columns by eluting with the proper concentration of sodium phosphate (Beland et al., 1979).

A radioimmunoassay for detection of nanogram amounts of the DNA-FAA adducts was developed with N-(deoxyguanosin-8-yl)-2-FAA as the immunogen (Poirier et al., 1977). This technique facilitated studies on the nature and rate of binding to DNA (Sage et al., 1979; Poirier et al., 1979).

The growing use of mass spectrometry, either alone or coupled with gas chromatography, to identify organic compounds has led to several useful studies on the fragmentation patterns which enable the identification of 2-FAA and various derivatives (Lhoest et al., 1976; Burchfield et al., 1977). One of these studies led to the conclusion that N-OH-FAA can exist in tautomeric forms (Lhoest et al., 1978).

III. METABOLISM

A. In Vivo

1. Ring Hydroxylation

The metabolism of FAA in vivo, reviewed in 1958 (Weisburger and Weisburger, 1958b), led to hydroxylation at the 1-, 3-, 5-, 7-, and 8-positions of FAA. Additionally, 6-OH-FAA was later identified as a metabolite (Weisburger et al., 1959a); thus most of the aromatic positions were affected. Hydroxylation at the aliphatic 9-position was also a metabolic pathway, but to only a small extent (Benkert et al., 1975). Appreciable species differences occurred in the amounts of hydroxyl compounds excreted (Weisburger et al., 1958; Weisburger and Weisburger, 1973). In turn, some minor portion of monohydroxylated derivatives was converted to even more water-soluble dihydroxy compounds (Weisburger et al., 1959b, c). Deacetylation also took place for the various aminofluorenols were identified as urinary metabolites (Weisburger et al., 1961c). Glucuronic acid or sulfuric acid conjugation of most of these hydroxylated derivatives served as a means to excrete them expeditiously.

Several groups have shown that FAA or its metabolites are excreted largely through the biliary pathway (cf., Weisburger and Weisburger, 1958b; Irving et al., 1967a; Levine, 1971; Miyata et al., 1972). Only a few of the many urinary metabolites have been identified in the bile, but biliary excretion often mirrors the urinary pattern for the main metabolites. Likewise, FAA or its metabolites were excreted in the prostatic secretion of both the rat and the dog (Smith et al., 1977).

The metabolism of FAA by newborn animals or by prenatal tissues represents a special class for such animals are usually more susceptible to FAA. One study showed a wide distribution of FAA or its metabolites throughout the fetus after administration to a pregnant mouse. N-OH-FAA was found in the fetuses; whether from the maternal circulation or through their own metabolic pathways was not well-defined (Takahashi and Yasuhira, 1975).

The relatively noncarcinogenic isomer 3-FAA was metabolized by rats to at least two monohydroxy derivatives and a dihydroxy derivative which were identified as urinary metabolites (Weisburger, 1961).

However, the ring-hydroxylated metabolites of FAA did not exhibit carcinogenic activity, even when tested under extreme conditions such as bladder implantation (Irving et al., 1963). These compounds represent detoxification products rather than activated metabolites. The considerable differences between species in the relative amounts of these products excreted (Table 1) are an indication that the enzymes involved vary from species to species. In this regard, relatively little attention has been paid to the mechanism of formation of the many ring-hydroxylated products from FAA. Although it has been postulated that ring hydroxylation of FAA results from a radical mechanism (Fukui et al., 1962), another explanation may involve formation of arene oxides as part of the metabolic process. Selective reaction of the arene oxides could account for the relatively large amounts of 7-OH-FAA and 5-OH-FAA and the much smaller quantities of 6- and 8-OH-FAA (Fig. 1).

TABLE 1 Species Differences in Hydroxylation of FAA

Species	Urinary excretion of major metabolites % of dose: N-OH-FAA	7-OH-FAA	5-OH-FAA
Cat	1.5	38	2.1
Dog	5.2	0.7	Small amount
Guinea pig	—	90	Trace
Hamster	5-6	28-35	4-5
Human	4-14	25-30	1.5
Mastomys	2.3	8.7	3-7
Monkey	0.6-2.7	7.2-18	—
Mouse	1.5-3.5	20-25	2.0-3.4
Rabbit	13[a]	28[a]	0[a]
Rainbow trout	0	3.0	0.21
Rat	0.3-15[b]	12	7
Steppe lemming	0.8	22	0.9

[a]After one dose.

[b]After repeated administration.

Sources: Data from Dyer et al. (1965), Weisburger and Weisburger (1973), and Weisburger (1980).

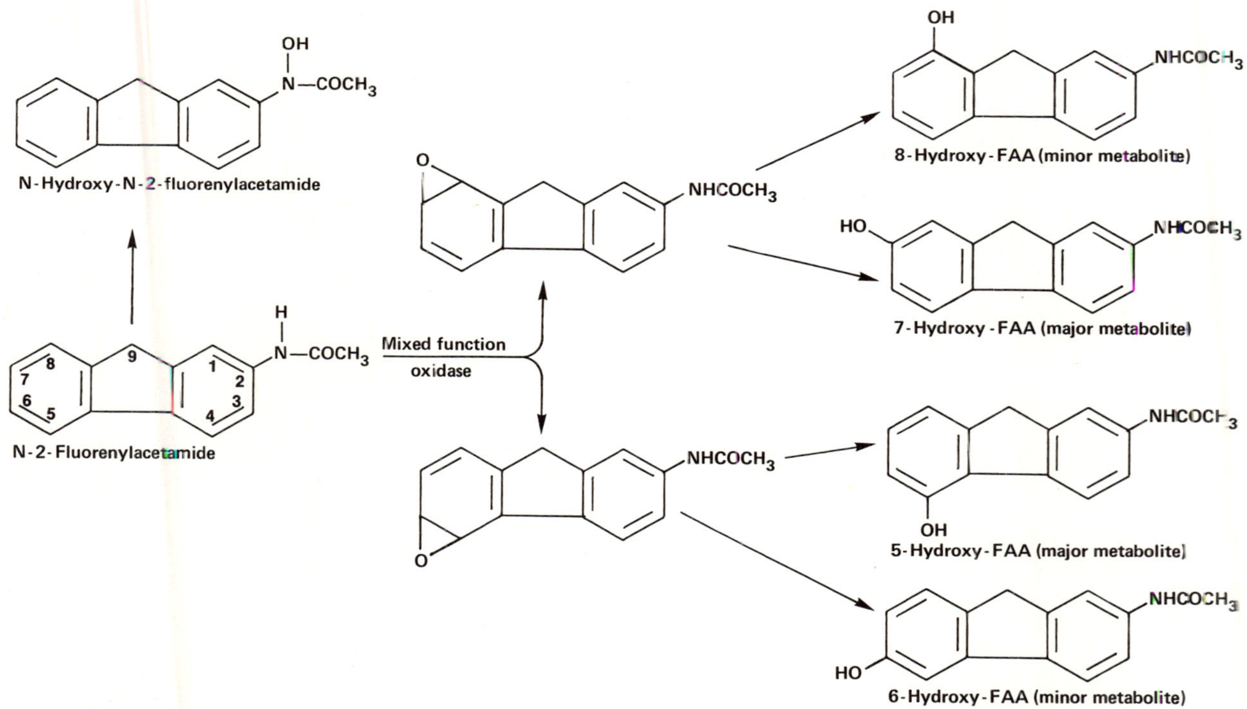

FIGURE 1 Possible mechanism of formation of 5-, 6-, 7-, and 8-hydroxy-2-fluorenylacetamide.

The formation of the 1- and 3-OH-FAA cannot be explained in this manner. The decrease in specific activity of the 1-OH- and 3-OH-FAA isolated as urinary metabolites from a combination of 9-^{14}C-FAA plus N-OH-FAA led to the conclusion that the o-amidophenols were formed by isomerization of N-OH-FAA (Miller and Miller, 1960). Studies with an inducible enzyme from rat liver confirmed this finding (Gutmann and Erickson, 1969, 1972). A report that tautomeric forms of N-OH-FAA exist may partially explain why both o-amidophenols are formed from N-OH-FAA (Lhoest et al., 1978).

Thus oxidation of FAA at various ring positions as well as the aliphatic type 9-position represents a major pathway for detoxication. Conjugation with glucuronic acid or sulfuric acid furnishes a means to solubilize and excrete the hydroxylated derivatives fairly rapidly. However, an appreciable portion of unidentified material remains. For example, arene oxides and glutathione conjugates of FAA have not yet been identified.

2. N-Hydroxylation

The discovery that hydroxylation of FAA also occurred on the nitrogen affording an activated metabolite led to an outpouring of research in this area. Various reviews have appeared on N-hydroxylation and the further metabolic reactions of the N-hydroxy derivative (Kiese, 1966; Miller and Miller, 1966, 1969b, 1976; Irving, 1970; Neumann, 1970; Weisburger and Weisburger, 1973; Kriek, 1974).

a. Species and strain differences

There are appreciable species differences in the extent of N-hydroxylation of FAA both in vivo and in vitro (Table 1). Usually there is a fair degree of correlation between N-hydroxylation in a given species and susceptibility to tumor induction by FAA. However, exceptions occur such as the monkey which apparently has not developed tumors from FAA, even though this species is capable of N-hydroxylation.

Appreciable strain differences in the response to FAA and degree of metabolic activation also occur. One study in rat strains correlated the level of N-hydroxylation with the effect in liver and mammary gland (Gutmann et al., 1972). In contrast, although most mouse strains are susceptible to FAA, the X/Gf mouse, which formed and excreted N-OH-FAA at a level comparable to the susceptible strains (Grantham et al., 1976), was resistant to the carcinogenicity of FAA (Goldfeder, 1974).

b. Effects of enzyme inducers on N-hydroxylation

The effect of simultaneous administration of FAA and various enzyme inducers such as phenobarbital or 3-methylcholanthrene generally has been to decrease the carcinogenicity of FAA by stimulation of ring hydroxylation (Cramer et al., 1960a; Miller and Miller, 1969a, b; Weisburger and Weisburger, 1973). Other compounds with a similar effect have been butylated hydroxytoluene (BHT) (Grantham et al., 1973; Ulland et al., 1973), acetanilide (Yamamoto et al., 1968), p-hydroxyacetanilide (Weisburger et al., 1973; Yamamoto et al., 1973; Mohan et al., 1976). Sodium cyclamate or sodium saccharin (Ershoff and Bajwa, 1974) and polychlorinated biphenyls (Makiura et al., 1974) also inhibited the carcinogenicity of FAA, although no studies were performed to ascertain the metabolic pattern. Although some of these compounds increased the level of N-OH-FAA excreted, they generally decreased the amount of carcinogen bound to DNA (Grantham et al., 1968).

Many factors can influence the levels of metabolites of FAA, through alterations in the activating or detoxifying enzymes. For example, a diet marginally deficient in the lipotropes choline, methionine, or folic acid changed the metabolic pattern. Although female rats were not affected, male rats fed FAA and a lipotrope-deficient diet had much lower levels of hepatic S-adenosylmethionine than normal. In such rats the urinary excretion of N-OH-FAA was higher and that of 5-OH-FAA was lower than usual. In female rats on the deficient diet N-OH-FAA levels were lower, while 5-OH-FAA was higher than in rats on normal diets. Excretion of 7-OH-FAA was not affected by the deficient diet. The altered metabolism of FAA apparently correlated well with the effects of the deficient diet on carcinogenesis by

FAA (Poirier et al., 1977). As an additional example of dietary effects, rats given corn oil excreted more N-OH-FAA glucuronide in the urine after an injection of FAA than did rats fed beef tallow (Castro et al., 1978).

Indole also decreased the toxic and carcinogenic action of FAA by lowering the production of N-OH-FAA (Hopp et al., 1976). The continued joint administration of indole and FAA protected the livers, thus allowing the animals to live longer and develop bladder carcinomas (Oyasu et al., 1963, 1970b, 1972).

Phenobarbital and BHT had biphasic effects for they inhibited the carcinogenicity of FAA if given simultaneously but enhanced the effect if administered after FAA (Peraino et al., 1973, 1977). Histochemical and autoradiographic studies showed that loss of glucose-6-phosphatase was the best indication of the transformation to abnormal cells after feeding FAA followed by phenobarbital (Pugh and Goldfarb, 1978). Feeding of phenobarbital prior to injection of labeled FAA reduced binding to DNA (Matsushima et al., 1972); if phenobarbital was fed after FAA treatment there was little effect on DNA binding (Mushlin and Peraino, 1974).

A single injection of piperonyl butoxide enhanced N-hydroxylation of FAA in hamster liver while binding to DNA or RNA was severalfold greater than in controls (Friedman and Woods, 1977). Piperonyl butoxide increased the toxicity of FAA and N-OH-FAA in newborn mice. There was no consistent influence on the carcinogenic effects; the incidence of FAA-hepatocarcinogenesis was not affected by the butoxide. However, in male mice given N-OH-FAA, piperonyl butoxide increased liver tumors somewhat (Fujii and Epstein, 1979).

Pretreatment of rats with 3-aminotriazole caused an increase in urinary excretion of both N- and ring-hydroxylated derivatives of FAA. Although ring hydroxylation by liver microsomes was decreased in the aminotriazole treated rats, esterification of N-OH-FAA was also inhibited (Lotlikar et al., 1973a).

c. Esterification and further activation of N-OH-FAA

It became evident that esterification of the N-hydroxy group of N-OH-FAA by acetate, phosphate, sulfate, or some other grouping was a necessary step in the activation process. Initially, in vivo experiments with excess sulfate (cf., Weisburger and Weisburger, 1973) and the presence of greater levels of a sulfotransferase enzyme in the livers of more susceptible male rats (Jackson and Irving, 1972) led to the thought that esterification with sulfate was necessary. However, the lack of sulfotransferase in other tissues affected by FAA or N-OH-FAA emphasized the probability that some other ester may also be involved. A study in rats fed FAA or N-OH-FAA showed that either Na_2SeO_3 or retinoic acid inhibited liver sulfotransferase levels by 50%. Conversely, glucuronyl transferase was increased, especially by the selenite (Daoud and Griffin, 1978). One would thus expect selenite or retinoic acid to have a protective effect against FAA or N-OH-FAA carcinogenesis.

The sulfotransferase enzyme has been separated from adult male rat liver and purified to 2000-fold the activity of the whole liver homogenate. Several steps, combining chromatography, gel filtration, and other procedures were needed to obtain a homogeneous preparation. A pH optimum of 6.3, activation by Mg^{2+}, an estimated molecular weight of 68,000, and stabilization by thiols were some of the physicochemical characteristics of this N-OH-FAA sulfotransferase (Wu and Straub, 1976).

In a parallel study the pH optimum for the sulfotransferase, dependent on 3'-phosphoadenosine 5'-phosphosulfate sulfonation of the N-OH group by hepatic cytosol, was 6.6 for N-OH-FAA, slightly higher than for the N-hydroxy derivative of monomethyl-4-aminoazobenzene. Hepatic cytosols from male rats had the greatest activity among the different species examined. Under conditions where certain other N-hydroxyarylamines served as substrates for the sulfotransferase, N-OH-FA did not react appreciably (Kadlubar et al., 1976).

Both N-O sulfation of N-OH-FAA and C-O sulfation of 7-OH-FAA were studied in fetal tissues from humans, monkeys, and guinea pigs and compared with results in adult rats. Rat liver was most efficient in forming the sulfate of N-OH-FAA, but certain human fetal tissues had measurable activity. Likewise, adult rat liver was preeminent with respect to forming a phosphate ester of N-OH-FAA. Human fetal liver had very high activity for making the sulfate ester of 7-OH-FAA, up to 10-12-fold that of fetal guinea pig liver (Namkung et al., 1977). Thus human fetal tissues have measurable levels of the enzymes involved in metabolism of FAA.

An independent investigation on binding of N-OH-FAA to tRNA in an isolated liver cell system showed that the acetyl group of N-OH-FAA was retained in the adduct. Furthermore, the degree of adduct formation was dependent on the sulfate concentration, an indication that the reaction probably was mediated through sulfate conjugation (King et al., 1976). The results reemphasize the fact that different tissues may have distinct activation pathways for arylhydroxamic acids. In addition, the liver sulfotransferase levels may be related to the degree of toxicity of N-OH-FAA (Irving, 1975). Thus several toxic actions, an acute effect, and a chronic effect (carcinogenicity), may be mediated through sulfotransferase.

An enzyme was also identified in rat liver which transferred the N-acetyl group of N-OH-FAA to the oxygen of the hydroxylamine, producing a very reactive and unstable N-acetoxyfluorenamine. The facile reaction of the intermediate with tRNA served as a measure of its reactivity. The enzyme, a sulfhydryl-dependent enzyme had a molecular weight of approximately 28,000 and was present in liver, kidney, stomach, small intestine, and colon with less activity in lung and spleen (King, 1974). An extensive study on the levels of acyltransferase in various strains and species showed that liver had the highest levels of all organs; rabbits, hamsters, and rats in descending order were the species with highest levels of enzyme (King and Olive, 1975). There was also evidence for a second type of acyltransferase in the small intestine of the rat, identified by immunological techniques and gel filtration (Olive and King, 1975). Cytosols from human small intestine, colon, or liver also showed acyltransferase capability, the small intestine being most active, indicating that humans would also be at risk from the arylhydroxamic acids (King et al., 1975). The enzyme was also present in lactating mammary glands of rats; Sprague-Dawley rats had twice the levels of Fischer rats (King et al., 1979).

In addition, the excretion of glucuronides of the arylhydroxamic acids in the urine and their possible reaction with bladder tissue, either as the glucuronides or as reactants formed on hydrolysis, led to investigation of such esters as activated forms of N-hydroxy arylamines. Treatment of hepatic microsomes from dogs, rats, or humans with uridine 5'-diphosphoglucuronic acid in the presence of various N-hydroxy amines or amides, including N-OH-FAA and N-OH-FA, led to water-soluble products, identified as the N-glucuronides. These glucuronides were relatively stable at neutral pH but at acid pH were rapidly hydrolyzed to reactive intermediates which bound to nucleic acids (Kadlubar et al., 1977). In contrast, the O-glucuronide of N-OH-FA, whether prepared chemically or by enzymic deacetylation of the corresponding glucuronide of N-OH-FAA, was quite unstable and rapidly formed nucleic acid adducts at neutral pH (Cardona and King, 1976). Thus, the presence of N-glucuronides in the bladder, combined with the acidity of the urine in species such as dogs and humans may enhance the formation of the ultimate carcinogens from the glucuronide.

Other possible mechanisms for the activation of arylhydroxamic acids have been delineated to some extent. One of these involves oxidation, probably by various peroxidases, to a free nitroxide radical which dismutates to form a nitrosoarene and an N-acetoxy-N-acetylaminoarene (Bartsch et al., 1972; Scribner and Naimy, 1973). Since peroxidases occur in various tissues (cf., Reigh et al., 1978), this is a feasible explanation for an activation pathway of FAA. Another report suggests that acethydroxamic acids, in the presence of certain rat liver proteins, act as donor for transfer of the acetyl group to the O-group of other aromatic hydroxylamines forming electrophilic N-acetoxyhydroxylamines (Bartsch et al., 1973). However, it is difficult to reconcile this concept with the fact that arylhydroxylamines are generally not very stable and may not exist as such in tissue, unless they are formed in situ by deacylation of the acethydroxamic acid. Under the latter circumstances such a mechanism may hold.

Physiological conditions under which N-OH-FAA might be activated through the free radical route have been studied. Cyanide did not inhibit a N-OH-FAA-horseradish peroxidase system, but ascorbate was oxidized preferentially if present. Besides nitrosofluorene and N-acetoxy-FAA, a third unidentified product was also formed (Floyd et al., 1976a). Linoleic acid hydroperoxide, in the presence of methemoglobin or hematin, also activated N-OH-FAA through the free radical route (Floyd et al., 1976b). Other hydroperoxides such as cumene hydroperoxide were effective (Floyd, 1976; Floyd and Soong, 1977b). A nitroxyl free radical was postulated as an obligatory intermediate in the oxidative activation of N-OH-FAA (Floyd and Soong, 1977a). The 2-nitrosofluorene produced in these reactions then reacted further with the lipids in cell membranes to produce a stable free nitroxide radical which became rigidly fixed in the cell membrane (Floyd et al., 1978).

Although phosphorylation of N-OH-FAA also yields a reactive intermediate (Lotlikar and Wasserman, 1970; Lotlikar and Luha, 1971), such esters have not yet been identified as metabolites of FAA in vivo.

It is apparent that several mechanisms are available by which N-OH-FAA can be activated further to a moiety capable of reacting with cellular macromolecules.

B. In Vitro

Metabolism studies in vitro offer several advantages over studies in animals. Tissue specificity can be determined as well as primary products without the complications of secondary metabolism or conjugating mechanisms. However, in vitro metabolism may not always reflect accurately the picture in vivo.

With FAA the main reactions studied in vitro include hydroxylation, deacetylation-acetylation, reduction of N-OH-FAA to FAA, and esterification of N-OH-FAA. Reviews on this subject have appeared (Irving, 1970; Weisburger and Weisburger, 1971, 1973).

The early work on hydroxylation of FAA by rat liver slices or homogenates has been reviewed (Weisburger and Weisburger, 1958b). Seal and Gutmann (1959) found that liver from hamster yielded the most active fractions, followed by guinea pig, rat, rabbit, and fowl and identified various ring-hydroxylated metabolites of FAA.

With the discovery of N-hydroxylation in vivo, this observation was extended to in vitro systems. Irving (1964) reported that with a NADPH generating system N-OH-FAA was formed from FAA by liver microsomes from hamsters, dogs, rabbits, chickens, and cats, in decreasing order. Because of their metabolic capability hamster microsomes were used as an adjunct in a transformation system to detect carcinogens such as FAA and derivatives (Poiley et al., 1979). Rat and mouse liver microsomes were active when NADPH was added, but guinea pig or human liver microsomes were not. These species variations were confirmed (Lotlikar et al., 1967). Pretreatment with 3-methylcholanthrene increased N-hydroxylation only slightly in rat liver microsomes, while in hamster liver microsomes there was a sizable increase. This effect held even when only low levels of FAA were used (Lotlikar et al., 1978). Likewise, there was a great variation in the level of N-hydroxylation by different samples of human liver (Enomoto and Sato, 1967; Dybing et al., 1979b). Both human and primate fetal and placental tissues had the capacity to oxidize FAA to the N- and C-hydroxy derivatives (Juchau et al., 1975; Juchau et al., 1976). 2,3,7,8-Tetrachlorodibenzo-p-dioxin administration to rats increased manyfold both N- and C-hydroxylation of FAA by maternal and fetal rat liver. There was no inducing effect on placental tissue (Berry et al., 1976).

Another report implies that N-hydroxylation of FAA in vitro with an NADPH generating system could be enhanced by lowering the amount of microsomal protein and substrate and using a HEPES buffer system (Baetcke et al., 1974); as much as 30% of FAA could be N-hydroxylated by mouse liver microsomes with this method.

The enzyme systems involved in N-hydroxylation of FAA have been investigated through differential induction and inhibition by 3-methylcholanthrene, phenobarbital, 3-aminotriazole, and carbon monoxide.

Since 3-methylcholanthrene pretreatment of hamsters did not alter N-oxide formation from incubation of liver microsomes with N,N-dimethylaniline whereas N-hydroxylation of

FAA was increased, it was concluded that a mixed function amine oxidase was not involved in N-hydroxylation (Lotlikar et al., 1973b).

N-Hydroxylation of FAA in liver microsomes from mice and hamsters was inhibited by carbon monoxide, by pretreatment of the animals with cobaltous chloride, and by an immune globulin against microsomal NADPH-cytochrome c reductase. These results led to the conclusion that N-hydroxylation was accomplished by a cytochrome P-450 dependent mixed function oxidase (Thorgeirsson et al., 1973). Since the degree of inhibition with carbon monoxide varied for the different positions hydroxylated, more than one P-450 may have been involved (Lotlikar and Zaleski, 1974). The electrophoretic separation of at least two polypeptides, which migrated near P-450, from livers of rats fed FAA tends to substantiate such a premise (Cameron et al., 1976a).

The presence or absence of induction of aryl hydrocarbon hydroxylase in mice could be correlated with N-hydroxylation of FAA in the livers after treatment with various microsomal enzyme inducers, indicating that a cytochrome P_1-450 was involved in N-hydroxylation (Thorgeirsson et al., 1975). The association between metabolism of xenobiotics and aryl hydrocarbon hydroxylase inducibility has been reviewed (Thorgeirsson and Nebert, 1976). The N-hydroxylase activity of genetically resistant mice could not be increased by partial hepatectomy and 3-methylcholanthrene treatment (Boobis et al., 1977). 3-Methylcholanthrene administration to rhesus monkeys led to six- or seven-fold increases in N-hydroxylation of FAA by liver microsomes, with a concurrent increase in hepatic cytochrome P-450, detected by electrophoresis as a polypeptide of molecular weight 54,000 (Thorgeirsson et al., 1978).

Both cytochrome P-450 and NADPH-cytochrome c reductase fractions of rat liver microsomes were required for optimum N- and ring-hydroxylation. Proteinase treatment and solubilization with Triton X-100 were important for partial purification of the cytochrome P-450 fraction (Lotlikar and Zaleski, 1975).

Various detergentlike molecules affected hydroxylation of FAA by hamster liver. Thus Triton X-100 inhibited N- and ring-hydroxylation appreciably in whole microsomal preparations while deoxycholate inhibited both hydroxylations completely. In a reconstituted microsomal system Triton X-100 increased N- more than ring-hydroxylation, whereas cholate and deoxycholate stimulated ring hydroxylation more than N-hydroxylation (Lotlikar and Dwyer, 1976). These results led to a study of the phospholipid requirement for the hydroxylase system. Removal of lipids from the microsomal powder of hamster liver decreased appreciably the level of hydroxylation, but activity was restored by adding back the extracted lipid, phosphatidylcholine, or dilauroyl phosphatidylcholine (Lotlikar et al., 1977).

The level of N-hydroxylase in rat liver microsomes was increased three- to 12-fold by pretreatment of rats with FAA. Although the system N-hydroxylating FAA is either a cytochrome P-450 or P_1-450, when FAA was injected, the content of P-450 or P_1-450 was not altered; neither were the activities of NADPH-cytochrome c reductase or NADPH-cytochrome P-450 reductase increased. Liver microsomal activity in mice fed FAA was also increased over that of mice given control diets (Lazear et al., 1978). Thus FAA may induce an unknown electron carrier associated with the hepatic mixed function oxidase (Malejka-Giganti et al., 1978). This self-induction by FAA of the enzymes increasing N-hydroxylation affords an explanation for the increase in N-OH-FAA with time as FAA is fed.

As mentioned previously, 9-OH-2-FAA is a relatively minor urinary metabolite of FAA in rats and guinea pigs. In a liver microsome system 9-OH-2-FAA could be isolated, as well as 9-oxo-FAA and N-(2-fluorenyl)glycolamide, indicating some differences between in vivo and in vitro metabolism (Benkert et al., 1975).

The oxidation of FAA-isomers has been investigated with 2-FAA and the marginal carcinogen 3-FAA, using the susceptible rat and the resistant guinea pig as experimental species. N-Hydroxylation of 2-FAA by hepatic microsomes from rats was 40- to 50-fold greater than was N-hydroxylation of 3-FAA. In guinea pig microsomes N-hydroxylation of 2-FAA was much lower than in the rat even though both 2- and 3-FAA were bound to the cytochrome P_1-450 of the guinea pig liver microsomes (Gutmann and Bell, 1977). Of interest was that liver microsomes from guinea pigs and rats converted 3-FAA to 9-OH-3-FAA which was an intermediate in formation of 9-oxo-3-FAA (Kaplan and Gutmann, 1979). 9-Hydroxylation was not increased by pretreatment with 3-methylcholanthrene, suggesting that a different microsomal hemoprotein from P-450 or P_1-450 was involved (Kaplan et al., 1978). These results also indicate a difference between the relative amounts of metabolites formed in vitro and in vivo (cf., Weisburger, 1961).

Intact dog bladder, microsomes, and bladder mucosa have been tested for their capability to N-oxidize various arylamines including 2-FA. However, the level of N-oxidation was very low, suggesting that N-oxidation occurs mostly in the liver and the role of the bladder is minimal (Brill, 1977).

Another reaction studied in vitro has been the acetylation of various arylamines, including 2-FA, by liver cytosol from various species. Although hamster had the highest activity, there was no correlation between rate of acetylation of 2-FA and susceptibility to carcinogenicity (Lower and Bryan, 1973). Regarding deacetylation of FAA by unfortified liver microsomes, hamster was most effective, followed by dog, mouse, rat, and guinea pig. 4-Acetylaminobiphenyl was a better substrate than FAA for dog liver microsomes (Lower and Bryan, 1976).

Isolated rat hepatocytes formed deacetylated, oxidized, and conjugated metabolites from FAA. Pretreatment of the animals with the inducer β-naphthoflavone increased the levels of C-hydroxy and conjugated derivatives appreciably but led to only a slight increase in deacetylation (Dybing et al., 1979a). The rate of acetylation of 2-fluorenamine by N-acetyltransferase isolated from rabbit or human liver showed variations depending on the genetic background of the tissue donors (Glowinski et al., 1978).

To summarize, oxidation of FAA apparently is mediated through an inducible enzyme of the P-450 family. There are indications, however, that other hemoproteins may be involved in some of these metabolic oxidations.

IV. EFFECTS OF FAA ON BIOLOGICAL SYSTEMS

The toxicity of FAA and its derivatives to lower forms of life, especially insects, was the factor which eventually led to the discovery of its carcinogenicity (cf., Weisburger and Weisburger, 1958b). The effect in insects was proposed as a short-term test for putative carcinogens. 2-FAA, N-OH-FAA, 2,7-fluorenediamine, and 7-fluoro-2-FAA all severely affected growth and development of the larvae of the housefly and inhibited pupation and adult emergence. Noncarcinogenic compounds such as fluorene were not effective (Shortino et al., 1963; Cantwell et al., 1966). However, FAA is also toxic to other species, from bacteria and flagellates (Moewus, 1960) to mammals. Embryonic development of zebrafish was retarded, partly due to decreased RNA content and impaired carbohydrate metabolism after administration of FAA (Hisaoka, 1958a, b). Developmental anomalies also occurred in mice exposed transplacentally (Izumi, 1962). Rats given a toxic dose of FAA showed a transient rise in the mitotic rate in adrenocortical cells; there was no correlation between organ weight and proliferative activity (Danz et al., 1976). Cyclic AMP in the adrenals was initially increased but then decreased to subnormal levels following FAA (Danz and Kittlick, 1977). With N-OH-FAA there were appreciable strain differences in the toxic effect in rats (Irving, 1975).

As noted with other aromatic amines, FAA caused anemia and formation of inclusion or Heinz bodies in the blood of mice treated with FAA (Martucci et al., 1961).

Administration of FAA has led to alterations in many components of biological systems, to be discussed in this section.

A. Lipids, Lipoproteins, Cholesterol, and Related Structures

A short-term feeding study as well as in vitro tests indicated that FAA was carried by serum lipoproteins (Avigan, 1959). Increases occurred in phospholipid levels per parenchymal cell of the liver during FAA feeding (Rees et al., 1962). Disk electrophoretic separation of serum lipoproteins from rats fed FAA revealed that a new peak representing a high density lipoprotein appeared during the first week of feeding. Changes in low density lipoprotein were not evident until after 15 or more weeks of feeding FAA (Narayan, 1967). In further investigations Narayan (1970) isolated the lipoproteins of rats by ultracentrifugation after intervals of up to 1 year on a diet containing FAA but deficient in essential fatty acids. These longer studies confirmed the sizable increases in both high-density and low-density lipoproteins in tumor-bearing rats.

Feeding FAA led to a loss of control of cholesterol synthesis in rat liver and wide variations from animal to animal (Horton and Sabine, 1971). In livers that had progressed to hyperplastic nodules or hepatomas after FAA, the uptake of an oral dose of cholesterol was almost equal to that in normal liver and severalfold that seen in transplantable hepatomas. In primary hepatomas the rate of cholesterol uptake was related to the degree of differentiation (Horton et al., 1973b). Further investigations showed that the lack of regulation of cholesterol synthesis as induced by FAA was probably the result of a defect in intracellular storage of cholesterol, rather than defective uptake (Horton et al., 1973a).

Although hyperplastic nodules had higher than normal levels of total, protein-bound, and ganglioside sialic acids, the total lipid content, the phospholipid distribution pattern, and the fatty acid composition of total lipids, neutral lipids, and/or polar lipids did not differ from control tissues. Free and esterified sterols were higher in the nodules (Merritt et al., 1976). Additional studies have delineated the pattern of the mono- and disialogangliosides in the livers of normal fetal, newborn, infant, weanling, and adult rats and in the livers of rats fed FAA. The monosialoganglioside pathway appeared to be repressed during adult development; during tumor development this pathway was restored and the disialoganglioside pathway was repressed (Merritt et al., 1978b). The activities of the biosynthetic enzymes involved in these pathways were correspondingly altered (Merritt et al., 1978a).

In a model system FAA bound to egg phosphatidylcholine, indicating it may be membrane bound (Tipping et al., 1979). Correspondingly, in rats fed FAA an increase in antioxidative activity of liver microsomal lipids was associated with an increase in phosphatidycholine and a decrease in phosphatidylethanolamine (Burlakova et al., 1978).

However, phospholipid levels as well as the phospholipid:cholesterol ratio were increased in preneoplastic and neoplastic liver membranes from rats fed FAA. The activity of 5'-nucleotidase was decreased but the various forms of ATPase were not affected in the liver membranes of the carcinogen-treated animals (Chandrasekhara and Narayan, 1970).

One of the initial actions of FAA in the liver was to induce cell proliferation, an effect which was reversible if FAA was discontinued (Laird and Barton, 1961). In addition, 2-FAA led to alterations in the granular endoplasmic reticulum, which became irreversible after long exposure, in the rat hepatocyte (Merkow et al., 1967; Flaks, 1968, 1970, 1971). In a model system FAA led to removal of the ribosomes from rat liver membranes when incubated with the membranes in the presence of NADPH and/or sodium sulfate (Williams and Parry, 1975).

In pancreatic exocrine cells 2-FAA also produced an irreversible lesion of the granular endoplasmic reticulum but did not induce neoplasms (Flaks and Moody, 1969). Of interest is that the noncarcinogenic analogue, 4-FAA, caused similar changes, along with mitochondrial damage and focal cytoplasmic degradation, although secretory protein synthesis was not significantly affected (Flaks and Lucas, 1972). The effects of 4-FAA persisted up to 12 months after cessation of feeding (Flaks and Lucas, 1973).

Lysosomes from rabbit liver were not disrupted by FA and only slightly by N-OH-FAA (Weissmann et al., 1968). However, in rats 2-FAA increased the size of hepatic lysosomes, involving increases in the specific activities and a redistribution of the enzymes β-glucuronidase and acid deoxyribonuclease (Berg and Christoffersen, 1974).

Although various hepatocarcinogens, including FAA, caused sizable swelling of rat liver mitochondria, structurally related noncarcinogens produced only small changes (Arcos et al., 1961). The four isomeric FAAs did not induce an adenosine triphosphate-energized change in mitochondrial volume (Hadler and Daniel, 1973). The corresponding N-hydroxy compounds were effective in agreement with their relative carcinogenicity in the rat. N-Acetoxy-FAA induced a delayed ATP energized increase in mitochondrial volume in vitro, probably through conversion to N-OH-FAA (Hadler and Demetriou, 1976).

Acute ethionine treatment of rats also leads to toxic effects on the liver with disaggregation of the polyribosomes and inhibition of protein synthesis. However, a combination of FAA with ethionine suppressed the effects on the polyribosomes and protein synthesis. Rats force-fed diets containing FAA and then an acute toxic dose of various other hepatocarcinogens showed variable responses, with respect to both protein synthesis and polyribosomal disaggregation (Sidransky and Verney, 1978).

A single intraperitoneal injection of N-OH-FAA led to numerous helical polysomes in the hepatic cytoplasm at 2 or 6 hr after treatment but not by 24 hr later. Polyribosome disaggregation occurred as well as inhibition of protein synthesis (Popp and Shinozuka, 1974). In partially hepatectomized rats N-OH-FAA caused dilation of the nuclear envelope and rough endoplasmic reticulum, vacuolization, and evagination of the perinuclear membranes. Furthermore, there was a dose-dependent inhibition of the incorporation of leucine into the nuclear membranes (Glazer and La Via, 1975).

There have been several other reports on the effects of FAA on the structures of cellular components. Electron microscopy was used to examine the fine structure of liver nuclei after FAA (Yasuzumi et al., 1970; Flaks and Basley, 1979). Similarly, after a 20-hr treatment period with 2-FA an increase in free ribosomes, disorganization of the cisternal endoplasmic reticulum, enlargement of the spongy endoplasmic reticulum, and an increase in glycogen occurred (Gustafsson and Afzelius, 1963). Some of these effects were not specific to FAA but also occurred after treatment with other carcinogens.

B. Enzymes

Administration of FAA leads to considerable alteration in certain enzymes, an effect that may not be specific but which may apply for various toxic or carcinogenic compounds.

1. Carbohydrate Metabolizing Enzymes

Addition of FAA to rat diaphragms incubated in a phosphate-saline medium caused only a slight decrease in glucose utilization and a sizable depression in glucose content (Gershbein, 1970). A more extensive study indicated that dietary induction of various carbohydrate-metabolizing enzymes of liver was lacking in livers of rats fed FAA for 2-4 weeks. Continued feeding of FAA increased only glucose-6-phosphate dehydrogenase; the levels of other enzymes seemingly were not affected (Poirier et al., 1969). Carbohydrate metabolizing enzymes of premalignant areas and hepatomas induced by FAA in rats have been followed (Sato et al., 1978). As the histological differentiation moved toward more malignant, glucose-6-phosphatase, fructose-1,6-bisphosphatase, and the isozymes of glucose-adenosine 5'-triphosphate phosphotransferase, pyruvate kinase, aldolase, and glycogen phosphorylase decreased gradually. In some cases the levels of the enzymes rose slowly in nonhepatic tissue. There were some differences in the variations from normal enzyme levels among the hepatomas induced by FAA, diethylnitrosamine and 3'-methyl-4-dimethylaminoazobenzene. However, increased biosynthesis of a muscle-type aldolase was observed in rat liver during administration of FAA (Silber et al., 1975). Similar results had been observed with muscle-type aldolase in rat liver after feeding the FAA derivative N,N',2,7-fluorenylenebisacetamide (Endo et al., 1970). Although gluconeogenic enzymes and xanthine oxidase decreased in host liver after feeding FAA, aspartate carbamoyltransferase increased. In the induced hepatocarcinoma, xanthine oxidase was not detected (Sapre et al., 1969).

Malic, isocitric, and glutamic dehydrogenases in rat liver generally decreased as the period of feeding FAA continued (Hou and Rees, 1961). Feeding FAA, in some cases with phenobarbital, led to tumors with new forms of aldehyde dehydrogenases which were detectable in areas of the liver where no tumor was detected by histological means (Feinstein et al., 1976). These isozymes, which were found only in the cytosol, were purified and characterized as existing as 105,000 dalton dimers composed of two subunits of 53,000 daltons (Lindahl and Feinstein, 1976). These hepatoma-specific isozymes were not the result of derepression of genes normally repressed in adult rat liver or other adult tissue (Lindahl, 1977). In hepatomas induced by FAA 15% of the total aldehyde dehydrogenase activity was identical immunochemically with normal liver cross-reacting material, but the other 85% was the hepatoma-specific type (Lindahl, 1978). In rat liver the isozyme pattern of pyruvate kinase changed during hepatocarcinogenesis from FAA from a predominance of isozyme L to K in hepatomas with the appearance of isozyme M in some hepatomas (Silber et al., 1978).

2. One-Carbon Enzymes

Feeding FAA to rats for periods up to 5 weeks led to significant decreases of various liver enzymes concerned with the metabolism of 1-carbon compounds, namely histidase, urocanase, N-formimino-L-glutamate:H_4-folate 5-formiminotransferase (FIGLU transferase), formylase, and methylene-H_4-folate dehydrogenase (Poirier and Pitot, 1969). Serine hydroxymethylase and dihydrofolate reductase were not affected (Poirier et al., 1972). Administration of a choline-deficient diet produced a similar pattern as did feeding FAA, indicating that either FAA or choline deficiency decreased the levels of the enzymes involved in the formylation of H_4-folate.

Baxter and Byvoet (1974a) found that histone methylation by an arginine methyltransferase from rat liver cytoplasm was inhibited by N-OH-FAA, N-acetoxy-FAA, and especially by N-OH-FA, which was the most effective inhibitor of all the carcinogens tested. It was theorized that N-OH-FA may be esterified in situ to an electrophile that may attack histone methylation sites. Likewise, N-OH-FA, N-OH-FAA, and N-acetoxy-FAA inhibited the methylation of histones by endogenous histone lysine methyltransferase, with N-OH-FA having the greatest effect (Baxter and Byvoet, 1974b). S-Adenosylmethionine synthetases gradually altered during FAA-hepatocarcinogenesis with the loss of the low K_m isozyme in the hepatocellular carcinomas (Liau et al., 1979).

3. Cyclic AMP

Cyclic AMP (adenosine 3',5'-monophosphate) plays an important role in the regulation of growth and differentiation, a property lost during carcinogenesis. The levels of cyclic AMP and the enzyme that catalyzes its formation, adenyl cyclase, were determined during the feeding of FAA to rats. Rats bearing hepatocarcinomas had increased levels of adenyl cyclase compared to controls. Adrenalin had very little stimulatory effect on cyclic AMP formation in tumor tissues in vitro, but adrenalin had a distinct stimulatory action in the premalignant livers. This change occurred before histological signs of malignancy appeared, and made the hormone stimulation pattern resemble that of immature liver (Christoffersen et al., 1972). The increased ability of liver from FAA-treated rats to produce cyclic AMP after adrenalin stimulation held both for homogenates and for liver slices where the cyclic AMP accumulated. However, cyclic AMP phosphodiesterase activity in the treated rats was not increased significantly (Christoffersen et al., 1974). The stimulatory effect on cyclic AMP formation held for isolated parenchymal liver cells from FAA-fed rats, in which the effect of isoprenalin was greater than that of adrenalin which surpassed that of phenylephrine (Christoffersen and Berg, 1975). FAA was most effective of various carcinogens examined for the cyclic AMP effect with adrenalin, followed by 3'-methyl-4-dimethylaminoazobenzene and 4-dimethylaminoazobenzene (Christoffersen, 1975).

4. Other Cellular Constituents and Enzymes

During feeding of FAA to rats, the excretion of N^1-methyl-2-pyridone-5-carboxamide (2-Py) increased gradually and reached a sustained plateau when hyperplastic nodules appeared. The formation of 2-Py in FAA-treated rat liver was higher than in control rat liver, while the activity of formation of N^1-methyl-4-pyridone-5-carboxamide (4-Py) decreased (Ohkubo et al., 1977). The enzymes involved were separated by diethylaminoethyl cellulose column chromatography and identified as N^1-methylnicotinamide oxidase I, producing 2-Py, and N^1-methylnicotinamide oxidase II, producing 4-Py. In the livers of rats fed FAA there was a shift toward oxidase I, while oxidase II was minimal or not detectable (Ohkubo and Fujimura, 1978).

FAA increased the activity of nicotine oxidase in rat liver. In turn, nicotine stimulated somewhat the activity of FAA-hydroxylase in liver microsomes (Yamamoto et al., 1966). Rats fed FAA excreted increased amounts of xanthurenic acid, rynurenic acid, and hydroxykynurenine after a challenge dose of L-tryptophan (Dyer and Morris, 1961). Similarly, FAA increased 2-hydroxylation of biphenyl in a fortified rat liver microsomal system (McPherson et al., 1976). 2-FA likewise had some activity as an inducer of zoxazolamine hydroxylase synthesis (Buu-Hoi and Hien, 1966). FAA inhibited the effect of neoepinephrine in isolated rat atria but not in guinea pig atria. There is no explanation for this difference (Gurkalo and Pliss, 1978). This effect illustrates the potent influence one drug can have on the action of another.

During a period of feeding FAA for 24 weeks certain enzymes involved in detoxification reactions increased. These included glucuronyl transferase, glutathione reductase, and uridine-diphosphate glucose dehydrogenase. Enzymes that N-demethylated morphine or hydroxylated acetanilide actually decreased (Trams et al., 1961).

Although FAA was inactive, FA was very active, more so than estradiol, in stimulating DPNH oxidation by horseradish and uterine peroxidase in the presence of Mn^{2+} (Williams-Ashman and Johnson, 1960).

FAA and other carcinogens had no definite effect on the sulfhydryl levels in mouse skin (Calcutt and Doxey, 1962). However, FAA caused an increase in -SH levels in rat liver (Calcutt et al., 1960). There were no outstanding differences in coproporphyrin, uroporphyrin, and protoporphyrin levels between control and FAA-treated rats (Zawirska et al., 1971). Feeding FAA did not influence the conjugation of cholic acid, a bile component, with taurine (Songster et al., 1963).

5. Proteases

Relatively few studies have been done on the effects of FAA on proteases and similar enzyme systems, perhaps because so many earlier studies showed relatively little effect. However, the effect of FAA, N-OH-FAA, and 1-OH-FAA on liver catalase and arginase was determined in rats fed the compounds in the diet for several weeks. Both FAA and N-OH-FAA treatment decreased catalase levels but had no effect on arginase, while 1-OH-FAA had no effect on either enzyme. The conclusion was that FAA or a metabolite did not bind to catalase (King and Gutmann, 1964).

Both glutathione (Neish, 1967) and glutathionase or γ-glutamyl transpeptidase (Fiala and Fiala, 1973) in liver were gradually increased on feeding 2-FAA to rats. Since liver glutathionase is generally elevated during carcinogenesis the activation may be related to the carcinogenic process (Fiala and Fiala, 1973). Liver nodules induced by FAA had a 20-30-fold increase in glutamyl transpeptidase activity over that of control liver. The altered foci in the liver were readily differentiated by histochemical techniques (Cameron et al., 1978). Cells isolated from the individual early lesions and carried in culture maintained the high γ-glutamyl transpeptidase levels. However, enzyme activity could not be increased in cultured normal hepatocytes by exposure to various carcinogens (Laishes et al., 1978a). A similar increase in γ-glutamyl transpeptidase was observed in hepatocytes of hyperplastic areas and nodules or in carcinomas induced by N-OH-FAA (Harada et al., 1976). Feeding a choline-devoid diet containing FAA to rats after a single dose of diethylnitrosamine led to many more foci of γ-glutamyl transpeptidase positive hepatocytes than did the FAA-diet adequate in choline (Shinozuka et al., 1979).

An intestinal arylamidase was isolated from the soluble $110{,}000 \times g$ supernatant fraction of rat small intestine, which was very active in hydrolyzing the butyramide of FA, with FAA being the next best substrate. The activity from different species fell in the order rat > mouse > guinea pig > rabbit > man > dog (none) (Nagasawa et al., 1976).

Initially, the livers from rats fed FAA had decreased ability to synthesize urea in vitro (Burke and Miller, 1960), but had greatly increased metabolic capacity for methionine over that of normal liver (Burke and Gangloff, 1965). Feeding FA led to a higher capacity of microsomes to incorporate amino acids into protein (Arrhenius and Hultin, 1962). However, this increase was thought to be a secondary effect and that the initial action was to inhibit amino acid incorporation. High dietary levels of vitamin E masked the inhibitory action of FA (Hultin and Arrhenius, 1965).

There was an apparent defect in aspartate metabolism in livers of rats fed FAA (Burke and Gangloff, 1965). Rats force-fed a diet of casein hydrolysate along with FAA did not have increases in liver ornithine transamidase and histidase, as did controls. Some other enzymes involved in amino acid metabolism, such as tryptophan pyrrolase, serine dehydratase, and tyrosine-α-ketoglutarate transaminase showed no or relatively little effect from FAA (Poirier and Pitot, 1969).

6. Hyperplastic Nodules

Of widespread interest is the composition of the hyperplastic nodules induced in rats by feeding FAA for a limited time. Such nodules have been investigated in many respects since their use as a tool in predictive and morphological studies was proposed (Epstein et al., 1967; Merkow et al., 1969). These nodules also afforded a model for defining the changes between the hyperplastic state and the hepatocellular carcinoma (Teebor and Becker, 1971). In some respects they appeared as a distinct new cell population (Slifkin et al., 1972). In one respect the hyperplastic nodules resembled normal hepatocytes in that they were not agglutinated by the plant lectin concanavalin A; the cells from primary hepatocellular carcinomas induced by FAA were agglutinated by this lectin (Becker and Shurgin, 1975). On the other hand, hepatocytes from nodules induced by FAA had some resistance to the delaying action on the mitotic cycle by L-asparaginase administration after partial hepatectomy. Aggregates of resistant cells occurred in a number of these nodules, but the resistance was not associated with gross chromosomal alteration (Becker and Klein, 1971). The altered hepatocytes resulting from limited FAA treatment were quite susceptible to further changes from a single dose of dimethylnitrosamine and progressed to a high incidence of hepatic nodules and carcinomas. However, a single dose of N-OH-FAA after the subcarcinogenic dose of FAA led to only a few such lesions (Becker, 1975).

Interestingly, Jackson and Irving (1973b) reported that FAA was hepatotoxic to partially hepatectomized female rats and caused abnormal nodular regeneration, but these nodules did not progress to carcinomas. The cellular proliferation caused by the hepatectomy appeared thus to have had a protective action. Additional studies on FAA-induced nodules indicated that corticosteroid-mediated enzyme-regulatory mechanisms still held in the hyperplastic nodules. Glucose-6-phosphatase activity was increased by 24-hr starvation, while steroid administration increased tyrosine transaminase and tryptophan pyrrolase levels (Teebor and Seidman, 1970). Phenylalanine hydroxylase activity was greatly decreased in the hyperplastic nodules (Terawaki et al., 1967).

A sequential study of hyperplastic areas, using both histochemical and radioautographic techniques, demonstrated deficiencies in β-glucuronidase and glucose-6-phosphatase, as well as canalicular ATPase and phosphorylase (Kitagawa, 1971a). However, the hyperplastic areas became almost equivalent to normal adult rat liver by 9 weeks later (Kitagawa and Sugano, 1973), and regulatory mechanisms held for several enzymes (Kitagawa and Pitot, 1975).

Several important metabolizing enzymes, such as cytochrome P-450 and arylhydrocarbon hydroxylase, were diminished in the hyperplastic nodules (Cameron et al., 1976b; Okita et al., 1976; Koblyakov and Kolyada, 1978). However, during the course of feeding FAA, NADPH-cytochrome reductase increased (Kobylakov and Kolyada, 1978). Likewise the enzymes D-T diaphorase and glucose-6-phosphate dehydrogenase increased six- or four-fold, respectively, over normal in the hyperplastic nodules (Schor et al., 1978). A hepatotoxic dose of N-OH-FAA also decreased cytochromes P-450 and b_5 but not cytochrome c reductase or glucose-6-phosphatase (Thorgeirsson et al., 1976).

The unique resistance of hyperplastic nodules to the cytotoxic effects of carcinogens has led to the use of the hyperplastic cells to analyze the sequence of events in hepatocarcinogenesis. The components of the system are an initiator or hepatocarcinogen, such as diethylnitrosamine (DEN), a selective growth inhibitor, usually FAA, and a generalized potent growth stimulus such as partial hepatectomy. As an example, rats were injected with DEN, 2 weeks later were fed FAA in the diet for 1 week, and then partially hepatectomized. This regimen led to tiny basophilic foci which enlarged and by 6 weeks were histologically similar to hyperplastic liver nodules (Solt and Farber, 1976; Solt et al., 1977; Ogawa et al., 1979). In a few cases Kupffer cell sarcomas were noted in rats on the nitrosamine-FAA-partial hepatectomy regimen rather than neoplastic nodules or hepatocellular carcinomas (Chopra et al., 1979). The cells in these nodules were relatively resistant to the acute necrogenic action of carbon tetrachloride and dimethylnitrosamine, whereas the surrounding liver was affected severely. The nodules had a decreased uptake of 9-^{14}C-FAA (Farber et al., 1976).

The hyperplastic nodules could be maintained in culture and used to determine the relative resistance to various hepatocarcinogens (Laishes et al., 1978b). It has been proposed that the technique could become a short-term test for hepatocarcinogens (Tatematsu et al., 1977b). Laishes and Farber (1978) have been able to transfer the isolated preneoplastic hepatocytes to syngeneic hosts by injection of the suspension into the hepatic portal vein. Partial hepatectomy of the host led to proliferation of the liver; in some cases large macroscopic colonies of altered hepatocytes were generated within 10 days with high levels of γ-glutamyl transpeptidase, which served as a marker. The technique may afford a means to observe the biologic features of single cells involved in the process of carcinogenesis.

7. Protein Binding

Although most emphasis has been placed on the binding of FAA to liver proteins in vivo (cf., Weisburger and Weisburger, 1958a; Miller and Miller, 1966), FAA or a metabolite binds to the proteins of other organs (Weisburger et al., 1961b; Hopp et al., 1977). In addition, FAA binds to rat serum albumin in vivo (Bahl and Gutmann, 1964). FAA or FA binds to proteins such as bovine serum albumin in the absence of any cellular constituents (Sahyun, 1964), probably by purely physicochemical means. Considerable effort has been expended on determining which conditions implement the covalent binding of FAA to cellular proteins in vitro.

Hultin (1959) found that binding of labeled FA to the microsomal proteins was predominant over that of proteins of other liver fractions when FA was incubated with rat liver slices. A TPNH-generating system enhanced binding, but ethionine, p-fluorophenylalanine, sulfhydryl reagents, glutathione, or cysteine inhibited binding, an indication that -SH groups may be involved. The fact that covalent binding was facilitated in the presence of microsomes (cf., Beije and Hultin, 1971; Hara et al., 1978) indicates that metabolism may be required for binding.

Despite the predominance of microsomal binding, FAA also bound to nuclear proteins of liver (Gronow and Lincoln, 1978) and was activated by nuclei (Kawajiri et al., 1979). Eventually there were changes in the liver nuclei and the ploidy of the nuclei due to the FAA (Irving et al., 1978). Tetraploid parenchymal nuclei from rat liver bound more N-OH-FAA than did diploid stromal or parenchymal nuclei (Tulp et al., 1978).

Various studies have been attempted to determine what metabolite of FAA was actually attached to the proteins. During the enzymic or chemical oxidation of aminofluorenols, quinone-imides and -imines derived from 1- and 3-OH-FAA or 1- and 3-OH-FA, respectively, were obtained which apparently bound readily to protein, either from rat liver slices or added bovine serum albumin (Nagasawa et al., 1958; Gutmann et al., 1958; Nagasawa and Gutmann, 1959; Nagasawa et al., 1959; Gutmann and Nagasawa, 1960; Gutmann and King, 1962; King et al., 1963b).

Deacetylation of 1-OH-FAA to the aminophenol seemed necessary for protein binding to occur in rat liver slices (Gutmann et al., 1960; Nagasawa and Osteraas, 1964), implying that a quinoneimine was the active intermediate. Protein binding to 1-OH-FAA did occur in vivo (Weisburger et al., 1959b; Irving and Williard, 1964). Furthermore, the quinoneimides bound readily to crystalline bovine serum albumin (Irving and Gutmann, 1959), indicating that a free amino or imino group was not required. In a model study 2-imino-1, 2-fluorenoquinone bound irreversibly to bovine liver catalase or arginase and thus inactivated both these enzymes (King et al., 1963a), contrary to the results in vivo in which arginase was not affected (King and Gutmann, 1964). N-OH-FAA did not interact in vitro with either catalase or arginase.

The activated derivative of FAA, N-acetoxy-FAA, reacted readily with ribonuclease, furnishing modified proteins. Separation of the protein followed by enzymatic hydrolysis afforded ε-N-acetyl-L-lysine. These results led to the conclusion that N-acetoxy-FAA is primarily an acetyl donor, although the possibility of arylamidation or of other reactions also exists (Barry and Gutmann, 1973). The analogue N-acetoxy-3-FAA was even more potent in acetylating ribonuclease than the 2-isomer (Barry and Gutmann, 1976).

In addition, the quinoneimides apparently were bound to protein through the ε-amino group of lysine (Irving and Gutmann, 1959). An amino acid, N^{ε}-(1-hydroxy-2-acetamido-4-fluorenyl)-dl-lysine, was synthesized as a model representing the binding of the imides to protein (Irving and Gutmann, 1961).

However, the concept that the quinoneimides (or -imines) derived from 1-OH- or 3-OH-FAA were important biological intermediates was apparently discarded on the basis of additional study. The model, 1, 2-fluorenoquinone-2-acetimide did not react with DNA and sRNA (King and Phillips, 1968), negating the importance of quinoneimides. Although the quinoneimides may be important for protein binding, they apparently are not the intermediates attaching to nucleic acids, a reaction generally considered most important in the process of carcinogenesis.

The liver proteins binding to FAA or its metabolites have also been characterized on the basis of their electrophoretic mobility. These proteins eventually decreased during hepatocarcinogenesis, and the tumors did not bind FAA to any measurable extent (Sorof et al., 1958). Although all electrophoretic classes of the soluble liver proteins bound the carcinogen, there were several peaks (g, fast h, and h_2) with appreciable concentrations of FAA or metabolites (Sorof et al., 1960). Similarly, all the cytoplasmic fractions of liver bound to FA in vitro, but binding was greater to microsomal or cell sap proteins (Hultin, 1959). Although 3-methylcholanthrene had an inhibitory action on carcinogenesis by FAA, the administration to rats then injected with labeled FAA had no significant effect on the level of FAA associated with liver cell components, including cell sap, light mitochondria, mitochondria, smooth and rough endoplasmic reticulum, nuclei, DNA, and RNA (McGregor, 1973).

Rats bearing transplantable hepatomas originally induced by various amides derived from FA had very little activity from either labeled FAA or N-OH-FAA bound to the h proteins. Instead most of the label was bound to the A and a_2 proteins (Sorof et al., 1966). Interestingly, N-OH-FAA did not bind specifically to an h protein (Sorof et al., 1969).

The soluble FAA-protein conjugates from rat liver or serum were separated on diethylaminoethylcellulose ion exchange columns (Seal and Gutmann, 1961) or by gel filtration on Sephadex (Barry and Gutmann, 1966). A weakly-basic protein from rat liver bound preferentially to FAA or a metabolite. Certain of the nuclear proteins binding to FAA were lysine-rich or arginine-rich histones (Barry et al., 1968).

A liver protein-FAA conjugate has also been resolved according to molecular size. The 7.5 S macromolecules (molecular weight ~150,000) had 40% of the soluble bound label from 9-^{14}C-FAA and also contained the fast h_2 and/or slow h_1 FAA-bound proteins. Molecular weights of the target proteins of other carcinogens such as aminoazo dyes or polycyclic aromatic hydrocarbons were considerably lower than that bound to FAA (Sorof et al., 1970).

The relationship, if any, between the FAA-binding proteins separated by the various research groups has not been considered. Logically, it seems that a combination of techniques used should lead to more definite advances than either alone. Thus, although there are clues to the composition of the binding proteins, these proteins have not been definitely characterized.

8. Antigens

The presence of an antigenic protein in hepatomas induced by 2-FAA in rats was demonstrated by ^{131}I-labeled antibodies or by fluorescein labeling (Day et al., 1960). These techniques demonstrated immunohistochemical differences among hepatomas induced by 2-FAA (Hiramoto et al., 1961, 1963). On the other hand, Dufour (1963) concluded that different experimental tumors including those induced by FAA and the transplantable Walker tumor had common immunological changes. Gel filtration, DEAE-cellulose chromatography, and specific adsorption and elution were used to purify the antibodies which localized in tumorous livers and in normal livers when injected (Isojima et al., 1965b). Antibodies from the microsomal and dense sediment fractions of hepatomas induced by 2-FAA differed somewhat in their localizing properties, although both localized mostly in hepatoma or normal liver (Isojima et al., 1965a). These antigens also bound to some of the 2-FAA (or a metabolite) in the liver microsomes (Kitagawa et al., 1966a). However, an anticarcinogen antibody specific for the 2-azo fluorenyl group localized in both the liver and kidney of rats fed 2-FAA (Kitagawa et al., 1966b). There was a lower concentration of FAA-binding components in nodules induced by feeding FAA than in the preneoplastic or normal liver. These FAA binding components were highly localized at the cell boundary and the perinuclear zone but were partially deleted in hyperplastic nodules and almost absent in hepatoma cells (Tanigaki et al., 1967).

Differences were noted, by means of the antibody technique, in the antigenic composition of microsomes from normal liver and FAA-induced rat hepatoma (Isojima et al., 1966). A specific study on the antigenic protein from microsomal membranes of hyperplastic liver nodules induced by FAA showed the antigen could be purified to a nearly homogeneous state. By means of deoxycholate solubilization of microsomes, this antigen could be detected in normal liver. However, the microsomes from hyperplastic nodules had four times as much of this antigen—which appeared to have a high tryptophan content and a subunit molecular weight of 52,000 $\pm$ 2000—than did normal microsomes (Griffin and Kizer, 1978). These two techniques thus substantiated the antigenic differences between normal and neoplastic liver. The antigenic components of rat hepatomas induced by FAA were even carried in cells cultured from the various hepatomas (Isojima et al., 1969). The tumors induced in rats by FAA, despite the presence of several antigenic factors, were usually lacking in immunogenicity in contrast to hepatomas induced by aminoazo dyes or diethylnitrosamine. This was the case for hepatomas, ear duct carcinomas, and mammary carcinomas (Baldwin and Embleton, 1969, 1971). These immunological aspects of FAA carcinogenesis have been reviewed by Kitagawa and Tanigaki (1968) and by Baldwin (1973).

Another type of protein produced by fetal tissues, an embryonic protein or α-fetoprotein (AFP), has been detected during certain stages of carcinogenesis by FAA (cf., Dufour, 1965; reviewed by Abelev (1971) and Kitagawa et al., 1973). The responses have often been variable, but in any event, FAA does not induce embryonic antigens to the extent that other hepatocarcinogens such as aflatoxin or some azo dyes do. Usually levels of FAA sufficient to cause an early AFP response, by 2 weeks after initiation of feeding in rats, were toxic, and only transient or nondetectable levels of AFP occurred at the usual dose level of FAA or N-OH-FAA (Kitagawa et al., 1972; Kroes et al., 1973). The strain and sex of the rats also influenced the appearance of AFP (Becker and Sell, 1974; Becker, 1976a). Mammary and ear duct carcinomas produced by FAA also expressed embryonic antigens (Baldwin and Vose, 1974). The localization of AFP could be followed by means of immunofluorescence techniques (Bannikov et al., 1977a). Although present in fetal liver and many hepatomas, AFP was not invariably found in hyperplastic nodules induced by FAA (Okita et al., 1974;

Tchipysheva et al., 1977). In a comparative test FAA-induced liver tumors were stronger inducers of AFP than liver tumors induced by N-OH-FAA (Kroes et al., 1975b). Furthermore, immunosuppression by a purified γ fraction of antilymphocytic serum did not enhance liver tumor induction by N-OH-FAA (Kroes et al., 1975a).

Mice fed FAA had no early elevation of AFP, and AFP did not rise until hepatocellular carcinomas developed (Becker and Sell, 1979a).

An intensive study on localization of AFP in livers of rats fed FAA on a cyclic basis showed that there were over 1000 neoplastic nodules per liver plus oval cells and atypical hyperplastic zones. About 1% of the oval cells had AFP as did cells from the zones of atypical hyperplasia (Sell, 1978). However, none of the neoplastic nodules and only a few or none of the normal hepatocytes had any AFP-producing cells (Sell, 1978; Bannikov et al., 1977b). These results led to the tentative conclusion that hepatocellular carcinomas may arise from premalignant neoplastic nodules, from oval cells, or from the atypical differentiation of hepatocytes (Sell, 1978). Investigation of the differences in AFP levels in rats after FAA or diethylnitrosamine led to the suggestion that neither hepatocyte injury alone nor hepatocyte gene derepression was responsible for the early AFP elevation with FAA. Rather, FAA stimulates a specific cell population to produce AFP (Becker and Sell, 1979b).

Besides these aforementioned antigens, two additional preneoplastic antigens have been detected in hyperplastic liver nodules or hepatocellular carcinomas induced by FAA (Okita and Farber, 1975; Okita et al., 1975). The preneoplastic antigen 1 was located mostly in the smooth and endoplasmic reticulum and persisted from the third week of feeding FAA throughout the evolution of nodules and hepatomas. The second antigen also appeared in the smooth endoplasmic reticulum after 13 weeks of feeding FAA and then disappeared when FAA was discontinued. These preneoplastic antigens which were not AFP (Lin et al., 1977) were not found in normal adult rat liver, fetal liver, adult rat serum, sera from rats with hyperplasias or hepatomas, or various normal rat tissues. However, the preneoplastic antigen has been identified as being identical with the enzyme epoxide hydrase (Levin et al., 1978). Thus, its association with the microsomal membranes (Griffin and Kizer, 1978) and its increase during FAA hepatocarcinogenesis are understandable.

Dufour (1965) concluded that during tumor development from FAA a two-stage process held, with a gamma globulin appearing in the initial stage. This was followed by a second antigenic factor, common to different tumors, similar to the results of Isojima and co-workers (1969). Dufour and co-workers (1968) also demonstrated that a β-glycoprotein of tumoral origin was present in variable concentration, depending on sex and environment, in lungs, spleen, bone marrow, and tumors of rats fed FAA.

An immunoelectrophoretic study of up to 14 plasma proteins synthesized by hepatic nodules and carcinomas induced by FAA showed that protein synthesis was first suppressed. In later stages production of protein was accelerated, but the pattern varied from nodule to nodule even within a single liver (Becker et al., 1972).

It appears that several new antigenic proteins form during the process of carcinogenesis by FAA. One of these, AFP, may be the expression of embryonic hepatocyte differentiation. The identification of one of the antigens as an enzyme involved in metabolic processes may be an expression of defense mechanisms against the toxic agent.

9. Nucleic Acid Enzymes

The stimulation of RNA synthesis by FAA was evidenced by the rapid incorporation of labeled uracil into the RNA of regenerating liver, preneoplastic liver and FAA-induced hepatoma, whereas normal liver utilized uracil to a very limited extent (Cantarow et al., 1958). However, administration of testosterone or growth hormone increased incorporation of uracil into the liver RNA of normal rats. Consequently, the effects of FAA on various uracil degrading enzymes were investigated. Uracil reductase, dihydrouracil hydrolase, and carbamoyl-α-alanine hydrolase all decreased in the livers of FAA-fed rats, but the effect on uracil reductase was most pronounced. Rats given FAA for 90 days only slowly recovered the usual enzyme activity (Fritzson and Efskind, 1965).

A study on many enzymes involved in the anabolism and catabolism of nucleic acid precursors showed the following: in the soluble fractions of livers from rats fed FAA for periods up to 3 months deoxyadenosine and uridine kinases were not affected. The levels of aspartate carbamoyl transferase; deoxycytidylate deaminase; deoxythymidylate kinase; deoxycytidine kinase; deoxythymidine kinase; the phosphohydrolases that dephosphorylate the 5'-monophosphates of deoxythymidine, deoxyuridine, deoxycytidine, uridine and cytidine; and acid phosphatase were all increased while alkaline phosphatase decreased (Eker et al., 1968). Adenosine deaminase and polynucleotide phosphorylase were also decreased (Rabbi et al., 1963). Polynucleotide ligase was increased in rat hepatomas induced by FAA (Tsukada et al., 1972). Although the level of adenylosuccinate lyase increased early in rats fed FAA, there was no rise in adenosine-5'-monophosphate deaminase. Adenylosuccinate synthetase decreased somewhat during the feeding period (Smith et al., 1979).

Male rats that were fed FAA showed a sharp increase of the activity of tRNA methyltransferases in the liver within a few days. Females had only a slight increase. Levels of these enzymes in colonic mucosa and spleen were not affected by feeding FAA (Wainfan et al., 1978). However, at 40-50 days of feeding FAA or 2-diacetylaminofluorene, tRNA methylase activity of liver was increased only slightly or moderately (Forrester and Hancock, 1978).

Although administration of FAA caused an apparent increase in the levels of ribonuclease in rat liver (Caldarera et al., 1962), latent ribonuclease in the supernatant fraction decreased (Wojnar and Roth, 1965). The level rose to normal after the FAA diet was stopped. Ribonuclease inhibitor activity increased up to a period of 12 weeks, but hyperplastic nodules induced by FAA had inhibitor activity comparable to that of controls (Wojnar and Roth, 1965). A more thorough study indicated that acid ribonuclease of liver (ribonuclease I) increased during feeding of FAA; the alkaline ribonucleases II and III increased during the first few weeks and then decreased to control levels at about 18-20 weeks after feeding with FAA began (Rahman et al., 1969).

The FAA derivative, N-acetoxy-FAA, inhibited DNA polymerase III holoenzyme from *Escherichia coli* severely, but had much less effect on polymerase III when deoxynucleoside triphosphates were present. The inhibitory action of N-acetoxy-FAA on DNA polymerase I was much less than on polymerase III (Berthold et al., 1978). RNA polymerases also were generally inhibited by FAA or N-OH-FAA (Glazer et al., 1975; Glazer, 1976, 1978; Herzog et al., 1975). Feeding FAA to rats caused the cytoplasmic alpha DNA polymerases, isolated from the livers, to be error prone. On the other hand, both the nuclear and cytoplasmic beta polymerases retained their fidelity (Chan and Becker, 1979).

Other enzymes of importance are the endonucleases, which attack damaged DNA during the repair process. Both N-acetoxy-FAA and N-OH-FA inhibited permanently 90% of rat liver mitochondrial 5'-endonuclease activity. Although FAA and N-OH-FAA had some effect, their continued presence was necessary (Morais et al., 1972). In rats fed FAA or FA for various time periods the liver mitochondrial 5'-endonuclease activity was not changed significantly from that in controls (Pilon et al., 1974). These results were confirmed by Teebor and co-workers (1977), who determined that the activities of two endonucleases that attack damaged DNA were not altered during feeding FAA to rats, indicating that suppression of excision repair did not occur during the process of hepatocarcinogenesis.

10. Nucleic Acid Interactions

Early attempts to show an effect of FAA on nucleic acids were generally negative, probably due to the insensitivity of the methods used (cf., Rodriguez et al., 1957). There were clues though that FAA had some action, for it led to a decrease in nucleotides and other constituents involved with cellular nucleic acids (Rabbi et al., 1962). It was found that FAA or 2,7-fluorenediamine bound to calf thymus DNA in vitro, probably through physicochemical forces, for there was no relationship between the degree of binding and carcinogenicity in the series of compounds tested (Dannenberg and Sonnenbichler, 1965).

With the development of better techniques to study nucleic acids, it was found that FAA and related compounds were covalently attached to nucleic acids in vivo. Various aspects of this topic have been discussed (Miller and Miller, 1969b; Weisburger and Weisburger, 1973; Irving, 1973; Kriek, 1974; Weinstein and Grunberger, 1974). The presumed steps in the process were activation of FAA to N-OH-FAA and subsequent esterification to a reactive intermediate(s) which actually bound to the nucleic acids.

a. Deoxyribonucleic acid

Many investigations have attempted to clarify the details and consequences of the binding process with DNA. The effect of FAA on DNA stability was compared with that of the hepatocarcinogenic aminoazo dye, 3'-methyl-4-dimethylaminoazobenzene (Yager and Potter, 1975). In contrast to the action of the dye, feeding FAA for 5 weeks to partially hepatectomized rats did not lead to a loss of prelabeled DNA (Albert et al., 1972; Yager and Potter, 1975), but after longer feeding periods there was some loss of the prelabeled DNA. However, both carcinogens had similar effects on the patterns of labeled thymidine incorporation (Yager and Potter, 1975). Thymidine uptake in the nuclear DNA of rats fed FAA was higher than in controls, but no peak of labeling occurred as in controls. Furthermore, there was a large variation in DNA labeling from animal to animal (Bushnell and Jeter, 1978). Thymidine uptake was increased in hepatocytes from FAA rats, but there was no dose-dependent response. However, pretreatment with 3-methylcholanthrene and then FAA led to a dose-dependent uptake of thymidine (Casciano et al., 1978). N-Acetoxy-FAA initially suppressed replicative synthesis of DNA in cultured lymphoid cells from mice, but eventually stimulated repair synthesis (Warren, 1978).

In mice injected only once with N-OH-FAA, single strand breaks began to appear in the DNA after 2 to 16 hr, but by 24 hr later DNA repair had already occurred (Szafarz, 1977). In mice FAA apparently did not cause strand breaks in DNA of liver cells (Schwarz et al., 1979). A few strand breaks appeared in phage DNA treated with N-acetoxy-FAA, but N-OH-FAA and FAA did not induce such lesions directly. However, the combination of N-acetoxy-FAA and alkali denaturation led to many strand breaks in phage DNA (Thielmann, 1977).

N-Acetoxy-FAA bound to DNA in both native and partially dehistonized chicken erythrocyte or native calf thymus chromatin. The proportion of the DNA reached by the FAA residue was 15-20% in native chromatin and about 55% in the dehistonized chromatin. Defects were noted in the DNA double helix, proportional to the level of DNA-bound carcinogen (Metzger and Daune, 1975). Modified duck erythrocyte chromatin had very few regions susceptible to a single-strand specific nuclease (Metzger et al., 1976).

The N-acetoxy-FAA modified DNA from duck erythrocytes and the chromatin reconstituted from this DNA had decreased ability to serve as a template for transcription with E. coli RNA polymerase. However, the modified DNA reacted with histones to form normal appearing nucleosome structures (Yamasaki et al., 1977a). N-Acetoxy-FAA modified DNA was methylated to only 47% of the usual level by a rat brain methyltransferase in the presence of S-adenosyl-L-methyl ^{3}H-methionine. The 7-iodo-N-acetoxy-FAA-DNA was methylated even less. Binding of the enzyme near or at the position of methylation may have been hampered by the presence of the FAA-guanine adduct (Salas et al., 1979).

Euchromatin prepared from rat liver nuclei after injection of labeled N-OH-FAA contained a 10-fold excess of label over the heterochromatin. About 80% of the N-OH-FAA was bound to the DNA of the chromatin and 20% to the protein. The euchromatin damage appeared to be repaired faster than heterochromatin damage (Moyer et al., 1977). By 10 days after a dose of N-OH-FAA the major portion of label was in the pelleted heterochromatic DNA and less than 5% of the original was in the eu- or heterochromatin (Schwartz and Goodman, 1979).

The physicochemical consequences of the binding of FAA or its metabolites to DNA have been followed, generally employing N-acetoxy-FAA to modify the nucleic acids. Although the major site affected was the C-8 in guanosine, there was evidence for attachment to the N-2 of guanosine (Westra et al., 1976). The ratio of products after hydrolysis of the modified DNA was 85% of N-(deoxyguanosin-8-yl)-FAA and 15% of 3-(deoxyguanosine-N-2-yl)-FAA. The pH during reaction of N-acetoxy-FAA with calf thymus DNA influenced the ratio of C-8 to N-2 substitution; thus at pH 4 the ratio was twice that at pH 9 (Kriek, 1979). Linear dichroism studies of FAA modified DNA provided information on the spatial relationships of the FAA to the guanine moiety, as well as an estimate that there were one to two FAA residues per 100 bases (Norden, 1978).

Endonuclease S-1 preferentially attacked the C-8 product (Yamasaki et al., 1977b). On this basis it was suggested that the C-8 adduct may cause major conformational changes in the double stranded helix of DNA while the N-2 adduct may not cause major distortions of the native DNA structure. The N-2 adduct or persistently bound form may be situated in the minor groove of the DNA and thus be relatively protected from attack by repair enzymes. A computer generated model also indicates that the N-2 adduct is situated within the minor groove of DNA, has very little freedom of rotation, and causes little helical distortion (Beland, 1978). Furthermore, investigation of the nuclease-accessible and nuclease-inaccessible regions of chromatin-DNA after treatment in vivo with 3-N-OH-FAA has emphasized the difference in half-life of the bound adducts (Ramanathan et al., 1976). Likewise, DNA modified by reaction with N-hydroxy-2-FA was hydrolyzed three times more slowly by endonuclease S_1 than N-acetoxy-FAA modified DNA. The regions of distortion introduced by 2-FA substitution apparently were smaller than those from FAA (Kriek and Spelt, 1979).

Further studies on the modified DNA showed that the modified bases were shifted outside the double helix while the carcinogen residue was inserted into the helix (Fuchs and Daune, 1972). Calf thymus DNA which had been modified by reaction with N-acetoxy-FAA had weak points, which made this DNA more susceptible to unwinding by formaldehyde than native DNA (Fuchs and Daune, 1974). The stability of the FAA-DNA adduct also differed depending on whether arylamidation or arylation had occurred. Native DNA was more likely to afford arylated bases, denatured DNA the arylamidation product (Fuchs, 1978). The modified DNA was a less effective primer-template and decreased the incorporation of thymidine triphosphate to less than normal levels in nuclei from normal and regenerating liver (Guzzo and Glazer, 1976).

Weinstein and Grunberger (1974) developed a computer-generated three-dimensional structure for the FAA-modified dinucleoside (A-G FAA), which depicted the spatial relationships of the bases in nucleic acid. The FAA-bound guanine was displaced from its normal coplanar relationship (Kapuler and Michelson, 1971). In addition, the guanine was rotated around the glycosidic bond from the usual anti to the syn conformation. Such conformational changes in the polynucleotide backbone could lead to a destabilization of the double-stranded DNA structure. This conclusion was confirmed by Deering et al. (1975). They found that supercoiled phage DNA after modification by acetoxy-FAA was sensitive to single-strand breakage by near ultraviolet light, proportional to the prior treatment with acetoxy-FAA. Binding of N-acetoxy-FAA to supercoiled SV 40 DNA led to unwinding of the DNA. However, on a molecular basis the effect was not as great as that of the activated metabolite of benzo(a)pyrene (Drinkwater et al., 1978). The rate and the extent of modification of denatured DNA (single stranded) by N-acetoxy-FAA were two to three times greater than with native calf thymus or salmon sperm DNA. The action of acetoxy-FAA on tRNA was intermediate between reactivity with the denatured and the native DNA (Levine et al., 1974). Modified phage DNA when transcribed by DNA-dependent RNA polymerase from E. coli led to a dose-dependent lesser rate of RNA synthesis than normal. Although there was relatively little effect on the RNA initiation rate, RNA chain length was greatly decreased and the number of chain termination sites was increased (Millette and Fink, 1975).

Boublik and co-workers (1975) made a study of the conformational properties of four 2'-5'-dinucleoside monophosphates modified by FAA and compared them with the corresponding 3'-5'-derivatives. The 2'-5'-derivatives showed sizable changes in circular dichroic spectra red shifts and changes in polarity, while the 3'-5' derivatives did not. The results may be related to the differences in the spatial arrangement of hydroxyl and phosphate groups, which in turn affect the phosphate-ribose backbone and the interaction with N-acetoxy-FAA.

However, from electric dichroism studies of modified DNA, Chang and co-workers (1974) concluded that the FAA residue was located outside the DNA helix, contrary to the conclusions of Fuchs and Daune (1972). Fuchs and co-workers (1976) concluded that the extreme conditions used by Chang et al. (1974) in preparation of the DNA may have been the cause of the discrepancy. Furthermore, Fuchs and co-workers (1976) showed that the fluorene ring of 7-fluoro-FAA or FAA was oriented similarly or perpendicular to the axis of the helix, but with 7-iodo-FAA the fluorene ring was lying along the phosphate-sugar backbone. In view of the differences in carcinogenicity of 7-fluoro- and 7-iodo-FAA, these results may be significant. A study of deoxytrinucleotides modified with the N-acetoxy derivatives of 7-iodo- and 7-fluoro-FAA led to the conclusion that 7-fluoro-FAA was inserted into the DNA structure while 7-iodo-FAA was lying outside the DNA. There was also some arylation on the 2-NH_2 group of C-3 of guanine by these compounds (Lefevre et al., 1978).

N-Acetoxy-FAA, N-OH-FAA, and FAA generally all increased the attachment of DNA and a synthetic polyribocytidylic-polyribo(G) to microsomal membranes and usually increased the density of the membrane-DNA complex (Kubinski and Kasper, 1971).

In rat hepatomas induced by FAA there was no difference in the rate of annealing or thermal lability of hybrid tumor RNA-tumor DNA versus tumor RNA-control DNA, indicating that gene amplification did not occur (Shearer, 1971). The binding of labeled FAA to the DNA of primary hepatomas induced by FAA was chiefly due to the 18S fraction and the polyadenylate-rich 10S and 5S fractions (Ivanov and Dzhioev, 1977).

Antibodies to the N-acetoxy-FAA-modified DNA have been produced, leading to detection by means of radioimmunoassay techniques (Poirier et al., 1977; Leng et al., 1978).

b. Ribonucleic acid

FAA and its derivatives have sizable effects on RNA; usually the level bound to RNA, although less than the amount bound to protein (Hara et al., 1978), was greater than the DNA level and was therefore easier to demonstrate. The degree of binding of FA and other compounds to isolated RNA from rat liver did not correlate with their biological effects (Brown and Ashton, 1962). FA inhibited somewhat the incorporation of ^{14}C-labeled adenine into the RNA of rat liver slices (Arrhenius and Hultin, 1961). FAA-fed rats showed no apparent peak in RNA labeling in either hepatocyte or "stromal" nuclei in the livers, contrary to the situation in controls (Bushnell and Jeter, 1978). However, a single dose of FAA led to the appearance in the cytoplasm of RNA types, which were usually present in the nucleus, probably because of loss of selection in transport of RNA to the cytoplasm (Shearer, 1974).

During the early stages of hepatocarcinogenesis FAA fed in the diet was preferentially attached to liver rRNA; even after 1 day there was almost four times more bound to tRNA than DNA. Binding to RNA seemed to correlate better with such factors as sex and inhibitory influences than DNA binding. Furthermore, administration of 3-methylcholanthrene (3-MC) decreased the binding to liver rRNA but increased that to tRNA. In view of the inhibition of FAA carcinogenesis by 3-MC, the binding to rRNA may be significant (Irving and Veazy, 1972).

Administration of N-OH-FAA to rats, with or without partial hepatectomy, led equally to inhibition of RNA synthesis in both normal and regenerating liver, but DNA synthesis was severely inhibited in regenerating but not in normal liver (Jackson and Irving, 1973a). Additional studies on normal and regenerating liver showed that N-OH-FAA was about eight-fold more effective than FAA as an inhibitor of nuclear ribosomal and heterogeneous RNA synthesis. The detoxification product 7-OH-FAA had no appreciable action on nuclear RNA synthesis while two other compounds, 2-FA and 2-diacetylaminofluorene were almost as active inhibitors as FAA itself (Glazer et al., 1974). Both N-OH-FAA and N-acetoxy-FAA inhibited RNA synthesis in isolated cell nuclei. In this system N-acetoxy-FAA also inhibited the template ability of DNA for RNA synthesis and the transcriptional ability of RNA polymerases I and II (Austin and Moyer, 1979). Although N-OH-FAA treatment of partially hepatectomized rats inhibited rRNA synthesis, it did not affect the labeling of poly(A) RNA except at high dose levels, an indication that rRNA synthesis was more sensitive to the inhibitory action of N-OH-

FAA (Glazer, 1977). N-OH-FAA treatment also modified RNA polymerase II, which transcribed base-pair transformation more than control enzyme (Glazer, 1978).

Administration of FAA or especially N-OH-FAA inhibited incorporation of labeled orotic acid into nuclear and cytoplasmic RNA (Zieve, 1972). Nuclear ribosomal and heterogonous RNA were affected about equally (Glazer et al., 1974, Glazer, 1974). N-OH-FAA and N-acetoxy-FAA depressed RNA polymerases in males, but N-OH-FAA did not affect polymerase levels in female rats. Various other compounds, including 1-OH-FAA, N-OH-3-FAA, N-OH-2-fluorenylbenzamide, 2-nitrosofluorene, and N-OH-acetanilide, had no inhibitory action on RNA polymerase; in fact, N-OH-3-FAA stimulated polymerase (Zieve, 1972). The results were interpreted as indicating that inhibition of RNA synthesis by N-OH-FAA is due to inactivation of the polymerases and not due to a decrease in the DNA available for transcription (Zieve, 1972; Glazer et al., 1975; Herzog et al., 1975).

A contrary view was supported by Grunberger and co-workers (1973), who concluded from studies in intact nuclei, in nucleoli, and in the nucleoplasmic fraction from rat liver that inhibition of RNA synthesis was due to impairment of nucleolar template function by N-OH-FAA rather than to RNA polymerase per se. In fact polymerase III was increased in the nuclear-free fraction but reduced in the nuclear-engaged fraction (Yu and Grunberger, 1976). Studies on hepatic nuclei from rats fed FAA for periods of 4 to 14 days confirmed this position, for RNA polymerase (polymerase I) increased progressively with time on the FAA diet, but the capacity for RNA synthesis remained constant (Adams and Goodman, 1976). The instability of polymerase I if an isotonic buffer was used in the isolation procedure may partially explain some of the differing results.

In only a few seconds N-acetoxy-FAA reduced the ability of rat liver DNA to act as a template for RNA synthesis in vitro. Treated DNA bound a 10-fold greater level of RNA polymerase than control DNA and was also more effective than control DNA in supporting the homopolymerization of adenylic acid by RNA polymerases. However, the N-acetoxy derivatives of 1-, 3-, or 4-FAA had no appreciable effect. It seemed that N-acetoxy-FAA inhibited RNA synthesis by preventing chain elongation but chain initiation was unaffected (Zieve, 1973). A reduction in chain elongation was also reported by Glazer (1976), who found differences in the capacity of the polymerases to transcribe a normal RNA product.

Exposure of cultures of rat liver epithelial cells to N-acetoxy-FAA inhibited uridine incorporation into total cellular RNA, especially the 45S ribosomal precursor. There was much less effect on synthesis of heterogeneous nuclear RNA (Kaplan and Weinstein, 1976).

The reaction of N-acetoxy-FAA with purified tRNA from _E. coli_ led to primary attachment at a guanosine residue at position 20 in the dihydrouridine loop (Fujimura et al., 1972). The major targets of N-acetoxy-FAA in yeast tyrosine tRNA were two residues in the dihydrouridine loop. In the absence of magnesium and potassium ions, binding increased and a modified tetranucleotide was formed in addition to the binding in the dihydrouridine loop (Pulkrabek et al., 1974). Reaction of pyridoxal 5'-phosphate with tRNA from either a human colon carcinoma cell line or _E. coli_ was competitively inhibited by N-acetoxy-FAA (Kopelovich and Wolfe, 1977).

A study with yeast sRNA, incubated with labeled N-OH-FAA and a peroxidase-H_2O_2 activation system, showed that the combination of the N-OH-FAA with the RNA was not due to the peroxidase activity since the binding was not affected by the presence of various peroxidase inhibitors (King et al., 1973). Radiolysis of N_2O saturated solutions of tRNA, to which were added N-OH-FAA, FAA, or the O-glucuronide of N-OH-FAA, led to adducts of the RNA with these compounds, but the best yields occurred with N-OH-FAA. Both the aromatic nucleus and the N-acetyl group were retained in the adducts, but their structures were not actually determined (Cardona et al., 1975).

The reactivities of the glucuronides of N-hydroxy derivatives of various carcinogenic aromatic amines were tested against tRNA, rRNA, DNA, poly(A), poly(G), poly(U), poly(C), poly(A, G), and poly(G, U). With only one exception, the glucuronide of N-OH-FAA showed greater reactivity with all the nucleic acids and polynucleotides than the other carcinogens (Irving, 1977). From a different viewpoint, of various synthetic polydeoxyribonucleotides tested with N-acetoxy-FAA, the alternating polymer poly(dG.dC).poly(dG.dC) was most reactive. The major product was 8-(N-2-fluorenylacetamide) guanosine (Harvan et al., 1977).

To summarize, activated carcinogens have many effects on nucleic acids. The physical conformation is altered, weak areas are introduced in the strands, and the functions of the nucleic acids are impaired. On the other hand, various processes act to remove much exogenous material from the nucleic acids. The possibility exists that what is not readily removed may be an initiator of the carcinogenic process.

11. DNA Repair

Studies on the mechanisms of DNA repair in human lymphocytes led to the finding that N-acetoxy-FAA, but not FAA itself, was quite effective in evoking unscheduled DNA synthesis, as measured by ^{3}H-thymidine incorporation in the presence of hydroxyurea (Lieberman et al., 1971a, b). Furthermore, in the presence of procarcinogens such as N-acetoxy- and N-OH-FAA, Ehrlich ascites cells and E. coli took up more radiolabeled DNA or RNA from the incubation medium than in the presence of nonultimate carcinogens such as FAA (Kubinski et al., 1976).

As a consequence, N-acetoxy-FAA has become of value in studying DNA repair in various systems, for although it induced repair, there was relatively little cellular damage from the compound (Lieberman et al., 1971a). Repair resulting from treatment with N-acetoxy-FAA was of the "long patch" type since up to 100 nucleotides were excised and replaced, in contrast to the action of methyl methanesulfonate which caused "short patch" repair (Regan and Setlow, 1974). Normal peripheral blood lymphocytes usually have a relatively low rate of repair of DNA damage induced by N-acetoxy-FAA unless previously stimulated by the mitogen concanavalin A. Human lymphoblastoid cells were more active in repair after N-acetoxy-FAA and also removed more of the bound carcinogen from the DNA than did the normal lymphocytes (Scudiero et al., 1976). The level of repair synthesis or chromosomal aberrations in human lymphocytes exposed to N-acetoxy-FAA correlated with the diastolic blood pressure of the individuals (Pero et al., 1976). Moreover, sex, age, and mortality rates were also correlated with the variations in the response of lymphocytes from different individuals (Pero et al., 1978).

The neoplastic human HeLa cell line has been proposed as a test system for carcinogens, measured by the induction of unscheduled DNA synthesis in these cells (Martin et al., 1978). In this system N-acetoxy-FAA, N-OH-FAA, and FAA were all active, the latter two compounds upon addition of a rat liver activation system to the HeLa cultures. The test was suggested as a mammalian system to verify results of bacterial mutagenicity trials. Some of the bacteria, such as E. coli, often used as tester strains in mutagenicity studies, also showed DNA excision repair after treatment with N-acetoxy-FAA (Thielmann, 1976). N-OH-FAA and FAA were much less effective (Thielmann and Gersbach, 1978). ATP was required, for without it endonucleolytic cleavage to initiate repair did not occur (Thielmann, 1976).

In primary cultures of rat hepatocytes, also suggested as a potential screening system, UV, N-OH-FAA, N-acetoxy-FAA, and to a lesser extent FAA all induced a repair response. This indicated that the cells could metabolize FAA to an active form (Yager and Miller, 1978).

The discovery that repair synthesis occurred in cells from various tissues or species upon exposure to N-acetoxy-FAA (Lieberman and Forbes, 1973) has been applied for development of putative short-term tests for chemical carcinogens. In rat liver epithelial cultures several carcinogens, including FAA, were active in this manner, indicating that the cells had retained the metabolic capacity of the liver (Williams, 1977). Treatment of rats with 3-methylcholanthrene prior to isolation of the hepatocytes and N-OH-FAA treatment to induce repair synthesis, apparently increased the sensitivity of this type of system (Casciano et al., 1978). Of interest was that feeding FAA to rats increased the capacity of liver to repair O^6-methylguanine, after a pulse dose of dimethylnitrosamine, over that seen in controls (Buckley et al., 1979).

When cells from hyperplastic liver nodules induced by feeding rats FAA in the diet were maintained in culture, the degree of unscheduled DNA synthesis after UV irradiation was variable among individual nodules or animals and also varied as a function of the time in culture. However, the level of repair synthesis in cells from hyperplastic nodules was always higher than or similar to that of normal liver cells (Kitagawa et al., 1975).

DNA damage in cells from newborn rats after exposure to various carcinogens, including FAA and N-OH-FAA, has also been proposed as an assay method for chemical carcinogens (Petzold and Swenberg, 1978).

FAA also stimulated DNA synthesis in mouse bladder epithelium, causing a peak in thymidine incorporation at 40 hr after a single oral dose. Feeding FAA to mice led to the greatest DNA synthesis in the bladder 1 week later, more than sufficient time for metabolism of the FAA to an activated form. However, in liver the peak of DNA synthesis occurred between 48 and 72 hr after a single oral dose of FAA (Lawson et al., 1970).

As for human cell systems, fibroblasts from xeroderma pigmentosum (XP) patients have been widely employed for investigations on DNA repair due to the deficiency in repair capability of such cells. When N-acetoxy-FAA was added to such cultures, unscheduled DNA synthesis was low, similar to the effect of ultraviolet irradiation (Setlow and Regan, 1972; Stich et al., 1972). Variations existed in the repair capacity of fibroblasts from different XP patients as well as in the ability to survive the cytotoxic effects of N-acetoxy-FAA or related compounds. The XP cells had a lower survival than normal cells, but conversely they had a higher dose-dependent mutation frequency, as measured by 8-azaguanine resistance (Maher and Wessel, 1975; Maher et al., 1975; Maher and McCormick, 1976). In addition, XP cells removed the bound carcinogen residues in the DNA to a much smaller extent than did normal human cells or cells from patients with Fanconi's anemia (Amacher and Lieberman, 1977). Despite the lower repair capability of XP cells, treatment of such cells with N-acetoxy-FAA, followed by keeping the cells for some time in a special storage medium, did not lead to more chromosomal aberrations in these cells (Tates, 1976). The removal of the bound carcinogen residue was not as rapid or extensive as removal of pyrimidine dimers after damage from UV light. By 48 hr after N-acetoxy-FAA treatment, 25-50% of the FAA residue was removed from the human cell DNA, while 80-90% of the dimers were removed. Mouse cells were less efficient than human cells in removing dimers, but they removed the FAA residue from DNA at about the same extent as human cells (Amacher et al., 1977).

Certain XP variants which were proficient in the excision repair of pyrimidine dimers were also proficient in the excision repair of lesions induced in their DNA by treatment with N-acetoxy-FAA. The time required though for the small sections of newly synthesized DNA to join into DNA of parental size by postreplication repair was relatively longer in the XP cells. In normal human cells N-acetoxy-FAA did not affect the process of postreplication repair (D'Ambrosio and Setlow, 1978).

However, study of damage and repair from carcinogens in normal human cells is probably more relevant to the general population than studies in neoplastic or abnormal cells. Thus, in normal human fibroblasts, it was found that N-acetoxy-FAA was active in inducing repair synthesis (Laishes and Stich, 1973; San and Stich, 1975). Although N-OH-FAA was somewhat effective, FAA had even less activity and various C-hydroxylated derivatives of FAA were inactive.

Similarly, in normal human diploid fibroblasts (WI-38 cells), N-acetoxy-FAA stimulated the incorporation of radioactivity from any one of the four labeled deoxyribonucleosides (thymidine, deoxycytidine, deoxyadenosine, or deoxyguanosine) into the DNA of the cells eight- to 45-fold (Lieberman and Poirier, 1973). The rate of repair after either N-acetoxy-FAA or UV damage was very similar except that the chemically treated cells showed a lag of about 30 min before active repair began (Poirier and De Cicco, 1977). Combined treatment of normal human fibroblasts with UV and N-acetoxy-FAA led to an additive effect. However, the rate-limiting steps and enzymatic paths concerned with the repair of the two types of damage appeared different (Ahmed and Setlow, 1977a). Combined treatment of XP-repair deficient cells led to a less than additive degree of repair or even an inhibition at saturating doses (Ahmed and Setlow, 1979a). This decrease was not due to cytotoxic effects or a cessation of repair synthesis (Ahmed and Setlow, 1979b). Repair synthesis in this combined system was stimulated by addition of ATP, inhibited by NaCl, and was only partially dependent upon the addition of the four deoxyribonucleoside 5'-triphosphates (Roberts and Lieberman, 1979).

In the same human cell system, three tumor promoters, namely, croton oil, 12-O-tetradecanoylphorbol-13-acetate, and anthralin, inhibited DNA repair synthesis after damage by N-acetoxy-FAA (Poirier et al., 1975). By means of autoradiographic techniques, it was determined that there was a twofold increase in carcinogen induced repair synthesis in the central nuclear area of these cells compared with the outer portion near the nuclear envelope (Harris et al., 1974).

The DNA of WI-38 cells was repaired to about the same extent in both the unique and repetitive sequences (Lieberman and Poirier, 1974a). The complementary undamaged strand served as a template for repair synthesis (Lieberman and Poirier, 1974b). In the chromatin which had been damaged by N-acetoxy-FAA, most of the repair synthesis occurred in nuclease-sensitive regions. Eventually much of the thymidine originally incorporated into these regions appeared in nuclease-resistant areas (Tlsty and Lieberman, 1978).

Various N-myristoyloxy derivatives of 2-FA induced repair synthesis in human fibroblasts to about the same extent as N-acetoxy-FAA (Bartsch et al., 1977).

In other cell types such as in cultured Balb/C 3T3 mouse cells, repair in both satellite and mainband DNA after treatment with N-acetoxy-FAA occurred to about the same extent (Lieberman and Poirier, 1974c).

Although FAA, N-OH-FAA, N-OH-FA, and 2-nitrosofluorene had no effect on DNA synthesis in cultured Chinese hamster cells, N-acetoxy-FAA led to synthesis of a lower molecular weight DNA, especially when caffeine was also present. However, caffeine did not influence incorporation of thymidine into the DNA of either control or N-acetoxy-FAA treated cells (Trosko et al., 1973). The damaged DNA was repaired by a postreplicative mechanism that required de novo protein synthesis for enhancement (D'Ambrosio and Setlow, 1976). Furthermore, treatment of Chinese hamster V-79 cells with both N-acetoxy-FAA and ultraviolet radiation was not additive in the level of repair. The V-79 cells were less proficient than human cells in excision repair of pyrimidine bases (Ahmed and Setlow, 1977b).

Despite the proposals to employ DNA repair synthesis as a short-term test for carcinogens, it is evident that there is a fair amount of variability among cell systems, similar to the situation in animals.

12. Mutagenicity

Although an early study indicated that 2-FAA was not mutagenic in Neurospora crassa (Barratt and Tatum, 1958), it was shown that 2-FAA can be mutagenic after metabolic activation (Ames et al., 1972, 1973; Durston and Ames, 1974; McCann et al., 1975; Rickard et al., 1978). Using Salmonella typhimurium as the indicator organism, without activation, 2-FAA was inactive, N-OH-FAA and N-acetoxy-FAA had some effect, while 2-nitrosofluorene was an extremely potent mutagen. The close analogue 2-nitrofluorene was also fairly mutagenic to S. typhimurium, but it was readily reduced by Bacteroides vulgatus to the less mutagenic 2-FA (Carter et al., 1979). The various ring-hydroxylated derivatives of 2-FAA were inactive. With metabolic activation as mediated by addition of mammalian liver fractions 2-FAA was effective, but N-OH-FAA and N-acetoxy-FAA were even more potent as mutagens. Structural requirements for the mutagenic activity of acylaminofluorenes in the S. typhimurium test system have been outlined (Nelson and Thorgeirsson, 1976). Ring-substituted derivatives, the 7-iodo-, 7-fluoro-N-OH-FAA, 7-iodo-, or 7-fluoro-N-acetoxy-FAA, were more mutagenic than the unsubstituted compounds at low concentrations. The iodo derivative was more mutagenic than the fluoro compound at low concentrations but toxic to the bacteria at higher levels (Santella et al., 1979).

Although various N-myristoyloxy derivatives of FA induced a high incidence of sarcomas after subcutaneous injection in rats, they were not mutagenic for S. typhimurium without tissue activation under conditions where N-acetoxy-FAA was highly mutagenic (Bartsch et al., 1977). The mutagenicities of various activated carcinogens, including N-acetoxy-FAA, toward S. typhimurium were correlated with their capacities to cause the unwinding of supercoiled SV40 DNA (Drinkwater et al., 1978).

McGregor (1975) investigated the mutagenic potential of 2-FAA and N-OH-FAA to S. typhimurium TA 1538 after addition of various liver fractions (nuclei, mitochondria, light mitochondria, smooth and rough endoplasmic reticulum, cell sap) from different species of animals. The greatest response came in the presence of liver from cotton rats, a species resistant to 2-FAA. Various human fetal and placental tissues and a human liver fraction also metabolized FAA to activated intermediates which produced mutations in Salmonella (Jones et al., 1977; Tang and Friedman, 1977). The metabolism of FA by rat hepatocyte nuclei led to 1200% more revertants than did metabolism of FAA. The hepatic postmitochondrial supernatant (S9) also showed more revertants with FA than FAA. Phenobarbital or 3-methylcholanthrene pretreatment altered the metabolic activity in each fraction (Stout and Becker, 1979).

Contrary to expectations addition of cofactors needed for sulfation decreased greatly the mutagenicity of N-OH-FAA to S. typhimurium (Mulder et al., 1977), indicating that the sulfate ester may react with other macromolecules before reaching the bacterial DNA. Further investigation on the cotton rat indicated that this species had all the known enzymes to activate FAA into an ultimate carcinogen or mutagen, but the activity of N-OH-FAA sulfotransferase in the livers of cotton rats was only one-third of that in susceptible Sprague-Dawley rats. Thus sulfotransferase did not appear important in mutagenic activation of N-OH-FAA (Schut and Thorgeirsson, 1978), contrary to its apparent importance in vivo.

The postmitochondrial and postmicrosomal fractions of livers from rats fed FAA on an intermittent schedule were tested with FAA or N-OH-FAA in S. typhimurium. During early exposure the S9 or postmitochondrial fraction from rats fed FAA produced more mutants than did that from controls, but the effect declined after several weeks. The S9 fraction prepared from nodules induced by FAA had only about half the activity of that from control livers. The activity of the postmicrosomal fraction remained near normal throughout the feeding period (Stout and Becker, 1978). Ascorbic acid gave anomalous results for it inhibited covalent binding of the enzymatically generated sulfate to DNA, but it also increased the mutagenicity of N-OH-FAA (Andrews et al., 1979).

Reducing agents such as cysteine, cysteamine, or glutathione inhibited the mutagenic activity of either N-acetoxy-FAA or N-OH-FAA if applied concurrently to S. typhimurium cultures (Rosin and Stich, 1978). There was no general pattern, however, of the ability of an antioxidant to inhibit mutagenicity (Rosin and Stich, 1979). Sodium selenite also inhibited the mutagenicity of FAA and its derivatives (Jacobs et al., 1977), as did retinol, especially for FA (Baird and Birnbaum, 1979). Diethylstilbestrol had a synergistic effect and increased the number of revertant colonies two- to fourfold over that noted with FAA or N-OH-FAA alone (Allaben et al., 1979). Inhibition of the mutagenic effect of N-OH-FAA to S. typhimurium in cultures containing rat or mouse liver fractions was also noted with paraoxon, adenosine 3'-phosphate 5'-phosphosulfate, vitamin E, BHT, vitamin C, cysteamine, or methionine (Sakai et al., 1978). Conversely, norharman and harman enhanced the mutagenicity of FAA, FA, and N-OH-FAA, but only in the presence of rat liver microsomal enzymes. Norharman and harman increased the mutagenicity of N-acetoxy-FAA without the liver enzymes (Umezawa et al., 1978).

Several groups of investigators have correlated the mutagenicity of N-OH-FAA in bacteria with deacylation by the mammalian liver preparation added to the culture. Apparently N-OH-FA was the primary mutagen formed from N-OH-FAA (Stout et al., 1976). The genetically mediated differences in inducibility of aryl hydrocarbon hydroxylase in mice were also associated with metabolic activation of FAA by liver fractions to a mutagen. Possible deacetylation of N-OH-FAA by a liver fraction also afforded a more active mutagen than if no mammalian enzyme were added to the N-OH-FAA-S. typhimurium system (Felton et al., 1976).

Similarly, a rat liver preparation of arylhydroxamic acid acyltransferase enhanced appreciably the mutagenicity of N-OH-FAA to S. typhimurium (TA 1538) (Weeks et al., 1978). Additional tests showed that 2-FA, which competes for the acyl group, or guanosine monophosphate which competes with nucleic acid for the electrophile generated from N-OH-FAA by acyltransferase, decreased formation of the acyltransferase-catalyzed nucleic acid-FA adduct, in the presence of tRNA, by 90 and 70%, respectively. However, 2-FA or guanosine monophosphate in the media had no effect on the acyltransferase-catalyzed mutagenicity of N-OH-FAA. It was concluded that the Salmonella strain used did not detect the reactive nucleophile N-acetoxy-2-FA formed from N-OH-FAA by N→O acyl transfer and that a metabolite of N-OH-FAA generated by acyl transfer may be the actual mutagen.

Sakai and co-workers (1978) studied the effects of various enzyme inhibitors on mutagenic activation of N-OH-FAA by liver cell fractions or the binding to nuclear nucleic acids and protein and reached a similar conclusion. The first step in either process was thought to be deacetylation, either by a membrane-bound amidase or by the N,O-acyltransferase in the supernatant fraction. Deacetylation was important, not only for activation by liver fractions, but also for kidney fractions, from both mouse and rat (Schut et al., 1978). Microsomal deacetylase was also involved in mutagenic activation of FAA by guinea pig liver homogenates, but activation by homogenates from induced mice or rats was thought to involve an additional enzyme (Okuno et al., 1979).

Several other organisms have been employed as indicators for the detection of the mutagenicity of FAA or its derivatives. Bacillus subtilis served as a DNA donor where the reduction in ability of the DNA to transform cells served as a measure of mutagenicity. With this system the O-glucuronide of N-OH-FA was a powerful mutagen, while that of N-OH-FAA was almost inactive (Maher and Reuter, 1973). Intracellular bacteriophage T4 of Escherichia coli was not affected by FAA, N-OH-FAA, FA, or polycyclic aromatic hydrocarbons. N-OH-FA was toxic but not mutagenic to phage T4, but N-acetoxy-FAA was a mutagen in this system (Corbett et al., 1970). On the other hand, 2,7-fluorenediamine, FA, FAA, and N-acetoxy-FAA were active mutagens for E. coli phage fd, even in the dark (Hobom and Braunitzer, 1967a, 1967b).

A DNA polymerase-deficient mutant of E. coli, proposed as a detection system for carcinogens, was not affected by N-acetoxy-FAA, N-OH-FAA, FAA, FA, or 2-nitrofluorene, indicating a lack of sensitivity (Fluck et al., 1976). Likewise, FAA was not detected by a micronucleus test (Trzos et al., 1978).

The yeast Saccharomyces cerevisiea has also been used in assays for mutagenicity. FAA was inactive in three strains tested but was effective after metabolic activation (Brusick and Andrews, 1974).

In the fruit fly Drosophila melanogaster 2-FAA and N-acetoxy-FAA did not induce point mutations. However, the latter compound did induce small chromosome deletions (Fahmy and Fahmy, 1970, 1972a). The effect apparently was mediated through the RNA-forming genes (Fahmy and Fahmy, 1972b).

Besides these studies in lower organisms, the mutagenicity and transforming ability of FAA, N-OH-FAA, and N-acetoxy-FAA have been determined in mammalian cells. N-Acetoxy-FAA was quite cytotoxic and highly mutagenic to Chinese hamster cells in culture (Huberman et al., 1972). Although combination treatment of such cells with both N-acetoxy-FAA and methyl methanesulfonate was detrimental to their survival, the mutant frequency of the cells was not increased (Myhr and DiPaolo, 1978a). Various N- and O-acyl derivatives of N-hydroxy-FA were examined in V79 cells. However, none of the N-myristoyloxy derivatives was definitely positive (Kuroki and Bartsch, 1979). Contrary to the situation with Syrian hamster embryo cells, caffeine did not enhance the mutagenic activity of N-acetoxy-FAA in the Chinese hamster V79 cell line, although it increased the lethal or toxic effect of N-acetoxy-FAA (Myhr and DiPaolo, 1978b). Sister chromatid exchanges were increased somewhat in Chinese hamster ovary cells treated with FA or FAA and definitely increased by N-OH-FAA or N-acetoxy-FAA. Addition of a rat liver activation system reduced the effectiveness of the fluorenylamine carcinogens (Takehisa and Wolff, 1977). High doses of N-OH-FAA were needed to show a slight effect in Chinese hamster cells, while FAA was nonmutagenic or had only very weak transforming activity (Huberman et al., 1972).

It was proposed that 10T 1/2 cells from a mouse fibroblast line be used to screen xenobiotics for possible mutagenic or carcinogenic hazards. The method involved induction of mutations to ouabain resistance in the mouse fibroblast; N-acetoxy-FAA was one of the more active compounds tested (Landolph and Heidelberger, 1979).

In Wistar rat hepatocyte cell lines FAA caused appreciable increases in mutations (San and Williams, 1977). Human fibroblasts were mutated by N-acetoxy-FAA, but the yield was only 2.5-3 detectable mutants/10,000 molecules FAA bound to the hypoxanthine-guanine-phosphoribosyl transferase locus (Huang and Lieberman, 1978).

13. Cell Transformation

A corollary of the various mutagenicity studies in bacteria was investigation of FAA and derivatives in vitro. Many such efforts have been proposed as short-term tests for carcinogenicity, in lieu of the expensive and time-consuming animal studies. One drawback is that isolated cell systems sometimes do not activate or metabolize procarcinogens to the ultimate carcinogens.

It has been proposed that 2-azidofluorene be used as a probe to study the effects of carcinogens without the need for metabolic activation. This nontoxic compound did not transform C3H 10T 1/2 mouse cells. However, when photolyzed while within the cells, its cytotoxicity was enhanced and transformed foci were obtained like those seen with N-acetoxy-FAA (Sarrif et al., 1978).

Suss and co-workers (1970) reported that DNA and RNA synthesis in HeLa or hamster embryo cell cultures were reduced more decidedly by N-acetoxy-FAA, N-OH-FAA, or FAA than was protein synthesis. Pulmonary explants from BALB/C mice after treatment with FAA in Trowell's medium, and implantation into the same strain of mice showed no evidence of neoplastic changes after several months (Flaks and Hamilton, 1970). In contrast, 3-methylcholanthrene caused adenomas and adenocarcinomatous formations under these conditions. Development of 1-cell mouse embryos was arrested by N-acetoxy-FAA, but 2-cell embryos were not affected and developed to blastulas (Ku and Voytek, 1976).

Epithelial-like cells from Fischer rat liver were transformed in culture when treated with N-OH-FAA (Williams et al., 1973; Williams, 1976b). The transformed cells yielded carcinomas upon injection into Fischer rats. Fischer rat embryo cells which were also injected with Rauscher leukemia virus did not transform when treated with FAA. However, N-OH-FAA, N-acetoxy-FAA, and FA all led to transformations (Freeman et al., 1973). These results indicate the cultured cells lacked the enzyme systems necessary to activate FAA. In contrast, FAA induced unscheduled DNA synthesis in hepatocytes from adult rat livers when the cells were grown on collagen membranes. Furthermore, fresh suspensions of hepatocytes elicited even higher levels of unscheduled DNA synthesis, an indication of the metabolic activity of the hepatocytes (Michalopoulos et al., 1978).

Cells from a primary adult rat liver line maintained hepatic function for 8-10 days after plating and metabolized FAA to N-OH-FAA and ring-hydroxylated metabolites. These cells responded markedly when hydrocortisone or insulin were added to the growth medium but other hormones were less effective (Leffert et al., 1977). Rat hepatocytes also metabolized FAA to a form with increased toxicity for rat fibroblasts (Wiebkin et al., 1978).

Low-passage fibroblast-like cells derived from 18-day rat embryos, when exposed to N-OH-2-FAA, N-OH-3-FAA, N-OH-2-fluorenylbenzamide, or their acetate esters in culture, showed signs of transformation such as changes in phenotype, growth in soft agar, agglutination with concanavalin A, some changes in karyotype and loss of diploidy (Sekely et al., 1973). However, none of the cell lines produced tumors after injection into isologous rats. The cells were thus transformed but not tumorigenic, indicating that transformation may be a multistep process (Kurzepa et al., 1978).

In a Syrian hamster embryo cell system N-acetoxy-FAA enhanced five- to sevenfold the transformation frequency if simian adenovirus 7 were added. Under similar conditions,

FAA was not effective (Casto et al., 1974, 1976). Previous treatment of hamster embryo cells in culture with methyl methanesulfonate enhanced the transformation frequency associated with various carcinogens, including N-acetoxy-FAA (DiPaolo et al., 1974). However, N-acetoxy-FAA had neither an additive nor synergistic action on UV-irradiation induced transformation of hamster cells (DiPaolo and Donovan, 1976). DiPaolo and Popescu (1974) found that treatment of human leukocyte or Syrian hamster embryonic cultures with N-acetoxy-FAA led to G-banding in the chromosomes. The effect may also have been due to nonspecific toxicity. Caffeine, although nonlethal or nontransforming at the concentrations added, enhanced up to fourfold the transformation induced by N-acetoxy-FAA. The effect was dependent on the concentration of caffeine, time of addition, and the length of exposure (Donovan and DiPaolo, 1974).

By viewing transformed foci of hamster embryo cells against a normal cell background observation of the changes was facilitated. N-Acetoxy-FAA treatment for 6 days led to many transformed foci, often of the round-cell type with nests of randomly oriented fibroblasts overlying the focus (Casto et al., 1977). The cells from these transformed foci formed tumors when inoculated into weanling hamsters.

Kidney cells from baby Syrian hamsters were not transformed by FAA but N-acetoxy-FAA was effective (Ishii et al., 1977). In fetal guinea pig cell cultures FAA did not induce transformation, and while N-acetoxy-FAA did, the cell lines so transformed were not tumorigenic on implantation in newborn guinea pigs (Evans and DiPaolo, 1975). An in vitro test with nonimmune leukocytes, and a test involving reactivity in guinea pig skin confirmed the nontumorigenicity of the acetoxy-FAA transformed line (Evans et al., 1975).

Sister-chromatid exchange production in human whole blood cultures was evoked by exposure to N-OH-FAA or sodium selenite. The combination of agents gave an 11-17% lower exchange rate than the sum of that produced individually (Ray et al., 1978).

V. CARCINOGENICITY OF FAA AND DERIVATIVES

A. FAA

FAA continues to be used as a model compound to investigate various aspects of tumor induction. Of interest is that monkeys that received total doses of 100-150 g of FAA in the diet showed no tumors, even after periods up to 15 years (Thorgeirsson et al., 1978). Whether this resistance holds for other primates is not known.

1. Species Response

Species susceptible to FAA or FA among the more usual laboratory animals are cats, dogs, hamsters, mice, rabbits, and rats (cf., Weisburger and Weisburger, 1973; Weisburger, 1980). Other more exotic species were bats (Heldt et al., 1974), chickens, guppies (Sato et al., 1973), tobacco callus cultures (Bednar and Linsmaier-Bednar, 1972), and certain types of bacteria (Lotlikar et al., 1972). However, other reports indicate that FAA did not inhibit the growth of E. coli, S. heidelberg, Staphylococcus epidermis, and other bacterial strains (Martinsen and Zachariah, 1978). Given subcutaneously FAA induced tumors in frogs but oral administration was ineffective (Khudoley, 1977).

Species resistant to FAA include cockroaches (Periplaneta americana) (Sutherland, 1969), steppe lemmings (Bolonina, 1965), X/Gf mice (Goldfeder, 1974), and monkeys (Dyer et al., 1966; Thorgeirsson et al., 1978). Guinea pigs were also resistant as reported previously (cf., Weisburger and Weisburger, 1958a; Lombard, 1962), but FAA did reduce leukocyte counts in treated animals (Lombard, 1961). Although the resistance of guinea pigs was explained by lack of the enzyme system forming N-OH-FAA, this reason was not valid for X/Gf mice and monkeys, which form and excrete N-OH-FAA (Enomoto et al., 1962; Dyer et al., 1966; Grantham et al., 1976). FAA and FA did not induce hyperplasia in newt skin (Neukomm and Luder-Huguenin, 1960) while rainbow trout had a minimal response to FAA.

Although neonatal male mice were quite sensitive to FAA so that a single dose usually led to liver tumors (Klein, 1959; Walters et al., 1967; Fujii and Takahashi, 1974), neonatal rats were not nearly as sensitive as newborn mice (Vasileva, 1968).

2. Hormonal Factors

Experimentally, the removal of endocrine organs, either surgically or by blocking their function, decreased the carcinogenicity of FAA in target organs such as the liver. For example, bilateral lesions in the hypothalamus, which has a role in pituitary control, completely inhibited liver lesions in rats fed FAA for 16 weeks (Toh, 1978). Removal of endocrine organs apparently blocked the initiation stage of FAA carcinogenesis (Goodall, 1965, 1966). On the other hand, administration of excess hormone along with FAA, often had no direct effect but led indirectly through the endocrine glands to increased neoplastic and nonneoplastic lesions (Toh, 1972). Various aspects of the role of hormonal factors on the carcinogenicity of FAA have been reviewed (Napalkov, 1958; Toh, 1973; Yamamoto and Weisburger, 1977).

3. Organ Systems

a. Bladder

Although implanting FA in mouse bladder did not cause tumors (Clayson et al., 1958), feeding FAA often led to such tumors. The incidence of the tumors in mice depended on the strain of mouse, method of administration, sex, and in some cases on the presence of a foreign body in the bladder. However, injection of an oil suspension of FAA into a bladder pouch did not produce tumors (Chapman, 1962). There was no apparent correlation between the early degree of hyperplasia and the ultimate development of a tumor (Wood, 1969). In a comparison between the action of 4-ethylsulfonylnaphthalene-1-sulfonamide (ENS) and FAA on mouse bladder, it was found that FAA caused little early proliferative change, whereas ENS led to increased cell proliferation, loss of organelles, loss of enzyme, and lysosome activity. However, FAA led to increased lysosomal activity and mitochondrial degeneration (Levi et al., 1971).

Bladder hyperplasia was seen in mice of certain strains fed FAA for only 90 days, and males were affected to a greater extent than females (Haley et al., 1974a, 1976). In fact, there was a dose-response relationship in males but not in females (Haley et al., 1974b). Various schedules of dosing BALB/c mice with FAA indicated that even a relatively short exposure to high levels resulted in bladder hyperplasia and carcinomas (Frith and Rule, 1978). The hyperplastic bladder epithelium showed a decrease in alkaline phosphatase, while the subepithelial stroma had an increase in enzyme levels (Highman et al., 1975, 1978).

When cells from bladder carcinomas induced by FAA in mice were grown in culture, the cells became polynucleate and grew in soft agar. They formed tumors when injected into syngeneic hosts and differed in morphology and other characteristics from normal bladder epithelium (Berky and Zolotor, 1977).

In rats gonadectomy did not influence the development of bladder tumors when a diet low in vitamin B_6 and containing FAA was fed (Veenema et al., 1964). To induce bladder tumors to any degree, both the deficient diet and the feeding of FAA had to be maintained for long periods (Melicow et al., 1964). The incidence of bladder tumors was higher, but the onset was later when indole was also fed with the FAA. However, as the level of indole was increased, benign liver tumors were more common and malignant liver tumors decreased (McDonald et al., 1962).

In rats fed FAA and indole or tryptophan (Dunning and Curtis, 1958; Dunning, 1967), regimens leading to bladder tumors, there were no consistent changes in urinary β-glucuronidase that could be correlated with the future development of tumors (Dyer et al., 1960). Administration of the β-glucuronidase inhibitor, 2,5-di-O-acetyl-D-glucosaccharo-(1→4)(6→3)-dilactone, to rats receiving a vitamin B_6 deficient diet along with FAA led to no bladder tumors, compared with an 18% incidence in a group fed the diet with FAA alone. However, in a tryptophan-FAA dietary study, concurrent feeding of 3-methylcholanthrene or the saccharolactone did not decrease bladder tumor incidence (Bradley, 1962; Miyakawa et al., 1973).

Various aspects of the use of FAA with indole to obtain bladder tumors in rats or hamsters have been investigated (Oyasu et al., 1963; Oyasu et al., 1968, 1970b, 1972). The bladder of the hamster is a vulnerable organ for tumors developed even after intratracheal instillation of a saline suspension of FAA (Oyasu et al., 1973). Mechanical irritation (Mobley et al., 1966; Cohen et al., 1968; El-Aaser et al., 1978) and infection with bladder parasites (Hashem and Boutros, 1961; Chapman, 1969) enhanced the action of FAA in the bladder, as did a single intraperitoneal dose of cyclophosphamide (Koss and Lavin, 1971). Sequential administration of FAA and three other bladder carcinogens to male Wistar rats led to a significant incidence of bladder cancer when each agent alone did not (Tatematsu et al., 1977a). Other combinations of the four agents were also tested and synergistic effects found (Tsuda et al., 1977).

FAA also induced bladder tumors in larger animals such as rabbits or dogs (Jabara, 1963). In rabbits the stasis of the urine was not a factor (Wood, 1970). Compared with FAA, N-OH-FAA was more toxic to rabbits and more carcinogenic at the injection site, but it was no more active than FAA as an inducer of bladder tumors in rabbits (Irving et al., 1967b). Rabbits that developed tumors from FAA had a greater uptake of tryptophan from the bladder than did those not developing tumors. However, the level of the metabolite N-OH-FAA in the urine did not differ appreciably in groups of rabbits with or without bladder tumors induced by FAA (Flanagan et al., 1975).

b. Mammary gland

The more common animal tumors induced by feeding FAA include mammary tumors in females; detailed reviews and reports on the histogenesis of such tumors in rats have appeared (Noble and Cutts, 1959; Middleton, 1965). Some of these tumors, when transplanted, showed a sudden loss of hormone dependence (Van Den Berghe and Verresen, 1963). Topical application of FAA to the mammary glands of adult female Sprague-Dawley rats led to a 30% incidence of mammary adenocarcinomas after 8-11 months (Malejka-Giganti et al., 1973). In monkeys long-term estrogen plus FA produced hyperplasia of the mammary gland but no malignant changes, a further indication of the resistance of monkeys (Geschickter and Hartman, 1959).

c. Liver

The most thoroughly investigated tumors induced by FAA are those of the liver. However, besides tumor induction, FAA had inhibitory effects on liver regeneration after partial hepatectomy (Gershbein, 1958). Several detailed reports on the progression of liver tumors induced by FAA and the histopathological description of the lesions have appeared (Maluguina, 1962; Gorski, 1965; Epstein et al., 1967; Svoboda and Higginson, 1968; Becker et al., 1973). Since male rats usually were more responsive than females (Sidransky et al., 1961), many of these studies employed males exclusively. An ultrastructural study of the nuclear inclusions in livers of rats fed FAA showed that heterochromatin was distributed throughout the nucleus after 3-4 months (Dobre et al., 1976). There were some differences in fine structure of FAA-induced hepatomas from those induced by the azo dyes (Pinchuk et al., 1967). However, various hepatocarcinogens, including FAA and 3'-methyl-4-dimethylaminoazobenzene, all caused the same changes in nuclei and nucleoli of rat liver cells, as observed by the light microscope (Sugihara et al., 1972). In the livers of rats fed FAA hyperplastic areas showed a decided increase in mitotic index after partial hepatectomy, whereas more advanced lesions had a moderate increase (Kitagawa, 1971b). Changes in certain marker enzymes aided in delineating hyperplastic areas (Kitagawa, 1976).

Prelabeling hepatic DNA with ^{3}H-thymidine enabled a study of cell loss and replacement in rats fed FAA. The data suggested that FAA produced an increase in the parenchymal liver cell replication rate that correlated with tumor incidence. When FAA feeding was stopped early enough so that tumors were not produced, very little original DNA was lost and the replication rate of the parenchymal cells was increased only slightly over that in control animals (Albert et al., 1972). FAA was more effective than aflatoxin B_1 and diethylnitrosamine in enhancing proliferative response, causing the loss of hepatic DNA, and increasing the parenchymal cell labeling index (Nishizumi et al., 1977). Chromosomal alterations in rat hepatocytes after ingestion of FAA were few and difficult to correlate with the patterns noted in the eventual hepatomas (Becker et al., 1971). Alterations in chromatin patterns also occurred during neoplasia (Becker, 1970b).

Dietary influences in hepatocarcinogenesis Many factors have been found to alter the induction of liver cancer by FAA, some rather drastically. Sugai and co-workers (1962) fed rats a level of FAA so low that practically no tumors developed. However, in rats also fed a fraction of thermally oxidized corn oil with FAA, there was a great increase in tumors of the liver, mammary gland, and ear duct. Although the study has not been repeated, other reports indicate that oxidized oils and fatty acids influence tumor induction by FAA. Readily oxidized unrefined sunflower oil enhanced somewhat the effect of FAA (Vysheslavova, 1969). When the fatty acids linolenic, linoleic, and oleic, were given in conjunction with FAA, linoleic acid enhanced tumorigenic action (Vysheslavova, 1972). On the other hand, Schramm (1961) reported that ethyl linolenate decreased the effect of FAA. A lipotrope-deficient high-fat diet enhanced hepatocarcinogenesis by FAA (Rogers, 1975). Likewise, the highest incidence of hepatomas from FAA was noted in rats fed high-fat, low-protein diets (Cheng et al., 1965). A choline-deficient diet also enhanced the development of tumors from FAA (Lombardi and Shinozuka, 1979).

Although not continued to the stage of frank neoplasia since mutagenicity was employed as a measure of activation, one study explored the effects of 5 and 20% levels of dietary beef tallow or corn oil on the activation of FAA in rats (Castro et al., 1978). Liver preparations from rats fed 20% corn oil and injected with FAA had very high capacity to mutate S. typhimurium. Long-term studies would be needed to substantiate these results, which indicate an increased effect of FAA under such conditions.

A magnesium-deficient diet plus FAA did not increase chronic myelogenous leukemia, reportedly induced by the deficient diet alone (Battifora et al., 1968). The incidence of hepatomas and hepatocellular carcinomas was similar in rats fed FAA in diets either deficient (1 ppm) or supplemented to excess (800 ppm) with cupric sulfate. However, the incidence of extrahepatic neoplasms was greater in rats on the deficient diet (Carlton and Price, 1973). A diet containing 2.5 ppm added sodium selenite protected rats fed 150 ppm FAA from early deaths, compared to diets containing 0.5, 0.1, or 0 ppm additional selenite. The onset of liver tumors was somewhat delayed by the higher selenite. However, the final mammary tumor incidence was comparable in all groups and liver tumor incidence was actually somewhat higher, probably due to better survival, in the high selenite group (Harr et al., 1972; Harr et al., 1973). Contrary to the situation with certain aminoazo dyes, feeding cupric acetate to rats had no inhibitory action on hepatoma incidence from FA (Goodall, 1964). However, cupric oxyacetate gave protection from the hepatotoxic effects of FAA (Fare, 1966). A low-pyridoxine diet delayed somewhat the appearance of liver tumors from FAA, but the overall incidence was not affected (Morris et al., 1963a).

On the other hand, the uptake of iron by rat liver was enhanced by administration of hepatotoxic agents, including FAA (Kent et al., 1963b). Relatively large areas of insoluble iron developed and hepatic acid phosphatase activity decreased. Ultrastructural studies showed that FAA caused an increase in pericanalicular bodies of low to intermediate density. The additional administration of iron-dextran also increased the number of pericanalicular bodies, and iron accumulated within them until they were packed to capacity (Kent et al., 1963a). A more detailed study on iron deposition in normal, preneoplastic, and neoplastic tissues of rats led to the conclusion that stainable iron was lacking in even the early liver lesions induced by FAA. Thus, iron stains permitted a sensitive and reliable means of detecting early hyperplastic or neoplastic lesions (Williams and Yamamoto, 1972; Williams et al., 1976). Kinetic studies of the development and reversion of the altered foci following limited courses of feeding FAA showed that by 24 weeks after removal of the FAA-diet 70% of the altered foci had disappeared (Williams and Watanabe, 1978).

Other synergistic and inhibitory effects Various attempts have been made to direct the action of FAA to a particular target through the use of specific agents. FAA enhanced the action of the Rous sarcoma virus in chickens when injected after virus but was inhibitory when given prior to virus (Engle and Groupe, 1969). Concurrent administration of FAA and carbon tetrachloride increased liver tumor incidence and decreased the latent period (Maltoni et al., 1968). The combination of FAA and dimethylnitrosamine (DMN) led to the same liver tumor incidence at other sites (Likhachev, 1969). FAA plus diethylnitrosamine led to multiple liver tumors (Makiura et al., 1974), but the effect was inhibited by a polychlorinated biphenyl (PCB). Partial hepatectomy and combined treatment with FAA and enzyme inducers such as PCB, phenobarbital, or β-naphthoflavone increased the number of hyperplastic nodules in the liver (Ito et al., 1978).

The hypoglycemic sulfonamide, tolbutamide, accelerated FA-induced liver changes in rats, while the hyperglycemic sulfonamide diazoxide slowed the process (Lacassagne and Hurst, 1969).

The simultaneous feeding of FAA plus Betatron irradiation checked the development of liver tumors, but vitamin B_{12} administration promoted the growth of liver tumors (Nicholson, 1958). Diener (1963) also noted the inhibitory action of radiation; in utero irradiation with 75 rad followed by postnatal feeding of FAA increased the usual tumors from FAA but 100-200 rads inhibited the development of neoplasms.

The administration of the toxin lasiocarpine at a dose sufficient to depress liver cell division after partial hepatectomy had no influence on the incidence of hyperplastic areas or hepatic carcinomas after feeding FAA in the diet (Rogers and Newberne, 1971).

Hamsters fed FAA developed cholangiocarcinomas with no male-female difference (Della Porta et al., 1959; cf., Maluguina, 1958; Weisburger and Weisburger, 1973). However, in castrated male hamsters treated with both FAA and diethylstilbestrol, no liver carcinomas or cirrhosis occurred, but there was cystic enlargement of the liver (Dontenwill and Mohr, 1961). Extension of this protocol to rats showed that castrated male rats fed FAA and injected thrice weekly with diethylstilbestrol developed an appreciable incidence of squamous carcinomas of the lung (Dontenwill and Mohr, 1962).

The hepatocarcinogenic action of FAA was accelerated by reserpine and protein or riboflavine deficiencies (Lacassagne and Hurst, 1967).

In general, phenobarbital when given along with FAA inhibited the hepatocarcinogenicity of FAA, but phenobarbital after a course of FAA enhanced the effect (Peraino et al., 1971, 1973, 1977). Apparently phenobarbital after FAA enhanced the persistence of altered foci in the liver and thus led to liver tumors (Watanabe and Williams, 1978). The pesticide DDT had an inhibitory effect (Peraino et al., 1975; Syrowatka et al., 1978), but amobarbital and diphenylhydantoin did not inhibit FAA. Pretreatment with ethionine or carbon tetrachloride increased the toxic effect of FAA but decreased the carcinogenicity of FAA plus indole (Oyasu, 1963).

The combination of FAA and 6-methylthiouracil led to an appreciable incidence of thyroid tumors in treated rats when either compound alone did not (Napalkov, 1959; Khristov, 1968).

Under the proper regimens many compounds can inhibit or delay the carcinogenicity of FAA. The structural analogues, acetanilide (Yamamoto et al., 1968), and p-hydroxyacetanilide (Weisburger et al., 1973; Yamamoto et al., 1973), toluidines, p-aminobenzoic acid, oxine (Hamamoto et al., 1970, 1971), and BHT (Ulland et al., 1973) all had some suppressive action. Several alkyl disulfones, although not tested for an inhibitory effect, decreased the excretion of N-OH-FAA in rats injected with FAA (Pliss et al., 1973). Thus such compounds might have an inhibitory action. Similarly, indole decreased the amount of N-OH-FAA excreted in the bile after a dose of FAA (Hopp et al., 1976) and thus decreased the toxicity of FAA. As mentioned, several pesticides had an inhibitory effect on the hepatocarcinogenicity of FAA (Hiasa et al., 1978).

Mechanistic studies showed that the enzyme inducer BHT caused increased excretion of glucuronides of the metabolites of FAA with a consequent decrease in the amount bound to liver protein or DNA (Grantham et al., 1973). Additionally BHT did not influence excision repair or postreplication repair of DNA. Thus BHT apparently acted at the anti-initiation level of FAA-induced DNA damage (Goodman et al., 1976).

Other factors inhibiting liver lesions or tumors from FAA or FA are alloxan diabetes (Bielschowsky and Bielschowsky, 1959), thiouracil (Truhaut et al, 1962), enzyme-inducing polycyclic hydrocarbons such as 3-methylcholanthrene (Miller et al., 1958; Marugami et al., 1967), and 1-naphthylisothiocyanate (Sidransky et al., 1966).

Tryptophan, indole, and indole acetic acid may protect the liver from FAA but often led to bladder tumors (Dunning and Curtis, 1958). Conversely, although trypan blue did not suppress liver carcinoma by FAA, when these toxic materials were given together, FAA did inhibit the reticulum cell sarcoma of the liver usually induced by the dye (Ito and Farber, 1966). Although p-hydroxypropiophenone inhibited the effect of ethionine or azo dyes, it did not inhibit the hepatocarcinogenicity of 2-FAA (Sidransky et al., 1963). Orotic acid, although inducing fatty livers, decreased the incidence of liver tumors from feeding FAA to rats (Sidransky and Verney, 1970).

The joint administration of FAA and 3-methylcholanthrene protected the adrenals from the usual action of FAA, but the mechanism was not investigated (Danz et al., 1977). Concurrent administration of β-naphthoflavone with FAA prevented the atrophy of the submaxillary gland duct usually induced by FAA (Stora, 1977).

Inhibition of protein synthesis by administration of cycloheximide almost completely protected against the liver necrosis usually induced by FAA, but did not prevent glycogen depletion (Flaks and Nicoll, 1974). Furthermore, single high doses of FAA had an autoprotective action and suppressed early liver injury, although some liver damage was evident after 5-7 days (Flaks and Nicoll, 1975).

d. Other tumors

Certain relatively unusual tumors have been induced by FAA. A low pyridoxine-FAA diet followed by diethylstilbestrol led to a high incidence of an infiltrating gingival carcinoma which arose in minor salivary glands or the odontogenic epithelium of the teeth (Zussman, 1965, 1966). Feeding both FAA and lead subacetate caused a higher than usual incidence of poorly differentiated malignant gliomas of the brain (Oyasu et al., 1970a). Alternate administration of FAA and DL-ethionine led to an intraocular tumor, probably a melanoma, in a female rat (Benson, 1962). Although none of the other rats had this lesion, mammary and ear duct tumors appeared earlier from the joint treatment (Benson, 1961). Cyclic use of ethionine and FAA caused changes suggestive of aging in certain tissues of female rats (Benson, 1964).

Lung tumors, although not often reported from treatment with FAA, were induced fairly rapidly either by feeding or by intraperitoneal injection of FAA in rats. Other more usual tumors were also observed (Fischer, 1959).

Direct injection of an oil solution of FAA into the thyroid did not yield thyroid cancer, only a foreign body reaction (Money and Rawson, 1965). In the submaxillary gland of rats, FAA led to atrophy of the serous ducts, instead of showing a carcinogenic effect (Lacassagne and Hurst, 1966).

B. Carcinogenicity of Analogs of FAA

Various positional isomers of FAA have been tested, but only 2-FAA had appreciable activity; 1-FAA and 3-FAA had minimal or no effect and 4-FAA was inactive. Interestingly, 7-iodo-FAA was inactive, while 7-chloro-FAA and 7-fluoro-FAA were carcinogenic. The 3-iodo-FAA caused many ear duct tumors in contrast to the inactivity of the 7-isomer. A fairly active carcinogen affecting several sites was 2,2,2-trifluoro-FAA; although less active, N-2-fluorenylsuccinamic acid was also carcinogenic (Morris et al., 1960). The various ring-substituted fluoro-FAAs were examined to probe ring positions that might be involved in the carcinogenicity of FAA. The 7-fluoro-FAA was especially potent; other analogs were less effective (Miller et al., 1962). An N-hydroxy derivative appeared to be the activated form of 7-fluoro-FAA for it affected more sites at a greater incidence than did 7-fluoro-FAA itself (Miller et al., 1966). Since 7-iodo-FAA, with a bulky substituent, was inactive, the requirement for a certain molecular configuration to fit into the activating system is indicated.

The o-methoxy derivatives of FAA were also tested; 1-methoxy-FAA and -FA were somewhat active as carcinogens while the corresponding 3-methoxy-FAA and -FA were inactive (Nagasawa and Gutmann, 1966). In contrast, the analogue 7-methoxy-FAA was a moderately potent carcinogen and led to mammary, ear duct, and liver tumors (Morris et al., 1960; Gutmann et al., 1968).

C. N,N'-2,7-Fluorenylenebisacetamide (2,7-DiFAA)

This compound became of interest when induction of stomach tumors in rats was noted (Morris et al., 1961; Stewart et al., 1961; Nagayo, 1968). Physiologically, 2,7-diFAA decreased secretion volume and acidity and pepsin secretion in the stomachs of rats, while FAA increased secretion volume (Bralow et al., 1967). 2,7-DiFAA led to atrophy and then hyperplasia of the gastric mucosa (Takayama, 1968a). Eventually hyperplastic nodules and hepatomas also developed in the liver besides the stomach tumors (Dyer et al., 1967b). The compound also induced atrophy and tumors of the salivary gland (Snell et al., 1961a) and some brain tumors (Snell et al., 1961b). Route of administration had relatively little effect on the incidence of the gastric tumors (Morris et al., 1962). Although given orally, 2,7-diFAA also induced skin tumors in rats (How and Snell, 1967). Other lesions induced by 2,7-diFAA included proliferation of the bile duct cells in mice (Kimura et al., 1972; Nishio, 1974) and in rats (Ito et al., 1973), and induction of liver tumors in mice (Takayama, 1968b). Spontaneously hypertensive rats were affected to a greater extent than normotensive animals. Female mice or males treated with estrogen were more sensitive than normal males (Nishio, 1974). In ICR mice the liver and lung were affected to a greater extent than the stomach (Takayama and Inui, 1967). Although reserpine inhibited the liver tumors in mice, females tended to show more of these tumors than males (Kozuka, 1970).

Up to 44% of rats fed 2,7-diFAA developed leukemia, generally of the chronic myelogenous type (Takayama et al., 1972; Takayama and Kamata, 1972, 1973). The leukemia incidence in rats increased in direct correlation with blood loss from repeated examination (Fujiwara and Takayama, 1976; Takayama and Fujiwara, 1978a, b).

Removal of the salivary gland had an inhibitory action on the mammary tumors induced in rats by 2,7-diFAA but not on other tumors (Hirano et al., 1976). Some of the variance in organs affected in the studies mentioned may have been due to strain differences. However, in Praomys (Mastomys), which had a high incidence of spontaneous gastric lesions, 2,7-diFAA led to tumors of the small intestine, pancreas, and bile duct with no stomach cancers (Hollander and Higginson, 1971). Likewise, half the Buffalo strain rats fed 2,7-diFAA had intestinal tumors, mostly in the ileum and colon (Yamada et al., 1971). Serotonin levels decreased in the cancerous intestinal mucosa arising from feeding 2,7-diFAA to rats (Thompson, 1969).

In view of the low actual incidence of stomach tumors induced in rats by 2,7-diFAA, various additional treatments have been devised to enhance the stomach tumor incidence. Castration and traumatic ulcer were ineffective in several cases (Nagayo, 1965; Nagayo and Ito, 1965). However, another trial did yield more stomach tumors when ulcers were present (Kowalewski and Todd, 1971; Kowalewski, 1973). Joint treatment with 7,12-dimethylbenz[a]anthracene, 4-nitroquinoline-1-oxide, or diethylnitrosamine increased somewhat the incidence of stomach tumors (Odashima, 1969), as did a combination of 2,7-diFAA and 3-methylcholanthrene (Stewart et al., 1965). Combined irradiation of the stomach and 2,7-diFAA increased stomach tumors (Nagayo et al., 1972), but hepatoma development was also accelerated (Nagayo et al., 1970). Carbon tetrachloride also enhanced the carcinogenic effect of 2,7-diFAA (Kozuka and Sassa, 1976).

A metabolism study with labeled 2,7-diFAA showed that after an oral dose most of the compound was excreted unchanged in the feces within 48 hr (Dyer et al., 1967a). The mitotic index and labeling index, after ^{3}H-thymidine, were decreased in the intestinal mucosa of rats fed the carcinogen for 3-5 months except for the proximal segment of the colon (Yamada et al., 1977). Nuclei from normal liver showed peaks of DNA in diploid or tetraploid ranges; adenomas induced in mouse liver by 2,7-diFAA also had a diploid range but with wider variation. In carcinoma cells the DNA value ranged from diploid to hyperhexaploid (Inui et al., 1971).

A single oral dose of the corresponding amine, 2,7-fluorenediamine in 50 to 55-day-old female Sprague-Dawley rats led to mammary carcinomas in almost 20% of the 6-month survivors. Under the same protocol N-OH-FAA led to a 27% mammary tumor incidence (Griswold et al., 1966). Administration of fluorenediamine in 10 oral doses to young female Sprague-Dawley rats led to many breast tumors at nine months (Griswold et al., 1968).

An in vitro study with labeled FA and 2,7-fluorenediamine indicated that more 2,7-fluorenediamine was deposited within rat stomach tissue than FA (Ray et al., 1965). This differential effect may be a partial explanation for the action of 2,7-diFAA as a carcinogen for the rat stomach.

An analog, N,N'-2,7-fluorenylenebis(2,2,2-trifluoro-)acetamide, had an action similar to but weaker than that of 2,7-diFAA (Morris et al., 1963b).

The use of 2,7-diFAA, reviewed by Snell and co-workers (1969) to induce carcinoma of the glandular stomach has been superseded by a more efficient agent, N-methyl-N-nitroso-N'-nitroguanidine (MNNG). MNNG is more specific as a gastric carcinogen, yields a higher incidence of tumors, and is easier to administer than 2,7-diFAA.

D. N-2-Fluorenyldiacetamide (2-DAF) (2-Diacetylaminofluorene)

This derivative of FAA also caused liver tumors in rats but in a somewhat more reproducible fashion than does FAA. The pathogenesis, morphology of the liver lesions, and the ultrastructural changes induced by 2-DAF have been described (Mikata and Luse, 1964; Reuber, 1965b, 1975a). The early effects were similar to those induced by FAA and other hepatocarcinogens. Transplantation of the small well-differentiated liver lesions was successful only when they were implanted intrahepatically. Poorly differentiated and large well-differentiated hepatocellular carcinomas grew in all transplantation sites (Reuber and Odashima, 1967). One of these transplantable carcinomas continued to secrete bile over several transplant generations (Reuber, 1961).

The influence of various hormonal factors on the carcinogenicity of 2-DAF has been explored. Among these are adrenocortical, androgenic, and anabolic hormones (Firminger and Reuber, 1961; Reuber and Firminger, 1962, 1963; Reuber, 1965b), thyroid hormones (Reuber, 1965c, 1966), growth hormone (Reuber, 1968a), and other drugs with hormonal activity (Reuber, 1960, 1969). Reviews have appeared lately on this subject (Toh, 1973; Yamamoto and Weisburger, 1977).

Younger male rats were more susceptible to the action of 2-DAF than females of the same age or older males (Reuber, 1975c). Although testosterone treatment of castrated young males fed 2-DAF increased the incidence of liver lesions over that in castrated males, in older castrated males testosterone had only a slight effect on 2-DAF hepatocarcinogenesis (Reuber, 1976a).

Hypophysectomy inhibited liver carcinogenesis by 2-DAF, similar to the case with FAA (O'Neal et al., 1958). Likewise, alloxan diabetes protected male rats against hepatic carcinomas from 2-DAF. Female rats were not very susceptible to the hepatocarcinogenic action of 2-DAF (Reuber, 1971).

As with FAA there were differences in response of various strains of rats to 2-DAF. Sprague-Dawley and NIH Black rats were most susceptible to development of liver carcinomas and cirrhosis, while Osborne-Mendel rats were the least susceptible (Reuber, 1976b). The severity and incidence of the hepatocellular carcinomas induced by 2-DAF was increased by removal of one kidney, which would cause a slower excretion of toxic metabolites (Reuber, 1975b). In hamsters 2-DAF caused cholangiofibrosis and cholangiocarcinomas, similar to the effect of FAA (Reuber, 1968b).

Thyroiditis, a toxic effect of 2-DAF, occurred in higher incidence in female rats. However, rats with this condition did not develop liver tumors (Reuber and Glover, 1973). In rats injected several times with carbon tetrachloride to induce cirrhosis, 2-DAF led to various degenerative lesions of the parathyroid, kidneys, and other tissues (Reuber, 1962).

Various enzyme systems have been followed histochemically in rat liver after feeding 2-DAF for 3 weeks. DPNH and TPNH diaphorases, succinic and choline dehydrogenase, esterase, glucose-6-phosphatase, ATPase, and acid phosphatase were all decreased. Alkaline phosphatase, β-glucuronidase, and 5'-nucleotidase were increased (Chang, 1960). These effects on enzymes were similar to that of FAA.

Administration of cigarette smoke tar along with 2-DAF decreased the severity of the early liver lesions but in long-term studies the effect vanished (Hoffman and Griffin, 1958). Administration of a high dose of chloramphenicol along with 2-DAF led to inhibition of the liver tumors and cirrhosis from the carcinogen proportional to the amount of chloramphenicol (Puron and Firminger, 1965). As occurred in other cases, protection of the liver led to an increase in other tumors, namely, the bladder (Oster et al., 1971). Investigation of the chloramphenicol effect showed that 2-DAF was metabolized in the same fashion as FAA, yielding N-OH-FAA, 3-, 5-, and 7-OH-FAA as urinary metabolites. Concurrent feeding of chloramphenicol actually increased the amount of N-OH-FAA excreted but decreased appreciably the level of binding to the proteins of liver, plasma, and red cells. Thus by competition chloramphenicol probably inhibits the binding of the carcinogen or an activated metabolite to an essential protein (Weisburger et al., 1967).

Impaired liver function in rats fed 2-DAF was correlated with the morphological changes induced (Morris et al., 1958). Increased retention of an i.v. dose of ^{144}Ce in the livers of rats fed 2-DAF, compared with rats on control diets, substantiated the impairment of liver function (Mahlum, 1967).

E. Fluorenylhydroxamic Acids

The increased carcinogenicity of N-OH-2-FAA, relative to the action of FAA, has been discussed previously (cf., Miller and Miller, 1969a; Weisburger and Weisburger, 1973). However, several types of tumors have been induced by application of N-OH-FAA in more unusual modes. Probably because N-OH-FAA was eluted very slowly from a cholesterol pellet implanted in mouse bladder (Bryan et al., 1964a), it induced bladder carcinomas in about 20% of the mice (Bryan et al., 1964b).

A single topical application of N-OH-2-FAA to the mammary glands of adult female Sprague-Dawley rats gave a 70% tumor incidence at the site; N-OH-3-FAA also was active in this fashion, but 3-FAA was not. Mammary gland microsomes did not N-hydroxylate 2- or 3-FAA, neither did they form N-sulfates of N-OH-2-FAA or N-OH-3-FAA, but they did form C-hydroxy derivatives of 2-FAA. Thus the hydroxamic acids, presumably formed elsewhere, may be the active agents in mammary neoplasia (Malejka-Giganti et al., 1973; Malejka-Giganti et al., 1977). The acetate esters of N-OH-2-FAA and N-OH-3-FAA were also carcinogenic in the same fashion as the parent compounds when applied topically to the mammary glands. However, upon topical application of N-OH-2-FAA, N-OH-3-FAA, or their acetate esters female F344 rats did not develop mammary tumors (Malejka-Giganti and Rydell, 1978). The acetate esters could be formed nonenzymatically when the hydroxamic acids were incubated with acetyl CoA (Malejka-Giganti et al., 1977).

Despite the lack of N-hydroxylation or N-sulfation by mammary gland tissue, the parenchymal cells contain a peroxidase which converted N-OH-FAA via a nitroxyl free radical. In turn, this dismutated to 2-nitrosofluorene and N-acetoxy-2-FAA (Reigh et al., 1978). This type of reaction may be one possible explanation for the unique carcinogenic action of N-OH-2-FAA.

In a comparison study, the relative reactivity of the various fluorenylhydroxamic acids and their esters with methionine, tRNA, guanosine, or adenosine was compared with the carcinogenicity of each, given by various routes. In each case N-OH-FAA > N-OH-3-FAA > N-OH-4-FAA. In fact, N-OH-4-FAA was only marginally carcinogenic at most. The N-acetoxy-2-FAA was most reactive toward nucleophiles; N-acetoxy-4-FAA reacted to some extent, but N-acetoxy-3-FAA did not react (Yost et al., 1975). These results tend to contradict the concept of electrophile-nucleophile reactivity in carcinogenicity.

In a comparative study in which N-OH-FAA was administered to infant rats or to weanlings on a comparable basis, more intestinal tumors were observed in those started as infants. Liver and a few other types of tumors were also noted (Weisburger et al., 1970). In *Praomis natalensis* (Mastomys) N-OH-FAA did not enhance the spontaneous stomach cancers of this species. Rather various liver lesions such as cholangiocarcinomas, bile duct adenomas, and cirrhosis were induced (Yamamoto et al., 1968). Liver damage in rats given graded doses of N-OH-FAA could be correlated with their sleeping time after pentobarbital (Weisburger et al., 1965), affording a "nondestructive" test to study various influences on liver damage from N-OH-FAA.

The action of N-OH-FAA could be inhibited by BHT (Ulland et al., 1973), acetanilide (Weisburger et al., 1973), and p-hydroxyacetanilide (Yamamoto et al., 1973). On the other hand, chronic administration of ethanol did not enhance appreciably the carcinogenicity of N-OH-FAA (Yamamoto et al., 1967). Joint feeding of the immunosuppressant azathioprine with N-OH-FAA also had no definitive enhancing action on hepatocarcinogenesis, although there was a potentiation of the toxic effects of N-OH-FAA (Frankel et al., 1970). The concerted action of additional pituitary hormones (from a transplantable pituitary tumor) enhanced somewhat the hepatocarcinogenicity of N-OH-FAA (Weisburger et al., 1964; Weisburger et al., 1968).

VI. SUMMARY AND CONCLUSIONS

Despite the extensive use of FAA in research on chemical carcinogenesis, the exact mechanism for its effect is still an elusive factor. Numerous hypotheses to account for its action have been proposed, but exceptions are discovered as research continues. Currently it appears that activation of FAA to an N-hydroxy derivative and binding to cellular macromolecules may be necessary but not sufficient conditions to express the carcinogenicity of FAA. Presently it is known that attachment of FAA leads to distortion of the usual DNA configuration and interferes with DNA function. However, repair processes are available to remove much of the FAA moiety. An unknown factor is the role of minor DNA-bound material, which is less likely to influence DNA configuration and function, as well as being less readily removed by repair processes. Likewise, the significance and consequences of attachment by FAA to RNA, proteins, and other cellular structures have not been thoroughly elucidated. Additional insight on the relevance of these factors may become available as new research techniques are developed. Eventually, by use of this fascinating model compound, greater insight into the processes involved in carcinogenesis will evolve.

ACKNOWLEDGMENT

The author is grateful for the dedicated secretarial assistance of Frances M. Williams and the bibliographic aid of L. M. Tahan.

REFERENCES

Abdurasulov, D. M., Nikolaev, A. I., and Gaziev, A. I. (1967). The effect of carcinogenic compounds on the content of free radicals in tissues of animals (Russian). Vopr. Onkol. 13(12):50-54.

Abelev, G. I. (1971). Alpha-fetoprotein in ontogenesis and its association with malignant tumors. Adv. Cancer Res. 14:295-358.

Adams, M. P., and Goodman, J. I. (1976). RNA synthesis and RNA polymerase activity in hepatic nuclei isolated from rats fed the carcinogen 2-acetylaminofluorene. Biochem. Biophys. Res. Commun. 68:850-857.

Ahmed, F. E., and Setlow, R. B. (1977a). Different rate-limiting steps in excision repair of ultraviolet- and N-acetoxy-2-acetylaminofluorene-damaged DNA in normal fibroblasts. Proc. Natl. Acad. Sci. USA 74:1548-1552.

Ahmed, F. E., and Setlow, R. B. (1977b). DNA repair in V-79 cells treated with a combination of ultraviolet radiation and N-acetoxy-2-acetylaminofluorene. Cancer Res. 37: 3414-3419.

Ahmed, F. E., and Setlow, R. B. (1979a). DNA repair in xeroderma pigmentosum cells treated with combinations of ultraviolet radiation and N-acetoxy-2-acetylaminofluorene. Cancer Res. 39:471-479.

Ahmed, F. E., and Setlow, R. B. (1979b). Kinetics of DNA repair in ultraviolet-irradiated and N-acetoxy-2-acetylaminofluorene-treated mammalian cells. Biophys. J. 24:665-675.

Albert, R. E., Burns, F. J., Bilger, L., Gardner, D., and Troll, W. (1972). Cell loss and proliferation induced by N-2-fluorenylacetamide in the rat liver in relation to hepatoma induction. Cancer Res. 32:2172-2177.

Allaben, W. T., Louie, S. C., and Lazear, E. J. (1979). Synergistic effect of diethylstilbestrol on the mutagenicity of 2-acetylaminofluorene and N-hydroxy-acetylaminofluorene in the Salmonella assay system. Cancer Lett. 7:109-114.

Amacher, D. E., Elliott, J. A., and Lieberman, M. W. (1977). Differences in removal of acetylaminofluorene and pyrimidine dimers from the DNA of cultured mammalian cells. Proc. Natl. Acad. Sci. USA 74:1553-1557.

Amacher, D. E., and Lieberman, M. W. (1977). Removal of acetylaminofluorene from the DNA of control and repair-deficient human fibroblasts. Biochem. Biophys. Res. Commun. 74:285-290.

Ames, B. N., Gurney, E. G., Miller, J. A., and Bartsch, H. (1972). Carcinogens as frameshift mutagens: Metabolites and derivatives of 2-acetylaminofluorene and other aromatic amine carcinogens. Proc. Natl. Acad. Sci. USA 69:3128-3132.

Ames, B. N., Lee, F. D., and Durston, W. E. (1973). An improved bacterial test system for the detection and classification of mutagens and carcinogens. Proc. Natl. Acad. Sci. USA 70:782-786.

Andrews, L. S., Fysh, J. M., Hinson, J. A., and Gillette, J. R. (1979). Ascorbic acid inhibits covalent binding of enzymatically generated 2-acetylaminofluorene-N-sulfate to DNA under conditions in which it increases mutagenesis in Salmonella TA-1538. Life Sci. 24:59-64.

Arcos, J. C., Gosch, H. H., and Zickafoose, D. (1961). Fine structural alterations in cell particles during chemical carcinogenesis. III. Selective action of hepatic carcinogens other than 3'-methyl-4-dimethylaminoazobenzene on different types of mitochondrial swelling. Effect of stimulated liver growth. J. Biophys. Biochem. Cytol. 10:23-36.

Arrhenius, E., and Hultin, T. (1961). The effect of 2-aminofluorene and related aromatic amines on the protein and ribonucleic acid metabolism of liver slices. Exp. Cell Res. 22:476-486.

Arrhenius, E., and Hultin, T. (1962). Effects of carcinogenic amines on amino acid incorporation by liver systems. I. Secondary increase in microsomal activity after aminofluorene treatment. Cancer Res. 22:823-834.

Austin, G. E., and Moyer, G. H. (1979). Inhibition of RNA synthesis by derivatives of the carcinogen 2-acetylaminofluorene. Proc. Soc. Exp. Biol. Med. 161:220-224.

Avigan, J. (1959). The interaction between carcinogenic hydrocarbons and serum lipoproteins. Cancer Res. 19:831-834.

Baetcke, K. P., Gough, D. J., and Shellenberger, T. E. (1974). Modified system in vitro for the metabolism of 2-acetylaminofluorene. Biochem. Pharmacol. 23:1745-1752.

Bahl, O. P., and Gutmann, H. R. (1964). On the binding of the carcinogen N-2-fluorenylacetamide to rat serum albumin in vivo. Biochim. Biophys. Acta 90:391-393.

Baird, M. B., and Birnbaum, L. S. (1979). Inhibition of 2-fluorenamine-induced mutagenesis in Salmonella typhimurium by vitamin A. J. Natl. Cancer Inst. 63:1093-1096.

Baldwin, R. W. (1973). Immunological aspects of chemical carcinogenesis. Adv. Cancer Res. 18:1-75.

Baldwin, R. W., and Embleton, M. J. (1969). Immunology of 2-acetylaminofluorene-induced rat mammary adenocarcinomas. Int. J. Cancer 4:47-53.

Baldwin, R. W., and Embleton, M. J. (1971). Tumor-specific antigens in 2-acetylaminofluorene-induced rat hepatomas and related tumors. Isr. J. Med. Sci. 7: 144-153.

Baldwin, R. W., and Vose, B. M. (1974). Embryonic antigen expression on 2-acetylaminofluorene induced and spontaneously arising rat tumours. Br. J. Cancer 30: 209-214.

Bannikov, G. A., Gel'shtein, V. I., and Tchipysheva, T. A. (1977a). Distribution of antigenic markers of differentiation—ligandin and alpha-fetoprotein at early stages of chemical carcinogenesis in the liver of rats. Vestn. Akad. Med. Nauk SSSR 3(3):39-41.

Bannikov, G. A., Gel'shtein, V. I., and Tchipysheva, T. A. (1977b). Evolution of the hepatocyte population in the process of chemical carcinogenesis. Vopr. Onkol. 23(4): 39-44.

Barratt, R. W., and Tatum, E. L. (1958). Carcinogenic mutagens. Ann. NY Acad. Sci. 71:1072-1084.

Barry, E. J., and Gutmann, H. R. (1966). Interaction of aromatic amines with rat liver proteins in vivo. I. Preferential labeling of a cytoplasmic protein or proteins by N-2-fluorenylacetamide-9-^{14}C. J. Biol. Chem. 241:4600-4609.

Barry, E. J., and Gutmann, H. R. (1973). Protein modifications by activated carcinogens. I. The acetylation of ribonuclease by N-acetoxy-2-fluorenylacetamide. J. Biol. Chem. 248:2730-2737.

Barry, E. J., and Gutmann, H. R. (1976). Protein modifications by activated carcinogens. II. The acetylation of ribonuclease by N-acetoxy-3-fluorenylacetamide. Chem. Biol. Interact. 13:47-55.

Barry, E. J., Ovechka, C. A., and Gutmann, H. R. (1968). Interaction of aromatic amines with rat liver proteins in vivo. J. Biol. Chem. 243:51-60.

Bartsch, H., Dworkin, C., Miller, E. C., and Miller, J. A. (1973). Formation of electrophilic N-acetoxyarylamines in cytosols from rat mammary gland and other tissues by transacetylation from the carcinogen N-hydroxy-4-acetylaminobiphenyl. Biochim. Biophys. Acta 304:42-55.

Bartsch, H., Malaveille, C., Stich, H. F., Miller, E. C., and Miller, J. A. (1977). Comparative electrophilicity, mutagenicity, DNA repair induction activity, and carcinogenicity of some N- and O-acyl derivatives of N-hydroxy-2-aminofluorene. Cancer Res. 37:1461-1467.

Bartsch, H., Miller, J. A., and Miller, E. C. (1972). N-Acetoxy-N-acetylaminoarenes and nitrosoarenes. One-electron nonenzymatic and enzymatic oxidation products of various carcinogenic aromatic acethydroxamic acids. Biochim. Biophys. Acta 273: 40-51.

Battifora, H. A., McCreary, P. A., Hahneman, B. M., Laing, G. H., and Hass, G. M. (1968). Chronic magnesium deficiency in the rat. Studies of chronic myelogenous leukemia. Arch. Pathol. 86:610-620.

Baumgarten, H. E., Staklis, A., and Miller, E. M. (1965). Reactions of amines. XIII. The oxidation of N-acyl-N-arylhyroxylamines with lead tetraacetate. J. Org. Chem. 30:1203-1206.

Baxter, C. S., and Byvoet, P. (1974a). Effects of carcinogens and other agents on histone methylation by a histone arginine methyltransferase purified from rat liver cytoplasm. Cancer Res. 34:1418-1423.

Baxter, C. W., and Byvoet, P. (1974b). Effects of carcinogens and other agents on histone methylation in rat liver nuclei by endogenous histone lysine methyltransferase. Cancer Res. 34:1424-1428.

Becker, F. F. (1975). Alteration of hepatocytes by subcarcinogenic exposure to N-2-fluorenylacetamide. Cancer Res. 35:1734-1736.

Becker, F. F. (1976a). Introductory remarks on AFP production during injury and chemical carcinogenesis. In Onco-Developmental Gene Expression, W. H. Fishman and S. Sell (Eds.). Academic Press, New York, pp. 207-208.

Becker, F. F. (1976b). Sequential phenotypic and biochemical alterations during chemical hepatocarcinogenesis. Cancer Res. 36:2563-2566.

Becker, F. F., Fox, R. A., Klein, K. M., and Wolman, S. R. (1971). Chromosome patterns in rat hepatocytes during N-2-fluorenylacetamide carcinogenesis. J. Natl. Cancer Inst. 46:1261-1269.

Becker, F. F., and Klein, K. M. (1971). The effect of L-asparaginase on mitotic activity during N-2-fluorenylacetamide hepatocarcinogenesis: Subpopulations of nodular cells. Cancer Res. 31:169-173.

Becker, F. F., Klein, K. M., and Asofsky, R. (1972). Plasma-protein synthesis by N-2-fluorenylacetamide-induced primary hepatocellular carcinomas and hepatic nodules. Cancer Res. 32:914-920.

Becker, F. F., Klein, K. M., Wolman, S. R., Asofsky, R., and Sell, S. (1973). Characterization of primary hepatocellular carcinomas and initial transplant generations. Cancer Res. 33:3330-3338.

Becker, F. F., and Sell, S. (1974). Early elevation of α-fetoprotein in N-2-fluorenylacetamide carcinogenesis. Cancer Res. 34:2489-2494.

Becker, F. F., and Sell, S. (1979a). α-Fetoprotein levels and hepatic alterations during chemical carcinogenesis in C57BL/6N mice. Cancer Res. 39:3491-3494.

Becker, F. F., and Sell, S. (1979b). Differences in serum α-fetoprotein concentrations during the carcinogenic sequences resulting from exposure to diethylnitrosamine or acetylaminofluorene. Cancer Res. 39:1437-1442.

Becker, F. F., and Shurgin, A. (1975). Concanavalin A agglutination of cells from primary hepatocellular carcinomas and hepatic nodules induced by N-2-fluorenylacetamide. Cancer Res. 35:2879-2883.

Bednar, T. W., and Linsmaier-Bednar, E. M. (1972). Induction of plant tissue neoplasms in vitro by substituted fluorenes. Chem. Biol. Interact. 4:233-238.

Beije, B., and Hultin, T. (1971). Oxidation and protein binding of aromatic amines by rat liver microsomes. Chem. Biol. Interact. 3:321-336.

Beland, F. A. (1978). Computer-generated graphic models of the N^2-substituted deoxyguanosine adducts of 2-acetylaminofluorene and benzo[a]pyrene and the O^6-substituted deoxyguanosine adduct of 1-naphthylamine in the DNA double helix. Chem. Biol. Interact. 22:329-339.

Beland, F. A., Dooley, K. L., and Casciano, D. A. (1979). Rapid isolation of carcinogen-bound DNA and RNA by hydroxyapatite chromatography. J. Chromatogr. 174:177-186.

Benkert, K., Fries, W., Kiese, M., and Lenk, W. (1975). N-(9-Hydroxy-9-H-fluoren-2yl)-acetamide and N-(9-oxo-9-H-fluoren-2yl)-acetamide: metabolites of N-(9H-fluoren-2yl)acetamide. Biochem. Pharmacol. 24:1375-1380.

Benson, W. R. (1961). The incidence of tumors after treatment with DL-ethionine and N-2-fluorenylacetamide. Am. J. Pathol. 39:491-498.

Benson, W. R. (1962). Intraocular tumor after ethionine and N-2-fluorenylacetamide. Arch. Pathol. 73:404-406.

Benson, W. R. (1964). Acceleration of aging changes in the exorbital lacrimal gland of the female rat. Am. J. Pathol. 45:587-597.

Berg, T., and Christoffersen, T. (1974). Early changes induced by 2-acetylaminofluorene in lysosomes in rat liver parenchymal cells. Biochem. Pharmacol. 23:3323-3329.

Berky, J. J., and Zolotor, L. (1977). Development and characterization of cell lines of normal mouse bladder epithelial cells and 2-acetylaminofluorene-induced urothelial carcinoma cells grown in monolayer tissue culture. In Vitro 13:63-75.

Berry, D. L., Zachariah, P. K., Namkung, M. J., and Juchau, M. R. (1976). Transplacental induction of carcinogen-hydroxylating systems with 2,3,7,8-tetrachlorodibenzo-p-dioxin. Toxicol. Appl. Pharmacol. 36:569-584.

Berthold, V., Thielmann, H. W., and Geider, K. (1978). Carcinogens inhibit DNA synthesis with isolated DNA polymerases from Escherichia coli. FEBS Lett. 86:81-84.

Bielschowsky, F., and Bielschowsky, M. (1959). Carcinogenesis in alloxan-diabetic rats. In Ciba Foundation Symposium on Carcinogenesis. Mechanisms of Action, G. E. Wolstenholme and M. O'Connor (Eds.). Churchill, London, pp. 95-104.

Bolonina, N. I. (1965). On resistance of the steppe lemming to some chemical carcinogenic agents and tumorigenic viruses (Russian). Vopr. Onkol. 11(5):80-83.

Boobis, A. R., Reinhold, C., and Thorgeirsson, S. S. (1977). Induction of aryl hydrocarbon (benzo[a]pyrene)hydroxylase and 2-acetylaminofluorene N-hydroxylase by polycyclic hydrocarbons in regenerating liver from inbred strains of mice. Biochem. Pharmacol. 26:1501-1505.

Boublik, M., Grunberger, D., and Lapidot, Y. (1975). Circular dichroism study of 2'-5'-dinucleoside monophosphates modified with N-2-acetylaminofluorene. Biochem. Biophys. Res. Commun. 62:883-890.

Bowman, M. C., and King, J. R. (1974). Analysis of 2-acetylaminofluorene: residues in laboratory chow and microbiological media. Biochem. Med. 9:390-401.

Bradley, H. J., Jr. (1962). Effect of a β-glucuronidase inhibitor and methylcholanthrene on the induction of bladder tumors in rats. J. Urol. 88:626-628.

Bralow, S. P., Brown, M., Gruenstein, M., and Shimkin, M. B. (1967). Effect of N,N'-2,7-fluorenylenebisacetamide and N-2-fluorenylacetamide on gastric secretion and cell population in rats. Gastroenterology 53:719-730.

Breeman, G. E., Kaspersen, F. M., and Westra, J. G. (1978). Non-specific tritiation of some carcinogenic aromatic amines. J. Labelled Comp. Radiopharmaceut. 14:741-750.

Brill, E. (1977). The role of dog bladder mucosa in the N-oxidation of arylamines. Res. Commun. Chem. Pathol. Pharmacol. 16:73-84.

Brown, R. A., and Ashton, F. T. (1962). The interaction of some carcinogens with rat liver RNA. Arch. Biochem. Biophys. 99:390-395.

Brusick, D., and Andrews, H. (1974). Comparison of the genetic activity of dimethylnitrosamine, ethyl methanesulfonate, 2-acetylaminofluorene and ICR-170 in Saccharomyces cerevisiae strains D_3, D_4 and D_5 using in vitro assays with and without metabolic activation. Mutat. Res. 26:491-500.

Bryan, G. T., Brown, R. R., Morris, C. R., and Price, J. M. (1964a). In vivo elution of tryptophan metabolites and other aromatic nitrogen compounds from cholesterol pellets implanted into mouse bladders. Cancer Res. 24:586-595.

Bryan, G. T., Brown, R. R., and Price, J. M. (1964b). Mouse bladder carcinogenicity of certain tryptophan metabolites and other aromatic nitrogen compounds suspended in cholesterol. Cancer Res. 24:596-602.

Buckley, J. D., O'Connor, P. J., and Craig, A. W. (1979). Pretreatment with acetylaminofluorene enhances the repair of O^6-methylguanine in DNA. Nature 281:403-404.

Burchfield, H. P., Storrs, E. E., and Green, E. E. (1977). Role of analytical chemistry in carcinogenesis. In Environmental Cancer, Advances in Modern Toxicology, Vol. 3, H. F. Kraybill and M. A. Mehlman (Eds.). Hemisphere, Washington, D.C., Wiley, New York, pp. 173-207.

Burke, W. T., and Gangloff, E. C. (1965). Metabolic profiles during carcinogenesis and related conditions in hepatic tissue. Cancer Res. 25:833-839.

Burke, W. T., and Miller, L. L. (1960). Biochemical changes during carcinogenesis. IV. Protein synthesis and urea production in perfused liver of rats fed 2-acetamidofluorene. Cancer Res. 20:658-660.

Burlakova, E. B., Dzhaliabova, M. I., Kobliakov, V. A., Koliada, A. I., and Molochkina, E. M. (1978). Disturbances in the lipid regulation of hepatic microsomal enzyme activity during chemical carcinogenesis (Russian). Dokl. Akad. Nauk SSSR 241:477-480.

Burtle, J. G., and Morath, R. J. (1965). An improved synthesis of fluorene-1, 2-quinone 2-acetimide. J. Chem. Soc. 5115-5116.

Bushnell, D. E., and Jeter, J. R., Jr. (1978). Effects of 2-acetylaminofluorene on diurnal oscillations in nucleic acid metabolism in two classes of nuclei isolated from rat liver. Cancer Res. 38: 2533-2538.

Buu-Hoi, N. P., and Hien, D.-P. (1966). Induction of zoxazolamine hydroxylase synthesis in rats by means of 6-aminochrysene. Naturwissenschaften 53: 435.

Buu-Hoi, N. P., Mangane, M., and Jacquignon, P. (1970). The orientation in the Ullmann-Fetvadjian acridine cyclizations with 2-aminofluorene. J. Heterocyclic Chem. 7: 155-157.

Calcutt, G., and Doxey, D. (1962). The effects of tumour initiating agents on mouse skin sulphydryl levels. Br. J. Cancer 16: 806-810.

Calcutt, G., Doxey, D., and Coates, J. (1960). The effects of some chemical carcinogens upon the -SH levels of target and non-target tissues. Br. J. Cancer 14: 746-757.

Caldarera, C. M., Budini, R., and Rabbi, A. (1962). Effect of administration of 4-dimethylaminoazobenzene (DAB) and of 2-acetamidofluorene (AAF) on the hepatic ribonuclease in the rat. Boll. Soc. Ital. Biol. Sper. 38: 1767-1769; Chem. Abst. 60: 2157b (1964).

Calder, I. C., and Williams, P. J. (1975). The thermal ortho-rearrangement of some carcinogenic N, O-diacetyl-N-arylhydroxylamines. Chem. Biol. Interact. 11: 27-32.

Cameron, R., Kellen, J., Kolin, A., Malkin, A., and Farber, E. (1978). γ-Glutamyltransferase in putative premalignant liver cell populations during hepatocarcinogenesis. Cancer Res. 38: 823-829.

Cameron, R., Sharma, R. N., Sweeney, G. D., Farber, E., and Murray, R. K. (1976a). A novel electrophoretic pattern of induction of rat liver microsomal membrane polypeptides by 2-acetylaminofluorene, nitrosamine and azo dye administration. Biochem. Biophys. Res. Commun. 71: 1054-1061.

Cameron, R., Sweeney, G. D., Jones, K., Lee, G., and Farber, E. (1976b). A relative deficiency of cytochrome P-450 and arylhydrocarbon [benzo(a)pyrene] hydroxylase in hyperplastic nodules induced by 2-acetylaminofluorene in rat liver. Cancer Res. 36: 3888-3893.

Cantarow, A., Williams, T. L., Melnick, I., and Paschkis, K. E. (1958). Influence of acetylaminofluorene, growth hormone, testosterone and hypothyroidism on incorporation of uracil-2-C^{14} in liver RNA in the rat. Cancer Res. 18: 818-821.

Cantwell, G. E., Shortino, T. J., and Robbins, W. E. (1966). The histopathological effects of certain carcinogenic 2-fluorenamine derivatives on larvae of the house fly. J. Invertebr. Pathol. 8: 167-174.

Cardona, R. A., and King, C. M. (1976). Activation of the O-glucuronide of the carcinogen N-hydroxy-N-2-fluorenylacetamide by enzymatic deacetylation in vitro: formation of fluorenylamine-tRNA adducts. Biochem. Pharmacol. 25: 1051-1056.

Cardona, R. A., King, C. M., and Redpath, J. L. (1975). Irradiation-induced adduct formation of RNA with carcinogenic arylamine derivatives. Cancer Res. 35: 2007-2014.

Carlton, W. W., and Price, P. S. (1973). Dietary copper and the induction of neoplasms in the rat by acetylaminofluorene and dimethylnitrosamine. Food Cosmet. Toxicol. 11: 827-840.

Carter, J. H., McLafferty, M. A., and Goldman, P. (1979). Effect of 2-nitrofluorene, 1, 2-dimethylhydrazine, and azoxymethane on Salmonella typhimurium mutants in the gastrointestinal tract of gnotobiotic rats. Cancer Res. 39: 2026-2030.

Casciano, D. A., Farr, J. A., Oldham, J. W., and Cave, M. D. (1978). 2-Acetylaminofluorene-induced unscheduled DNA synthesis in hepatocytes isolated from 3-methylcholanthrene treated rats. Cancer Lett. 5: 173-178.

Casto, B. C., Janosko, N., and DiPaolo, J. A. (1977). Development of a focus assay model for transformation of hamster cells in vitro by chemical carcinogens. Cancer Res. 37: 3508-3515.

Casto, B. C., Pieczynski, W. J., and DiPaolo, J. A. (1974). Enhancement of adenovirus transformation by treatment of hamster embryo cells with diverse chemical carcinogens. Cancer Res. 34:72-78.

Casto, B. C., Pieczynski, W. J., Janosko, N., and DiPaolo, J. A. (1976). Significance of treatment interval and DNA repair in the enhancement of viral transformation by chemical carcinogens and mutagens. Chem. Biol. Interact. 10:105-125.

Castro, C. E., Felkner, I. C., and Yang, S. P. (1978). Dietary lipid-dependent activation of the carcinogen N-2-fluorenylacetamide in rats as monitored by Salmonella typhimurium. Cancer Res. 38:2836-2841.

Chan, J. Y., and Becker, F. F. (1979). Decreased fidelity of DNA polymerase activity during N-2-fluorenylacetamide hepatocarcinogenesis. Proc. Natl. Acad. Sci. USA 76:814-818.

Chandrasekhara, N., and Narayan, K. A. (1970). Studies on liver plasma membranes of rats fed N-2-fluorenylacetamide. Cancer Res. 30:2876-2880.

Chang, C.-T., Miller, S. J., and Wetmut, J. G. (1974). Physical studies of N-acetoxy-N-2-acetylaminofluorene-modified deoxyribonucleic acid. Biochemistry 13:2142-2148.

Chang, J. P. (1960). Histochemical study of enzymatic behavior in cells of rat livers during the early stage of carcinogenesis induced by 3'-methyl-4-dimethylaminoazobenzene and N-2-fluorenyldiacetamide. In Cell Physiology of Neoplasia, 14th Annual Symposium Fundamental Cancer Research, M. D. Anderson Tumor Institute, University of Texas Press, Austin, pp. 471-499.

Chapman, W. H. (1962). A method for producing bladder tumors in mice, with a technique allowing easy interpretation of the difference between hyperplasia and true tumor. J. Urol. 88:518-526.

Chapman, W. H. (1969). Infection with Trichosomoides crassicauda as a factor in the induction of bladder tumors in rats fed 2-acetylaminofluorene. Invest. Urol. 7:154-159.

Cheng, Y.-S., Chiang, C.-M., and Chen, Y. (1965). The effects of diet and dosage of carcinogen on the induction of liver tumors in rats fed 2-acetylaminofluorene. Acta Biol. Exp. Sinica 10:92-105.

Chopra, P., Manga, A., and Nayak, N. C. (1979). Kupffer cell sarcoma in rats after exposure to small doses of dimethylnitrosamine and N-2-acetylaminofluorene during hepatic regeneration. J. Natl. Cancer Inst. 62:1089-1095.

Christoffersen, T. (1975). Effect of treatment of rats with some chemical carcinogens on the stimulatory effect of adrenaline on cyclic AMP accumulation in liver slices. Acta Pharmacol. Toxicol. 37:233-236.

Christoffersen, T., and Berg, T. (1975). Altered hormone control of cyclic AMP formation in isolated parenchymal liver cells from rats treated with 2-acetylaminofluorene. Biochim. Biophys. Acta 381:72-77.

Christoffersen, T., Bronstad, G. O., Walstad, P., and Oye, I. (1974). Cyclic AMP metabolism in rat liver during 2-acetylaminofluorene carcinogenesis. Biochim. Biophys. Acta 372:291-303.

Christoffersen, T., Morland, J., Osnes, J.-B., and Elgjo, K. (1972). Hepatic adenyl cyclase: alterations in hormone response during treatment with a chemical carcinogen. Biochim. Biophys. Acta 279:363-366.

Clayson, D. B., Jull, J. W., and Bonser, G. M. (1958). The testing of o-hydroxy amines and related compounds by bladder implantation and a discussion of their structural requirements for carcinogenic activity. Br. J. Cancer 12:222-230.

Cohen, A. E., McCombs, H. L., and Gershoff, S. N. (1968). Cocarcinogenic effect of diet and foreign body insertion on urinary bladder neoplasia in the rat. Invest. Urol. 5:602-608.

Commoner, B., Woolum, J. C., Senturia, B. H., Jr., and Ternberg, J. L. (1970). The effects of 2-acetylaminofluorene and nitrite on free radicals and carcinogenesis in rat liver. Cancer Res. 30:2001-2007.

Corbett, T. H., Heidelberger, C., and Dove, W. F. (1970). Determination of the mutagenic activity to bacteriophage T_4 of carcinogenic and noncarcinogenic compounds. Mol. Pharmacol. 6:667-679.

Cramer, J. W., Miller, J. A., and Miller, E. C. (1960a). The hydroxylation of the carcinogen 2-acetylaminofluorene by rat liver: stimulation by pretreatment in vivo with 3-methylcholanthrene. J. Biol. Chem. 235:250-256.

Cramer, J. W., Miller, J. A., and Miller, E. C. (1960b). N-Hydroxylation: a new metabolic reaction observed in the rat with the carcinogen 2-acetylaminofluorene. J. Biol. Chem. 235:885-888.

D'Ambrosio, S. M., and Setlow, R. B. (1976). Enhancement of postreplication repair in Chinese hamster cells. Proc. Natl. Acad. Sci. USA 73:2396-2400.

D'Ambrosio, S. M., and Setlow, R. B. (1978). Defective and enhanced postreplication repair in classical and variant xeroderma pigmentosum cells treated with N-acetoxy-2-acetylaminofluorene. Cancer Res. 38:1147-1153.

Dannenberg, H., and Sonnenbichler, J. (1965). Untersuchungen zur Wechselwirkung zwischen aromatischen Kohlenwasserstoffen und Aminen mit Desoxyribonucleinsäure. Z. Krebsforsch. 67:127-134.

Danz, M., and Kittlick, P. D. (1977). Action of a single toxic dose of 2-acetylaminofluorene or allylic alcohol on adrenals. 2. Effect on adrenal cyclic 3',5'-adenosine monophosphate concentration during 1st and 2nd day. Exp. Pathol. 13:139-144.

Danz, M., Urban, H., Jäger, A., and Trautvetter, P. (1976). Action of a single toxic dose of 2-acetylaminofluorene or allylic alcohol on adrenals. 1. Behaviour of organ weight and mitotic activity of adrenocortical cells. Exp. Pathol. 12:301-308.

Danz, M., Urban, W., and Schmidt, A. (1977). Prevention of 2-acetylaminofluorene-induced extrahepatic short-term effects by 3-methylcholanthrene. Exp. Pathol. 13: 262-267.

Daoud, A. H., and Griffin, A. C. (1978). Effects of selenium and retinoic acid on the metabolism of N-acetylaminofluorene and N-hydroxyacetylaminofluorene. Cancer Lett. 5:231-237.

Dardas, A., and Carraz, G. (1974). Marquage de l'amino-2-fluorene par un radical libre. Comportement du signal en presence de sang. Eur. J. Med. Chem. 9:458-461.

Davey, J., Keene, B. R., and Mannering, G. (1967). The synthesis and ionisation constants of some fluorenamines. J. Chem. Soc. (C) 120-123.

Day, E. D., Planinsek, J. A., and Pressman, D. (1960). Localization of radioiodinated antibodies in rats bearing tumors induced by N-2-fluorenylacetamide. J. Natl. Cancer Inst. 25:787-802.

Deering, R. A., Taylor, W. D., and Burns, L. R. (1975). Near-ultraviolet light-induced strand breaks in DNA pretreated with the carcinogen, N-acetoxy-2-acetylaminofluorene. Biophys. J. 15:181-190.

Della Porta, G., Shubik, P., and Scortecci, V. (1959). The action of N-2-fluorenylacetamide in the Syrian golden hamster. J. Natl. Cancer Inst. 22:463-467.

Diener, E. (1963). Die Beeinflussung der Cancerogenese durch Anwendung ionisierender Strahlen wahrend der Embryonalentwicklung. Z. Krebsforsch. 65:607-619.

DiPaolo, J. A., and Donovan, P. J. (1976). In vitro morphologic transformation of Syrian hamster cells by U.V.-irradiation is enhanced by x-irradiation and unaffected by chemical carcinogens. Int. J. Radiat. Biol. 30:41-53.

DiPaolo, J. A., Donovan, P. J., and Casto, B. C. (1974). Enhancement by alkylating agents of chemical carcinogen transformation of hamster cells in culture. Chem. Biol. Interact. 9:351-364.

DiPaolo, J. A., and Popescu, N. C. (1974). Chromosome bands induced in human and Syrian hamster cells by chemical carcinogens. Br. J. Cancer 30:103-108.

Dobre, M. A., Moraru, I., Cotutiu, C., and Motoc, F. (1976). Nuclear inclusions and other ultrastructural aspects in the liver of animals treated with N-2-acetylaminofluorene. Pathol. Eur. 11:63-68.

Dobrescu, F., Kohn, D., Martin, A., Zalman, M., and Frasinel, N. (1966). Quartäre Ammoniumsalze von 2-Amino und 2.7-Diaminofluoren. Pharmazie 21:214-216.

Dobrescu, F., Mercea, C., and Nartea, E. (1971). Neue Schiffsche Basin des 2-Aminofluorens. Pharmazie 26:467-469.

Donahue, E. V., McCann, J., and Ames, B. N. (1978). Detection of mutagenic impurities in carcinogens and noncarcinogens by high pressure liquid chromatography and the Salmonella/microsome test. Cancer Res. 38:431-438.

Donovan, P. J., and DiPaolo, J. A. (1974). Caffeine enhancement of chemical carcinogen-induced transformation of cultured Syrian hamster cells. Cancer Res. 34:2720-2727.

Dontenwill, W., and Mohr, U. (1961). Cystische Leberdystrophie beim Goldhamster im Experiment. Klin. Wochenschr. 39:593-594.

Dontenwill, W., and Mohr, U. (1962). Über die unterschiedliche carcinogene Wirkung von Acetaminofluoren in der Ratten-und Hamsterlunge. Klin. Wochenschr. 40:212-213.

Drinkwater, N. R., Miller, J. A., Miller, E. C., and Yang, N.-C. (1978). Covalent intercalative binding to DNA in relation to the mutagenicity of hydrocarbon epoxides and N-acetoxy-2-acetylaminofluorene. Cancer Res. 38:3247-3255.

Duchesne, J., Lion, Y., and Van De Vorst, A. (1969). Cancerisation chimique et radicaux libres. C. R. Acad. Sci. [D] (Paris) 269:1562-1563.

Dufour, D. (1963). Modifications immunologiques communes a differentes tumeurs experimentales. Laval Med. 34:831-833.

Dufour, D. (1965). Distinction de deux phases dans les modifications immunologiques au cours de la cancerisation au 2-acetylaminofluorene. Pathol. Biol. 13:385-387.

Dufour, D., Tremblay, A., and Lemieux, S. (1968). Influence du sexe, de la carcinogenese et de la vie en milieu exempt de germe sur la concentration tissulaire en une β-proteine. Experientia 24:1271-1272.

Dunning, W. F. (1967). The role of indole and its metabolites in the incidence of induced bladder cancer in rats. In Bladder Cancer, A Symposium, K. F. Lampe (Ed.). Aesculapius, Birmingham, Ala., pp. 122-128.

Dunning, W. F., and Curtis, M. R. (1958). The role of indole in incidence of 2-acetylaminofluorene-induced bladder cancer in rats. Proc. Soc. Exp. Biol. Med. 99:91-95.

Durston, W. E., and Ames, B. N. (1974). A simple method for the detection of mutagens in urine: Studies with the carcinogen 2-acetylaminofluorene. Proc. Natl. Acad. Sci. USA 71:737-741.

Dybing, E., Søderlund, E., Haug, L. T., and Thorgeirsson, S. S. (1979a). Metabolism and activation of 2-acetylaminofluorene in isolated rat hepatocytes. Cancer Res. 39:3268-3275.

Dybing, E., von Bahr, C., Aune, T., Glaumann, H., Levitt, D. S., and Thorgeirsson, S. S. (1979b). In vitro metabolism and activation of carcinogenic aromatic amines by subcellular fractions of human liver. Cancer Res. 39:4206-4211.

Dyer, H. M., Kelly, M. G., and O'Gara, R. W. (1966). Lack of carcinogenic activity and metabolic fate of fluorenylacetamide in monkeys. J. Natl. Cancer Inst. 36:305-322.

Dyer, H. M., Lueders, K. K., and Morris, H. P. (1967a). Recovery of radioactivity of N,N'-2,7-fluorenylenebisacetamide-9-C^{14} from rats. J. Natl. Cancer Inst. 38:93-101.

Dyer, H. M., Lueders, K. K., and Reuber, M. D. (1967b). Early effects of N,N'-2,7-fluorenylenebisacetamide on the gastric mucosa of the rat. J. Natl. Cancer Inst. 38:103-110.

Dyer, H. M., and Morris, H. P. (1961). An effect of N-2-fluorenylacetamide on the metabolism of tryptophan in rats. J. Natl. Cancer Inst. 26:315-329.

Dyer, H. M., Morris, H. P., and Maupin, G. E. (1960). A study of urinary β-glucuronidase activity in the production of bladder tumors in rats. J. Natl. Cancer Inst. 24:181-196.

Dyer, H. M., Sherwin, B. E., and Morris, H. P. (1965). Observations on the metabolism of N-2-fluorenylacetamide in dogs and rats. J. Natl. Cancer Inst. 34:363-370.

Eker, P., Fritzson, P., Spaeren, U., and Efskind, J. (1968). Effect of dietary 2-acetylaminofluorene on rat liver enzymes involved in the anabolism and catabolism of nucleic acid precursors. Scand. J. Clin. Lab. Invest. 22 (Supp.) 106: 65-77.

El-Aaser, A. A., Hassanein, S. M., El-Bolkainy, M. N., Omar, S., El-Sebai, I., and El-Merzabani, M. M. (1978). Bladder carcinogenesis using bilharzia-infested Swiss mice. Eur. J. Cancer 14: 645-648.

Endo, H., Eguchi, M., and Yanagi, S. (1970). Irreversible fixation of increased level of muscle type aldolase activity appearing in rat liver in the early stage of hepatocarcinogenesis. Cancer Res. 30: 743-752.

Engle, C. G., and Groupe, V. (1969). Effect of chemical carcinogens on virus-induced Rous sarcoma. Cancer Res. 29: 1345-1349.

Enomoto, M., Lotlikar, P., Miller, J. A., and Miller, E. C. (1962). Urinary metabolites of 2-acetylaminofluorene and related compounds in the rhesus monkey. Cancer Res. 22: 1336-1342.

Enomoto, M., and Sato, K. (1967). N-Hydroxylation of the carcinogen 2-acetylaminofluorene by human liver tissue in vitro. Life Sci. 6: 881-887.

Epstein, S. M., Ito, N., Merkow, L. P., and Farber, E. (1967). The cellular analysis of liver carcinogenesis: the induction of large hyperplastic nodules in the liver with 2-fluorenylacetamide or ethionine and some aspects of their morphology and glycogen metabolism. Cancer Res. 27: 1702-1712.

Ershoff, B. H., and Bajwa, G. S. (1974). Inhibitory effect of sodium cyclamate and sodium saccharin on tumor induction by 2-acetylaminofluorene in rats. Proc. Soc. Exp. Biol. Med. 145: 1293-1297.

Evans, C. H., Cooney, A. M., and DiPaolo, J. A. (1975). Colony inhibition mediated by nonimmune leukocytes in vitro and skin reactivity in vivo as indices of tumorigenicity of guinea pig cultures transformed by chemical carcinogens. Cancer Res. 35: 1045-1052.

Evans, C. H., and DiPaolo, J. A. (1975). Neoplastic transformation of guinea pig fetal cells in culture induced by chemical carcinogens. Cancer Res. 35: 1035-1044.

Fahmy, O. G., and Fahmy, M. J. (1970). Gene elimination in carcinogenesis: reinterpretation of the somatic mutation theory. Cancer Res. 30: 195-205.

Fahmy, O. G., and Fahmy, M. J. (1972a). Mutagenic properties of N-acetyl-2-aminofluorene and its metabolites in relation to the molecular mechanisms of carcinogenesis. Int. J. Cancer 9: 284-298.

Fahmy, O. G., and Fahmy, M. J. (1972b). Mutagenic selectivity for the RNA-forming genes in relation to the carcinogenicity of alkylating agents and polycyclic aromatics. Cancer Res. 32: 550-557.

Farber, E., Parker, S., and Gruenstein, M. (1976). The resistance of putative premalignant liver cell populations, hyperplastic nodules, to the acute cytotoxic effects of some hepatocarcinogens. Cancer Res. 36: 3879-3887.

Fare, G. (1966). The effect of cupric oxyacetate on rat liver damage associated with five poisons of unrelated chemical structure. Br. J. Cancer 20: 569-581.

Feinstein, R. N., Fry, R. J., Cameron, E. C., Peraino, C., and Morris, H. P. (1976). New aldehyde dehydrogenase isozymes in chemically induced liver tumors in the rat. Proc. Soc. Exp. Biol. Med. 152: 463-468.

Felton, J. S., Nebert, D. W., and Thorgeirsson, S. S. (1976). Genetic differences in 2-acetylaminofluorene mutagenicity in vitro associated with mouse hepatic aryl hydrocarbon hydroxylase activity induced by polycyclic aromatic compounds. Mol. Pharmacol. 12: 225-233.

Fiala, S., and Fiala, E. S. (1973). Activation by chemical carcinogens of γ-glutamyl transpeptidase in rat and mouse liver. J. Natl. Cancer Inst. 51: 151-158.

Firminger, H. I., and Reuber, M. D. (1961). Influence of adrenocortical, androgenic, and anabolic hormones on the development of carcinoma and cirrhosis of the liver in A × C rats fed N-2-fluorenyldiacetamide. J. Natl. Cancer Inst. 27: 559-595.

Fischer, W. (1959). Über Tumoren, die durch Azetylaminofluoren hervorgerufen werden, insbesondere über Lungentumoren bei Ratten. Zentralbl. Allg. Pathol. 99:392-401.

Flaks, A., and Hamilton, J. M. (1970). In vitro effects of chemical carcinogens. Eur. J. Cancer 6:151-153.

Flaks, B. (1968). Permanent changes in the fine structure of rat hepatocytes following prolonged treatment with 2-acetylaminofluorene. Eur. J. Cancer 4:297-304.

Flaks, B. (1970). Changes in the fine structure of rat hepatocytes during the early phases of chronic 2-acetylaminofluorene intoxication. Chem. Biol. Interact. 2:129-150.

Flaks, B. (1971). Fine structure of rat hepatocytes during the late phase of chronic 2-acetylaminofluorene intoxication. Chem. Biol. Interact. 3:157-176.

Flaks, B., and Basley, W. A. (1979). Acute fine structural changes in rat hepatocytes induced by a single large dose of 2-acetylaminofluorene. Virchows Archiv. [Cell Pathol] 29:309-320.

Flaks, B., and Lucas, J. (1972). Fine structural changes in rat pancreatic cells during prolonged treatment with 4-acetylaminofluorene. Chem. Biol. Interact. 5:217-225.

Flaks, B., and Lucas, J. (1973). Persistent ultrastructural changes in pancreatic acinar cells induced by 4-acetylaminofluorene. Chem. Biol. Interact. 6:91-98.

Flaks, B., and Moody, J. A. (1969). Ultrastructural alterations of the cytomembranes of rat pancreatic exocrine cells induced by treatment with 2-acetylaminofluorene. Eur. J. Cancer 5:231-238.

Flaks, B., and Nicoll, J. W. (1974). Modification of toxic liver injury in the rat. I. Effect of inhibition of protein synthesis on the action of 2-acetylaminofluorene, carbon tetrachloride, 3'-methyl-4-dimethylaminoazobenzene and diethylnitrosamine. Chem. Biol. Interact. 8:135-150.

Flaks, B., and Nicoll, J. W. (1975). Modification of toxic liver injury in the rat. II. Protective effect of cycloheximide on ethionine-induced damage and autoprotective effects of high doses of ethionine, 3'-methyl-4-dimethylaminoazobenzene, and 2-acetylaminofluorene. Toxicol. Appl. Pharmacol. 32:603-620.

Flanagan, M. J., Ekbal, S., Coogan, P. S., Kalin, G., and Hass, G. M. (1975). Tryptophan urinary bladder absorption and bladder cancer. Invest. Urol. 13:17-19.

Fletcher, T. L. (1968). Use of dimethyl sulfoxide as a solvent and (or) reactant in selected reactions. Q. Rep. Sulfur Chem. 3:107-112.

Fletcher, T. L., and Namkung, M. J. (1961). Improved Schiemann reactions with tetrahydrofuran. Chem. Ind. 179-180.

Fletcher, T. L., and Namkung, M. J. (1970). Derivatives of fluorene. XXXIII. Synthesis and reactions of hydrazofluorenes and related compounds. J. Org. Chem. 35:4231-4234.

Fletcher, T. L., Namkung, M. J., and Pan, H.-L. (1967). Derivatives of fluorene. XXIII. New thiofluorenes related to metabolism of the carcinogen N-2-fluorenylacetamide. J. Med. Chem. 10:936-941.

Fletcher, T. L., Namkung, M. J., Pan, H.-L., and Wetzel, W. H. (1960a). Derivatives of fluorene. VIII. Fluorofluorenes. II. J. Org. Chem. 25:996-1000.

Fletcher, T. L., Namkung, M. J., Wetzel, W. H., and Pan, H.-L. (1960b). Derivatives of fluorene. X. Fluorofluorenes. III. J. Org. Chem. 25:1342-1348.

Fletcher, T. L., and Pan, H.-L. (1959). Azomethine and α-bromoamine formation in the aralkylation of certain weak aromatic amines in dimethyl sulfoxide. J. Org. Chem. 24:141-142.

Fletcher, T. L., and Wetzel, W. H. (1960). Derivatives of fluorene. XI. New nitrogen mustards. J. Org. Chem. 25:1348-1354.

Fletcher, T. L., Wetzel, W. H., and Namkung, M. J. (1966). Derivatives of fluorene. XXII. Nitrogen mustards. II. J. Med. Chem. 9:593-598.

Fletcher, T. L., Wetzel, W. H., Namkung, M. J., and Pan, H.-L. (1959). Derivatives of fluorene. VI. Fluorofluorenes. I. J. Am. Chem. Soc. 81:1092-1094.

Floyd, R. A. (1976). Microsome catalyzed conversion of N-hydroxy-N-acetyl-2-aminofluorene by cumene-hydroperoxide. Life Sci. 18:189-195.

Floyd, R. A., and Soong, L. M. (1977a). Obligatory free radical intermediate in the oxidative activation of the carcinogen N-hydroxy-2-acetylaminofluorene. Biochim. Biophys. Acta 498:244-249.

Floyd, R. A., and Soong, L. M. (1977b). Spin trapping in biological systems. Oxidation of the spin trap 5,5-dimethyl-1-pyrroline-1-oxide by a hydroperoxide-hematin system. Biochem. Biophys. Res. Commun. 74:79-84.

Floyd, R. A., Soong, L. M., and Culver, P. L. (1976a). Horseradish peroxidase/hydrogen peroxide-catalyzed oxidation of the carcinogen N-hydroxy-N-acetyl-2-aminofluorene as effected by cyanide and ascorbate. Cancer Res. 36:1510-1519.

Floyd, R. A., Soong, L. M., Stuart, M. A., and Reigh, D. L. (1978). Free radicals and carcinogenesis. Some properties of the nitroxyl free radicals produced by covalent binding of 2-nitrosofluorene to unsaturated lipids of membranes. Arch. Biochem. Biophys. 185:450-457.

Floyd, R. A., Soong, L. M., Walker, R. N., and Stuart, M. (1976b). Lipid hydroperoxidase activation of N-hydroxy-N-acetylaminofluorene via a free radical route. Cancer Res. 36:2761-2767.

Fluck, E. R., Poirier, L. A., and Ruelius, H. W. (1976). Evaluation of a DNA polymerase-deficient mutant of E. coli for the rapid detection of carcinogens. Chem. Biol. Interact. 15:219-231.

Forrester, P. I., and Hancock, R. L. (1978). Hepatocarcinogen-induced tRNA methylase activity in rat liver. Physiol. Chem. Phys. 10:115-123.

Frankel, H. H., Yamamoto, R. S., Weisburger, E. K., and Weisburger, J. H. (1970). Chronic toxicity of azathioprine and the effect of this immunosuppressant on liver tumor induction by the carcinogen N-hydroxy-N-2-fluorenylacetamide. Toxicol. Appl. Pharmacol. 17:462-480.

Freeman, A. E., Weisburger, E. K., Weisburger, J. H., Wolford, R. G., Maryak, J. M., and Huebner, R. J. (1973). Transformation of cell cultures as an indication of the carcinogenic potential of chemicals. J. Natl. Cancer Inst. 51:799-808.

French, C. M., and Pritchard, R. (1961). The magnetochemistry of some carcinogens and related compounds. Arch. Biochem. Biophys. 93:598-604.

Friedman, M. A., and Woods, S. (1977). Effects of piperonyl butoxide on hydroxylation of 2-acetylaminofluorene in hamster liver. Res. Commun. Chem. Pathol. Pharmacol. 17:623-630.

Frith, C. H., and Rule, J. E. (1978). The effects of discontinuing administration of high levels of 2-acetylaminofluorene on the transitional epithelium of the mouse urinary bladder. J. Environ. Pathol. Toxicol. 1:581-585.

Fritzson, P., and Efskind, P. (1965). The effect of dietary 2-acetylaminofluorene on the uracil-degrading enzymes in rat liver. Cancer Res. 25:703-707.

Fuchs, R., and Daune, M. (1972). Physical studies on deoxyribonucleic acid after covalent binding of a carcinogen. Biochemistry 11:2659-2666.

Fuchs, R. P. (1978). Arylamidation and arylation by the carcinogen N-2-fluorenylacetamide: a sensitive and rapid radiochemical assay. Anal. Biochem. 91:663-673.

Fuchs, R. P., and Daune, M. P. (1974). Dynamic structure of DNA modified with the carcinogen N-acetoxy-N-2-acetylaminofluorene. Biochemistry 13:4435-4440.

Fuchs, R. P., Lefevre, J.-F., Pouyet, J., and Daune, M. P. (1976). Comparative orientation of the fluorene residue in native DNA modified by N-acetoxy-N-2-acetylaminofluorene and two 7-halogeno derivatives. Biochemistry 15:3347-3351.

Fujii, K., and Epstein, S. S. (1979). Effects of piperonyl butoxide on the toxicity and hepatocarcinogenicity of 2-acetylaminofluorene and 4-acetylaminobiphenyl, and their N-hydroxylated derivatives, following administration to newborn mice. Oncology 36: 105-112.

Fujii, K., and Takahashi, H. (1971). Tumor induction with a single administration of N-2-fluorenylacetamide or N-hydroxy-2-fluorenylacetamide to newborn mice: Effect of age after birth. Gan. 63:354-349.

Fujimura, S., Grunberger, D., Carvajal, G., and Weinstein, I. B. (1972). Modifications of ribonucleic acid by chemical carcinogens. Modification of Escherichia coli formyl methionine transfer ribonucleic acid with N-acetoxy-2-acetylaminofluorene. Biochemistry 11:3629-3635

Fujiwara, M., and Takayama, S. (1976). Influence of blood collection on incidence of 2,7-FAA induced rat leukemia. Acta Pathol. Jpn. 26:139-145.

Fukui, K., Nagata, C., Imamura, A., Yonezawa, T., and Tagashira, Y. (1962). Relationship between the electronic structure and carcinogenic activity of acetamidofluorene and related compounds. Gan. 53:25-40.

Fullerton, F. R., and Jackson, C. D. (1976). Determination of 2-acetylaminofluorene and its metabolites in urine by high pressure liquid chromatography. Biochem. Med. 16: 95-103.

Gershbein, L. L. (1958). Effect of carcinogenic and noncarcinogenic hydrocarbons and hepatocarcinogens on rat liver regeneration. J. Natl. Cancer Inst. 21:295-310.

Gershbein, L. L. (1970). Effect of carcinogens on rat diaphragm carbohydrate metabolism. Trans. Ill. State Acad. Sci. 63:341-343.

Geschickter, C. F., and Hartman, C. G. (1959). Mammary response to prolonged estrogenic stimulation in the monkey. Cancer 12:767-781.

Glazer, R. I. (1974). Inhibition by N-hydroxy-2-acetylaminofluorene of incorporation of [5-^{3}H]orotic acid into RNA of two classes of nuclei from normal and regenerating liver. Biochim. Biophys. Acta 361:361-366.

Glazer, R. I. (1976). Alterations in the transcriptional capacity of hepatic DNA-dependent RNA polymerase I and II by N-hydroxy-2-acetylaminofluorene. Cancer Res. 36:2282-2289.

Glazer, R. I. (1977). The action of N-hydroxy-2-acetylaminofluorene on the synthesis of ribosomal and poly(a)-RNA in normal and regenerating liver. Biochim. Biophys. Acta 475:492-500.

Glazer, R. I. (1978). Comparisons of the fidelity of transcription of RNA polymerase I and II following N-hydroxy-2-acetylaminofluorene treatment. Nucleic Acids Res. 5:2607-2616.

Glazer, R. I., Glass, L. E., and Menger, F. M. (1975). Modification of hepatic ribonucleic acid polymerase activities by N-hydroxy-2-acetylaminofluorene and N-acetoxy-2-acetylaminofluorene. Mol. Pharmacol. 11:36-43.

Glazer, R. I., and La Via, M. F. (1975). Biochemical and morphological changes in hepatic nuclear membranes produced by N-hydroxy-2-acetylaminofluorene. Cancer Res. 35:2511-2519.

Glazer, R. I., Nutter, R. C., Glass, L. E., and Menger, F. M. (1974). 2-Acetylaminofluorene and N-hydroxy-2-acetylaminofluorene inhibition of incorporation of orotic acid-5-^{3}H into nuclear ribosomal and heterogeneous RNA in normal and regenerating liver. Cancer Res. 24:2451-2458.

Glowinski, I. B., Radtke, H. E., and Weber, W. W. (1978). Genetic variation in N-acetylation of carcinogenic arylamines by human and rabbit liver. Mol. Pharmacol. 14:940-949.

Goldfeder, A. (1974). Characterization of X/Gf mice with respect to their resistance to oncogenesis. Trans. NY Acad. Sci. 36:50-77.

Goodall, C. M. (1964). Failure of copper to inhibit carcinogenesis by 2-aminofluorene. Br. J. Cancer 18:777-781.

Goodall, C. M. (1965). Restoration by iodide of hepatic reactions to 2-aminofluorene in thyroidectomized rats. Endocrinology 76:1027-1032.

Goodall, C. M. (1966). Hepatic carcinogenesis in thyroidectomized rats: apparent blockade at the stage of initiation. Cancer Res. 26:1880-1883.

Goodman, J. I. (1976). Separation of the products of the reaction of deoxyguanosine with N-acetoxy-2-acetylaminofluorene by high pressure liquid chromatography. Anal. Biochem. 70:203-207.

Goodman, J. I., Trosko, J. E., and Yager, J. D., Jr. (1976). Studies on the mechanism of inhibition of 2-acetylaminofluorene toxicity by butylated hydroxytoluene. Chem. Biol. Interact. 12:171-182.

Gorrod, J. W. (1968). Oxidation of aromatic amines by peracetic acid. Tetrahedron Lett. 6155-6158.

Gorski, T. (1965). The induction of neoplastic growth with 2-acetylaminofluorene. Pol. Med. J. 4:334-338.

Grantham, P. H. (1967). Separation of the urinary metabolites of N-2-fluorenylacetamide on columns of DEAE-cellulose anion exchanger. Biochem. Pharmacol. 16:429-440.

Grantham, P. H., Mohan, L. C., and Weisburger, E. K. (1976). Metabolism of N-2-fluorenylacetamide in X/Gf mice: lack of a correlation between biochemical interaction and carcinogenicity. J. Natl. Cancer Inst. 56:649-651.

Grantham, P. H., Mohan, L. C., Yamamoto, R. S., Weisburger, E. K., and Weisburger, J. H. (1968). Alteration of the metabolism of the carcinogen N-2-fluorenylacetamide by acetanilide. Toxicol. Appl. Pharmacol. 13:118-130.

Grantham, P. H., Weisburger, E. K., and Weisburger, J. H. (1961). Ionization constants of derivatives of fluorene and other polycyclic compounds. J. Org. Chem. 26:1008-1017.

Grantham, P. H., Weisburger, J. H., and Weisburger, E. K. (1973). Effect of the antioxidant butylated hydroxytoluene (BHT) on the metabolism of the carcinogens N-2-fluorenylacetamide and N-hydroxy-N-2-fluorenylacetamide. Food Cosmet. Toxicol. 11:209-217.

Griffin, M. J., and Kizer, D. E. (1978). Purification and quantitation of preneoplastic antigen from hyperplastic nodules and normal liver. Cancer Res. 38:1136-1141.

Griswold, D. P., Jr., Casey, A. E., Weisburger, E. K., and Weisburger, J. H. (1968). The carcinogenicity of multiple intragastric doses of aromatic and heterocyclic nitro or amino derivatives in young female Sprague-Dawley rats. Cancer Res. 28:924-933.

Griswold, D. P., Jr., Casey, A. E., Weisburger, E. K., Weisburger, J. H., and Schabel, F. M., Jr. (1966). On the carcinogenicity of a single intragastric dose of hydrocarbons, nitrosamines, aromatic amines, dyes, coumarins, and miscellaneous chemicals in female Sprague-Dawley rats. Cancer Res. 26:619-625.

Gronow, M., and Lincoln, J. C. (1978). The binding of ^{14}C-labelled acetylaminofluorene to nuclear proteins and DNA. Cancer Lett. 5:269-275.

Grunberger, G., Yu, F.-L., Grunberger, D., and Feigelson, P. (1973). Mechanism of N-hydroxy-2-acetylaminofluorene inhibition of rat hepatic ribonucleic acid synthesis. J. Biol. Chem. 248:6278-6281.

Gurkalo, V. K., and Pliss, G. B. (1978). Influence of chemical carcinogens on the physiological effects of adrenomimetics. Vopr. Onkol. 24(4):49-53.

Gustafsson, R. G., and Afzelius, B. A. (1963). Comparative effects on rat liver cells after dimethylnitrosamine, 2-fluorenamine, or prednisolone treatment studied by electron microscopy. J. Natl. Cancer Inst. 30:1045-1075.

Gutmann, H. R. (1964). The oxidation of 2-fluorenamine and 4-aminobiphenyl by peracetic acid. Experientia 20:128-129.

Gutmann, H. R. (1974). Isolation and identification of the carcinogen N-hydroxy-2-fluorenylacetamide and related compounds by liquid chromatography. Anal. Biochem. 58:469-478.

Gutmann, H. R., and Bell, P. (1974). Route to the tritiation of carbon atom-9 of carcinogenic fluorenylhydroxamic acids. J. Labelled Comp. 10:255-270.

Gutmann, H. R., and Bell, P. (1977). N-Hydroxylation of arylamides by the rat and guinea pig. Evidence for substrate specificity and participation of cytochrome P_1-450. Biochim. Biophys. Acta 498:229-243.

Gutmann, H. R., Burtle, J. G., and Nagasawa, H. T. (1958). Protein binding of model quinone imides. I. The synthesis of some fluorenoquinone imides. J. Am. Chem. Soc. 80:5551-5555.

Gutmann, H. R., and Erickson, R. R. (1969). The conversion of the carcinogen N-hydroxy-2-fluorenylacetamide to o-amidophenols by rat liver in vitro. An inducible enzymatic reaction. J. Biol. Chem. 244:1729-1740.

Gutmann, H. R., and Erickson, R. R. (1972). The conversion of the carcinogen N-hydroxy-2-fluorenylacetamide to o-amidophenols by rat liver in vitro. Substrate specificity and mechanism of the reaction. J. Biol. Chem. 247:660-666.

Gutmann, H. R., Galitski, S. B., and Foley, W. A. (1968). The carcinogenicity of the o-methoxy derivatives of N-2-fluorenylacetamide and of related compounds in the rat. Cancer Res. 28:234-244.

Gutmann, H. R., and King, C. M. (1962). Protein labeling by 2-imino-1,2-fluorenoquinone, a metabolite in vitro of the carcinogen N-(2-fluorenyl)acetamide. Biochim. Biophys. Acta 56:394-396.

Gutmann, H. R., Malejka-Giganti, D., Barry, E. J., and Rydell, R. E. (1972). On the correlation between the hepatocarcinogenicity of the carcinogen, N-2-fluorenylacetamide, and its metabolic activation by the rat. Cancer Res. 32:1554-1561.

Gutmann, H. R., Malejka-Giganti, D., and McIver, R. (1975). Identification of carcinogenic acetates of fluorenylhydroxamic acids by high-pressure liquid chromatography. J. Chromatogr. 115:71-78.

Gutmann, H. R., and Nagasawa, H. T. (1960). The oxidation of o-aminophenols by cytochrome c and cytochrome oxidase. III. 2,3-Fluorenoquinone from 2-amino-3-fluorenol and binding of quinoid oxidation products to bovine serum albumin. J. Biol. Chem. 235:3466-3471.

Gutmann, H. R., Seal, U. S., and Irving, C. C. (1960). Mechanisms of protein binding of N-2-fluorenylacetamide. Deacetylation of N-(1-hydroxy-2-fluorenyl)acetamide and the effect of ethionine. Cancer Res. 20:1072-1978.

Guzzo, G. J., and Glazer, R. I. (1976). Effects of N-acetoxy-2-acetylaminofluorene and N-methyl-N'-nitro-N-nitroso-guanidine on nuclear DNA synthesis in rat liver. Cancer Res. 36:1041-1048.

Hadler, H. I., and Daniel, B. G. (1973). A correlation between the carcinogenicity of isomeric N-hydroxy-N-acetylaminofluorenes and their in vitro effect on mitochondria. Cancer Res. 33:117-122.

Hadler, H. I., and Demetriou, J. M. (1976). The disturbance of oxidative phosphorylation by N-acetoxy-N-acetyl-2-aminofluorene, a model ultimate carcinogen. J. Antibiot. (Tokyo) 28:809-818.

Haley, T. J., Farmer, J., Jaques, W. E., Frith, C., Sprowls, R. W., and Schieferstein, G. (1976). Dose-response hyperplasia from feeding N-2-fluorenylacetamide (2-FAA) to BALB/c mice for varying time intervals. Proc. Soc. Exp. Biol. Med. 152:156-159.

Haley, T. J., Schieferstein, G., Harmon, J. R., Dooley, K. L., Jaques, W. E., Frith, C., and Farmer, J. H. (1974a). Ninety day subchronic toxicity of N-2-fluorenylacetamide (2-FAA) in C57BL/6j and BALB/cStCr/BR mice. Proc. Soc. Exp. Biol. Med. 146:648-651.

Haley, T. J., Schieferstein, G., Jaques, W. E., Farmer, J., Frith, C., and Sprowls, R. W. (1974b). Dose-response predictability of urinary bladder hyperplasia by N-2-fluorenylacetamide feeding in mice: Its modification by sex. J. Pharm. Sci. 63:1940-1947.

Hara, E., Yonekawa, H., Kawajiri, K., Masuda, A., and Tagashira, Y. (1978). In vitro binding of 2-acetaminofluorene to RNA and protein with rat liver microsomes. Gan. 69:533-538.

Harada, M., Okabe, K., Shibata, K., Masuda, H., Miyata, K., and Enomoto, M. (1976). Histochemical demonstration of increased activity of γ-glutamyl transpeptidase in rat liver during hepatocarcinogenesis. Acta Histochem. Cytochem. 9:168-179.

Harr, J. R., Exon, J. H., Weswig, P. H., and Whanger, P. D. (1973). Relationship of dietary selenium concentration; chemical cancer induction; and tissue concentration of selenium in rats. Clin. Toxicol. 6:487-495.

Harr, J. R., Exon, J. H., Whanger, P. D., and Weswig, P. H. (1972). Effect of dietary selenium on N-2-fluorenylacetamide (FAA) induced cancer in vitamin E supplemented selenium deficient rats. Clin. Toxicol. 5:187-194.

Harris, C. C., Connor, R. J., Jackson, F. E., and Lieberman, M. W. (1974). Intranuclear distribution of DNA repair synthesis induced by chemical carcinogens or ultraviolet light in human diploid fibroblasts. Cancer Res. 34:3461-3468.

Harvan, D. J., Hass, J. R., and Lieberman, M. W. (1977). Adduct formation between the carcinogen N-acetoxy-2-acetylaminofluorene and synthetic polydeoxyribonucleotides. Chem. Biol. Interact. 17:203-210.

Hashem, M., and Boutros, K. (1961). The influence of bilharzial infection on the carcinogenesis of the mouse bladder. An experimental study. J. Egypt. Med. Assoc. 44: 598-606.

Heldt, L. V., Rowe, N. H., and Spain, J. D. (1974). Response at fifteen weeks of the big brown bat (*Eptesicus fuscus*) to intraperitoneal injections of N-2-acetylaminofluorene. Cancer Res. 34:2807-2809.

Herzog, J., Serroni, A., Briesmeister, B. A., and Farber, J. L. (1975). N-Hydroxy-2-acetylaminofluorene inhibition of rat liver RNA polymerases. Cancer Res. 35: 2138-2144.

Hiasa, Y., Ohshima, M., Ohmori, T., and Murata, Y. (1978). Effect of α-benzene hexachloride on 2-fluorenylacetamide carcinogenesis in rats. Gan. 69:423-426.

Highman, B., Frith, C. H., and Littlefield, N. A. (1975). Alkaline phosphatase activity in hyperplastic and neoplastic urinary bladder epithelium of mice fed 2-acetylaminofluorene. J. Natl. Cancer Inst. 54:257-261.

Highman, B., Frith, C. H., and Littlefield, N. A. (1978). Sequential alkaline phosphatase changes in hyperplastic and neoplastic urothelium of mice fed 2-acetylaminofluorene. Environ. Pathol. Toxicol. 1:223-231.

Hiramoto, R., Bernecky, J., Jurandowski, J., and Pressman, D. (1961). Immunohistochemical staining properties of the N-2-FAA rat hepatoma. Cancer Res. 21:1372-1376.

Hiramoto, R., Jurand, J., Bernecky, J., and Pressman, D. (1963). Immunohistochemical differences among N-2-fluorenylacetamide-induced rat hepatomas. Cancer Res. 23: 109-111.

Hirano, T., Morris, H. P., Jackson, C. M., and Lewis, J. W. (1976). An inhibitory effect of salivary gland extirpation on the induction of mammary tumors in rats by N,N'-2,7-fluorenylenebisacetamide. Acta Pathol. Jpn. 26:341-356.

Hisaoka, K. K. (1958a). The effects of 2-acetylaminofluorene on the embryonic development of the zebrafish. I. Morphological studies. Cancer Res. 18:527-535.

Hisaoka, K. K. (1958b). The effects of 2-acetylaminofluorene on the embryonic development of the zebrafish. II. Histochemical studies. Cancer Res. 18:664-667.

Hobom, G., and Braunitzer, G. (1967a). Virusproteine. I. Isolierung von Mutanten des Phagen fd mit proteinchemischen Methoden. Hoppe-Seyler's Z. Physiol. Chem. 348: 783-796.

Hobom, C., and Braunitzer, G. (1967b). Virusproteine. II. Untersuchung polycyclischer aromatischer Amine auf ihre mutagene Wirkung am Phagen fd. Hoppe Seylers Z. Physiol. Chem. 348:797-803.

Hoffman, H. E., and Griffin, A. C. (1958). Action of cigarette tar and smoke on chemically induced carcinogenesis. Tex. Rep. Biol. Med. 16:333-345.

Hollander, C. F., and Higginson, J. (1971). Spontaneous cancers in *Praomys (Mastomys) natalensis*. J. Natl. Cancer Inst. 46:1343-1355.

Hong, S.-J., and Piette, L. H. (1976). Electron spin resonance spin-label studies of intercalation of ethidium bromide and aromatic amine carcinogens in DNA. Cancer Res. 36:1159-1171.

Hopp, M. L., Matsumoto, M., Lee, C., and Oyasu, R. (1977). Absorption and protein binding of N-2-fluorenylacetamide and its metabolites in the bladder of the rabbit. J. Natl. Cancer Inst. 58:281-285.

Horton, B. J., Horton, J. D., and Pitot, H. C. (1973a). Abnormal cholesterol uptake, storage, and synthesis in the livers of 2-acetylaminofluorene-fed rats. Cancer Res. 33:1301-1305.

Horton, B. J., Mott, G. E., Pitot, H. C., and Goldfarb, S. (1973b). Rapid uptake of dietary cholesterol by hyperplastic liver nodules and primary hepatomas. Cancer Res. 33:460-464.

Horton, B. J., and Sabine, J. R. (1971). Metabolic controls in precancerous liver: defective control of cholesterol synthesis in rats fed N-2-fluorenylacetamide. Eur. J. Cancer 7:459-465.

Hou, C. T., and Rees, K. R. (1961). Correlations of histological and biochemical changes in the livers of rats during prolonged administration of acetylaminofluorene. Br. J. Cancer 15:624-629.

How, S.-W., and Snell, K. C. (1967). Skin tumors induced in rats by the dietary administration of N,N'-2,7-fluorenylenebisacetamide. J. Natl. Cancer Inst. 38:407-434.

Huang, S. L., and Lieberman, M. W. (1978). Induction of 6-thioguanine resistance in human cells treated with N-acetoxy-2-acetylaminofluorene. Mutat. Res. 57:349-358.

Huberman, E., Donovan, P. J., and DiPaolo, J. A. (1972). Mutation and transformation of cultured mammalian cells by N-acetoxy-N-2-fluorenylacetamide. J. Natl. Cancer Inst. 48:837-840.

Hultin, T. (1959). Reactions of 2-aminofluorene and related aromatic amines with liver proteins in vitro. Exp. Cell Res. 18:112-125.

Hultin, T., and Arrhenius, E. (1965). Effects of carcinogenic amines on amino acid incorporation by liver systems. III. Inhibition by aminofluorene treatment and its dependence on vitamin E. Cancer Res. 25:124-131.

Ikan, R., Kirson, I., and Bergmann, E. D. (1965). Thin-layer chromatography of 2-substituted fluorenes. J. Chromatogr. 18:526-529.

Inagaki, A., Uno, S., Yoneda, M., and Ohkawa, K. (1976). 2,7-Fluorenediamine and 2,5-fluorenediamine as peroxidase reagents for blood smears. J. Lab. Clin. Med. 88:334-338.

Inui, N., Takayama, S., and Kuwabara, N. (1971). DNA measurement on cell nucleus of normal liver, adenoma, and hepatoma in mice: histologic features. J. Natl. Cancer Inst. 47:47-58.

Irving, C. C. (1964). Enzymatic N-hydroxylation of the carcinogen 2-acetylaminofluorene and the metabolism of N-hydroxy-2-acetylaminofluorene-9-^{14}C in vitro. J. Biol. Chem. 239:1589-1596.

Irving, C. C. (1970). Conjugates of N-hydroxy compounds. In _Metabolic Conjugation and Metabolic Hydrolysis_, Vol. I, W. H. Fishman (Ed.). Academic Press, New York, pp. 53-119.

Irving, C. C. (1973). Interaction of chemical carcinogens with DNA. In _Methods in Cancer Research_, Vol. VIII, H. Busch (Ed.). Academic Press, New York, pp. 189-244.

Irving, C. C. (1975). Comparative toxicity of N-hydroxy-2-acetylaminofluorene in several strains of rats. Cancer Res. 35:2959-2961.

Irving, C. C. (1977). Influence of the aryl group on the reaction of glucuronides of N-arylacethydroxamic acids with polynucleotides. Cancer Res. 37:524-528.

Irving, C. C., and Gutmann, H. R. (1959). Protein binding of model quinone imides. II. Interaction of some o-quinone imides with crystalline bovine serum albumin. J. Biol. Chem. 234:2878-2884.

Irving, C. C., and Gutmann, H. R. (1961). Protein binding of model quinone imides. III. Preparation of N$^{\varepsilon}$-(1-hydroxy-2-acetamido-4-fluorenyl)-DL-lysine. J. Org. Chem. 26:1859-1861.

Irving, C. C., Gutmann, H. R., and Larson, D. M. (1963). Evaluation of the carcinogenicity of aminofluorenols by implantation into the bladder of the mouse. Cancer Res. 23:1782-1791.

Irving, C. C., Roszell, J. A., and Fredi, J. L. (1978). Effects of chronic feeding of 2-acetylaminofluorene on nuclear populations in rat liver. Adv. Enzyme Regul. 16: 365-377.

Irving, C. C., and Veazy, R. A. (1972). Preferential binding of 2-acetylaminofluorene to rat liver rRNA during early stages of hepatocarcinogenesis. Biochem. Biophys. Res. Commun. 47:1159-1164.

Irving, C. C., and Williard, R. F. (1964). On the in vivo protein binding of 1-hydroxy-2-acetylaminofluorene-1-C^{14} in the rat. Cancer Res. 24:77-82.

Irving, C. C., Wiseman, R., Jr., and Hill, J. T. (1967a). Biliary excretion of the O-glucuronide of N-hydroxy-2-acetylaminofluorene by the rat and rabbit. Cancer Res. 27:2309-2317.

Irving, C. C., Wiseman, R., Jr., and Young, J. M. (1967b). Carcinogenicity of 2-acetylaminofluorene and N-hydroxy-2-acetylaminofluorene in the rabbit. Cancer Res. 27:838-848.

Ishii, Y., Elliott, J. A., Mishra, N. K., and Lieberman, M. W. (1977). Quantitative studies of transformation by chemical carcinogens and ultraviolet radiation using a subclone of BHK_{21} clone 13 Syrian hamster cells. Cancer Res. 37:2023-2029.

Ishikawa, N., and Okazaki, M. (1958). Studies on the fluorene derivatives. II. Nitration of 2-methoxyfluorene. Yuki Gosei Kagaku Kyokai Shi 16:467-471.

Isojima, S., Bernecky, J., Planinsek, J., Yagi, Y., and Pressman, D. (1965a). Differences between antibodies against the dense sediment and microsome fractions of the N-2-fluorenylacetamide-induced rat hepatoma. Cancer Res. 25:968-975.

Isojima, S., Planinsek, J., Yagi, Y., and Pressman, D. (1966). Differences between the microsomes of normal rat liver and of N-2-fluorenylacetamide-induced rat hepatoma as determined by the paired label antibody technic. Cancer Res. 26:1527-1533.

Isojima, S., Yagi, Y., Planinsek, J., and Pressman, D. (1965b). Purification of localizing antibodies formed against microsomes of the N-2-fluorenylacetamide-induced rat hepatoma. Cancer Res. 25:962-967.

Isojima, S., Yagi, Y., and Pressman, D. (1969). Antigens common to rat hepatomas induced with 2-acetylaminofluorene. Cancer Res. 29:140-144.

Ito, M., Masuko, K., Matsuyama, M., Suzuki, H., Nagayo, T., and Aoki, K. (1973). Proliferation of bile ductular cells in the spontaneously hypertensive rat fed N,N'-2,7-fluorenylenebisacetamide. J. Natl. Cancer Inst. 50:699-706.

Ito, N., and Farber, E. (1966). Effects of trypan blue on hepatocarcinogenesis in rats given ethionine or N-2-fluorenylacetamide. J. Natl. Cancer Inst. 37:775-785.

Ito, N., Tatematsu, M., Hirose, M., Nakanishi, K., and Murasaki, G. (1978). Enhancing effect of chemicals on production of hyperplastic liver nodules induced by N-2-fluorenylacetamide in hepatectomized rats. Gan. 69:143-144.

Ivanov, S. D., and Dzhioev, F. K. (1977). Binding of 9-^{14}C-acetylaminofluorene with rat liver nucleic acids during hepatocarcinogenesis and in primary hepatomas. Biull. Eksp. Biol. Med. 83:332-334.

Izumi, T. (1962). Developmental anomalies in offspring of mice induced by administration of 2-acetylaminofluorene during pregnancy. Acta Anat. Nippon 37:239-249.

Jabara, A. G. (1963). A comparison of the pathological effects of 2-acetylaminofluorene, 4-acetylaminobiphenyl, and 2-acetylaminobiphenyl in the dog. Cancer Res. 23:921-927.

Jackson, C. D., and Irving, C. C. (1972). Sex differences in cell proliferation and N-hydroxy-2-acetylaminofluorene sulfotransferase levels in rat liver during 2-acetylaminofluorene administration. Cancer Res. 32:1590-1594.

Jackson, C. D., and Irving, C. C. (1973a). Effect of N-hydroxy-2-acetylaminofluorene on ribonucleic acid and deoxyribonucleic acid synthesis. Biochem. Pharmacol. 22: 1247-1249.

Jackson, C. D., and Irving, C. C. (1973b). Effects of 2-acetylaminofluorene on liver cell proliferation after partial hepatectomy of female rats. Cancer Res. 33:397-401.

Jacobs, M. M., Matney, T. S., and Griffin, A. C. (1977). Inhibitory effects of selenium on the mutagenicity of 2-acetylaminofluorene (AAF) and AAF derivatives. Cancer Lett. 2:319-322.

Jones, A. H., Fantel, A. G., Kocan, R. A., and Juchau, M. R. (1977). Bioactivation of procarcinogens to mutagens in human fetal and placental tissues. Life Sci. 21:1831-1835.

Juchau, M. R., Berry, D. L., Zachariah, P. K., Namkung, M. J., and Slaga, T. (1976). Prenatal biotransformation of benzo[a]pyrene and N-2-fluorenylacetamide in human and subhuman primates. In Carcinogenesis, vol. I, Polynuclear Aromatic Hydrocarbons: Chemistry, Metabolism and Carcinogenesis, R. I. Freudenthal and P. W. Jones (Eds.). Raven Press, New York, pp. 23-34.

Juchau, M. R., Namkung, M. J., Berry, D. L., and Zachariah, P. K. (1975). Oxidative biotransformation of 2-acetylaminofluorene in fetal and placental tissues of humans and monkeys. Correlations with aryl hydrocarbon hydroxylase activities. Drug Metab. Dispos. 3:494-501.

Kadlubar, F. F., Miller, J. A., and Miller, E. C. (1976). Hepatic metabolism of N-hydroxy-N-methyl-4-aminoazobenzene and other N-hydroxy arylamines to reactive sulfuric acid esters. Cancer Res. 36:2350-2359.

Kadlubar, F. F., Miller, J. A., and Miller, E. C. (1977). Hepatic microsomal N-glucuronidation and nucleic acid binding of N-hydroxy arylamines in relation to urinary bladder carcinogenesis. Cancer Res. 37:805-814.

Kaplan, E., and Gutmann, H. R. (1979). Microsomal metabolism of arylamides by the rat and guinea pig. II. Oxidation of 3-fluorenylacetamide at carbon atom 9. Formation of 3-acetamido-9-fluorenone. Biochem. Pharmacol. 28:1609-1614.

Kaplan, E., Gutmann, H. R., and Emory, T. H. (1978). Microsomal metabolism of arylamides by the rat and guinea pig. I. Oxidation of N-3-fluorenylacetamide at carbon-atom-9—a major metabolic reaction. Biochem. Pharmacol. 27:1581-1589.

Kaplan, L. A., and Weinstein, I. B. (1976). Preferential inhibition of the synthesis of 45S ribosomal RNA precursor by N-acetoxyacetylaminofluorene in rat liver epithelial cultures. Chem. Biol. Interact. 12:99-108.

Kapuler, A. M., and Michelsen, A. M. (1971). The reaction of the carcinogen N-acetoxy-2-acetylaminofluorene with DNA and other polynucleotides and its stereochemical implications. Biochim. Biophys. Acta 232:436-450.

Kawajiri, K., Yonekawa, H., Hara, E., and Tagashira, Y. (1979). Activation of 2-acetylaminofluorene in the nuclei of rat liver. Cancer Res. 39:1089-1093.

Kent, G., Minick, O. T., Volini, F. I., Orfei, E., and de la Huerga, J. (1963a). Iron storage in N-2-fluorenylacetamide-induced hepatic injury. Lab. Invest. 12:1102-1112.

Kent, G., Volini, F. I., Orfei, E., Minick, O. T., and de la Huerga, J. (1963b). Effect of hepatic injuries upon iron storage in the liver. Lab. Invest. 12:1094-1101.

Khristov, K. (1968). Experimental tumors of the thyroid gland in rats treated with acetylaminofluorene and methylthiouracil. Onkologiya 5:49-60; Chem. Abst. 70:2320y.

Khudoley, V. V. (1977). Tumor induction by carcinogenic agents in anuran amphibian Rana temporaria. Arch. Geschwulstforsch. 47:385-395.

Kiese, M. (1966). The biochemical production of ferrihemoglobin-forming derivatives from aromatic amines, and mechanism of ferrihemoglobin formation. Pharmacol. Rev. 18: 1091-1161.

Kiese, M., and Wiedemann, I. (1968). Elimination of N-hydroxy arylamines from the blood of guinea pigs. Biochem. Pharmacol. 17:1151-1158.

Kimura, I., Sakuma, F., Ito, Y., Nishio, O., and Yasukawa, S. (1972). Unusual proliferation of bile-duct cells in ICR female mice given 2,7-fluorenylbisacetamide while nursing sucklings. Gan. 63:507-508.

King, C. M. (1974). Mechanism of reaction, tissue distribution, and inhibition of arylhydroxamic acid acyltransferase. Cancer Res. 34:1503-1515.

King, C. M., Bednar, T. W., and Linsmaier-Bednar, E. M. (1973). Activation of the carcinogen N-hydroxy-2-fluorenylacetamide: insensitivity to cyanide and sulfide of the peroxidase-H_2O_2 induced formation of nucleic acid adducts. Chem. Biol. Interact. 7:185-188.

King, C. M., Chang, S. F., and Gutmann, H. R. (1963a). The oxidation of o-aminophenols by cytochrome c and cytochrome oxidase. V. Inactivation of catalase and arginase by 2-imino-1,2-fluorenoquinone. J. Biol. Chem. 238:2206-2212.

King, C. M., and Gutmann, H. R. (1964). The action of the carcinogen N-(2-fluorenyl)acetamide on rat liver catalase and arginase in vivo. Cancer Res. 24:770-779.

King, C. M., Gutmann, H. R., and Chang, S. F. (1963b). The oxidation of o-aminophenols by cytochrome c and cytochrome oxidase. IV. Interaction of 2-imino-1,2-fluorenoquinone and of 2-imino-2,3-fluorenoquinone with bovine serum albumin. J. Biol. Chem. 238: 2199-2205.

King, C. M., and Olive, C. W. (1975). Comparative effects of strain, species, and sex on the acyltransferase- and sulfotransferase-catalyzed activations of N-hydroxy-N-2-fluorenylacetamide. Cancer Res. 35:906-912.

King, C. M., Olive, C. W., and Cardona, R. A. (1975). Activation of carcinogenic arylhydroxamic acids by human tissues. J. Natl. Cancer Inst. 55:285-287.

King, C. M., and Phillips, B. (1968). The non-reactivity of 1,2-fluorenoquinone-2-acetimide with deoxyribonucleic acid and soluble ribonucleic acid. Biochem. Pharmacol. 17:833-835.

King, C. M., Traub, N. R., Cardona, R. A., and Howard, R. B. (1976). Comparative adduct formation of 4-aminobiphenyl and 2-aminofluorene derivatives with macromolecules of isolated liver parenchymal cells. Cancer Res. 36:2374-2381.

King, C. M., Traub, N. R., Lortz, Z. M., and Thissen, M. R. (1979). Metabolic activation of arylhydroxamic acids by N-O-acyltransferase of rat mammary gland. Cancer Res. 39:3369-3372.

Kitagawa, M., and Tanigaki, N. (1968). Carcinogen-bound protein in liver. In Gann Monograph #4, Y. Yamamura, T. Aoki, and M. Muramatsu (Eds.). Maruzen, Tokyo, pp. 155-173.

Kitagawa, M., Tanigaki, N., Yagi, Y., Planinsek, J., and Pressman, D. (1966a). Carcinogen-binding antigens in rat liver microsomes. Cancer Res. 26:752-756.

Kitagawa, M., Yagi, Y., Planinsek, J., and Pressman, D. (1966b). In vivo localization of anticarcinogen antibody in organs of carcinogen treated rats. Cancer Res. 26:221-228.

Kitagawa, T. (1971a). Histochemical analysis of hyperplastic lesions and hepatomas of the liver of rats fed 2-fluorenylacetamide. Gan. 62:207-216.

Kitagawa, T. (1971b). Responsiveness of hyperplastic lesions and hepatomas to partial hepatectomy. Gan. 62:217-224.

Kitagawa, T. (1976). Sequential phenotypic changes in hyperplastic areas during hepatocarcinogenesis in the rat. Cancer Res. 36:2534-2539.

Kitagawa, T., Michalopoulos, G., and Pitot, H. C. (1975). Unscheduled DNA synthesis in cells from N-2-fluorenylacetamide-induced hyperplastic nodules of rat liver maintained in a primary culture system. Cancer Res. 35:3682-3692.

Kitagawa, T., and Pitot, H. C. (1975). The regulation of serine dehydratase and glucose-6-phosphatase in hyperplastic nodules of rat liver during diethylnitrosamine and N-2-fluorenylacetamide feeding. Cancer Res. 35:1075-1084.

Kitagawa, T., and Sugano, H. (1973). Combined enzyme histochemical and radioautographic studies on areas of hyperplasia in the liver of rats fed N-2-fluorenylacetamide. Cancer Res 33:2993-3001.

Kitagawa, T., Yokochi, T., and Sugano, H (1972). α-Fetoprotein and hepatocarcinogenesis in rats fed 3'-methyl-4-(dimethylamino)azobenzene or N-2-fluorenylacetamide. Int. J. Cancer 10:368-381.

Kitagawa, T., Yokochi, T., and Sugano, H. (1973). α-Fetoprotein and hepatocarcinogenesis in rats. In Gann Monograph #14, H. Hirai and T. Miyaji (Eds.). University Park Press, Baltimore, pp. 249-268.

Klein, M. (1959). Influence of low dose of 2-acetylaminofluorene on liver tumorigenesis in mice. Proc. Soc. Exp. Biol. Med. 101:637-638.

Koblyakov, V. A., and Kolyada, A. Y. (1978). The state of the enzymatic system of microsomal oxidases after repeated administration of 2-acetylaminofluorene (Russian). Vopr. Med. Khim. 24:113-118.

Kopelovich, L., and Wolfe, G. (1977). Modification of ribonucleic acid by vitamin B_6. 1. Specific interaction of pyridoxal 5'-phosphate with transfer ribonucleic acid. Biochemistry 16:3721-3726.

Koss, L. G., and Lavin, P. (1971). Studies of experimental bladder carcinoma in Fischer 344 female rats. I. Induction of tumors with diet low in vitamin B_6 containing N-2-fluorenylacetamide after single dose of cyclophosphamide. J. Natl. Cancer Inst. 46:585-595.

Kowalewski, K. (1973). Relationship between vagotomy, peptic ulcer and gastric adenocarcinoma in rats fed 2,7-diacetylaminofluorene. Can. J. Surg. 16:210-217.

Kowalewski, K., and Todd, E. F. (1971). Carcinogenic action of 2,7-diacetylaminofluorene on the stomach of rats with experimental gastric ulcer. Scand. J. Gastroenterol. 6:323-328.

Kozuka, S. (1970). Inhibiting effect of reserpine and female sensitivity in hepatic tumor induction with 2,7-diacetamidofluorene in SMA/M_S strain mice. Cancer Res. 30:1384-1386.

Kozuka, S., and Sassa, R. (1976). Acceleration of hepatocarcinogenesis of 2,7-bis(acetamido)fluorene by carbon tetrachloride and time relation of treatment. Gan. 67:141-145.

Kriek, E. (1974). Carcinogenesis by aromatic amines. Biochim. Biophys. Acta 355:177-203.

Kriek, E. (1979). Effect of pH on the ratio of substitution products in DNA after reaction with the carcinogen N-acetoxy-2-acetylaminofluorene. Cancer Lett. 7:141-146.

Kriek, E., and Spelt, C. E. (1979). Differential excision from DNA of the C-8 deoxyguanosine reaction products of N-hydroxy-2-aminofluorene and N-acetoxy-N-acetyl-2-aminofluorene by endonuclease S_1 from Aspergillus oryzae. Cancer Lett. 7:147-154.

Kroes, R., Berkvens, J. M., and Weisburger, J. H. (1975a). Immunosuppression in primary liver and colon tumor induction with N-hydroxy-N-2-fluorenylacetamide and azoxymethane. Cancer Res. 35:2651-2656.

Kroes, R., Sontag, J. M., Sell, S., Williams, G. M., and Weisburger, J. H. (1975b). Elevated concentrations of serum α-fetoprotein in rats with chemically induced liver tumors. Cancer Res. 35:1214-1217.

Kroes, R., Williams, G. M., and Weisburger, J. H. (1973). Early appearance of serum α-fetoprotein as a function of dosage of various hepatocarcinogens. Cancer Res. 33:613-617.

Ku, K. Y., and Voytek, P. (1976). The effects of U.V.-light, ionizing radiation and the carcinogen N-acetoxy-2-fluorenylacetamide on the development in vitro of one- and two-cell mouse embryos. Int. J. Radiat. Biol. 30:401-408.

Kubinski, H., Morin, N. R., and Zeldin, P. E. (1976). Increased attachment of nucleic acids to eukaryotic and prokaryotic cells induced by chemical and physical carcinogens and mutagens. Cancer Res. 36:3025-3033.

Kubinski, K., and Kasper, C. B. (1971). Carcinogen and microsomal membrane interactions: changes in membrane density and ability to bind nucleic acids. Science 171:201-203.

Kuroki, T., and Bartsch, H. (1979). Mutagenicity of some N- and O-acyl derivatives of N-hydroxy-2-aminofluorene in V79 Chinese hamster cells. Cancer Lett. 6:67-72.

Kurzepa, H., Gutmann, H. R., Malejka-Giganti, D., Krauss, A., Cervenka, J., Vosika, G. J., and Rydell, R. E. (1978). Studies on the transformation of rat embryo cells of low passage by carcinogenic fluorenylhydroxamic acids and their acetate esters. In Vitro 14:261-270.

Lacassagne, A., and Hurst, L. (1966). Action du 2-acetaminofluorene (AAF) sur les tubes sereux de la glande sousmaxillaire du rat. C. R. Acad. Sci. [D] (Paris) 263:2059-2061.

Lacassagne, A., and Hurst, L. (1967). Quelques elements de comparaison de l'action hepatocancerogene du 2-acetaminofluorene chez le rat avec celles du p-dimethylaminoazobenzene et de la diethylnitrosamine. Bull. Cancer 54:171-184.

Lacassagne, A., and Hurst, L. (1969). Influence de sulfamides hypo- ou hyperglycemiants sur la cancerisation du foie du rat par le 2-acetylaminofluorene. Bull. Cancer 56: 397-410.

Laird, A. K., and Barton, A. D. (1961). Cell proliferation in precancerous liver: relation to presence and dose of carcinogen. J. Natl. Cancer Inst. 27:827-839.

Laishes, B. A., and Farber, E. (1978). Transfer of viable putative preneoplastic hepatocytes to the livers of syngeneic host rats. J. Natl. Cancer Inst. 61:507-512.

Laishes, B. A., Ogawa, K., Roberts, E., and Farber, E. (1978a). Gamma-glutamyl transpeptidase: a positive marker for cultured rat liver cells derived from putative premalignant and malignant lesions. J. Natl. Cancer Inst. 60:1009-1016.

Laishes, B. A., Roberts, E., and Farber, E. (1978b). In vitro measurement of carcinogen-resistant liver cells during hepatocarcinogenesis. Int. J. Cancer 21:186-193.

Laishes, B. A., and Stich, H. F. (1973). Relative DNA damage induced in cultured human skin fibroblasts by exposure to the precarcinogen 2-acetylaminofluorene, the proximate carcinogen N-hydroxy-2-acetylaminofluorene, and the ultimate carcinogen N-acetoxy-2-acetylaminofluorene. Can. J. Biochem. 51:990-994.

Landolph, J. R., and Heidelberger, C. (1979). Chemical carcinogens produce mutations to ouabain resistance in transformable C3H/10T 1/2 Cl 8 mouse fibroblasts. Proc. Natl. Acad. Sci. USA 76:930-934.

Lawson, T. A., Dawson, K. M., and Clayson, D. B. (1970). Acute changes in nucleic acid and protein synthesis in the mouse bladder epithelium induced by three bladder carcinogens. Cancer Res. 30:1586-1592.

Lazear, E. J., Louie, S. C., Shaddock, J. G., Barren, P. R., and Norvell, M. (1978). The effects of dietary protein, fat and 2-acetylaminofluorene on the microsomal activity levels of liver from BALB/c mice. Toxicol. Lett. 2:345-350.

Lefevre, J.-F., Fuchs, R. P., and Daune, M. P. (1978). Comparative studies on the 7-iodo and 7-fluoro derivatives of N-acetoxy-N-2-acetylaminofluorene: binding sites on DNA and conformational change of modified deoxytrinucleotides. Biochemistry 17: 2561-2567.

Leffert, H. L., Moran, T., Boorstein, R., and Koch, K. S. (1977). Procarcinogen activation and hormonal control of cell proliferation in differentiated primary adult rat liver cell cultures. Nature 267:58-61.

Leng, M., Sage, E., Fuchs, R. P., and Daune, M. P. (1978). Antibodies to DNA modified by the carcinogen N-acetoxy-N-2-acetylaminofluorene. FEBS Lett. 92:207-210.

Levi, P. E., Knowles, J. C., Cowen, D. M., Wood, M., and Cooper, E. H. (1971). Disorganization of mouse bladder epithelium induced by 2-acetylaminofluorene and 4-ethylsulfonylnaphthalene-1-sulfonamide. J. Natl. Cancer Inst. 46:337-352.

Levin, W., Lu, A. Y. H., Thomas, P. E., Ryan, D., Kizer, D. E., and Griffin, M. J. (1978). Identification of epoxide hydrase as the preneoplastic antigen in rat liver hyperplastic nodules. Proc. Natl. Acad. Sci. USA 75:3240-3243.

Levine, A. F., Fink, L. M., Weinstein, I. B., and Grunberger, D. (1974). Effect of N-2-acetylaminofluorene modification on the conformation of nucleic acids. Cancer Res. 34:319-327.

Levine, W. G. (1971). Metabolism and biliary excretion of N-2-fluorenylacetamide and N-hydroxy-2-fluorenylacetamide. Life Sci. II 10:727-735.

Lhoest, G., Razzouk, C., and Mercier, M. (1976). Biological implications of the reaction possibilities of the proximate carcinogenic compound, N-hydroxy-2-fluorenylacetamide. Biomed. Mass Spectrom. 3:21-27.

Lhoest, G., Roberfroid, M., and Mercier, M. (1978). The proximodistal carcinogen N-hydroxy-2-fluorenylacetamide, toxification and detoxification routes due to electrophilic and combined nucleophilic and electrophilic tautomerism effects. Biomed. Mass Spectrom. 5:38-43.

Liau, M. C., Chang, C. F., and Becker, F. F. (1979). Alteration of S-adenosylmethionine synthetases during chemical hepatocarcinogenesis and in resulting carcinomas. Cancer Res. 39:2113-2119.

Lieberman, M. W., Baney, R. N., Lee, R. E., Sell, S., and Farber, E. (1971a). Studies on DNA repair in human lymphocytes treated with proximate carcinogens and alkylating agents. Cancer Res. 31:1297-1306.

Lieberman, M. W., and Forbes, P. D. (1973). Demonstration of DNA repair in normal and neoplastic tissues after treatment with proximate chemical carcinogens and ultraviolet radiation. Nature New Biol. 241:199-201.

Lieberman, M. W., and Poirier, M. C. (1973). Deoxyribonucleoside incorporation during DNA repair of carcinogen-induced damage in human diploid fibroblasts. Cancer Res. 33:2097-2103.

Lieberman, M. W., and Poirier, M. C. (1974a). Distribution of deoxyribonucleic acid repair synthesis among repetitive and unique sequences in the human diploid genome. Biochemistry 13:3018-3023.

Lieberman, M. W., and Poirier, M. C. (1974b). Base-pairing and template specificity during deoxyribonucleic acid repair synthesis in human and mouse cells. Biochemistry 13:5384-5388.

Lieberman, M. W., and Poirier, M. C. (1974c). Intragenomal distribution of DNA repair synthesis: repair in satellite and mainband DNA in cultured mouse cells. Proc. Natl. Acad. Sci. USA 71:2461-2465.

Lieberman, M. W., Rutman, J. Z., and Farber, E. (1971b). Thymidine labeling of pyrimidine isostichs from human lymphocyte DNA during repair after damage with N-acetoxy acetylaminofluorene or nitrogen mustard. Biochim. Biophys. Acta 247: 497-501.

Likhachev, A. Y. (1969). Blastomogenesis in rats in the combined effect of N-2-fluorenylacetamide and N-nitrosodimethylamine (Russian). Vopr. Onkol. 15(9):65-69.

Lin, J.-C., Hiasa, Y., and Farber, E. (1977). Preneoplastic antigen as a marker for endoplasmic reticulum of putative premalignant hepatocytes during liver carcinogenesis. Cancer Res. 37:1972-1981.

Lindahl, R. (1977). Aldehyde dehydrogenase in 2-acetaminofluorene-induced rat hepatomas. Ontogeny and evidence that the new isoenzymes are not due to normal gene de-repression. Biochem. J. 164:119-123.

Lindahl, R. (1978). Aldehyde dehydrogenase in 2-acetylaminofluorene-induced rat hepatomas. Characterization of antigens recognized by anti-hepatoma aldehyde dehydrogenase sera. Biochim. Biophys. Acta 525:9-17.

Lindahl, R., and Feinstein, R. N. (1976). Purification and immunochemical characterization of aldehyde dehydrogenase from 2-acetylaminofluorene-induced rat hepatomas. Biochim. Biophys. Acta 452:345-355.

Lombard, C. (1961). Chute du nombre des globules sanguins chez les cobayes traites par le 2-acetylaminofluorene (2-AAF). C. R. Soc. Biol. (Paris) 155:141-142.

Lombard, C. (1962). Cancerisation du cobaye par le 2-acetylaminofluorene. C. R. Soc. Biol. (Paris) 156:1165-1167.

Lombardi, B., and Shinozuka, H. (1979). Enhancement of 2-acetylaminofluorene liver carcinogenesis in rats fed a choline-devoid diet. Int. J. Cancer 23:565-570.

Lotlikar, P. D., and Dwyer, E. N. (1976). Effect of detergents on N- and ring-hydroxylation of 2-acetamidofluorene by hamster liver microsomal preparations. Biochem. J. 160:821-824.

Lotlikar, P. D., Dwyer, E. N., Baldy, W. J., and Nyce, J. (1977). Phospholipid requirement for 2-acetamidofluorene N- and ring-hydroxylation by hamster liver microsomal cytochrome P-450 enzyme system. Biochem. J. 168:571-574.

Lotlikar, P. D., Enomoto, M., Miller, J. A., and Miller, E. C. (1967). Species variations in the N- and ring-hydroxylation of 2-acetylaminofluorene and effects of 3-methylcholanthrene pretreatment. Proc. Soc. Exp. Biol. Med. 125:341-346.

Lotlikar, P. D., Fukuda, S., and Yamamoto, N. (1972). Effects of the carcinogen 2-acetylaminofluorene and its derivatives on bacteria and bacteriophages. Mol. Pharmacol. 8:645-650.

Lotlikar, P. D., Hong, Y. S., and Baldy, W. J. (1978). Effect of 3-methylcholanthrene pretreatment on 2-acetylaminofluorene N-hydroxylation and ring-hydroxylation by rat and hamster liver microsomes. Toxicol. Lett. 2:135-139.

Lotlikar, P. D., and Luha, L. (1971). Acylation of carcinogenic hydroxamic acids by carbamoyl phosphate to form reactive esters. Biochem. J. 124:69-74.

Lotlikar, P. D., Scribner, J. D., Miller, J. A., and Miller, E. C. (1966). Reaction of esters of aromatic N-hydroxy amines and amides with methionine in vitro: a model for in vivo binding of amine carcinogens to protein. Life Sci. 5:1263-1269.

Lotlikar, P. D., and Wasserman, M. B. (1970). Reactive phosphate ester of the carcinogen 2-(N-hydroxy)acetamidofluorene. Biochem. J. 120:661-665.

Lotlikar, P. D., Wasserman, M. B., and Luha, L. (1973a). Effect of 3-amino-1,2,4-triazole pretreatment on N- and ring-hydroxylation of 2-acetylaminofluorene by the rat. Proc. Soc. Exp. Biol. Med. 144:445-449.

Lotlikar, P. D., Wertman, K., and Luha, L. (1973b). Role of mixed-function amine oxidase in N-hydroxylation of 2-acetamidofluorene by hamster liver microsomal preparations. Biochem. J. 136:1137-1140.

Lotlikar, P. D., and Zaleski, K. (1974). Inhibitory effect of carbon monoxide on the N- and ring-hydroxylation of 2-acetamidofluorene by hamster hepatic microsomal preparations. Biochem. J. 144:427-430.

Lotlikar, P. D., and Zaleski, K. (1975). Ring- and N-hydroxylation of 2-acetamidofluorene by rat liver reconstituted cytochrome P-450 enzyme system. Biochem. J. 150:561-564.

Lower, G. M., Jr., and Bryan, G. T. (1973). Enzymatic N-acetylation of carcinogenic aromatic amines by liver cytosol of species displaying different organ susceptibilities. Biochem. Pharmacol. 22:1581-1588.

Lower, G. M., Jr., and Bryan, G. T. (1976). Enzymic deacetylation of carcinogenic arylacetamides by tissue microsomes of the dog and other species. J. Toxicol. Environ. Health 1:421-432.

Maher, V. M., Birch, N., Otto, J. R., and McCormick, J. J. (1975). Cytotoxicity of carcinogenic aromatic amides in normal and xeroderma pigmentosum fibroblasts with different DNA repair capabilities. J. Natl. Cancer Inst. 54:1287-1294.

Maher, V. M., and McCormick, J. J. (1976). Effect of DNA repair on the cytotoxicity and mutagenicity of UV irradiation and of chemical carcinogens in normal and xeroderma pigmentosum cells. In Biology of Radiation Carcinogenesis, J. M. Yuhas, R. W. Tennant, and J. D. Regan (Eds.). Raven Press, New York, pp. 129-145.

Maher, V. M., and Reuter, M. A. (1973). Mutations and loss of transforming activity of DNA caused by the O-glucuronide conjugate of the carcinogen N-hydroxy-2-aminofluorene. Mutat. Res. 21:63-71.

Maher, V. M., and Wessel, J. E. (1975). Mutations to azaguanine resistance induced in cultured human diploid fibroblasts by the carcinogen N-acetoxy-2-acetylaminofluorene. Mutat. Res. 28:277-284.

Mahlum, D. D. (1967). Influence of hepatocarcinogen feeding on the retention of cerium-144 by the liver. Toxicol. Appl. Pharmacol. 11:585-590.

Makiura, S., Aoe, H., Sugihara, S., Hirao, K., Arai, M., and Ito, N. (1974). Inhibitory effects of polychlorinated biphenyls on liver tumorigenesis in rats treated with 3'-methyl-4-dimethylaminoazobenzene, N-2-fluorenylacetamide and diethylnitrosamine. J. Natl. Cancer Inst. 53:1253-1257.

Malejka-Giganti, D., Gutmann, H. R., and Rydell, R. E. (1973). Mammary carcinogenesis in the rat by topical application of fluorenylhydroxamic acids. Cancer Res. 33:2489-2497.

Malejka-Giganti, D., McIver, R. C., Glasebrook, A. L., and Gutmann, H. R. (1978). Induction of microsomal N-hydroxylation of N-2-fluorenylacetamide in rat liver. Biochem. Pharmacol. 27:61-69.

Malejka-Giganti, D., and Rydell, R. E. (1978). Lack of susceptibility of F344 rats to mammary tumor induction by topically applied fluorenylacetohydroxamic acids and their acetates. J. Natl. Cancer Inst. 60:433-435.

Malejka-Giganti, D., Rydell, R. E., and Gutmann, H. R. (1977). Mammary carcinogenesis in the rat by topical application of fluorenylhydroxamic acids and their acetates. Cancer Res. 37:111-117.

Maltoni, C., Peretti, S., and Ghetti, G. (1968). Sinergismo d'azione oncogena della 2-N-fluorenilacetamide e del tetracloruro di carbonio sul fegatto di ratto. Cancro 21:63-72.

Maluguina, L. L. (1958). Tumors produced by 2-acetylaminofluorene in hamsters (Russian). Vopr. Onkol. 4(3):279-283.

Maluguina, L. L. (1962). On pretumorous changes provoked in the liver of rats by means of 2-acetylaminofluorene (2AAF) (Russian). Vopr. Onkol. 8(5):6-13.

Martin, C. N., McDermid, A. C., and Garner, R. C. (1978). Testing of known carcinogens and noncarcinogens for their ability to induce unscheduled DNA synthesis in HeLa cells. Cancer Res. 38:2621-2627.

Martinsen, C. S., and Zachariah, P. K. (1978). Growth of various bacteria on polycyclic aromatic hydrocarbons and N-2-fluorenylacetamide. J. Appl. Bacteriol. 44:365-371.

Martucci, E., Di Toro, R., and Rigillo, N. (1961). Anemia emolitica con formazione di corpi inclusi in topi trattati con 2-acetamidofluorene. Pediatria (Napoli) 69:836-840.

Marugami, M., Ito, N., Konishi, Y., Hiasa, Y., and Farber, E. (1967). Influence of 3-methylcholanthrene on liver carcinogenesis in rats ingesting DL-ethionine, 3'-methyl-4-dimethylaminoazobenzene, and N-2-fluorenylacetamide. Cancer Res. 27:2011-2109.

Matsushima, T., Grantham, P. H., Weisburger, E. K., and Weisburger, J. H. (1972). Phenobarbital-mediated increase in ring- and N-hydroxylation of the carcinogen N-2-fluorenylacetamide and decrease in amounts bound to liver deoxyribonucleic acid. Biochem. Pharmacol. 21:2043-2051.

McCann, J., Choi, E., Yamasaki, E., and Ames, B. N. (1975). Detection of carcinogens as mutagens in the Salmonella/microsome test: Assay of 300 chemicals. Proc. Natl. Acad. Sci. USA 72:5135-5139.

McDonald, J. H., Oyasu, R., and Hass, G. M. (1962). The relation of liver neoplasms to bladder tumors produced by 2-acetylaminofluorene. J. Urol. 87:381-390.

McGregor, D. (1973). Effects of methylcholanthrene on 2-acetamidofluorene association with liver cell components. Biochem. Pharmacol. 22:3136-3139.

McGregor, D. (1975). The relationship of 2-acetamidofluorene mutagenicity in plate tests with its in vivo liver cell component distribution and its carcinogenic potential. Mutat. Res. 30:305-316.

McPherson, F. J., Bridges, J. W., and Parke, D. V. (1976). Studies on the nature of the in vitro enhancement of biphenyl 2-hydroxylation provoked by some chemical carcinogens. Biochem. Pharmacol. 25:1345-1350.

Meindl, P., Bodo, G., and Tuppy, H. (1976). Synthetische niedermolekulare Induktoren von Interferon I. Mitteilung: Derivates des Diaminofluoren-9-ons, Diaminobenzophenons und Diaminobiphenyls. Arzneim. Forsch. 26:312-316.

Melicow, M. M., Uson, A. C., and Price, T. D. (1964). Bladder tumor induction in rats fed 2-acetamidofluorene (2-AAF) and a pyridoxine-deficient diet. J. Urol. 91:520-529.

Merkow, L. P., Epstein, S. M., Caito, B. J., and Bartus, B. (1967). The cellular analysis of liver carcinogenesis: ultrastructural alterations within hyperplastic liver nodules induced by 2-fluorenylacetamide. Cancer Res. 27:1712-1721.

Merkow, L. P., Epstein, S. M., Farber, E., Pardo, M., and Bartus, B. (1969). Cellular analysis of liver carcinogenesis. III. Comparison of the ultrastructure of hyperplastic liver nodules and hepatocellular carcinomas induced in rat liver by 2-fluorenylacetamide. J. Natl. Cancer Inst. 43:33-63.

Merritt, W. D., Keenan, T. W., and Morre, D. J. (1976). Gangliosides and other lipids of hyperplastic liver nodules induced by N-2-fluorenylacetamide. Cancer Biochem. Biophys. 1:179-185.

Merritt, W. D., Morre, D. J., and Keenan, T. W. (1978a). Gangliosides of liver tumors induced by N-2-fluorenylacetamide. II. Alterations in biosynthetic enzymes. J. Natl. Cancer Inst. 60:1329-1337.

Merritt, W. D., Richardson, C. L., Keenan, T. W., and Morre, D. J. (1978b). Gangliosides of liver tumors induced by N-2-fluorenylacetamide. I. Ganglioside alterations in liver tumorigenesis and normal development. J. Natl. Cancer Inst. 60:1313-1327.

Metzger, G., and Daune, M. P. (1975). In vitro binding of N-acetoxy-N-2-acetylaminofluorene to DNA in chromatin. Cancer Res. 35:2738-2742.

Metzger, G., Wilhelm, F. X., and Wilhelm, M. L. (1976). Distribution along DNA of the bound carcinogen N-acetoxy-N-2-acetylaminofluorene in chromatin modified in vitro. Chem. Biol. Interact. 15:257-265.

Michalopoulos, G., Sattler, G. L., O'Connor, L., and Pitot, H. C. (1978). Unscheduled DNA synthesis induced by procarcinogens in suspensions and primary cultures of hepatocytes on collagen membranes. Cancer Res. 38:1866-1871.

Middleton, P. J. (1965). The histogenesis of mammary tumours induced in the rat by chemical carcinogens. Br. J. Cancer 19:830-839.

Mikata, A., and Luse, S. A. (1964). Ultrastructural changes in the rat liver produced by N-2-fluorenyldiacetamide. Am. J. Pathol. 44:455-479.

Miller, E. C., Fletcher, T. J., Margreth, A., and Miller, J. A. (1962). The carcinogenicities of derivatives of fluorene and biphenyl: fluoro derivatives as probes for active sites in 2-acetylaminofluorene. Cancer Res. 22:1002-1014.

Miller, E. C., Lotlikar, P. D., Pitot, H. C., Fletcher, T. L., and Miller, J. A. (1966). N-Hydroxy metabolites of 2-acetylaminophenanthrene and 7-fluoro-2-acetylaminofluorene as proximate carcinogens in the rat. Cancer Res. 26:2239-2247.

Miller, E. C., and Miller, J. A. (1960). A mechanism of ortho-hydroxylation of aromatic amines in vivo. Biochim. Biophys. Acta 40:380-382.

Miller, E. C., and Miller, J. A. (1966). Mechanisms of chemical carcinogenesis. Nature of proximate carcinogens and interactions with macromolecules. Pharmacol. Rev. 18:805-838.

Miller, E. C., and Miller, J. A. (1969a). Studies on the mechanism of activation of aromatic amines and amide carcinogens to ultimate carcinogenic electrophilic reactants. Ann. NY Acad. Sci. 163:731-750.

Miller, E. C., and Miller, J. A. (1976). The metabolism of chemical carcinogens to reactive electrophiles and their possible mechanisms of action in carcinogenesis. In Chemical Carcinogens, C. E. Searle (Ed.). ACS Monograph 173, American Chemical Society, Washington, D.C., pp. 737-762.

Miller, E. C., Miller, J. A., Brown, R. R., and MacDonald, J. C. (1958). On the protective action of certain polycyclic aromatic hydrocarbons against carcinogenesis by aminoazo dyes and 2-acetylaminofluorene. Cancer Res. 18:469-477.

Miller, J. A., and Miller, E. C. (1969b). The metabolic activation of carcinogenic aromatic amines and amides. Prog. Exp. Tumor Res. 11:273-301.

Millette, R. L., and Fink, L. M. (1975). The effect of modification of T7 DNA by the carcinogen N-2-acetylaminofluorene: termination of transcription in vitro. Biochemistry 14:1426-1432.

Miyakawa, M., Yoshida, O., Harada, T., and Kato, T. (1973). The effect of urinary β-glucuronidase inhibitor on the induction of tumors with 2-acetylaminofluorene in rats. Invest. Urol. 10:256-261.

Miyata, K., Noguchi, Y., and Enomoto, M. (1972). Biliary excretion of metabolites of 2-acetamidofluorene by mouse and guinea pig in vivo and in isolated perfused rat liver. Jpn. J. Exp. Med. 42:483-489.

Mobley, T. L., Coyle, J. K., Al-Hussaini, M., and McDonald, D. F. (1966). The role of chronic mechanical irritation in experimental urothelial tumorigenesis. Invest. Urol. 3:325-333.

Moewus, F. (1960). Enhancement of mitotic activity by fluorene derivatives. J. Natl. Cancer Inst. 24:1299-1308.

Mohan, L. C., Grantham, P. H., Weisburger, E. K., Weisburger, J. H., and Idoine, J. B. (1976). Mechanisms of the inhibitory action of p-hydroxyacetanilide on carcinogenesis by N-2-fluorenylacetamide or N-hydroxy-N-2-fluorenylacetamide. J. Natl. Cancer Inst. 56:763-768.

Money, W. L., and Rawson, R. W. (1965). Intrathyroid implantation of chemical carcinogens in the rat. Arch. Pathol. 79:470-474.

Morais, R., Poirier, L. A., and Dupuis, C. (1972). Inhibition of mitochondrial 5'-endonuclease activity by carcinogenic amines and their N-oxidized products. Chem. Biol. Interact. 5:391-399.

Morris, H. P., Sidransky, H., and Wagner, B. P. (1963a). Influence of a diet low in pyridoxine on tumorigenesis in rats ingesting N-2-fluorenylacetamide. Tumori 49: 159-171.

Morris, H. P., Velat, C. A., Wagner, B. P., Dahlgard, M., and Ray, F. E. (1960). Studies of carcinogenicity in the rat of derivatives of aromatic amines related to N-2-fluorenylacetamide. J. Natl. Cancer Inst. 24:149-180.

Morris, H. P., Wagner, B. P., and Lombard, L. S. (1958). A comparison of impaired function with morphological changes occurring in livers of rats ingesting N-2-fluorenyldiacetamide. J. Natl. Cancer Inst. 20:1-35.

Morris, H. P., Wagner, B. P., Ray, F. E., Snell, K. C., and Stewart, H. L. (1961). Comparative study of cancer and other lesions of rats fed N,N'-2,7-fluorenylenebisacetamide or N-2-fluorenylacetamide. Natl. Cancer Inst. Monogr. 5: 1-53.

Morris, H. P., Wagner, B. P., Ray, F. E., Stewart, H. L., and Snell, K. C. (1962). Comparative carcinogenic effects of N,N'-2,7-fluorenylenebisacetamide by intraperitoneal and oral routes of administration to rats, with particular reference to gastric carcinoma. J. Natl. Cancer Inst. 29:977-1011.

Morris, H. P., Wagner, B. P., Ray, F. E., Stewart, H. L., and Snell, K. C. (1963b). Carcinogenic effects of N,N'-2,7-fluorenylenebis-2,2,2-trifluoroacetamide (2,7-FAA-F_6) administered orally to Buffalo strain rats. J. Natl. Cancer Inst. 30:143-161.

Moyer, G. H., Gumbiner, B., and Austin, G. E. (1977). Binding of N-hydroxy acetylaminofluorene to eu- and heterochromatin fractions of rat liver in vivo. Cancer Lett. 2:259-266.

Mulder, G. J., Hinson, J. A., Nelson, W. L., and Thorgeirsson, S. S. (1977). Role of sulfotransferase from rat liver in the mutagenicity of N-hydroxy-2-acetylaminofluorene in Salmonella typhimurium. Biochem. Pharmacol. 25:1356-1358.

Mushlin, P. S., and Peraino, C. (1974). Effects of dietary phenobarbital on the binding of 2-acetylaminofluorene to rat liver nuclear DNA. Proc. Soc. Exp. Biol. Med. 145: 859-862.

Myhr, B. C., and DiPaolo, J. A. (1978a). Mutagenesis of Chinese hamster cells in vitro by combination treatments with methyl methanesulfonate and N-acetoxy-2-acetylaminofluorene. Cancer Res. 38:2539-2543.

Myhr, B. C., and DiPaolo, J. A. (1978b). Mutagenesis by N-acetoxy-2-acetylaminofluorene of Chinese hamster V79 cells is unaffected by caffeine. Chem. Biol. Interact. 21:1-18.

Nagasawa, H. T., and Gutmann, H. R. (1959). The oxidation of o-aminophenols by cytochrone c and cytochrome oxidase. I. Enzymatic oxidations and binding of oxidation products to bovine serum albumin. J. Biol. Chem. 234:1593-1599.

Nagasawa, H. T., and Gutmann, H. R. (1966). o-Methoxy derivatives of the carcinogen, N-2-fluorenylacetamide. Potent latent biological arylating agents. J. Med. Chem. 9: 719-725.

Nagasawa, H. T., Gutmann, H. R., and Morgan, M. A. (1959). The oxidation of o-aminophenols by cytochrome c and cytochrome oxidase. II. Synthesis and identification of oxidation products. J. Biol. Chem. 234:1600-1604.

Nagasawa, H. T., Kuo, T. H., Shirota, F. N., and Alexander, C. S. (1976). An intestinal arylamidase that selectively hydrolyzes certain aromatic amides. Biochem. Pharmacol. 25:853-858.

Nagasawa, H. T., Morgan, M. A., and Gutmann, H. R. (1958). The enzymic oxidation of o-aminophenols. Biochim. Biophys. Acta 28:665-666.

Nagasawa, H. T., and Osteraas, A. J. (1964). The biological arylation of proteins in vitro by a metabolite of the carcinogen N-2-fluorenylacetamide. Biochem. Pharmacol. 13: 713-723.

Nagayo, T. (1965). Effect of oral administration of N,N'-2,7-fluorenylenebisacetamide combined with traumatic ulcers of the glandular stomach of Buffalo rats. J. Natl. Cancer Inst. 35:829-840.

Nagayo, T. (1968). Gastro-intestinal carcinomas of Buffalo rats fed N,N'-2,7-fluorenylenebisacetamide. Gann Monograph #3, R. Kinosita, T. Nagayo, and T. Tanaka (Eds.). Maruzen, Tokyo, pp. 105-107.

Nagayo, T., and Ito, M. (1965). Pathological studies on the induced cancers of the gastro-intestinal tracts in the Buffalo rats fed N,N'-2,7-fluorenylenebisacetamide. Nagoya Med. J. 11:19-30.

Nagayo, T., Ito, M., and Yamada, S. (1970). Accelerated induction of hepatoma in rats fed N,N'-2,7-fluorenylenebisacetamide by x-irradiation to the target area. Gan. 61: 81-83.

Nagayo, T., Ito, M., and Yamada, S. (1972). Histogenesis and autoradiography of adenocarcinoma of the glandular stomach in rats induced by oral administration of N,N'-2,7-fluorenylenebisacetamide combined with irradiation to the stomach region. Gan. 63: 143-151.

Namkung, M. J., and Fletcher, T. L. (1960). Derivatives of fluorene. VII. New mono- and dinitro-compounds and some of their reactions. J. Org. Chem. 25:740-744.

Namkung, M. J., and Fletcher, T. L. (1961). Derivatives of fluorene. XV. Fluorofluorenes. IV. J. Org. Chem. 26:2243-2244.

Namkung, M. J., and Fletcher, T. L. (1967). Derivatives of fluorene. XXV. Fluorofluorenes. VI. Can. J. Chem. 45:2569-2575.

Namkung, M. J., and Fletcher, T. L. (1968a). Derivatives of fluorene. XXVI. Anomalous substitution in the deactivated fluorene nucleus: use of dimethyl sulphoxide with an ylid to promote bromination. Chem. Ind. 1486-1487.

Namkung, M. J., and Fletcher, T. L. (1968b). Derivatives of fluorene. XXVII. New thiofluorenes related to the metabolism of the carcinogen N-2-fluorenylacetamide. J. Med. Chem. 11:1235-1236.

Namkung, M. J., and Fletcher, T. L. (1969). Synthesis and reactions of 2,2'-hydrazofluorene and related compounds. J. Chem. Soc. [D[1052-1053.

Namkung, M. J., Fletcher, T. L., and Wetzel, W. (1965). Derivatives of fluorene. XX. Fluorofluorenes, V. New difluoro-2-acetamidofluorenes for the study of carcinogenic mechanisms. J. Med. Chem. 8:551-554.

Namkung, M. J., Zachariah, P. K., and Juchau, M. R. (1977). O-Sulfonation of N-hydroxy-2-fluorenylacetamide and 7-hydroxy-N-2-fluorenylacetamide in fetal and placental tissues of humans and guinea pigs. Drug Metab. Dispos. 5:288-294.

Napalkov, N. P. (1058) Experimental tumors of the thyroid gland (Russian). Vopr. Onkol. 4:738-750.

Napalkov, N. P. (1959). Experimental thyroid tumors induced by 6-methylthiouracil in combination with 2-acetylaminofluorene. Vopr. Onkol. 5(7):25-33.

Narayan, K. A. (1967). Serum lipoproteins during chemical carcinogenesis. Biochem. J. 103:672-676.

Narayan, K. A. (1970). Serum lipoproteins of rats fed an essential fatty acid-deficient diet and N-2-fluorenylacetamide. Cancer Res. 30:1185-1191.

Neish, W. J. P. (1967). Liver glutathione and polyamines in hepatocarcinogen-treated rats. Biochem. Pharmacol. 16:163-173.

Nelson, W. L., and Thorgeirsson, S. S. (1976). Structural requirements for mutagenic activity of 2-acylaminofluorenes in the Salmonella test system. Biochem. Biophys. Res. Commun. 71:1201-1206.

Neukomm, S., and Luder-Huguenin, M. (1960). Investigations on the neoplastic power of chemical compounds in newt. Oncologia 13:294-303.

Neumann, H.-G. (1967). Uber die Darstellung von carcinogenen Aminen aus hydrierbaren Vorstuffen und die Stabilitat der eingefuhrten Wasserstoff-Atome gegen Austauschreaktionen. Z. Physiol. Chem. 348:313-318.

Neumann, H.-G. (1970). Uber die Aktivierung krebserzeungender aromatischer Amine im Stoffwechsel. Klin. Wochenschr. 48:959-967.

Nicholson, M. L. (1958). Krebsentstehung nach Verfutterung von 2-Azetylaminofluoren an Ratten mit gleichzeitiger fraktionierter 31-MeV-Bestrahlung sowie Vit. B_{12}-Behandlung. Strahlentherapie 105:512-523.

Nishio, O. (1974). Influences of factors on the rapid production of hepatocyte hyperplasia and unusual proliferation of bile duct cells in ICR mice which were given 2,7-fluorenylbis acetamide. J. Nara Med. Assoc. 25:355-366.

Nishizumi, M., Albert, R. E., Burns, F. J., and Bilger, L. (1977). Hepatic cell loss and proliferation induced by N-2-fluorenylacetamide, diethylnitrosamine, and aflatoxin B_1 in relation to hepatoma induction. Br. J. Cancer 36:192-197.

Noble, R. L., and Cutts, J. H. (1959). Mammary tumors of the rat: a review. Cancer Res. 19:1125-1139.

Norden, B. (1978). Structural evidence on DNA carcinogen interactions. N-Acetoxy-N-2-acetylaminofluorene binding to DNA. Biophys. Chem. 8:385-391.

Odashima, S. (1969). Experimental carcinoma of the glandular stomach in rats. I. Effect of 7,12-dimethylbenz[a]anthracene or 4-nitroquinoline 1-oxide placed on glandular stomach combined with oral administration of N,N'-(2,7-fluorenylene)bisacetamide or N-nitrosodiethylamine. Gan. 60:211-222.

Ogawa, K., Medline, A., and Farber, E. (1979). Sequential analysis of hepatic carcinogenesis: a comparative study of the ultrastructure of preneoplastic, malignant, prenatal, postnatal and regenerating liver. Lab. Invest. 41:22-35.

Ohkawa, K., Antakly, R. W., Tanaka, S., and Sugai, N. (1976). New techniques for cytochemical localization of exogenous peroxidase activity with 2,7-fluorenediamine and 2,5-fluorenediamine as hydrogen donors. Ann. Histochim. 21:353-363.

Ohkubo, M., and Fujimura, S. (1978). Loss of activity of an N^1-methyl-4-pyridone-5-carboxamide-forming N^1-methylnicotinamide oxidase in livers of rats fed 2-acetylaminofluorene. Cancer Res. 38:697-702.

Ohkubo, M., Shimizu, M., Kubo, A., and Fujimura, S. (1977). Increased urinary excretion of 1-methyl-2-pyridone-5-carboxamide in rats administered 2-acetylaminofluorene. Chem. Biol. Interact. 18:101-110.

Okita, K., and Farber, E. (1975). An antigen common to preneoplastic hepatocyte populations and to liver cancer induced by N-2-fluorenylacetamide, ethionine, or other hepatocarcinogens. Gann Monograph #17, Univ. Tokyo Press, Tokyo, pp. 283-299.

Okita, K., Gruenstein, M., Klaiber, M., and Farber, E. (1974). Localization of α-fetoprotein by immunofluorescence in hyperplastic nodules during hepatocarcinogenesis induced by 2-acetylaminofluorene. Cancer Res. 34:2758-2763.

Okita, K., Kligman, L. H., and Farber, E. (1975). A new common marker for premalignant and malignant hepatocytes induced in the rat by chemical carcinogens. J. Natl. Cancer Inst. 54:199-202.

Okita, K., Noda, K., Fukumoto, Y., and Takemoto, T. (1976). Cytochrome P-450 in hyperplastic liver nodules during hepatocarcinogenesis with N-2-fluorenylacetamide in rats. Gan. 67:899-902.

Okuno, S., Takeishi, K., and Seno, T. (1979). Differential effect of a microsomal deacetylase inhibitor on the mutagenicity in Salmonella typhimurium of 2-acetylaminofluorene by liver homogenates of guinea pigs, mice and rats. Cancer Lett. 6:1-5.

Olive, C. W., and King, C. M. (1975). Evidence for a second arylhydroxamic acid acyl-transferase species in the small intestine of the rat. Chem. Biol. Interact. 11:599-604.

O'Neal, M. A., Hoffman, H. E., Dodge, B. G., and Griffin, A. C. (1958). Role of the pituitary in N-2-fluorenyldiacetamide carcinogenesis. J. Natl. Cancer Inst. 21:1161-1168.

Oster, W. F., Firminger, H. I., and Morrison, D. M. (1971). Inhibition of N-2-fluorenyldiacetamide induced hepatic carcinogenesis in rats by chloramphenicol: a dose related phenomenon with reduced protein binding of carcinogen. Yale J. Biol. Med. 43: 297-306.

Oyasu, R. (1963). Effect of pretreatment with hepatotoxic substances on 2-acetamidofluorene and indole tumorigenesis in rat. Effect of carbon tetrachloride and ethionine. Gan. 54:339-351.

Oyasu, R., Battifora, H. A., Clasen, R. A., McDonald, J. H., and Hass, G. M. (1970a). Induction of cerebral gliomas in rats with dietary lead subacetate and 2-acetylaminofluorene. Cancer Res. 30:1248-1261.

Oyasu, R., Battifora, H. A., Eisenstein, R., McDonald, J. H., and Hass, G. M. (1968). Enhancement of tumorigenesis in the urinary bladder of rats by neonatal administration of 2-acetylaminofluorene. J. Natl. Cancer Inst. 40:377-388.

Oyasu, R., Kitajima, T., Hopp, M. L., and Sumie, H. (1972). Enhancement of urinary bladder tumorigenesis in hamsters by coadministration of 2-acetylaminofluorene and indole. Cancer Res. 32:2027-2033.

Oyasu, R., Kitajima, T., Hopp, M. L., and Sumie, H. (1973). Induction of bladder cancer in hamsters by repeated intratracheal administrations of 2-acetylaminofluorene. J. Natl. Cancer Inst. 50:503-506.

Oyasu, R., Miller, D. A., McDonald, J. H., and Hass, G. M. (1963). Neoplasms of rat urinary bladder and liver. Rats fed 2-acetylaminofluorene and indole. Arch. Pathol. 75:184-190.

Oyasu, R., Sumie, H., and Burg, H. E. (1970b). Neoplasms of urinary bladders of hamsters treated with 2-acetylaminofluorene and indole. J. Natl. Cancer Inst. 45: 853-860.

Pan, H.-L., and Fletcher, T. L. (1960). Derivatives of fluorene. IX. 4-Hydroxy-2-fluorenamine; new 3,4-benzocoumarin derivatives. J. Org. Chem. 25:1106-1109.

Pan, H.-L., and Fletcher, T. L. (1962). Derivatives of fluorene. XVII. Alkyl phosphates, phosphites and phosphonates with lithium halides or alkyl halides in the N-alkylation of fluorenamines. J. Org. Chem. 27:3639-3643.

Pan, H.-L., and Fletcher, T. L. (1964). Derivatives of fluorene. XVIII. New halogeno-fluorenes. I. Potential antitumor agents. J. Med. Chem. 7:31-38.

Pan, H.-L., and Fletcher, T. L. (1968). A facile preparation of sulphydryl compounds in dimethyl sulphoxide. Chem. Ind. 546.

Pan, H.-L., and Fletcher, T. L. (1972). Derivatives of fluorene. 35. Hydrazine-hydrate and Raney-nickel reduction of nitrofluorenones to aminofluoren-9-ols. Int. J. Meth. Synthet. Org. Chem. 4:192-194.

Pan, H.-L., Namkung, M. J., and Fletcher, T. L. (1968). Derivatives of fluorene XXVIII. New thiofluorenes related to metabolism of the carcinogen N-2-fluorenylacetamide. III. J. Med. Chem. 11:1236-1237.

Peraino, C., Fry, R. J., and Staffeldt, E. (1971). Reduction and enhancement by phenobarbital of hepatocarcinogenesis induced in the rat by 2-acetylaminofluorene. Cancer Res. 31:1506-1512.

Peraino, C., Fry, R. J., and Staffeldt, E. (1977). Effects of varying the onset and duration of exposure to phenobarbital on its enhancement of 2-acetylaminofluorene-induced hepatic tumorigenesis. Cancer Res. 37:3623-3627.

Peraino, C., Fry, R. J., Staffeldt, E., and Christopher, J. P. (1975). Comparative enhancing effects of phenobarbital, amobarbital, diphenylhydantoin, and dichlorodiphenyltrichloroethane on 2-acetylaminofluorene-induced hepatic tumorigenesis in the rat. Cancer Res. 35:2884-2890.

Peraino, C., Fry, R. J., Staffeldt, E., and Christopher, J. P. (1977). Enhancing effects of phenobarbitone and butylated hydroxytoluene on 2-acetylaminofluorene-induced hepatic tumorigenesis in the rat. Food Cosmet. Toxicol. 15:93-96.

Peraino, C., Fry, R. J., Staffeldt, E., and Kisieleski, W. E. (1973). Effects of varying the exposure to phenobarbital on its enhancement of 2-acetylaminofluorene-induced hepatic tumorigenesis in the rat. Cancer Res. 33:2701-2705.

Pero, R. W., Bryngelsson, C., Mitelman, F., Kornfalt, R., Thulin, T., and Norden, A. (1978). Interindividual variation in the responses of cultured human lymphocytes to exposure from DNA damaging chemicals. Interindividual variation to carcinogen exposure. Mutat. Res. 53:327-341.

Pero, R. W., Bryngelsson, C., Mitelman, F., Thulin, T., and Norden, A. (1976). High blood pressure related to carcinogen-induced unscheduled DNA synthesis, DNA carcinogen binding, and chromosomal aberrations in human lymphocytes. Proc. Natl. Acad. Sci. USA 73:2496-2500.

Petzold, G. L., and Swenberg, J. A. (1978). Detection of DNA damage induced in vivo following exposure of rats to carcinogens. Cancer Res. 38:1589-1594.

Pilon, R., Dupuis, C., and Morais, R. (1974). Studies on liver mitochondrial 5'-endonuclease activity in rats fed carcinogenic amines and on their binding to mitochondrial proteins. Chem. Biol. Interact. 8:371-378.

Pinchuk, V. G., Zotikov, L. A., and Monastyrskaya, B. D. (1967). Fine structure of hepatomas induced in rats fed 2-acetylaminofluorene (Russian). Vopr. Onkol. 13(11): 66-72.

Pliss, G. B., Gurkalo, V. K., and Petrov, A. S. (1973). The influence of alkyl disulfones on the formation of a carcinogenic metabolite of 2-acetylaminofluorene (Russian). Vopr. Onkol. 19(11):43-47.

Poiley, J. A., Raineri, R., and Pienta, R. J. (1979). Use of hamster hepatocytes to metabolize carcinogens in an in vitro bioassay. J. Natl. Cancer Inst. 63:519-524.

Poirier, L. A., Grantham, P. H., and Rogers, A. E. (1977). The effects of a marginally lipotrope-deficient diet on the hepatic levels of S-adenosylmethionine and on the urinary metabolites of 2-acetylaminofluorene in rats. Cancer Res. 37:744-748.

Poirier, L. A., and Pitot, H. C. (1969). Dietary induction of some enzymes of amino acid metabolism during 2-acetylaminofluorene feeding. Cancer Res. 29:464-469.

Poirier, L. A., Poirier, M. C., and Pitot, H. C. (1969). Dietary induction of some enzymes of carbohydrate metabolism during 2-acetylaminofluorene feeding. Cancer Res. 39:470-474.

Poirier, M. C., and De Cicco, B. T. (1977). Kinetics of excision repair synthesis induced by N-acetoxy-2-acetylaminofluorene and ultraviolet irradiation in human diploid fibroblasts. J. Natl. Cancer Inst. 59:339-343.

Poirier, M. C., De Cicco, B. T., and Lieberman, M. W. (1975). Nonspecific inhibition of DNA repair synthesis by tumor promoters in human diploid fibroblasts damaged with N-acetoxy-2-acetylaminofluorene. Cancer Res. 35:1392-1397.

Poirier, M. C., Dubin, M. A., and Yuspa, S. H. (1979). Formation and removal of specific acetylamino-DNA adducts in mouse and human cells measured by radioimmunoassay. Cancer Res. 39:1377-1381.

Poirier, M. C., Miller, J. A., and Miller, E. C. (1965). The carcinogenic activities of N-hydroxy-2-acetylaminofluorene and its metal chelates as a function of retention at the injection site. Cancer Res. 25:527-533.

Poirier, M. C., Poirier, L. A., and Lepage, R. (1972). The hepatic activities of 1-carbon enzymes during the chronic administration of diethylnitrosamine, 2-acetylaminofluorene, and N,N-dimethyl-4-aminoazobenzene to rats. Cancer Res. 32:1104-1107.

Poirier, M. C., Yuspa, S. H., Weinstein, I. B., and Blobstein, S. (1977). Detection of carcinogen-DNA adducts by radioimmunoassay. Nature 270:186-188.

Popp, J. A., and Shinozuka, H. (1974). Inhibition of protein synthesis and induction of helical polysomes in rat liver by N-hydroxy-2-fluorenylacetamide. Chem. Biol. Interact. 9:37-43.

Pugh, T. D., and Goldfarb, S. (1978). Quantitative histochemical and autoradiographic studies of hepatocarcinogenesis in rats fed 2-acetylaminofluorene followed by phenobarbital. Cancer Res. 38:4450-4457.

Pulkrabek, P., Grunberger, D., and Weinstein, I. B. (1974). Effects of the ionic environment on modification of yeast tyrosine transfer ribonucleic acid with N-acetoxy-2-acetylaminofluorene. Biochemistry 13:2414-2419.

Puron, R., and Firminger, H. I. (1965). Protection against induced cirrhosis and hepatocellular carcinoma in rats by chloramphenicol. J. Natl. Cancer Inst. 35:29-37.

Rabbi, A., Caldarera, C. M., and Barbiroli, B. (1962). Effects of administration of liver-cancer inducing compounds on free nucleotides of rat liver. Boll. Soc. Ital. Biol. Sper. 38:1909-1912; Chem. Abst. 60:4591b (1964).

Rabbi, A., Caldarera, C. M., and Rossoni, C. (1963). Ricerche su alcuni aspetti del metabolismo nucleotidico nel fegato di ratto trattato con 4-dimetilaminoazobenzene (DAB) e 2-acetilaminofluorene (AAF). Boll. Soc. Ital. Biol. Sper. 39:1825-1828.

Rahman, Y. E., Cerny, E. A., and Peraino, C. (1969). Studies on rat liver ribonucleases. IV. Liver ribonucleases in developing 2-acetylaminofluorene fed and partially hepatectomized rats. Biochim. Biophys. Acta 178:68-73.

Raineri, R., Poiley, J. A., Ernst, M. K., Hillesund, T., and Pienta, R. J. (1978). A high pressure liquid chromatography procedure for the separation of metabolites of 2-acetylaminofluorene from cells in culture. J. Liquid Chromatogr. 1:457-467.

Ramanathan, R., Rajalakshmi, S., and Sarma, D. S. (1976). Nonrandom nature of in vivo interaction of ^{3}H-N-hydroxy-2-acetylaminofluorene and its subsequent removal from rat liver chromatin-DNA. Chem. Biol. Interact. 14:375-377.

Ray, F. E., Rivers, F. T., and Hoch-Ligeti, C. (1965). Uptake by rat stomach of 2-aminofluorene-^{3}H hydrochloride and 2,7-diaminofluorene-^{3}H hydrochloride in vitro. Br. J. Cancer 19:560-564.

Ray, J. H., Altenburg, L. C., and Jacobs, M. M. (1978). Effect of sodium selenite and methyl methanesulfonate or N-hydroxy-2-acetylaminofluorene co-exposure on sister-chromatid exchange production in human whole blood cultures. Mutat. Res. 57:359-368.

Razzouk, C., Lhoest, G., Roberfroid, M., and Mercier, M. (1977). Subnanogram estimation of the proximate carcinogen N-hydroxy-2-fluorenylacetamide by gas-liquid chromatography. Anal. Biochem. 83:194-203.

Rees, K. R., Rowland, G. F., and Ross, H. F. (1962). The metabolism of isolated rat-liver nuclei during chemical carcinogenesis. 2. 2-Acetamidofluorene, α-naphthylisothiocyanate and 2',4'-dimethyl-4-dimethylaminoazobenzene. Biochem. J. 82:347-352.

Regan, J. D., and Setlow, R. B. (1974). Two forms of repair in the DNA of human cells damaged by chemical carcinogens and mutagens. Cancer Res. 34:3318-3325.

Reigh, D. L., Stuart, M., and Floyd, R. A. (1978). Activation of the carcinogen N-hydroxy-2-acetylaminofluorene by rat mammary peroxidase. Experientia 34:107-108.

Reuber, M. D. (1960). Endometrial sarcomas of the uterus and carcinosarcomas of the submaxillary salivary gland in castrated A X C strain female rats receiving N,N-fluorenyldiacetamide and norethandrolone. J. Natl. Cancer Inst. 25:1141-1153.

Reuber, M. D. (1961). A transplantable bile-secreting hepatocellular carcinoma in the rat. J. Natl. Cancer Inst. 26:891-897.

Reuber, M. D. (1962). Parathyroid hyperplasia, multicystic kidneys, osteitis fibrosa generalisata and metastatic calcification in cirrhotic rats fed N-2-fluorenyldiacetamide. Am. J. Pathol. 41:645-659.

Reuber, M. D. (1965a). Role of the adrenal glands in the development of lesions of the liver in rats ingesting N-2-fluorenyldiacetamide. J. Natl. Cancer Inst. 34:587-594.

Reuber, M. D. (1965b). Development of preneoplastic and neoplastic lesions of the liver in male rats ingesting 0.025 percent N-2-fluorenyldiacetamide. J. Natl. Cancer Inst. 34:697-724.

Reuber, M. D. (1965c). The thyroid gland and N-2-fluorenyldiacetamide carcinogenesis and cirrhosis of the liver in Wistar male rats. J. Natl. Cancer Inst. 35:959-966.

Reuber, M. D. (1966). Importance of thyroid hormone and testosterone in the induction of carcinoma and cirrhosis of the liver in female Wistar rats ingesting N-2-fluorenyldiacetamide. J. Natl. Cancer Inst. 36:775-781.

Reuber, M. D. (1968a). Effect of growth hormone on hepatic carcinogenesis and cirrhosis in A x C rats given N-2-fluorenyldiacetamide. Cancer Res. 28:2177-2179.

Reuber, M. D. (1968b). Histogenesis of cholangiofibrosis and well-differentiated cholangiocarcinoma in Syrian hamsters given 2-acetamidofluorene or 2-diacetamidofluorene. Gan. 59:239-246.

Reuber, M. D. (1969). Influence of hormones on N-2-fluorenyldiacetamide-induced hyperplastic hepatic nodules in rats. J. Natl. Cancer Inst. 43:445-452.

Reuber, M. D. (1971). Effect of alloxan diabetes on hepatic carcinogenesis and cirrhosis in A x C rats given 2-diacetamidofluorene. Gan. 62:157-161.

Reuber, M. D. (1975a). Evolution of hyperplasia, hyperplastic nodules and carcinomas of the liver in rats ingesting N-2-fluorenyldiacetamide. In Gann Monograph #17, S. Odashima, S. Takayama, and H. Sato (Eds.). University of Tokyo Press, Tokyo, pp. 303-342.

Reuber, M. D. (1975b). Carcinoma and cirrhosis of the liver in A x C male rats with one kidney ingesting 0.025% N-2-fluorenyldiacetamide. Pathol. Microbiol. 42:119-126.

Reuber, M. D. (1975c). Influence of age and sex on carcinoma and cirrhosis of the liver in A x C strain rats ingesting 0.025% N-2-fluorenyldiacetamide. Pathol. Microbiol. 43:31-37.

Reuber, M. D. (1976a). Effect of age and testosterone on the induction of hyperplastic nodules, carcinomas and cirrhosis of the liver in rats ingesting N-2-fluorenyldiacetamide. Eur. J. Cancer 12:137-141.

Reuber, M. D. (1976b). Various degrees of susceptibility of different stocks of rats to N-2-fluorenyldiacetamide hepatic carcinogenesis. J. Natl. Cancer Inst. 57:111-114.

Reuber, M. D., and Firminger, H. I. (1962). Effect of progesterone and diethylstilbestrol on hepatic carcinogenesis and cirrhosis in A x C rats fed N-2-fluorenyldiacetamide. J. Natl. Cancer Inst. 29:933-943.

Reuber, M. D., and Firminger, H. I. (1963). Morphologic and biologic correlation of lesions obtained in hepatic carcinogenesis in A x C rats given 0.025 percent N-2-fluorenyldiacetamide. J. Natl. Cancer Inst. 31:1407-1429.

Reuber, M. D., and Glover, E. L. (1973). Chronic thyroiditis in Buffalo-strain rats ingesting 3'-methyl-4-dimethylaminoazobenzene or N-2-fluorenyldiacetamide. Pathol. Microbiol. 39:383-388.

Reuber, M. D., and Odashima, S. (1967). Further studies on the transplantation of lesions in hepatic carcinogenesis in rats given 2-(diacetamido)fluorene. Gan. 58:513-520.

Rickard, R. W., Dorough, H. W., and Pan, S. H. (1978). Metabolic capabilities of the Salmonella mutagenicity test system. J. Agric. Food Chem. 26:141-146.

Roberts, J. D., and Lieberman, M. W. (1979). Deoxyribonucleic acid repair synthesis in permeable human fibroblasts exposed to ultraviolet radiation and N-acetoxy-2-(acetylamino)fluorene. Biochemistry 18:4499-4505.

Rodriguez, N. M., Rodriguez, B. M., and Cerecedo, L. R. (1957). Effect of 2-acetylaminofluorene on the nucleic acids in certain tissues of the Swiss mouse. Exp. Med. Surg. 15: 68-74.

Rogers, A. E. (1975). Variable effects of a lipotrope-deficient, high-fat diet on chemical carcinogenesis in rats. Cancer Res. 35: 2469-2474.

Rogers, A. E., and Newberne, P. M. (1971). Lasiocarpine: factors influencing its toxicity and effects on liver cell division. Toxicol. Appl. Pharmacol. 18: 356-366.

Rosin, M. P., and Stich, H. F. (1978). Inhibitory effect of reducing agents on N-acetoxy- and N-hydroxy-2-acetylaminofluorene-induced mutagenesis. Cancer Res. 38: 1307-1310.

Rosin, M. P., and Stich, H. F. (1979). Assessment of the use of the Salmonella mutagenesis assay to determine the influence of antioxidants on carcinogen-induced mutagenesis. Int. J. Cancer 23: 722-727.

Sage, E., Fuchs, R. P., and Leng, M. (1979). Reactivity of the antibodies to DNA modified by the carcinogen N-acetoxy-N-acetyl-2-aminofluorene. Biochemistry 18: 1328-1332.

Sahyun, M. R. (1964). Enthalpy of binding of aromatic amines to bovine serum albumin. Nature 203: 1045-1046.

Sakai, S., Reinhold, C. E., Wirth, P. J., and Thorgeirsson, S. S. (1978). Mechanism of in vitro mutagenic activation and covalent binding of N-hydroxy-2-acetylaminofluorene in isolated liver cell nuclei from rat and mouse. Cancer Res. 38: 2058-2067.

Salas, C. E., Pfohl-Leszkowicz, A., Lang, M. C., and Dirheimer, G. (1979). Effect of modification by N-acetoxy-N-2-acetylaminofluorene on the level of DNA methylation. Nature 278: 71-72.

San, R. H., and Stich, H. F. (1975). DNA repair synthesis of cultured human cells as a rapid bioassay for chemical carcinogens. Int. J. Cancer 16: 284-291.

San, R. H., and Williams, G. M. (1977). Rat hepatocyte primary cell culture-mediated mutagenesis of adult rat liver epithelial cells by procarcinogens. Proc. Soc. Exp. Biol. Med. 156: 534-538.

Santella, R. M., Fuchs, R. P., and Grunberger, D. (1979). Mutagenicity of 7-iodo and 7-fluoro derivatives of N-hydroxy and N-acetoxy-N-2-acetylaminofluorene in the Salmonella typhimurium assay. Mutat. Res. 67: 85-87.

Sapre, N. N., Gothoskar, S. V., and Bhide, S. V. (1969). Biochemical studies on the host-liver and hepatocarcinoma induced by N-2-fluorenylacetamide (N-2-FAA). Indian J. Cancer 6: 219-227.

Sarrif, A. M., White, W. E., Jr., and DiVito, N. (1978). Photolysis of 2-azidofluorene in situ as a probe in chemical carcinogenesis: bypass of requirement for metabolic activation. Biochem. Biophys. Res. Commun. 83: 506-512.

Sato, K., Takaya, S., Imai, F., Hatayama, I., and Ito, N. (1978). Different deviation patterns of carbohydrate-metabolizing enzymes in primary rat hepatomas induced by different chemical carcinogens. Cancer Res. 38: 3086-3093.

Sato, S., Matsushima, T., Tanaka, N., Sugimura, T., and Takashima, F. (1973). Hepatic tumors in the guppy (Lebistes reticulatus) induced by alfatoxin B_1, dimethylnitrosamine, and 2-acetylaminofluorene. J. Natl. Cancer Inst. 50: 765-778.

Schmeltz, I., and Hoffmann, D. (1977). Nitrogen-containing compounds in tobacco and tobacco smoke. Chem. Rev. 77: 295-311.

Schor, N. A., Ogawa, K., Lee, G., and Farber, E. (1978). The use of the D-T diaphorase for the detection of foci of early neoplastic transformation in rat liver. Cancer Lett. 5: 167-171.

Schramm, T. (1961). Einfluss von Fettsauren auf die Carcinogenese. III. Einfluss von Linolensaureathylester auf die durch 2-Acetylaminofluoren induzierte Carcinogenese. Acta Biol. Med. Ger. 7: 75-86.

Schut, H. A., and Thorgeirsson, S. S. (1978). In vitro metabolism and mutagenic activation of 2-acetylaminofluorene by subcellular liver fractions from cotton rats. Cancer Res. 38: 2501-2507.

Schut, H. A., Wirth, P. J., and Thorgeirsson, S. S. (1978). Mutagenic activation of N-hydroxy-2-acetylaminofluorene in the Salmonella test system: the role of deacetylation by liver and kidney fractions from mouse and rat. Mol. Pharmacol. 14:682-692.

Schwartz, E. L., and Goodman, J. T. (1979). Quantitative and qualitative aspects of the binding of N-hydroxy-2-acetylaminofluorene to hepatic chromatin fractions. Chem. Biol. Interact. 20:287-303.

Schwarz, M., Hummel, J., Appel, K. E., Rickart, R., and Kunz, W. (1979). DNA damage induced in vivo evaluated with a nonradioactive alkaline elution technique. Cancer Lett. 6:221-226.

Scribner, J. D. (1977). Conversion of the carcinogen N-acetoxy-2-acetamidofluorene to 4-hydroxy-2-acetamidofluorene. J. Am. Chem. Soc. 99:7383-7384.

Scribner, J. D., and Naimy, N. K. (1973). Reactions of esters of N-hydroxy-2-acetamidophenanthrene with cellular nucleophiles and the formation of free radicals upon decomposition of N-acetoxy-N-arylacetamides. Cancer Res. 33:1159-1164.

Scudiero, D., Norin, A., Karran, P., and Strauss, B. (1976). DNA excision-repair deficiency of human peripheral blood lymphocytes treated with chemical carcinogens. Cancer Res. 36:1397-1403.

Seal, U. S., and Gutmann, H. R. (1959). Metabolism of the carcinogen N-(2-fluorenyl)acetamide by liver cell fractions. J. Biol. Chem. 234:648-654.

Seal, U. S., and Gutmann, H. R. (1961). On the mechanism of protein binding of the carcinogen N-2-fluorenylacetamide by rat liver. Ion exchange chromatography of the soluble fraction. Arch. Biochem. Biophys. 95:1-11.

Sekely, L. I., Malejka-Giganti, D., Gutmann, H. R., and Rydell, R. E. (1973). Malignant transformation of rat embryo fibroblasts by carcinogenic fluorenylhydroxamic acids in vitro. J. Natl. Cancer Inst. 50:1337-1345.

Sell, S. (1978). Distribution of α-fetoprotein- and albumin-containing cells in the livers of Fischer rats fed four cycles of N-2-fluorenylacetamide. Cancer Res. 38:3107-3113.

Setlow, R. B., and Regan, J. D. (1972). Defective repair of N-acetoxy-2-acetylaminofluorene-induced lesions in the DNA of xeroderma pigmentosum cells. Biochem. Biophys. Res. Commun. 46:1019-1024.

Shearer, R. W. (1971). DNA of rat hepatomas: search for gene amplification. Biochem. Biophys. Res. Commun. 43:1324-1328.

Shearer, R. W. (1974). Specificity of chemical modification of ribonucleic acid transport by liver carcinogens in the rat. Biochemistry 13:1764-1767.

Shinozuka, H., Sells, M. A., Katyal, S. L., Sell, S., and Lombardi, B. (1979). Effects of a choline-devoid diet on the emergence of γ-glutamyltranspeptidase-positive foci in the liver of carcinogen-treated rats. Cancer Res. 39:2515-2521.

Shortino, T. J., Cantwell, G. E., and Robbins, W. E. (1963). Effect of certain carcinogenic 2-fluorenamine derivatives on larvae of the house fly, Musca domestica Linnaeus. J. Insect. Pathol. 5:489-497.

Sidransky, H., Clark, S., and Baba, T. (1963). Influence of p-hydroxypropiophenone on liver tumorigenesis in rats ingesting ethionine and N-2-fluorenylacetamide. J. Natl. Cancer Inst. 30:999-1013.

Sidransky, H., Ito, N., and Verney, E. (1966). Influence of α-naphthyl-isothiocyanate on liver tumorigenesis in rats ingesting ethionine and N-2-fluorenylacetamide. J. Natl. Cancer Inst. 37:677-686.

Sidransky, H., and Verney, E. (1970). Influence of orotic acid on liver tumorigenesis in rats ingesting ethionine, N-2-fluorenylacetamide, and 3'-methyl-dimethylaminoazobenzene. J. Natl. Cancer Inst. 44:1201-1215.

Sidransky, H., and Verney, E. (1978). Acute effects of selected hepatocarcinogens on polyribosomes and protein synthesis in the livers of rats fed purified diets containing hepatocarcinogens. Cancer Res. 38:1166-1172.

Sidransky, H., Wagner, B. P., and Morris, H. P. (1961). Sex differences in liver tumorigenesis in rats ingesting N-2-fluorenylacetamide. J. Natl. Cancer Inst. 26:151-187.

Sieglitz, A. (1964). Uber 2.3.7-Derivate des Fluorens. Chem. Ber. 97:3392-3396.

Silber, D., Checinska, E., Rabczynski, J., Kasprzak, A. A., and Kochman, M. (1978). Isozyme pattern of pyruvate kinase during hepatocarcinogenesis induced by 2-acetylaminofluorene in rat liver. Eur. J. Cancer 14:729-739.

Silber, D., Checinska, E., Rabczynski, J., and Kochman, M. (1975). Isozyme pattern of fructose diphosphate aldolase during hepatocarcinogenesis induced by 2-acetylaminofluorene in rat liver. Int. J. Cancer 16:675-681.

Slifkin, M., Merkow, L. P., Epstein, S. M., and Pardo, M. (1972). The cellular analysis of liver carcinogenesis. VI. Growth and ultrastructural characteristics of N-2-fluorenylacetamide hyperplastic liver nodule cells grown in vitro. Arch. Pathol. 94: 1-10.

Smith, E. R., Hagopian, M., and Reister, H. C. (1977). The uptake and secretion of 2-acetylaminofluorene by the rat and dog prostate. Toxicol. Appl. Pharmacol. 40: 185-191.

Smith, L. D., Emerson, R. L., and Nixon, L. K. (1979). Effect of hepatocarcinogens on the adenine purine nucleotide cycle during the initiation phase of carcinogenesis. Cancer Res. 39:2132-2138.

Snell, K. C., Stewart, H. L., and Morris, H. P. (1969). The sequential development of atrophy, precancerous lesions, and cancer of the glandular stomach and other organs and tissues of rats ingesting N,N'-2,7-fluorenylenebisacetamide. In Gann Monograph #8, Japanese Cancer Assoc. (Ed.). Maruzen, Tokyo, pp. 125-142.

Snell, K. C., Stewart, H. L., Morris, H. P., Wagner, B. P., and Ray, F. E. (1961a). Atrophy, proliferative lesions, and tumors of the salivary glands of rats ingesting N-2-fluorenylacetamide or N,N'-2,7-fluorenylenebisacetamide. Natl. Cancer Inst. Monogr. 5:55-83.

Snell, K. C., Stewart, H. L., Morris, H. P., Wagner, B. P., and Ray, F. E. (1961b). Intracranial neurilemmoma and medulloblastoma induced in rats by the dietary administration of N,N'-2,7-fluorenylenebisacetamide. Natl. Cancer Inst. Monogr. 5:85-103.

Solt, D., and Farber, E. (1976). New principle for the analysis of chemical carcinogenesis. Nature 263:701-703.

Solt, D. B., Medline, A., and Farber, E. (1977). Rapid emergence of carcinogen-induced hyperplastic lesions in a new model for the sequential analysis of liver carcinogenesis. Am. J. Pathol. 88:595-618.

Songster, C. L., Schochet, S. S., Jr., and Farber, E. (1963). Metabolism of bile components during carcinogenesis. I. Conjugation of cholic acid in vitro in experimental liver carcinogenesis. Cancer Res. 23:1069-1076.

Sorof, S., Young, E. M., Coffey, C. B., and Morris, H. P. (1966). On protein binding of fluorenyl carcinogens by minimal deviation hepatomas. Cancer Res. 26:81-88.

Sorof, S., Young, E. M., and Fetterman, P. L. (1960). Electrophoretic distribution of derivatives of 2-acetylaminofluorene-9-^{14}C bound to soluble proteins of rat liver in vivo. Exp. Cell Res. 20:253-256.

Sorof, S., Young, E. M., McBride, R. A., and Coffey, C. B. (1970). On protein targets of chemical carcinogens: dissimilar molecular sizes of the principal protein conjugates. Cancer Res. 30:2029-2034.

Sorof, S., Young, E. M., McBride, R. Z., Coffey, C. B., and Luongo, L. (1969). Increased selectivity of interaction between fluorenylamine carcinogens and liver proteins during hepatocarcinogenesis. Mol. Pharmacol. 5:625-639.

Sorof, S., Young, E. M., and Ott, M. G. (1958). Soluble liver h proteins during hepatocarcinogenesis by aminoazo dyes and 2-acetylaminofluorene. Cancer Res. 18:33-46.

Stewart, H. L., Snell, K. C., and Morris, H. P. (1965). The combined effect of 3-methylcholanthrene and N,N'-2,7-fluorenylenebisacetamide on the induction of cancer of the glandular stomach of the rat. J. Natl. Cancer Inst. 34:157-174.

Stewart, H. L., Snell, K. C., Morris, H. P., Wagner, B. P., and Ray, F. E. (1961). Carcinoma of the glandular stomach of rats ingesting N,N'-2,7-fluorenylenebisacetamide. Natl. Cancer Inst. Monogr. 5:105-139.

Stich, H. F., San, R. H., Miller, J. A., and Miller, E. C. (1972). Various levels of DNA repair synthesis in xeroderma pigmentosum cells exposed to the carcinogens, N-hydroxy and N-acetoxy-2-acetylaminofluorene. Nature New Biol. 238:9-10

Stora, C. (1977). Utilisation de l'atrophie des tubes sereux de la glande sous-maxillaire du rat sous acetaminofluorene pour eprouver le pouvoir detoxifiant de la beta naphtoflavone. C. R. Acad. Sci. [D] (Paris) 285:1271-1274.

Stout, D. L., Baptist, J. N., Matney, T. S., and Shaw, C. R. (1976). N-Hydroxy-2-aminofluorene: the principal mutagen produced from N-hydroxy-2-acetylaminofluorene by a mammalian supernatant enzyme preparation. Cancer Lett. 1:269-274.

Stout, D. L., and Becker, F. F. (1978). Alteration of the ability of liver microsomes to activate N-2-fluorenylacetamide to a mutagen of _Salmonella typhimurium_ during hepatocarcinogenesis. Cancer Res. 38:2274-2278.

Stout, D. L., and Becker, F. F. (1979). Metabolism of 2-aminofluorene and 2-acetylaminofluorene to mutagens by rat hepatocyte nuclei. Cancer Res. 39:1168-1173.

Sugai, M., Witting, L. A., Tsuchiyama, H., and Kummerow, F. A. (1962). The effect of heated fat on the carcinogenic activity of 2-acetylaminofluorene. Cancer Res. 22:510-519.

Sugihara, R., Hiasa, Y., and Ito, N. (1972). Ultrastructural changes in nuclei and nucleoli of rat liver cells treated with hepatocarcinogens. Gan. 63:419-426.

Suss, R., Kinzel, V., Volm, M., Wayss, K., and Scribner, J. (1970). Effect of acetamidofluorene and activated derivatives on "macromolecular synthesis" in single cell cultures. Z. Krebsforsch. 74:338-343.

Sutherland, D. J. (1969). Effects of certain carcinogens on _Periplaneta americana_ (L.). Natl. Cancer Inst. Monogr. 31:433-445.

Suzuki, K., Weisburger, E. K., and Weisburger, J. H. (1959). Nitration of 1- and 3-fluorofluorene. J. Org. Chem. 24:1511-1517.

Suzuki, K., Weisburger, E. K., and Weisburger, J. H. (1961a). Replacement and elimination of bromine in bromonitrofluorenones. The preparation of 2,3- and 1,2,3-substituted fluorenes and fluorenones. J. Org. Chem. 26:2236-2239.

Suzuki, K., Weisburger, E. K., and Weisburger, J. H. (1961b). Derivatives of 3-fluorofluorene by the Pschorr synthesis. J. Org. Chem. 26:2239-2242.

Svoboda, D., and Higginson, J. (1968). A comparison of ultrastructural changes in rat liver due to chemical carcinogens. Cancer Res. 28:1703-1733.

Syrowatka, T., Jurek, A., and Nazarewicz, T. (1978). Influence of DDT on the hepatotoxicity of 2-acetylaminofluorene in Wistar rats. Rocz. Panstw. Zakl. Hig. 29:57-64.

Szafarz, D. (1977). An improved method for DNA alkaline gradient analysis and its application to the effect of carcinogens on mouse liver DNA. Biochimie 59:775-778.

Takahashi, G., and Yasuhira, K. (1975). Macroautoradiographic assays in pregnant mice and their fetuses given N-acetyl-9-[^{14}C]-2-aminofluorene and p-[^{14}C]-dimethylaminoazobenzene. Cancer Res. 35:2126-2131.

Takayama, S. (1968a). Induction of adenomatous hyperplasia of the glandular stomach in mice fed N,N'-(2,7-fluorenylene)bisacetamide. In _Gann Monograph #3_, R. Kinosita, T. Nagayo, and T. Tanaka (Eds.). Maruzen, Tokyo, pp. 97-103.

Takayama, S. (1968b). Induction of transplantable liver tumors in DBF_1 mice after oral administration of N,N'-2,7-fluorenylenebisacetamide. J. Natl. Cancer Inst. 40:629-641.

Takayama, S., and Fujiwara, M. (1978a). Hematogenous development of rat mature granulocytic leukemia—comparison of 2,7-FAA-induced and transplanted leukemia. Acta Pathol. Jpn. 28:523-529.

Takayama, S., and Fujiwara, M. (1978b). Site of origin of 2,7-FAA-induced rat leukemia. Acta Pathol. Jpn. 28:531-539.

Takayama, S., and Inui, N. (1967). Induction of malignant tumors in mice fed N,N'-(fluoren-2,7-ylene)bis-acetylamine. Gan. 58:193-198.

Takayama, S., and Kamata, S. (1972). Initial changes of leukemia in rats fed 2,7-diacetylaminofluorene. Acta Pathol. Jpn. 22:477-487.

Takayama, S., and Kamata, S. (1973). Classification of initial leukemic changes in rats fed N,N'-2,7-fluorenylenebisacetamide. Acta Pathol. Jpn. 23:755-768.

Takayama, S., Yamada, T., and Kamata, S. (1972). Chronic myelogenous leukemia in rats fed 2,7-diacetylaminofluorene. Acta Pathol. Jpn. 22:309-319.

Takehisa, S., and Wolff, S. (1977). Induction of sister chromatid exchanges in Chinese hamster cells by carcinogenic mutagens requiring metabolic activation. Mutat. Res. 45:263-270.

Tang, T., and Friedman, M. A. (1977). Carcinogen activation by human liver enzymes in the Ames mutagenicity test. Mutat. Res. 46:387-394.

Tanigaki, N., Kitagawa, M., Yagi, Y., and Pressman, D. (1967). The reaction of specific antibody with 2-acetylaminofluorene fixed in liver cells. Cancer Res. 27:747-752.

Tatematsu, M., Miyata, Y., Mizutani, M., Hananouchi, M., Hirose, M., and Ito, N. (1977a). Summation effect of N-butyl-N-(4-hydroxybutyl) nitrosamine, N-[4-(5-nitro-2-furyl)-2-thiazolyl] formamide, N-2-fluorenylacetamide, and 3,3'-dichlorobenzidine on urinary bladder carcinogenesis in rats. Gan. 68:193-202.

Tatematsu, M., Shirai, T., Tsuda, H., Miyata, Y., Shinohara, Y., and Ito, N. (1977b). Rapid production of hyperplastic liver nodules in rats treated with carcinogenic chemicals: a new approach for an in vivo short-term screening test for hepatocarcinogens. Gan. 68:499-507.

Tates, A. D. (1976). A search for storage effects on chromosome aberrations induced in normal type- and xeroderma pigmentosum fibroblasts by tetraethylene-imino-1,4-benzo chinon and N-acetoxy-N-2-acetylaminofluorene. Mutat. Res. 34:299-312.

Tchipysheva, T. A., Guelstein, V. I. (Gel'shtein), and Bannikov, G. A. (1977). α-Fetoprotein-containing cells in the early stages of liver carcinogenesis induced by 3'-methyl-4-dimethylaminoazobenzene and 2-acetylaminofluorene. Int. J. Cancer 20: 388-393.

Teebor, G. W., and Becker, F. F. (1971). Regression and persistence of hyperplastic hepatic nodules induced by N-2-fluorenylacetamide and their relationship to hepatocarcinogenesis. Cancer Res. 31:1-3.

Teebor, G. W., Duker, N. J., and Becker, F. F. (1977). Normal endonuclease activities for damaged DNA during hepatocarcinogenesis. Biochim. Biophys. Acta 477:125-131.

Teebor, G. W., and Seidman, I. (1970). Retention of metabolic regulation in the hyperplastic hepatic nodule induced by N-2-fluorenylacetamide. Cancer Res. 30:1095-1101.

Terawaki, A., Sato, M., Yamanouchi, M., Fukuyama, T., Ito, N., and Nakajima, S. (1967). Phenylalanine hydroxylase activity in isolated, perfused liver of rats bearing rhodamine sarcoma, hepatoma and nodular hyperplasia. Gan. 58:185-191.

Thielmann, H. W. (1976). Carcinogen-induced DNA repair in nucleotide-permeable Escherichia coli cells. Analysis of DNA repair induced by the carcinogens N-acetoxy-N-2-acetylaminofluorene and 7-bromomethylbenz[a]anthracene. Eur. J. Biochem. 61: 501-513.

Thielmann, H. W. (1977). Detection of strand breaks in PH1CH1174 RF1 and PM2 DNA reacted with ultimate and proximate carcinogens. Z. Krebsforsch. 90:37-69.

Thielmann, H. W., and Gersbach, H. (1978). The nucleotide-permeable Escherichia coli cell, a sensitive DNA repair indicator for carcinogens, mutagens, and antitumor agents binding covalently to DNA. Z. Krebsforsch. 92:177-214.

Thompson, J. H. (1969). N,N'-2,7-fluorenylenebisacetamide (2,7-FAA)-induced rat bowel cancer. Ir. J. Med. Sci. [7] 2:565-583.

Thorgeirsson, S. S., Felton, J. S., and Nebert, D. W. (1975). Genetic differences in the aromatic hydrocarbon-inducible N-hydroxylation of 2-acetylaminofluorene and acetaminophen-produced hepatotoxicity in mice. Mol. Pharmacol. 11:159-165.

Thorgeirsson, S. S., Jollow, D. J., Sasame, H. A., Green, I., and Mitchell, J. R. (1973). The role of cytochrome P-450 in N-hydroxylation of 2-acetylaminofluorene. Mol. Pharmacol. 9:398-404.

Thorgeirsson, S. S., Mitchell, J. R., Sasame, H. A., and Potter, W. Z. (1976). Biochemical changes after hepatic injury by allyl alcohol and N-hydroxy-2-acetylaminofluorene. Chem. Biol. Interact. 15:139-147.

Thorgeirsson, S. S., and Nebert, D. W. (1976). The Ah locus and the metabolism of chemical carcinogens and other foreign compounds. Adv. Cancer Res. 25:149-193.

Thorgeirsson, S. S., and Nelson, W. L. (1976). Separation and quantitative determination of 2-acetylaminofluorene and its hydroxylated metabolites by high pressure liquid chromatography. Anal. Biochem. 75:122-128.

Thorgeirsson, S. S., Sakai, S., and Adamson, R. H. (1978). Induction of monooxygenases in rhesus monkeys by 3-methylcholanthrene: metabolism and mutagenic activation of N-2-acetylaminofluorene and benzo[a]pyrene. J. Natl. Cancer Inst. 60:365-369.

Tipping, E., Ketterer, B., and Christodoulides, L. (1979). Interactions of small molecules with phospholipid bilayers. Binding to egg phosphatidylcholine of some uncharged molecules (2-acetylaminofluorene, 4-dimethylaminoazobenzene, oestrone and testosterone) that bind to ligandin and aminoazo-dye-binding protein A. Biochem. J. 180:319-326.

Tlsty, T. D., and Lieberman, M. W. (1978). Distribution of DNA repair synthesis in chromatin and its rearrangement following damage with N-acetoxy-2-acetylaminofluorene. Nucleic Acids Res. 5:3261-3273.

Toh, Y.-C. (1972). Systematic effect of testosterone on rat liver tumor induction by N-2-fluorenylacetamide. J. Natl. Cancer Inst. 48:113-118.

Toh, Y. C. (1973). Physiological and biochemical reviews of sex differences and carcinogenesis with particular reference to liver. Adv. Cancer Res. 18:155-209.

Toh, Y. C. (1978). Inhibitory effect of hypothalamic lesions on liver tumor induction by N-2-fluorenylacetamide in male rats. Cancer Res. 38:42-51.

Trams, E. G., Inscoe, J. K., and Resnik, R. A. (1961). Liver enzymes during hepatic carcinogenesis. J. Natl. Cancer Inst. 26:959-968.

Trosko, J. E., Frank, P., Chu, E. H., and Becker, J. E. (1973). Caffeine inhibition of postreplication repair of N-acetoxy-2-acetylaminofluorene-damaged DNA in Chinese hamster cells. Cancer Res. 33:2444-2449.

Truhaut, R., deClercq, M., and Loisillier, F. (1962). Action de pyrimidines de synthese sur le developpement de cancers du foie provoques chez des rats par l'acetylamino-2-fluorene. Rev. Fr. Etude. Clin. Biol. 7:298-303.

Trzos, R. J., Petzold, G. L., Brunden, M. N., and Swenberg, J. A. (1978). The evaluation of sixteen carcinogens in the rat using the micronucleus test. Mutat. Res. 58:79-86.

Tsuda, H., Miyata, Y., Murasaki, G., Kinoshita, H., Fukushima, S., and Ito, N. (1977). Synergistic effect of urinary bladder carcinogenesis in rats treated with N-butyl-N-(4-hydroxy-butyl)nitrosamine, N-[4-(5-nitro-2-furyl)-2-thiazolyl]formamide, N-2-fluorenylacetamide, and 3,3'-dichlorobenzidine. Gan. 68:183-192.

Tsukada, F., Hokari, S., Hayasaki, N., and Ito, N. (1972). Increased activity of polynucleotide ligase from rat hepatoma induced by N-2-fluorenylacetamide. Cancer Res. 32:886-888.

Tulp, A., Welagen, J. J., and Westra, J. G. (1978). Binding of the chemical carcinogen N-hydroxy-acetylaminofluorene to ploidy classes of rat liver nuclei as separated by velocity sedimentation at unit gravity. Chem. Biol. Interact. 23:293-303.

Ulland, B. M., Weisburger, J. H., Yamamoto, R. S., and Weisburger, E. K. (1973). Antioxidants and carcinogenesis: butylated hydroxytoluene, but not diphenyl-p-phenylenediamine, inhibits cancer induction by N-2-fluorenylacetamide and by N-hydroxy-N-2-fluorenylacetamide in rats. Food Cosmet. Toxicol. 11:199-207.

Umezawa, K., Shirai, A., Matsushima, T., and Sugimura, T. (1978). Comutagenic effect of norharman and harman with 2-acetylaminofluorene derivatives. Proc. Natl. Acad. Sci. USA 75:928-930.

Van Den Berghe, H., and Verresen, H. (1963). La progression tumorale dans deux carcinomes mammaires du rat provoques par l'acetylaminofluorene. Bull. Assoc. Fr. Etude. Cander 50:291-303.

Vasileva, I. A. (1968). Significance of age of rats for sensitivity to blastomogenic action of 2-acetylaminofluorene. Vopr. Onkol. 14(8):58-63.

Veenema, R. J., Fingerhut, B., and Tannenbaum, M. (1964). The effect of gonadectomy on the experimental production of bladder carcinoma in the Fischer rat (F/Fu). Invest. Urol. 1:587-592.

Vysheslavova, M. Y. (1969). The effect of sunflower oil with various degrees of oxidation on induction of rat tumors by 2-acetylaminofluorene (Russian). Vopr. Onkol. 15(4): 66-70.

Vysheslavova, M. Y. (1972). The effect of fatty acids (linolenic, linoleic, and oleic) on the development of 2-acetylaminofluorene-induced tumors in rats. Vestn. Akad. Med. Nauk. SSSR 27(2):22-27.

Wainfan, E., Randle, S. S., Relyea, N. M., and Balis, M. E. (1978). Effects of acetylaminofluorene on transfer RNA methyltransferases of rat organs. Cancer Res. 38: 1852-1856.

Walters, M. A., Roe, F. J., Mitchley, B. C., and Walsh, A. (1967). Further tests for carcinogenesis using newborn mice: 2-naphthylamine, 2-naphthylhydroxylamine, 2-acetylaminofluorene and ethyl methane sulphonate. Br. J. Cancer 21:367-372.

Warren, J. R. (1978). Damage of proliferating lymphoid cell deoxyribonucleic acid by methyl methanesulfonate and N-acetoxy-2-acetylaminofluorene. Cancer Lett. 5:253-260.

Watanabe, K., and Williams, G. M. (1978). Enhancement of rat hepatocellular-altered foci by the liver tumor promoter phenobarbital: evidence that foci are precursors of neoplasms and that the promoter acts on carcinogen-induced lesions. J. Natl. Cancer Inst. 61:1311-1314.

Weeks, C. E., Allaben, W. T., Louie, S. C., Lazear, E. J., and King, C. M. (1978). Role of arylhydroxamic acid acyltransferase in the mutagenicity of N-hydroxy-N-2-fluorenylacetamide in Salmonella typhimurium. Cancer Res. 38:613-618.

Weinstein, I. B., and Grunberger, D. (1974). Structural and functional changes in nucleic acids modified by chemical carcinogens. In Chemical Carcinogenesis, Part A, P. O. T'so and J. A. DiPaolo (Eds.). Marcel Dekker, New York, pp. 217-235.

Weisburger, E. K. (1961). New metabolites of N-3-fluorenylacetamide. J. Natl. Cancer Inst. 27:1451-1463.

Weisburger, E. K. (1980). Species specific biochemical pathways of malignant growth. In Pathologic Growth in Plants, Animals and Man, H. E. Kaiser (Ed.). Williams & Wilkens, Baltimore, pp. 335-350.

Weisburger, E. K., Grantham, P. H., and Benjamin, T. (1978). Separation and analysis of various carcinogenic aromatic amines and their metabolites. In Prevention and Detection of Cancer, Vol. 2, H. E. Nieburgs (Ed.). Marcel Dekker, New York, pp. 1961-1972.

Weisburger, E. K., and Weisburger, J. H. (1958a). A new route to 3- and 2,6-substituted fluorenes. J. Org. Chem. 23:1193-1198.

Weisburger, E. K., and Weisburger, J. H. (1958b). Chemistry, carcinogenicity, and metabolism of 2-fluorenamine and related compounds. Adv. Cancer Res. 5:331-431.

Weisburger, J. H., Grantham, P. H., Morris, H. P., and Weisburger, E. K. (1961a). Chromatographic separation of the urinary metabolites of the carcinogen N-2-fluorenylacetamide into free compounds, sulfuric acid, and glucuronic acid esters. Cancer Res. 21:949-955.

Weisburger, J. H., Grantham, P. H., Morris, H. P., and Weisburger, E. K. (1961b). On the in vitro and in vivo protein-binding of N-2-fluorenylacetamide and related compounds. J. Natl. Cancer Inst. 27:153-171.

Weisburger, J. H., Grantham, P. H., and Weisburger, E. K. (1963). Metal ion complexing properties of carcinogen metabolites. Biochem. Pharmacol. 12:179-191.

Weisburger, J. H., Klein, M., Weisburger, E. K., Glass, R. M., Woodard, G. M., and Cronin, M. T. I. (1970). A comparison of the effect of the carcinogen N-hydroxy-N-2-fluorenylacetamide in infant and weanling rats. J. Natl. Cancer Inst. 45:29-35.

Weisburger, J. H., Pai, S. R., and Yamamoto, R. S. (1964). Pituitary hormones and liver carcinogenesis with N-hydroxy-2-fluorenylacetamide. J. Natl. Cancer Inst. 32: 881-904.

Weisburger, J. H., Pai, S. R., Yamamoto, R. S., Korzis, J., and Weisburger, E. K. (1968). Pituitary hormones and the mechanism of induction of liver cancer with N-hydroxy-N-2-fluorenylacetamide. Isr. J. Med. Sci. 4:1223-1230.

Weisburger, J. H., Schmehl, E. A., and Pai, S. R. (1965). Liver damage by the carcinogen N-hydroxy-N-2-fluorenylacetamide. Pentobarbital sleeping time and liver morphology. Toxicol. Appl. Pharmacol. 7:579-587.

Weisburger, J. H., Shirasu, Y., Grantham, P. H., and Weisburger, E. K. (1967). Chloramphenicol, protein synthesis, and the metabolism of the carcinogen N-2-fluorenyldiacetamide in rats. Inhibition by chloramphenicol of carcinogen binding. J. Biol. Chem. 242:372-378.

Weisburger, J. H., and Weisburger, E. K. (1971). N-Oxidation enzymes. In Handbook of Experimental Pharmacology, Vol. 28, Concepts in Biochemical Pharmacology, Part II, B. B. Brodie and J. R. Gillette (Eds.). Springer-Verlag, Berlin, pp. 312-333.

Weisburger, J. H., and Weisburger, E. K. (1973). Biochemical formation and pharmacological, toxicological, and pathological properties of hydroxylamines and hydroxamic acids. Pharmacol. Rev. 25:1-66.

Weisburger, J. H., Weisburger, E. K., Grantham, P. H., and Morris, H. P. (1959a). N-(6-Hydroxy-2-fluorenyl)acetamide, a urinary metabolite after intraperitoneal injection of N-2-fluorenylacetamide into rats. J. Biol. Chem. 234:2138-2140.

Weisburger, J. H., Weisburger, E. K., Grantham, P. H., and Morris, H. P. (1959b). The biosynthetic preparation of C^{14}-labeled N-(1- and 3-hydroxy-2-fluorenyl)acetamides, and their metabolism in rats and guinea pigs. J. Natl. Cancer Inst. 22:825-844.

Weisburger, J. H., Weisburger, E. K., Madison, R. M., Wenk, M. L., and Klein, D. S. (1973). Effect of acetanilide and p-hydroxyacetanilide on the carcinogenicity of N-2-fluorenylacetamide and N-hydroxy-N-2-fluorenylacetamide in mice, hamsters, and female rats. J. Natl. Cancer Inst. 51:235-240.

Weisburger, J. H., Weisburger, E. K., and Morris, H. P. (1958). Differences in the metabolism of N-2-fluorenylacetamide in the guinea pig and the rat. Cancer Res. 18: 1039-1047.

Weisburger, J. H., Weisburger, E. K., and Morris, H. P. (1959c). The biosynthesis of N-(7-hydroxy-2-fluoren-9-C^{14}-yl)acetamide from N-2-fluoren-9-C -ylacetamide and its metabolism in the rat and in the guinea pig. Arch. Biochem. 80:187-198.

Weisburger, J. H., Weisburger, E. K., and Morris, H. P. (1961c). Aminofluorenols as urinary metabolites of N-2-fluorenylacetamide. J. Natl. Cancer Inst. 27:145-152.

Weissmann, G., Troll, W., van Duuren, B. L., and Sessa, G. (1968). Studies on lysosomes. X. Effects of tumor-promoting agents upon biological and artificial membrane systems. Biochem. Pharmacol. 17:2421-2434.

West, R. W., and Oller, W. L. (1978). Analysis of 2-acetylaminofluorene in laboratory animal chow by reverse phase liquid chromatography. J. Liquid Chromatogr. 1:181-185.

Westra, J. G., Kriek, E., and Hittenhausen, H. (1976). Identification of the persistently bound form of the carcinogen N-acetyl-2-aminofluorene to rat liver DNA in vivo. Chem. Biol. Interact. 15:149-164.

Wiebkin, P., Fry, J. R., and Bridges, J. W. (1978). Metabolism-mediated cytotoxicity of chemical carcinogens and noncarcinogens. Biochem. Pharmacol. 27:1849-1851.

Williams, D. J., and Parry, G. (1975). Endoplasmic membrane as a source and a target for chemically reactive metabolic intermediate. Biochem. Soc. Trans. 3:69-72.

Williams, G. M. (1976a). Functional markers and growth behavior of preneoplastic hepatocytes. Cancer Res. 36:2540-2543.

Williams, G. M. (1976b). The use of liver epithelial cultures for the study of chemical carcinogenesis. Am. J. Pathol. 85:739-753.

Williams, G. M. (1977). Detection of chemical carcinogens by unscheduled DNA synthesis in rat liver primary cultures. Cancer Res. 37:1845-1851.

Williams, G. M., Elliott, J. M., and Weisburger, J. H. (1973). Carcinoma after malignant conversion in vitro of epithelial-like cells from rat liver following exposure to chemical carcinogens. Cancer Res. 33:606-612.

Williams, G. M., Klaiber, M., Parker, S. E., and Farber, E. (1976). Nature of early appearing, carcinogen-induced liver lesions resistant to iron accumulation. J. Natl. Cancer Inst. 57:157-165.

Williams, G. M., and Watanabe, K. (1978). Quantitative kinetics of development of N-2-fluorenylacetamide-induced, altered (hyperplastic)hepatocellular foci resistant to iron accumulation and of their reversion or persistence following removal of carcinogen. J. Natl. Cancer Inst. 61:113-121.

Williams, G. M., and Yamamoto, R. S. (1972). Absence of stainable iron from preneoplastic and neoplastic lesions in rat liver with 8-hydroxyquinoline-induced siderosis. J. Natl. Cancer Inst. 49:685-692.

Williams-Ashman, H. G., and Johnson, M. K. (1960). Aromatic amines as hydrogen carriers for the peroxidase-catalyzed oxidation of reduced pyridine nucleotides. Enzymologia 22:327-331.

Wojnar, R. J., and Roth, J. S. (1965). Ribonuclease inhibitor and latent ribonuclease in rat liver during feeding of 2-acetamidofluorene. Cancer Res. 25:1913-1918.

Wood, M. (1969). Factors influencing the induction of tumours of the urinary bladder and liver by 2-acetylaminofluorene in the mouse. Eur. J. Cancer 5:41-47.

Wood, M. (1970). Aetiology of tumours of the urinary bladder. Induction of tumours in the urinary tract of the rabbit by aromatic amines. Ind. Med. Surg. 39:82-88.

Woolum, J. C., and Commoner, B. (1970). Isolation and identification of a paramagnetic complex from the livers of carcinogen-treated rats. Biochim. Biophys. Acta 201: 131-140.

Wu, S.-C., and Straub, K. D. (1976). Purification and characterization of N-hydroxy-2-acetylaminofluorene sulfotransferase from rat liver. J. Biol. Chem. 251:6529-6536.

Yager, J. D., Jr., and Miller, J. A., Jr. (1978). DNA repair in primary cultures of rat hepatocytes. Cancer Res. 38:4385-4394.

Yager, J. D., Jr., and Potter, V. R. (1975). A comparison of the effects of 3'-methyl-4-dimethylaminoazobenzene, 2-methyl-4-dimethylaminoazobenzene, and 2-acetylaminofluorene on rat liver DNA stability and new synthesis. Cancer Res. 35: 1225-1234.

Yamada, S., Ito, M., and Nagayo, T. (1971). Histological and autoradiographical studies on intestinal tumors of rat induced by oral administration of N,N'-2,7-fluorenylenebisacetamide. Gan. 62:471-478.

Yamada, S., Ito, M., Nagayo, T., and Okumura, Y. (1977). Kinetics of preneoplastic epithelia of the intestinal mucosa induced in Buffalo rats by oral administration of N,N'-2,7-fluorenylenebisacetamide. Gan. 68:805-811.

Yamamoto, I., Nagai, K., Kimura, H., and Iwatsubo, K. (1966). Nicotine and some carcinogens in special reference to the hepatic drug-metabolizing enzyme. Jpn. J. Pharmacol. 16:189-190.

Yamamoto, R. S., Frankel, H. H., and Weisburger, J. H. (1970). The effects of isomers of acetotoluidide and aminobenzoic acid on the toxicity and carcinogenicity of N-2-fluorenylacetamide. Toxicol. Appl. Pharmacol. 17:98-106.

Yamamoto, R. S., Glass, R. M., Frankel, H. H., Weisburger, E. K., and Weisburger, J. H. (1968). Inhibition of the toxicity and carcinogenicity of N-2-fluorenylacetamide by acetanilide. Toxicol. Appl. Pharmacol. 13:108-117.

Yamamoto, R. S., Korzis, J., and Weisburger, J. H. (1967). Chronic ethanol ingestion and the hepatocarcinogenicity of N-hydroxy-N-2-fluorenylacetamide. Int. J. Cancer 2: 337-343.

Yamamoto, R. S., Pai, S. R., Korzis, J., and Weisburger, J. H. (1968). The carcinogenicity of N-hydroxy-N-2-fluorenylacetamide and the metabolism of N-2-fluorenylacetamide in Praomis (Mastomys) natalensis. Br. J. Cancer 22:769-775.

Yamamoto, R. S., and Weisburger, E. K. (1977). Role of hormones on digestive and urinary tract carcinogenesis. Recent Prog. Horm. Res. 33:617-653.

Yamamoto, R. S., Williams, G. M., Frankel, H. H., and Weisburger, J. H. (1971). 8-Hydroxyquinoline: chronic toxicity and inhibitory effect on the carcinogenicity of N-2-fluorenylacetamide. Toxicol. Appl. Pharmacol. 19:687-698.

Yamamoto, R. S., Williams, G. M., Richardson, H. L., Weisburger, E. K., and Weisburger, J. H. (1973). Effect of p-hydroxyacetanilide on liver cancer induction by N-hydroxy-N-2-fluorenylacetamide. Cancer Res. 33:454-457.

Yamasaki, H., Leffler, S., and Weinstein, I. B. (1977a). Effect of N-2-acetylaminofluorene modification on the structure and template activity of DNA and reconstituted chromatin. Cancer Res. 37:684-691.

Yamasaki, H., Pulkrabek, P., Grunberger, D., and Weinstein, I. B. (1977b). Differential excision from DNA of the C-8 and N^2 guanosine adducts of N-acetyl-2-aminofluorene by single strand-specific endonucleases. Cancer Res. 37:3756-3760.

Yasuzumi, G., Sugihara, R., Ito, N., Konishi, Y., and Hiasa, Y. (1970). Fine structure of nuclei as revealed by electron microscopy. VII. Hyperplastic liver nodules in rat induced by 3'-methyl-4-dimethylaminoazobenzene, 2-fluorenylacetamide and DL-ethionine. Exp. Cell Res. 63:83-95.

Yost, Y. (1969). Oxidation of fluorenamines and preparation of 2,2'- and 4,4'-azofluorene. J. Med. Chem. 12:961-970.

Yost, Y., Gutmann, H. R., and Rydell, R. E. (1975). The carcinogenicity of fluorenylhydroxamic acids and N-acetoxy-N-fluorenylacetamides for the rat as related to the reactivity of the esters towards nucleophiles. Cancer Res. 35:447-459.

Young, P. R., and McNair, H. M. (1976). High-pressure liquid chromatography of aromatic amines. J. Chromatogr. 119:569-579.

Yu, F.-L., and Grunberger, D. (1976). Multiple sites of action of N-hydroxy-2-acetylaminofluorene in rat hepatic nuclear transcription. Cancer Res. 36:3629-3633.

Zawirska, B., Medras, K., and Sosnik, K. H. (1971). Die Pyrrolfarbstoffe der Organe wahrend der mit 2-Amino-N-Acetylfluoren bei Ratten induzierten Karzinogenese. Zentrabl. Allg. Pathol. 114:41-50.

Zieve, F. J. (1972). Inhibition of rat liver ribonucleic acid polymerase by the carcinogen N-hydroxy-2-fluorenylacetamide. J. Biol. Chem. 247:5987-5995.

Zieve, F. J. (1973). Effects of the carcinogen N-acetoxy-2-fluorenylacetamide on the template properties of deoxyribonucleic acid. Mol. Pharmacol. 9:658-669.

Zussman, W. V. (1965). Salivary and sebaceous gland alterations in rats ingesting N-2-fluorenylacetamide. Arch. Pathol. 80:278-284.

Zussman, W. V. (1966). Infiltrating gingival carcinoma in rats ingesting N-2-fluorenylacetamide. Cancer Res. 26 (Part 1):544-549.

15

Ionizing Radiation

GEORGE W. CASARETT / University of Rochester School of Medicine, Rochester, New York

This paper is based on work performed under contract with the U.S. Department of Energy at the University of Rochester Department of Radiation Biology and Biophysics and has been assigned Report No. UR-3490-1368.

I. INTRODUCTION

Before presenting information on radiation exposures from various natural and human-made radiation sources, several sections of the chapter are presented to provide some general perspective concerning concepts and quantities relating to: radiation dose, qualities, linear energy transfer (LET), relative biological effectiveness (RBE), and quality factor (QF); radiation protection guidelines; doses in the United States; internal emitters; radiation cancerogenesis and general dose-effect relationships; the influence of dose size, dose rate, and LET on the relationships and the RBE; estimation of cancerogenic risks; and some available numerical risk estimates.

It is not within the scope of the chapter, or possible with the paucity of available data, to attempt to provide reliable numerical risk estimates for any and every radiation source and exposure circumstance to be discussed in the chapter. However, although the radiation cancerogenic risk is largely a matter of dose, LET, and spatial and temporal distribution of dose to target tissues or cells—influenced by biological variables such as age and sex—the presented available risk estimates per unit dose based on linear extrapolation or interpolation to exposure levels of practical interest in radiation protection (permitting as it does the neglect of influence of dose size and dose rate), could be applied by the reader to various exposure and dose circumstances to derive very crude "upper limit" risk estimates as averages for the exposed population.

The scope and intent of this chapter are: (1) to discuss ionizing radiation as a carcinogen; (2) to present information on sources of human radiation exposure; (3) to discuss the scientific knowledge of radiation cancerogenesis with the required qualifications; and (4) to describe the necessarily pragmatic and prudent approaches and assumptions in cancerogenic risk estimation for purposes of radiation protection and the resulting risk estimates for human radiation cancerogenesis.

II. RADIATION EXPOSURE AND DOSE

The Roentgen (R) is a unit of exposure of X or gamma radiation based on the ionization that these radiations produce in air. An exposure of 1 Roentgen results in 2.584×10^{-4} coulombs per milligram of air, or 1 electrostatic unit per cc of air at standard temperature and pressure.

The rad is the unit of absorbed dose of ionizing radiation, one rad corresponding to the absorption of 0.01 joule of energy per kilogram of the tissue concerned. One rad is also equal to 100 ergs absorbed per gram of any substance.

The incidence of cancer induced by a given absorbed dose of radiation in a given tissue, all other conditions being equal, is similar for radiations of low linear energy transfer (LET), for example, X rays or beta or gamma radiation, regardless of whether the energy is delivered to the tissues from radiation sources outside the body or from radioactive materials deposited within the body. For certain types of radiation, however, for example, for neutrons and for the alpha radiation emitted by some radioactive materials, the incidence of cancer induction in a given tissue for a given absorbed dose—all other conditions being equal—is greater, often by a factor of 5 to 20 or greater, depending on dose size and dose rate, than that from the same dose of X rays or beta or gamma radiation, because of the greater linear energy transfer (LET) of neutrons and alpha particles.

Linear energy transfer (LET) is the average energy released per unit track length, usually expressed in keV per micrometer of track length. Within limits, the relative biological effectiveness (RBE) depends on the LET.

Relative biological effectiveness (RBE) is a factor expressing the relative effectiveness of radiations with different LET in producing a given biological effect, in terms of the ratio of the required dose of the radiation in question to that of a standard reference radiation, usually 250 keV X rays. This unit is now limited to use in radiobiology and is not used directly in radiation protection.

Quality factor (QF or Q) is another name for a linear energy transfer dependent factor, selected on the basis of RBE values for purposes of radiation protection, by which absorbed doses are to be multiplied to account for the varying effectiveness of different radiations.

The rem has been the dose equivalent unit in radiation protection. Numerically, the rem is equal to the absorbed radiation dose (in rad) multiplied by the appropriate effectiveness modifying factors such as the radiation quality factor (QF), the dose distribution factor (DF), and any other necessary modifying factors. This unit has enabled the summation of doses from various kinds of radiation, with various RBE values, as a measure of potential effect. It has also been used, on the basis of the assumption that effect is proportional to dose regardless of dose size and dose rate, to sum the total dose to a population ("collective dose"), calculate the average per capita individual dose in populations, or estimate individual or collective dose commitments for the future, as a measure of potential effect. The collective dose is the product of the number of people in the exposed population and their average dose.

There are two types of exposure assessment serving different purposes: (1) the individual-related assessment, which would indicate the potential risk to individuals; and (2) the radiation source-related assessment, which could be used to indicate the total potential risk or consequences from given sources. The individual dose assessment may be related to a time period ranging from the time of a single exposure to a lifetime, depending on the circumstances and purpose. Continued practices involving radionuclides inevitably give rise to accumulations of radioactivity in the human body or in the environment until a steady state is reached. For such situations, the dose commitment from, for example, 1 year of practice, could be assessed as the sum of the individual's future annual doses. This summation may be applied also to the average individual in a population and extended over generations.

On the assumption of proportionality between radiation dose and individual risk within the range of doses encountered, the collective dose is a quantity that is proportional to the potential radiation risk. To assess the total potential risk of a given practice that may result in worldwide exposure, the global collective dose is appropriate. For the assessment of the total potential radiation risk from worldwide exposure, including future dose contributions committed by the practice, collective dose commitments are calculated as the sum of the annual global collective doses over all future years. The collective dose commitment may be related also to a more limited amount of a practice.

III. MAXIMUM PERMISSIBLE DOSE EQUIVALENTS (NCRP)

To provide perspective on maximum permissible radiation exposure, this section presents briefly some of the current nonemergency dose-limiting recommendations of the National Council on Radiation Protection and Measurements (NCRP). The indicated values are for the limited scope of this chapter. NCRP Report No. 39 (1971) should be consulted for more complete information. The recommendations refer to radiation exposures other than those from natural sources and medical applications.

The recommended maximum permissible dose equivalent (MPD) for individuals of the general public, or occasionally exposed individuals, is 0.5 rem in any given year. The recommended MPD for the population annually is 0.17 rem average per capita. The recommended MPD values for combined whole-body occupational exposure are (1) 5 rems in any 1 year for the prospective annual limit; (2) 10-15 rems in any 1 year for the retrospective annual limit; and (3) (N-18) × 5 rems (where N is age in years) for long-term accumulation. The recommended MPD values for occupational exposure of parts of the body are: (1) for skin 15 rems in any 1 year; (2) for hands 75 rems in any 1 year (25 rems/quarter); (3) for forearms 30 rems in any 1 year (10 rems/quarter); and (4) for other organs, tissues, and organ systems 15 rems in any 1 year (5 rems/quarter). The recommended occupational MPD for fertile women (with respect to fetus) is 0.5 rem in the gestation period.

Present radiation protection policies also include the principle of eliminating any exposures which are not necessary and of keeping all the doses as low as is reasonably achievable. The effect of these precautions is that exposure at the limit is rare and that the dose contributions are such that the average dose in each group of persons to which a limit applies is much lower than the limit.

IV. ANNUAL WHOLE-BODY DOSE RATES IN THE UNITED STATES (1970)

To provide perspective on the annual whole-body dose rates in the United States, estimates from the 1972 National Academy of Sciences BEIR committee report (1972) on annual whole-body dose rates in the United States in 1970 are summarized in Table 1.

V. BODY DISTRIBUTION OF RADIONUCLIDES (INTERNAL EMITTERS)

The cancerogenic effects of radiations from internal emitters on given tissues are essentially similar qualitatively to those produced by radiations from external sources, and quantitative differences are usually due to differences in radiation dose, dose rate, microdistribution of dose, LET, and RBE, biological and other variables being equal. An exception may be that large amounts of some internal radionuclides could also exert chemical influence on cells and tissues in ways not yet fully appreciated.

The distribution of radiation doses to body tissues from an internal emitter depends on several factors, including: (1) route of entry (percutaneous absorption, ingestion, inhalation, various routes of injection); (2) physical and chemical nature of the radionuclide and its compound as these affect metabolism (deposition, translocation, excretion); (3) rate of physical decay (physical half-life); (4) rate of excretion, which, together with physical decay, determines biological half-life; and (5) qualities of radiations emitted.

Some radioisotopes that become widely distributed in the body are tritium and those of carbon, potassium, cesium, sodium, and phosphorus. Some of the radioisotopes that have an affinity for erythrocytes are those of iron, cobalt, tellurium, polonium, and chromium. Among the radioisotopes that show preferential deposition in the mineral component of bone are those of calcium, strontium, radium (Ra-226), uranium, magnesium, and lead. Radioisotopes that tend to deposit considerably in liver, kidney, bone marrow, or osteoid tissue (bone surface) are those of yttrium, the rare earths, polonium, radium (Ra-224), plutonium, thorium, and other actinides. The radioactive gaseous elements, such as radon-222, xenon-133, and krypton-85, are inhaled and distributed widely in the body. The radioisotopes of iodine have a marked affinity for the thyroid gland.

VI. RADIATION CANCEROGENESIS

A. General Aspects (Casarett, 1965, 1973, 1978)

The most important latent somatic effect of low doses of radiation is the occasional induction of malignant diseases.

In some of the epidemiologic studies of the cancerogenic effects of radiation in humans it has been possible to obtain some crude indication of the dose-effect (incidence) relationships for some types of malignancy. In general, however, the human epidemiologic evidence is too limited and imprecise to establish clearly the mathematical forms of the dose-effect relationships, or the influence of various physical and biological variables on them, or to contribute much to the understanding of mechanisms of radiation cancerogenesis.

Experimental animal research has been of great importance in revealing the types of tumor induced by radiation in different species, the dose-incidence relationships, the influence of dose rate and LET on the RBE and effectiveness per unit dose, the influence of other physical and biologic variables, and aspects of mechanisms, under conditions in which reliable estimates are made of the incidence, the doses and dose rates are known, and variables are

TABLE 1 Estimates of Annual Whole-Body Dose Rates in the United States (1970)

Radiation source	Average whole-body dose rate per capita (mrem/year)	Annual person-rems (in millions)
Environmental		
Natural	102	20.91
Global fallout (nuclear weapons)	4	0.82
Nuclear power	0.003	0.0007
Subtotals	106	21.73
Medical		
Diagnostic X rays	72	14.8
Radiopharmaceuticals	1	0.2
Subtotals	73	15.0
Occupational	0.8	0.16
Miscellaneous	2	0.5
Subtotals	2.8	0.66
Totals	182	37.4

Source: From NAS-BEIR (1972).

controlled. Experimental studies in animals have been of great value also in establishing the greater cancerogenic effectiveness per rad of neutrons and of alpha radiation than low-LET radiations, and in showing how and why the shapes of the dose-effect relationships differ between low-LET and high-LET radiations.

Most if not all types of cancer apparently result from multistage or multievent mechanisms, including cellular initiating events that confer neoplastic potential upon cells and promotional events that act to permit or to stimulate the potentiated cells to proliferate as neoplastic cells. It is apparent that there are two general classes of mechanisms of cancerogenesis, depending on whether or not the required promotional tissue changes are located largely in the same locale as the potentiated cells that will originate the cancer.

None of the many types of changes that radiation can cause in cells or tissues is unique for radiation; these changes can be caused by a variety of agents or conditions, including many of those known or suspected to be cancerogenic or cocancerogenic, that is, promotional. Therefore radiation-induced changes of cancerogenic significance may be additive or synergistic with the cancerogenic effects of other agents or conditions.

Radiation can cause all the changes required to induce a particular cancer in an individual, or it may contribute only some of the required changes, presumably even as little as one single hit event, the remainder of the required changes being contributed by causes other than the particular radiation dose in question. Relatively small doses can cause genic changes or chromosomal aberrations, some of which may be associated with cell transformation or cancerogenic initiation; larger doses are required to cause the chronic tissue or organ pathology and disfunctions that have been implicated as cancerogenic-promoting factors and to cause these changes considerably earlier than they would otherwise develop as a result of other pathology occurring with increasing age.

The cancerogenic effect of radiation exposure may be either to cause earlier appearance of the cancer (that is, temporal advancement) in individuals who would have had the cancer eventually without the radiation exposure, or to absolutely induce the cancer in individuals who would not have had the cancer otherwise. The difference between temporal advancement and absolute induction of cancer by radiation exposure involves all grades of contribution of radiation to the total mechanism of the cancer and cannot be fully appreciated statistically without thorough ascertainment of the differences in total lifetime incidence as well as in age-adjusted incidences, between exposed and appropriate nonexposed control populations.

In addition to the period of time from the completion of a cancerogenic mechanism to the detectability of the growing cancer, there is a period of time between the delivery of the effective radiation dose (induction dose) to an individual and the completion of the consequent course of pathological processes required to fulfill the cancerogenic mechanism. In practice the latent period often refers to these two periods combined. For many cancers there is a tendency for the latent period after brief radiation exposure to increase as dose decreases. Obviously, the life expectancy of the individual at the time of the radiation exposure in relation to the required latent period for a cancer is one of the determining factors in the dose required to insure the development of that cancer within his lifetime.

The typical latent period for various human malignancies induced by irradiation may vary from approximately 1 decade (leukemia) to 2 or 3 decades for other cancers.

In regard to the question of dose threshold for radiation cancerogenesis, the radiation dose required to temporally advance or absolutely induce a particular cancer in an individual (that is, his or her individual threshold dose) depends on the extent to which the rest of the cancerogenic mechanism will have been completed by causes other than the particular exposure in question, before, during, or after this exposure and within his or her after-survival time.

For practical purposes the term "threshold dose" for radiation cancerogenesis has real meaning only in terms of the radiation dose required to cause the effect in an individual or, if a population is being considered, only in terms of the dose required for the most susceptible individual in that particular population.

There is a finite probability, however small, that exposure to the smallest quantity of ionizing radiation could cause a change in a cell, for example, a point mutation, which could contribute a part of the complex mechanism of carcinogenesis. Whether or not this change would result in the temporal advancement or absolute induction of the cancer would depend on whether or not it occurred in an individual in whom the balance of the mechanism will have been provided by other means within his or her after-survival time.

On logical or theoretical grounds it may be erroneous to assume the existence of an absolute threshold dose for radiation induction of cancer of any kind in populations of unlimited size and heterogeneity with respect to genetics, environment, clinical history, age, sex, etc., even if the probability of completion of a cancerogenic mechanism by the smallest amount of radiation in an individual is extremely small and even though one or another sample of the population were to show an observed ("practical") threshold dose of substantial size.

A practical threshold ascribed to insufficient life span is only another way to indicate for a particular population sample the absence of individuals of sufficiently low threshold for a particular cancer to accommodate the required latent period for a low radiation dose within their after-survival time. The practical threshold may differ between different samples of the population according to size of sample (as it affects statistics) and actual differences in distribution of individual thresholds (and ages) at the lower exposure levels.

B. General Aspects of Dose-Effect Relationships (Casarett, 1965, 1973, 1978)

It is the distribution of the individual radiation dose thresholds for a cancer in any particular population that determines the shape, as well as the intercept, of the dose-incidence curve for a given radiation quality.

An observed dose-incidence curve that involves only parts or combined fragments of the potential total curve, may be fairly linear or nonlinear (concavely or convexly). Portions or combined fragments of an observed nonlinear curve may be fairly linear. Any of these types of observed curves may or may not suggest a practical threshold directly or by extrapolation, and none of them excludes the possibility of lack of absolute threshold in a larger or more heterogenous population.

Experimental data over a wide range of single doses of low-LET radiation, or data from composites of several different experiments comprising a wide range of single doses, with

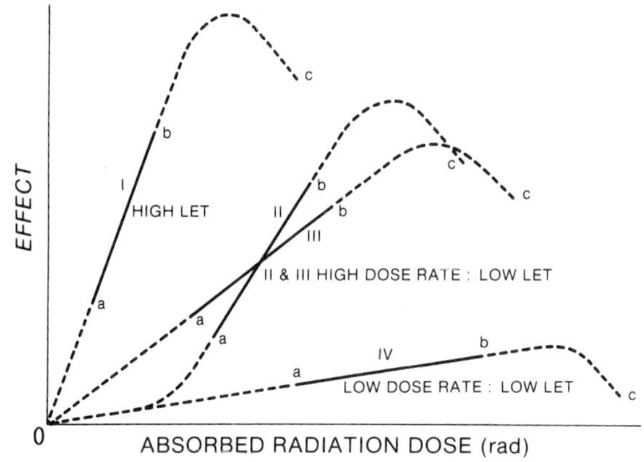

FIGURE 1 Schematic representation of various arithmetic radiation cancerogenic dose-effect curves for high-LET (linear energy transfer) radiation (curve I) and for low-LET radiation (curves II, III, and IV) at high dose rate (curves II and III) or low dose rate (curve IV). In the curves the solid portions (a-b) represent linear fits to observed data points in the rapidly rising portions of the curves, the dashed lines (a-o) represent regions for which no reliable data are available and paths of extrapolation from a-b to zero dose and effect, and the dashed lines b-c represent the generally known convex-upward portions of the dose-effect curves at high doses (peaking or plateauing of effect followed by decline of effect). Although not depicted, the effect may decline further from c with further increase in dose.

ascertainment of absolute lifetime excess incidence of cancers, are often compatible with a general sigmoid curve, as may be represented by the general shape of curve II in Fig. 1. There is a zone of uncertainty at very low dose levels in which no concrete data exist, and in which theoretically the curve may be fairly linear but with low slope, followed by a more rapidly rising nonlinear (concave upward) portion where the slope (effect per unit dose) increases with dose (or dose rate), followed by a convex upward portion (b-c, Fig. 1) leading to a peak or plateau and then a falling portion with further increase in dose.

The decline in rate of increase in incidence at high dose levels, first represented by the development of the peak (or plateau) incidence levels, then by a fall in the curve at still higher dose levels (b-c, Fig. 1), has been attributed in experimental work to degrees of tissue destruction, cell killing and sterilization, which are excessive for efficient cancer induction, and in some instances, for example, with whole-body irradiation, to shortening of life span from other radiation effects, leaving inadequate latency accommodation for efficient cancer induction.

For various types of cancers in various species or strains of experimental animals the range of single doses involved in such a sigmoid dose-incidence curve may vary greatly, and the length and steepness of various parts of the curve may vary greatly depending on the distribution of individual thresholds for the after-survival involved. This distribution can skew the curve in various ways. It can be inferred that decreased steepness of the rising portion of a curve indicates more effective cellular repair.

At low doses and/or dose rates of low-LET radiation, the dose-effect curve is nearly linear (curve IV, Fig. 1), but with a much lower slope than would be derived by linear extrapolation or interpolation on dose from data at high doses and/or dose rates. For example, in Fig. 1 curve III may be used to depict a linear fit (a-b) of observed data (a-b) in curve II for the purpose of linear extrapolation to zero dose and effect, with the result that the effect at low dose levels may be overestimated. The statistical uncertainties in human epidemiological data often allow such a procedure for purposes of conservative radiation protection.

The dose-effect curves for high-LET radiations, for example, neutrons or alpha particles, tend to rise more steeply in the lower dose range than those for low-LET radiations, are more linear through the low and intermediate dose ranges before the high dose plateau and decline occur, and are much less dependent on the dose size or dose rate in the rising region of the curve (curve I, Fig. 1).

Experimental investigation has shown that marked reduction of overall radiation dose rate from intense exposure down to low rates by protraction of exposure or by fractionation of exposure over extended periods of time permits less interaction among the total ionizing events and permits more recovery of cells and tissues from radiation injury, to a much greater extent in the case of low-LET radiations than in the case of high-LET radiations.

Substantial reduction of the overall dose rate for a low-LET or high-LET radiation dose that, as an intense exposure, is in excess of the optimal dose to cause maximal cancerogenic effect may increase the cancerogenic effect or effectiveness by reducing the counterproductive excessive damage of tissue or the life-shortening effect of intensive exposure. Substantial reduction of overall dose rate of a low-LET radiation dose that, as an intense exposure, is optimal or below optimal for maximum cancerogenic effect may reduce the cancerogenic effect or effectiveness, but this is not usually the case for high-LET radiation.

Under circumstances of prolonged protraction or fractionation of radiation dose there is some uncertainty as to how much of the total accumulated dose is required for the induction of the cancer and how much is superfluous or wasted. A particular induction dose takes a relatively long time to accumulate at a relatively low dose rate, and this longer time is taken at the expense of time available for the latent period even if the dose rate does not influence the required size of the induction dose. To the extent that reduced dose rate does reduce the cancerogenic effect, the required induction doses may be larger at the lower dose rates and still take more time to accumulate at still greater expense of the available latent period.

Nonuniformity of microdistribution of dose within the tissue of interest and among individuals of the study group with respect to this tissue, and the associated problems of dosimetry and expression of relevant target dose, also cause considerable uncertainty as to relevant induction dose. The existence of hot spots of radioactive isotopes in tissues, for example, alpha particle emitting isotopes, is a particularly notable example. There is uncertainty as to whether the relative induction dose for cancerogenesis in individuals is more closely related to doses in or closely around the "hot spots" or in more distant regions of more diffuse distribution of the radiation.

As the effect of high-LET radiation is proportional to dose (linear) and relatively independent of dose rate, the RBE of that radiation increases as the dose and/or dose rate decrease, not that the effectiveness of the high-LET radiation changes, but because the effectiveness of the low-LET reference radiation decreases with reduction of dose and/or dose rate.

In regard to any requirement for a minimum amount of radiation energy deposited within a small volume to initiate a biological effect, the probability of low-LET radiation producing the effect with a single track or "hit" is small, and the probability increases with increasing LET to a point above which the efficiency in terms of energy per unit mass may decrease with increase of energy deposition that is superfluous or "wasted" in terms of production of the specified effect. Thus, the RBE may increase with increasing LET to a peak at an intermediate LET, often observed to be from about 100 to 300 keV μm, and then decrease as LET rises further, without dependence on size of dose and dose rate (Kellerer and Rossi, 1972).

In general, the experimentally observed shapes of the dose-effect relationships for low-LET radiations, and their dependence on dose size and dose rate, support the conclusion that simple linear extrapolation or interpolation on dose from effects observed at intermediate to high doses and dose rates—that is, on the rising portions of the observed curves, without accounting for the influence of dose size, dose rate, and other influencing variables—tends to systematically overestimate the overall risks at low doses and low dose rates.

The overall effectiveness per rad of low-LET radiation is generally reduced with decrease in dose size as well as decrease in dose rate, so that it is possible that the effectiveness of very low doses at very low dose rates, such as those encountered in radiation protection situations, may be very much smaller than that at high doses and high dose rates. However, as the degrees of reduction for various tumors have not yet been estimated with confidence, only conservative effectiveness reducing factors for these variables have been proposed so far, and these have been applied to the risk estimates derived on the basis of the linear hypothesis.

The difficulty in formulating complete and precise dose-effect relationship models for estimation of radiation risks to human beings, or to experimental animals, resides not only in the paucity and fragmentary nature of the available data on effects, but importantly also on the incompleteness of knowledge of the details of the mechanisms of radiation induction of the effects.

It should be noted that however well the sigmoid curve may represent the probability of the low-LET radiation induction of a cancer in groups of experimental animals, which are usually relatively homogenous (with respect to age at irradiation, genetic background, environmental conditions and care, diet, treatments and procedures within experimental and control subgroups, etc.), the distribution of individual thresholds in a population that is highly heterogenous in these respects, such as the human population, may often be different, not to mention the great uncertainties concerning dose to relevant target tissues, dose rate, appropriateness of control populations, and incomplete follow-up and ascertainment of absolute excess incidence in human population studies.

Under these circumstances it is not surprising that the fragmentary epidemiologic data on correlation of radiation exposure (usually high doses and dose rates) with excess incidence of one or another kind of cancer are compatible with linear relationships, though not necessarily incompatible with or excluding other relationships in the same or in lower dose ranges. Furthermore, the analysis of epidemiologic data often involves the selection of single values and/or integration of inhomogeneous organ or individual doses to characterize radiation exposure of collective subgroups as the significant dose parameter under conditions of non-uniform exposure and exposure rate, with neglect of dose rate. These procedures tend to preimpose linearity on the data and contribute a presumption of linearity, since the linear hypothesis is the only one that normally permits these procedures.

Theoretically, for an effect that can be produced by the action of a single radiation track or "hit" in relation to the pertinent biological target, the dose-effect relationship should be linear (proportional) over a certain range of dose levels, other conditions being unchanged during irradiation. For effects requiring two or more tracks or hits on a target or multiple targets, the increase in effect would theoretically be related to some power function of dose greater than unity. Available data indicate that chemical and biological amplification of the random radiation-induced initial molecular changes into manifest cellular and tissue damage and lesions is influenced by balance and interactions between the production of injury and the repair of injury. These interacting processes, as well as the probability that a single hit can cause a given effect, apparently depend on the type of effect, the radiation quality (LET), the spatial and temporal distribution of dose, and the physiological condition or phase of the relevant cells undergoing irradiation. Even if the radiation effect in question is the result of at least one event in a single target, this does not mean that all hits produce the effect. Mammalian cells can repair damaging events that are essentially single hit in character.

Recent efforts to formulate a unifying biophysical theory of the relationship between radiation quality and biological effectiveness have been reported by Rossi (1970) and Kellerer and Rossi (1971, 1972). These authors observed that the RBE of neutrons for various biological effects varies inversely with the square root of the neutron dose, and postulated that this is a general radiobiological relationship.

According to their hypothesis, biological effect of radiation results from impairment at two sites within a single target in the cell nucleus and that the yield of such impairments for a given LET is proportional to the mean value of the square of the specific energy and therefore proportional to a quadratic function of the absorbed dose; that is, $Y = aD + bD^2$, where Y is the yield, D the absorbed dose, and a and b are coefficients. The coefficient of the linear term (aD) is a function of the LET and the size of the site. The coefficient of the square term (bD^2) depends on the probability of interactions between radiation effects and/or their repair. This coefficient may be from 0 to 1 depending on the dose rate and time for repair.

For high-LET radiations in practical dose ranges, the coefficient of the linear term is greatly predominant over the coefficient of the square term. For low-LET radiations the coefficient of the linear term is so low that it is important only at low doses and the quadratic term becomes more important at higher doses. The biological effect of low-LET radiation is usually smaller at low dose rate because of repair. The square term does not contribute to the effect of low-LET radiation at low dose levels at which the effect is independent of dose rate. Under this condition the linear term alone represents the dose-effect relationship (see curve IV, Fig. 1). As the effect of high-LET radiation is linear with dose and independent of dose rate, the RBE increases at low doses and low dose rates because the effectiveness of the low-LET radiation decreases at such dose and dose rate levels.

Although the yield of radiation effect for many effects in diploid mammalian cells or in experimental animals in response to low-LET radiation may be represented, at first approximation, by the expression $Y = aD + bD^2$, or, as is often used, E (effect) $= aD + bD^2$, there are very few available sets of data sufficient to enable statistically vigorous derivation of the numerical values for the constants. In the case of sets of data which are uncertain statistically, as in many sets of human epidemiological data as compared with well-designed and controlled experiments, it has often been impossible statistically to exclude completely the alternative linear dose-effect relationship for the observed sets of data. It should be noted that neither the linear nor the square or quadratic equation can be expected to hold for cancerogenic effects of large doses at high dose rates at which the yield of effect per unit dose decreases from that at dose levels in the rapidly rising portion of the dose-effect curve.

The relative contributions of the linear and square or other required high-power dose terms should be expected to vary with type of effect and among individuals, depending on the influence of several biological variables. Available dose-effect data for a variety of radiation effects in mammalian systems indicate that the single dose (high dose rate) level at which the contributions of the linear and dose square terms might be roughly equal would be seldom likely to be less than 50 rad, and that a weighted average of 100 rad, that is, $a/b = 100$ rad, does not seem unreasonable. If $a/b = 100$ rad, the contribution of the quadratic term, for low LET, high dose rate irradiation would be four times as large as that from the linear term at 400 rad and one-tenth that of the linear term at 10 rad, for example. As the effectiveness of the radiation per unit dose (rad) varies with dose (and dose rate) in the contribution of the quadratic term, the effectiveness of single dose, high dose rate, low-LET radiation would be nearly five times larger at 400 rad than at 10 rad, if $a/b = 100$ rad. If a/b were less than 100 rad for some effects, the contribution of the quadratic term would be larger at a given dose and there would be a more marked departure from linearity. If a/b were equal to 50 rad, for example, the effectiveness of the radiation just specified would be nearly eight times higher at 400 rad than at 10 rad, unless at the high dose level the effectiveness were in a declining phase for an effect counteracted by excessive cell killing or other damage.

Under these circumstances, and considering that most of the available data on human radiation cancerogenesis is related to doses from 100 to a few hundred rad and sometimes less, it should not be surprising if the very limited available human data, especially when subjected to the assumptions of the linear hypothesis in curve construction and fitting for extrapolation to zero dose-effect for risk estimation for radiation protection, have failed to reveal evidence of marked dose rate dependence.

The foregoing generalization, concerning the expression $Y = aD + bD^2$ and the dose levels for equivalent or predominating contributions of the linear and dose square terms to effect, is undoubtedly greatly oversimplified as to cancerogenic effects, in view of the complexity of cancerogenic mechanisms and effects, for which dose-effect relationships are poorly defined, and the variability among cancerogenic effects in various tissues. It may be more valid for overall cancerogenic effect than for every individual cancer type.

In summary, the available scientific evidence for the influence of dose size, dose rate, and LET on the effectiveness of ionizing radiation strongly supports the repeatedly stated conclusion (ICRP, 1969; NCRP, 1971; NAS-BEIR, 1972; UNSCEAR, 1972; NCRP, 1975; ICRP, 1977) that the use of the linear hypothesis to estimate the potential risks of low-LET irradiation at the low levels of dose and dose rate of general concern in radiation protection by extrapolation from available observations at higher doses and higher dose rates, without correcting for the influence of dose size, dose rate, and LET, is likely to overestimate the risks at the low levels of dose and dose rate. Risk estimates obtained in this way for purposes of radiation protection have been justified as prudent—because the error is on the conservative side—on pragmatic grounds because of the difficulty of doing otherwise with the human data, and on the basis that such estimates may provide some indication of the upper limits of hypothetical risks. However, such estimates do not provide precise indication of the actual risks of low-level, low-LET irradiation. The extent to which they may be overestimates could lead to unnecessarily restrictive and costly control regulations and to societal decisions between alternative means to common ends that might result in greater societal hazards and economic burdens than those avoided, as has been emphasized in other reports (e.g., NAS-BEIR, 1972; NCRP, 1975; ICRP, 1977). Although the information needed for more precise and detailed assessment of risks at low levels of irradiation is gradually accumulating, it will be necessary for radiation protection purposes, for a considerable time to come, to estimate such risks by extrapolation on the basis of tentative assumptions.

VII. CANCEROGENIC RISK ESTIMATION

A. Available Data

It is necessary to estimate not only the total risk of all malignancies due to whole-body irradiation at various dose levels, but also the risks to individual organs, which vary in their susceptibility to radiation cancerogenesis. Often, single organs or groups of organs are selectively irradiated, for example, in medical exposure or in the inhalation or ingestion of radionuclides which deposit selectively in certain tissues or organs.

Several epidemiologic studies of human populations for radiation cancerogenesis have now been made and continued for relatively long periods of time. The most important of these studies is that of the atomic bomb (A-bomb) survivors at Hiroshima and Nagasaki. This irradiated population involves brief, substantially uniform whole-body irradiation of large numbers of people of all ages who have now been closely studied for about 30 years. The irradiation at Hiroshima included a substantial contribution from neutrons as well as gamma radiation. Approximate estimates of the cancerogenic risk of whole-body irradiation and irradiation of various organs have been derived from this study.

Some evidence on the radiation cancerogenic risk for the thyroid gland has also been derived from a study of populations of two Pacific islands after exposure in 1954 to radiation from external sources and radioiodine concentration in the gland from fallout from a nuclear weapon.

Extensive information on radiation induction of lung cancer has also been obtained in a number of studies of uranium miners who inhaled radon and daughter products (alpha emitters) in the course of their work.

Cancerogenic risk estimates have been obtained also from several studies of patients who have received frequent diagnostic radiologic examinations or radiotherapy for various diseases. Female patients with pulmonary tuberculosis who have received substantial radiation exposures to the chest from diagnostic X-ray examinations have been found to develop mammary cancer in excess of normal expectation. Excess incidence of cancers in various locally irradiated organs has been observed in studies of patients irradiated with X rays to the spine for ankylosing spondylitis, to the pelvis for diseases of the uterus, to the breast for diseases of the mammary glands, or to the head and neck region for ringworm of the scalp, pharyngeal infections, or supposed enlargement of the thymus gland. Excess incidence of various cancers has also been observed in irradiated tissues in studies of patients who received radium preparations for the treatment of spinal or other conditions, or thorium compounds as diagnostic radiological contrast media. It has also been observed that the mothers of children who have died of childhood malignancies had had diagnostic X-ray exposure of the fetus in greater incidence than mothers of children who had not died of childhood malignancies.

These studies have yielded approximate estimates of the cancerogenic risks of radiation for several tissues, and have excluded any high risk for others. Reasonably consistent risk estimates have been obtained from several different studies for thyroid, female mammary glands, lung, bone, and bone marrow (as regards induction of acute and chronic myleogenous leukemia). The risk estimates for brain, salivary glands, stomach and other parts of the gastrointestinal tract, urinary bladder, lymphoid tissues, and liver are still less reliable, apparently lower. The radiation cancerogenic risks for muscle, adipose tissue, the prostate gland, or many other tissues not mentioned here are apparently very low, since no unequivocal evidence of risk has been found for these tissues. None of the epidemiologic studies has detected any induction of chronic lymphatic leukemia.

In general, it appears that the radiation cancerogenic risks are relatively high for the female mammary glands and for the thyroid, although the mortality rate from the thyroid cancers is low. The risks for lung and for leukemia are somewhat lower, and those for other organs for which risk estimates have been obtained appear to be still lower (UNSCEAR, 1977).

The cancerogenic risk of whole-body irradiation cannot be derived reliably by adding the risks of all body organs, especially when some are not known with any precision. Several sources of information (UNSCEAR, 1977), however, indicate that the total risk for all fatal malignancies as an average for both sexes and all ages is likely to be in the region of five times that for leukemia alone.

B. Linear Extrapolation

Under radiation exposure conditions at the low doses and low dose rates usually encountered in radiation protection situations, no significant and unequivocal evidence of radiation induction of cancer has been observed in humans or experimental animals. On the other hand, the possibility that occasional cancers could be caused in some incidence, however small, by such low levels of radiation dose cannot be dismissed on theoretical grounds.

Radiation protection policy during the past 20 years or so has been based partly on the possibility of no threshold doses for cancerogenic effects. Because of the lack of data on such effects at the low-radiation levels of interest, and in view of the practical improbability of ever obtaining reliable human data at such levels, the estimation of radiation risks at radiation levels within or approaching the radiation protection guide limits for the general population can be made only by extrapolation or interpolation from observations of effects at much higher doses and dose rates. Such extrapolation or interpolation necessarily involves assumptions concerning the nature of the effect, the dose-effect relationships below observational levels, the mechanisms of induction of the effect, the relative susceptibility of populations at risk and control populations, the influence of biological and environmental variables, and the influence of physical variables such as spatial and temporal distributions of dose, radiation quality (LET), and changing relative biological effectiveness of high-LET radiation with changes in dose size and dose rate.

The linear (proportional) nonthreshold dose-effect relationship, with its independence of dose size and dose rate, and with relative neglect of other biological and physical variables, has often been chosen for extrapolation or interpolation on dose, even for low-LET radiations, arbitrarily and pragmatically, as a prudent conservative approach to risk estimation for cancerogenic effects. This hypothesis allows the use of mean doses, integrated partial organ doses, and the neglect of dose rate.

In general, the experimentally observed shapes of the dose-effect relationships for low LET radiations, and their dependence on dose size and dose rate, support the conclusions that simple linear extrapolation or interpolation on dose from effects observed at intermediate to high doses and dose rates—that is, on the rising portions of the observed curves, without accounting for the influence of dose size, dose rate, and other influencing variables—tends to systematically overestimate the overall risks at low doses and low dose rates.

C. Some Available Numerical Risk Estimates

The NAS-BEIR committee (1972), in estimating risks for radiation induction of cancers at the low doses and dose rates to which populations are exposed, chose to base the estimates exclusively on available human data, and therefore data at relatively high doses and/or dose rates, but acknowledging the data, principles, and theories derived from experiments on animals that would tend to oppose this approach scientifically.

This committee assumed a linear (proportional) nonthreshold dose-incidence relationship for extrapolating from the observed data at high doses and/or dose rates, fitting the curves to the observed data and interpolating them to pass through the intercept at the zero dose-zero effect point, using data on A-bomb survivors in Japan, certain groups of patients irradiated for medical reasons, and certain groups occupationally exposed.

These risk estimates involved extrapolations by factors greater than 1000 in dose size and from 100 million to a billion in dose rate. The body of the BEIR report indicates the factors that might invalidate this linear extrapolation, but justified the approach on pragmatic grounds. The committee cited the cogent radiobiological reasons, both theoretical and factual, for doubting that the dose-incidence relationship remains constant despite changes in dose and dose rate and population at risk. The committee recognized that at least for low-LET radiation the cancerogenic effectiveness probably decreases with decreasing dose and dose rate, that there may be a linear component at low dose and/or dose rate, and that the slope of that linear component would probably be lower than the overall linear slope employed for extrapolation from high dose, high dose rate data.

The BEIR committee also recognized in their report that their treatment of the neutron component in the data from the Hiroshima A-bomb studies, which are a major basis for the committee's risk estimates, might seriously underestimate the neutron RBE and overestimate the gamma radiation cancer induction risk at low doses and dose rates, but stated that firm data enabling other approaches were lacking. The committee concluded that it was impractical at the time to use other than the linear hypothesis for estimating risks in support of public policy on radiation protection.

The BEIR committee recognized that estimates of risks at low doses and dose rates based on linear extrapolation from observed effects at high doses and dose rates in the range of rapidly rising incidence—that is, before the curve reaches the very high doses at which there is a decline in cancerogenic effectiveness attributable to excessive cell killing—may well be overestimates of risks for low-LET radiation, and stated that, therefore, these estimates should be considered only as upper limits of risk for low-LET radiation at low levels of exposure, and that the lower limit could be considerably smaller (0 not excluded by the data).

The BEIR committee's overall risk estimates for various specific malignancies, in terms of cancer deaths (or cases for thyroid cancer) per 10^6 persons exposed, per year, per rem, were approximately as follows:

Leukemia, 1-2
Thyroid cancer cases after irradiation of children, 2.5-9.3 (with lesser risk in irradiated adults)
Lung cancer, 1
Breast cancer in women, 3
Skeletal cancer, 0.2

Cancer of the gastrointestinal tract, 1
Cancers at other sites combined, possibly 1

These rates are annual averages over the period of time after irradiation during which an excess of the incidence of the neoplasms has been evident.

The BEIR committee estimated that the overall excess mortality from cancer (including leukemia) in irradiated populations can be largely accounted for by specific types of neoplasms for which risk estimates were given. In the Japanese A-Bomb survivors, this excess mortality was estimated to approximate 2.5 deaths per 10^6 exposed persons per year per rem, averaged over the period in which the excess has been observed.

Some studies of diagnostic in utero radiation effects have suggested that prenatal irradiation might increase the overall juvenile cancer mortality at the rate of 50 cases per 10^6 per year per rem, averaged over the first 10 years of life. The BEIR committee pointed out, however, that a possibility still exists that the excess incidence observed in these studies may be dependent on factors other than radiation.

The BEIR committee has pointed out that to estimate the actual total risk of cancer attributable to a particular increase in the level of exposure of the general population to radiation, would require systematic information of the effects of lifelong, low-dose irradiation that is not available. However, the committee made an approximate calculation at the level of mortality on the basis of the data from the 25-year follow-up studies on A-bomb survivors and on patients treated with intensive spinal irradiation for ankylosing spondylitis. The rates of radiation-induced excess mortality from all forms of malignancy were extrapolated linearly to low dose and dose rate levels. On this basis, exposure of the U.S. population of about 200 million persons to, for example, 100 mrem (equal to annual average background radiation dose equivalent) during 1 year could be expected to cause 1350-3300 deaths from cancer during the 25 years after irradiation, or about 50-130 deaths per year in the United States. On the basis of proportionality (linear hypothesis), the total cancer death risk for the 25 years after whole-body irradiation can thus be calculated as approximately 63-163 per million exposed persons per rem. Continued exposure of the population to an additional 100 mrem/year could be expected ultimately to cause 1350-3300 deaths annually, provided the effect of a given increment of dose did not persist beyond 25 years after exposure. The rate per million persons on this basis would be about 7-17 at 100 mrem/year.

An estimation of the complete cumulative experience of an entire population requires more specific attention to age at exposure, duration of latency, size and duration of effect, age and sex distribution in the population, age-specific mortality from the various malignancies, and other factors influencing the effect. Because of these influential factors, the BEIR committee considered it advisable to illustrate the great uncertainty that necessarily characterizes its estimates of the effect of a particular level of low-dose and low-dose-rate radiation exposure on the entire population. Choosing a range of values for each parameter entering into such estimates, the committee estimated that the annual number of cancer deaths associated with an increase in radiation exposure of the whole U.S. population by 100 mrem/year ranges from about 2000-9000. Much weight was given to these estimates by the high risk estimates for juvenile cancer mortality from prenatal irradiation, based on the suggested risks from epidemiological studies of prenatal diagnostic irradiation, which are still questionable as to the degree of contribution of radiation to the effect, and which have not been confirmed in studies of the Japanese A-bomb populations. The committee considered that the most likely estimate from this approach is about 3000-4000 cancer deaths or roughly about 1% of the annual cancer death rate in the U.S. population.

On the basis of the NAS-BEIR (1972) risk estimates it can be calculated that 100 mrem/year to the population could cause up to about 7 to 45 cancer deaths per million exposed persons per year, depending on the risk model used, with the lower limit possibly much lower for low-LET radiations, zero risk not excluded by the data.

The recent report of the United Nations Scientific Committee on the Effects of Atomic Radiation (UNSCEAR, 1977) gives some more recent linearly derived total risk estimates for radiation induction of various cancers in human beings, without extrapolation to low radiation levels. This report indicates that the risk estimates obtainable for individual organs or tissues cannot be determined with great accuracy, but that for several tissues, such as bone marrow and the thyroid gland, approximate estimates are obtainable from several different sources and are mutually consistent with the accuracy of their determination. The report states that it is thus becoming possible to classify different body tissues into groups with different degrees of sensitivity to induction of malignancies by radiation. The report emphasizes, however, that such classifications, and the values for the induction rates themselves, are derived from the results of exposure at high dose levels, ordinarily in excess of 100 rad of low-LET radiation, and that the corresponding rates per unit absorbed dose at doses of a few rad, while unlikely to be higher, may be substantially lower.

The thyroid and the female breast appear to have relatively high risks of cancer induction by radiation at levels usually in excess of 100 rad, at least for certain ages at exposure. Average total risk rates for all ages appear to be in the region of 100×10^{-6} induced cancers per rad absorbed dose of low-LET radiation. The low mortality rate for radiation-induced thyroid cancer and the moderately low mortality rate for breast cancers probably bring the corresponding average risk for fatal cancer induction for these two tissues to about 10×10^{-6} and 50×10^{-6} per rad, respectively (UNSCEAR, 1977).

The radiation cancerogenic risk for lung was stated to be high for males over 35 years of age, on the basis of a value derived from data on uranium miners, and probably also for females at these ages. Rates at other ages were said to be difficult to establish, but seemed clearly to be lower, and the mean rate for all ages in the region of 25 to 50×10^{-6} per rad of low-LET radiation was deemed probable (UNSCEAR, 1977).

The risk of radiation induction of leukemia (acute and chronic granulocytic types) was said to range probably from about 50×10^{-6} per rad at moderately high doses to about 20×10^{-6} per rad at the lower dose levels in observed data. For radiation-induced leukemia, the mean interval between exposure and death is the region of 10 years, much shorter than the mean interval for other malignancies, which typically appears to be 25 years or more. Therefore, the total induced mortality from leukemia could be estimated with greater confidence in most surveys than could be done for other malignancies (UNSCEAR, 1977).

The risk rates for stomach, liver, and large intestine were reported to be less reliably determined, but appeared to be substantially lower, probably in the region of 10 - 15×10^{-6} per rad for fatal cancers. For the brain, quantitative information is scanty, but the rate for all tumors that may prove fatal in this situation was regarded as possibly similar. The salivary glands were said to appear to have an induction rate of about this range also, but the risk rate for fatal cancers is likely to be lower (UNSCEAR, 1977).

For bone, esophagus, small intestine, urinary bladder, pancreas, rectum, and the lymphatic tissues, risks of radiation induction of cancer were said to be identifiable, but appear to be still lower, with values probably in the region of 2 to 5×10^{-6} per rad. The risk for the mucosa of cranial sinuses appeared to be similar. No good estimate is available for skin cancer induction, but the induction of fatal cancers of skin appears also to be low (UNSCEAR, 1977).

The UNSCEAR report (1977) gives evidence that suggests tentatively that the total of all fatal malignancies that may ultimately result from a given uniform whole-body exposure may be in the region of 4 to 6 times that for leukemia alone. The report indicates that the total rate of all fatal solid cancers for the various tissues or organs for which some estimate has been made amounts to about 200×10^{-6} per rad for moderately high doses, for example, a hundred to a few hundred rad of low-LET radiation. If leukemia is induced with a rate of 50×10^{-6} per rad at these dose levels, the final ratio of all fatal malignancies to leukemias could thus be in the region of 6 (UNSCEAR, 1977).

The UNSCEAR report goes on to say that it is to be expected that low-LET radiation is likely to be less cancerogenic per unit absorbed dose at doses of a few rads than at levels of 100 rad or a few hundred rads. For dose levels at which a leukemia induction rate of 15 to 25×10^{-6} per rad may apply, a ratio of 4 to 6 between the frequency of other induced fatal malignancies and the frequency of leukemia would imply a total for all fatal induced malignancies of about 100×10^{-6} per rad at such dose levels. The report reemphasizes that such a value is derived essentially from mortalities induced at doses in excess of 100 rad, and that the value appropriate to the much lower dose levels involved in occupational exposure and even more so in environmental exposures to radiation, may well be substantially less; and this reservation applies also to values quoted for individual organs or tissues.

The UNSCEAR Report (1977) indicated that some epidemiologic studies have suggested that malignancies may be induced in the fetus by exposure in utero at average absorbed doses in the range 0.2 to 20 rad from diagnostic X rays, and that the induction rate of fatal malignancies per unit of absorbed dose is difficult to determine with any confidence. On the assumption that the radiation is the sole or major cause, the total risk was estimated as being in the region of 200 to 250×10^{-6} per rad.

VIII. NATURAL RADIATION SOURCES, NORMAL AND ENHANCED EXPOSURES

A. Normal Exposure

Radiation exposure due to natural sources, both terrestrial and cosmic irradiation, varies somewhat with altitude and terrestrial radionuclide distribution, and is the largest contributor to the collective dose of the world population. Humans have always been exposed to ionizing radiation from various natural sources everywhere in the world, at a relatively constant rate for many centuries, although even the normal natural exposure varies considerably with geographic location or even within a small location, such as a building.

Natural radiation sources include external sources, such as cosmic rays and radioactive substances in the ground and building materials, and internal sources in the form of naturally occurring radioactive substances in the human body, particularly potassium-40 and radon-222 and its daughters, but also other nuclides, including tritium, radon-222, beryllium-7, carbon-14, sodium-22, rubidium-87, and radionuclides of the uranium and thorium series (uranium, thorium, radium, and long-lived decay products of radon-222).

The average contribution of natural sources to the radiation exposure of human populations living in areas of normal radiation background, in terms of the annual per capita dose, has been assessed by the UNSCEAR (1977) for four tissues: the gonads, the whole lung, the cells lining the bone surfaces, and the red bone marrow, with the contribution from all types of radiation included. In those tissues the annual dose from normal exposure to natural sources has been estimated to be of the order of 100 mrad. Because of the inhalation of radon-222 and its daughter products, the dose in the lung is 20-45% higher than the dose in the other tissues, and about 31% of this lung dose is owing to alpha radiation, whereas beta and gamma radiations cause more than 90% of the dose in the other tissues. An annual dose of the order of 200 mrad is received by the epithelial cells of the tracheobronchial tree, mainly from alpha particles. The variability among individuals in dose from potassium-40 in the body is small. However, there is large variation in lung dose among individuals due to varying concentrations of radon and its daughter products in air. The normal variation of the lung dose contribution from radon-222 and its short-lived decay products ranges from 4 to 400 mrad/year. In indoor air the average concentration of radon at a given emanation rate from the building, basement, or tap water depends on the ventilation rate.

Populations at high altitudes or in regions of high natural terrestrial radiation receive much higher doses from external sources, and some populations receive higher internal emitter doses from ingestion of food with relatively high concentrations of internal emitters or from living in houses with low ventilation rates as in colder climates.

According to the UNSCEAR (1977), the annual collective dose from natural radiation sources to the world population (global collective dose) is of the order of 3×10^8 man rad for most of the body tissues, but about 30 percent higher for the whole lung.

B. Enhanced Exposures

1. Introduction

It is very probable that the examples presented in this section do not represent the complete picture of enhanced natural irradiation. According to the UNSCEAR (1977), technologically enhanced natural irradiation does not add significantly to the collective dose on the global scale but may give rise in localized areas or for people exposed under extreme conditions to appreciable increases in individual doses from natural irradiation. The present state of knowledge does not allow an accurate estimate of the collective dose from technologically enhanced natural irradiation.

Exposure to natural radiation may be enhanced by human activities such as high-altitude flights, construction of buildings using natural materials of high radionuclide content, reduction of ventilation rate in homes, and boring deep wells into radon-rich water, among other activities to be discussed now. Enhanced exposures to natural radiation are also variable, ranging from slight increases to those of orders of magnitude.

2. Passengers in Aircraft

According to the UNSCEAR (1977), there is an annual air travel total of about 10^9 passenger hours. Under average solar conditions, the dose rate for subsonic flights is about 0.3 mrad/hr, and the annual collective dose contributed by air travel is about 3×10^5 man rad. The risk of high dose rates from cosmic radiation at high altitude due to large solar flares has made it necessary to equip supersonic aircraft with radiation monitors in order to warn the pilot when a solar flare is developing. Although the radiation of solar flare origin does not contribute significantly to the average dose rate, the dose rate at high altitudes during the occasional intense solar flare may increase by several orders of magnitude. However, such occasions are infrequent and do not add significantly to the collective dose to the world population.

The prospect of large-scale development of supersonic aircraft transport systems necessitates consideration of dose rates and persons exposed at high altitudes to the ever-present galactic cosmic rays, which vary in intensity by a factor of about 2 during the sun's 11-year solar cycle, and the occasional large, short-term increases in the radiation due to solar protons from solar flares. The doses to human tissues in a given flight will depend markedly on the duration of the flight and on the altitude and geomagnetic latitude of the flight.

According to the UNSCEAR (1977), during the time of minimum solar activity, when cosmic ray flux densities are at maximum, the absorbed dose rates are, at 12 km altitude, 300 μrad/hr from the ionizing component and 20 μrad/hr from neutrons, and, at 20 km altitude, 600 μrad/hr from the ionizing component, and 30 μrad/hr from the neutron component.

3. Coal-Fired Power Plants

The burning of coal enhances radiation exposure to naturally occurring radionuclides, particularly radium, thorium, uranium, and lead. According to the UNSCEAR (1977), tentative estimates indicate that lead-210, thorium-228, and thorium-232 appear to be the most important contributors to the collective dose commitment due to atmospheric release. Most of the dose is due to alpha radiation. The concentrations of the significant radionuclides have been measured both in coal of various origins and in slag and fly ash. The collective dose commitment per megawatt year production of electric energy (MW(e)y) due to the deposition of fly ash has been found to be small, between 0.002 and 0.02 man rad per MW(e)y in the various body tissues from discharged material deposited on the ground, and also between 0.002 and 0.02 man rad per MW(e)y from the material inhaled.

Klein and co-workers (1975) have estimated that the annual world coal consumption is approaching 3×10^9 tons; the burning of about 3×10^3 tons of coal is required to produce 1 megawatt-year of electrical energy.

4. Building Materials

Some building materials, such as blocks, plasterboard, cement, rock, and so on, considerably enhance radiation exposure levels indoors, because of radium-226 and other nuclides. These building materials are either of natural origin, such as pumice stone, granite, or concrete from alum shale, or by-products of industrial processes, such as slag or phosphogypsum. According to the UNSCEAR (1977), if all the phosphogypsum derived from 1 ton of marketable phosphate ore were used in the building industry, the resulting collective dose commitment might be a few man rad per ton of rock. The dose rates in air from gamma radiation in buildings constructed from such materials may be substantially higher than the average normal dose rate from terrestrial radiation. The radon levels would also be considerably enhanced for a given ventilation rate. Changes in the ventilation in a poorly ventilated room influence the radon level considerably. The ventilation rate in houses varies in different countries depending on climate, heating systems, and building standards.

Other by-products that have been shown to contain relatively high concentrations of naturally occurring radionuclides and which may be used in building are red slime, a waste product of aluminum mills, and blast furnace slag, a by-product of iron manufacture (Kolb and Schmier, 1975).

The UNSCEAR (1977) pointed out that the average dose rates in air measured in buildings using building materials with higher than average radioactivity are much lower than that which would be expected from the radioactive content of the materials considered, because materials that are usually less active are also used in the same buildings.

Waste products of the uranium and radium industries have also been used as building materials; for example, in Grand Junction, Col. tailings from uranium mills were used during 1952-1966 as fill material under houses and as building materials (U.S. Congress, 1971).

5. Phosphate Fertilizers

According to the UNSCEAR (1977), mineral phosphate deposits usually contain relatively high concentrations of radioactive nuclides of the uranium-238 decay series. Very large quantities of phosphate rock are mined; some of the material is converted to fertilizers and some is disposed of as waste. Both the fertilizer and waste may lead to exposure of the public, as well as the by-product, chemical gypsum, which may be used as a building material. The assessment of the collective dose commitment per ton of marketable phosphate rock shows that the contribution from phosphate fertilizers is small, of the order of 3×10^{-4} man rad/ton of fertilizer. For a worldwide annual use of 10^8 tons of phosphate fertilizers, the collective dose commitment from a year's use of these fertilizers is of the order of 3×10^4 man rad.

6. Natural Gas

Natural gas used for kitchen ranges and space heaters is a source of radon in buildings. The radon produced in the ground diffuses from the geological formations into the natural gas wells. This source of radon, however, is found to be insignificant in comparison with the other sources of radon (UNSCEAR, 1977).

There are very few data on radon levels caused by natural gas consumption in homes. Making various assumptions concerning many factors the resultant annual doses to the basal cells of the bronchial epithelium has been estimated to be 0.6-1.5 mrad (UNSCEAR, 1977). If the radon daughters are in equilibrium with the radon in the gas the equilibrium factor of the radon daughters in the air would be higher, so that the corresponding doses will be about twice as great.

The doses caused by the gas consumed in space heaters has not been calculated specifically because a typical individual could not be defined, but by indirect methods the average individual annual dose to the bronchial epithelium was estimated to be 5.4 mrad (Jonassen and Hayes, 1974).

The occupational exposure to radon-222 and its decay products in the natural gas industry have been examined by external radiation surveys in nine gas processing plants of the United States (Gesell, 1975). Exposure rates obtained at the equipment surfaces ranged from background level up to 8 milliroentgens/hr at the surface of the various product pumps. As the equipment is in low-occupancy areas the tissue dose rates would be less than 2 mrad/hr. The long-lived decay products of radon-222, which are likely to be concentrated on the inner surfaces of the pumps, do not contribute to the external absorbed dose while the pumps remain closed, but if the pumps are open for repair or maintenance, an opportunity exists for inhalation of lead-210 and polonium-210.

IX. RADIATION-EMITTING CONSUMER PRODUCTS

A wide variety of consumer products contain radioactive nuclides that have been deliberately incorporated for specific purposes. These may be classified in six categories as follows: (1) radioluminous products; (2) electronic and electrical devices; (3) antistatic devices; (4) gas and aerosol (smoke) detectors; (5) ceramic, glassware, alloys, and so on, containing uranium or thorium; and (6) other devices including scientific instruments. In addition, some electronic products, such as television sets, may emit X rays. The most widespread radiation-emitting consumer products are radioluminescent timepieces, compasses, luminous signs, smoke detectors, antistatic devices, and television sets. National regulations on exposures to radiation from consumer products varies. The most commonly used radionuclides in consumer products are tritium, krypton-85, and promethium-147, the use of which involves trivial amounts of penetrating radiation (UNSCEAR, 1977).

Many millions of units of various types of consumer products containing deliberately incorporated radionuclides are used daily throughout the world. Estimates of doses in individuals resulting from the use of such products show that in all cases these doses are small. The highest calculated whole-body doses result from the wearing of radioluminous watches, the radioactive consumer product in most widespread use.

Until the 1960s radium-226 was the most common nuclide in radioluminescent paint and therefore also in watches, alarm clocks, and other radioluminescent instruments. The average radium-activated wristwatch gives the wearer a gonad dose of a few mrad per year. This external radiation source is eliminated by the present use of tritium for the same purpose, but some tritium may escape from watches and cause internal irradiation producing a whole-body dose of about 0.5 mrad/year. The present use of radioluminescent paint in the watch industry may cause a collective dose to the world population of the order of 10^6 man rad in 1 year. It also causes some occupational exposure. Luminizers have been among the groups of workers receiving higher than average radiation doses. The collective dose from the occupational exposures are small in comparison with those from the exposure of the public, but high individual doses may still occur (UNSCEAR, 1977).

Household color television receivers have been the most common consumer product that could expose the public to X rays. However, since the extensive adoption of solid-state circuitry the X ray emission from the recently built color television receivers is probably negligible under normal conditions of operation and servicing.

The assessment of the global collective dose from consumer products containing deliberately incorporated radionuclides is made difficult by insufficient knowledge of radioactivities involved, the number of products in use, and disposal of the products. It is likely that the average annual per capita gonad dose due to the use of consumer products is less than 1 mrad, almost entirely due to radioluminous timepieces (UNSCEAR, 1977).

The NCRP (1977) issued a report on radiation exposure from consumer products. The values given here have been derived from that report and summarized by Casarett (1978).

Some consumer products emit low-LET radiations beyond their confines, and these penetrating radiations can result virtually in whole-body radiation, while in the case of other products the radiation to tissue consists mainly of the high-LET alpha particles which penetrate tissue only shallowly and close to the products.

There are some radiation-emitting consumer products that are in such widespread use in the United States that large numbers of people are irradiated by them. Some of these products may irradiate on the order of 10^6 - 10^8 people to average annual whole-body or gonadal dose equivalents varying for different products over a range of the order of 1-10 mrem, such as some television receivers, timepieces with radium-containing dials, gas and aerosol detectors, and building and road construction materials. On the order of 10^4 people may be irradiated by vacuum high-voltage switches to 30 mrem or from electron microscopes to 300 mrem average annual whole-body or gonadal dose equivalent.

Smaller annual whole-body or gonadal dose equivalents, of the order of less than 1 μrem to 1 mrem, may be received by many people (10^4 to 10^8) from cold cathode gas discharge tubes, X-ray airport inspection systems, timepieces with dials containing tritium or promethium-147, radioisotopic check sources, static eliminators, and radioactive materials in transport in commercial passenger aircraft.

Small or unknown numbers of people receive annual whole-body or gonadal radiation dose equivalents of the order of tens to hundreds of mrem from products such as personnel scanning systems and shoe-fitting fluroscopes, or dose equivalents from a small fraction of a mrem to a few mrem from products such as radium-containing dials of old aircraft instruments and spark gap irradiators.

Certain other consumer products may locally irradiate certain tissues of many people (10^7 to 10^8) to relatively high annual dose equivalents, of the order of a few millirem to tens of rem. Such sources include: natural radioisotopes (polonium-210 and lead-210) in tobacco smoke and radioisotopes in fossil fuels, irradiating tissues of the respiratory tract; radioisotopes in dental prosthetics irradiating oral mucous membranes; and radioisotopes in ophthalmic glass lenses irradiating the cornea and contiguous structures. There are also raw materials that are contaminated with radioisotopes, for example, precious metals used to make jewelry, which may result in highly localized irradiation to relatively small numbers of people to dose equivalents up to thousands of rem over long periods of time.

It is conceivable that large numbers of people in the general public could accumulate, from combinations of many of the commonly used consumer product sources of radiation exposure, average annual whole-body or gonadal dose equivalents in the tens of millirem and additional considerable doses to respiratory tract tissues, oral mucosa, and cornea.

X. EXPOSURES FROM NUCLEAR (FISSION) POWER GENERATION (UNSCEAR, 1977)

The total installed nuclear electric generating capacity in the world in 1976 was 79.8 GW(e) from 188 reactors operating in 19 countries. The predicted capacity for the year 2000 is about 2000 GW(e).

The nuclear fuel cycle consists of the processes of mining and milling of uranium, conversion to fuel material, usually including enrichment in the isotope uranium-235, fabrication of fuel elements, utilization of the fuel in nuclear reactors, reprocessing of spent fuel and recycling for use of recovered fissile materials, transportation of materials between fuel cycle installations, and disposal of radioactive waste.

Almost all of the radioactive material in the fuel cycle is present in reactors, stored spent fuel, or in well-contained fractions separated from the fuel during the reprocessing operations. However, releases of small quantities of radioactive material into the environment may occur at various stages of the fuel cycle. Most of the radionuclides released into the environment are of concern only locally or regionally because their half-lives are short relative to the time needed for their dispersion to greater distances. Some radionuclides can become globally distributed because of their longer half-lives or more rapid dispersion.

In addition to the small releases of radioactive material during a normal operation, the possibility exists that additional amounts of radioactive materials may be accidentally discharged.

The total collective dose commitment to the world population has been assessed by estimating the contribution from four components: the occupationally exposed group, the local population, the regional or intermediate population, and the world population.

There is a special problem in presenting collective dose to the world population for a few radionuclides with very long half-lives, especially uranium-238 (4.5×10^9 years) and iodine-129 (1.6×10^7 years). Although these radionuclides would not accumulate in sufficient quantities in the biosphere to cause a dose rate of more than 1 mrad/year, even if nuclear power production with current technology were continued for 500 years at a rate of 2000 GW(e) per year (GW(e)y), the exposure over many millions of years would make the collective dose commitments high and unrealistic. The accumulation of a global collective dose of one man rad per MW(e)y from these radionuclides would require that a world population of 10^{10} people would have to be exposed, in the case of uranium-238, for about 10 million years, or in the case of iodine-129, about 10 thousand years. Because of the small annual doses, the exposures from these nuclides were not included in the assessments of global collective dose commitments.

Carbon-14, although presenting a similar problem, has a much shorter half-life (5730 years). The collective dose commitment from release of carbon-14 from light water reactors and related reprocessing plants was estimated to be about 5 man rad per MW(e)y in soft tissues and 14 man rad per MW(e)y in bone lining cells and red bone marrow, with half of the collective dose delivered within 5700 years and as much as one-fourth of the collective dose delivered within 500 years. With nuclear industry operating at a constant rate for 500 years the maximum future annual collective dose would be about 1 man rad per MW(e)y in soft tissues and 3 man rad per MW(e)y in bone-lining cells and red bone marrow.

The following are the contributions to the exposure of the personnel and the public from the various steps of nuclear energy production, in terms of collective dose commitment (man rad) per MW(e)y (UNSCEAR, 1977).

Mining, milling, and fuel fabrication (occupational exposure)	0.2-0.3
Reactor operation (occupational exposure)	1.0
Reactor operation (local and regional population exposure	0.2-0.4
Reprocessing (occupational exposure)	1.2
Reprocessing (local and regional population exposure)	0.1-0.6
Reprocessing (global population exposure)	1.1-3.3
Research and development (occupational exposure)	1.4
Whole industry	5.2-8.2

The occupational contributions dominate. However, the contribution of 1.2 man rad per MW(e)y from reprocessing would not be representative of a closed fuel cycle for the whole nuclear industry, nor would research and development be expected to contribute highly in the developed industry. Therefore, the total collective dose commitment in the future with existing technology would not be expected to exceed 3 to 6 man rad per MW(e)y.

The available data (UNSCEAR, 1977) indicate that more than 50% of the collective dose commitment to the world population from nuclear power production is due to the global dispersion of the long-lived radionuclides carbon-14, krypton-85, and tritium.

The collective dose commitments to various organs for the production of 1 MW(e)y range from about 2 to 4 man rad. For the current installed capacity of about 80 GW(e), and assuming a utilization factor of 70%, the whole-body collective dose commitment per year of electric energy production was estimated to be about 1.3×10^5 man rad, corresponding to about 3.5 hr of natural radiation exposure.

In addition to the local collective dose commitments from effluents from mining and milling and from uranium fuel fabrication, there are local and regional collective dose commitments from the effluents of reactor operation, including fission noble gases, activation gases, tritium, carbon-14, iodine, particulates in airborne effluents, and radionuclides in liquid effluents. There are also local and regional collective dose commitments from effluents in fuel reprocessing, including krypton-85, tritium, carbon-14 and radioactive cesium, ruthenium, strontium, iodine, plutonium, americium, and curium. Miscellaneous contributions to dose commitment are made from transportation of radionuclides and from radionuclides used in nuclear laboratories.

Although accidents in any stage of the fuel cycle may release radioactive material or cause personnel exposure, reactor accidents have been of most concern because the potential consequences for the general public of some reactor accidents are much greater than those from accidents at other stages in the fuel cycle. Reactor accidents are low-probability, high-risk events.

In the several hundred reactor-years of operation to 1978, there has not been an accident in a commercial power reactor that has lead to any exposure of the public. In the whole nuclear industry, including research and development, accidents involving radioactivity have been very infrequent; most of those that have occurred have been at experimental or pilot plants, and of these only a few have involved exposure of members of the public. In view of this record, accident analysis in the nuclear industry is based on considerations of probability and reliability.

The most comprehensive nuclear reactor accident analysis so far (USAEC, 1975) was based on the detailed study of events or faults that might lead to release of radioactivity, and expressed its main conclusions in terms of the probabilities of different accident releases per reactor-year of operation of large light-water reactors. The doses and collective doses that would result from a given release were assessed by the use of a consequence model, also stochastic in nature, which took account of different weather conditions and population distributions. The probability of incurring an accidental collective dose of a given value or within a given range can be obtained from the convolution of the functions representing a release model and the consequence model. For large light-water reactors (1000 MW(e)), this approach gives a value of about 250 man rad/reactor-year, implying a normalized accident collective dose commitment of 0.25 man rad/MW(e)y (UNSCEAR, 1977).

The UNSCEAR (1977) pointed out that the value just given includes individual doses for which proportionality of dose and risk does not apply, such as doses causing acute effects, and that, therefore, it is not possible to assess the relative detriment by comparing this accident collective dose to the collective dose from normal operations.

Predictions of expected lifetime doses for workers who spend 40 years at the same job were made, usually on the basis of linear extrapolation from accumulative doses to workers with 5-15 years of employment. Most of the information from which predictions could be made related to the nuclear power industry, and the situation varied greatly from one country to another. The highest lifetime dose estimates were for fuel reprocessing workers in the United Kingdom and the United States, with a reasonable probability that some workers will receive accumulative lifetime doses exceeding 100 rad, although practically none will be expected to receive more than 200 rad. Workers at power reactors and other jobs associated with the nuclear industry appear more likely to receive maximum lifetime doses of 50 to 100 rad, but only a few specialized workers will be in this category.

It can be seen in the foregoing list that the portions of the nuclear fuel cycle which contribute the majority of collective occupational dose per unit energy generated are reactors, fuel reprocessing, and the associated research and development. Uranium mining, milling, and fuel fabrication together with transportation of both irradiated and nonirradiated fuel, contribute a collective whole-body dose of only 0.2 man rad per MW(e)y, plus additional collective dose of 0.1 man rad per MW(e)y to the lungs of uranium miners.

The production of nuclear power is subject to national regulations usually based on internationally agreed principles. The global dose commitment corresponds to 0.6 days of natural radiation exposure for 1 year of energy production at the present installed capacity of 80 GWe. Assuming that the present nuclear technology remains the same, 1 year of energy production at the projected nuclear installed capacity in the year 2000 (2000 GWe) would lead to a global dose commitment equivalent to about 15 days of natural radiation exposure (UNSCEAR, 1977).

XI. NUCLEAR EXPLOSIONS (UNSCEAR, 1977)

The total global dose commitment from all nuclear explosions occurring before 1976 ranges from about 100 millirad (in the gonads) to about 200 millirad (in bone-lining cells). The values are about 50% higher in the northern temperate zone and about 50% lower in the southern temperate zone. About 70 mrad of the global dose commitment for all tissues are contributed by external exposures from cesium-137 and short-lived gamma-emitting nuclides. The majority of the internal exposure is contributed by the relatively long-lived (about 30 years) nuclides cesium-137 and strontium-90 in the skeleton. The much shorter-lived ruthenium-106 and cerium-144 contribute significantly to the exposure of the lung. Other radionuclides contributing to internal irradiation are tritium, carbon-14, manganese-54, iron-55, krypton-85, strontium-89, iodine-131, barium-140, and plutonium.

The highest dose commitment is due to carbon-14, about 120 mrad for the gonads and lungs and 450 mrad for the bone-lining cells and the red bone marrow. However, because these doses will be delivered over a period of many thousands of years, they are not included in the estimates of the dose commitments given in the previous paragraph.

The total global collective dose commitment in different tissues from nuclear test explosions is 4×10^8 to 8×10^8 man rad if the carbon-14 contribution is not included. This commitment is equivalent to 16 to 24 months of normal exposure to irradiation from natural sources. If the carbon-14 contribution is included the collective dose commitment is doubled.

For a few weeks after a nuclear explosion short-lived iodine-131 is an important contributor to the exposure of the thyroid. The highest doses have been found in infants who consume fresh milk, and annual thyroid doses from a few millirad to about 200 mrad have been estimated. The thyroid dose in adults is about one-tenth that in infants.

The UNSCEAR (1977) presented a summary of dose commitments to various tissues from radionuclides produced in all nuclear tests carried out before 1976. The radiations involved are external radiations from short-lived nuclides and cesium-137, and radiations from the internal emitters H-3, C-14, Mn-54, Fe-55, Sr-90, Sr-89, Ru-106, Cs-137, Ce-144, and Pu-239. The totals in the northern temperate zone for the four tissues under consideration are as follows (in millirad): gonads 150, bone marrow 260, bone-lining cells 290, and lung 260. The values are roughly a third of these in the southern temperate zone and intermediate for the whole world population. In regard to these radionuclides, the radiation exposure to which the world population was committed by nuclear tests up to 1975 is already largely completed for all except cesium-137 (external and internal), H-3, C-14, Sr-90, and Pu-239. Therefore, only these five nuclides need to be considered for current annual doses. Cesium-137 makes major age-independent contributions to dose for all body tissues, but the further substantial contribution to dose from Sr-90 in bone marrow and bone-lining cells is strongly dependent on age. Comparatively, the contributions to annual doses from H-3, C-14, and Pu-239 are very small (UNSCEAR, 1977).

XII. MEDICAL IRRADIATION

Medical applications of radiation contribute the largest human-made per capita doses in the population and cause the highest individual organ doses except for accidental exposures. Medical irradiation is usually given at high dose rates and usually involves irradiation of limited regions of the body. A special feature is that the patients who are irradiated may expect to benefit directly from the radiation procedures.

According to a NAS-BEIR committee report (1972), the average per capita annual dose to members of the U.S. population from medical irradiation (largely diagnostic) is about 70 mrad, with an annual collective dose equivalent of about 15 million person-rems.

The patient's dose in various organs and tissues may vary from insignificant doses up to high doses which cause local tissue damage near treatment areas, depending on the purpose. Therefore, the per capita doses from medical irradiations comprise a large variety of dose levels and dose distributions in the individual cases. However, the largest contributions to the per capita dose come from diagnostic X-ray examinations involving large numbers of individuals. In such cases the per capita annual doses to the tissues of interest are roughly similar in magnitude and in many technologically developed countries are in the range of 50-100 mrad, the genetically significant dose often being about half of the per capita gonad dose. The annual collective dose for medical practices is in the range of 5×10^4 to 10^5 man rad per million persons in countries with developed radiological facilities and about 10^3 man rad per million persons in countries with limited facilities. The occupational exposure of radiation workers in the medical field has been estimated to give an annual collective dose of the order of only 10^2 man rad per million persons. The annual global collective dose for medical procedures has been estimated to be of the order of 5×10^7 man rad for the contribution made by those countries with developed radiological facilities and 2×10^6 man rad for the contribution of those countries with limited facilities. The highest human contribution to the global collective radiation dose is that of the medical uses of radiation, in particular diagnostic X-ray procedures (UNSCEAR, 1977).

In a survey of ionizing radiation doses in the United States (Klement et al., 1972) it was stated that the most tenuous estimate developed in the study was the mean annual dose to nonfederal employees exposed during the use of radiation in diagnostic and therapeutic medical and dental radiology. The data available consisted of information from three states, Maine in 1965, Wisconsin in 1969, and Illinois in 1970. On the basis of these data, Klement and co-workers (1972) assigned an average annual dose of 0.32 rad per nonfederal medical X-ray worker.

In a study of personnel occupationally exposed in radium therapy in Wisconsin (Klement et al., 1972), it was estimated that there may be up to 38,000 individuals occupationally exposed in radium treatment in the United States who are not otherwise reported, that the average occupational dose was 0.5 rad per treatment, and that the average annual per capita dose was 0.54 rad for the 740 medical workers in Wisconsin. This average was assumed to apply nationally. The medical use of radium sources is decreasing.

Brodsky (1976) has estimated the average annual dose to nuclear medicine workers in the United States to be 0.5 to 0.6 rad, leading to a total annual collective dose of 7000 man rad.

According to the UNSCEAR (1977), on the basis of the available data, which is fragmentary and may be biased toward countries where doses are generally relatively low, lifetime doses to medical workers are unlikely to exceed 50 rad based on current practices. Lifetime doses to workers now reaching the end of their working lives may be considerably greater, but much of the dose will have been received using techniques that are no longer acceptable.

The UNSCEAR (1977) pointed out the difficulty in comparing the risk of medical irradiation with the risk from other sources of human-made exposure or from natural background radiation. The diagnostic radiation doses to organs vary greatly, from a few millirads to a few tens of rads, and are usually given at high dose rates compared with other human-made and natural radiation sources. Since the production of various effects of radiation, including cancerogenesis, depends on the dose, the body part irradiated, the dose rate, and the total duration of exposure, detailed risk estimation for medical exposure is highly complex. In its risk estimation the UNSCEAR (1977) has used the concept of collective dose based on simple assumptions concerning dose-effect relationships in order to use the product of the number of persons in a subgroup and the dose received by a particular organ as a measure of the relative radiation detriment. It was pointed out, however, that in radiotherapeutic practice, as compared with diagnostic practice, higher doses are given to smaller groups of patients, and since the dose-effect relationship is likely to be different, the risks from the two practices should not be summed.

In therapeutic radiology with external beams and sealed sources, radiation doses up to 1000 or 2000 rad have been used for treatment of nonneoplastic benign diseases, mostly skin diseases for which low energy, relatively low-penetration radiation has been used. Radiation doses up to 6000 or 7000 rads of highly penetrating radiation are used in the treatment of various kinds of malignant neoplastic diseases. In such cases large radiation doses are also received by some of the normal tissues within the treatment volume or in the path of the radiation beams. However, the life-threatening aspect of the malignancy makes the consideration of effects of irradiation in normal tissues long after successful treatment of secondary importance. Similar considerations apply to the therapeutic uses of radiopharmaceuticals, which include treatment with iodine-131 for hyperthyroidism, heart disease, and thyroid cancer, and the use of P-32 for the treatment of polycythemia vera.

There is little information on the radiation doses received by the public from releases from waste disposal (mainly liquid waste) of medically used radiopharmaceuticals. Those at greatest risk are the families of the patients, who would also receive external radiation exposure directly from the activity remaining in the patients. Therapeutically applied radiopharmaceuticals result in considerable waste activity in urine, particularly from the use of iodine-131. In the diagnostic use of radiopharmaceuticals, much of the short-lived radionuclides decays rapidly so that little remains to be disposed of as waste.

According to the UNSCEAR (1977), diagnostic radiology in many technically developed countries has been expanding at a rate between 5 and 15% annually, and the growth rate in developing countries is likely to be greater. The diagnostic use of radiopharmaceuticals has been expanding rapidly in the last decade, many countries reporting a doubling of the number of tests every 3 to 5 years. Less radiotherapy is being used for nonmalignant diseases, and radiotherapy for malignant diseases now usually involves high energy radiation from accelerators or teletherapy units. In general, the doses to various organs from diagnostic use of radiopharmaceuticals are of the same order or smaller than those from diagnostic X-ray examinations of the same organs or functions.

XIII. CONCLUSION

The UNSCEAR (1977) has summarized estimated global whole-body dose commitments for 1 year of the different sources and practices discussed, and have expressed these as the durations of exposure (in days) of the world population to natural radiation which would cause the same dose commitments. Of course, it would take 365 days of exposure of the world population to natural radiation sources to reach the annual collective dose of the order of 3×10^8 man rad for most of the body tissues (about 30% higher for lung). On the basis of 1 year of exposure to the sources or practices and the days of natural radiation exposure commercial air travel would be equivalent to 0.4 day of natural irradiation; production of phosphate fertilizer at the present production rate, 0.04 day; global production of electric energy by coal-fired power plants at the present global installed capacity, 10^6 MW(e), 0.02 day; radiation-emitting consumer products, 3 days; nuclear power at the present installed capacity, 8×10^4 MW(e), 0.6 day; residual radiation exposure related to nuclear explosions, averaged over the period 1951 to 1976, 30 days; and the use of radiation in medical diagnosis, 70 days.

Under the assumption of proportionality between increments in dose and risk, the relative contribution of the total radiation detriment from each of the various sources would be roughly in proportion to the global dose commitments indicated. The UNSCEAR (1977) stresses, however, that comparisons based on the values given in this summary would be misleading if the appropriate qualifications were not taken into account; in particular, the dose commitments from future practices are dependent on technological developments and on the evolution of relevant regulations, both of which are difficult to predict.

The UNSCEAR (1977) identified specific occupations with respect to levels of radiation exposure. The groups most liable to overexposure are industrial radiographers working with radionuclide sources. Klement and co-workers (1972) estimated for 31,424 industrial workers an average annual per capita dose of 0.19 rad. Estimates of lifetime doses to industrial workers are also based on scanty data but again appear unlikely to exceed 50 rad. Medical workers handling radium sources are also liable to receive high doses, but the use of these sources is decreasing. Other medical workers receive very low doses in some countries and comparatively large doses in others. Some groups of workers at nuclear power reactors receive relatively high doses, particularly those engaged in maintenance and health physics work. The highest average dose to groups of workers of moderate numbers were recorded for fuel reprocessing workers. Lung doses to miners are high but appear to be decreasing.

In considering occupational radiation doses in relation to statutory or regulatory obligations (ICRP, 1966) regarding doses to individuals, the UNSCEAR (1977) has defined a "reference distribution" of dose in terms of the following properties: (1) log-normal distribution of annual doses; (2) mean of annual dose distribution = 0.5 rad, that is, 0.1 of the ICRPs (1966) maximum permissible annual whole-body dose; and (3) proportion of workers exceeding this maximum permissible annual dose of 5 rad is 0.1%. The UNSCEAR concluded that a dose distribution with these characteristics would comply well with the intent of the ICRP's system of dose limitation for occupational exposure to radiation. The parameters used to determine whether or not a given occupational group receives radiation doses that are consistent with the defined reference distribution are the average annual dose $\bar{D}$ and the relative proportion Ω of the annual collective dose due to annual doses exceeding 1.5 rad. For the reference distribution, $\bar{D} = 0.5$ rad and $\Omega = 1$.

According to the UNSCEAR (1977), groups of workers for which $\bar{D}$ is equal to or greater than 1.0 rad <u>or</u> Ω is equal to or greater than 2.0 include industrial radiographers, luminizers, radiotherapy workers, some nuclear reactor workers, nuclear fuel reprocessing workers, workers in the manufacture of radiopharmaceuticals and industrial radiation sources, miners, and staff of jet aircraft. According to the UNSCEAR (1977), if the general practice of radiation protection is satisfactory and the limits of the parameters are correctly defined, the parameters for most groups of occupational workers should fall within the range $\bar{D} = 0.1$ to 1.0 rad and $\Omega = 0.1$ to 2.0. Included among these groups are medical workers in the use of diagnostic X rays and in nuclear medicine, most workers at most nuclear reactors, nuclear fuel manufacture workers, and workers in nuclear power research. Workers in groups for which both $\bar{D}$ and Ω are equal to or less than 0.1 are highly unlikely to receive annual doses greater than 1.5 rad, and the annual average dose is very low, while some workers in groups for which $\bar{D}$ is equal to or less than 0.1 rad, but Ω is greater than 0.1, are more likely to receive annual doses greater than 1.5 rad despite the extremely low average dose. Finally, although no such distribution has been found, workers in a group for which $\bar{D}$ is greater than 0.1 and Ω is equal to or less than 0.1, would have nearly the same annual dose, very few workers would receive doses in excess of 1.5 rad, and the fraction receiving low doses would be less than that in the reference distribution.

REFERENCES

Brodsky, A. (1976). Personal communication cited in UNSCEAR 1977.

Casarett, G. W. (1965). Experimental radiation carcinogenesis. In *Progress in Experimental Tumor Research*, Vol. 7, F. Homburger (Ed.). Karger, New York, pp. 49-82.

Casarett, G. W. (1973a). Pathogenesis of radionuclide-induced tumors. In *Radionuclide Carcinogenesis*, C. L. Sanders, R. H. Busch, J. E. Ballou, and D. D. Mahlum (Eds.). USAEC Office of Information Services, Washington, D.C., pp. 1-14.

Casarett, G. W. (1973b). Possible effects of relatively low levels of radiation. Monograph in *Current Problems in Radiology*, Vol. III, No. 2. Year Book Medical Publishers. Chicago, Ill.

Casarett, G. W. (1978). Biological effects of low levels of radiation exposure. In *Radioactivity in Consumer Products*, U.S. Nuclear Regulatory Commission, Washington, D.C., pp. 184-198.

Gesell, T. F. (1975). Occupational radiation exposure due to radon-222 in natural gas and natural gas products. Health Phys. 29: 681-687.

ICRP (1966). Recommendations of the International Commission on Radiological Protection. ICRP Publication 9, Pergamon, Oxford, England.

ICRP (1969). Radiosensitivity and spatial distribution of dose. Pergamon, New York.

ICRP (1977). Recommendations of the International Commission on Radiological Protection. ICRP Publication 26, Pergamon, Oxford, England.

Jonassen, N., and Hayes, E. I. (1974). The measurement of low concentrations of the short-lived radon-222 daughters in the air by alpha spectroscopy. Health Phys. 26: 104-110.

Kellerer, A. M., and Rossi, H. H. (1971). RBE and the primary mechanisms of radiation action. Radiat. Res. 47:153-84.

Kellerer, A. M., and Rossi, H. H. (1972). The theory of dual radiation action. Curr. Top. Radiat. Res. 8:85-158.

Klein, D. H., Andren, A. W., and Carter, J. A. (1975). Pathways of thirty-seven trace elements through coal-fired power plants. Environ. Sci. Technol. 9:973-979.

Klement, A. W., Miller, C. R., and Minx, R. P. (1972). Estimates of ionizing radiation doses in the United States 1960-2000. U.S. Environmental Protection Agency Report ORP/CSD72-1, Washington, D.C.

Kolb, W., and Schmier, H. (1975). Building material induced radiation exposure of the population. Proceedings of Third European Congress of the International Radiation Protection Association. Cited in UNSCEAR 1977.

NAS-BEIR (National Academy of Sciences, Advisory Committee on the Biological Effects of Ionizing Radiation) (1972). The effects on populations of exposure to low levels of ionizing radiation. National Academy of Sciences-National Research Council, Washington, D.C.

NCRP (1971). Basic radiation protection criteria, NCRP Report No. 39. National Council on Radiation Protection and Measurements, Washington, D.C.

NCRP (1975). Review of the current state of radiation protection philosophy. NCRP Report No. 43, NCRP, Washington, D.C.

NCRP (1977). Radiation exposure from consumer products and miscellaneous sources. NCRP Report No. 56, NCRP, Washington, D.C.

Rossi, H. H. (1970). The effects of small doses of ionizing radiation. Phys. Med. Biol. 15:255-262.

UNSCEAR (1972). Ionizing radiation: levels and effects. United Nations, New York.

UNSCEAR (1977). Sources and effects of ionizing radiation. United Nations, New York.

USAEC (1975). Reactor Safety Study. An assessment of accident risks in U.S. commercial power plants. U.S. Atomic Energy Commission Report WASH-1400 (NUREG 75/014), USAEC, Washington, D.C.

United States Congress (1971). Use of uranium mill tailings for construction purposes. Joint Committee on Atomic Energy, Washington, D.C.

Author Index

Numbers in parentheses are reference numbers and indicate that an author's work is referred to although his name is not cited in the text. Underlined numbers give the page on which the complete reference is listed.

B

C

D

E

H

I

L

M

N

S

U

V

Y

Z

Subject Index

B

D

E

N

O

P